PLEURAL DISEASE

LUNG BIOLOGY IN HEALTH AND DISEASE

Executive Editor

Claude Lenfant
Director, National Heart, Lung, and Blood Institute
National Institutes of Health
Bethesda, Maryland

1. Immunologic and Infectious Reactions in the Lung, *edited by C. H. Kirkpatrick and H. Y. Reynolds*
2. The Biochemical Basis of Pulmonary Function, *edited by R. G. Crystal*
3. Bioengineering Aspects of the Lung, *edited by J. B. West*
4. Metabolic Functions of the Lung, *edited by Y. S. Bakhle and J. R. Vane*
5. Respiratory Defense Mechanisms (in two parts), *edited by J. D. Brain, D. F. Proctor, and L. M. Reid*
6. Development of the Lung, *edited by W. A. Hodson*
7. Lung Water and Solute Exchange, *edited by N. C. Staub*
8. Extrapulmonary Manifestations of Respiratory Disease, *edited by E. D. Robin*
9. Chronic Obstructive Pulmonary Disease, *edited by T. L. Petty*
10. Pathogenesis and Therapy of Lung Cancer, *edited by C. C. Harris*
11. Genetic Determinants of Pulmonary Disease, *edited by S. D. Litwin*
12. The Lung in the Transition Between Health and Disease, *edited by P. T. Macklem and S. Permutt*
13. Evolution of Respiratory Processes: A Comparative Approach, *edited by S. C. Wood and C. Lenfant*
14. Pulmonary Vascular Diseases, *edited by K. M. Moser*
15. Physiology and Pharmacology of the Airways, *edited by J. A. Nadel*
16. Diagnostic Techniques in Pulmonary Disease (in two parts), *edited by M. A. Sackner*
17. Regulation of Breathing (in two parts), *edited by T. F. Hornbein*
18. Occupational Lung Diseases: Research Approaches and Methods, *edited by H. Weill and M. Turner-Warwick*
19. Immunopharmacology of the Lung, *edited by H. H. Newball*
20. Sarcoidosis and Other Granulomatous Diseases of the Lung, *edited by B. L. Fanburg*
21. Sleep and Breathing, *edited by N. A. Saunders and C. E. Sullivan*
22. *Pneumocystis carinii* Pneumonia: Pathogenesis, Diagnosis, and Treatment, *edited by L. S. Young*
23. Pulmonary Nuclear Medicine: Techniques in Diagnosis of Lung Disease, *edited by H. L. Atkins*

24. Acute Respiratory Failure, *edited by W. M. Zapol and K. J. Falke*
25. Gas Mixing and Distribution in the Lung, *edited by L. A. Engel and M. Paiva*
26. High-Frequency Ventilation in Intensive Care and During Surgery, *edited by G. Carlon and W. S. Howland*
27. Pulmonary Development: Transition from Intrauterine to Extrauterine Life, *edited by G. H. Nelson*
28. Chronic Obstructive Pulmonary Disease: Second Edition, *edited by T. L. Petty*
29. The Thorax (in two parts), *edited by C. Roussos and P. T. Macklem*
30. The Pleura in Health and Disease, *edited by J. Chrétien, J. Bignon, and A. Hirsch*
31. Drug Therapy for Asthma: Research and Clinical Practice, *edited by J. W. Jenne and S. Murphy*
32. Pulmonary Endothelium in Health and Disease, *edited by U. S. Ryan*
33. The Airways: Neural Control in Health and Disease, *edited by M. A. Kaliner and P. J. Barnes*
34. Pathophysiology and Treatment of Inhalation Injuries, *edited by J. Loke*
35. Respiratory Function of the Upper Airway, *edited by O. P. Mathew and G. Sant'Ambrogio*
36. Chronic Obstructive Pulmonary Disease: A Behavioral Perspective, *edited by A. J. McSweeny and I. Grant*
37. Biology of Lung Cancer: Diagnosis and Treatment, *edited by S. T. Rosen, J. L. Mulshine, F. Cuttitta, and P. G. Abrams*
38. Pulmonary Vascular Physiology and Pathophysiology, *edited by E. K. Weir and J. T. Reeves*
39. Comparative Pulmonary Physiology: Current Concepts, *edited by S. C. Wood*
40. Respiratory Physiology: An Analytical Approach, *edited by H. K. Chang and M. Paiva*
41. Lung Cell Biology, *edited by D. Massaro*
42. Heart–Lung Interactions in Health and Disease, *edited by S. M. Scharf and S. S. Cassidy*
43. Clinical Epidemiology of Chronic Obstructive Pulmonary Disease, *edited by M. J. Hensley and N. A. Saunders*
44. Surgical Pathology of Lung Neoplasms, *edited by A. M. Marchevsky*
45. The Lung in Rheumatic Diseases, *edited by G. W. Cannon and G. A. Zimmerman*
46. Diagnostic Imaging of the Lung, *edited by C. E. Putman*
47. Models of Lung Disease: Microscopy and Structural Methods, *edited by J. Gil*
48. Electron Microscopy of the Lung, *edited by D. E. Schraufnagel*
49. Asthma: Its Pathology and Treatment, *edited by M. A. Kaliner, P. J. Barnes, and C. G. A. Persson*
50. Acute Respiratory Failure: Second Edition, *edited by W. M. Zapol and F. Lemaire*
51. Lung Disease in the Tropics, *edited by O. P. Sharma*

52. Exercise: Pulmonary Physiology and Pathophysiology, *edited by B. J. Whipp and K. Wasserman*
53. Developmental Neurobiology of Breathing, *edited by G. G. Haddad and J. P. Farber*
54. Mediators of Pulmonary Inflammation, *edited by M. A. Bray and W. H. Anderson*
55. The Airway Epithelium, *edited by S. G. Farmer and D. Hay*
56. Physiological Adaptations in Vertebrates: Respiration, Circulation, and Metabolism, *edited by S. C. Wood, R. E. Weber, A. R. Hargens, and R. W. Millard*
57. The Bronchial Circulation, *edited by J. Butler*
58. Lung Cancer Differentiation: Implications for Diagnosis and Treatment, *edited by S. D. Bernal and P. J. Hesketh*
59. Pulmonary Complications of Systemic Disease, *edited by J. F. Murray*
60. Lung Vascular Injury: Molecular and Cellular Response, *edited by A. Johnson and T. J. Ferro*
61. Cytokines of the Lung, *edited by J. Kelley*
62. The Mast Cell in Health and Disease, *edited by M. A. Kaliner and D. D. Metcalfe*
63. Pulmonary Disease in the Elderly Patient, *edited by D. A. Mahler*
64. Cystic Fibrosis, *edited by P. B. Davis*
65. Signal Transduction in Lung Cells, *edited by J. S. Brody, D. M. Center, and V. A. Tkachuk*
66. Tuberculosis: A Comprehensive International Approach, *edited by L. B. Reichman and E. S. Hershfield*
67. Pharmacology of the Respiratory Tract: Experimental and Clinical Research, *edited by K. F. Chung and P. J. Barnes*
68. Prevention of Respiratory Diseases, *edited by A. Hirsch, M. Goldberg, J.-P. Martin, and R. Masse*
69. *Pneumocystis carinii* Pneumonia: Second Edition, *edited by P. D. Walzer*
70. Fluid and Solute Transport in the Airspaces of the Lungs, *edited by R. M. Effros and H. K. Chang*
71. Sleep and Breathing: Second Edition, *edited by N. A. Saunders and C. E. Sullivan*
72. Airway Secretion: Physiological Bases for the Control of Mucous Hypersecretion, *edited by T. Takishima and S. Shimura*
73. Sarcoidosis and Other Granulomatous Disorders, *edited by D. G. James*
74. Epidemiology of Lung Cancer, *edited by J. M. Samet*
75. Pulmonary Embolism, *edited by M. Morpurgo*
76. Sports and Exercise Medicine, *edited by S. C. Wood and R. C. Roach*
77. Endotoxin and the Lungs, *edited by K. L. Brigham*
78. The Mesothelial Cell and Mesothelioma, *edited by M.-C. Jaurand and J. Bignon*

79. Regulation of Breathing: Second Edition, *edited by J. A. Dempsey and A. I. Pack*
80. Pulmonary Fibrosis, *edited by S. Hin. Phan and R. S. Thrall*
81. Long-Term Oxygen Therapy: Scientific Basis and Clinical Application, *edited by W. J. O'Donohue, Jr.*
82. Ventral Brainstem Mechanisms and Control of Respiration and Blood Pressure, *edited by C. O. Trouth, R. M. Millis, H. F. Kiwull-Schöne, and M. E. Schläfke*
83. A History of Breathing Physiology, *edited by D. F. Proctor*
84. Surfactant Therapy for Lung Disease, *edited by B. Robertson and H. W. Taeusch*
85. The Thorax: Second Edition, Revised and Expanded (in three parts), *edited by C. Roussos*
86. Severe Asthma: Pathogenesis and Clinical Management, *edited by S. J. Szefler and D. Y. M. Leung*
87. *Mycobacterium avium*–Complex Infection: Progress in Research and Treatment, *edited by J. A. Korvick and C. A. Benson*
88. Alpha 1–Antitrypsin Deficiency: Biology • Pathogenesis • Clinical Manifestations • Therapy, *edited by R. G. Crystal*
89. Adhesion Molecules and the Lung, *edited by P. A. Ward and J. C. Fantone*
90. Respiratory Sensation, *edited by L. Adams and A. Guz*
91. Pulmonary Rehabilitation, *edited by A. P. Fishman*
92. Acute Respiratory Failure in Chronic Obstructive Pulmonary Disease, *edited by J.-P. Derenne, W. A. Whitelaw, and T. Similowski*
93. Environmental Impact on the Airways: From Injury to Repair, *edited by J. Chrétien and D. Dusser*
94. Inhalation Aerosols: Physical and Biological Basis for Therapy, *edited by A. J. Hickey*
95. Tissue Oxygen Deprivation: From Molecular to Integrated Function, *edited by G. G. Haddad and G. Lister*
96. The Genetics of Asthma, *edited by S. B. Liggett and D. A. Meyers*
97. Inhaled Glucocorticoids in Asthma: Mechanisms and Clinical Actions, *edited by R. P. Schleimer, W. W. Busse, and P. M. O'Byrne*
98. Nitric Oxide and the Lung, *edited by W. M. Zapol and K. D. Bloch*
99. Primary Pulmonary Hypertension, *edited by L. J. Rubin and S. Rich*
100. Lung Growth and Development, *edited by J. A. McDonald*
101. Parasitic Lung Diseases, *edited by A. A. F. Mahmoud*
102. Lung Macrophages and Dendritic Cells in Health and Disease, *edited by M. F. Lipscomb and S. W. Russell*
103. Pulmonary and Cardiac Imaging, *edited by C. Chiles and C. E. Putman*
104. Gene Therapy for Diseases of the Lung, *edited by K. L. Brigham*
105. Oxygen, Gene Expression, and Cellular Function, *edited by L. Biadasz Clerch and D. J. Massaro*
106. Beta$_2$-Agonists in Asthma Treatment, *edited by R. Pauwels and P. M. O'Byrne*

107. Inhalation Delivery of Therapeutic Peptides and Proteins, *edited by A. L. Adjei and P. K. Gupta*
108. Asthma in the Elderly, *edited by R. A. Barbee and J. W. Bloom*
109. Treatment of the Hospitalized Cystic Fibrosis Patient, *edited by D. M. Orenstein and R. C. Stern*
110. Asthma and Immunological Diseases in Pregnancy and Early Infancy, *edited by M. Schatz, R. S. Zeiger, and H. N. Claman*
111. Dyspnea, *edited by D. A. Mahler*
112. Proinflammatory and Antiinflammatory Peptides, *edited by S. I. Said*
113. Self-Management of Asthma, *edited by H. Kotses and A. Harver*
114. Eicosanoids, Aspirin, and Asthma, *edited by A. Szczeklik, R. J. Gryglewski, and J. R. Vane*
115. Fatal Asthma, *edited by A. L. Sheffer*
116. Pulmonary Edema, *edited by M. A. Matthay and D. H. Ingbar*
117. Inflammatory Mechanisms in Asthma, *edited by S. T. Holgate and W. W. Busse*
118. Physiological Basis of Ventilatory Support, *edited by J. J. Marini and A. S. Slutsky*
119. Human Immunodeficiency Virus and the Lung, *edited by M. J. Rosen and J. M. Beck*
120. Five-Lipoxygenase Products in Asthma, *edited by J. M. Drazen, S.-E. Dahlén, and T. H. Lee*
121. Complexity in Structure and Function of the Lung, *edited by M. P. Hlastala and H. T. Robertson*
122. Biology of Lung Cancer, *edited by M. A. Kane and P. A. Bunn, Jr.*
123. Rhinitis: Mechanisms and Management, *edited by R. M. Naclerio, S. R. Durham, and N. Mygind*
124. Lung Tumors: Fundamental Biology and Clinical Management, *edited by C. Brambilla and E. Brambilla*
125. Interleukin-5: From Molecule to Drug Target for Asthma, *edited by C. J. Sanderson*
126. Pediatric Asthma, *edited by S. Murphy and H. W. Kelly*
127. Viral Infections of the Respiratory Tract, *edited by R. Dolin and P. F. Wright*
128. Air Pollutants and the Respiratory Tract, *edited by D. L. Swift and W. M. Foster*
129. Gastroesophageal Reflux Disease and Airway Disease, *edited by M. R. Stein*
130. Exercise-Induced Asthma, *edited by E. R. McFadden, Jr.*
131. LAM and Other Diseases Characterized by Smooth Muscle Proliferation, *edited by J. Moss*
132. The Lung at Depth, *edited by C. E. G. Lundgren and J. N. Miller*
133. Regulation of Sleep and Circadian Rhythms, *edited by F. W. Turek and P. C. Zee*
134. Anticholinergic Agents in the Upper and Lower Airways, *edited by S. L. Spector*
135. Control of Breathing in Health and Disease, *edited by M. D. Altose and Y. Kawakami*

136. Immunotherapy in Asthma, *edited by J. Bousquet and H. Yssel*
137. Chronic Lung Disease in Early Infancy, *edited by R. D. Bland and J. J. Coalson*
138. Asthma's Impact on Society: The Social and Economic Burden, *edited by K. B. Weiss, A. S. Buist, and S. D. Sullivan*
139. New and Exploratory Therapeutic Agents for Asthma, *edited by M. Yeadon and Z. Diamant*
140. Multimodality Treatment of Lung Cancer, *edited by A. T. Skarin*
141. Cytokines in Pulmonary Disease: Infection and Inflammation, *edited by S. Nelson and T. R. Martin*
142. Diagnostic Pulmonary Pathology, *edited by P. T. Cagle*
143. Particle–Lung Interactions, *edited by P. Gehr and J. Heyder*
144. Tuberculosis: A Comprehensive International Approach, Second Edition, Revised and Expanded, *edited by L. B. Reichman and E. S. Hershfield*
145. Combination Therapy for Asthma and Chronic Obstructive Pulmonary Disease, *edited by R. J. Martin and M. Kraft*
146. Sleep Apnea: Implications in Cardiovascular and Cerebrovascular Disease, *edited by T. D. Bradley and J. S. Floras*
147. Sleep and Breathing in Children: A Developmental Approach, *edited by G. M. Loughlin, J. L. Carroll, and C. L. Marcus*
148. Pulmonary and Peripheral Gas Exchange in Health and Disease, *edited by J. Roca, R. Rodriguez-Roisen, and P. D. Wagner*
149. Lung Surfactants: Basic Science and Clinical Applications, *R. H. Notter*
150. Nosocomial Pneumonia, *edited by W. R. Jarvis*
151. Fetal Origins of Cardiovascular and Lung Disease, *edited by David J. P. Barker*
152. Long-Term Mechanical Ventilation, *edited by N. S. Hill*
153. Environmental Asthma, *edited by R. K. Bush*
154. Asthma and Respiratory Infections, *edited by D. P. Skoner*
155. Airway Remodeling, *edited by P. H. Howarth, J. W. Wilson, J. Bousquet, S. Rak, and R. A. Pauwels*
156. Genetic Models in Cardiorespiratory Biology, *edited by G. G. Haddad and T. Xu*
157. Respiratory-Circulatory Interactions in Health and Disease, *edited by S. M. Scharf, M. R. Pinsky, and S. Magder*
158. Ventilator Management Strategies for Critical Care, *edited by N. S. Hill and M. M. Levy*
159. Severe Asthma: Pathogenesis and Clinical Management, Second Edition, Revised and Expanded, *edited by S. J. Szefler and D. Y. M. Leung*
160. Gravity and the Lung: Lessons from Microgravity, *edited by G. K. Prisk, M. Paiva, and J. B. West*
161. High Altitude: An Exploration of Human Adaptation, *edited by T. F. Hornbein and R. B. Schoene*
162. Drug Delivery to the Lung, *edited by H. Bisgaard, C. O'Callaghan, and G. C. Smaldone*

163. Inhaled Steroids in Asthma: Optimizing Effects in the Airways, edited by R. P. Schleimer, P. M. O'Byrne, S. J. Szefler, and R. Brattsand
164. IgE and Anti-IgE Therapy in Asthma and Allergic Disease, edited by R. B. Fick, Jr., and P. M. Jardieu
165. Clinical Management of Chronic Obstructive Pulmonary Disease, edited by T. Similowski, W. A. Whitelaw, and J.-P. Derenne
166. Sleep Apnea: Pathogenesis, Diagnosis, and Treatment, edited by A. I. Pack
167. Biotherapeutic Approaches to Asthma, edited by J. Agosti and A. L. Sheffer
168. Proteoglycans in Lung Disease, edited by H. G. Garg, P. J. Roughley, and C. A. Hales
169. Gene Therapy in Lung Disease, edited by S. M. Albelda
170. Disease Markers in Exhaled Breath, edited by N. Marczin, S. A. Kharitonov, M. H. Yacoub, and P. J. Barnes
171. Sleep-Related Breathing Disorders: Experimental Models and Therapeutic Potential, edited by D. W. Carley and M. Radulovacki
172. Chemokines in the Lung, edited by R. M. Strieter, S. L. Kunkel, and T. J. Standiford
173. Respiratory Control and Disorders in the Newborn, edited by O. P. Mathew
174. The Immunological Basis of Asthma, edited by B. N. Lambrecht, H. C. Hoogsteden, and Z. Diamant
175. Oxygen Sensing: Responses and Adaptation to Hypoxia, edited by S. Lahiri, G. L. Semenza, and N. R. Prabhakar
176. Non-Neoplastic Advanced Lung Disease, edited by J. R. Maurer
177. Therapeutic Targets in Airway Inflammation, edited by N. T. Eissa and D. P. Huston
178. Respiratory Infections in Allergy and Asthma, edited by S. L. Johnston and N. G. Papadopoulos
179. Acute Respiratory Distress Syndrome, edited by M. A. Matthay
180. Venous Thromboembolism, edited by J. E. Dalen
181. Upper and Lower Respiratory Disease, edited by J. Corren, A. Togias, and J. Bousquet
182. Pharmacotherapy in Chronic Obstructive Pulmonary Disease, edited by B. R. Celli
183. Acute Exacerbations of Chronic Obstructive Pulmonary Disease, edited by N. M. Siafakas, N. R. Anthonisen, and D. Georgopoulos
184. Lung Volume Reduction Surgery for Emphysema, edited by H. E. Fessler, J. J. Reilly, Jr., and D. J. Sugarbaker
185. Idiopathic Pulmonary Fibrosis, edited by J. P. Lynch III
186. Pleural Disease, edited by D. Bouros

ADDITIONAL VOLUMES IN PREPARATION

Therapy for Mucus-Clearance Disorders, *edited by B. K. Rubin and C. P. van der Schans*

Oxygen/Nitrogen Radicals: Lung Injury and Disease, *edited by V. Vallyathan*

Interventional Pulmonary Medicine, *edited by J. F. Beamis, P. N. Mathur, and A. C. Mehta*

Lung Development and Regeneration, *edited by D. J. Massaro, G. Massaro, and P. Chambon*

The opinions expressed in these volumes do not necessarily represent the views of the National Institutes of Health.

PLEURAL DISEASE

Edited by

Demosthenes Bouros
*Demokritos University of Thrace Medical School
and University Hospital of Alexandroupolis
Alexandroupolis, Greece*

MARCEL DEKKER, INC.   NEW YORK · BASEL

Although great care has been taken to provide accurate and current information, neither the author(s) nor the publisher, nor anyone else associated with this publication, shall be liable for any loss, damage, or liability directly or indirectly caused or alleged to be caused by this book. The material contained herein is not intended to provide specific advice or recommendations for any specific situation.

Trademark notice: Product or corporate names may be trademarks or registered trademarks and are used only for identification and explanation without intent to infringe.

Library of Congress Cataloging-in-Publication Data
A catalog record for this book is available from the Library of Congress.

ISBN: 0-8247-4027-0

This book is printed on acid-free paper.

Headquarters
Marcel Dekker, Inc., 270 Madison Avenue, New York, NY 10016, U.S.A.
tel: 212-696-9000; fax: 212-685-4540

Distribution and Customer Service
Marcel Dekker, Inc., Cimarron Road, Monticello, New York 12701, U.S.A.
tel: 800-228-1160; fax: 845-796-1772

Eastern Hemisphere Distribution
Marcel Dekker AG, Hutgasse 4, Postfach 812, CH-4001 Basel, Switzerland
tel: 41-61-260-6300; fax: 41-61-260-6333

World Wide Web
http://www.dekker.com

The publisher offers discounts on this book when ordered in bulk quantities. For more information, write to Special Sales/Professional Marketing at the headquarters address above.

Copyright © 2004 by Marcel Dekker, Inc. All Rights Reserved.

Neither this book nor any part may be reproduced or transmitted in any form or by any means, electronic or mechanical, including photocopying, microfilming, and recording, or by any information storage and retrieval system, without permission in writing from the publisher.

Current printing (last digit):
10 9 8 7 6 5 4 3 2 1

PRINTED IN THE UNITED STATES OF AMERICA

In memory of my father

INTRODUCTION

The Lung Biology in Health and Disease series has published a very large number of volumes focused on a wide variety of disorders of the respiratory system. These works have discussed basic science and clinical investigations related to many aspects of lung diseases. However, very little has been presented regarding pleural disease. Yet, one need only attend a pulmonary disease clinic to become well aware of the prevalence of pleural disorders: they have protean manifestations and many degrees of severity.

All the best textbooks of respiratory medicine have many entries about pleural disease, often columns and columns of them in the index. Surprisingly, however, the sum of pages covering these entries is often quite limited compared with entries about some diseases of lesser prevalence. Why this should be the case is open to speculation. Less interest? Less knowledge? Less ... whatever! Surely, it cannot be said that the pleura is an organ of no importance. In some ways, albeit with significant differences, it may be compared to the pericardium, whose alterations and disorders have great significance. Obviously, no explanation for this situation is readily forthcoming (at least to this writer!).

However, the appearance of *Pleural Disease*, edited by Demosthenes Bouros, may change all that. Comprising 51 chapters, this volume is one of the most comprehensive presentations about the pleura ... in health *and* in disease!

It would be presumptuous to claim that all aspects of pleural disease are included (indeed, how could one say?), but this is truly a presentation of all that is known today. The large number of contributors from many countries is evidence of the volume's comprehensiveness, and the multinationality of the authors further ensures the breadth of the discussions.

Pleural Disease may have been long in coming, but it surely was worth the wait. I am indebted to Dr. Bouros for favoring the Lung Biology in Health and Disease series with his contribution. The authors, as well, deserve much credit and gratitude.

Claude Lenfant, M.D.
Bethesda, Maryland

PREFACE

Pleural diseases present a frequent problem in everyday clinical practice. It is estimated that about 25% of the consultations of a pulmonary service concern pleural diseases. Various medical specialists, including pneumonologists, thoracic surgeons, radiologists, internists, cardiologists, pediatricians, and oncologists, deal with their diagnosis and treatment. However, relatively few scientists and clinicians through their excellent and continuous work have contributed to the advancement of our understanding of the basic and clinical aspects of the pleura in health and disease.

The aim of this book is to provide a comprehensive, authoritative, state-of-the-art presentation of all aspects of pleural diseases by the world's leading authorities. Authors from many countries and renowned institutions contributed to this 51-chapter book, resulting in an international approach to current diagnosis and treatment of pleural diseases, both benign and malignant. I believe that these contributors have given the book a lively flavor, putting the future of the field in an exciting perspective.

Newer techniques, including medical thoracoscopy, pleural lavage, intrapleural fibrinolytics, image-guided small-bore catheters, video-assisted thoracoscopic surgery (VATS), pleuroperitoneal shunt, and extrapleural pneumonectomy are presented in detail. Recent advances in the anatomy, physiology, and pathophysiology of the pleura are presented by experts. The increasing role of imaging techniques, both radiological and ultrasound, in the diagnosis and management of the various pleural diseases is extensively detailed. Interventional techniques for the diagnosis and treatment of pleural diseases, including pleural thoracentesis and closed biopsy, chest tube insertion, pleural lavage, medical thoracoscopy, and VATS, are also elucidated. A critical evaluation of the various diagnostic tests for discrimination between transudates and exudates is elegantly presented. The differentiation of a benign from a malignant pleural effusion is an everyday clinical problem. The importance of clinical evaluation in the differential diagnosis of a pleural effusion is nicely illustrated.

A great deal of this volume is dedicated to pleural infection. A number of experts present their experience in the current diagnosis and management of parapneumonic and surgical pleural infections from both the medical and surgical points of view. The role of newer medical techniques, such as intrapleural instillation of fibrinolytics, the insertion of new, small, image-guided catheters, and medical thoracoscopy are extensively described. Also, the evolution of VATS as a high-priority surgical technique is described and updated.

Tuberculous pleuritis continues to be a major health problem in developing countries and a frequent diagnostic problem in clinical practice. Malignant pleural effusions, primary or metastatic, are an important cause of morbidity, and the various aspects of this condition are presented here. The current understanding and management of mesothelioma and benign asbestos-related pleural disease are presented, together with the interesting technique of extrapleural pneumonectomy.

The specific characteristics and methods of diagnosis and management of different organ diseases with concomitant pleural disease are also presented in this volume. Pleural effusions in the ICU, in children, and related to drug consumption are included as well. All aspects of pneumothorax, hemothorax, and chylothorax/pseudochylothorax, which represent a continuing challenge to clinicians, are presented. Other chapters deal with undiagnosed persistent pleural effusion, the pleural space in patients having undergone organ transplantation, the pharmacokinetics and pharmacodynamics of the pleural fluid, and animal research models in pleural investigation. Some overlap between the chapters was encouraged, which allowed for an uninterrupted flow of ideas and helped to achieve detailed coverage of the diverse topics.

This book would have been impossible to produce without the help and support of all the distinguished authors, to whom I am profoundly indebted for their contributions. Finally, I am most grateful to my family—Stella, Efrosini, Evangelos, Calliope, Caroline—for their forbearance and continuous support.

Demosthenes Bouros

CONTRIBUTORS

Gerald F. Abbott, M.D. Assistant Professor, Department of Diagnostic Imaging, Brown Medical School, and Rhode Island Hospital, Providence, Rhode Island, U.S.A.

Michael G. Alexandrakis, M.D. Assistant Professor, Department of Hematology, University of Crete Medical School, and University Hospital of Heraklion, Heraklion, Crete, Greece

Katerina Antoniou, M.D. Department of Pneumonology, University of Crete Medical School, and University Hospital of Heraklion, Heraklion, Crete, Greece

Veena B. Antony, M.D. Dr. Calvin H. English Professor, Department of Medicine, Indiana University School of Medicine, Indianapolis, Indiana, U.S.A.

Philippe Astoul, M.D., Ph.D. Professor, Department of Pulmonary Diseases, University of the Mediterranean, and Hôpital Sainte-Marguerite, Marseille, France

Petros Bakakos, M.D. Consultant, Department of Respiratory and Critical Care Medicine, Sotiria Chest Diseases Hospital, Athens, Greece

Robert P. Baughman, M.D. Professor, Department of Internal Medicine, University of Cincinnati, Cincinnati, Ohio, U.S.A.

Michael H. Baumann, M.D., F.C.C.P. Professor, Division of Pulmonary, Critical Care, and Sleep Medicine, Department of Medicine, University of Mississippi Medical Center, Jackson, Mississippi, U.S.A.

Semra Bilaçeroğlu, M.D., F.C.C.P. Associate Professor, Department of Thoracic Medicine, Izmir Training and Research Hospital for Thoracic Medicine and Surgery, Izmir, Turkey

Chris T. Bolliger, M.D., Ph.D. Professor, Lung Unit, Department of Internal Medicine, University of Stellenbosch, and Tygerberg Hospital, Capetown, South Africa

Demosthenes Bouros, M.D., F.C.C.P. Professor, Department of Pneumonology, Demokritos University of Thrace Medical School, and Head, Department of Pneumonology, University Hospital of Alexandroupolis, Alexandroupolis, Greece

Philippe Camus, M.D. Professor, Department of Pulmonary Diseases and Critical Care Medicine, University of Bourgogne Medical School, and University Medical Center le Bocage, Dijon, France

Paula Carvalho, M.D. Associate Professor, Division of Pulmonary and Critical Care Medicine, Department of Medicine, University of Washington, Seattle, Washington, and Medical Director, Intensive Care Unit, VA Medical Center, Boise, Idaho, U.S.A.

Kristina Crothers, M.D. Senior Fellow, Department of Pulmonary and Critical Care Medicine, University of California, San Francisco, San Francisco, California, U.S.A.

Peter D. O. Davies, D.M. F.R.C.P. Tuberculosis Research Unit, The Cardiothoracic Centre, Liverpool NHS Trust, Liverpool, England

Andreas H. Diacon, M.D. Department of Internal Medicine, University of Stellenbosch, and Tygerberg Hospital, Capetown, South Africa

Dean M. Donahue, M.D. Assistant Professor, Division of Thoracic Surgery, Department of Surgery, Harvard Medical School, and Massachusetts General Hospital, Boston, Massachusetts, U.S.A.

Pierre Fournel, M.D. Department of Pneumonology–Thoracic Oncology, University Hospital of Saint-Etienne, Saint-Etienne, France

Contributors

Marios E. Froudarakis, M.D. Lecturer, Department of Pneumonology, University of Crete Medical School, and University Hospital of Heraklion, Heraklion, Crete, Greece

Dimitris Georgopoulos, M.D. Professor, Department of Medicine, and Director, Department of Intensive Care Medicine, University of Crete, and University Hospital of Heraklion, Heraklion, Crete, Greece

Peter Goldstraw, F.R.C.S. Consultant, Department of Thoracic Surgery, Royal Brompton Hospital, and Imperial College School of Medicine, London, England

E. Brigitte Gottschall, M.D., M.S.P.H. Assistant Professor, Division of Environmental and Occupational Health Sciences, Department of Medicine, National Jewish Medical and Research Center, University of Colorado School of Medicine, Denver, Colorado, U.S.A.

Kostas I. Gourgoulianis, M.D. Professor, Department of Pneumonology, Medical School, University of Thessaly, Larissa, Greece

Elpis Hatziagorou, M.D. Clinical and Research Fellow, Third Department of Pediatrics, Aristotelian University of Thessaloniki, and Hippokration General Hospital, Thessaloniki, Greece

John E. Heffner, M.D. Professor, Department of Medicine, Medical University of South Carolina, Charleston, South Carolina, U.S.A.

Gunnar Hillerdal, M.D. Assistant Professor, Department of Medicine, Karolinska Institute, and Department of Pulmonary Medicine, Karolinska Hospital, Uppsala, Sweden

Laurence Huang, M.D. Associate Professor, Department of Medicine, University of California, San Francisco, San Francisco, California, U.S.A.

Michael A. Jantz, M.D., F.C.C.P. Assistant Professor, Division of Pulmonary and Critical Care Medicine, Department of Medicine, University of Florida Health Sciences Center, Gainesville, Florida, U.S.A.

Philippe G. Jorens, M.D., Ph.D. Professor, Department of Intensive Care Medicine, University of Antwerp, and University Hospital of Antwerp, Edegem, Antwerp, Belgium

Marc A. Judson, M.D. Professor, Division of Pulmonary and Critical Care Medicine, Department of Medicine, Medical University of South Carolina, Charleston, South Carolina, U.S.A.

Ok Hwa Kim, M.D., Ph.D. Professor, Department of Radiology, Ajou University Medical Center, Suwon, South Korea

Epaminondas N. Kosmas, M.D., Ph.D., F.C.C.P. Senior Registrar, Department of Respiratory Medicine, University of Athens, and Sotiria Chest Diseases Hospital, Athens, Greece

Ioannis Kottakis, M.D. Assistant Professor, Department of Pneumonology, Demokritos University of Thrace Medical School, and University Hospital of Alexandroupolis, Alexandroupolis, Greece

Despina S. Kyriakou, M.D., Ph.D. Assistant Professor, Department of Hematology, University of Thessalia Medical School, and University Hospital of Larissa, Larissa, Thessalia, Greece

George Ladas, F.E.T.C.S. Consultant, Department of Thoracic Surgery, Royal Brompton Hospital, and Imperial College School of Medicine, London, England

Ioannis Liapakis, M.D. Department of Surgery, University Hospital of Alexandroupolis, Alexandroupolis, Greece

Richard W. Light, M.D. Professor, Department of Medicine, Vanderbilt University, and Saint Thomas Hospital, Nashville, Tennessee, U.S.A.

Joseph A. LoCicero III, M.D. Professor and Chair, Department of Surgery, The University of South Alabama, Mobile, Alabama, U.S.A.

Eugene J. Mark, M.D. Associate Professor, Department of Pathology, Harvard Medical School, and Massachusetts General Hospital, Boston, Massachusetts, U.S.A.

Gilbert Massard, M.D., F.E.C.T.S. Professor, Department of Thoracic Surgery, Université Louis Pasteur, and Hôpitaux Universitaires de Strasbourg, Strasbourg, France

Douglas J. Mathisen, M.D. Professor and Chief, Division of Thoracic Surgery, Department of Surgery, Harvard Medical School, and Massachusetts General Hospital, Boston, Massachusetts, U.S.A.

Theresa C. McLoud, M.D. Professor and Associate Radiologist in Chief, Department of Radiology, Harvard Medical School, and Massachusetts General Hospital, Boston, Massachusetts, U.S.A.

Contributors

Ioanna Mitrouska, M.D. Consultant, Department of Respiratory Medicine, University of Crete, and University Hospital of Heraklion, Heraklion, Crete, Greece

John F. Murray, M.D., D.Sc.(hon), F.R.C.P. Professor Emeritus, Division of Pulmonary and Critical Care Medicine, Department of Medicine, University of California, San Francisco, San Francisco, California, U.S.A.

Lee S. Newman, M.D., M.A., F.C.C.P. Professor, Department of Medicine, National Jewish Medical and Research Center, University of Colorado School of Medicine, Denver, Colorado, U.S.A.

Marc Noppen, M.D., Ph.D. Professor, Respiratory Department, Free University of Brussels, and Academic Hospital AZ-VUB, Brussels, Belgium

Michael W. Owens, M.D. Associate Professor, Division of Pulmonary and Critical Care Medicine, Department of Medicine, Louisiana State University Health Sciences Center, Shreveport, Louisiana, U.S.A.

Spyridon A. Papiris, M.D., F.C.C.P., F.A.C.A. Associate Professor, Division of Pulmonary and Critical Care Medicine, Department of Internal Medicine, National and Capodistrian University of Athens, Athens, Greece

Kyung Joo Park, M.D. Professor, Department of Radiology, Ajou University Medical Center, Suwon, South Korea

D. Keith Payne, M.D. Professor, Division of Pulmonary and Critical Care Medicine, Department of Medicine, Louisiana State University Health Sciences Center, Shreveport, Louisiana, U.S.A.

Ming-Jen Peng, M.D. Senior Visiting Staff, Chest Division, Department of Medicine, Mackay Memorial Hospital and Taipei Medical University, Taipei, Taiwan

Maria Plataki, M.D. Department of Pneumonology, University Hospital of Heraklion, Heraklion, Crete, Greece

Vlasis S. Polychronopoulos, M.D., F.C.C.P. Director, Third Chest Department, Sismanoglion General Hospital, Athens, Greece

Luis Puente-Maestu, M.D., Ph.D. Chief, Division of Lung Function and Bronchoscopy, Department of Pulmonology, Hospital General Universitario Gregorio Marañón, Madrid, Spain

Antonis Rasidakis, M.D. Head, Department of Respiratory and Critical Care Medicine, Sotiria Chest Diseases Hospital, Athens, Greece

Francisco Rodriguez-Panadero, M.D. Head, Respiratory Endoscopy Section, Respiratory Disease Unit, Hospital Universitario Virgen del Rocío, Sevilla, Spain

Charis Roussos, M.D., M.Sc, Ph.D. M.R.S., F.R.C.P.(C) Professor and Chair, Division of Pulmonary and Critical Care Medicine, Department of Internal Medicine, National and Capodistrian University of Athens, Athens, Greece

Steven A. Sahn, M.D. Professor, Division of Pulmonary and Critical Care Medicine, Department of Medicine, Medical University of South Carolina, Charleston, South Carolina, U.S.A.

Sophia E. Schiza, M.D. Department of Pneumonology, University Hospital of Heraklion, Heraklion, Crete, Greece

Patrique Segers, M.D. Department of Thoracic and Vascular Surgery, University of Antwerp, and University Hospital of Antwerp, Edegem, Antwerp, Belgium

Sally Seymour, M.D. Clinical Fellow, Department of Internal Medicine, University of Cincinnati, Cincinnati, Ohio, U.S.A.

Charlie Strange, M.D. Associate Professor, Division of Pulmonary and Critical Care Medicine, Department of Medicine, Medical University of South Carolina, Charleston, South Carolina, U.S.A.

David J. Sugarbaker, M.D. Chief, Division of Thoracic Surgery, Department of Surgery, Brigham & Women's Hospital, Boston, Massachusetts, U.S.A.

Pascal Thomas, M.D., F.E.T.C.S. Professor, Department of Thoracic Surgery, Sainte Marguerite University Hospital of Marseille, Marseille, France

Michael Toumbis, M.D. Department of Pneumonology, Sotiria Chest Diseases Hospital, Athens, Greece

John N. Tsanakas, M.D., M.R.C.P.C.H.(UK) Associate Professor, Third Department of Pediatrics, Aristotelian University of Thessaloniki, and Hippokration General Hospital, Thessaloniki, Greece

Nikolaos E. Tzanakis, M.D., Ph.D. Assistant Professor, Department of Pneumonology, University of Crete Medical School, and University Hospital of Heraklion, Heraklion, Crete, Greece

Paul E. Van Schil, Ph.D. Professor, Department of Thoracic and Vascular Surgery, University of Antwerp, and University Hospital of Antwerp, Edegem, Antwerp, Belgium

Demetrios A. Vassilakis, M.D. Consultant, Department of Pneumonology, Rethymnon General Hospital, Rethymnon, Crete, Greece

Johny A. Verschakelen, M.D., Ph.D. Professor, Department of Radiology, University Hospitals, Gasthuisberg, Leuven, Belgium

Victoria Villena, Ph.D. Respiratory Unit, Hospital Universitario 12 de Octubre, Madrid, Spain

Nai-San Wang, M.D., Ph.D. Professor, Department of Pathology, Chungtai Institute of Health Sciences and Technology, Taichung, Taiwan

Athol U. Wells, M.D., M.B.Ch.B., F.R.C.P., F.R.A.C.P. Consultant in Respiratory Medicine, Royal Brompton Hospital, London, England

Mark Woodhead, B.Sc., D.M., F.R.C.P. Department of Respiratory Medicine, Manchester Royal Infirmary, Manchester, England

Cameron D. Wright, M.D. Associate Professor, Division of General Thoracic Surgery, Department of Surgery, Harvard Medical School, and Massachusetts General Hospital, Boston, Massachusetts, U.S.A.

Jean-Claude Yernault, M.D., Ph.D. Professor, Department of Respiratory Medicine, Free University of Brussels, and Medical Director, Erasme University Hospital, Brussels, Belgium

Lambros S. Zellos, M.D., M.P.H. Department of Thoracic Surgery, Harvard Medical School, and Brigham & Women's Hospital, Boston, Massachusetts, U.S.A.

CONTENTS

Introduction Claude Lenfant   *v*
Preface   *vii*
Contributors   *ix*

1. The History of Pleural Disease   **1**
Jean-Claude Yernault

    I. Introduction   1
    II. From Hippocrates to the Nineteenth Century   3
    III. The Nineteenth Century   8
    IV. Conclusion   14
    References   15

2. Anatomy of the Pleura   **23**
Ming-Jen Peng and Nai-San Wang

    I. Introduction   23
    II. Embryology   24
    III. The Pleura and Pleural Cavity   24
    IV. Gross and Light Microscopic Findings of the Pleura   26

V.	The Fine Structure of Mesothelial Cells	26
VI.	The Microvillus and Lubricating Membrane	28
VII.	The Blood Supply of the Pleura	29
VIII.	Innervation	30
IX.	Pleural Fluid and Contents	30
X.	Transport Across the Mesothelial Cell and Pleura	31
XI.	Lymphatics	32
XII.	Pleuro-Lymphatic Communication	33
XIII.	Regional Differences	36
XIV.	Dispute Over the Existence of Stomas	37
XV.	Pleuro-Peritoneal Communication and Diaphragmatic Defects	38
XVI.	Resting and Reactive Mesothelial Cells	38
XVII.	Subclinical Alterations and Repair of the Pleura	39
XVIII.	Summary	40
	References	40

3. Physiology of the Pleura — 45
Kostas I. Gourgoulianis

I.	Functional Anatomy	45
II.	Pleural Fluid Pressure and Dynamics	46
III.	Pleural Lymphatic Flow	48
IV.	Water and Ion Transportation	49
V.	Pathophysiology	49
	References	50

4. Pathophysiology of the Pleura — 53
Veena B. Antony

I.	Defense Mechanisms of the Pleura	53
II.	Cytokine Networks in the Pleural Space	54
III.	Changes in Pleural Cell Populations	56
IV.	Pleural Effusion Formation During Inflammation	59
V.	Resolution of Pleural Inflammation	60
VI.	Therapeutic Strategies Based on Pathophysiology of Pleural Disease	60
	References	61

5. Respiratory Function in Pleural Effusion — 65
Ioanna Mitrouska and Dimitris Georgopoulos

I.	Theoretical Considerations	66
II.	Respiratory System Mechanics	67
III.	Respiratory Muscles	70
IV.	Gas Exchange	71

V.	Conclusion	75
	References	75

6. Imaging of the Pleura — 79
Theresa C. McLoud and Gerald F. Abbott

I.	Pleural Effusion	79
II.	Pneumothorax	86
III.	Focal Pleural Disease	86
IV.	Diffuse Pleural Disease: Fibrothorax	95
V.	Malignant Pleural Disease	98
VI.	Thoracic Splenosis	106
	References	106

7. The Role of Ultrasonography in the Evaluation of Pleural Diseases — 111
Ok Hwa Kim and Kyung Joo Park

I.	Introduction	111
II.	Technique of Pleural Ultrasonography	112
III.	Normal Pleura and Artifacts of Pleural Ultrasonography	112
IV.	Pleural Effusion	114
V.	Pleural Tumors	123
VI.	Pneumothorax	125
VII.	Ultrasonography-Guided Thoracentesis and Catheter Drainage	125
VIII.	Ultrasonography-Guided Pleural Biopsy	127
	References	128

8. Pleural Thoracentesis and Biopsy — 131
Andreas H. Diacon and Chris T. Bolliger

I.	Introduction	131
II.	Indications, Contraindications	132
III.	Technique	133
IV.	Processing of Material	141
V.	Complications	142
VI.	Yield of Pleural Thoracentesis and Biopsy	143
VII.	Limitations	146
	References	147

9. Chest Tubes — 153
Michael H. Baumann

I.	Introduction	153
II.	Chest Tube Placement Technique and Complications	154

III.	Specific Chest Tube–Related Questions	156
IV.	The Pleural Drainage Unit	161
V.	Selected Applications	162
VI.	Summary	170
	References	170

10. Pleural Lavage as a Diagnostic and Research Tool 175
Marc Noppen

I.	Introduction	175
II.	Pleural Lavage as a Research Tool in Animals	176
III.	Pleural Lavage as a Research Tool in Humans	177
IV.	Pleural Lavage as a Diagnostic Tool in Humans	179
V.	Conclusions	180
	References	180

11. Medical Thoracoscopy 183
Philippe Astoul

I.	Introduction	183
II.	Equipment and Technique	184
III.	Complications and Contraindications	188
IV.	Clinical Applications	190
V.	Conclusion	204
	References	204

12. Diagnostic Video-Assisted Thoracoscopic Surgery in Pleural Disease 209
George Ladas

I.	Background	209
II.	Historic Overview	209
III.	Indications	210
IV.	Contraindications	211
V.	Instrumentation and Technique	211
VI.	Results	213
	References	214

13. Therapeutic Use of Thoracoscopy for Pleural Diseases 215
Gilbert Massard and Pascal Thomas

I.	Introduction	215
II.	Potential Indications for Therapeutic Thoracoscopy	216
III.	Preliminary Remarks	216
IV.	Video-Assisted Thoracic Surgery Management of Empyema	217

	V. VATS Management for Spontaneous Pneumothorax	221
	VI. Conclusion	231
	References	231

14. Discrimination Between Transudative and Exudative Pleural Effusions: Evaluating Diagnostic Tests in the Pleural Space   237
John E. Heffner

I.	Introduction	237
II.	Approaches to Diagnosis and Available Tests	237
III.	Derivation and Clinical Use of Diagnostic Tests	239
IV.	Measures of Diagnostic Accuracy	239
V.	Diagnostic Performance of Pleural Fluid Tests	247
VI.	Limitations of Pleural Fluid Tests	248
VII.	Conclusions	249
	References	249

15. Differentiating Between Benign and Malignant Pleural Effusions   253
D. Keith Payne and Michael W. Owens

I.	Introduction	253
II.	Clinical Manifestations of Benign and Malignant Pleural Effusion	254
III.	Diagnostic Approaches	254
IV.	Summary	261
	References	261

16. Clinical Evaluation of the Patient with a Pleural Effusion   267
Steven A. Sahn

I.	Introduction	267
II.	Value of Pleural Fluid Analysis	267
III.	Symptoms with Pleural Effusions	268
IV.	Physical Examination	269
V.	Laboratory Tests	270
	References	281

17. Transudate Pleural Effusions   287
Paula Carvalho

I.	Introduction	287
II.	Causes of Transudative Pleural Effusions	288
III.	Management of Transudative Pleural Effusions	297
	References	298

18.	**Interventional Radiology of Pleural Disease** *Johny A. Verschakelen*	**305**
	I. Introduction	305
	II. Imaging Guidance Modalities	305
	III. Percutaneous Drainage of Thoracic Fluid and Air Collections	307
	IV. Imaging of Complications	311
	V. Video-Assisted Thoracic Surgery	311
	References	312
19.	**Drug-Induced Pleural Diseases** *Philippe Camus*	**317**
	I. Introduction	317
	II. Diagnostic Criteria	318
	III. Drug-Induced Pleural Involvement	319
	IV. Pleural Involvement Following Chest Radiation Therapy	339
	V. Complications of Intrapleural Delivery of Drugs	344
	VI. Pleural Disease in Drug Abusers	344
	VII. Conclusion	344
	References	344
20.	**Parapneumonic Pleural Effusions and Empyema** *Demosthenes Bouros, Maria Plataki, and Sophia E. Schiza*	**353**
	I. Introduction	353
	II. Definitions	353
	III. Epidemiology	354
	IV. Pathophysiology	356
	V. Classification of Parapneumonic Effusion	358
	VI. Etiology of PPE/PE	362
	VII. Clinical Picture	362
	VIII. Diagnosis	363
	IX. Imaging Techniques	363
	X. Pleural Fluid Analysis	368
	XI. Differential Diagnosis	369
	XII. Treatment Strategy	369
	XIII. Methods for Treatment of PPE/PE	373
	XIV. Summary	381
	References	382
21.	**Postsurgical Pleural Infection** *Joseph A. LoCicero III*	**391**
	I. Postoperative Changes in the Pleura	391
	II. Residual Space Following Surgical Intervention	392

III.	Development of Space Infection	394
IV.	Management of Postoperative Pleural Infection	394
	References	396

22. Surgical Management of Empyema   399
Dean M. Donahue and Douglas J. Mathisen

I.	Introduction	399
II.	Empyema Without BPF	400
III.	Empyema with BPF	404
IV.	Management of the Pleural Space	406
V.	Conclusion	408
	References	409

23. Malignant Pleural Effusions   411
Steven A. Sahn

I.	Introduction	411
II.	Pathogenesis of Metastasis and Effusions	412
III.	Clinical Features	414
IV.	Radiological Findings	415
V.	Diagnosis	418
VI.	Management	420
VII.	Prognosis	430
VIII.	Conclusion	430
	References	431

24. Pleural Effusion in Lung Carcinoma   439
Marios E. Froudarakis and Pierre Fournel

I.	Introduction	439
II.	Pathogenesis	440
III.	Diagnostic Approach	440
IV.	Therapeutic Approach	445
	References	447

25. Benign Tumors of the Pleura   457
Cameron D. Wright and Eugene J. Mark

I.	History	457
II.	Incidence	458
III.	Etiology	458
IV.	Demographics	458
V.	Clinical Features	458
VI.	Laboratory Features	459
VII.	Radiographic Features	459

VIII.	Pathology	467
IX.	Malignant Fibrous Tumor of the Pleura	471
X.	Calcifying Fibrous Pseudotumor of the Pleura	475
	References	476

26. Pleurodesis   479
Francisco Rodríguez-Panadero

I.	Pleurodesis in Malignant Pleural Effusions	479
II.	Definition of Success or Failure of Pleurodesis in MPE	483
III.	Pleurodesis in Pneumothorax	486
IV.	Pleurodesis in Benign Effusions	487
V.	Technical Aspects of Pleurodesis	488
VI.	Mechanisms of Pleurodesis	490
VII.	Side Effects and Complications of Pleurodesis	494
VIII.	Alternatives to Talc Pleurodesis	496
IX.	Other Alternatives to Pleurodesis	498
	References	498

27. Pleuroperitoneal Shunts in Malignant Effusions   505
George Ladas and Peter Goldstraw

I.	Introduction	505
II.	The Evolution of Pleuroperitoneal Shunts	507
III.	Surgical Technique	510
IV.	The Royal Brompton Experience	513
V.	Conclusion	515
	References	516

28. Mesothelioma: Benign and Malignant   517
Gunnar Hillerdal

I.	"Benign" Mesotheliomas	517
II.	Malignant Pleural Mesothelioma	518
	References	527

29. Extrapleural Pneumonectomy for Early-Stage Diffuse Malignant Pleural Mesothelioma   531
Lambros S. Zellos and David J. Sugarbaker

I.	Introduction	531
II.	Clinical Presentation	532
III.	Diagnosis	532
IV.	Staging	533

V.	EPP Versus Pleurectomy/Decortication	535
VI.	EPP with Adjuvant Systemic Chemoradiation	537
VII.	EPP with Adjuvant Regional Modalities	539
VIII.	Conclusions	540
	References	540

30. Benign Asbestos-Related Pleural Disease — 545
E. Brigitte Gottschall and Lee S. Newman

I.	Introduction	545
II.	History	545
III.	Pathogenesis	546
IV.	Pleural Plaques	547
V.	Diffuse Pleural Thickening	553
VI.	Benign Asbestos Pleural Effusion	556
VII.	Rounded Atelectasis	558
	References	562

31. Pleural Manifestations of Interstitial Lung Disease — 571
Robert P. Baughman and Sally Seymour

I.	Introduction	571
II.	New Onset of ILD and Pleural Effusion	573
III.	Chronic ILD of Unknown Cause	573
IV.	Clinical Evaluation of Pleural Disease in ILD	585
	References	587

32. Immunological Diseases of the Pleura — 595
Demetrios A. Vassilakis, Athol U. Wells, and Demosthenes Bouros

I.	Introduction	595
II.	Rheumatoid Arthritis	596
III.	Systemic Lupus Erythematosus	600
IV.	Systemic Sclerosis	604
V.	Polymyositis/Dermatomyositis	604
VI.	Sjögren's Syndrome	605
VII.	Ankylosing Spondylitis	605
VIII.	Mixed Connective Tissue Disease	606
IX.	Eosinophilia-Myalgia Syndrome	606
X.	Angio-Immunoblastic Lymphadenopathy	607
XI.	Churg-Strauss Syndrome	608
XII.	Wegener's Granulomatosis	609
XIII.	Miscellaneous Diseases	609
	References	610

33. **Pleural Effusions in Blood Diseases** — 621
  Despina S. Kyriakou, Michael G. Alexandrakis, and Demosthenes Bouros

  I. Non-Hodgkin's Lymphomas and Hodgkin's Disease — 621
  II. Acute Leukemias — 623
  III. Bone Marrow Transplantation — 625
  IV. Myelodysplastic Syndromes — 626
  V. Chronic Leukemias — 626
  VI. Pleural Effusions Related to the Treatment of Hematological Malignancies — 627
  VII. Multiple Myeloma — 628
  VIII. Thalassemias — 629
  IX. Anemias and Coagulation Disorders — 629
  References — 630

34. **Pleural Effusions in HIV** — 639
  Kristina Crothers and Laurence Huang

  I. Introduction — 639
  II. Epidemiology of Pleural Effusion in Hospitalized HIV-Infected Patients — 640
  III. Outcome of HIV-Infected Patients with Pleural Effusion — 642
  IV. Diagnostic Evaluation of the HIV-Infected Patient with Pleural Effusion — 642
  V. Infectious Causes of Pleural Effusion in HIV-Infected Patients — 643
  VI. Malignant Pleural Effusions in HIV-Infected Patients — 650
  VII. Causes of Transudative Effusions in HIV-Infected Patients — 653
  VIII. Conclusion — 654
  References — 654

35. **Pneumothorax** — 661
  Charlie Strange and Michael A. Jantz

  I. Introduction — 661
  II. Traumatic Pneumothorax — 662
  III. Iatrogenic Pneumothorax — 662
  IV. Primary Spontaneous Pneumothorax — 662
  V. Secondary Spontaneous Pneumothorax — 664
  VI. Bronchopleural Fistula — 665
  VII. Tension Pneumothorax — 668
  VIII. Therapy — 669
  IX. Observation — 669

X.	Aspiration	670
XI.	Chest Thoracostomy Tubes	670
XII.	Chest Thoracostomy Tube Pleurodesis	671
XIII.	Thoracoscopy and Pleuroscopy	671
XIV.	Thoracotomy	672
XV.	Timing of Interventions	672
XVI.	Future Research	673
	References	673

36. Tuberculous Pleuritis 677
Peter D. O. Davies

I.	Introduction	677
II.	Definition	677
III.	Epidemiology	678
IV.	Tuberculous Pleurisy and HIV	679
V.	Pathophysiology	679
VI.	Case Study 1: A Breathless Man	681
VII.	Case Study 2: A Febrile Immigrant with an Effusion	682
VIII.	Case Study 3: A Breathless Woman	685
IX.	Case Study 4: A Case of Empyema	686
X.	Case Study 5: Untreated Tuberculous Pleuritis Leads to Something Worse	688
XI.	Diagnosis	688
XII.	Management of Tuberculous Pleural Effusion	692
XIII.	Management of Complications of Pleural Tuberculosis	693
	References	694

37. Pleural Effusions in Children 699
John N. Tsanakas and Elpis Hatziagorou

I.	Introduction	699
II.	Clinical Presentation	700
III.	Investigation	701
IV.	Diagnostic and Therapeutic Approach	704
V.	Summary	716
	References	716

38. Pleural Effusions in Cardiac Disease 721
John F. Murray

I.	Introduction	721
II.	Prevalence	722
III.	Pathogenesis	722
IV.	Congestive Heart Failure	724
V.	Pericarditis	728

VI.	Postcardiac Injury Syndrome	729
VII.	Coronary Artery Revascularization	730
VIII.	Other Causes	731
IX.	Summary	732
	References	733

39. Pleural Effusions in Pregnancy and Gynecological Diseases — 737
Nikolaos E. Tzanakis and Katerina Antoniou

I.	Introduction	737
II.	Pleural Effusion in Gynecology	738
III.	Pregnancy-Related Pleural Effusion	742
	References	750

40. Pleural Disease in the Intensive Care Unit — 757
Spyridon A. Papiris and Charis Roussos

I.	Pleural Effusions in the Intensive Care Unit	757
II.	Pneumothorax and Related Conditions Secondary to Pulmonary Barotrauma in the ICU	769
	References	780

41. Pleural Effusions in Gastrointestinal Tract Diseases — 783
Epaminondas N. Kosmas and Vlasis S. Polychronopoulos

I.	General Considerations	783
II.	Transudative Pleural Effusion	784
III.	Exudative Pleural Effusion	788
IV.	Metastatic Pleural Effusions	802
	References	803

42. Pleural Effusions in Pulmonary Embolism — 811
Luis Puente-Maestu and Victoria Villena

I.	Introduction	811
II.	Mechanisms	812
III.	Clinical Picture	814
IV.	Diagnosis	817
V.	Conclusion	828
	References	829

43. Pleural Effusions Secondary to Fungal, Nocardial, and Actinomycotic Infection — 837
Mark Woodhead

I.	Introduction	837
II.	*Aspergillus* Species	838

III.	*Candida* and *Torulopsis* Species	841
IV.	*Pneumocystis carinii*	841
V.	*Cryptococcus* Species	842
VI.	*Mucor* Species	842
VII.	*Histoplasma capsulatum*	842
VIII.	*Blastomyces dermatitidis*	843
IX.	*Coccidioides immitis*	843
X.	*Paracoccidioides brasiliensis*	844
XI.	*Sporothrix schenkii*	844
XII.	*Actinomyces israelii*	844
XIII.	*Nocardia* Species	846
	References	847

44. Pleural Effusions in Parasitic Infections 851
Semra Bilaçeroğlu

I.	Introduction	851
II.	Amebiasis	852
III.	Echinococcosis	859
IV.	Paragonimiasis	871
V.	Pneumocystosis	876
VI.	Nematode (Roundworm) Infections	878
VII.	Parasitoses with Unlocated Parasites	882
VIII.	Schistosomiasis	883
IX.	Incidentally Found Parasites in the Pleura	884
X.	Miscellaneous Parasitoses Rarely Causing Pleural Effusion	885
	References	886

45. Iatrogenic and Rare Pleural Effusions 897
Maria Plataki and Demosthenes Bouros

I.	Iatrogenic Pleural Effusions	897
II.	Yellow Nail Syndrome	900
III.	Uremia	902
IV.	Trapped Lung	903
V.	Therapeutic Radiation Exposure	904
VI.	Drowning	905
VII.	Amyloidosis	905
VIII.	Milk of Calcium Pleural Collections	906
IX.	Pleural Effusion in Electrical Injury	906
X.	Mediastinal Cysts	907
XI.	Whipple's Disease	907
XII.	Syphilis	907
	References	908

46.	**Management of the Undiagnosed Persistent Pleural Effusion** *Richard W. Light*	**915**
	I. Introduction	915
	II. Diseases That Cause Undiagnosed Persistent Pleural Effusions	915
	III. Tests to Consider for Patients with Persistent Undiagnosed Pleural Effusion	924
	References	928
47.	**Hemothorax** *Paul E. Van Schil, Philippe G. Jorens, and Patrique Segers*	**931**
	I. Introduction	931
	II. Etiology	932
	III. Clinical Presentation	934
	IV. Diagnosis	934
	V. Treatment	935
	VI. Conclusion	940
	References	940
48.	**Chylothorax and Pseudochylothorax** *Petros Bakakos, Michael Toumbis, and Antonis Rasidakis*	**943**
	I. Chylothorax	943
	II. Pseudochylothorax	955
	References	958
49.	**The Pleural Space and Organ Transplantation** *Marc A. Judson and Steven A. Sahn*	**963**
	I. Introduction	963
	II. Bone Marrow Transplantation	963
	III. Heart Transplantation	969
	IV. Liver Transplantation	972
	V. Kidney Transplantation	975
	VI. Lung and Heart-Lung Transplantation	979
	VII. Summary	985
	References	985
50.	**Pharmacokinetics and Pharmacodynamics in Pleural Fluid** *Ioannis Liapakis, Ioannis Kottakis, Richard W. Light, and Demosthenes Bouros*	**999**
	I. Introduction	999
	II. Pharmacokinetics in Pleural Fluid	1000
	III. Pharmacodynamics in Pleural Fluid	1004

	IV.	Conclusion	1005
		References	1006
51.	\multicolumn{2}{l}{**Animal Models in Pleural Investigation**}	**1009**

51. **Animal Models in Pleural Investigation** — 1009
    Richard W. Light

I.	Pleural Inflammation	1009
II.	Hypersensitivity Reactions	1012
III.	Pleurodesis	1013
IV.	Asbestos	1016
V.	Tuberculosis	1017
VI.	Empyema	1018
VII.	Malignancy	1021
VIII.	Asbestos and Mesothelioma	1025
	References	1027

Index — *1035*

PLEURAL DISEASE

1

The History of Pleural Disease

JEAN-CLAUDE YERNAULT

Free University of Brussels
and Erasme University Hospital
Brussels, Belgium

I. Introduction

Before considering the history of pleural disease, clarification of the meaning of terms previously used in the literature is needed. The Greek word *pleuron* means side and/or rib (1,2). Consequently, for the ancients, any disease in the chest wall was called pleuritis, especially if accompanied by pain in the side (3). Thoracic pain was already recognized in Egyptian medicine, as suggested in the *Ebers Papyrus* (ca. 1550 B.C), which mentions a patient suffering "from pain under the ribs" (4), and pleural disease certainly did exist at the time, as shown by autopsies of mummies finding pleural lesions alone (5) or accompanying pulmonary lesions (6). A similar allusion to thoracic pain can be found in the annals of Assyro-Babylonian medicine (7): "when a man, after falling in water, feels pain which diffuses now in one side now in the other one, according to whether he breathes in a way or another."

The pleural membrane was not known by Hippocrates (460–337 B.C.) but Aristotle (384–322 B.C.) recognized that all the organs are surrounded by a membrane (8). Pliny (23–79) emphasized that the "foreseeing nature" contained all the main thoracic viscera, in particular membranes he called, "*membranae propriae*" (9).

Aretaeus the Cappadocian, who lived in Alexandria about the second century A.D. (10), stated that "under the ribs, the spine, and in the internal part of the thorax, there is stretched a thin but strong membrane, adhering to the bone, which is called succingens " (11,12). He further stressed the fact that the lung is insensible to pain, but that pain is present if any of the membranes surrounding the lung is inflamed.

Galen (129–200 A.D.) (13,14) wrote: "nature created another structure of the same substance as peritoneum and performing for the organs of pneuma as does the peritoneum for the organs of assimilation.... It is called the undergirder since it undergirds the inside of the ribs.... It has two designations, being called membrane by some and coat by others, membrane from its substance, coat from its function. It is made of two leaves, one covering the whole lung, the other one covering the ribs and the mediastinum; it prevents the lungs from striking the nude ribs during the respiratory act."

The term "pleurisy" (from the Greek *pleuresis* and the French *pleurésie*) was customarily used to describe any inflammation of the pleura (1,15)—with (wet pleurisy) or without (dry pleurisy) effusion. Some authors recommended reserving the term "pleuritis" for an inflammation without effusion (1,15,16) and "pleurisy" for cases with effusion (16). Much confusion existed in the field between dry and wet pleurisy: doctors as prominent as Boerhaave (17), Buchan (18), and Tissot (19) spoke of dry pleurisy in cases without sputum and of wet pleurisy in cases with sputum.

The term "empyema" (from the Greek *en* = in and *puon* = pus) in hippocratic texts refers to any collection of pus in the thorax (20) or even more generally to any suppuration (2), not differentiating between an abscess in the lung or a purulent effusion in the thoracic cavity, the latter also being called "pyothorax," a more specific term than empyema (21). Further confusion has arisen from a broader use of the word empyema to describe any collection of liquid in the pleural cavity (22) or even the operation to evacuate such liquid: "when I speak of empyema, I mean a wound made at the lower part of the breast to give issue to the matter distributed in its cavity" (23). Such an operation was also called thoracic paracentesis (from the Greek *para* = on the side and *kentein* = to prick, to pierce), a term that appeared in the sixteenth century (24). To describe the removal of fluid from the chest, whether by aspiration or by drainage (25), the term "thoracentesis" was created to replace thoracic paracentesis.

The term "pleurodynia" (from the Greek *odyno* = pain), which literally means pain in the side (1,15), is sometimes used to describe a rheumatic pain that has its seat in the intercostal muscles and may mimic pleurisy (22).

Marrotte (26) made a distinction between the method of empyema, which allows free entrance of air into the pleural cavity, and thoracentesis, which prevents air from penetrating inside the thorax and favors reexpansion of the lung.

II. From Hippocrates to the Nineteenth Century

Hippocrates noted that the three disease states of the chest he called pleurisy, peripneumony, and pain occur chiefly in winter (27), and that another cause of pleurisy was excessive intake of strong drink of (e.g., wine) (28). He insisted that in some subjects the pain could be felt in the shoulder, the clavicle, and the armpit. He described a fourth state, empyema, that could be recognized in all cases by the following signs (29):

A constant fever—slight in the daytime, higher at night
Copious sweat
A desire to cough, but slight or no expectoration

Empyema may be associated with several classical physical signs (30–32): digital hippocratism ("the nails of the hands are bent, the extremities of the fingers are hot, there are swellings in the feet"), hippocratic succussion ("shaking the patient by the shoulders, you listen [to hear in] which side a splashing sound can be heard"). Sometimes no noise can be heard because of the density and quantity of the fluid (33), and eventually local redness or swelling occurs before spontaneous external evacuation of pus. By direct auscultation, Hippocrates also identified pleural rub, a leathery sound audible at the stage of dry pleurisy (30–34).

The possible association of empyema with digestive symptoms was mentioned in The Aphorisms (27): those who are subject to acid eructations are seldom attacked by pleurisy; when diarrhea accompanies pleurisy, it is unfavorable.

Several therapeutic approaches are mentioned in the hippocratic writings, rib trephination, intercostal incision, and cautery among them (21,30,33): "what drugs will not cure, the knife will; what the knife will not cure, the cautery will; what the cautery will not cure will be considered incurable" (35). The incision should be performed as low as possible, so that the pus may flow out more easily. It was also recommended that the cauterization or the incision be done before pus stayed too long; however in the latter case the patient recovers nearly always. The wound should be packed with a linen or cotton cloth, which allows the fluid to escape around it, but prevents the free inflow of air (36). Much like Hippocrates did not consistently distinguish between pleurisy and peripneumony, neither did he differentiate between empyema and lung abscess (37,38).

By the term pleurisy, Aristotles meant the "coagulation or thickening of liquid matter" (9). Diocles of Carystos (ca. 350 B.C.), who wrote the first book of anatomy, may well have been the first to distinguish between pleurisy and pneumonia (39,40). Asklepiades of Bithynia (124 B.C.) called pleurisy a "flow of liquid matter in the internal lateral portions of the body, of short duration and acute, with fever and inflammation" (9). Apollonius (81–58 B.C.) suggested that pleurisy is not necessarily limited to the pleural membrane: "pleurisy is generally an acute disease of short duration in the pleural membranes, and in the fleshy parts connected with these membranes; it also occurs at times in parts of the lung" (9).

Celsus (25 B.C. to 50 A.D.) considered pleurisy an acute pernicious disease characterized by pain in the side, fever, and cough, sometimes dry, which can, however, be accompanied by pituitous (limited disease) or bloody (more severe disease) sputum (41,42). He advocated applying a hot iron to the side where there is the greatest swelling until it reaches the pus and the matter is drawn off. Occasionally the abscess would drain spontaneously or rupture in the bronchial tree. Bloodletting and the application of sharp mustard on the chest were among the recommended remedies.

Soranus (9) described pleurisy as a severe affliction in the internal lateral parts of the body with acute fever and a cough in which fluid of varying character is produced. It is more common in old than in young men, in women than in men, and in the wintertime.

Aretaeus gave a classic description (3) of pleurisy and its possible conversion to empyema (11,12). He underlined the importance of pain, which "stresses to all its adhesions at the shoulders and clavicles, and in certain cases even to the back and shoulder blade ('dorsal pleurisy' of the Ancients)"(12). Accompanying symptoms are dyspnea, insomnolency, dry cough, "difficult expectoration of phlegm, or bilious, or deeply tinged with blood, or yellowish"(12).

Aretaeus included empyema among the chronic diseases; he defined it as an abscess of matter that forms in cavities above or along the region of chest, or in those below the diaphragm. He noticed that it is a wonder how "from a thin, slender membrane, having no depth like that which lines the chest, so much pus should flow."(12) Rather than true pain, heaviness is a common symptom. Swelling of the feet and fingers can be observed, as well as distension of the thorax.

For the cure of pleurisy, Aretaeus (44) proposed several remedies, except in the case of pleuritis from peripneumonia, where recovery readily takes place. In many cases there was "no time for procrastination nor for putting off the great remedy: we must by all means open a vein." Aretaeus also recommended applying to the side "soft oil with the healing ointment of rue, and the decoction of dill—also a very soothing fomentation." As far as treatment is concerned, "ptisan is to be preferred.... It will be calculated to moisten and warm, and able to dissolve and clear away phlegm, to evacuate upwards without pain such matters as should be brought up, and also readily evacuate the bowels downwards." Cold water was not recommended for pleuritics.

Galen (45,46) described the inflammation of the pleural membrane as causing pain with dyspnea, an acute fever, and a special pulse. When the upper parts of the membrane are affected, pain irradiates towards the clavicles; when the inferior parts are affected, pain irradiates towards the hypochondrium. Pain may be due to forced movements of the diaphragm during respiration, and hepatic pain can be transmitted to the pleura.

Coelius Aurelianus (ca. 400) described the following symptoms of pleurisy (9):

Acute fever

Coughing with severe pain in the side reaching up to the collarbone and the shoulder blade of affected side, in some cases also touching the arm, chest, and iliac region

Pricking, throbbing, and burning pain, continuous or intermittent, persistently adhering to the same place, or else moving about, returning and changing; accompanied by sighing, difficulty in breathing (Greek dyspnea)

Cough, dry in some cases but frequently with fluid discharges, at first frothy, then bloody, then bilious, and then "sanious"

Patients are able to lie on affected side.

In a case of pleurisy on the verge of turning into pneumonia, all the characteristics are aggravated and intensified, with the sole exception of the pain. When it is becoming empyema, pain becomes fixed in one place and remains there, becoming less severe; new symptoms appear: trembling recurring at regular or irregular intervals, dyspnea, a rapid pulse.

In the sixth century Alexander of Tralles (525–605) gave an accurate clinical picture of pleurisy (10), and Aetius of Amida (ca. 540) also gave an account of pleurisy (43).

In the eleventh century, Avicenna (980–1037) described the symptoms of simple pleurisy (20) as follows:

Constant fever

Violent pain felt under the ribs, sometimes becomes only obvious when the patient breathes

Difficult and fast breathing

Weak and hasty pulse

Cough, first dry, then accompanied by expectoration, indicating lung involvement.

In the twelfth century, a few surgeons manifested a renewed interest for the therapy of empyema. Lanfranchi (1295) did not hesitate to operate (43), and Henri de Mondeville (1260–1320) recommended in cases that had ruptured drainage via an intercostal incision in the lower chest (33). Later Fabricius of Aquapendente (1537–1619) was also a supporter of the operation (33); he attributed the poor prognosis to the lack of surgeons who knew anatomy and could incise with safety.

Paracelsus (1493–1541) was of the opinion (47) that diseases in themselves are not apprehensible by the sense and that their presence must be deduced from the symptoms—for example, in pleurisy from side pain, dyspnea, fever, pulse, and sputum. Goeurot (1546) described four major signs in cases of "pleuresie:" a great burning fever, sore ribs within as if they were pricked continuously with needles, a short breath, a strong cough (48,49).

Ambroise Paré (1517–1590), a surgeon, defined "pleurisie" as an inflammation of the membranes investing the ribs that commonly infers a pricking pain, a fever, and difficulty in breathing. According to Paré, when the disease tends to suppuration or turns into an empyema, the "chirurgeon may make a vent between the third and fourth true and legitimate ribs, with an actual or potential cautery, or with a sharp knife drawn upwards, but not downwards. If the patient shall have a large body, chest and ribs, you may divide and perforate the ribs themselves with a trepan. The pus and matter must be evacuated by little and little at several times, and the capacity of the chest cleansed by a detergent injection of bailey water and honey of rose" (50–53).

Intending to create a new classification of diseases, Sydenham (1624–1689) focused on epidemic diseases and defined "intercurrent" fevers as those that could occur in any year, among them pleurisy (54): "The patient is seized with a sharp, pricking pain, in the side or in the region of the ribs, which shoots sometimes towards the shoulder-blades, sometimes towards the spine, sometimes towards the front of the chest. . . . The cough is accompanied by so much pain, that the patient holds his breath. . . . The matter brought up by expectoration is, at the onset of the disease, scanty and thin, and frequently streaked with particles of blood. . . . At times the disease gains strength (venesection having been omitted)."

Sydenham (54) argued against the practice of medicine by unqualified people when pus is effused in the cavity of the thorax: "This form of mischief arises from the unreasonable and preposterous use of over-heating medicines, which are the favorite prescription of certain women of rank, whose charity and benevolence would be better employed in feeding the poor than in physicking them." As far as therapy is concerned, his "sheet-anchor is venesection, but immediately after the blood letting the following draught is to be taken (popywater, sal prunella & symp of violets)," whereas meat altogether is forbidden.

For Lowe (1654) the signs of "pleurisie" were "great dolor, from the shoulder unto the nethermost rib, punction in the side, continual fever, difficulty of respiring, hard pulse, great alteration with want of appetite, evil favored breath heaviness and ponderosity of the sides, great fever chiefly in the night, little sleep, some sweats which happen through great pain" (48).

Willis (1621–1675) emphasized that "pleuresie and peripneumonia" have a great affinity, but that they exist separately, that the seat of sense of pain is in the pleura, and that difficult breathing occurs by reason of the action of the muscular fibers being impaired (55).

Le Clerc (1696) advocated drainage of an empyema through an intercostal incision below the angle of the scapula, four fingerbreadths from the spine, between the 2nd and 3rd false ribs (counting from the bottom); then the finger should be inserted and adhesions separated. A wick or tent of linen or lint, impregnated with some ointment should be inserted, and the whole covered with a cloth dressing (36).

Boerhaave's (1668–1738) aphorisms include a description of pleural pain modulation by breathing movements (17): "The patient is afflicted with an acute inflammatory pain and stitch, which are much increased upon breathing in the air, and milder in the breathing out, or while the patient gently keeps in his breath, gentler also when he performs breathing without moving the chest, but chiefly by the repeated raising and lowering of the belly.... He coughs almost incessantly, which because of the violent pain it causes, he strives to suppress. When the patient spits.... it is a moist pleuresie; when that is wanting, 'tis a dry pleuresie." Boerhaave called paraphrenitis a pleurisy that invades the pleura which surrounds the diaphragm and emphasized on the intolerable pain it causes.

The year 1761 stands as one of the great dates in medicine, with the publication of Morgagni's (56) "The seats and causes of the diseases investigated by anatomy" and Auenbrugger's (57) "Inventum novum ex percussione thoracis humani." Dissecting the bodies of men and women having died of various diseases, Morgagni (56) was surprised by the frequency of adherences between the lungs and the thoracic wall; in a case of a left hydrothorax, he compared the macroscopic appearance of the serum it contained to that of the urine of horses.

Auenbrugger (57) introduced chest percussion to evaluate diseases of the thoracic cavity. "If a sonorous region of the chest appears, on percussion, entirely destitute of the natural sound—that is, if it yields only a sound like that of a fleshy limb when struck—disease exists in that region." His 12th observation concerns a disease he called "dropsy of the chest," corresponding to a collection of water in the cavity of the chest between the pleura costalis and the lungs. Among the 15 general symptoms that he enumerated were difficult and laborious breathing, a cough at intervals which is dry or only attended by sputa of a thin watery nature, a sense of breathlessness and suffocation on the slightest motion, and the inability to lie down. If the chest is half-filled, a louder sound will be obtained over the parts to which the fluid does not extend; and, in this case, the resonance will be found to vary according to the position of the patient and the consequent level that the liquid attains.

In the 18th century, however, Auenbrugger's technique did not gain wide acceptance (58), as illustrated by Cullen's assertion: "I have not had occasion or opportunity to observe the method proposed by Auenbrugger." Although he recognized that pleurisy is accompanied by a "pungitive" pain increasing during inspiration, Cullen expressed the view that no sign could establish the precise seat of a thoracic disease. He thought that the most decisive symptom in the recognition of hydrothorax was fluctuation of water in the chest, perceived by the patient himself or by the physician upon certain movement of the body (59).

Buchan (1729–1805) distinguished between "true" and "spurious or bastard" pleurisy (18). In the latter case the pain is more external and chiefly affects the muscles between the ribs. Buchan recognized two kinds of true pleurisy: moist, where the patient spits freely, and dry, where the patient spits little or not at all. According to him, pleurisy prevailed among laborers and was most frequent in the spring. He considered the following symptoms characteristic of pleurisy:

> "[A] violent pricking pain in one of the sides among the rib, most violent when the patient draws in his breath, which extents sometimes towards the back bone, sometimes towards the sore part of the breast, and the other times towards the shoulderblades"
>
> "[S]pittle at first thin, but afterwards grosser and often streaked with blood"
>
> "[T]he crisis or height of fever is sometimes attended with very alarming symptoms difficulty of breathing, irregular pulse, convulsive motions"

Several therapeutic approaches were proposed by Buchan (18), starting with bloodletting in large quantities. Local therapies applied to the affected side included emollient fomentations, a bladder filled with warm milk and water, soft poultices or cataplasms (wheat bread and milk, softened with oil or fresh butter), and leaves of various plants. Sharp, oily, and mucilaginous medicines were recommended to promote spitting. Having a bath of warm milk and water in which emollient vegetables were boiled was considered of benefit.

According to Tissot (1728–1797)a pleurisy had four characteristics (19): high fever, difficulty in breathing, cough, and a sharp pain in the thoracic wall. The pain due to pleurisy was not differentiated from that due to pneumonia, except perhaps in that it was more external. The patient could lie more easily on the affected than on the healthy side. A dry pleurisy was a pleurisy without sputum.

According to Sharp (1761) a bloody pleural effusion should not be evacuated because its removal would increase the bleeding, whereas the bleeding might be stopped by the pressure of the accumulated fluid.

Stoll (1742–1787) emphasized that a wet pleurisy frequently accompanies peripneumonia; he distinguished between true and false pleurisy, the latter involving the muscles rather than the pleural membrane (60). Baillie (1761–1825) recognized that the pleural liquid is frequently a mixture of serous fluid and coagulable lymph and that in empyema pus could accumulate in the entire cavity or be confined to a part of it by adhesions between the lungs and pleura (61).

III. The Nineteenth Century

By the turn of the eighteenth century, whether pleurisy could be clearly differentiated from peripneumony remained unsettled. In 1787, at the Paris Academy of Sciences, Portal presented an "observation that proves that pleurisy is not a disease differing essentially from peripneumony." However, in 1798, Pinel strongly supported this essential distinction (62,63).

The physiology of the serous membranes was clearly described by Bichat (1771–1802) in his *A Treatise on the Membranes* (64). He emphasized that "the serous membranes are characterized by the lymphatic fluid, which incessantly lubricates them, and that every serous membrane represents a sack without an opening spread over the respective organs which it embraces. Their first function is doubtless to form about the essential organs a boundary, which separates them from those of their vicinity—a second office is to facilitate the moving of the organs."

The nineteenth century witnessed the development of the clinical method and physical examination. Landré-Beauvais (65) called attention to the measurement of the frequency of breathing, which accelerates both during hydrothorax and chest inflammation; he also noticed that in some cases of pleurisy the inspiration can be so distressing that the patient is forced to exhale promptly (*expiratio celer*). Movements of the arm or the trunk can accentuate pain when it arises in the parietal muscles (pleurodynia), whereas pressing the intercostal spaces accentuates the shooting pain of pleurisy. Double (66) recognized the role of percussion, an obscure or dull sound indicating extravasation of liquid in the chest, but he was far from recommending the procedure in every patient: "chest percussion not only in some cases can bless patients' sense of decency, but can also tire them out or become painful, if one would insist too much on this sort of search." Double (67) also attempted to distinguish pain finding its origin in the intercostal or parietal muscles from pleural pain, suggesting that a parietal pain is not constant, but imprecise and superficial, that it can be aggravated by mechanical means, but ceases after parietal compression or massage.

Corvisart's translation of and comments on Auenbrugger's work (68) did much to popularize percussion among the medical community, in France first and then rapidly abroad. He maintained that it is the best means to detect a liquid effusion in the chest. He supported percussion with a open hand, its strength being proportionate to the thickness of the muscles and teguments. He added to the percussion the tactile sense of using the fingertips (68–70).

With the introduction of the stethoscope and indirect auscultation, Laennec (71–73) revolutionized the practice of medicine; pleural diseases did not escape his clearsightedness. His systematic anatomo-pathological correlations allowed him to recognize the signs of pure pleural disease and to separate them from those of peripneumonia. He emphasized that "the symptoms of acute pleuritis are generally pretty well marked, though not unequivocally so, but that in chronic pleurisy it is not, for the most part, till after many weeks and months that the real nature of the disease is suspected" (74). As soon as an effusion takes place, the natural sound fails over the whole space occupied by the liquid. If effusion is inconsiderable, it tends to the posterior or inferior parts of the chest; in the course of a few hours, the dull sound exists over the whole affected side. When the cylinder is applied to the chest, a great diminution or absence of respiratory sounds is observed, except in the space of three fingers' breadth along the vertebral column. With copious effusion, the loss of sound is complete, whereas the respiration becomes puerile on the other side. When the effusion begins to diminish, the intensity of the sound first augments along the spine, then along the anterior superior part of the chest and top of the shoulder. The resonance takes longer to be restored, percussion yielding a dull sound long after the reappearance of respiration under the stethoscope.

Laennec described egophonism as a pathognomonic sign when it exists, which always indicates a moderate degree of effusion. Egophonism is perceived at the upper and thinnest part of the effused fluid; it is accompanied generally by bronchial respiration and bronchophonism. As already described by Hippocrates in cases of empyema, the affected side becomes larger, which can be perceived after 2 days of illness, more evidently in lean fat persons, but becomes indistinct in women with large mammae. When measuring the thoracic dimensions with a piece of rubber, the affected size is never as enlarged as perceived by the eye. Sometimes over time the affected size becomes narrower than before the disease.

Laennec suggested practicing hippocratic succussion in the following manner: "having placed the patient in a firm seat, cause his hands to be held by an assistant, and then shake him by the shoulder, in order to hear on which side the disease shall produce a sound." He recognized that fluctuation indicates the coexistence of pneumothorax with a liquid effusion.

A follower of Laennec, Stokes (75) gave a description of pleurisy that would for the most part still be valuable today. He insisted on the vocal quality: "Egophonia is a strong reverberation of the voice, which seems shrill, interrupted, and quivering like that of a goat. It always appears to indicate the existence of a small quantity of liquid in the cavity of the pleura, or the occurrence of thick pseudomembranes yet in a soft state." The phenomenon ceases when the effusion becomes abundant, and returns when it diminishes. Proof of an effusion is given by the dullness of sound on percussion and absence of the respiratory murmur. Early symptoms include a pain in the side, below the breast, followed by a dry cough and oppression; inspirations are short and frequent. Pain is increased by percussion, intercostal pressure, cough, and respiratory motion. The dullness is at its maximum laterally and posteriorly, where the respiratory murmur is inaudible. In cases of chronic pleuritis, the affected side becomes more voluminous than the other. It may contract, giving the patient a crooked or bent appearance, the chest becoming evidently narrower, with a lower shoulder, and the ribs brought nearer to one another. In measuring the thorax, the patient is stripped of all clothing and made to sit upright, with his arms in the same relative position. "The semi-circumference is to be taken by a string, from the spinous process to the middle of the sternum; and then turning the string without moving its extremity from the spinous process, we are to measure the opposite side in the same manner."

Louis (76,77) was struck by the frequency of pleural adhesions, not only in the cases of phthisis he autopsied, but also in other diseases (35 adherences in 112 subjects). A type of pleural lesion was suggested to be specific to phthisis, the semi-cartilaginous pleural layer covering the top of the lungs. The association between phthisis and pleural adhesions had already been made by Bayle

(78), who remarked that it should not, however, be deduced that pleurisy is the determinant of the lung lesions. Baron (79) had also been surprised at the extent of disease that dissection frequently shows among the thoracic viscera, even when the signs generally supposed to denote its presence were scarcely observable.

Piorry (80) introduced indirect percussion and claimed that the plessimeter allowed recognition of differences in percussion better than direct percussion, stating that the plessimeter discovered half a pint of serous liquid, whereas breathing still could be heard clearly. He also insisted on the possible existence of partial or circumscribed pleural effusions, such as interlobar, diaphragmatic, mediastinal, or costopulmonary effusion. He remarked on the limited value of some signs described by Laennec, such as the change in level of dullness with change in posture, and on the difficulty in eliciting the egophonism sign. Gerhard (81) also believed egophony to be of secondary importance.

In the first edition of their classical textbook, Barth and Roger (82) insisted on the semiological value of an abolished respiration when it is auscultated in the lower half or two thirds of the chest, together with a percussed dullness; for them such an association is nearly pathognomonic of a thoracic effusion. They emphasized that Reynaud (83) had been the first (after Hippocrates!) to point out the ascending and descending character of the pleural rub. They had little confidence in egophonia as an efficient diagnostic sign. Reynaud (83) also proposed placing a hand under each scapula to detect a pleuritic effusion by absence of vibration over a dull portion of the thorax.

Skoda (84,85) noticed that in cases of massive but incomplete pleural effusion, a tympanic sound is heard above the upper level of the effusion, where the lung is nevertheless partially deprived of air, which, he thought, was opposed to the laws of physics. This more than expected resonant note over the lung above an ipsilateral pleural effusion is still called skodaic resonance; it is in fact a strong argument in favor of the cage resonance theory rather than the topographic percussion theory of genesis of the percussion notes (86). Trousseau (87) described skodaic resonance as a special, "half-tympanic" sound, better heard under the clavicle near the sternum.

Damoiseau (88) was the first to recognize that the top border of dullness over a pleural effusion is not horizontal, but rather follows a semi-elliptic form, being highest in the axilla; soon later Stillé (89) made the same observation. This phenomenon, known as Damoiseau's curve in Europe, was rediscovered by Ellis in the United States, where it remains described as the letter S curve of Ellis. By contrast in cases of hydropneumothorax the upper limit of dullness remains strictly horizontal. Near the top of an effusion and next to the spine persists a small area of relative resonance known as Garland's triangle, whereas a right-angle triangle of dullness is found over the posterior part of the chest opposite a large pleural effusion; the latter, known as Grocco's triangle, was first described by Koranyi in 1897 (86).

The course of a pleurisy was well described by Walshe (90). At the outset is a dry stage, with a grazing friction-sound and a limitation of the expansion of the hemithorax, the percussion note being not diminished. Increased frequency of breathing is a constant symptom. At the stage of plastic exudation, the resonance becomes less clear and a sensation of resistance is perceived in the finger applied on the intercostal space; a rubbing vibration can be perceived but the resonance of the voice remains unchanged. Some cough is present in the majority of cases, usually dry. At the effusive stage the vocal fremitous is abolished, the vesicular murmur is suppressed or very weak, and there is a loss of resonance together with a rise of pitch of the percussion note and an increased parietal resistance. A tubular or amphoric resonance is heard at the upper front of the affected side. The limits of toneless and resonance part may be changed by altering the posture. Egophony is found in a minority of cases. After effusion has occurred, the patient lies on his back, the affected side, or diagonally between both, whereas in the dry and plastic stages he commonly lies on the sound side or the back.

If the effusion progresses, the affected side looks bulged and a lateral detrusion of the heart occurs. The vocal vibration disappears, and the respiratory sounds are suppressed, except close to the spine and at the apex; the dullness is absolute. In case of recovery, the thoracic enlargement gradually disappears, the friction sound and vocal vibration return, the percussion sound recovers and the vesicular murmur is gradually restored. The healed side may even contract, drawing down the shoulder (91–93). In cases of phrenic pleurisy, the pain is usually severe, agonizing under the influence of full inspiration, varying in amount inexplicably from time to time. Hiccup and vomiting are occasionally observed. Risus sardonicus has not fallen under Walshe's observation; orthopnea with trunk bent forwards is, however, frequent.

Citing Rokitansky, von Niemeyer (94) insisted on the changes occurring in consequence of extensive effusion: "the thorax is dilated in a manner more or less apparent, the intercostal spaces are widened and prominent, the diaphragm is forced down into the abdomen, the mediastinum and heart are displaced to other side." However, to appreciate correctly the circumference of the thorax, it should be measured directly (95). A pleurisy with little fibrinous exudation is accompanied by a severe piercing pain when a breath is drawn; coughing and sneezing are especially painful. A pressure upon the ribs and intercostal muscles increases the pain. The respiration is shallow and cautious, and the body is generally bent towards the affected side. Some patients have a distinct sensation of friction or of scratching at some point of the thorax. The friction sounds are heard more distinctly when the stethoscope is pressed rather firmly on the thoracic wall; they are not altered by a cough, unlike the buzzing ronchus which it may resemble. A true pleural friction sound can sometimes be produced by the heart beating (89,95).

In his series of 78 cases of pleurisy, Blakiston (96) noticed that the patient laid on the affected side in 46 cases, on the opposite side in 4, and indifferently in 28 cases. He considered vocal resonance as one of the least valuable signs and heard a pure beating sound rarely. The only sign that was never absent in his experience was a hurried respiration. His findings contradict Andral's opinion

(97) that the evocation of the vocal fremitus is the best way to evaluate the height of a pleural effusion. Flint (98,99) also stated that the abolition of the normal fremitus is the more significant sign of effusion; on the other hand, he was repeatedly disappointed in seeking for egophony, which led him to "distrust its availability." Beau (100) noticed that cough, like voice, at times could have a bleating character. A proposal by Baccelli, quoted by Woillez (101), attracted some interest. He suggested that the whispered voice could be transmitted through a serous exudate, but would pass with difficulties, or not all, through a purulent fluid. His proposal was accepted by Gueneau de Mussy, but not by Tripier (101); however, it did not gain wide acceptance and was no longer judged as sufficient to make a differential diagnosis between purulent and serous effusions (102,103). Landouzy (104) suggested that egophony is rather a sign suggestive of a recent effusion, whereas in older cases an amphoric voice can be auscultated; he noticed that in some cases the beating sound remains after draining off of the liquid. This amphoric breathing can be found in purulent and serous effusions and probably indicates the presence of false membranes. The coupling of egophony, dullness, and absence of thoracic vibrations was taken by Dieulafoy (105) as a symptomatic triad that never misleads.

Since no clinical sign was able to definitely confirm the presence of a pleural effusion, and even less its nature, the development of the technique of pleural puncture was a major advance in respiratory medicine. Davies (106,107) proposed the needle as an instrument to prove the existence of fluid but with little pain and no danger; it was about 1 1/2 inches long, pointed like a trocar, and had a groove running nearly to its end. Trousseau in France (108,109) and Hughes and Cock in England (110,111) proposed a trocar for the diagnosis and drainage of a pleural effusion, prolonged with a cannula, which external end was placed in a glass of fluid to prevent air from entering the chest (112). Among their followers were Allbutt (113) and Bowditch (114–116), who insisted on the safety of paracentesis, which in his view should be performed much more frequently.

Potain (117) devised a cannula permitting the introduction of a pointed mandrin rendering the penetration of tissues easier and to connect it, by means of a long rubber tube with thick walls, to a flask in which a vacuum was maintained. The underwater seal drainage was supported by von Bülau (118) and Hewitt (119). The apparatus devised by Mosler (120) consisted of a needle connected through a three-way tap to a glass syringe with a brass top and nozzle, providing for the slow action of a piston rod in the form of a male screw. The pneumatic aspirator of Dieulafoy (105,121) allowed for air-tight aspiration of the body fluids, whereas other devices permitted drainage as well as irrigation of the pleural cavity (122,123). The question of the deleterious effect of air penetration in the pleural cavity was solved by Fraentzl, who definitely showed that air does no harm if not charged with infectious germs (112).

Advances in microscopy and in bacteriology made it possible to recognize the etiology of the serous and purulent pleural effusions. Bowditch (116) was among the first to examine the abstracted pleural fluid microscopically. Ehrlich

(124–126) identified the carcinomatous nature of some pleurisies, the relation of the hemorrhagic puerperal pleuritis to microorganisms and septicopyema, and the main bacteria responsible for an empyema, among which were the tuberculous bacilli (127). Netter (128) confirmed that streptococci and pneumococci are among the most frequently found bacilli. Fowler (129) stated that "to form a trustworthy opinion as to the nature of a pleural effusion, it is necessary to know its naked eye appearances, the results of its microscopical examination (drawn with an oil immersion lens) and the effects of inoculation." The cytological examination was stressed by Widal (130) and his coworker Ravaut (131). They found that acute serofibrinous pleuritis is characterized by the quasi-exclusive presence of small lymphocytes and the absence of epithelial cells and insisted on the importance of inoculating the pleural liquid into a guinea pig peritoneum.

The discovery of x-rays by Roentgen (132) was very soon followed by their application to radioscopy of the chest. In France the first results of thoracic radioscopy were presented on the August 6, 1896, at a meeting in Nancy by Oudin and Barthélémy (133). Bouchard (134,135) noticed that the pleural effusions were less transparent to x-rays than the normal lung and frequently pushed the mediastinum away. Repeating the examination in the same patient he observed that, as the percussed height decreased, its fluoroscopic opacity diminished (136). Bergonié (137,138) noticed that the outline of the liquid effusion changes when the patient changes position, which was confirmed by Williams in the United States (139–141). Williams further emphasized that "the outline of the diaphragm is less well defined, or obliterated altogether, according to the amount of fluid present" and the "greater opacity of pleural fluid along the lateral chest wall." For him, the mediastinal shift was frequently underestimated by percussion. He also pointed out the horizontal airfluid interface of an hydropneumothorax. Béclère (142,143) described the x-ray appearance of localized interlobar and diaphragmatic effusions.

Direct access to the pleural cavity was made possible by Jacobaeus (144,145), who first used the cystoscope to explore the pleural cavity and developed thoracoscopy. He may well have been preceded, however, (146) by Gordon (147), who observed the thoracic cavity with a binocular instrument in a case of purulent effusion and noticed that the pleura showed a granular surface and that the lung was neither much reduced in size nor compressed against the spine.

IV. Conclusion

Although a clear nosology of lung diseases did not yet exist at the time and the pleural membrane was not known, Hippocrates gave the first description of signs and symptoms of pleurisy and of empyema; he also promoted their therapeutic approach. Aretaeus and Aurelianus were among his greatest followers. An excellent description of pleural pain was given by Boerhaave, but it was the invention of chest percussion by Auenbrugger that led to the physical diagnosis of pleurisy.

Laennec, with his stethoscope, allowed a further advance in the clinical recognition of pleural effusion. The next step was taken by Davies, who introduced the needle to puncture the thoracic cavity. Advances in microscopic examination and in microbiology which made possible etiological diagnosis of pleural diseases were ultimately followed by roentgenology and thoracoscopy. At the beginning of the twentieth century, the clinician had in his hands the major tools to make the diagnosis of pleurisy.

References

1. Bossy J. La Grande Aventure du Terme Médical. Filiation et Valeurs Actuelles. Montpellier: Sauramps, 1999.
2. Haubrich WS. Medical Meanings. A Glossary of Word Origins. Philadelphia: American College of Physicians, 1997.
3. Penso G. La Médecine Romaine. Paris: Dacosta, 1984.
4. Leca AP. La Médecine Égyptienne au Temps des Pharaons. Paris: Dacosta, 1971.
5. Estes JW. The Medical Skills of Ancient Egypt. Canton, MA: Watson, 1993.
6. Shaw AFP. Histological study of the mummy of Har Mose, the singer of the XVIIIth dynasty. J Path Bact 1938; 47:115–123.
7. Thorwald J. La Médecine Assyro-Babylonnienne. In: Daussy Trad H, ed. Histoire de la Médecine dans l' Antiquité. Paris: Hachette, 1966:106–176.
8. Geoffroy J. L'Anatomie et la Physiologie d'Aristote. Paris: Mulot et Henry, 1878.
9. Aurelianus C. Pleurisy. In: Drabkin IE, ed. Treatise on Acute Diseases. Book II. Chicago: University of Chicago Press, 1950:181–227.
10. Guthrie D. A History of Medicine. London: Nelson, 1945.
11. Major RH. Classic Descriptions of Disease. Springfield, IL: Charles C Thomas, 1932.
12. Adams F. On pleurisy. The Extant Works of Aretaeus, the Cappadocian. London: Sydenham Society, 1856:255–258.
13. Singer C. Galen on Anatomical Procedures. Oxford: Oxford University Press, 1999.
14. Galien. Des organes respiratoires. In: Pichot A, ed. De l'Utilité des Parties du Corps Humain. Oeuvres Médicales Choisies I. Trad C Daremberg. Paris: Gallimard, 1994:99–156.
15. Delamare J, ed. Dictionnaire des Termes de Médecine. 22e éd. Paris: Maloine, 1989.
16. Manuila L, Manuila A, Nicoulin M. Dictionnaire Médical. 7e éd. Paris: Masson, 1996.
17. Boerhaave. Of a pleuresie. In: Boerhaave's Aphorisms: Concerning the Knowledge and Cure of Diseases. Transl by J Delacoste. London: Cowse and Innys, 1715: 220–235.
18. Buchan W. Of the pleurisy. In:Domestic Medicine or the Family Physician. Philadelphia: Aitken, 1774:120–127.
19. Tissot S. De la pleurésie. In: Teysseire D, Verry-Jolivet C, eds. Avis au Peuple sur sa Santé (1782). Paris: Quai Voltaire, 1993:99–104.

20. Castiglioni A. Histoire de la Médecine. Trans J Bertrand et F Gidon. Paris: Payot, 1931.
21. Ellis H. Thoracic and vascular surgery. A History of Surgery. London: Greenwich Medical Media Ltd, 2001:211–235.
22. Littré E, Robin C. Dictionnaire de Médecine 14e éd. Paris: Baillière, 1878.
23. Dionis P. Démonstrations Chirurgicales: Cours d'Opérations sur l'Anatomie de l'Homme. Paris: d'Houry, 1695.
24. Capron L. Mots & Maux. Jeux de Mots d' Omicron. Paris: Baillière, 2001.
25. Hurt R. Pioneers in the emergence of thoracic surgery as a speciality. In: The History of Cardiothoracic Surgery from Early Times. New York: Parthenon, 1996:25–35.
26. Marrotte. Rapport sur la paracentése du thorax. Bull Soc Méd Hôp. Paris: Tome Deuxième, 1853:165–172.
27. Hippocrates. The Aphorisms. Transl T Coar. London: Longman and Co, T and G Underwood, Cox and Son, 1822.
28. Hippocrate. De l'art médical. In: Gourevitch D, ed. Trad E Littré; présentation. Paris: Le Livre de Poche, 1994:567–572.
29. Hippocrate. Pronostic. In: Jouanna J, Magdelaine C, eds. L'Art de la Médecine. Paris: Flammarion, 1999:187–207.
30. Hippocrate. Des maladies. In: Debru A, ed. La Consultation. Trad E Littré. Paris: Hermann, 1986:211–233.
31. Hoerni B. Histoire de l'Examen Clinique d' Hippocrate à nos Jours. Paris: Immothep/Maloine, 1996.
32. Fabre J. The Hippocratic Doctor: Ancient Lessons for the Modern World. London: R Soc Med Press, 1997.
33. Hurt R. The diagnosis and treatment of empyema. In: The History of Cardiothoracic Surger from Early Times. New York: Parthenon, 1996:153–182.
34. Bariéty M, Coury C. Histoire de la Médecine. Paris: Fayard, 1963.
35. Jackson R. Doctors and Diseases in the Roman Empire. London: British Museum Publications, 1988.
36. Meade RH. Empyema. In: A History of Thoracic Surgery. Springfield, IL: Charles C Thomas, 1961:234–256.
37. Grmek MD. Les inflammations purulentes communes. In: Les Maladies à l'Aube de la Civilisation Occidentale. Paris: Payot, 1983:179–198.
38. Souques A. La pleurésie et l'empyéme hippocratiques. Presse Méd 1938; 46:425–427.
39. Colin A. Dictionnaire de Noms Illustres en Médecine. Bruxelles: Prodim, 1994.
40. Major RH. A history of Medicine. Springfield, IL: Charles C Thomas, 1954.
41. Celse. Traité de Médecine. Trad Ninnin. Paris: Delahays, 1855.
42. Celse. De Medicina. Transl WG Spencer. London: Heinemann, 1938.
43. Garrison FH. An Introduction to the History of Medicine. 2d ed. Philadelphia: Saunders, 1917.
44. Adams F. Cure of pleurisy. In: The Extant Works of Aretaeus, the Cappadocian. London: Syndenham Society, 1856:410–416.
45. Galien. Des lieux affectés. In: Pichot A, ed. Oeuvres Médicales Choisies II. Trad C Daremberg. Paris: Gallimard, 1994:123–274.
46. Daremberg C. Des lieux affectés. In: Oeuvres Anatomiques, Physiologiques et Médicales de Galen. Vol II. Paris: Baillière, 1854:468–705.

47. Pagel W. Paracelsus. An Introduction to Philosophical Medicine in the Era of Renaissance. 2d ed. Basel: Karger, 1982.
48. Balaban C, Erlen J, Siderits R, eds. The Skilful Physician. [1656]. Amsterdam: Harwood, 1997.
49. Goeurot J. The Regiment of Life, Whereunto Is Added a Treatyse of the Pestilences. London, 1546.
50. Keynes G. The Apologie and Treatise of Ambroise Paré. London: Falcon, 1951.
51. Paré A. Livre I: Introduction pour parvenir à la connaissance de la chirurgie. In: Guerrand RH, De Bissy F, eds. Oeuvres Complètes. Paris: Union Latine d' éditions, 1973:49–108.
52. Paré A. Livre IV: Des parties vitales. In: Guerrand RH, De Bissy F, eds. Oeuvres Complètes. Paris: Union Latine d' édition, 1973:184–200.
53. Paré A. Livre VIII: Des tumeurs en particulier. In: Guerrand RH, De Bissy F, eds. Oeuvres Complètes. Paris: Union Latine d' éditions, 1973:287–323.
54. Sydenham T. Pleurisy. In: The Works of Thomas Sydenham, M.D. Transl RG Latham. London: Sydenham Society, 1848:244–250.
55. Willis T. Pharmaceutice Rationalis: or an Exercitation of the Operations of Medicines in Humane Bodies. London: Dring Harper, and Leigh, 1679.
56. Morgagni JB. Letter the sixteenth. Treats of respiration being injured from causes within the thorax and principally from the dropsy of the thorax, and pericardium. In: The Seats and Causes of Diseases Investigated by Anatomy. Transl B Alexander. London: A Millar, T Cadell, Johnson and Payne, 1769:378–426.
57. Sigerist HE. On percussion of the chest being a translation of Auenbrugger's original treatise entitled Inventum novum ex percussione thoracis humani, ut signo abstrusos interni pectoris morbos detegendi [Vienna, 1761], by John Forbes [London 1824]. Bull Inst Hist Med 1936; 4:373–403.
58. Nicolson M. Giovanni Battista Morgagni and eighteenth-century physical examination. In: Lawrence C, ed. Medical Theory, Surgical Practice. London: Routledge, 1992:101–134.
59. Cullen M. De la pneumonie ou de la fluxion de poitrine. In: Eléments de Médecine Pratique. Trad Bosquilon M. Vol I. Paris: Barrois, 1785:244–271.
60. Stoll M. Médecine Pratique avec les Aphorismes de Stoll et Boerhaave. Trad Mahon. Paris: Delahays, 1855:364–369.
61. Baillie M. Diseases appearances in the cavity of the thorax. In: The Morbid Anatomy of Some of the Most Important Parts of the Human Body. London: Johnson and Nicol, 1793:33–41.
62. May E. La Médecine. Son Passé—Son Présent—Son Avenir. Paris: Payot, 1957.
63. Pinel P. Nosographie Philosophique. Paris, 1798
64. Bichat X. A Treatise on the Membranes. New edition by M Husson, 1802. Transl JG Goffin. Boston: Cummings and Hilliard, 1813.
65. Landré-Beauvais AJ. Des signes tirés de la respiration. In: Séméiotique ou Traité des Signes des Maladies. Paris, 1809:61–87.
66. Double FJ. Signes tirés de la percussion de la poitrine. In: Sémiologie Générale, ou Traité des Signes et de leur Valeur dans les Maladies. Vol I. Paris: Croullebois, 1811:367–378.
67. Double FJ. Signes fournis par la respiration. In: Séméiologie Générale, ou Traité des Signes et de leur Valeur dans les Maladies. Vol II. Paris: Croullebois, 1817:12–69.

68. Corvisart JN. Nouvelles Méthodes pour Reconnaître les Maladies Internes de la Poitrine par la Percussion de Cette Cavité, par Avenbrugger. Paris: Migneret, 1808.
69. Baron Corvisart, Busquet P, ed. Aphorismes de Médecine Clinique, Recueillis par FV Mérat. Paris: Masson, 1929.
70. Hechemann L. Corvisart et la Percussion. Thése Paris: Michalon, 1906.
71. Laennec RTH. De l'Auscultation Médiate. Paris: Brosson and Chaudé, 1819.
72. Laennec RTH. Traité de l'Auscultation Médiate et des Maladies des Poumons et du Coeur. 2d ed. Paris: Asselin, reissued 1879.
73. Laennec RTH. A Treatise on the Diseases of the Chest and on Mediate Auscultation. Transl J Forbes. New York: Samuel Wood and Sons, 1830.
74. Jarcho S. A review of John Forbes' translation of Laennec. Am J Cardiol 1962; 10:859–863.
75. Stokes W. An Introduction to the Use of the Stethoscope. Edinburgh: Machlachlan and Stewart, 1825.
76. Louis PCA. Des plèvres. In: Recherches Anatomico-Pathologiques sur la Phtisie. Paris: Gabon, 1825:39–43.
77. Louis PCA. Des plévres. In: Recherches Anatomiques, Pathologiques et Thérapeutiques sur la Phtisie. 2e ed. Paris: Baillière, 1843:42–46.
78. Bayle GL. Complications de la Phtisie avec Diverses Maladies. In: Recherches sur la physie pulmonaire. Paris: Gabon, 1810:64–80.
79. Baron J. An Enquiry Illustrating the Nature of Tuberculated Accretions of Serous Membranes. London: Longman, Hurst, Reees, and Brown, 1819.
80. Piorry PA. Des maladies de la plévre. In: De la Percussion Médiate et des Signes Obtenus à l'Aide de ce Nouveau Moyen d'Exploration dans les Maladies des Organes Thoraciques et Abdominaux. Paris: Chaudé et Baillière, 1828:62–95.
81. Gerhard WW. Pleurisy. In: On the Diagnosis of Diseases of the Chest; Based upon the Comparison of their Physical and General Signs. Philadelphia: Key and Biddle, 1836:126–139.
82. Barth, Roger H. Traité Pratique d'Auscultation. Paris: Béchet jeune et Labé, 1841.
83. Reynaud M. Mémoire sur Quelques Faits et Aperçus Nouveaux, Relatifs à l' Auscultation de la Poitrine. J Hebd Méd 1829; 5:563–596.
84. Skoda J. Abhandlung über Perkussion und Auskultation. 6 ed. Wien: Seidel & Sohn, 1864.
85. Major RH. Skodaic resonance. Josef Skoda. In: Classic Descriptions of Disease. Springfield, IL: Charles C Thomas, 1932:520–522.
86. McGee SR. Percussion and physical diagnosis: separating myth from science. Dis Mon 1995; 41:645–692.
87. Trousseau A. Pleurésie-Paracentése de la poitrine. In: Clinique Médicale de l' Hôtel-Dieu de Paris. 6e éd par M Peter. Paris: Baillière, 1882:732–831.
88. Damoiseau H. Recherches cliniques sur plusieurs points du diagnostic des épanchements pleurétiques. Arch Gén Méd 1843; IVe sér-tome III:131–156.
89. Stillé E. Physical signs in diseases of the respiratory apparatus. In: Elements of General Pathology. A Practical Treatise. Philadelphia: Lindsay and Blakiston, 1848:379–404.
90. Walshe WH. Pleurisy. In: A Practical Treatise on the Diseases of the Lung: Including the Principles of Physical Diagnosis. 3d ed. Am ed. Philadelphia: Blanchard and Lea, 1860:204–251.
91. Bowditch HI. Physical signs of pleurisy. In: The Young Stethoscopist. 2d ed. New York: SS & W Wood, 1858:74–80.

92. Landouzy H. Nouvelles données sur le diagnostic de la pleurésie et les indications de la thoracentèse. Arch Gén Méd 1856; t.VIII:513–531 & 690–705.
93. Addison T. On the difficulties and fallacies attending physical diagnosis in diseases of the chest. In: Wilks, Daldy, eds. A Collection of the Published Writings of the Late Thomas Addison. London: New Sydenham Society, 1868:65–98.
94. von Niemeyer F. Diseases of the pleura. In: A Text-book of Practical Medicine. 7th ed. Transl GH Humpheys and CE Hackey. Vol. I. New York: Appleton and Co, 1869: 253–285.
95. Woillez EJ. Pleurésie. In: Traité Clinique des Maladies Aiguës des Organes Respiratoires. Paris: Delahaye, 1872:278–530.
96. Blakiston P. Chronic pleurisy. In: Practical Observations on Certain Diseases of the Chest, and on the Principles of Auscultation. Philadelphia: Lea and Blanchard, 1848:266–279.
97. Andral M. Affections de la plèvre. In: Traité de l'Auscultation Médiate, et des Maladies des Poumons et du Coeur, par RTH Laennec 4e éd. Paris: Chaudé, 1837:401–699.
98. Flint A. Acute pleuritis—chronic pleuritis—empyema—pleuralgia. In: Physical Exploration and Diagnosis of Diseases Affecting the Respiratory Organs. Philadelphia: Blanchard and Lea, 1856:538–587.
99. Flint A. A treatise on the Principles and Practice of Medicine. Philadelphia: Lea, 1866.
100. Beau JHS. Pleurésie. In: Traité Expérimental et Clinique d'Auscultation. Paris: Baillière, 1856:187–191.
101. Woillez EJ. Pleurésie. In: Traité Théorique et Clinique de Percussion et d'Auscultation. Paris: Delahaye, 1879:515–554.
102. Powell RD. On Diseases of the Lungs and Pleurae Including Consumption. 3rd ed. New York: W Wood & Co, 1886.
103. Eichhorst H. Diagnostic physique des maladies de la plèvre. In: Traité de Diagnostic Médical. Trad Marfan AB, Weiss F. Paris: Steinheil, 1890: 359–362.
104. Landouzy H. De la Valeur de l'Égophonie dans la Pleurésie. Arch Gén Méd 1861; tome XVIII, Vol II:669–678.
105. Dieulafoy G. Traité de l'Aspiration de Liquides Morbides. Paris: Masson, 1873.
106. Davies T. Lectures on the Diseases of the Lungs and Heart. London: Longmans, 1835.
107. Davies AT. A note on Thomas Davies, introducer of the exploring needle. Proc R Soc Med 1923; 16:19–22.
108. Trousseau A. De la paracentése dans la période extrême de la pleurésie aiguë. Bull Acad Méd 1843; 9:138.
109. Trousseau A. Paracentesis thoracis in acute pleurisy. Lancet 1844; 1:755–756.
110. Hughes HM, Cock E. On paracentesis thoracis with cases. Guys Hospital Reports 1844; 2:48–104.
111. Jarcho S. Hughes and Cock on thoracentesis (1844). Am J Cardiol 1963; 12:853–859.
112. Hochberg LA. Empyema thoracis. In: Thoracic Surgery Before the 20th Century. New York: Vantage, 1960:239–322.
113. Allbutt TC. On thoracentesis. Practitioner 1872; 9:75–80.
114. Bowditch HI. On pleuritic effusions, and the necessity of paracentesis for their removal. Am J Med Sci 1852; 23:320–350.

115. Bowditch HI. Paracentesis thoracis: a resume of twelve years experience. Am J Med Sci 1863; 89:2–21.
116. Jarcho S, Henry I. Bowditch on pleuritic effusion and thoracentesis (1852). Am J Cardiol 1965; 15:832–836.
117. Potain H. Thoracentèse. Gaz Hôp 1872; 45:725–772, 734–735.
118. von Bülau G. Für die Heber Drainage bei Behandlung des Empyems. Z Klin Med 1891; 18:31–45.
119. Hewitt C. Thoracentesis: the plea for continuous aspiration. Br Med J 1876; 1:317.
120. Mosler F. Zur Thoracentese mit Aspiration. Wien Med Presse 1879; 20:464–470, 503–509.
121. Dieulafoy G. De l' Aspiration Pneumatique Sous-Cutanée. Méthode de Diagnostic et de Traitement. Paris: Masson, 1870.
122. Carson J. The operation of paracentesis thoracis. Lancet 1847; 1:114–117.
123. Quincke H. Zur Behandlung der Pleuritis. Berl klin Wchnschr 1872; 9:65–68, 89–92.
124. Ehrlich P. Beiträge zur Ätiologie und Histologie pleuritischer Exsudate (1882). In: Himmelweit F. ed. The Collected Papers of Paul Ehrlich. Vol. I. London: Pergamon, 1956:290–310.
125. Ehrlich P. Über pleuritis (1887). In: Himmelweit F, ed. The Collected Papers of Paul Ehrlich. London: Pergamon, 1956:340–341.
126. Ehrlich P. Über Empyem (1888). In: Himmelweit F, ed. The Collected Papers of Paul Ehrlich. London: Pergamon, 1956:342–343.
127. Koch R. Die Aetiologie der Tuberkulose. Berl Klin Wochenschr 1882; 19:221–230.
128. Netter R. Maladies de la plèvre. In: Charcot, Bouchard, Brissaud, eds. Traité de Médecine. Paris: Masson, 1893:973–1070.
129. Fowler JK. Acute inflammation of the pleura. In: Fowler JK, Godlee RJ, eds. The Diseases of the Lungs. London: Longmans, Green and Co, 1898: 543–575.
130. Widal F. Cytologie des épanchements pleuraux. In: Fernand Widal, ed. Oeuvre Scientifique. Paris: Masson, 1932:175–199.
131. Ravaut. Le diagnostic de la nature des épanchements séro-fibrineux de la plèvre. Thèse de Paris, 1900.
132. Roëntgen WK. On a new kind of rays. Transl A Stanton. Nature 1896; 53:274–276.
133. Pallardy G, Pallardy MJ, Wackenheim A. Histoire Illustrée de la Radiologie. Paris: Dacosta, 1989.
134. Bouchard C. La pleurésie de l' homme étudiée à l' aide des rayons de Röntgen. C R Acad Sci 1896; 123:967–968.
135. Bouchard C. Application de la radioscopie au diagnostic des maladies du thorax. Rev Tuberc 1896; 4:273–277.
136. Heitzman ER, Greene R. Chest radiology. In: Gagliardi RA, McClennan BL, eds. A History of the Radiological Sciences. Reston, VA: Radiology Centennial, 1996:131–172.
137. Bergonié J. Nouveaux faits de radioscopie de lésions intrathoraciques. C R Acad Sci 1896; 123:1268–1269.
138. Bergonié J, Carriére. Etude fluoroscopique des épanchements pleurétiques. Arch Electricité Méd 1899; 7:301–332.
139. Williams FH. The roentgen rays in thoracic diseases. Am J Med Sci 1897; 114: 665–687.

140. Williams FH. The Roentgen Rays in Medicine and Surgery. New York: Macmillan, 1901.
141. Greene R. Imaging the respiratory system in the first few years after discovery of the x-ray: Contributions of Francis H. Williams, M.D. Am J Roentgenol 1992; 159:1–7.
142. Béclère A. Les Rayons de Röntgen et le Diagnostic de la Tuberculose. Paris: Masson, 1898.
143. Béclère A. Les Rayons de Roentgen et le Diagnostic des Affections Thoraciques. Paris: Alcan, 1901.
144. Jacobaeus HC. Über die Möglichkeit die Zystoskopie bei Untersuchung seröser Höhlungen Anzuwenden. München Med Wochenschr 1910; 57:2090–2092.
145. Jacobaeus HC. The practical importance of thoracoscopy in surgery of the chest. Surg Gynecol Obstetr 1922; 34:289–296.
146. Hurt R. Examination and investigation of the chest. In: The History of Cardiothoracic Surgery from Ancient Times. New York: Parthenon, 1996:37–61.
147. Gordon S. Clinical reports of rare cases. Dublin Q J Med Soc 1866; 41:83–99.

2
Anatomy of the Pleura

MING-JEN PENG

MacKay Memorial Hospital
and Taipei Medical University
Taipei, Taiwan

NAI-SAN WANG

Chungtai Institute of Health Sciences
and Technology
Taichung, Taiwan

I. Introduction

In vertebrates, including humans, all vital organs are located within the body cavity, which is surrounded and protected by a body wall formed by ribs, vertebrae, and layers of thick muscle. The body cavity is divided into thoracic, cardiac, and abdominal compartments. The thoracic cage is constructed like a vertical cone-shaped bellows, with the diaphragm as the moving part in the lowermost and widest end for the best protection and function of the lung. Within the limited protected cavity space, the lung moves and changes volume constantly.

The lung expands at inhalation and deflates at exhalation. To decrease the friction generated between the lung and the thoracic wall, the inner surface of the thoracic cage and the outer surface of the lung are covered by a serous, elastic membrane with a smooth and lubricating surface: the pleura. The pleural cavity is almost like a sealed wet and stretchable elastic bag inserted between the lung and the thoracic wall.

The pleura and the pleural cavity are therefore crucial for the efficient function of the lung, as are the pericardium and the pericardial cavity for the heart. This arrangement is so important that in the embryo a primitive body cavity (coelom) lined by a serous membrane is formed, and the measures needed to maintain the cavity open are implemented before all vital organs develop.

II. Embryology

The mesothelium (the lining cell) and its supporting connective tissues of the serous membrane, including the pleura, pericardium, and peritoneum, are all derived from the primitive mesoderm of the embryo. In the human embryo, the primitive mesoderm on both sides of the notochord divides first into the medial segmented and lateral nonsegmented plates. The medial segmented plates later develop into the protecting skull and vertebrae, the brain and spinal cord, and the ribs and thick muscles of the dorsal or back parts of the body wall.

The lateral nonsegmented plates, on the other hand, split into the internal splanchnopleure (the precursor of internal organs) and the lateral or external somatopleure (the precursor of the anterior and lateral body wall) to form a pair of slit-like cavities. These two lateral cavities with splanchnopleure and somatopleure extend cephalocaudally along the length of the embryo, and ventrally or anteriorly, out and over the surface of the yolk sac. The fusion of the left and right somatopleure and two cavities ventrally, i.e., the fusion and closure of the ventral wall, creates an intraembryonic coelom, a primitive body cavity, at the 7th week of gestation (1). At this time the cavity is already completely covered by a layer of serous membrane with mesothelial cells on the surface (2).

With the shrinkage of the yolk sac, the coelom expands, and all internal organs that constantly move and change in size and shape, including the lung, heart, liver, and bowel, protrude as they develop into the body cavities. They are enveloped by the layer of serous membrane that covers the inner surface of the cavities. In the meanwhile, the coelom divides into the pleural and peritoneal cavities by the fusion of the transverse septum arising from the ventral, as well as left and right pleuroperitoneal folds from the dorsal walls. When the two pleuroperitoneal folds fuse, the two pleural cavities are completely separated from each other and from the pericardial cavity (2). This arrangement lends flexibility to the organs to expand, retract, deform, or displace each other, as they develop and grow in the limited space of the three body cavities.

III. The Pleura and Pleural Cavity

The part of the pleura that covers the entire surface of the lung, including the interlobar fissures, is the visceral pleura; that which covers the rest of the thoracic cavity, including the inner surface of the thoracic cage, mediastinum, and diaphragm, is the parietal pleura. The visceral and parietal pleurae, which merge with each other at the hilum of the lung, originate from the same serous membrane of the early embryonic cavity. They later differentiate, influenced by the substructures they cover.

Anatomy of the Pleura

Different names have been given to the parietal pleura at different parts of the thoracic cavity. Those include the costal pleura, which lines the inner surfaces of the ribs and intercostal muscles; the diaphragmatic pleura, which covers the convex surface of the diaphragm; the cervical pleura, which rises into the neck, over the summit of the lung; and the mediastinal pleura, which covers the mediastinal viscera (3).

The pleural cavity is an expandable space that is formed between the visceral pleura and the parietal pleura (4). The right and left pleural cavities are completely separated from each other and from the mediastinum and the pericardial cavity between them. The dome, or cupola, of the pleural cavity extends above the first rib for 2–3 cm along the medial one third of the clavicle behind the sternocleidomastoid muscles. Manipulations, such as the insertion of a central venous pressure (CVP) catheter, surgical dissection of lymph nodes, or accidental injuries of the anterior lower neck, therefore, may inadvertently enter the pleural cavity and induce a pneumothorax.

In the lower mediastinum, the dorsal and ventral mediastinal parietal pleurae are pulled into the chest cavity as the lung develops and may persist vertically from the hilum of the lung to the diaphragm to form back-to-back layers of parietal pleura called the pulmonary ligament. This ligament may divide the pleural space below the hilum of the lung into anterior and posterior compartments (5). This ligament may contain large lymphatic vessels. Rarely, incomplete ligation of, or damage to, these lymphatic vessels during surgical procedures may result in postoperative pleural effusion (6).

The pleurae reflect usually at the lower or caudal boundaries of the thoracic cage but may extend beyond the costal margins at the right infrasternal and bilateral costovertebral angles. In a radiological study, the lung lies at or below the level of the 12th rib ventrally in 80% of the patients, and in 18% the lung reaches the level of the body of the L1 vertebra adjacent to bilateral costovertebral angles dorsally (7).

At deep inspiration, the lung fills the pleural cavity completely. During expiration, or quiet breathing, because of the retraction of the lung, the most caudal or distal reflected sites of the parietal pleura that extend beyond the costal margins may be in direct contact with each other to form the recess. Excess fluid in the pleural cavity often accumulates first in the recess. Attempts to aspirate fluids in the recess or approaching the liver, adrenals, or kidneys posteriorly during medical or surgical procedures may inadvertently damage the lung and pleura, causing pneumothorax or hemothorax (7).

The visceral pleurae extend into the interlobar space; each lobe, therefore, may expand or collapse individually without affecting the others. Abnormal divisions of lobes and segments are, however, common (4), and interlobar fissures may be incompletely or completely separated by septa. These altered fissures may appear as linear shadows or "vanishing tumors" radiologically when they trap fluid that may come and go in conditions such as heart failure (8).

The major fissure of the lung extends obliquely downward from posterior to anterior, roughly paralleling the sixth rib. Thus, a chest tube placed through the fifth, sixth, or seventh intercostal space may enter the pleural cavity near the major fissure, and, if it is directed centrally, can enter and be trapped within the fissure resulting in ineffective drainage (9).

IV. Gross and Light Microscopic Findings of the Pleura

The normal pleural surface is smooth, wet and glistening, and semitransparent. By light microscopy, the pleura is generally divided into five layers. From the pleural surface, the layers are: (a) a single layer of mesothelial cells; (b) a thin submesothelial connective tissue layer, including a basal lamina; (c) a thin superficial elastic layer; (d) a loose connective tissue layer; and (e) a deep fibroelastic layer. However, the thickness of each layer is quite varied between species and also between regions in the same animals (4,10–14), as will be discussed in Section XIII.

The human mesothelial cells range from 16.4 ± 6.8 to 41.9 ± 9.5 μm in diameter and from 1 to 4 μm in thickness (10,14). The mesothelial cells, therefore, may appear flattened like endothelial cells or cuboidal like epithelial cells. The shape and size of the mesothelial cells usually reflect the substructure of the pleura (see Sec. XIII) or the functional status of the cells (see Sec. XVI).

The thickness and boundaries of the superficial connective and elastic fiber layers (the second and third layers) are usually imprecise. The loose fourth connective tissue layer contains adipose tissue, vessels, nerves, and lymphatics and often serves as the cleavage plane at pleurectomy. The fifth, deep fibroelastic layer often adheres tightly to or is fused with the parenchyma of the lung, mediastinum, diaphragm, or the chest wall.

V. The Fine Structure of Mesothelial Cells

As described in the previous section, a single layer of polygonal mesothelial cells covers the surface of both parietal and visceral pleurae. The most striking characteristic of the mesothelial cell is the bushy surface microvilli, best shown by transmission and scanning electron microscopy (Figs. 1 and 2). The microvillus is approximately 0.1 μm in diameter and up to 3 or more μm in length. Many microvilli are often aggregated with each other and appear wavy [10, 14–17].

The microvilli presumably contribute to the formation and absorption as well as the organization of the lubricating surface film of the pleural fluid (see Sec. VI). Pinocytotic vesicles are numerous and are often associated with microvilli on the cell membrane of mesothelial cells, especially on the pleural surface.

The nucleus of a mesothelial cell is ovoid and shows a prominent nucleolus. The cytoplasm may appear thin and scarce, or thick and abundant, but always contains a moderate to abundant amount of organelles including mitochondria, rough and smooth endoplasmic reticulum, and dense bodies

Anatomy of the Pleura

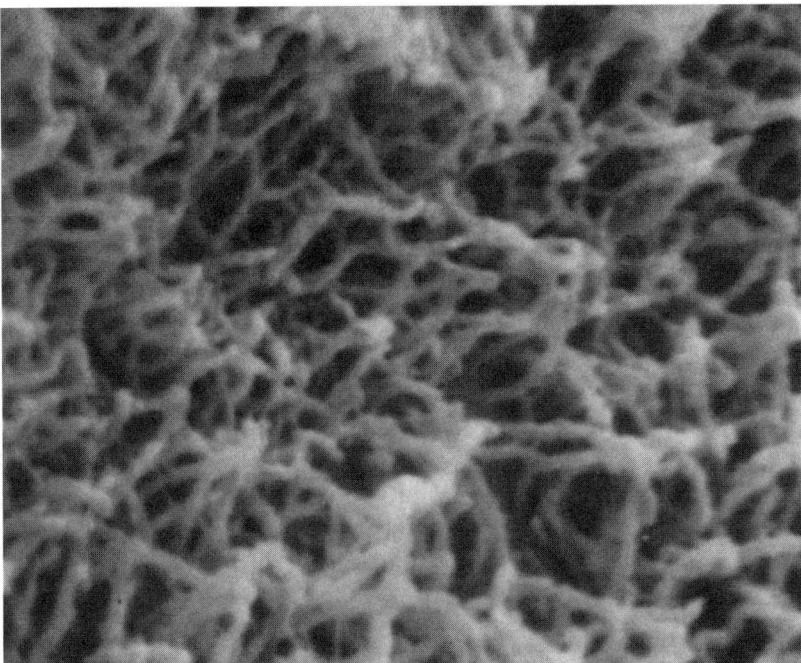

Figure 1 Bushy surface microvilli of the mesothelial cell are best appreciated by scanning electron microscopy. In average, there are 300 microvilli on a 100 μm^2 surface area of a mesothelial cell. (Rabbit visceral pleura, SEM ×20,000.)

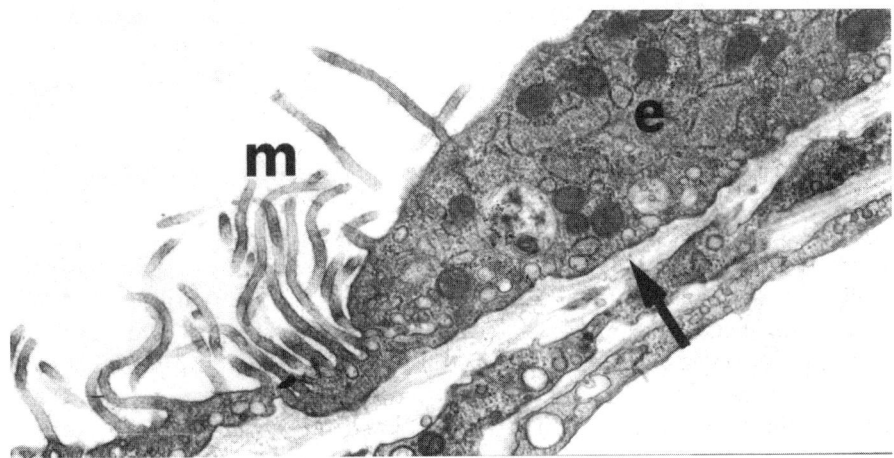

Figure 2 The distribution of microvilli is uneven within the same cell. The microvilli (m) are bushy with a length-to-diameter ratio of usually over 10. Even the flattened mesothelial cell shows many mitochondria and abundant endoplasmic reticulum (e). (Rabbit visceral pleura, TEM ×21,100.) (From Ref. 19.)

(Fig. 2). Polyribosomes, intermediate (prekeratin) fibrils, Golgi apparatus, and glycogen granules are also well developed, suggesting that the mesothelial cell is an active cell (18) (see Secs. XVI and XVII).

A tight junction is always present between mesothelial cells at the apical portion. The presence of intermediate and desmosome junctions are, however, less consistent (19). The basal portions of two adjacent mesothelial cells are often overlapped but not attached to each other and are without intercellular junctions. The overlap disappears when the lung is at full inspiration (19). This suggests that the mesothelial cells stretch, and their cell bodies slide over with each other during respiratory movements. The basal lamina is always present beneath the mesothelial cells and beneath the overlapped cytoplasmic processes.

The intramembranous organization—the dots and lines that glue the two layers of cell membranes together—of the junctional complexes between parietal mesothelial cells is as loose as that of the venular endothelium (19,20). This finding suggests that the parietal mesothelial layer is as labile and leaky as the endothelial layer of the small vein.

The intramembranous organization of the junctional complexes of the visceral mesothelial cell, however, is more complex than that of the parietal one in mice (19,20). This probably suggests that the visceral mesothelial layer is less likely to leak or is normally subjected to more tensile stretching than the parietal side.

VI. The Microvillus and Lubricating Membrane

Microvilli are present diffusely over the entire pleural surface but are distributed unevenly. The density of microvilli ranges from less than a few to more than 600 (average 300) per 100 μm^2 (Fig. 1) [11,14–16]. Generally, more microvilli are found in the caudal than in the cranial portion of the lung or chest wall, and more are found on the visceral than on the parietal pleurae at the same part of the thorax [11,14]. They are least concentrated on the ribs.

The function of microvilli is not completely certain. The microvilli increase the surface area of the cell and presumably also increase the cell membrane–dependent functions, including the number of a variety of receptors for ligands and the production of enzymes, such as metalloproteinases. The association of microvilli and pinocytotic vesicles may be important in transcellular transport (21). The most important function of the bush-like microvilli, however, seems to involve surrounding glycoproteins rich in hyaluronic acid to lubricate the pleural surface and lessen the friction between the lung and thorax (14,15).

The microvilli and hyaluronic acid are most abundant in the lower thoracic cavity where the contraction and relaxation of the diaphragm, the expansion and retraction of the lung and the thoracic cage, namely, the most actively moving parts of the bellows of respiration, are. The hyaluronic acid is secreted by the mesothelial cell and also by mesenchymal cells in the submesothelial interstitial tissue. Hyaluronic acid is demonstrable by alcian blue or colloidal iron stains by light microscopy (LM) and electron microscopy (EM) (14).

VII. The Blood Supply of the Pleura

A. The Blood Supply of the Parietal Pleura

The arterial blood supplies of the parietal pleura are very rich and come from multiple branches of many adjacent systemic arteries: the costal pleura, from the intercostal and internal mammary arteries; the mediastinal pleura, from the bronchial, upper diaphragmatic, internal mammary, and mediastinal arteries; the cervical pleura, from the subclavian arteries, and their collaterals; the diaphragmatic pleura, from the superior phrenic branches of the internal mammary arteries, the posterior mediastinal arteries from the thoracic aorta, and the inferior phrenic arteries of the abdominal aorta [3,4,13].

The veins of the parietal pleura follow their arteries, and most of them drain into the azygos vein, and then into the superior vena cava. The venous blood of the diaphragm, however, drains either caudally into the inferior vena cava through the inferior phrenic veins, or cranially into the superior vena cava through the superior phrenic veins, which run parallel with the internal mammary artery, and then into the brachiocephalic trunk.

B. The Blood Supply of the Visceral Pleura

Contrary to the parietal pleura, the arterial blood supply to the visceral pleura is often compromised and still controversial in humans. In animals with thick pleurae, such as horses, pigs, or sheep, the blood supply of the visceral pleura originates from the bronchial arteries. In those with thin pleurae, such as mice, rats, and rabbits, the blood supply to the visceral pleura originates from the pulmonary circulation. Albertine and coworkers have demonstrated that in young adult sheep the bronchial artery supplies the visceral pleura, completely and exclusively (10).

Humans have thick visceral pleura. Therefore, the systemic bronchial circulation should supply the human visceral pleura, but this is not completely certain (22). All investigators agree that the bronchial artery supplies most of the pleura facing the mediastinum, the pleura covering the interlobular surfaces, and a part of the diaphragmatic surface. The blood supply for the remaining portions of the visceral pleura, that is, the entire convex costal lung surface and the greater part of the diaphragmatic surface, is less certain (23). For some authors (4), this part of the visceral pleura is supplied by pulmonary arteries that arise beneath the pleura from the pulmonary parenchyma. Milne and Pistolesi, with particular reference to the techniques used to delineate pulmonary and bronchial vessels, concluded that the visceral pleural circulation is derived from and is continuous with the pulmonary circulation (24). At least in humans, this disagreement about the blood supply to the visceral pleura is not completely clarified (see Sec. VII.C).

The greater part of the venous return from the bronchial artery in the visceral pleura is drained through the pulmonary veins, except for a small area around the hilum where the pleural veins drain into the bronchial veins.

C. Shunting and Other Aging or Pathological Changes

In human lungs, shunts between the systemic and pulmonary arteries and veins exist, probably less than 5%, normally, but increase with age and any chronic lung diseases (4). In aged human lungs, the bronchial arteries in the visceral pleura, especially those far away from the hilum, are often sclerotic and obliterated. It is likely that the pulmonary circulation with some functional impairment would compensate the portion of pleura deprived of the original bronchial blood supply. This is most apparent in bullae of the lung.

On the other hand, in the aged lung, and in many chronic lung and pleural diseases, the bronchial arterial system proliferates around the airway, in the lobular septum, or even into the pleura with fibrosis. In pleural inflammation and fibrosis, especially when adhesions between the lung and the chest wall develop, systemic arteries often invade into the visceral pleura from the parietal side. The changing of the types of vascular supply and the problem of shunting in the lung and pleura require careful evaluation in the management of pleura and lung diseases.

VIII. Innervation

The costal pleura and the peripheral part of diaphragmatic pleura are innervated by somatic intercostal nerves (3,13). When either of these areas is irritated, pain is referred to the adjacent chest wall. In contrast, the phrenic nerve innervates the central portion of the diaphragm. With irritation of this portion of the diaphragmatic pleura, pain is referred to the ipsilateral shoulder.

The visceral pleura is extensively innervated by pulmonary branches of the vagus nerve and sympathetic trunk. The visceral pleura contains no pain fibers and may be manipulated without causing unpleasant sensation. Therefore, the presence of pleuritic chest pain always indicates inflammation or irritation of the parietal pleura.

IX. Pleural Fluid and Contents

The normal amount of pleural fluid is small. One can collect approximately 0.2 mL of fluid from a pleural cavity of the normal rabbit and less than 1 mL from a human (25). In another study, the volume of the pleural liquid collected from a pleural cavity was 0.98 mL in the rabbit and 2.35 mL in the dog (26).

The pleural fluid forms a thin layer, at least 10 μm thick, between the visceral and parietal pleurae (27,28). The layer of liquid is thick enough to prevent the visceral and parietal pleural surfaces from touching each other (29). Experimentally, Albertine et al. could not demonstrate direct contact between visceral and parietal mesothelial cells across the costal pleural space of sheep (30).

The normal pleural fluid contains 1–2 g of protein per 100 mL, similar to the concentration detected in the interstitial fluid of animals and humans (25,31). However, levels of large molecular weight proteins, such as lactate dehydrogenase (LDH) (molecular weight 134,000), in the pleural fluid are less than half of that found in the serum. There are 1400–4500 cells in 1 μL of pleural fluid in normal animals and humans (25,26,31). They are mostly macrophages with a few lymphocytes and red blood cells. These data indicate that the amount of fluid is closely regulated and the barrier for molecular and cellular passage is tightly restricted in the pleural cavity.

The pleural fluid originates from the systemic circulation, mostly from the parietal pleura in the less dependent region of the pleural cavity where the blood vessels are close to the mesothelial surface. Reabsorption is through the lymphatics in the most dependent part of the pleural cavity, mainly in the parietal pleura, on the diaphragmatic surface and in the mediastinal regions (32) (see Sec. X).

Interchange of fluid between the alveolar or pulmonary interstitial and pleural spaces is anatomically restricted, as described earlier (see Sec. V). However, in pathological conditions, such as congestive heart failure (CHF) or adult respiratory distress syndrome (ARDS) with high permeability lung edema, the barriers are broken and alveolar and pulmonary interstitial fluid may move towards the pleural space. In such conditions, the pleural space is considered as one of the main exits for the evacuation of lung edema (33).

X. Transport Across the Mesothelial Cell and Pleura

The water filters in and out of the pleura according to the net hydrostatic-oncotic pressure gradient (33). Because the fluid in the pleural space alters transpleural forces respiration, it is closely maintained at the optimal volume and thickness (34).

Water and small molecules of 4 nm can pass freely between the mesothelial cells. Intrapleural injections of hypo- and hypertonic fluids induce an increase in the number and sizes of pinocytotic and cytoplasmic vesicles in the mesothelial cell (35). Intrapleural injection of ferritin (11 nm), carbon particles (20–50 nm), and polystyrene particles (up to 1000 nm) also appear in the cytoplasmic vesicles of the mesothelial cells (19). Some of the smaller particles are later found in mesenchymal cells in the pleural wall (19). These findings suggest that the transcytoplasmic transport is also active in the mesothelial cell.

Particles of 1000 nm in size, however, are engulfed by the mesothelial cell but are not transported across the basal lamina. Although the parietal mesothelial cell layer may be labile or leaky, effective removal of large particles or cells through the pleura is unlikely, unless the basal lamina and the deeper layers of the pleura have been damaged.

However, uncomplicated hemothorax resolves itself, and intrapleurally injected, labeled, red blood cells can be recovered intact in the systemic circulation (36,37). Furthermore, large molecular weight proteins and iso-osmotic fluid in the pleural space are absorbed rapidly through the lymphatics (38). Therefore, a larger and faster communication route than the cytoplasmic passage must exist between the pleural cavity and the circulation system (see Sec. XII).

XI. Lymphatics

The lymphatics within the lung are divided into two systems: the superficial or pleural plexus localized in the subpleural connective tissue layer of the visceral pleura, and the deep plexus located in the bronchovascular bundles, including peribronchial, peripulmonary vascular, and interlobular septum or connective tissue. Communications between the two plexuses exist only at the junction of the pleura and the interlobular septum (4,13).

The pleural space, which may be considered a potential and expandable interstitial space, lies between the above-mentioned superficial pulmonary pleural plexus and the parietal pleural lymphatic system. These two types of lymphatic circulation play important but different roles in the formation and removal of pleural fluid in normal and altered conditions (23,33). Their structures and roles are discussed further below.

A. Lymphatic Circulation of the Visceral Pleura

The superficial lymphatic plexus of the visceral pleura is composed of lymph capillaries and collecting lymph vessels. The larger collecting lymph vessels are arranged mainly along the margin of the pleural bases of the respiratory lobules, forming a polyhedral and widely meshed network. Smaller blind-ending side branches and capillaries are distributed unevenly from the meshed network (23).

Although lymph may flow in any direction governed by the pressure gradient, the larger lymphatic vessels of the visceral pleura are equipped with one-way valves, directing flow towards the hilum of the lung. Therefore, all lymph from the visceral pleura eventually reaches the lung root, either by entering the lymph vessels in the lobular and lobar septa of the lung or by flowing a long distance on the pleural surface of the lung. Anatomically, most large and small lymphatic vessels in the visceral pleura are located closer to the alveolar than the pleural cavity side and drain their contents into the vessels in the lobular septum.

B. Lymphatic Circulation of the Parietal Pleura

In humans, lymphatic plexuses of the costal pleura are mainly confined to intercostal spaces and are absent or minimal over the ribs (23). The lymph collected in the costal pleura drains ventrally towards nodes along the internal mammary artery or dorsally toward the internal intercostal lymph nodes near the heads of the ribs.

The lymphatic vessels of the mediastinal pleura are most increased in areas with abundant fat tissue; the collected lymph drains to the tracheobronchial and mediastinal lymph nodes. In the caudal portion of the mediastinum, these lymphatics are often associated with Kampmeier's foci (see Sec. XII.D). The lymphatic vessels of the diaphragmatic pleura drain into parasternal, middle phrenic, and posterior mediastinal nodes.

Similar to the arterial and venous system of the parietal pleura, the parietal lymphatics are richer in number and less restricted in their directions and passages of drainage than their counterparts in the visceral pleura. The parietal lymphatics, therefore, play a major role in the removal of the pleural content in normal conditions as well as in pleural effusion. This removal is sustained by the pleuro-lymphatic communications (see next section).

XII. Pleuro-Lymphatic Communication

The existence of anatomical communication large enough for red blood cells to traverse between the serous cavity, especially the peritoneal cavity, and the lymphatic channels was recognized many years before morphological confirmation (36). These connections were hypothesized by von Recklinghausen in 1863 (39) and Dybkowsky in 1866 (40) and have been clearly demonstrated by ultrastructural studies since the 1970s (41,42). The pleuro-lymphatic communication consists of the following structures.

A. Stomas

Ovoid or round openings of 2–6 µm in diameter (sometimes larger) have been found in selected areas on the pleural surface of the anterior lower chest wall, mediastinum, and diaphragm in rabbits and mice (41,42). They are not easily located, may be single and isolated (Fig. 3), but are most often found in groups. Shinohara found about 1000 lymphatic stomas in a thoracic hemisphere of a golden hamster (43). In his hamsters, about 15% of lymphatic stomas are distributed in the ventro-cranial regions of the thoracic wall and about 85% in the dorsocaudal region. In the ventro-cranial region, lymphatic stomas are found along the costal margin, and in the dorsocaudal, predominantly in the pre- and para-vertebral fatty tissue. In addition, he has described some small mesothelial pores and gaps, but claims that no lymphatic stomas open on the pleural surface of the diaphragm.

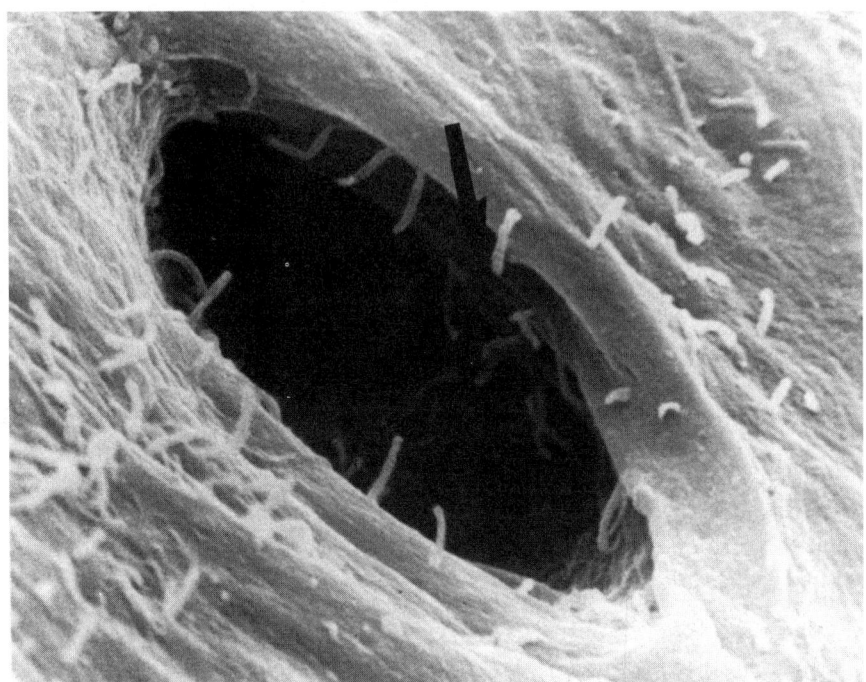

Figure 3 Microvilli (arrow) of a mesothelial cell extend into a stoma on the pleural surface. The stoma ranges from 2 to 12 μm in size and serve as a communication site between the pleural cavity and the lymphatic channel. (SEM ×25,800.) (From Ref. 19.)

Nevertheless, stomas have been found in the parietal and diaphragmatic pleura and are especially abundant on the parietal peritoneum in many animal species and in humans (41,42,44). Contrary to this, to date, stomas have not been convincingly documented on the visceral pleural side in all animals studied.

B. Membrana Cribriformis (Cribriform Lamina)

The substructure of the portion of the parietal pleura with stomas is a loosely knit layer of interweaving connective tissue bundles (Fig. 4) (45,46). The membrana cribriformis forms the roof of a lymphatic lacuna (see below). A layer of mesothelial cells covers the pleural surface of this connective tissue bundle network, and a layer of lymphatic endothelial cells covers the opposite surface (Fig. 5) (41). The membrana cribriformis, therefore, is reminiscent of a Japanese shoji (framed paper screen). A stoma presumably is formed where lining cells on both surfaces do not cover the space between the connective tissue bundles.

The membrana cribriformis has also not been found in the visceral pleura in either humans or any other species of animals studied.

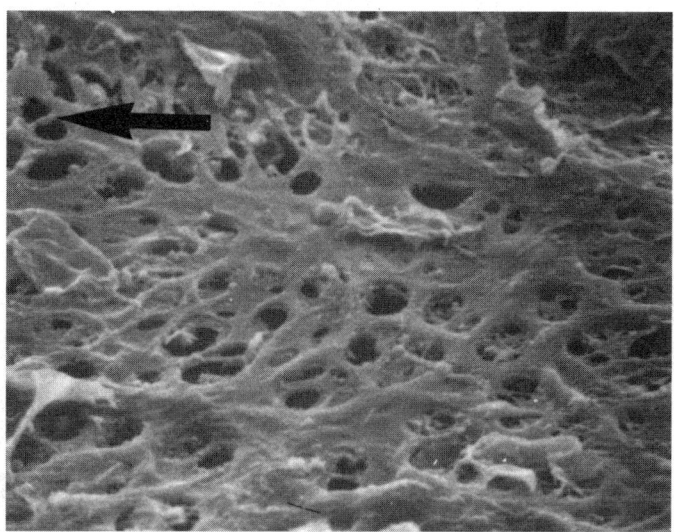

Figure 4 Multiple irregular fenestrations are present on the parietal pleura of a human autopsy case exposing the membrana cribriformis. (SEM ×1100.) (From Ref. 19.)

C. Lacuna and Lymphatic Channels

Beneath the stomas and the membrana cribriformis is a lacuna that is the terminal dilatation of a lymphatic channel. The lacuna has a number of small stomas open to the pleural cavity at one end and an out-draining lymphatic channel with checking valves at the other (41).

The respiratory movements alter the rate of removal of particles, red blood cells, and fluid from the pleural cavity (34,36,41). At inspiration, the chest wall is stretched and the intercostal spaces are widened; the stomas are also pulled open. At the same time, the fluid and particles in the pleural cavity are sucked into the lacuna by a negative pressure or pushed into it by the expanding lung. At expiration, the diameters of stomas decrease when the chest wall shrinks. The lacuna is compressed, and the fluid and particles in it are propelled into the lymphatic channel. At the next inspiration, the lacuna and stomas are dilated again, but retrograde flow of the fluid and particles in the lymphatic channel is prevented by the lymphatic valves. Stomas and lacunae appear to function similarly on the peritoneal side of the diaphragm (46,47).

D. Kampmeier's Foci

As early as 1928, Kampmeier discovered small milky spots in the dorsal and caudal portion of the mediastinum and occasionally in other locations in the parietal pleural of rats and humans (48,49). By scanning electron microscopy, the foci appear as irregularly elevated mound-like structures (19). These foci are covered by modified, cuboidal mesothelial cells with stomas and have an

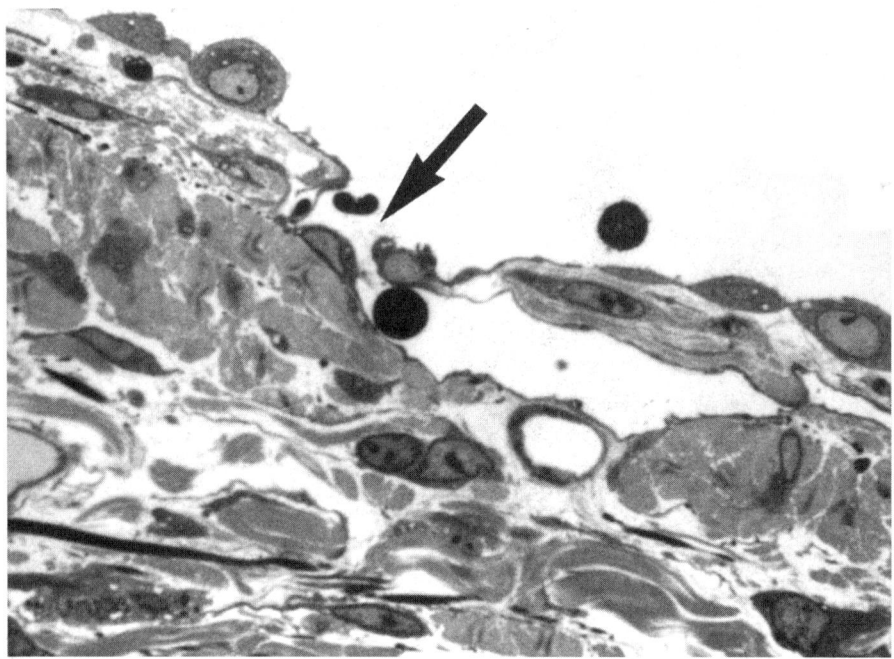

Figure 5 A red blood cell is present at the stoma (arrow) of a lacuna. The diameters of the two mononuclear (dark) cells appear larger than the narrowest portion of the stoma. The stoma is completely covered by mesothelial and lymphatic endothelial cells. Rabbits, lower thoracic wall. (Light microscopy ×1000.) (From Ref. 41.)

aggregate of lymphocytes, histiocytes, plasma cells, and other mononuclear cells around the centrally located lymphatic or vascular vessels. Mesothelial cells of these foci appear to have increased cytoplasmic mass and granules, and presumably have been adapted to offer a defense mechanism. Similar foci are later found in the thoracic cavity of the dog and in the mesentery of many species of mammals (49). They possibly represent structures of local defense, a function similar to the tonsils of the oropharynx. Infectious agents or other noxious particles in the pleural cavity may trespass or bypass the Kampmeier's foci to reach the parasternal lymph nodes (50).

XIII. Regional Differences

Substantial morphological differences exist in different regions of the pleura. They include the size and shape as well as the density of surface microvilli, the mesothelial cells, the substructure of mesothelial cells, and the number of the pleurolymphatic communications including the focal specialization of Kampmeier's foci (11,14,48).

Anatomy of the Pleura

As briefly stated earlier, the mesothelial cells on the pleural surface may appear either cuboidal and bumpy or flattened. The cuboidal and bumpy mesothelial cells are found over pleura with loose substructures. Those loose substructures are found in most of the visceral and mediastinal pleurae, the pleural recesses, and the subcostal portions of the parietal pleura.

The flattened mesothelial cells are most obvious over the ribs, somewhat less so in the tendinous portion of the diaphragm, and even less frequently over most of the muscular portions of the parietal pleura and diaphragm. It is quite possible that most cuboidal and flattened mesothelial cells covering the loose substructures are similar. Their size and shape, however, change constantly, reflecting the stretching of their substructures. The flattened mesothelial cells over the rib, however, do not have this flexibility.

The visceral pleura is relatively thin in the cranial or apical, statically expanded, portion of the lung, with relatively flattened mesothelial cells showing sparse microvilli. The pleura covering the actively moving and stretching caudal or basal portion of the lung is thicker and has cuboidal mesothelial cells showing increased microvilli (14). The basal lamina and the deeper three layers are often difficult to discern in the visceral pleura, especially towards the apex of the lung where systemic arterial supply is often replaced by a pulmonary one (see Sec. VII.B). Blebs or bullae may be formed, even in healthy, young, tall adults, on the relatively thin pleura of the upper lung, and more often so in patients with chronic obstructive lung diseases. The bullae may rupture spontaneously, resulting in acute pneumothorax.

On the parietal side, the pleura over the rib has a layer of flattened mesothelial cells with sparse microvilli and relatively thin second, third, and fourth layers. The fifth dense fibroelastic layer fuses with the perichondrium or periosteum of the rib.

In the portions of parietal pleura over loose structures, the mesothelial cells are cuboidal and prominent. The second and third layers are usually well defined and the fourth layer is often merged with the deeper and wider interstitial space, containing a poorly formed or completely absent fifth layer. This loose fourth layer often serves as the cleavage plane in pleurectomy.

The pleura over skeletal muscle cells, e.g., that over the intercostal muscle and the diaphragm, is somewhere between the aforementioned two types of pleura in layering and thickness. In general, the cellular and noncellular components of the pleura are modified because of the substructure the pleura covers.

XIV. Dispute Over the Existence of Stomas

Although the existence of stomas connecting the pleural cavity with the lymphatics has been clearly demonstrated in animals and in humans (41–44), skeptics still exist. This is understandable because of the sparsity of the stomas and the limited availability of good human tissues for study (51). Focal collections of fibrin, macrophages, red blood cells, and tissue debris could further obscure the stoma (41).

Stomas are easily found in the peritoneal cavity (41,47,52). Why there are so many on the peritoneal side of the diaphragm but so few on the pleural side is not completely clear. The stomas are probably similar to the draining holes of a sink: they are made as required and placed where they are needed. Normally, the pleural cavity is completely secluded from the external world, and few cells are discharged into, and thus need to be removed from, the pleural cavity. The peritoneal cavity, on the other hand, is much more likely to be directly or indirectly affected by the ailments of the gastrointestinal tract. In females, ovulation or ascending infection from gynecological sources generate cells and fluid in the peritoneal cavity that need to be cleared.

Additional stomas, therefore, may be recruited in both peritoneal and pleural cavities in disease or when more tissue debris needs to be removed. Those thin and fragile mesothelial and lymphatic lining cells over the lamina cribriformis appear easily broken during inflammation or chronic pleural effusion (41). Stomas may also increase in number and size with age or with wear and tear, somewhat similar to the relationship of interalveolar pores of Kohn and fenestrae (>15 µm in diameter) in the alveolus. Incidentally, large pleural stomas are also named fenestrae.

XV. Pleuro-Peritoneal Communication and Diaphragmatic Defects

Communication between the two lymphatic plexuses on the pleural and peritoneal surfaces is rare or poorly formed. This is important and understandable because fluid or inflammatory infiltrates in the peritoneal cavity should not readily reach the pleural cavity to interfere with the vital respiratory function.

However, different sized diaphragmatic defects are probably much more common than clinically suspected. The defects could be congenital or acquired. The acquired ones are likely from thinning and separation of the taut collagenous fibers of the tendinous portion of the diaphragm, such as that seen in the late stages of chronic obstructive lung disease. All such defects might cause an accumulation of pleural fluid in diseases such as hepatic hydrothorax (53) and Meig's syndrome and also during the process of continuous ambulatory peritoneal dialysis.

Even without diaphragmatic defects, excessive accumulation of fluid in the peritoneal cavity may reach the pleural cavity or, rarely, vice versa, from insufficiency of the thoracic duct and its major lymphatic attributes.

XVI. Resting and Reactive Mesothelial Cells

The resting mesothelial cells are cuboidal or flattened, and their enzymes are predominantly those of the pentose pathway (54). Mesothelial cells are, however, susceptible to and stimulated by a variety of lymphokines and thrombin (14,55,56). The stimulated, activated, or reactive mesothelial cells may become large cuboidal, or even columnar, in shape with increased microvilli (14). These reactive cells have mainly the enzymes of the oxidative pathway (57). Surface membrane– or mitochondria-associated enzymes, including $5'$-nucleotidase, alkaline phosphatases, ATPase, and cytochrome oxidase, are also increased. The fibrinolytic activities and synthesis of prostacyclins (58), a variety of lymphokines, and hyaluronic acid–rich glycoproteins (59,60) are also enhanced.

In inflammation, the rate of the proliferation of mesothelial cells is increased, probably as a response to the action of a variety of growth and proliferate factors. It has been shown that mesothelial cells from rats have receptors for platelet-derived growth factors (PDGF) and that human mesothelial cells in culture show increased growth in response to PDGF and to transforming growth factor-beta (TGF-β). Co-expression of cytokeratin and vimentin by subserosal cells in reactive processes is also present, suggesting an inward migration of the proliferating mesothelial cells (61).

The proliferative response of mesothelial cells is common and nonspecific and occurs in the subacute phase of several types of lung injury. The response may be prolonged when pleural fibrosis develops.

XVII. Subclinical Alterations and Repair of the Pleura

Pleuritis or pleural effusion frequently develops in patients with pneumonia, pulmonary infarction, or heart failure. Most of these pleural changes may regress without intrapleural intervention (62). How these pleural changes regress is not completely clear. In experimental animal studies, mesothelial cells proliferate and become reactive, as described above, in response to injuries. The mesothelial reaction apparently assists in the removal of fibrin and inflammatory debris and helps to repair the surface to maintain the patency of the pleural cavity as well as the pathways of drainage (59,63,64). The degree of damage to the basal lamina, as in other epithelial injury and repair, appears to be the decisive factor in a complete recovery or development of fibrosis in the pleural cavity (65).

Recent computed tomography (CT) and magnetic resonance imaging (MRI) studies suggest that unsuspected pleural lesions are common, especially in smokers (66). Pleural changes may occur in patients with lung cancer or myocardial ischemia without clinical or radiological evidence of pleural disease (62). This type of minor damage of the pleura is almost constantly incurred and repaired without clinical symptoms or signs. The pleural cavity is probably not as exclusively protected from the external world as we previously assumed. Without the reactive or reparative mesothelial cells, the patency of the serous cavity and the function of the lung and heart could be quickly compromised.

XVIII. Summary

The lung and heart, the vital organs, have to be well protected, but they also have to move and change volume continuously to function. For the best protection and function of the lung, the thoracic cage is constructed like a vertical cone-shaped bellows with the diaphragm as the moving part in the lowermost and widest end. Furthermore, the outer surface of the lung and the inner surface of the protective thoracic cage are covered by an elastic, serous, and lubricating membrane to form the pleural cavity. This is almost like inserting a sealed, wet, and stretchable plastic bag between the lung and the thoracic wall and diaphragm to decrease friction. The lubrication is accomplished by the facing mesothelial cells that have bushy surface microvilli enmeshing hyaluronic acid–rich glycoproteins. The amount of fluid in the pleural cavity is regulated by the hydrostatic-osmotic pressure relationship and pleuro–lymphatic drainage. Excess fluid, large particles, and cells in the pleural cavity are removed through preformed stomas and assisted by respiratory movements. The stoma is mainly found in the anterior lower thoracic wall and diaphragm and is like the drain of a sink. Finally, clinical and subclinical injuries of the pleura appear to occur often. Reactive mesothelial cells constantly repair the damage and keep the pleural cavity open. Without mesothelial cells, the lung cannot function properly and the pleural cavity will be quickly obliterated by fibrosis.

References

1. Patten BM, Carlson BW. Foundations of Embryology. 3d ed. New York: McGraw-Hill, 1974.
2. Hesseldahl H, Larsen JF. Ultrastructure of human yolk sac: endoderm, mesenchyme, tubules and mesothelium. Am J Anat 1969; 126:315–335.
3. Clemente CD. Anatomy of the Human Body. 30th American ed. Philadelphia: Lea and Febiger, 1985.
4. Von Hayek H. The Parietal Pleura and the Visceral Pleura. New York: Hafner, 1960.
5. Rabinowitz JG, Cohen BA, Mendelson DS. Symposium on nonpulmonary aspects in chest radiology. The pulmonary ligament. Radiol Clin North Am 1984; 22:659–672.
6. Collins JD, Disher AC, Shaver ML, Miller TQ. Imaging the hepatic lymphatics: experimental studies in swine. J Natl Med Assoc 1993; 85:185–191.
7. Morrissey BM, Bisset RA. The right inferior lung margin: anatomy and clinical implication. Br J Radiol 1993; 66:503–505.
8. Satoh K, Sato A, Kobayashi T, Kawase Y, Takahashi K, Mitani M, Fujiwara N, Takahashi H, Ohkawa M, Tanabe M. Septal structure of incomplete interlobar fissures of the lung. Acad Radiol 1996; 3:475–478.
9. Webb WR, La Berge JM. Radiographic recognition of chest tube malposition in the major fissure. Chest 1984; 85:81–83.
10. Albertine KH, Wiener-Kronish JP, Roos PJ, Staub NC. Structure, blood supply,

and lymphatic vessels of the sheep's visceral pleura. Am J Anat 1982; 165:277–294.
11. Mariassay AT, Wheeldon EB. The pleura: a combined light microscopic, scanning, and transmission electron microscopic study in the sheep. I. Normal pleura. Exp Lung Res 1983; 4:293–314.
12. Michailova KN. The serous membranes in the cat. Electron microscopic observations. Anat Anz 1996; 178:413–424.
13. Nagaishi C. Pulmonary pleura. Functional Anatomy and Histology of the Lung. Tokyo: Igaku Shoin, 1972.
14. Wang NS. The regional difference of pleural mesothelial cells in rabbits. Am Rev Respir Dis 1974; 110:623–633.
15. Andrews PM, Porter KR. The ultrastructural morphology and possible functional significance of mesothelial microvilli. Anat Rec 1973; 177:409–426.
16. Legrand M, Pariente R, Andre J, Chretien J, Brouet G. Ultrastructure de la pleure parietale humaine. Presse Med 1971; 55:2515–2520.
17. Odor DL. Observations of the rat mesothelium with electron and phase microscopes. Am J Anat 1954; 95:433–446.
18. Inoue T, Osatake H. Three dimensional demonstration of the intracellular structures of mouse mesothelial cells by scanning electron microscopy. J Submicrosc Cytol Pathol 1989; 21:215–227.
19. Wang NS. Mesothelial cells in situ. In: Chretien J, Bignon J, Hirsch A, eds. The Pleura in Health and Disease. New York: Marcel Dekker, 1985:23–42.
20. Simionescu M, Simionescu N. Organization of cell junctions in the peritoneal mesothelium. J Cell Biol 1977; 74:98–110.
21. Madison LD, Bergstrom-Porter B, Torres AR, Shelton E. Regulation of surface topography of mouse peritoneal cells: formation of microvilli and vesiculated pits on omental mesothelial cells by serum and other proteins. J Cell Biol 1979; 82:783–797.
22. Davila RM, Crouch EC. Anatomic organization and function of the human pleura. Semi Respir Crit Care Med 1995; 16:261–268.
23. Bernaudin J-F, Fleury JY. Anatomy of the blood and lymphatic circulation of the pleural serosa. In: Chretien J, Bignon J, Hirsch A, eds. The Pleura in Health and Disease. New York: Marcel Dekker, 1985:101–124.
24. Milne ENC, Pistolesi M. Reading the Chest Radiograph: A Physiologic Approach. St. Louis: Mosby, 1993.
25. Yamada S. Über die serose Flussigkeit in der Pleurahohle der gesunden Menschen. Z Ges Exp Med 1933; 90:342–348.
26. Miserocchi G, Agostoni E. Contents of the pleural space. J Appl Physiol 1971; 30:208–213.
27. Agostoni E, Miserocchi G, Bonanni MV. Thickness and pressure of the pleural liquid in some mammals. Respir Physiol 1969; 6:245–256.
28. Butler JP, Huang J, Loring SH, Lai-Fook SJ, Wang PM, Wilson TA. Model for a pump that drives circulation of pleural fluid. J Appl Physiol 1995; 78:23–29.
29. Murray JF. The Normal Lung. Phildelphia: W.B. Saunders.
30. Albertine KH, Wiener-Kronish JP, Bastacky J, Staub NC. No evidence for mesothelial cell contact across pleural space of sheep. J Appl Physiol 1991; 70:123–134.
31. Sahn SA, Willcox ML, Good JT Jr, Potts DE, Filley GF. Characteristics of normal rabbit pleural fluid: physiologic and biochemical implications. Lung 1979; 146:63–69.

32. Miserocchi G. Physiology and pathophysiology of pleural fluid turnover. Eur Respir J 1997; 10:219–225.
33. Staub NC. New concepts about the pathophysiology of pulmonary edema. J Thorac Imaging 1988; 3:8–14.
34. Miserocchi G, Venturoli D, Negrini D, Del Fabbro M. Model of pleural fluid turnover. J Appl Physiol 1993; 75:1798–1806.
35. Shumko JZ, Feinberg RN, Shalvoy RM, DeFouw DO. Responses of rat pleural mesothelium to increased intrathoracic pressure. Exp Lung Res 1993; 19:283–297.
36. Wilson JL, Herrod CM, Searle GL. The absorption of blood from the pleural space. Surgery 1960; 48:766–774.
37. Courtice FC, Simmonds WT. Physiological significance of lymph drainage of serous cavities and lungs. Physiol Rev 1954; 34:419–448.
38. Pistolesi M, Miniati M, Giuntini C. Pleural liquid and solute exchange. Am Rev Respir Dis 1989; 140:825–847.
39. Von Recklinghausen FV. Zur Fettresorption. Virchow Arch (Pathol Anat) 1863; 26:172–208.
40. Dybkowsky. Ueber Aufsaugung und Absonderung der Pleurawand. Ber Kgl Sachs Gesellsch Wissensch Math-physik Kl 1866; 18:191–218.
41. Wang N. The preformed stomas connecting the pleural cavity and the lymphatics in the parietal pleura. Am Rev Respir Dis 1975; 111:12–20.
42. Wheeldon EB, Mariassay AT. The pleura: a combined light microscopic, scanning, and transmission electron microscopic study in the sheep. II. Response to injury. Exp Lung Res 1983; 5:125–140.
43. Shinohara H. Distribution of lymphatic stomata on the pleural surface of the thoracic cavity and the surface topography of the pleural mesothelium in the golden hamster. Anat Rec 1997; 249:16–23.
44. Li J. Ultrastructural study on the pleural stomata in human. Funct Develop Morph 1993; 3:277–280.
45. Kihara T. The extravascular fluid passway system. Ketsuekigaku Togikai Hokoku 1950; 3:118.
46. Miura T, Shimada T, Tanaka K, Chujo M, Uchida Y. Lymphatic drainage of carbon particles injected into the pleural cavity of the monkey, as studied by video-assisted thoracoscopy and electron microscopy. J Thorac Cardiovasc Surg 2000; 120:437–447.
47. Tsilibary EC, Wissig SL. Absorption from the peritoneal cavity: SEM study of the mesothelium covering the peritoneal surface of the muscular portion of the diaphragm. Am J Anat 1977; 149:127–133.
48. Cooray GH. Defensive mechanisms in the mediastinum with special reference to the mechanics of pleural absorption. J Pathol Bacteriol 1949; 61:551–567.
49. Lang J, Liebich HG. Über eigenartige Kapillarkonvolute der Pleura parietalis. III. Elektronenmikroskopische Untersuchungen. Z Mikrosk-Anat Forsch 1976; 90:1074–1092.
50. Burke HE, Wilson JA. A new method for establishing the diagnosis of pleural disease—parasternal lymph node biopsy. Am Rev Respir Dis 1966; 93:201–208.
51. Gaudio E, Rendina EA, Pannarale L, Ricci C, Marinozzi G. Surface morphology of the human pleura: a scanning electron microscopic study. Chest 1988; 93:149–153.
52. Negrini D, Del Fabbro M, Gonano C, Mukenge S, Miserocchi G. Distribution of diaphragmatic lymphatic lacunae. J Appl Physiol 1992; 72:1166–1172.
53. Lieberman FL, Hidemura R, Peters RL, Reynolds TB. Pathogenesis and

treatment of hydrothorax complicating cirrhosis with ascites. Ann Int Med 1966; 64:341–351.
54. Whitaker D, Papadimitriou JM, Walters M N-I. The mesothelium: a histochemical study of resting mesothelial cells. J Pathol 1980; 132:273–284.
55. Hotts JW, Sparks JA, Godbey SW, Antony VB. Mesothelial cell response to pleural injury: thrombin-induced proliferation and chemotaxis of rat mesothelial cells. Am J Respir Cell Mol Biol 1992; 6:421–425.
56. Light RW. Pleural Diseases. 2d ed. Philadelphia: Lea & Febiger, 1990.
57. Whitaker D, Papadimitriou JM, Walters M N-I. The mesothelium: a cytochemical study of "activated" mesothelial cells. J Pathol 1982; 136:169–179.
58. Coene MC, Van Hove C, Claeys M, Herman AG. Arachidonic acid metabolism by cultured mesothelial cells. Biochim Biophys Acta 1982; 710:437–445.
59. Ryan GB, Grobety J, Majino G. Mesothelial injury and recovery. Am J Pathol 1973; 71:93–112.
60. Whitaker D, Papadimitriou JM, Walters M N-I. The mesothelium: its fibrinolytic properties. J Pathol 1980; 136:291–299.
61. Adamson IYR, Bakowska J, Bowden DH. Mesothelial cell proliferation: a nonspecific response to lung injury associated with fibrosis. Am J Respir Cell Mol Biol 1994; 10:23–28.
62. Peng MJ, Wang NS, Vargas FS, Light RW. Subclinical surface alterations of human pleura: a scanning electron microscopic study. Chest 1994; 106:351–353.
63. Watters WB, Buck RC. Scanning electron microscopy of mesothelial regeneration in the rat. Lab Invest 1972; 26:604–609.
64. Whitaker D, Papadimitriou JM. Mesothelial healing: morphological and kinetic investigations. J Pathol 1985; 145:159–175.
65. Davila RM, Crouch EC. Role of mesothelial and submesothelial stromal cells in matrix remodeling following pleural injury. Am J Pathol 1993; 142:547–555.
66. Kohda E, Suzuki K, Tanaka M, Taki Y, Kobayashi K, Kanazawa M, Yamaguchi K. Radiological approach to the pleura and pleural cavity with CT and MRI. Nippon Kyobu Shikkan Gakkai Zasshi 1994; 32:148–154.

3

Physiology of the Pleura

KOSTAS I. GOURGOULIANIS

University of Thessaly
Larissa, Greece

The pleura consists of two membranes: the visceral covering the lung and the parietal pleura covering the diaphragm and the chest wall. The main function of the pleura is to allow extensive movement of the lung to the chest wall. The visceral pleura also contributes to the shape of the lung, provides a limit to expansion, and contributes to the work of deflation (1,2). Pleural space is a protecting mechanism against the development of alveolar edema and pneumothorax. Pleural space provides a route by which edema escapes the lung. The continuous submesothelial tissue with the connective tissue of the lung parenchyma prevents the overdistension of alveoli at the pleura surface (3).

I. Functional Anatomy

After development from the embryonic mesoderm, the pleural mesothelia differentiate into the visceral and the parietal pleura by the third week of gestational age. By 9 weeks the pleural cavity has become separated from pericardial space. The pleural membranes are smooth and overlying with a single cell layer of mesothelial cells flat or cuboid in shape with a maximum body thickness of 4 μm and a maximum diameter of 40 μm. Mesothelial cells synthesize and secrete several macromodules of the pleural matrix, such as elastin, fibronectin, glycoproteins and collagen, and phagocytose particles and neutrophil chemotactic factors. Both visceral and parietal mesothelial cells present microvilli protruding into the pleural space. Microvilli are more dense over the visceral than the parietal pleura and in caudal than in cranial regions. Microvilli increase the area for metabolic functions. Mesothelial cells connect to each other with tight junctions (4,5).

Pleural lymphatics are connected to the pleural cavity via lacunas or stomas in the mesothelial surface. These stoma are numerous in the lower portion of the mediastinal and costal pleura and over the diaphragmatic portion of parietal pleura. Efferent lymphatic vessels from parietal pleura drain to parasternal and paravertebral nodes, whereas the lymphatics drain into tracheo-bronchial nodes (6). The lymphatic network is very rich within the parietal pleura. Lymphatics of the visceral do not communicate with the pleural cavity and are parts of the pulmonary lymphatic system (7).

The parietal pleura is supplied by intercostal arteries and the visceral pleura by the bronchial systemic circulation. Both pleura therefore have a systemic circulation, although the visceral circulation may have a slightly lower pressure because of its drainage into a lower pressure venous system (8).

Pleural membranes have some histological similarities and important anatomical differences. The submesothelial connective tissue layer of the parietal is thicker than its visceral pleura. The visceral pleura lacks innervation, and its blood supply is more complex than parietal pleura. An active lymphatic system exists only in parietal pleura (9).

II. Pleural Fluid Pressure and Dynamics

The parietal and visceral pleura are separated by a thin layer, about 20 μm, of fluid. Normally pleural fluid volume is 0.1 mL/kg of body weight—approximately 10 mL in a healthy adult man. Despite the small volume of fluid present in the pleural space, the rate of pleural fluid filtration and reabsorption exceeds 1 L per day. In pleural fluid, glucose concentration is similar to that of plasma, whereas the concentration of macromolecules such as albumin is lower than in the blood (10,11).

Movement of fluid within pleural membranes is based on the balance of hydrostatic and oncotic pressures between the microvasculature and the pleural space (12,13). Fluid exchange across the pleural membranes is described by Starling's law:

$$\text{Fluid movement} = L \times S \left[(P_{cap} - P_{pl}) - \sigma(\Pi_{cap} - \Pi_{pl}) \right]$$

where P and Π are the hydrostatic and osmotic pressures, respectively, within the capillaries (cap) and pleural space (pl), L is the hydraulic conductivity of the membrane, S is the surface area, and σ is the osmotic coefficient for proteins (Fig. 1). At the parietal pleura there is fluid filtration from systemic capillaries into the adjacent interstitium and from the latter across the mesothelium to

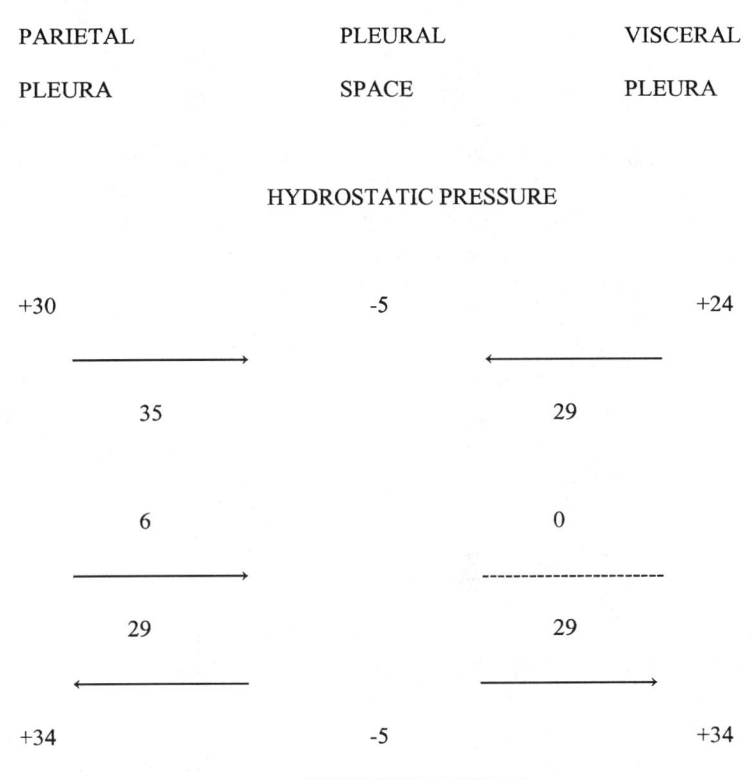

Figure 1 Pressures (cmH$_2$O) that normally influence the movement of fluid in and out of the pleural space.

pleural space. The actual pleural pressure in humans is approximately -5 cmH$_2$O at functional residual capacity and -30 cmH$_2$O at total lung capacity. According to this model of pressure gradients, net transmembrane Starling pressure moves fluid from pleural space to visceral pleura and then to pulmonary capillaries (14,15).

Recently there have been conflicting data concerning the entry and exit of pleural fluid normally. Pressure gradients are not the only explanation of the fluid turnover. First, the pleural space is analogous to any interstitial space of the body. Because intrapleural pressure is lower than interstitial pressure, this pressure difference constitutes a gradient for fluid movement into but not out of the pleural cavity. Second, the normal protein concentration (10 g/L) in pleural fluid is low, which implies sieving of the proteins across a high pressure gradient such as from the high-pressure systemic vessels. Third, erythrocytes instilled into pleural space are absorbed intact and in almost the same proportion as the fluid and protein. This indicates that the major route of exit is via the lymphatic stomas of the parietal pleura (16–19).

III. Pleural Lymphatic Flow

Lymphatics have a large capacity for absorption. When fluid was instilled into the pleural space of awake sheep, the exit rate increased to about 30 times the baseline exit rate (20). Our previous data showed that about one out of four women had pleural effusion during labor and possibly in the third trimester of pregnancy (21). The conditions of labor appear to favor the development of pleural effusion. We speculate that obstruction of lymphatic stomas of parietal pleura during Valsalva maneuvers is the main reason for this phenomenon. Other minor reasons are the increased pressure in systemic circulation, the decreased oncotic pressures, and possibly changes in hormonal status. According to Starling's equation, all these pressure changes increase the fluid influx into the pleural cavity. Additionally, the lymphatics lose their large capacity for absorption, which results in the accumulation of fluid during labor (21,22).

The ability of the lymphatics of the diaphragm to drain fluid at subatmospheric pressure has been demonstrated in spontaneously breathing rabbits. Lymphatic flow is based on an intrinsic mechanism (myogenic activity of the lymphatic wall) and an extrinsic mechanism (movement of the tissues surrounding the lymph channels) (23). Labor seems to influence the extrinsic mechanism and to decrease dramatically the pleural fluid efflux.

A recent study from our research group showed that amiloride increased the transepithelial resistance of only parietal pleura, although ouabain, an inhibitor of the Na^+-K^+ pump and nitroprusside sodium, a nitric oxide donor, had the same effect on parietal and visceral pleura. This amiloride effect is most serious in the basolateral, diaphragmatic membrane, than in the apical pleural membrane (24). Amiloride is a drug known to impair smooth muscle contractility (25). Negrini et al. estimated that about 40% of total pleural lymphatic flow depends on an intrinsic mechanism (7,8). Our data are in agreement with Negrini et al. because the amiloride effect occurred only in sites with stomas (parietal pleura, especially diaphragmatic) (26,27). The real increase in parietal pleura resistance is from 20 to about 22 Ω/cm^2. This small increase of parietal resistance may induce difficulties in pleural fluid exit (24,28).

Lymphatic stomas do not offer any restriction to the passage of molecules as large as protein, and so fluid drainage leaves the protein concentration unaffected, which depends on the sieving offered by pleural tissues. Normally about 80% of the total fluid leaves the pleural cavity via lymphatics. Lymphatics have the ability to increase flow when pleural fluid or pressure increases. Lymphatics represent a regulatory system. If the lymphatic conductance decreases significantly (labor) and the filtration coefficient is normal, only a small increase in pleural fluid results (benign postpartum pleural effusion). If the filtration coefficient increases significantly (inflammation), the lymphatic conductance increases lymph flow to maximum. When the filtration rate exceeds the maximum flow rate, lymphatic drainage is insufficient to counterbalance filtration rates, which results in pleural fluid accumulation (parapneumonic pleural effusion) (29).

IV. Water and Ion Transportation

Mesothelial cells have not been shown to generate an electrical potential difference as would be expected if there were active transport across them (30). Pleural fluid is alkaline with a higher bicarbonate than plasma. If the mesothelial cells were leaky, it is difficult to explain how a bicarbonate gradient could be maintained. Recently, indirect evidence was provided to support active electrocyte transport by mesothelial cells. Zocchi et al. showed the occurrence of solute-coupled liquid absorption from the pleural cavity using inhibitors for the Na^+/Cl^-, Na^+/H^+, Cl^-/HCO_3^- double exchange or for the Na^+/K^+ pump (31,32). Evidence for a small, active transport of Na^+ from the serosal to the interstitial side of the dog parietal pleura in vitro was found by D'Angelo et al. (12).

Our recent experiments showed active transport across both visceral and parietal pleura (24)—more specifically, an increase in the transepithelial electrical resistance when (a) ouabain, an inhibitor of Na^+-K^+ pump, was added to the mucosal surface of visceral pleura, (b) amiloride, an inhibitor of Na^+ channels and Na^+/H^+ exchanger, was added to the serosal solution in parietal pleura, and (c) sodium nitroprusside, a nitric oxide donor, was added to the serosal surface of parietal pleura and to the serosal or mucosal solutions of visceral pleura. We suggest the occurrence of two kinds of cells in the pleural mesothelium. The first type has double exchanger or Na^+ channels on the serosal side. These cells should transport Na^+ (and hence water) out of the pleural space. The second kind of cell is likely to be provided by the Na^+-K^+ pump on the serosal side and would be involved in recycling K^+. Nitric oxide increases resistance. This phenomenon suggests an effect on either pleural mesothelium or endothelium of lymphatic stomas or both (33).

Because pleural fluid is filtered and reabsorbed through the parietal pleura, a useful description of pleural fluid turnover can be attempted by a model considering four compartments, capillaries parietal or visceral, interstitium, pleural space, and mesothelial cells parietal or visceral, separated by two resistances—endothelium of capillaries and mesothelium of pleura and an outflow lymphatic system draining from parietal pleura. Most experiments showed that the Starling mechanism determines flow production through the endothelium of capillaries. Recently, evidence was provided to support active electrolyte and water transport through mesothelial cells (34–36).

V. Pathophysiology

For pleural fluid accumulation, either the entry rate of liquid must increase to more than 30 times normal to exceed the lymphatic removal capacity, or the exit rate of fluid must decrease, or both rates must change. The increase in capillary filtration leads to hypooncotic pleural effusion (transudate). More transudates result from congestive heart failure and were thought to originate from the pleural capillaries. In these patients with interstitial pulmonary edema, fluid may come from the pulmonary interstitium across the leaky visceral pleura. When interstitial edema is formed, interstitial pressure increases from -10 to about 6 cmH$_2$O. Over a 3-hour period, no fluid flux occurred across the visceral pleura to the pleural cavity. This finding is in agreement with the clinical observation that pulmonary edema is rarely complicated with pleural effusion. These data suggest that pleural effusion in interstitial edema is the final status when liquid influx exceeds lymphatic drainage (37,38). Other transudates, from nephrotic syndrome or pulmonary atelectasis, may be formed because of pressure changes across the pleural capillaries.

Hyperoncotic fluid (exudates) occurs when the protein permeability is increased. Exudates arise from injured capillaries due to inflammation or malignancy. Although many clinicians are unsure about the role of lymphatics in pleura physiology, the disturbances of the lymphatic system (benign post-partum pleural effusion, yellow nail syndrome), the infiltration of draining parasternal lymph nodes (malignancies), and elevation of the systemic venous pressure into which the lymph drains (heart failure) are causes of pleural fluid accumulation (39).

Despite previous conflicting theories, lymphatic drainage is the major route of pleural fluid efflux. Our data, based on clinical observations such as benign postpartum pleural effusion and electrophysiological experiments in pleura, showed a major role of lymphatic stoma activities in pleural physiology.

Acknowledgments

We thank Professor P. A. Molyvdas for his useful comments and Smaragda Efremidou for assistance in the preparation of the manuscript.

References

1. Gray SW, Skandalakis JE. Development of the pleura. In: Chretien J, Bignon DJ, Hirsh A, eds. The Pleura in Health and Disease. New York: Marcel Dekker, 1985:3–18.
2. Albertine KH, Wiener-Kronish JP, Staub NC. The structure of the parietal pleura and its relationship to pleural liquid dynamics in sheep. Anat Rec 1984; 208:401–409.
3. Miserocchi G, Agostoni E. Contents of the pleural space. Respir Physiol 1971; 30: 208–218.
4. Marlassy TA, Wheeldon EB. The pleura: a combined light microscopic, scanning, and transmission electron microscopic study of the pleura. Exp Lung Res 1983; 4:293–313.
5. Staub NC, Wiener-Kronish JP, Albertine KH. Transport through the pleura:

physiology of normal liquid and solute exchange in the pleural space. In: The Pleura in Health and Disease. New York: Marcel Dekker, 1977:169–193.
6. Wang NS. The performed stomas connecting the pleura cavity and the lymphatics in the parietal pleura. Am Rev Respir Dis 1975; 111:12–20.
7. Negrini D, Del Fabbro M, Gonano C, Mukenges S, Miserocchi G. Distribution of diaphragmatic lymphatic lacunae. J Appl Physiol 1993; 74:1779–1784.
8. Negrini D, Mukenge S, Del Fabbro M, Gonano C, Miserocchi G. Distribution of diaphragmatic lymphatic stomata. J Appl Physiol 1991; 70:1544–1549.
9. Wang NS. The preformed stomas connecting the pleural cavity and the lymphatics in parietal pleura. Am Rev Respir Dis 1974; 110:623–633.
10. Agostoni E, Zocchl L. Solute-coupled liquid absorption from the pleural space. Respir Physiol 1990; 81:19–27.
11. Albertine KH, Wiener-Kronish JP, Staub NC. The structure of the parietal pleura and its relationship to pleural liquid dynamics in sheep. Anat Rec 1984; 208:401–409.
12. D'Angelo E, Helsler N, Agostoni E. Acid-base balance of pleural liquid in dogs. Respir Physiol 1979; 37:137–149.
13. Kinasewitz GT, Fishman AP. Influence of alterations in starling forces on visceral pleural fluid movement. J Appl Physiol 1981; 51:671–677.
14. Kinasewitz GT, Groome LJ, Marshall RP, Diana JN. Permeability of the canine visceral pleura. J Appl Physiol 1983; 55:121–130.
15. Payne DK, Kinasewitz GT, Gonzalez E. Comparative permeability of canine visceral and parietal pleura. J Appl Physiol 1988; 65:2558–2564.
16. Albertine KH, Wiener-Kronish JP, Roos PI, Staub NC. Structure, blood supply, and lymphatic vessels of the sheep's visceral pleura. Am J Anat 1982; 165:277–294.
17. Engelberg J, Radin J. Tracheal-vascular and vascular-pleural potential in the rat lung. Respir Physiol 1977; 30:253–263.
18. Frazier HS. The electrical potential profile of the isolated toad bladder. J Gen Physiol 1962; 45:515–528.
19. Fromter I, Diamond JM. Route of passive ion permeation in epithelia. Nat New Biol 1972; 235:9–13.
20. Leak LV, Rahil K. Permeability of the diaphragmatic mesothelium: the ultrastructural basis for "stomata". Am J Anat 1978; 151:557–564.
21. Gourgoulianis KI, Karantanas AH, Diminikou G, Molyvdas PA. Benign postpartum pleural effusion. Eur Respir J 1995; 8:1748–1750.
22. Tsilibary EC, Wissing SL. Lymphatic absorption from peritoneal cavity: regulation of patent of mesothelial stoma. Microvasc Res 1983; 25:22–39.
23. Miserocchi G. Effect of diaphragmatic contraction or relaxation on size and shape of lymphatic stomata on the peritoneal surface in anesthetized rabbits. Proc Physiol Soc 1989; 417:132P.
24. Hatzoglou CH, Gourgoulianis KI, Molyvdas PA. Effects of SNP ouabain and amiloride on electrical potential profile of isolated sheep pleura. J Appl Physiol 2001; 90:1565–1569.
25. Ding JW, Dickie J, O'Brodovich H, Shintani Y, Rafii B, Hackam D, Marunaka Y, Rotstein OD. Inhibition of amiloride-sensitive sodium-channel activity in distal lung epithelial cells by nitric oxide. Am J Physiol Lung Cell Mol Physiol 1998; 274:L378–L387.
26. Diamond JM. Transport of salt and water in rabbit and guinea pig gall bladder. J Gen Physiol 1964; 48:1–14.

27. Lewis SA, Diamond JM. Na^+ transport by rabbit urinary bladder, a tight epithelium. J Membr Biol 1976; 28:1–40.
28. Lucky J, Chen XJ, Brown LA, Eaton DC. Nitric oxide inhibits lung sodium transport through a cGMP-mediated inhibition of epithelial cation channels. Am J Physiol Lung Cell Mol Physiol 1998; 274:L475–L484.
29. Kim K, McElroy Critz A, Crandall E. Transport of water and solutes across sheep visceral pleura. Am Rev Respir Dis 1979; 120:883–892.
30. Bernaudin JF, Jaurand MC, Fleury J, Bignon DJ. Mesothelial cells. In: Crystal RG, West JB, eds. The Lung: scientific Foundations. New York: Raven, 1991:631–638.
31. Zocchi L, Agostoni E, Cremaschi D. Electrolyte transport across the pleura of rabbits. Respir Physiol 1991; 86:125–138.
32. Zocchi L, Agostoni E, Cremaschi D. Liquid volume, Na^+ and mannitol concentration in hypertonic mannitol-Ringer hydrothorax. Respir Physiol 1992; 89:341–351.
33. Guo V, Duvall MD, Crow JP, Matalon S. Nitric oxide inhibits Na^+ absorption across cultured alveolar type II monolayers. Am J Physiol Lung Cell Mol Physiol 1998; 274:L369–L377.
34. Basset G, Bouchonnet F, Crone C, Sammon G. Potassium transport across rat alveolar epithelium: evidence for an apical Na^+-K^+ pump. J Physiol (Lond) 1988; 400:529–543.
35. Zocchi L, Agostoni E, Cremaschi D. Electrolyte transport across the pleura of rabbits. Respir Physiol 1991; 86:125–138.
36. Gourgoulianis KI, Karantanas AH, Molyvdas PA. Peripartum pleural effusion. Chest 1997; 111:1467–1468.
37. Agostoni E. Mechanics of the pleural space. Physiol Rev 1972; 52:57–128.
38. Miserocchi G, Negrini D, Gonado C. Direct measurement of interstitial pulmonary pressure in in-situ lungs with intact pleural space. J Appl Physiol 1990; 69:2168–2174.
39. Light RW. Physiology of the pleural space. In: Pleural Diseases. 4th ed. Philadelphia: Lippincott Williams and Wilkins, 2001:8–20.

4

Pathophysiology of the Pleura

VEENA B. ANTONY

Indiana University School of Medicine
Indianapolis, Indiana, U.S.A.

I. Defense Mechanisms of the Pleura

The pleura is a monolayer of mesothelial cells intricately connected with the underlying lung and tissues through a network of balancing cellular and humoral factors that allow for host defense of the pleural space. The pleural membrane not only serves a barrier function, but also has multiple other defense mechanisms which are focused on maintaining the homeostatic balance of the pleural space. Since the pleura encircles a closed potential space, it does not interface with the external environment as does the lung (1). Changes in the delicate homeostatic balance of the pleural space can be initiated by the presence of foreign cells, proteins, or microbes. Even the presence of air in the pleural space changes this balance.

Innate immunity of the pleura is seen early during inflammation, within the first few hours following an insult to the pleural space (2). A significant proportion of the innate immunity of the pleura is provided by the pleural mesothelial cell, a multipotent cell that completely lines the pleural space. The pleural mesothelial cell must not only recognize the offending organism, it must initiate the process of responses and coordinate the perpetuation of the inflammatory changes. These responses may differ, depending on the invading microbe or cell. Malignant cells must be recognized as foreign in spite of their development of multiple factors that allow them to present themselves as innocuous and allow them to enter the pleural space as a Trojan horse.

The free surface of the mesothelium is covered by glycoconjugates, which consist of pleural mesothelial cell–associated sialomucins (3). These are strong anionic sites that coat the pleural surface with a negative charge and act to repulse the presence of abnormal particles and organisms. Thus, not only do these glycoproteins mechanically repel (because of their strong negative charge) the opposing pleural membrane, they also provide a second level of mechanical repulsion to invading cells, microbes, and particulates (4). The presence of these sialomucins on the surface of the mesothelium allow it to function mechanically as "teflon" rather than "velcro." Epithelial surfaces that have been stripped of their sialomucins are far more susceptible to damage. Mesothelial cells also have multiple pattern recognition receptors, which recognize the carbohydrate residua of microbial metabolism. The innate immune system of the mesothelial cell also recognizes pathogen-associated molecular patterns, which then can initiate multiple levels of defense mechanisms (5). Some of these pattern recognition receptors include CD 14, integrins, and the mannose receptor. The inflammatory responses initiated by the pleural mesothelial cell include release of chemokines to recruit neutrophils, mononuclear cells, and lymphocytes and the release of factors such as interleukin (IL)-1, IL-6, and interferons, which function as co-stimulators of T cells. T-cell–independent mesothelial responses following phagocytosis of asbestos particles, microbes, etc., lead to the release of IL-12 and tumor necrosis factor (TNF)-α. These cytokine responses perpetuate the proinflammatory loop.

Acquired immunity is the specific immune system of lymphocytes, both T and B lymphocytes, that allows for expression of distinct antigenic receptors (6). Activated T lymphocytes orchestrate specific immune responses in the pleural space. Mesothelial cells contribute to the cytokines that allow for an undifferentiated T cell to become a T-helper (Th)1 or Th2 type cell that leads to different responses in the pleural space (7). Thus, the defense mechanisms of the pleura include functions starting from providing a mechanical barrier to invasion as well as a sophisticated, multilayered, and coordinated system of cytokines and recruited cells.

II. Cytokine Networks in the Pleural Space

Cytokines are polypeptide structures with multiple biological functions and are key ingredients for the process of initiation, perpetuation, and resolution of the inflammatory response of the pleura. Cytokines do not act alone, but form a multitiered, connecting network that establishes communication between cells and allows for an orchestrated inflammatory cascade of events critical to the inflammatory response (8). The accumulation of inflammatory cells and fluid in the pleural space is a classic response of pleural inflammation. The mesothelial cell is known to produce multiple chemokines from the chemokine family (9).

The chemokine family is named according to the location of the amino-terminal cystine residue with a C, C-C, C-X-C, or CCXXXC motif. Pleural mesothelial cells are known to release chemokines from all the member family groups. The C-X-C chemokines, such as IL-8, have been well characterized. These chemokines are critical for neutrophil chemotactic and activating properties. The C-X-C chemokines themselves include those that contain an amino acid residue that precedes the first N-terminal cysteine residue. These amino acids are GLU-LEU-ARG, otherwise known as the ELR motif. The presence or absence of the GLU-LEU-ARG (ELR) motif appears to be critical and is defined by logical activities noted among the C-X-C chemokines. The factors that lack the ELR motif are not potent neutrophil chemotaxins and also have angiostatic properties, while those containing an ELR motif, such as IL-8, are chemotactic for neutrophils and are also angiogenic (10). The C-C group of chemokines is defined by the position of the first two end-terminal cysteines. These include macrophage inflammatory protein-1α, β, γ; MCP-1, 2, 3, and 4; and RANTES. The C chemokine lymphotaxin is important for the recruitment of lymphocytes to the pleural space. Mesothelial cells have also been described to produce fractalkine.

A. Cytokine Networks During Acute Infections

A characteristic feature of parapneumonic effusions is the accumulation of neutrophils and mononuclear phagocytes. IL-8, an 8.3 kDa protein, is found in significant quantities in pleural fluids obtained from patients who develop parapneumonic effusions. The pleural fluid from both patients with uncomplicated parapneumonic effusions as well as empyema is chemotactic for neutrophils and contains higher levels of IL-8 when compared to pleural effusions of patients with malignancy, tuberculosis, or heart failure (11). In patients with uncomplicated parapneumonic effusions, a significantly higher correlation of neutrophil to chemokine level is seen with epithelial neutrophil activating protein-78 (ENA-78) than with IL-8. This chemokine is also known to have specific chemotactic activity for neutrophils. Broaddus et al. (12), using an endotoxin model for pleurisy, demonstrated that inhibition of neutrophil entry into the pleural space was mediated by antibodies to rabbit IL-8. Other early mediators released by mesothelial cells include IL-1β and TNF-α. The early responses of the pleural mesothelial cell in acute inflammation lead to a widening of the inflammatory changes with the recruitment of several phagocytic cells that may themselves release cytokines and thus communicate with the resident mesothelial cell. In the exudative stage of parapneumonic effusions, the pleural fluid is still free flowing. However, during the fibrinopurulent stage, as there is further movement of inflammatory cells and bacteria into the pleura space, other cytokine networks appear to be initiated.

Pleural mesothelial cells release growth factors such as platelet-derived growth factor, transforming growth factor (TGF)-β, and fibroblast growth factor. These factors are known to be mitogenic for fibroblasts and are also angiogenic. The goal appears to be walling off of the pleural space in a fibrous peel for the development of new capillaries and revascularization of the injured mesothelium. This allows for an increased influx of inflammatory cells into the area to prevent further spread of the infection to other areas. In effect, the pleural space is transformed into an abscess cavity.

B. Cytokine Networks in Granulomatous Disease of the Pleura

Tuberculosis is a classic example of a pleural granulomatous response. This includes the development of cytokine networks that drive the Th1/Th2 responses. Early during the course of granulomatous disease there is a neutrophil predominant response (13), but the most persistent response is that of mononuclear phagocytes that engulf mycobacteria, resulting in a coalescing of mononuclear cells into granulomas. Mesothelial cells release members of the C-C chemokine family, including MCP-1. MCP-1 is a protein member of the supergene family that has been demonstrated in tuberculous pleural fluids. These fluids have also been described to contain MIP-1α, a specific chemokine for monocytes. Interferon (IFN)-γ, a critical cytokine for the recruitment of mononuclear cells, is also present in pleural fluids of patients with granulomatous inflammation (14). Mesothelial cells produce IL-12, which drives the Th response towards the Th1 cytokines, including IL-4. Neutralization of the IFN-γ response in the pleural space causes abrogation of the development of granulomas. IFN-γ augments cytokine and chemokine production by local cells and allows for a significant increase in MCP-1 and MIP-1 production by mesothelial cells.

Interferon-γ upregulates microbicidal, phagocytic, and T cell–activating functions as well as nitric oxide release by mesothelial cells (15). Nitric oxide is part of a microbicidal mechanism of mesothelial cells that results in the killing of mycobacteria as well as increased production of other oxidants such as H_2O_2 and superoxide anion. IFN-γ itself is regulated by other cytokines, such as TNF-α, which synergize with IFN-γ in macrophage activation. IL-12 also functions with TNF-α, IL-1β, IL-15, and IL-18 to achieve optimal IFN-γ expression. In patients with human immunodeficiency (HIV) infection, there is a disruption of the cytokine network in the pleural space with disastrous results for the patients. Cytokines such as IL-10 are present in significant quantities in the pleural fluid of patients with disseminated tuberculosis and can prevent critical Th1 type responses from functioning. This leads to poor granuloma formation and dissemination of the disease.

III. Changes in Pleural Cell Populations

The pleural mesothelial cell is the single most common cell of the pleural space. It is also the primary cell that initiates responses to noxious stimuli (16,17). The mesothelial cell is a metabolically active cell that maintains a dynamic state of homeostasis in the pleural space until provoked. It is actively phagocytic and is capable of producing several cytokines, as mentioned above (8). Mesothelial cells are ciliated, as described in Chapter 2, and have multiple tight intercellular adherens junctions as well as focal adhesions that anchor the mesothelial cell onto the extracellular membrane via integrins (7). When injured, mesothelial cells respond via proliferation and chemotaxis to cover areas of denuded extracellular matrix. This proliferative and chemotactic response is mediated in part by an autocrine response to the production of chemokines in the local area of injury. Mesothelial cells also maintain both juxtacrine and paracrine communications between cells to allow for a rapid response during inflammation.

A. Neutrophils

Neutrophils are the first cells to respond during inflammation (18). Neutrophils are produced in the bone marrow, where they evolve from pluripotent stem cells that also give rise to other cells of the granulocytic series, including eosinophils. During inflammation, these cells move from the vascular compartment into the pleural space and form the first line of inflammatory cell defense against invading organisms or particulates such as asbestos (19). A significantly large number of neutrophils are found in the lung vasculature. During inflammation, neutrophils move out of the vascular compartment and into the pleural space using the adhesion molecule ICAM-1 on mesothelial surfaces to interdigitate with the CD-11/CD-18 ligands on their surfaces (20). The primary function of neutrophils in the pleural space are phagocytosis and bacterial killing (21). They have potent antibacterial defense mechanisms such as release of oxidants and proteases (6,22). Neutropenic animals with empyema are unable to clear bacteria and develop disseminated disease. The eventual fate of neutrophils in the pleural space during acute inflammatory events such as empyema is unclear. Neutrophils are cleared from the pleural space by macrophages that engulf apoptotic cells. Mesothelial cells regulate the process of apoptosis of neutrophils via production of granulocyte-macrophage colony-stimulating factor (GM-CSF), thus manipulating the life span of the neutrophil in the pleural space (23–25).

B. Lymphocytes

The mesothelial cell releases several chemokines, which are directed at lymphocytes. Both B- and T-cell lymphocytes are found during inflammatory disease. Lymphocytes are common in granulomatous disease, while both T and B lymphocytes are found in malignant pleural effusions and in effusions caused by abnormal of immune responses such as lupus erythematosus and rheumatoid disease (26). Pleural fluid from patients with tuberculosis contain natual killer (NK) cells as well as gamma-delta T cells, which are critical for responses against mycobacteria. The T lymphocytes are divided into CD4 and CD8 lymphocytes. The CD4 lymphocytes predominate in diseases such as tuberculosis, while CD8 lymphocytes predominate in diseases such as lymphoma. Activated T lymphocytes release multiple cytokines, including IFN-γ and a host of other cytokines

(27). CD8 T lymphocytes can function as specific cytotoxic cells, while NK cells can regulate B-cell function. B-cell immunoglobulin production is displayed on its surface as an IgM molecule. They can exhibit specific markers and make immunoglobulins with specificity for a single antigen.

C. Pleural Fibroblasts

Pleural fibroblasts, though not present in large numbers under normal conditions, are often exposed to the environment of the pleural space when there is denudation of the mesothelium. The pleural fibroblast is a spindle-shaped elongated cell with a large oval nucleus with one or more nucleoli. The cytoplasm consists of abundant rough endoplasmic reticulum with well-developed Golgi apparatus and numerous mitochondria. Fibroblasts are known to produce collagen and can release several cytokines such as chemokines, which can then perpetuate the inflammatory process. The proliferation of fibroblasts is determined by the environment that is present in the pleural milieu. Potent mitogens for fibroblasts include PDGF, FGF, and EGF. Inhibitors of fibroblast growth include PGE2, which also can be produced by pleural mesothelial cells (28). IFN-γ may have either an inhibitory or a stimulatory effect on the growth of pleural fibroblasts. Fibroblasts derived from different tissue sites display distinct morphological, structural, and functional characteristics. Pleural fibroblasts appear to have specific functions and demonstrate specific behavior in response to injury of the overlying extracellular matrix and cells (29).

D. Malignant Cells

The presence of malignant cells in the pleural space is abnormal. Certain malignant cells demonstrate a greater predilection for the pleural space than elsewhere. Cancers of the lung, breast, stomach, and ovary following metastasis are seen in greater frequency in the pleural space than at other sites. The presence of a malignant cell in the pleural space indicates that the malignant cell has overcome the pleural defense mechanisms to localize in the pleural space. Malignant cells have a large armamentarium of mechanisms whereby they can present themselves as innocuous cells to the mesothelial cellular environment (30). Malignant cells may use a host of factors such as receptors for CD44 (31), whose ligand is hyaluron, which is produced in significant quantities by the pleural mesothelial cell to interdigitate with the mesothelial cell (32). This allows for proteolytic digestion of large molecular weight hyaluron, leaving smaller fragments, which are both chemotactic for the malignant cells and angiogenic.

Angiogenesis is critical for the ability of the malignant cells to develop an environment surrounded by blood vessels through which it is fed and can grow. Malignant cells can produce multiple cytokines including VEGF and bFGF, which are angiogenic and increase the permeability of the tissues around it to allow for growth of new capillaries, leading to vascularization of the pleural surface. This leads to the eventual seeding of the pleural surface and independent growth of the tumor by eluding the defense mechanisms of the pleura. Malignant cells can also produce autocrine growth factors.

IV. Pleural Effusion Formation During Inflammation

One of the signatures of an inflammatory process in the pleural space is the development of an exudative pleural effusion. Whether it is movement of leukocytes from the vascular compartment into the pleural space or malignant cells moving from the vascular or lymphatic space, a critical barrier provided by the mesothelial monolayer has been breached. Individual pleural mesothelial cells are linked together into a tight membrane by connecting intracellular proteins at key areas called adherens junctions. Pleural mesothelial cell adherens junction transmembrane, cell-to-cell connecting, homophilic proteins are responsible for maintaining pleural barrier function. Activation of the pleural mesothelial monolayer by malignant cells, bacteria, or cytokines causes a breach in the integrity of the pleura and results in altered shape, gap formation between mesothelial cells, and leakage of protein, fluids, and movement of phagocytic cells out into the pleural space. Vascular permeability factor (VPF) (33), also commonly known as vascular endothelial growth factor (VEGF), is upregulated in mesothelial cells when they are activated. VEGF has been found in large quantities in parapneumonic effusions as well as malignant pleural effusions. VEGF is a 35–45 kDa dimeric polypeptide expressed in several isoforms resulting from alternative mRNA splicing of a single gene and is now recognized to be a pivotal permeability and angiogenic factor mediating neovascularization under many conditions (34). VEGF is also known to play a central role in the formation of ascites in animal models. Adherens junction proteins, namely cadherins and catenins, are transmembrane proteins that function as a zipper between cells, allowing a change in permeability to occur via signaling mechanisms that lead to contraction of the intracellular actin cytoskeletal filaments leading to gap formation between cells (35). A major cadherin in pleural mesothelial cells is neural cadherin (n-cadherin). When adherens junctions are stabilized as in tightly confluent cells, the majority of n-cadherin loses tyrosine phosphorylation and combines with plakoglobin and actin (36). However, when cells have weakened junctions, n-cadherin is heavily phosphorylated in tyrosine, and there is decreased expression of β-catenin as well (37). Thus, n-cadherin and β-catenin are critical determinants of mesothelial paracellular permeability. This interaction is a dynamic one, since this permeability is also reversible. VEGF induces tyrosine phosphorylation of adherens junction proteins to allow paracellular permeability. During the formation of a pleural effusion, not only can cells migrate via the interaction of surface ligands for intercellular molecules expressed on mesothelial cells, but this also allows proteins of high molecular weight to leak across the pleural membrane. Exposure of pleural mesothelial monolayers to malignant cells or organisms leads to a rapid drop-off in electrical resistance across the pleural membrane and a transfer of protein.

V. Resolution of Pleural Inflammation

The resolution of a pleural inflammatory process is dependent on multiple factors, but primarily on the neutralization of the inciting agent. In infections secondary to bacteria, mycobacteria, viruses, etc., death of the organism and eventual clearance of the bacterial cell products from the pleural space is associated with resolution. However, in diseases such as malignant pleural effusions, this may not occur on its own without the use of chemotherapeutic options. For example, in diseases such as metastatic small-cell carcinoma, chemotherapy can cause a rapid decrease and resolution of malignant pleural effusions, while in diseases such as mesothelioma or non–small-cell lung cancer, effective resolution of the pleural effusion is much more difficult. Interestingly, the pleural mesothelial cell plays a role during the process of resolution of acute inflammatory diseases such as empyema. GM-CSF is known to prolong the life span of leukocytes by inhibition of apoptosis (23). GM-CSF is found in high levels in parapneumonic effusions and in empyema (24). Mesothelial cells are also shown to undergo apoptosis when stimulated with live bacteria, but not dead organisms.

Inflammation of the pleural surface may resolve with fibrosis or without fibrosis. The cytokine networks that move the resolution of inflammation towards fibrosis are not clear. However, it is apparent that resolution without fibrosis requires regeneration of a normal mesothelial surface following injury and denudation, while repair with fibrosis involves the production and proliferation of fibroblasts.

VI. Therapeutic Strategies Based on Pathophysiology of Pleural Disease

A. Gene Therapy

Gene therapy in the pleural space uses exogenous cDNA to manipulate the mesothelial cell to achieve a certain therapeutic effect. Gene therapy has been used in the pleural space primarily to counteract mesothelioma. Gene therapy against mesothelioma has used both viral-based vectors, such as adenovirus or adeno-associated virus–based systems, as well as non–viral-based systems. These include liposomes where cationic lipids are mixed with neutral lipids, which combine with DNA. The rationale for the administration of a replication-deficient recombinant adenovirus that has been genetically engineered to contain the herpes simplex virus thymidine kinase gene is the hope that delivery of this gene into the pleural cavity of patients with mesothelioma would transduce the tumor cells enabling them to express viral thymidine kinase and convey sensitivity to the nontoxic antiviral drug ganciclovir. Phase 1 studies of both this drug as well as the γ-interferon gene have been partially successful, and the outcomes of these studies are as yet unclear and undergoing further clarification (38).

B. Pleurodesis

Pleurodesis implicates the obliteration of the pleural space and absence of defining surfaces between the parietal and visceral pleura. All pleurodesis agents aim at initiating an inflammatory response that eventually results in the development of pleural fibrosis. Talc has been demonstrated to cause release of several fibroblast growth factors by the pleural mesothelial cells. These include bFGF and PDGF (39). Initiation of an inflammatory response that allows for the directed movement of the inflammation to resolve with fibrosis has been the goal. Interestingly, if malignant disease is advanced to the point where the pleural mesothelial surface is covered by malignant deposit so that the talc or other sclerosing agent has little interaction with the normal pleural mesothelial surface, the fibrotic response has been found to be attenuated with decreases in the amount of pleural fluid fibroblast growth factors. This finding emphasizes the important role played by the mesothelial cell in the process of pleural fibrosis.

References

1. Wang N. Mesothelial cells in situ. In: Chretien j, Bignon J, Hirsch A, eds. The Pleura in Health and Disease. New York: Marcel Dekker, 1985:23–42.
2. Medzhitov R, Janeway CA Jr. Innate immunity: impact on the adaptive immune response. Curr Opin Immunol 1997; 9:4–9.
3. Ohtsuka A, Yamana S, Murakami T. Localization of membrane-associated sialomucin on the free surface of mesothelial cells of the pleura, pericardium, and peritoneum. Histochem Cell Biol 1997; 107:441–447.
4. Sassetti C, Van Zante A, Rosen SD. Identification of endoglycan, a member of the CD34/podocalyxin family of sialomucins. J Biol Chem 2000; 275:9001–9010.
5. Gorbach S, Bartlett J, Blacklow N. Infectious diseases. In: Gorbach S, Bartlett J, Blacklow N, eds. Host Factors. Philadelphia: Saunders, 1992:37.
6. Burton DR, Woof JM. Human antibody effector function. Adv Immunol 1992; 51:1–84.
7. Mohammed KA, Nasreen N, Ward MJ, Antony VB. Induction of acute pleural inflammation by *Staphylococcus aureus*. I. CD4+ T cells play a critical role in experimental empyema. J Infect Dis 2000; 181:1693–1699.
8. Jonjic N, Peri G, Bernasconi S, Sciacca F, Colotta F, Pelicci P, Lanfrancone L, Mantovani A. Expression of adhesion molecules and chemotactic cytokines in cultured human mesothelial cells. J Exp Med 1992; 176:1165–1174.
9. Antony VB, Hott JW, Kunkel SL, Godbey SW, Burdick MD, Strieter RM. Pleural mesothelial cell expression of C-C (monocyte chemotactic peptide) and C-X-C (interleukin 8) chemokines. Am J Respir Cell Mol Biol 1995; 12:581–588.

10. Strieter RM, Koch AE, Antony VB, Fick RB Jr, Standiford TJ, Kunkel SL. The immunopathology of chemotactic cytokines: the role of interleukin-8 and monocyte chemoattractant protein-1. J Lab Clin Med 1994; 123:183–197.
11. Antony VB, Godbey JB, Kunkel SL, Hott JW, Hartman DL, Burdick MD, Strieter RM. Recruitment of inflammatory cells to the pleural space chemotactic cytokinesis IL-8 and MCP-1 in human pleural fluids. J Immunol 1993; 15:7216–7233.
12. Broaddus VC, Boylan AM, Hoeffel JM, Kim KJ, Sadick M, Chuntharapai A, Hebert CA. Neutralization of IL-8 inhibits neutrophil influx in a rabbit model of endotoxin-induced pleurisy. J Immunol 1994; 152:2960–2967.
13. Antony VB, Sahn SA, Antony AC, Repine JE. Bacillus Calmette-Guerin-stimulated neutrophils release chemotaxins for monocytes in rabbit pleural spaces and in vitro. J Clin Invest 1985; 76:1514–1521.
14. Ellner JJ, Barnes PF, Wallis RS, Modlin RL. The immunology of tuberculous pleurisy. Semin Respir Infect 1988; 3:335–342.
15. Owens MW, Milligan SA, Grisham MB. Nitric oxide synthesis by rat pleural mesothelial cells: induction by growth factors and lipopolysaccharide. Exp Lung Res 1995; 21:731–742.
16. Chen JY, Chiu JH, Chen HL, Chen TW, Yang WC, Yang AH. Human peritoneal mesothelial cells produce nitric oxide: induction by cytokines. Perit Dial Int 2000; 20:772–777.
17. Owens MW, Grisham MB. Nitric oxide synthesis by rat pleural mesothelial cells: induction by cytokines and lipopolysaccharide. Am J Physiol 1993; 265:L110–L116.
18. Malech H. Phagocytic cells: Egress from marrow and diapedesis. In: Gallin JG IM, Snyderman R, eds. Inflammation: Basic Principles and Clinical Correlates. New York: Raven Press, 1988:297–308.
19. Broaddus VC, Yang L, Scavo LM, Ernst JD, Boylan AM. Asbestos induces apoptosis of human and rabbit pleural mesothelial cells via reactive oxygen species. J Clin Invest 1996; 98:2050–2059.
20. Nasreen N, Hartman D, Mohammed K, Antony V. Talc induces pleural mesothelial cell expression of proinflammatory cytokines and intracellular adhesion molecule-1 (ICAM-1). Am J Respir Crit Care Med 1998; 158:971–978.
21. Spitznagel J. Non-oxidative antimicrobial reactions of leukocytes. Contemp Top Immunobiol 1984; 14:283.
22. Ganz T, Selsted ME, Szklarek D, Harwig SS, Daher K, Bainton DF, Lehrer RI. Defensins. Natural peptide antibiotics of human neutrophils. J Clin Invest 1985; 76:1427–1435.
23. Cox G, Gauldie J, Jordana M. Bronchial epithelial cell-derived cytokines (G-CSF and GM-CSF) promote the survival of peripheral blood neutrophils in vitro. Am J Respir Cell Mol Biol 1992; 7:507–513.
24. Nasreen N, Mohammed KA, Sanders KL, Hardwick J, VanHorn RD, Loghmani F, Lundine, Antony VB. Differential expression of C-phos, C-June, and apoptosis in pleural mesothelial cells exposed to *Stap. aureus*. Am J Respir Crit Care Med 2001; 163:A772.
25. Payne CM, Glasser L, Tischler ME, Wyckoff D, Cromey D, Fiederlein R, Bohnert O. Programmed cell death of the normal human neutrophil: an in vitro model of senescence. Microsc Res Tech 1994; 28:327–344.
26. Sahn SA. State of the art. The pleura. Am Rev Respir Dis 1988; 138:184–234.
27. Mantovani A, Garlanda C. Novel pathways for negative regulation of inflammatory cytokines centered on receptor expression. Dev Biol Stand 1999; 97:97–104.

28. Hott JW, Godbey SW, Antony VB. Mesothelial cell modulation of pleural repair: thrombin stimulated mesothelial cells release prostaglandin E2. Prostaglandins Leukot Essent Fatty Acids 1994; 51:329–335.
29. Rennard S, Jaurand M, Bignon J, Ferrans V, Crystal R. Connective tissue matrix of the pleura. In: Chretien J, Bignon J, Hirsch A, eds. The Pleura in Health and Disease. New York Marcel Dekker, 1985; 5:69–85.
30. Antony VB. Pathogenesis of malignant pleural effusions and talc pleurodesis. Pneumologie 1999; 53:493–498.
31. Ponta H. The CD44 protein family. Int J Biochem Cell Biol 1998; 30:299–305.
32. Bourguignon LY, Lokeshwar VB, Chen X, Kerrick WG. Hyaluronic acid-induced lymphocyte signal transduction and HA receptor (GP85/CD44)-cytoskeleton interaction. J Immunol 1993; 151:6634–6644.
33. Becker PM, Alcasabas A, Yu AY, Semenza GL, Bunton TE. Oxygen-independent upregulation of vascular endothelial growth factor and vascular barrier dysfunction during ventilated pulmonary ischemia in isolated ferret lungs. Am J Respir Cell Mol Biol 2000; 22:272–279.
34. Thickett DR, Armstrong L, Millar AB. Vascular endothelial growth factor (VEGF) in inflammatory and malignant pleural effusions. Thorax 1999; 54:707–710.
35. Corada M, Liao F, Lindgren M, Lampugnani MG, Breviario F, Frank R, Muller WA, Hicklin DJ, Bohlen P, Dejana E. Monoclonal antibodies directed to different regions of vascular endothelial cadherin extracellular domain affect adhesion and clustering of the protein and modulate endothelial permeability. Blood 2001; 97:1679–1684.
36. Blankesteijn WM, van Gijn ME, Essers-Janssen YP, Daemen MJ, Smits JF. Beta-catenin, an inducer of uncontrolled cell proliferation and migration in malignancies, is localized in the cytoplasm of vascular endothelium during neovascularization after myocardial infarction. Am J Pathol 2000; 157:877–883.
37. Antony VB, Loddenkemper R, Astoul P, Boutin C, Goldstraw P, Hott J, Rodriguez Panadero F, Sahn SA. Management of malignant pleural effusions. Eur Respir J 2001; 18:402–419.
38. Dejana E. Endothelial adherens junctions: implications in the control of vascular permeability and angiogenesis. J Clin Invest 1996; 98:1949–1953.
39. Antony V, Kamal M, Godbey S, Loddenkemper F. Talc induced pleurodesis: role of basic fibroblast growth factor (bFGF). Eur Respir J 1997; 10:403S.

5

Respiratory Function in Pleural Effusion

IOANNA MITROUSKA and DIMITRIS GEORGOPOULOS

University of Crete
and University Hospital of Heraklion
Heraklion, Crete, Greece

The pleural space is approximately 10–20 μm wide and encompasses the area between the mesothelium of the parietal and visceral pleura (the two layers of the pleura) (1). The pleural space actually contains a tiny amount of fluid (0.3 mL/kg body mass) with a low concentration of protein (~1 g/dL). The surface pressure of the visceral pleura together with alveolar pressure set the transpulmonary pressure, while the surface pressure of the parietal pleura sets the transthoracic pressure (2). These surface pressures usually differ from the pleural liquid pressure, due to the presence of contacts between the lung and chest wall and the additional distortions that result (3,4). In upright humans the vertical gradient of pleural surface pressure is approximately 0.25 cmH_2O/cm height, whereas within the liquid column the gradient is somewhat greater (~1 cmH_2O/cm height) (5). In normal humans the difference between surface and liquid pleural pressure is relatively small in the bottom of the lung and increases higher up, with liquid pressure becoming more negative than surface pressure.

The pressures of the pleural space are important determinants of the mechanical properties of the lung and chest wall and, thus, of the total respiratory system (6). This is because the distending pressure of the lung and chest wall is critically dependent on the relevant pressures of the pleural space (7). Any distortion of the pressures of pleural space affects the distending pressures of the lung and chest wall and thus the relevant volumes, which in turn influences the gas exchange properties of the lung via several mechanisms (8). It follows that pleural effusion, which alters both the liquid and surface pleural pressures, affects the mechanical properties of the respiratory system as well as the gas exchange properties (9).

Interpretation of the effects of pleural effusion on the respiratory system is rather complicated for several reasons. First, it is difficult to find and study patients with "pure" pleural effusion without lung disease. Second, the validity of esophageal pressure measurement in patients with pleural disease is questionable (10,11). Indeed, in the presence of pleural effusion esophageal pressure might not reflect pressure of the pleural space, and thus the calculation of transpulmonary and transthoracic pressures may be misleading. In which case measuring mechanical properties of respiratory system is complicated. Thirdly, data form studies that use animal models of pleural effusion may not be applicable in humans, because there are considerable differences in pleural anatomy between species (12). All these factors should be taken into account when the effects of pleural effusion on respiratory system function are considered.

I. Theoretical Considerations

A pure increase in the amount of fluid in the pleural space causes an increase in pleural pressure (surface and liquid). This increase results in an alteration in distending pressures of chest wall and lung. The distending pressure of the chest wall increases while that of the lung decreases. As a result, all else being the same, the volume of chest wall and lung is increased and decreased, respectively (13). It follows that with pleural effusion an uncoupling between the volume of lung and chest wall occurs; the volume of chest wall is no longer equal with that of the lung, a situation that is broadly similar to that encountered in pneumothorax. The differences between these two conditions are mainly due to the enhanced gravitational gradient of pleural pressure due to the presence of liquid and the fact that the pleural effusion usually does not occupy the entire pleural space, creating local alteration in pleural pressure. Nevertheless, although above the effusion normal pleural pressure may apply, there would still be a tendency toward chest wall enlargement because of the rib cage stability, which would be opposed by the lung elastic recoil. Theoretical considerations predict that pleural effusion should cause a restrictive ventilatory defect characterized by a reduction in vital capacity, functional residual capacity and total lung capacity.

Accumulation of fluid in the pleural space may also affect the function of respiratory muscles mainly because of an increase in chest wall volume. The force-length relationship of respiratory muscles dictates that for a given neural activation the pressure developed by the muscles decreases with a decrease in their length (14). An increase in chest wall volume decreases the length of inspiratory muscles, mainly that of the diaphragm, and increases the length of expiratory muscles. It follows that with pleural effusion, all else being the same, for a given neural activation, pressure developed by the inspiratory and expiratory muscles should decrease and increase, respectively.

The above analysis is oversimplified because it ignores the secondary effect of pleural effusion on the pressure-volume (P-V) curve of the chest wall and lung and the interaction between the two hemithoraces. However, it is useful as a framework to explain the animal and human data regarding the effects of pleural effusion on respiratory system.

Gas exchange properties of the lung may be also affected by pleural effusion. The decrease in functional residual capacity (FRC) may force the lung volume at the end of expiration to operate near or even below the closing volume, a situation clearly associated with hypoxemia (15–18). This should be further aggravated by assuming the supine position (15,–17,19). Finally, under certain circumstances large pleural effusion may impede the filling of the right heart, and by decreasing the cardiac output an exaggerated effect of ventilation/perfusion inequalities and right to left shunt on PO_2 occurs (20–22).

II. Respiratory System Mechanics

The effect of pleural effusion on respiratory system mechanics may be studied either by instillation of fluid into the pleural space or by removing fluid from pleural space. Obviously the first method is used in animals, while the second is the only practical way to study pleural effusion effects in humans (23–30).

Animal data indicate that a pure increase in the amount of fluid in the pleural space causes an increase and a decrease in the chest wall and lung volumes, respectively. Krell and Rodarte (27) have shown in head-up dogs that lung volume decreased by about one third the saline volume added to the pleural space at FRC and one fifth at total lung capacity (TLC) (Fig. 1). Consequently, chest wall volume increased by two thirds at FRC and four fifths at TLC. The pressure-volume curve showed an apparent increase in lung elastic recoil and a decrease in chest wall elastic recoil with the addition of saline. These authors further showed that the reduction in lung volume was mainly due to a reduction in lower lobe with minimal change in upper lobe volume. As a result, an increase of the vertical gradient in regional lung volumes with increasing effusion volumes was observed. These results indicate that pleural effusion produces a nonuniform alteration in pleural pressure, which in turn affects the regional lung and chest wall volumes.

The static changes induced by pleural effusion may also alter the dynamic properties of respiratory system. Dechman et al. (25) infused normal saline into the pleural space of dogs and using multiple regression analysis calculated dynamic elastance and resistance of respiratory system, lung, and chest wall. Pleural effusion caused a marked increase in respiratory system elastance and resistance due to alteration in dynamic properties of the lung, while the dy-

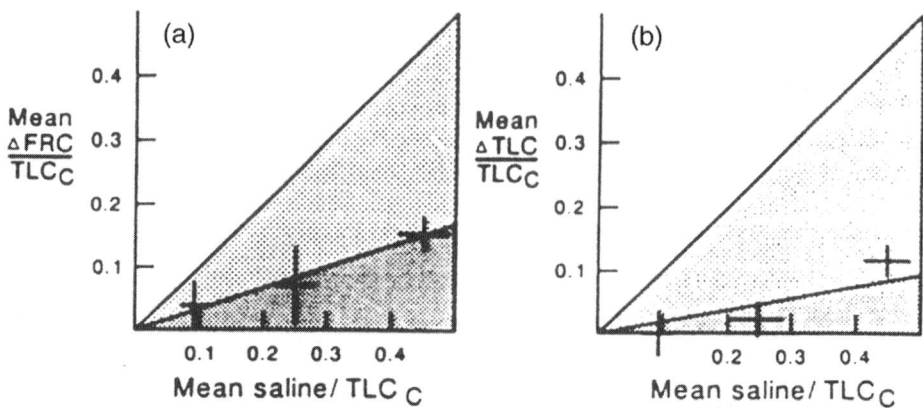

Figure 1 Changes in lung volume with saline effusions in a dog model of pleural effusion. (a) Decrease in functional residual capacity as a function of saline volume added to pleural space (mean±SD). The change in FRC and the volume of saline were expressed as a fraction of control total lung capacity ($\Delta FRC/TLC_c$ and saline/TLC_c, respectively). (b) Similar graph for mean decrease in total lung capacity ($\Delta TLC/TLC_c$) as a function of saline volume added to pleural space (saline/TLC_c). Line delineating stippled area, line of identity. Because sum of decrease in lung volume and increase in chest wall volume must equal added saline volume, light stippled area represents increase in chest wall volume for each value of saline. Increase of chest wall volume would be overestimated by amount equal to volume of intrathoracic blood displaced by addition of saline. Decrease in lung volume is about one third, and increase in chest wall volume is about two thirds the added saline volume. Note change in lung volume is about one-fifth the volume of saline added. (From Ref. 27.)

namic elastance and resistance of the chest wall decreased. Similar results have been observed by Sousa et al. in rats (29). The changes in dynamic properties of the lung were partially reversed by deep inflation, suggesting that airway closure may be an important determinant of these alterations (25). These secondary effects of pleural effusion on lung function should be considered when therapy is planned for patients.

Several studies in humans have examined the effects of pleural effusion on respiratory system function (8,23–27). The interpretation of the results, however, is complicated mainly due to the underlying lung diseases. Indeed, it has been found that pleural effusion is not always associated with an increase in pleural pressure. Light et al. (31) measured directly pleural pressure in a large number of patients with pleural effusion and observed values between −21 to +8 cmH_2O. In a subsequent study, the same group showed that the increase in vital capacity as a result of removing an amount of pleural fluid was related both to the initial value of pleural pressure as well as with its change during aspiration; a markedly negative initial pressure or a large change during aspiration was associated with a relatively small increase in vital capacity (VC) (28). These results presumably may be explained by the underlying disease, which caused a poorly compliant lung. Pleural thickening and the resulting low chest wall compliance may also underlie the observed changes in some patients. These findings have also been confirmed by other investigators (24,32).

Notwithstanding the difficulties in separating the effects of pleural effusion from those of the underlying diseases, several studies have shown that aspiration of pleural fluid is associated with increases in static lung volume, which are less than the volume of fluid removed (24,26,32). This observation indicates that pleural effusion causes a decrease in lung volume and a chest wall expansion in accordance with the theoretical prediction. Estenne et al. (32) measured respiratory mechanics 2 hours after removal a mean fluid volume of 1800 mL and observed that mean total lung capacity, vital capacity, and FRC increased by 640, 300, and 460 mL, respectively. They also demonstrated that the static pressure-volume curve of the lung was shifted upward and to the left, so for a given lung volume elastic recoil pressure was lower after thoracocentesis (Fig. 2). Therefore, it appears that pleural effusion may alter the lung

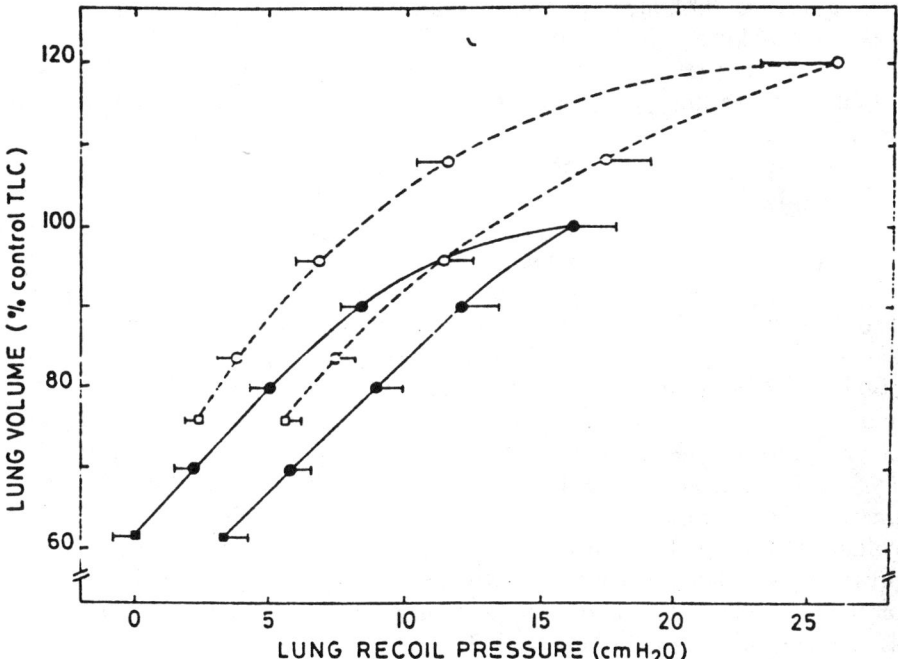

Figure 2 Static inspiratory and expiratory pressure-volume curve of the lung before (closed circles) and after (open circles) thoracocentesis. Lung volume was expressed as a percentage of total lung capacity (TLC) before thoracocentisis. The squares indicate the position of functional residual capacity. Each bar represents ±SE. (From Ref. 32.)

compliance. Decompression of the lung with reopening of some air spaces and a decrease in the surface tension of the alveolar lining fluid layer, due to breathing at higher lung volumes, are the most plausible mechanisms that mediate the change in lung compliance. Gilmartin et al. (26) studied seven patients 24 hours after removal of pleural fluid (0.8–2.5 L) and observed that in addition to static lung volume increase, FEV_1 was also increased. Furthermore, they analyzed the forced flow-volume curves, and the obtained information indicated that the lung emptied slightly faster in the presence of effusion. Indeed, the time-constant of forced expiration derived from the slope of expired volume/flow relationship was significantly less before aspiration. The authors explained this finding by accepting that pleural effusion reduces the number of functioning compliant lung units, while airway size remains inappropriate large for the reduced lung volume. This assumption is in accordance with the results of Estenne et al. (32), who found that pleural effusion has an effect on lung compliance. Animal data also indicate that pleural effusion, apart from the changes in static lung volume, may also have secondary effects on lung mechanics (27).

In a landmark study, Anthonisen and Martin (23) used ^{133}Xe gas distribution and studied regional lung volume and ventilation in patients with small to moderate sized pleural effusion and no evidence of other respiratory system disease. Although regional lung volume at the base with the effusion was reduced, lung expansion at the site of effusion did not differ from that the other side. These results suggest that, at least with small to moderate sized pleural effusion, the lung may actually float on the effusion rather than be compressed. It appears that the amount of pleural effusion may be a critical factor for the observed change in respiratory system mechanics.

III. Respiratory Muscles

The effect of pleural effusion on respiratory muscle function has been studied by Estenne et al. (32). They measured minimal pleural pressure-volume curves obtained during static maximal inspiratory efforts at different volumes before and after removal of pleural fluid and found that for a given lung volume pleural pressure was approximately 20 cm lower after thoracocentesis (Fig. 3). This finding indicates that either the power of inspiratory muscles increased or their efficiency improved. The authors estimated the change in chest wall volume following the fluid aspiration and observed that if minimal pleural pressure was related to chest wall volume, the pressures generated by the inspiratory muscles before and after thoracocentesis fall on the same curve (Fig. 4). These results strongly suggest that pleural effusion, by increasing the chest wall volume, decreases the length of inspiratory muscles and thus reduces their effectiveness. The effects of pleural effusion on expiratory muscles are not known, but according to the above results it is reasonable to conclude that in the presence of pleural effusion the efficiency of expiratory muscles would probably be increased.

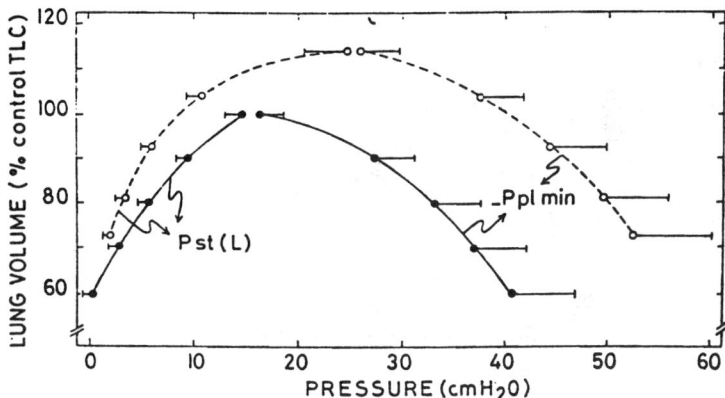

Figure 3 Pressure-volume of lung recoil pressure (Pst(L)) and maximal static inspiratory pleural pressure (Ppl min) versus lung volume, before (closed circles) and after (open circles) thoracocentesis. Lung volume was expressed as a percentage of total lung capacity (TLC) before thoracocentesis. Each bar represents ±SE. (From Ref. 32.)

IV. Gas Exchange

Although pleural effusion is thought to contribute to hypoxemia (33), studies in humans have demonstrated contradictory results (34). Oxygenation has been shown to improve, remain unchanged, or even worsen after thoracocentesis (34,35). The underlying lung disease and the occurrence of interstitial edema due to reexpansion of the lung after thoracocentesis complicates the interpretation of these results. In an attempt to resolve this issue, Nishida et al. (18) created graded increasing bilateral pleural effusion in anesthetized pigs. At each pleural volume, intravascular volume was altered to normal, low, or high to investigate the interaction between oxygenation, hemodynamics and pleural effusion. They observed that pleural effusion caused an acute decrease in PaO_2 the magnitude of which depended on the volume of pleural effusion. The hypoxemia was mainly due to calculated intrapulmonary right-to-left shunt, which increased proportionally to the volume of the instilled pleural fluid (Fig. 5). At highest volume of pleural effusion, mixed venous O_2 was reduced, and this may also contribute to hypoxemia, particularly in the presence of increased shunt. All these changes were reversed by aspirating the pleural fluid without any evidence of hysteresis. The intravascular volume status did not appear to influence PaO_2 significantly. Although this model has several limitations, these data suggest that even moderately sized pleural effusions may be an important contributor to arterial hypoxemia, particularly in the presence of respiratory failure. It is possible that under these circumstances removal of the pleural fluid either by thoracocentesis or using negative fluid balance could have potential benefits in term of oxygenation. Talmor et al. (36) inserted a chest tube in a subset of mechanically ventilated patients with acute respiratory failure and

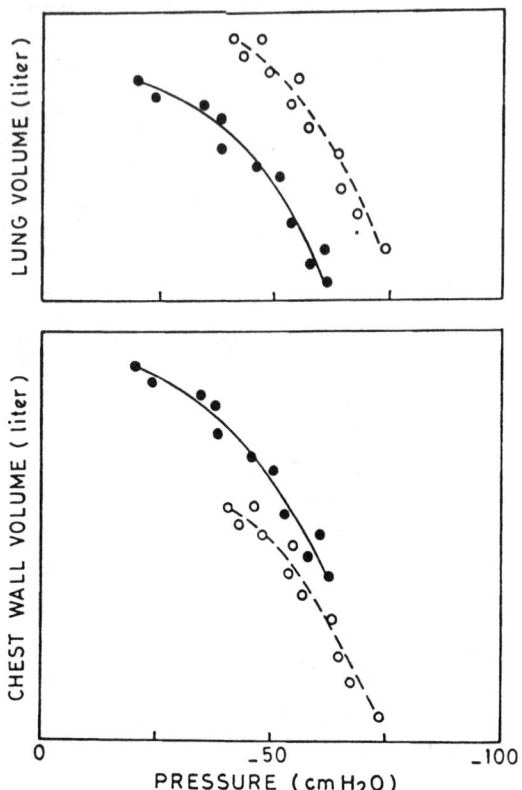

Figure 4 Proposed mechanism of the more negative pleural pressures generated by the inspiratory muscles after removal of 1500 mL of pleural fluid. Total lung capacity increased by 350 mL after fluid removal. Closed circles represent data obtained before thoracocentesis; open circles represent data obtained after thoracocentesis. In the top panel, pleural pressures are expressed as a function of lung volume; in the bottom panel, they are expressed as a function of total chest wall volume. (From Ref. 32.)

pleural effusion who had a poor response to positive end-expiratory pressure (PEEP) and observed that oxygenation and respiratory system compliance improved immediately after chest tube drainage. These results should be interpreted with caution, however. The risk: benefit ratio of this procedure is not well established. Furthermore, several studies in patients with acute respiratory distress syndrome (ARDS) have shown that mortality, the main outcome variable, is not related to the level of hypoxemia (37). It has been suggested that improvement in oxygenation may be a cosmetic effect. At present, insertion of a chest tube is not recommended as routine procedure in these patients. In selected patients with large pleural effusion and refractory hypoxemia, in whom other measures to increase oxygenation have failed, chest tube drainage may be beneficial.

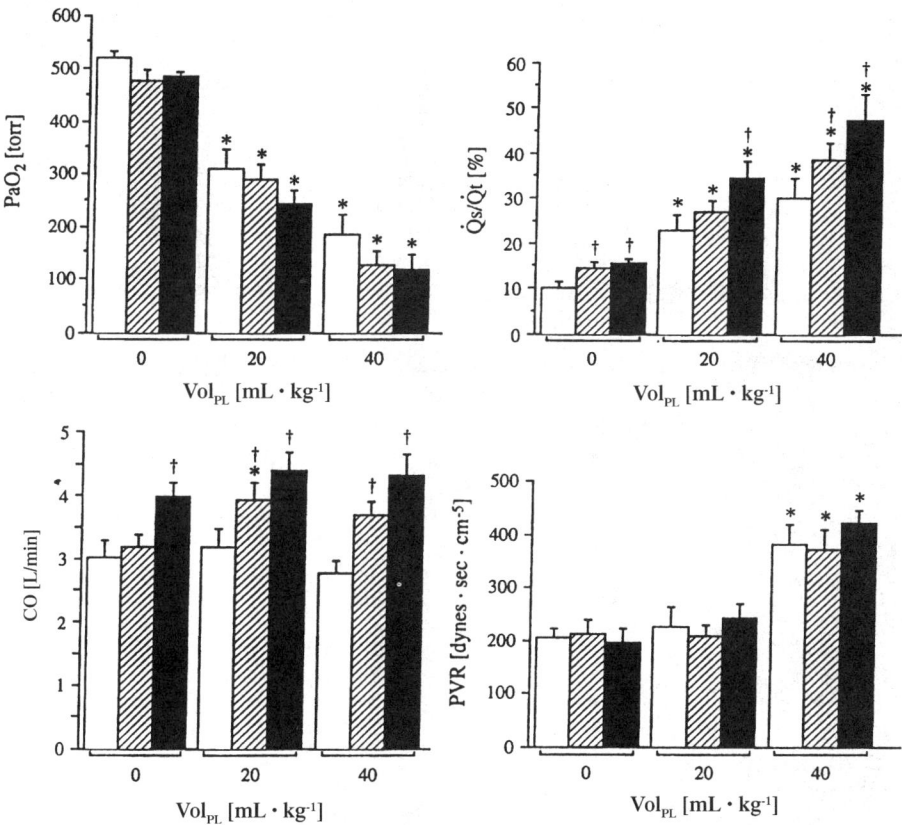

Figure 5 Effects of intrapleural volume (Vol_{PL}) and intravascular volume (Vol_{vasc}) on PaO_2 (top left), calculated intrapulmonary shunt (Qs/Qt) (top right), cardiac output (CO) (bottom left) and pulmonary vascular resistance (PVR) (bottom right) in a pig model of pleural effusion. Open bars, low Vol_{vasc}; hatched bars, normal Vol_{vasc}; solid bars, high Vol_{vasc}. *$p < 0.05$ vs. $Vol_{PL} = 0$ mL/kg. †$p < 0.05$ vs. low Vol_{vasc}. (From Ref. 18.)

Agusti et al. (38) used the multiple inert gas elimination technique (MIGET) (39) to study the distribution of ventilation-perfusion ratios as well as the effects of thoracocentesis in patients with pulmonary effusion. The results of this study showed that the intrapulmonary shunt was the main mechanism underlying arterial hypoxemia, in line with the animal data (18). Withdrawing approximately 700 mL of pleural fluid caused a significant decrease in pleural pressure (from 3.6 to -7.1 cmH$_2$O) without a significant effect on PaO_2, shunt, and alveolar-arterial difference for PO_2 (Figs. 6,7). A significant, although small, increase in blood flow perfusing low V/Q' units was observed after thoracocentesis, indicating that either some degree of lung

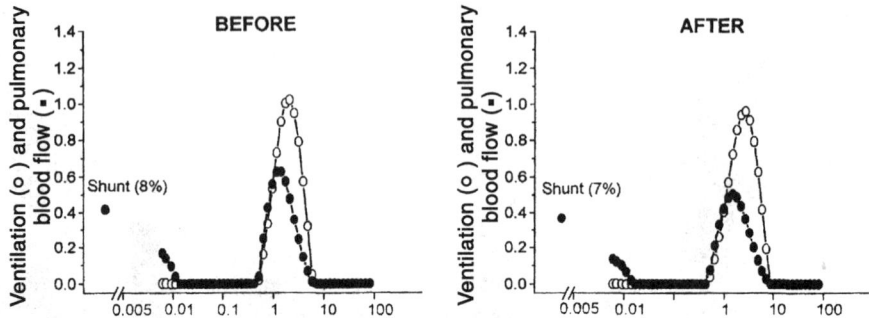

Figure 6 Distribution of ventilation-perfusion (VA/Q) ratios in representative patient, before (left panel) and after (right panel) thoracocentesis studied with the MIGET technique. (From Ref. 38.)

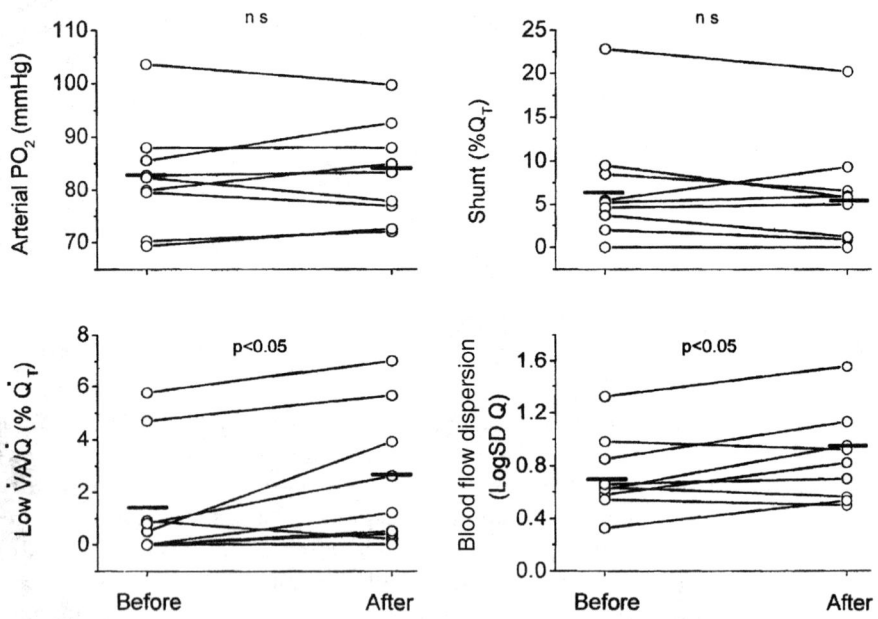

Figure 7 Individual (open circles) and mean (solid bars) values of arterial PaO_2, low VA/Q ratios, shunt, and blood flow dispersion before and 30 minutes after draining pleural effusion by thoracocentesis. (From Ref. 38.)

reexpansion or acute interstitial pulmonary edema occurred as a result of pleural pressure decrease. Nevertheless, despite the relatively large pleural fluid drainage, the changes in gas exchange properties of the lung were quite small, suggesting that the effects of pleural effusion on oxygenation indices are long-lasting, possibly due to delayed pulmonary volume reexpansion after fluid drainage (24,40,41) with or without the coexistence of ex vacuo pulmonary edema (41–43).

The effect of pleural effusion on cardiac function, although beyond the scope of this review, deserves some comments. It has been shown in dogs that large pleural effusion may compromise the right heart function by inducing diastolic collapse of the right ventricle, which is associated with a decrease in cardiac output (44). This condition is similar to cardiac tamponade. This may aggravate hypoxemia, particularly in the presence of increased right-to-left shunt. It is of interest to note that this complication may occur when pleural pressure is about 4 cmH_2O, a value frequently seen in patients (21). Indeed, compromised cardiac function documented by echocardiography has been reported in patients with large pleural effusion (22). Therapeutic thoracocentesis may be lifesaving in these patients by increasing both cardiac output and oxygenation (32).

V. Conclusion

The accumulation of pleural fluid causes a restrictive ventilatory effect. Pure pleural effusion is associated with chest wall volume expansion, and this reduces the efficiency of inspiratory muscles. Drainage of pleural fluid usually results in an increase in static lung volume, which is considerably less that the amount of aspirated fluid. Pleural effusion is invariably associated with hypoxemia due to an increase in right-to-left shunt, effect that an at least in humans, is not readily reversible upon fluid aspiration.

References

1. Light RW. Anatomy of the pleura. In: Light RW, ed. Pleural Diseases. Vol. 1. Philadelphia, PA: Lippincot Williams & Wilkins, 2001:1–7.
2. Light RW. Physiology of the pleural space. In: Light RW, ed. Pleural Diseases. Vol. 1. Philadelphia: Lippincot Williams & Wilkins, 2001:8–20.
3. Agostoni E. Mechanics of the pleural space. Resp Physiol 1972:57–128.
4. Lee KF, Olak J. Anatomy and physiology of the pleural space. Chest Surg Clin North Am 1994; 4:391–403.
5. Milic-Emili J, Henderson JAM, Dolovich MB, Trop D, Kanelo K. Regional distribution of inspired gas in the lung. J Appl Physiol 1966; 21:749–759.
6. Fenn WO. The pressure-volume diagram of the breathing mechanism. In: W BM, ed. Respiratory Physiology in Aviation: Rundolph Field, USAF School of Aviation Medicine, 1954:19–27.

7. Ward ME RC, Macklem PT. Respiratory mechanics. In: Murray JF, ed. Textbook of Respiratory Medicine. Vol. 1. Philadelphia: WB Saunders, 1994:90–138.
8. Lai-Fook SJ, Rodarte JR. Pleural pressure distribution and its relationship to lung volume and interstitial pressure. J Appl Physiol 1991; 70:967–978.
9. Agostoni E, D'Angelo E. Pleural liquid pressure. J Appl Physiol 1991; 71:393–403.
10. Milic-Emili JMJ, Turner JM, Glauser EM. Improved technique for estimating pleural pressure from esophageal balloons. J Appl Physiol 1964; 19:207–211.
11. Villena V, Lopez-Encuentra A, Pozo F, De-Pablo A, Martin-Escribano P. Measurement of pleural pressure during therapeutic thoracentesis. Am J Respir Crit Care Med 2000; 162:1534–1538.
12. Tenney SMBDF. Comparative mammalian respiratory control. In: Cherniak NSWJ, ed. The Respiratory System. Vol. 2. Bethesda, MD: American Physiological Society, 1986:833–855.
13. Agostoni EHER. Static behavior of the respiratory system. A FP, ed. Handbook of Physiology. Vol. 3. Bethesda, MD: American Physiological Society, 1986:113–130.
14. Younes M, Riddle W. A model for the relation between respiratory neural and mechanical outputs. I. Theory. J Appl Physiol 51:963–978.
15. Craig DB, Wahba WM, Don HF, Couture JG, Becklake MR. "Closing volume" and its relationship to gas exchange in seated and supine positions. J Appl Physiol 1971; 31:717–721.
16. Blair EHJ. The effect of change in body position on lung volume and intrapulmonary gas mixing in normal subjects. J Clin Invest 1955; 34:383–398.
17. Kaneko K, Milic-Emili J, Dolovich MB, Dawson A, Bates DV. Regional distribution of ventilation and perfusion as a function of body position. J Appl Physiol 1966; 21:767–777.
18. Nishida O, Arellano R, Cheng DC, DeMajo W, Kavanagh BP. Gas exchange and hemodynamics in experimental pleural effusion. Crit Care Med 1999; 27:583–587.
19. Neagley SR, Zwillich CW. The effect of positional changes on oxygenation in patients with pleural effusions. Chest 1985; 88:714–717.
20. Negus RA, Chachkes JS, Wrenn K. Tension hydrothorax and shock in a patient with a malignant pleural effusion. Am J Emerg Med 1990; 8:205–207.
21. Kisanuki A, Shono H, Kiyonaga K, et al. Two-dimensional echocardiographic demonstration of left ventricular diastolic collapse due to compression by pleural effusion. Am Heart J 1991; 122:1173–1175.
22. Kaplan LM, Epstein SK, Schwartz SL, Cao QL, Pandian NG. Clinical, echocardiographic, and hemodynamic evidence of cardiac tamponade caused by large pleural effusions. Am J Respir Crit Care Med 1995; 151:904–908.
23. Anthonisen NR, Martin RR. Regional lung function in pleural effusion. Am Rev Respir Dis 1977; 116:201–207.
24. Brown NE, Zamel N, Aberman A. Changes in pulmonary mechanics and gas exchange following thoracocentesis. Chest 1978; 74:540–542.
25. Dechman G, Sato J, Bates JH. Effect of pleural effusion on respiratory mechanics, and the influence of deep inflation, in dogs. Eur Respir J 1993; 6:219–224.
26. Gilmartin JJ, Wright AJ, Gibson GJ. Effects of pneumothorax or pleural effusion on pulmonary function. Thorax 1985; 40:60–65.
27. Krell WS, Rodarte JR. Effects of acute pleural effusion on respiratory system mechanics in dogs. J Appl Physiol 1985; 59:1458–1463.
28. Light RW, Stansbury DW, Brown SE. The relationship between pleural pressures

and changes in pulmonary function after therapeutic thoracentesis. Am Rev Respir Dis 1986; 133:658–661.
29. Sousa AS, Moll RJ, Pontes CF, Saldiva PH, Zin WA. Mechanical and morphometrical changes in progressive bilateral pneumothorax and pleural effusion in normal rats. Eur Respir J 1995; 8:99–104.
30. van Noord JA, Demedts M, Clement J, Cauberghs M, Van de Woestijne KP. Effect of rib cage and abdominal restriction on total respiratory resistance and reactance. J Appl Physiol 1986; 61:1736–1740.
31. Light RW, Jenkinson SG, Minh VD, George RB. Observations on pleural fluid pressures as fluid is withdrawn during thoracentesis. Am Rev Respir Dis 1980; 121:799–804.
32. Estenne M, Yernault JC, De Troyer A. Mechanism of relief of dyspnea after thoracocentesis in patients with large pleural effusions. Am J Med 1983; 74:813–819.
33. Mattison LE, Coppage L, Alderman DF, Herlong JO, Sahn SA. Pleural effusions in the medical ICU: prevalence, causes, and clinical implications. Chest 1997; 111:1018–1023.
34. Dobyns EL. Pleural effusions and hypoxemia. Crit Care Med 1999; 27:472.
35. Chang SC, Shiao GM, Perng RP. Postural effect on gas exchange in patients with unilateral pleural effusions. Chest 1989; 96:60–63.
36. Talmor M, Hydo L, Gershenwald JG, Barie PS. Beneficial effects of chest tube drainage of pleural effusion in acute respiratory failure refractory to positive end-expiratory pressure ventilation. Surgery 1998; 123:137–143.
37. Luhr OR, Karlsson M, Thorsteinsson A, Rylander C, Frostell CG. The impact of respiratory variables on mortality in non-ARDS and ARDS patients requiring mechanical ventilation. Intensive Care Med 2000; 26:508–517.
38. Agusti AG, Cardus J, Roca J, Grau JM, Xaubet A, Rodriguez-Roisin R. Ventilation-perfusion mismatch in patients with pleural effusion: effects of thoracentesis. Am J Respir Crit Care Med 1997; 156:1205–1209.
39. Evans JW, Wagner PD. Limits on VA/Q distributions from analysis of experimental inert gas elimination. J Appl Physiol 1977; 42:889–898.
40. Perpina M, Benlloch E, Marco V, Abad F, Nauffal D. Effect of thoracentesis on pulmonary gas exchange. Thorax 1983; 38:747–750.
41. Doerschuk CM, Allard MF, Oyarzun MJ. Evaluation of reexpansion pulmonary edema following unilateral pneumothorax in rabbits and the effect of superoxide dismutase. Exp Lung Res 1990; 16:355–367.
42. Trapnell DH, Thurston JG. Unilateral pulmonary oedema after pleural aspiration. Lancet 1970; 1:1367–1369.
43. Brandstetter RD, Cohen RP. Hypoxemia after thoracentesis. A predictable and treatable condition. JAMA 1979; 242:1060–1061.
44. Vaska K, Wann LS, Sagar K, Klopfenstein HS. Pleural effusion as a cause of right ventricular diastolic collapse. Circulation 1992; 86:609–617.

6

Imaging of the Pleura

THERESA C. McLOUD

Harvard Medical School
and Massachusetts General Hospital
Boston, Massachusetts, U.S.A.

GERALD F. ABBOTT

Brown Medical School
and Rhode Island Hospital
Providence, Rhode Island, U.S.A.

A variety of imaging techniques can be used to evaluate the pleura and the pleural space. Standard radiographs are the most common. Sonography, computed tomography (CT), and magnetic resonance imaging (MRI) have assumed an increasing and important role in the diagnosis of pleural disease. This chapter will discuss a variety of diffuse and focal pleural processes and the contribution of each of these imaging techniques to diagnosis and management.

I. Pleural Effusion

Pleural effusions develop when an imbalance occurs in the rates of pleural fluid production and resorption. Clinically, pleural effusions are classified as transudates or exudates by analysis of their specific gravity and determination of their protein and lactic acid dehydrogenase (LDH) content (1). Transudates are commonly bilateral and develop due to physical factors that affect the rate of pleural fluid formation and resorption (e.g., increased hydrostatic pressure, decreased osmotic pressure). Exudates occur when the pleura is pathologically altered with associated impairment of lymph flow or increase in permeability.

Pleural effusion has many causes, the most frequent being (in order of decreasing incidence) left ventricular failure, pneumonia, malignancy, pulmonary embolism, cirrhosis, pancreatitis, collage vascular disease, and tuberculosis.

On chest radiographs of erect subjects, a moderate-size pleural effusion typically manifests as a homogeneous lower zone opacity with a well-defined curvilinear upper border and concave surface abutting the lung. Free pleural fluid may extend into the interlobar fissures and produce opacities that vary with the shape and orientation of the fissure and the direction of the x-ray beam (2). Focal collections within fissures may form mass-like opacities ("pseudotumor") (Fig. 1). Incomplete interlobar fissures may manifest as curvilinear sharp interfaces in the presence of pleural effusions (3) (Fig. 2). Focal accumulation of fluid at the lateral aspect of the minor fissure produces the thorn sign, formed by converging concave interfaces extending medially from the lateral pleural surface to form a thorn-like point (4).

Small effusions may not be apparent on posterior anterior (PA) and lateral radiographs. Lateral decubitus views may detect as little as 5 mL of fluid. Ultrasonography and CT are also more sensitive than the chest radiograph in detecting small pleural effusions and may reveal septations and loculations suggestive of an exudate. Transudates are typically anechoic on ultrasonography and without associated pleural thickening. Exudates are often associated with pleural thickening, and ultrasonography may also demonstrate septation, stranding, and adjacent parenchymal lung disease. CT may be useful in detecting and characterizing effusions as free or loculated, differentiating pleural from parenchymal disease, and facilitating percutaneous biopsy (5–7).

Large effusions may opacify the entire hemithorax and characteristically produce contralateral shift of the mediastinal structures (Fig. 3). Occasionally, effusions may accumulate in a subpulmonic location and produce unique imaging features. The convex upper edge of a subpulmonic effusion mimics the contour of the hemidiaphragm. The apparent hemidiaphragm appears "elevated" with the peak of its convexity shifted laterally. The fluid is usually mobile and will relocate to the most dependent part of the pleural space on lateral decubitus radiographs (8).

Hemothorax usually occurs as a result of trauma but may be a manifestation of coagulopathy, infection, vascular abnormalities, or other causes. The radiographic features of acute hemothorax are indistinguishable from other pleural effusions. On CT, acute collections may show areas of hyperintensity. Subsequently, loculations may form and extensive pleural thickening may occur (fibrothorax) (9,10).

Empyema is defined and diagnosed by a variety of criteria including grossly purulent fluid, positive Gram stains or cultures, a pH of < 7 or a glucose level of < 40 mg/mL, and a white blood cell count in the pleural fluid of $> 5 \times 10^9$ cells per liter. Most empyemas are associated with pneumonia, surgery, trauma, or an infectious process occurring below the diaphragm. Empyemas evolve through exudative, fibrinopurulent, and organizing stages. In the early exudative stage, empyemas are indistinguishable from noninfectious pleural effusions. Empye-

Imaging of the Pleura

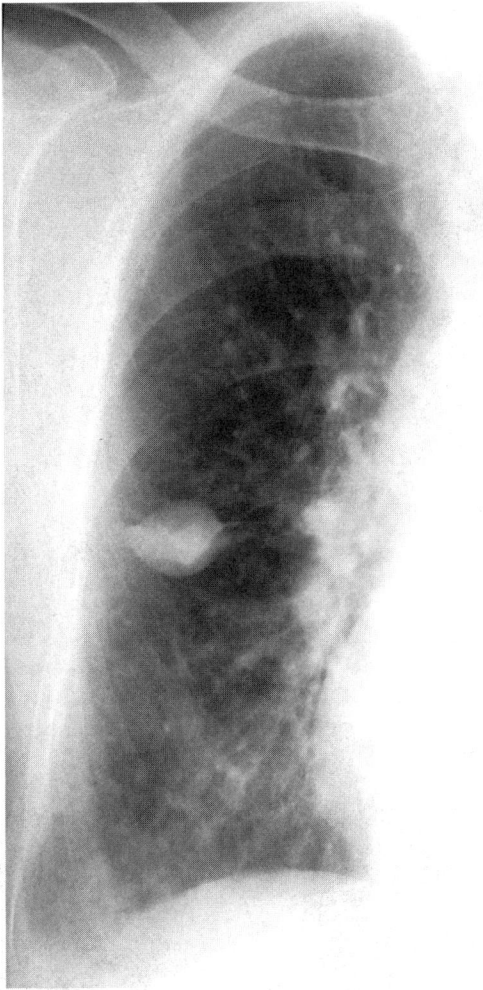

Figure 1 Pseudotumor: PA chest radiograph (detail) demonstrates an elliptical opacity in the right hemithorax with tapering medial and later margins that merge with the minor fissure.

mas that progress to the fibrinopurulent stage tend to form loculations, and ultrasonography often demonstrates septations within such collections. The final organizing stage is characterized by extensive pleural thickening ("peel"), which encases the lung. In this advanced stage there may be communication with the lung (bronchopleural fistula), or the fluid may drain through the chest wall (empyema necessitatis) (9).

The fibrinopurulent effusions of empyema have a tendency to loculate and will not fall to the most dependent portion of the pleural cavity on radiographs

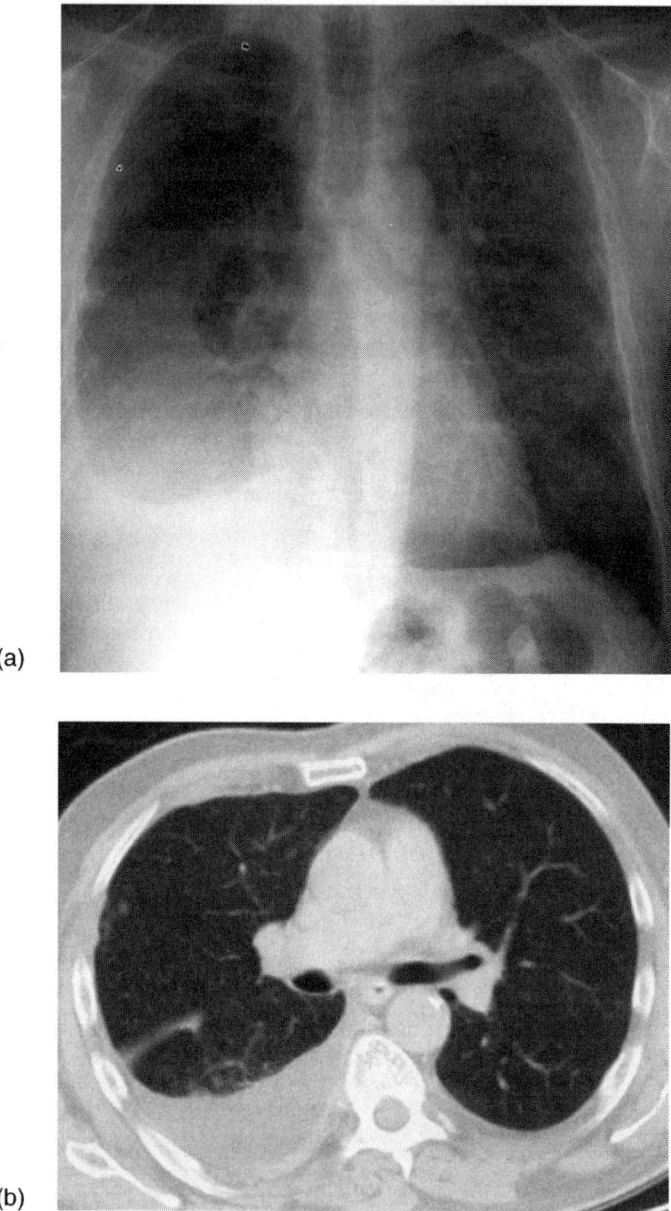

Figure 2 Incomplete interlobar fissures: (a) PA radiograph demonstrates a right pleural effusion that obscures the lower half of the hemithorax and forms a sharply defined curvilinear interface in the perihilar region; (b) CT (lung window) shows pleural effusion extending into an incomplete interlobar fissure.

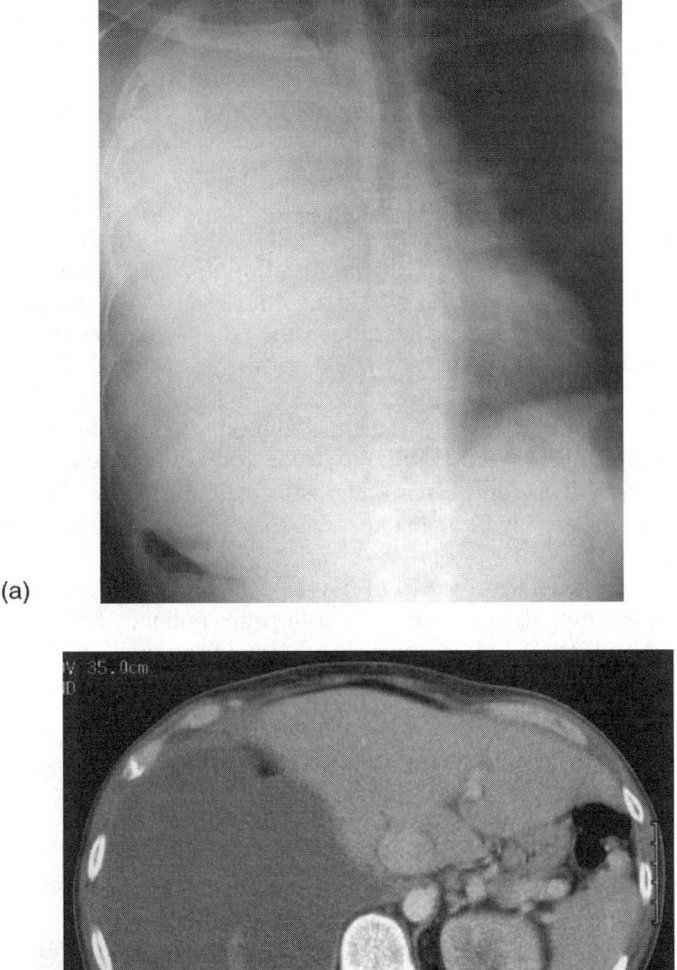

Figure 3 Hemothorax: (a) PA radiograph demonstrates opacification of the right hemithorax with shift of the mediastinal structures to the contralateral side, inferomedial displacement of the right mainstem bronchus, and inferolateral displacement of gas within the hepatic flexure of the colon; (b) CT demonstrates a large pleural effusion that inverts the right hemidiaphragm.

taken in various positions. Such fixed collections typically manifest as oval, lenticular, or round opacities. The margins of these collections are sharply defined when in profile to the x-ray beam, but some margins may be indistinct or imperceptible. Air-fluid levels may be apparent on the chest radiograph if a bronchopleural fistula is present. The appearance of air-fluid levels in abscesses and empyema differs. Typically, a lung abscess is spherical in shape, and if an air/fluid interface is demonstrated within the abscess, it will appear roughly equal in length on orthogonal radiographic views. By contrast, empyemas are often lenticular, forming obtuse angles with the chest wall. An airfluid interface within an empyema will often be disparate in length on orthogonal radiographs, e.g., demonstrating a short length on a frontal radiograph and a longer length on a lateral radiograph (11). When multiple air-fluid levels are demonstrated in an empyema, they may extend across lung zones that would normally be interrupted, in the case of parenchymal diseases, by the presence of interlobar fissures (Fig. 4).

Ultrasound and CT are the most useful modalities for demonstrating and characterizing empyema and may be useful in providing guidance for percutaneous drainage. Ultrasound often demonstrates septations within such collections. The septations may be so extensive as to preclude tube thoracostomy (12) (Fig. 5).

CT does not demonstrate septations within an empyema but is a very useful tool in defining the extent of such collections and may help in distinguishing pleural collections from lung abscesses. One of the most useful and specific

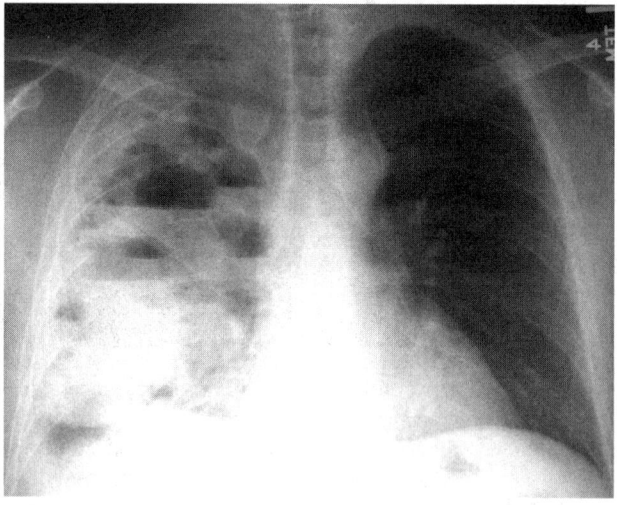

Figure 4 Empyema: PA chest radiograph demonstrates multiple air-fluid levels extending throughout the right hemithorax. The numerous air-fluid levels do not appear to be impeded by interlobar fissures, a feature suggesting their location in the pleural space.

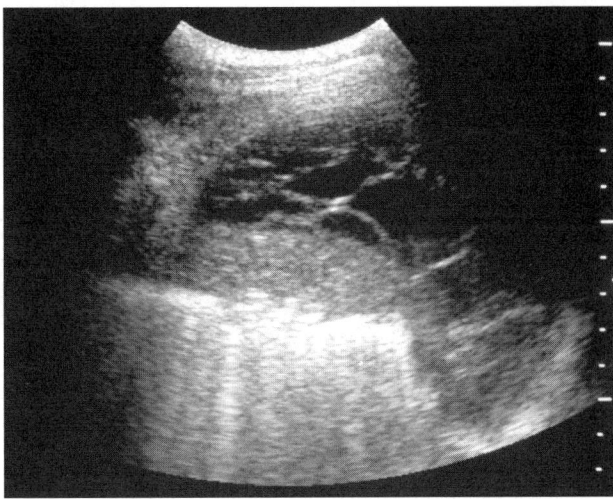

Figure 5 Empyema with septations: ultrasound demonstrates multiple septations within a loculated empyema.

signs is the demonstration of a "split pleura," which is noted on contrast-enhanced studies. The thickened pleura appears uniform in thickness, with smooth inner and outer margins. The thickened parietal and visceral pleura brightly enhance and are separated by the pleural fluid collection (Fig. 6).

Pleural effusions can be distinguished from abdominal ascites by several CT criteria. On axial CT images, pleural effusion will lie peripheral to the

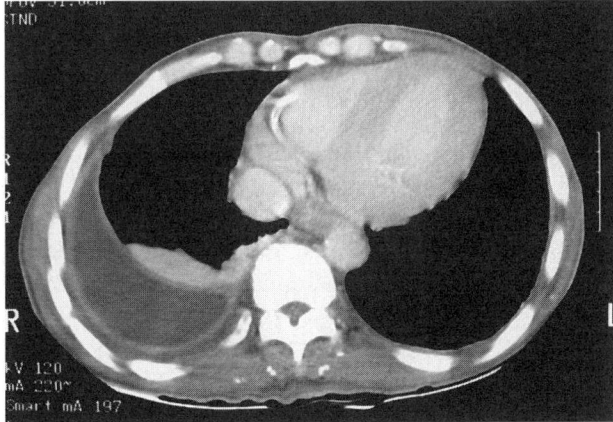

Figure 6 Empyema with "split pleura" sign: contrast-enhanced CT demonstrates uniformly thickened visceral and parietal pleura separated by a pleural fluid collection in the posterolateral aspect of the right hemithorax.

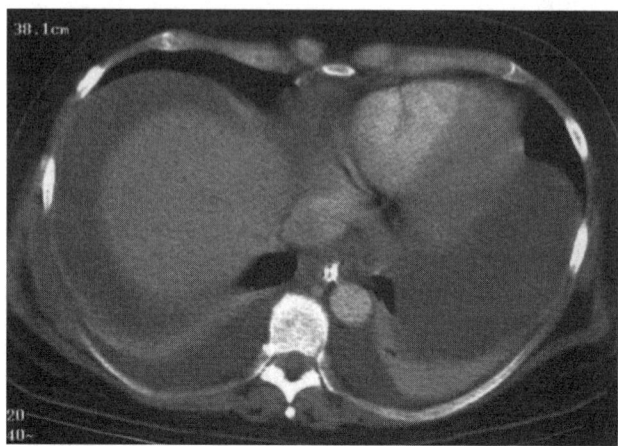

Figure 7 Pleural effusion and ascites: CT demonstrates ascites and bilateral pleural effusions. The pleural effusions, shown in the posterior costophrenic sulci, are "outside" of (posterior to) the hemidiaphragm and displace the diaphragmatic crura anteromedially. Ascites lies "within" the diaphragmatic contours and obscures the hepatic surface.

diaphragm and displace the crus medially; ascites will manifest as fluid density bounded laterally by the diaphragm. Furthermore, the surface of the bare area of the liver will be obscured by ascites, but unaffected by pleural effusion (13–15) (Fig. 7).

II. Pneumothorax

Pneumothorax is an abnormal collection of air in the pleural space. In contradistinction to free pleural effusions, which gravitate to the most dependent portions of the involved thorax, air will rise to the most nondependent portion of the thorax unless pleural adhesions obliterate the pleural space. In the erect subject, such air collections characteristically manifest as abnormal lucency in the pulmonary apex, displacing the sharp well-defined visceral pleural line. In the supine patient pneumothorax collects in the anterior costophrenic sulcus, producing hyperlucency over the upper abdomen and the deep costophrenic sulcus sign (Fig. 8). The presence of pneumothorax can be confirmed by decubitus or upright chest radiographs (16).

III. Focal Pleural Disease

Focal pleural abnormalities include asbestos-related pleural plaques, localized pleural tumors, and direct invasion of the pleura by lung carcinoma.

Imaging of the Pleura 87

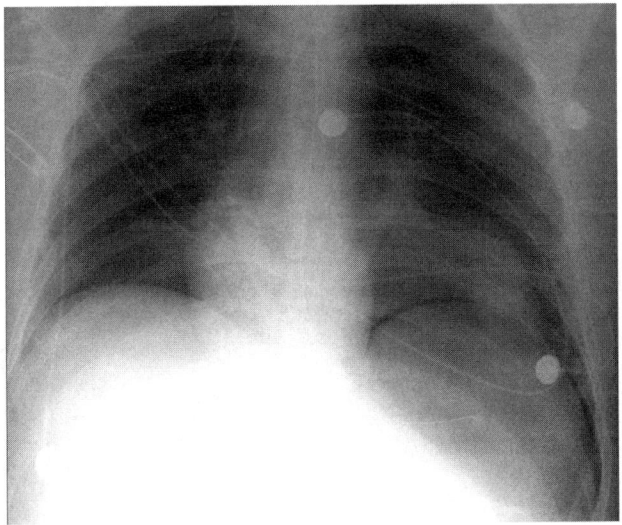

Figure 8 Deep sulcus sign: AP chest radiograph of a supine patient demonstrates abnormal lucency overlying the left hemidiaphragm and extending into the left costophrenic sulcus, which appears "deep" in comparison with the contralateral sulcus.

A. Pleural Plaques

Pleural plaques are the most common manifestation of asbestos exposure. They are localized collection of dense collagenous connective tissue (17,18). They serve as a marker of exposure and may be seen with brief or slight exposure. Generally, plaques do not appear until 20 or more years after initial exposure (19,20). In and of themselves they do not produce any symptoms, and they are often incidentally discovered at the time of the chest radiograph. Pleural plaques are usually localized to the posterior and lateral aspects of the pleura. They tend to spare the lung apices and costophrenic angles. They arise from the parietal pleura but occasionally can be seen in the visceral pleura in the interlobar fissures (18,21). In approximately 25% of cases (22–24) plaques are unilateral.

The chest radiograph is the principal imaging modality for the detection of asbestos-related pleural plaques. Plaques appear as localized, limited, plateau-like, smooth, and nodular areas of pleural thickening (19,25) (Fig. 9). On a posteroanterior (PA) radiograph, a well-developed pleural plaque has either a "profile" or en face presentation (19,25). A plaque seen in profile appears as a sharply marginated, dense band of soft tissue density, ranging from 1 to 10 mm in thickness, paralleling the inner margin of the lateral thoracic wall. Plaques are usually bilateral, often symmetrical, and more prominent in the lower half of the thorax between the 6th and 9th ribs (19,25). When seen en face, a pleural plaque appears as a faint, ill-defined, veil-like opacity with irregular edges (19,26).

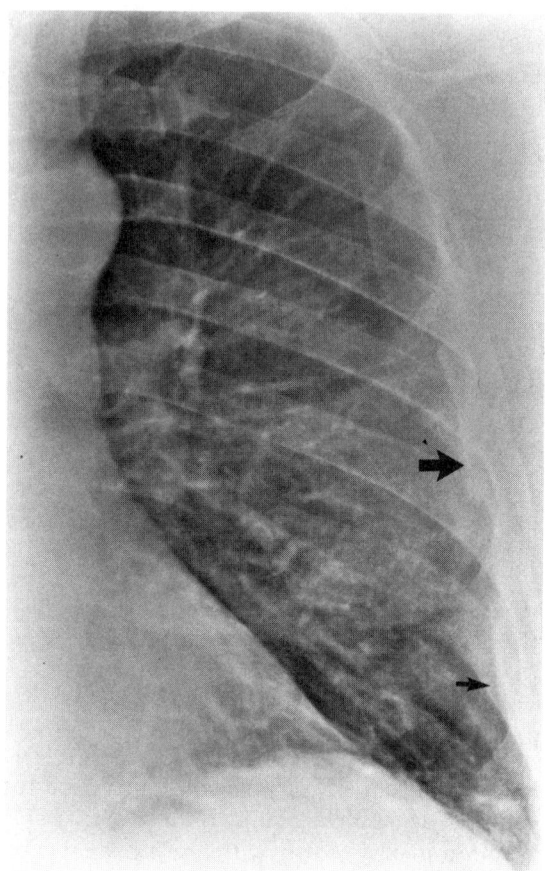

Figure 9 Pleural plaques: PA radiograph (left lung) shows multiple pleural plaques (arrows). They are interrupted, smooth areas of pleural thickening with sharp margins paralleling the chest wall.

In addition to the standard PA chest radiograph, oblique views are helpful not only to confirm suspected pleural plaques, but also to detect additional plaques unsuspected on the PA projection (19,27).

Pleural calcification generally does not develop until at least 20 years after exposure to asbestos; however, it is most frequently seen after 30–40 years. Calcification usually occurs in localized pleural plaques but may also occur in diffuse pleural thickening. Calcifications can be identified along the chest wall, diaphragm, or cardiac border. They are often small and are easily overlooked unless systematically sought after. When viewed en face, they have an irregular unevenly dense pattern likened to the fringe of a holly leaf (19,25) (Fig. 10).

Imaging of the Pleura

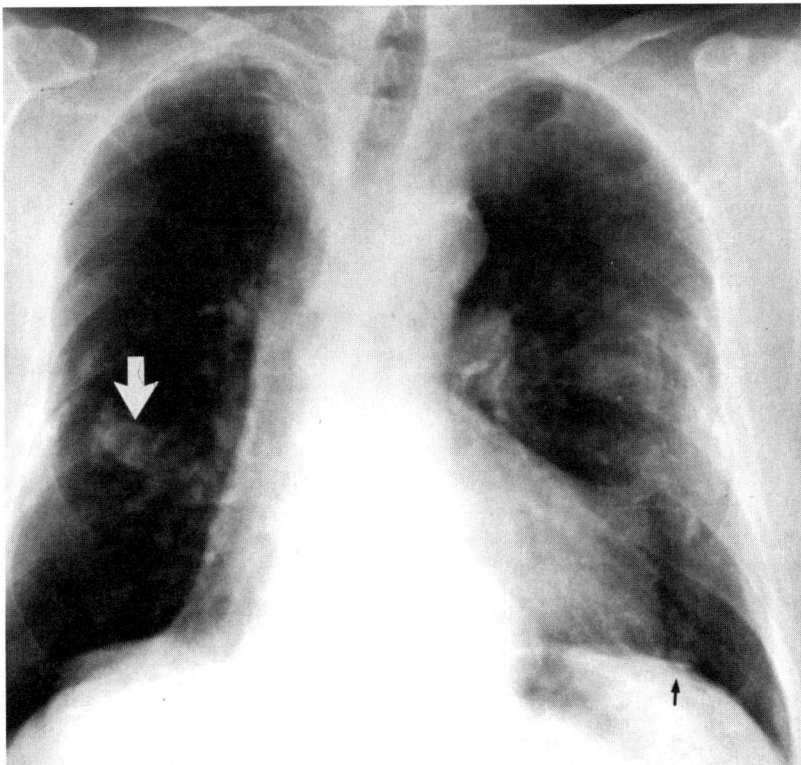

Figure 10 Calcified pleural plaques: calcified plaques are seen along the diaphragm and chest wall (black arrow). En face plaques appear as dense geometric opacities superimposed on the lung parenchyma (white arrow).

The diagnostic accuracy of radiography in the detection of pleural plaques depends upon the disease prevalence in the sample population and the presence or absence of calcification (18,22,28). With the use of criteria recommended by the International Labor Office (ILO) (29) Classification of the Pneumoconioses, the sensitivity of radiography for the detection of pleural plaques ranges from 30 to 80% and the specificity ranges from 60 to 80% (18,22,24,30–32). The low specificity of chest radiography in the diagnosis of pleural plaques is related to the difficulty in distinguishing plaques from normal muscle, fat, and companion shadows of the chest wall (9,33). Radiological findings that are suggestive of extrapleural fat are a bilateral location along the mid-lateral chest wall and a symmetrical distribution (34).

CT has been shown to be more sensitive in the detection of pleural plaques than standard radiography (35,36). Both the demand for and the cost of CT as well as the radiation dosage make it an unrealistic choice as a screening examination in persons who have been exposed to asbestos. However, it can be extremely helpful in differentiating pleural plaques from lung nodules and in resolving equivocal findings on standard radiographs (6) (Fig. 11). The lack of superimposition of structures and the greater contrast resolution of CT and particularly high-resolution CT allow improved sensitivity in the detection of pleural abnormalities and easy distinction of plaques from extrapleural fat (18). Pleural plaques on CT appear as circumscribed areas of pleural thickening separated from the underlying rib and extrapleural soft tissues by a thin layer of fat (18).

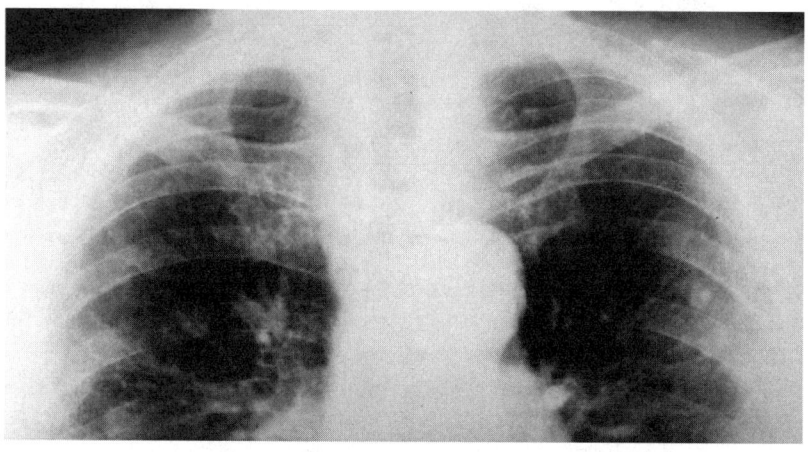
(a)

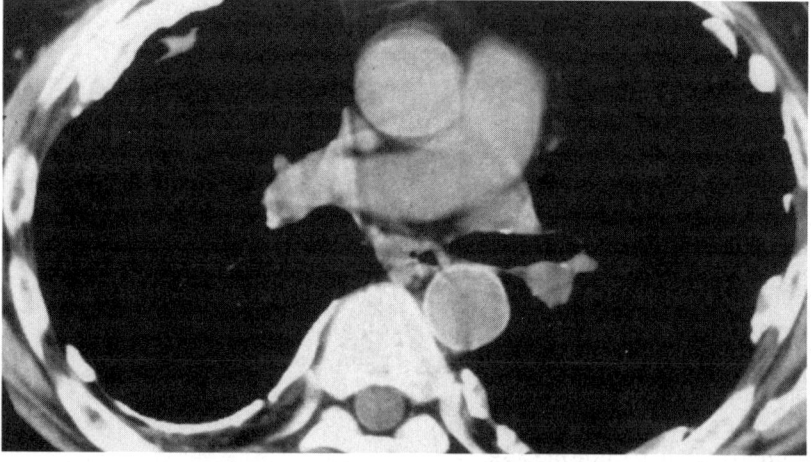
(b)

Figure 11 Pleural plaques simulating pulmonary nodules: patient with long smoking history and asbestos exposure. (a) Cone-down view of upper thorax demonstrates multiple modular opacities. (b, c) CT scan shows multiple plaques seen en face on the standard radiograph. Most are calcified.

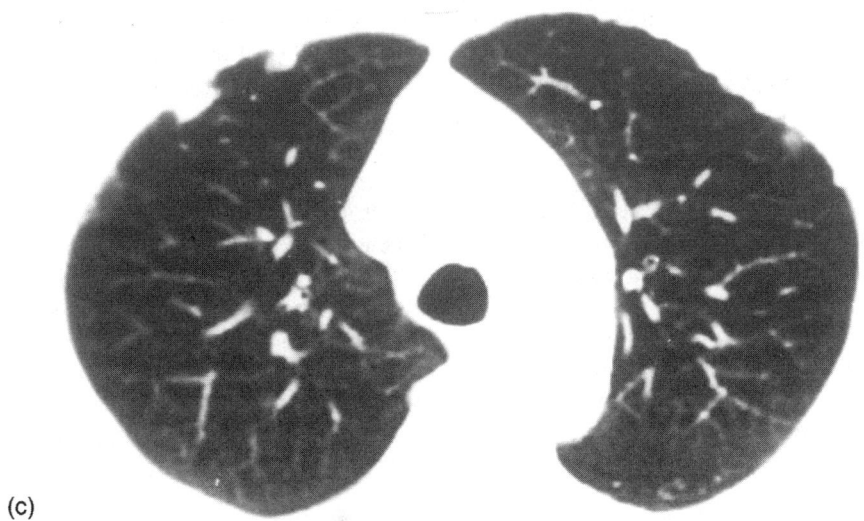

(c)

Figure 11 Continued.

B. Localized Pleural Tumors

Focal pleural tumors include fibrous tumors of the pleura, lipomas, liposarcomas, and localized invasion of the pleura by lung carcinoma. Occasionally, malignant pleural disease such as malignant mesothelioma and pleural metastases may cause focal abnormalities, but they are more commonly associated with diffuse pleural disease. Most localized pleural tumors with the exception of invasive lung cancer are relatively uncommon.

C. Fibrous Tumor of the Pleura

Fibrous tumors of the pleura are the most common focal pleural tumors, although they are generally an uncommon neoplasm and account for less than 5% of all pleural tumors (37). These tumors have a peak incidence over the age of 50 and are seen with equal frequency in men and women. They are not related to asbestos exposure (38). Approximately 60% of these tumors are considered benign, and 40% are malignant (38). However, both the benign and malignant varieties are associated with long survival after surgical resection (18,38). The malignant variety is characterized by the presence of pleural effusion and occasional chest wall invasion and the tendency to recur after surgical resection. Approximately 40% of localized pleural fibromas are attached to the visceral pleura by a pedicle (38). These tumors may reach enormous size, and tumors as large as 40 cm have been reported (9,38). Calcification is present in 5% of cases. These tumors may have a high incidence of associated of hypertrophic pulmonary osteoarthopathy (9) and hypoglycemia is present in 4–5% of cases (38,39). Radiographic findings include a well-delineated mass, which may form obtuse angles with the chest wall and mediastinum and which displaces the adjacent lung parenchyma (Fig. 12). Frequently the upper edge of the lesion may tend to fade into the lung parenchyma. If the lesion has a pedicle, it may be mobile and change position with different patient posture (9,18,40). These lesions may also occur in the interlobar fissures.

CT findings include a well-delineated often lobulated soft tissue mass in close relation to the pleural surface (19). Although an obtuse angle of the mass with respect to the pleural surface may not be identified in every case, a smoothly tapering margin is characteristic and may indicate a pleural location (41) (Fig. 12). Displacement of adjacent lung parenchyma with compressive atelectasis and bowing of the bronchi and pulmonary vessels around the mass is often noted. Enhancement of the tumor following administration of contrast material is frequent and may be homogeneous or heterogeneous (42). In the malignant variety of this tumor, CT may demonstrate local invasion of the chest wall with associated rib destruction. Larger lesions (≥ 10 cm in diameter) are more likely to be malignant.

Magnetic resonance imaging may be helpful in the diagnosis of these lesions. In cases in which there is a fairly high collagen content, fibrous tumors of the pleura may exhibit low single intensity on both T1- and T2-weighted images and enhancement with intravenously administered gadolinium contrast agent (43) (Fig. 13). This is in contradistinction to most tumors, which will demonstrate increased signal intensity on T2-weighted images because of high water content.

D. Pleural Lipoma and Liposarcoma

Pleural lipomas and liposarcomas are rare tumors (44–47). Lipomas are usually asymptomatic and are discovered incidentally on chest radiographs. A definitive diagnosis is usually not possible on standard films. However, CT clearly delineates the pleural origin of these lesions in the majority of cases and their fatty composition (-50 to -150 Houndsfield units) (48) (Fig. 14). Benign lipomas have completely uniform fatty density, although linear soft tissue strands due to fibrous stroma may be present. On the other hand, thymolipomas, angiolipomas, and teratomas are characterized by islands of soft tissue density interspersed with fat (49,50). Liposarcomas can be differentiated from lipomas easily by a higher and heterogeneous density (51).

Lipomas may be totally intrathoracic, i.e., within the ribs, or transmural with extension into the chest wall (44). Pleural lipomas on MR scanning can be identified readily by their signal characteristics. Such lesions are of bright signal intensity on T1-weighted images and also moderately bright on T2-weighted

---

Figure 12 Fibrous tumor of the pleura: (a) large elliptical mass filling most of the lower half of the right chest; (b) CT demonstrates a partially enhancing mass abutting the pleura but without an obtuse angle with the chest wall.

Imaging of the Pleura

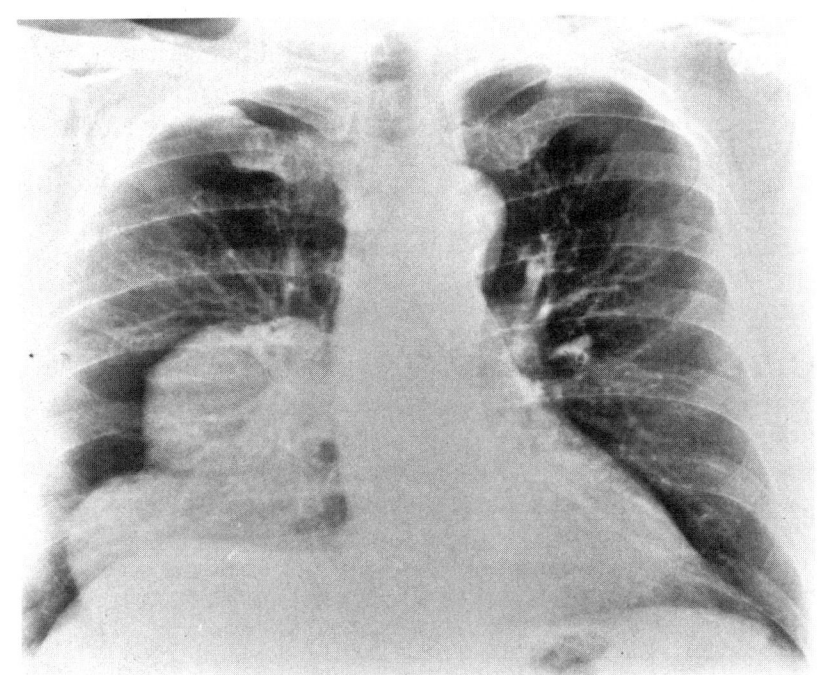
(a)

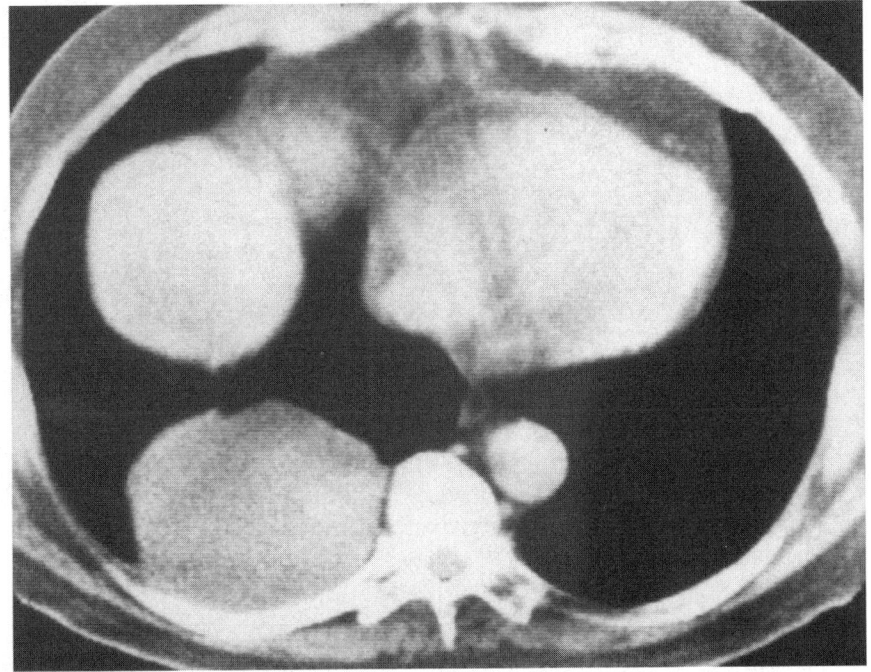
(b)

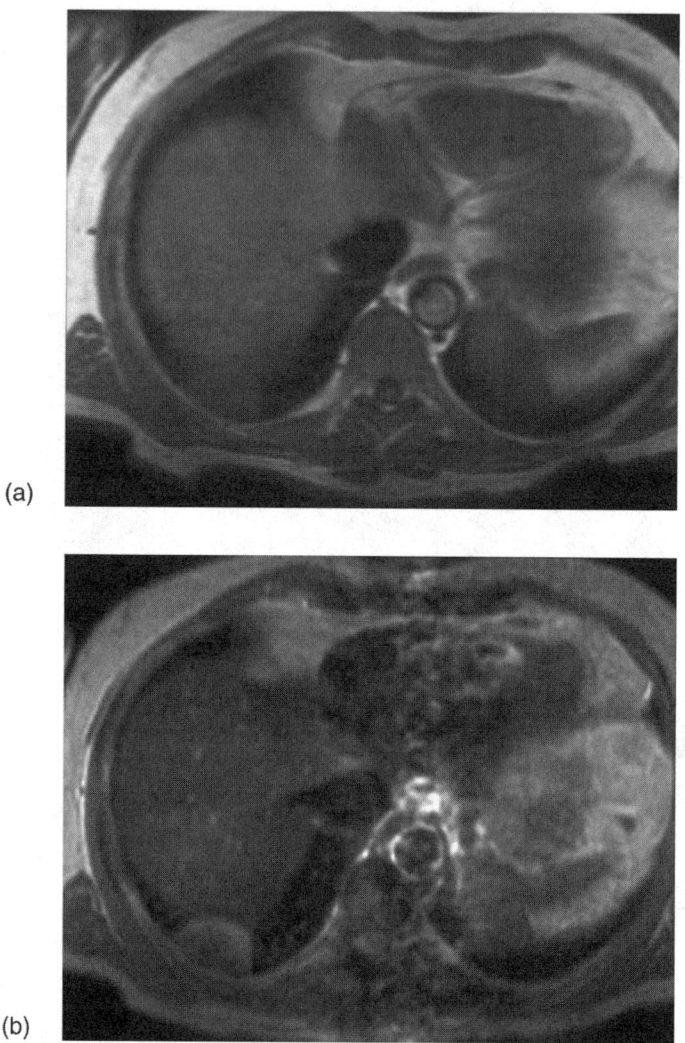

Figure 13 MRI fibrous tumor of the pleura: (a) T1-weighted image demonstrates a posterior inferior mass of low signal intensity; (b) T2-weighted image. The mass exhibits mostly low signal intensity.

images. However, CT is usually diagnostic, and MRI is not required for diagnosis.

E. Local Extension of Lung Cancer

Lung cancers that invade the parietal pleura and chest wall are designated T3 tumors and are potentially resectable. Surgical treatment, however, requires en

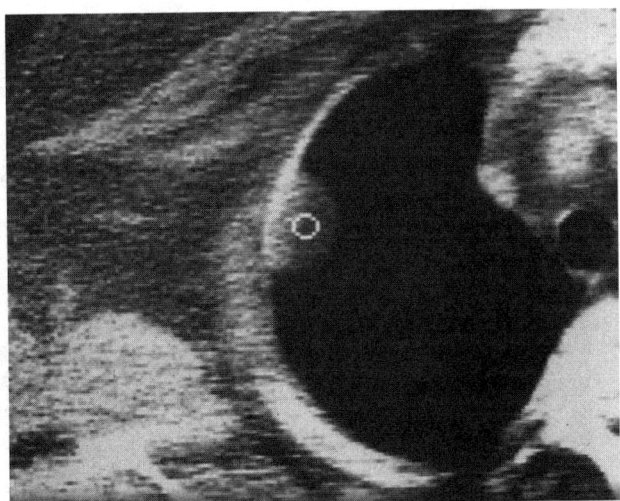

Figure 14 Lipoma: well-defined peripheral mass of homogeneously low attenuation (H.U. = −60).

bloc resection of the pulmonary malignancy and the contiguous chest wall and is associated with slightly increased morbidity and mortality (52). In selecting patients as operative candidates, it may be desirable to determine preoperatively whether chest wall invasion is present. The value of CT scanning in the determination of chest wall invasion is limited. The only CT findings with high positive predictive values are bone destruction adjacent to the lung mass or obvious extension of the mass beyond the ribs into the chest wall (53). Pleural thickening contiguous to the tumor is a nonspecific finding and may be caused by local fibrous adhesions or invasion of the parietal pleura by tumor. Inspiratory and expiratory CT scans have been used to evaluate respiratory shift (i.e., a change in the relative location between the peripheral lung tumor and the chest wall during respiration). The presence of such a shift is a reliable indicator of the lack of parietal pleural invasion by tumor in the lower half of the chest (54). MRI has a slight advantage over CT in the evaluation of chest wall invasion. T1- and T2-weighted sequences may show direct tumor extension, and the yield is improved with the use of gadolinium contrast (55) (Fig. 15).

IV. Diffuse Pleural Disease: Fibrothorax

Fibrothorax or diffuse pleural thickening involving most of the pleural space may develop as the result of previous hemothoraces, tuberculous effusions and other types of empyema, benign asbestos pleurisy, and occasionally other processes.

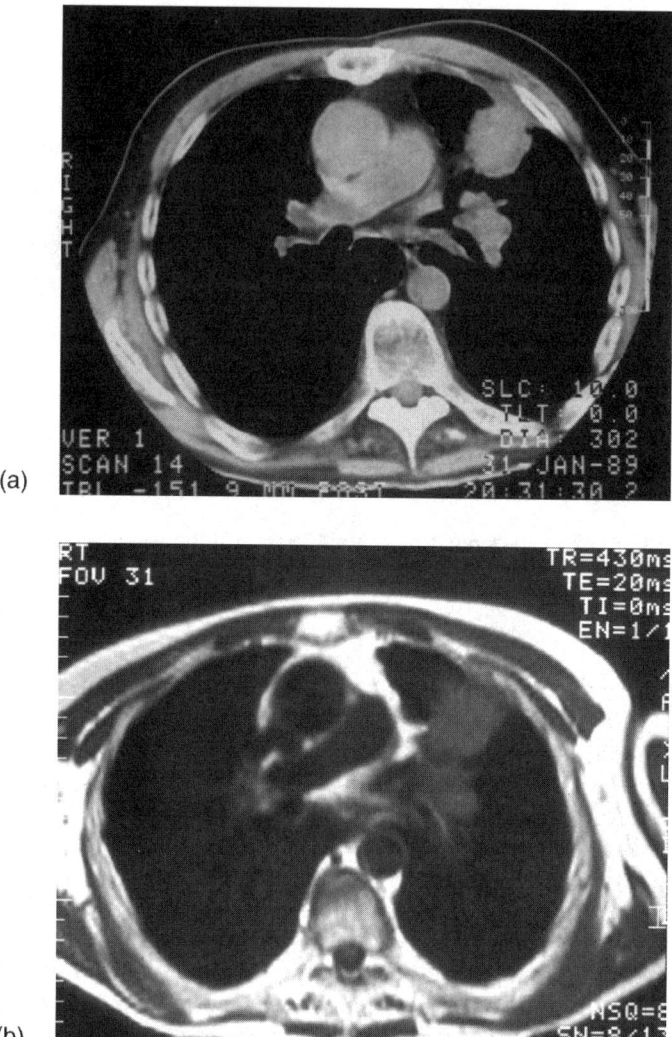

Figure 15 Lung cancer invading chest wall: (a) CT scan demonstrates a peripheral mass with adjacent pleural thickening. CT is indeterminate for chest wall or parietal pleural thickening; (b) T1 weighted images demonstrates tongue-like extensions of low signal intensity due to tumor invading the extrapleural fat of the chest wall.

Diffuse pleural thickening is often associated with a decrease in volume of the ipsilateral lung. Bilateral pleural thickening may be associated with a severe restrictive defect on pulmonary functioning testing. Diffuse pleural thickening secondary to asbestos exposure is seen less frequently than pleural plaques. It is characterized by uniform homogeneous density with smooth contours and frequently by obliteration of the costophrenic angle (19,27) (Fig. 16). Diffuse

Imaging of the Pleura

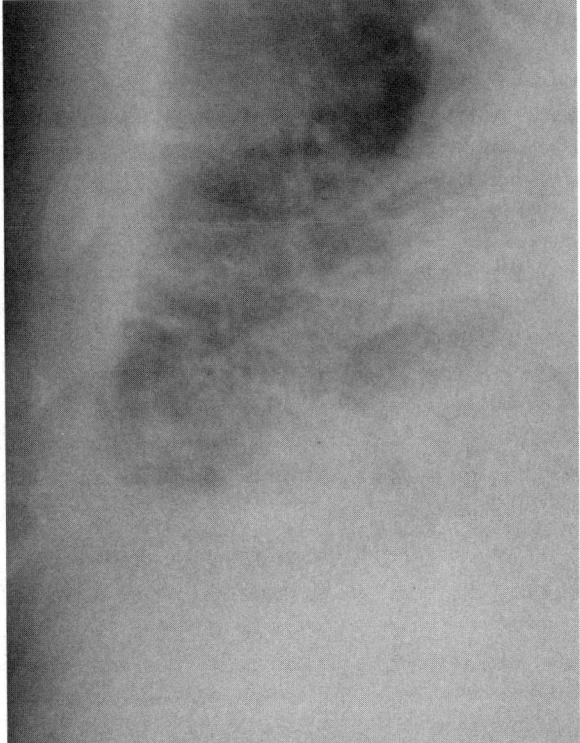

Figure 16 Asbestos pleural thickening: There is diffuse pleural thickening on the right, which is smooth and extends to the costophrenic angle. The underlying lung is involved with asbestosis.

pleural thickening is most often the result of a previous benign asbestos effusion (19,56). Asbestos-related pleural thickening usually involves the visceral pleura and is frequently associated with restrictive lung function (17).

CT may be extremely helpful in both the identification of diffuse pleural thickening and its characterization (Fig. 17). Characteristics of fibrothorax include smoothly contoured pleural thickening without nodularity, thickness of < 1 cm, and lack of involvement of the mediastinal pleura (57) (Fig. 17). CT may also be useful in determining the etiology of fibrothorax. For example, evidence of underlying parenchymal disease is often seen in patients who have had previous tuberculosis (9,18). If pleural calcification is extensive, it favors previous tuberculosis, hemothorax, or empyema. Calcification may be seen in asbestos pleural thickening, but is less common (58). Diffuse asbestos pleural thickening, although most frequently unilateral, may be associated with pleural abnormalities on the opposite side such as pleural plaques.

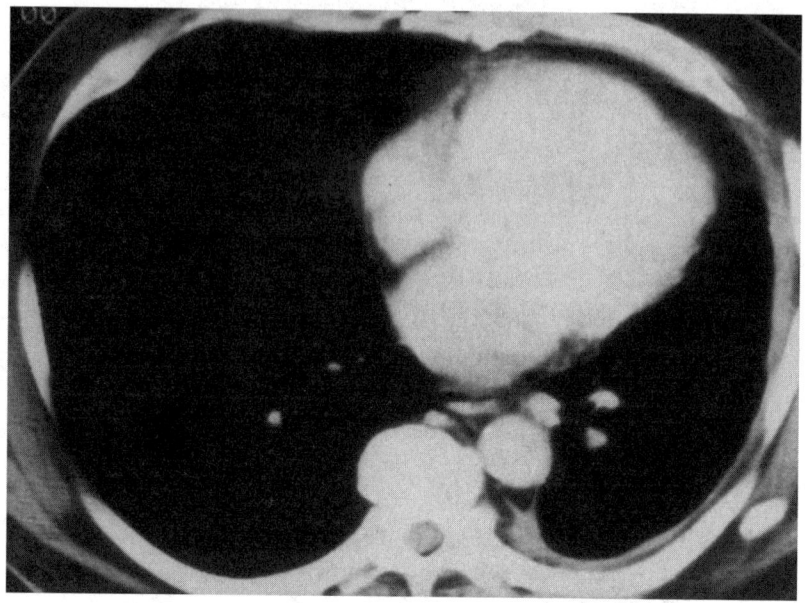

Figure 17 Fibrothorax: CT demonstrates diffuse, smooth pleural thickening 3 mm in thickness involving the lateral and posterior pleura.

CT may also be helpful in determining the extent of pleural thickening and to evaluate the underlying parenchyma particularly in patients with asbestos exposure where the pleural thickening prevents adequate parenchymal lung evaluation (59). CT can eliminate superimposition of opacities, thus allowing better evaluation of the lung parenchyma in the presence of asbestos pleural disease.

V. Malignant Pleural Disease

A. Malignant Mesothelioma

Malignant mesothelioma is a rare primary malignant tumor of the pleura. The majority of affected patients (80%) have a history of occupational exposure to asbestos. Occupations with the greatest risk include shipyard work, building construction and demolition, brake-lining manufacture, and heating trades. Approximately 2000–3000 new cases of mesothelioma occur in the United States each year (60). There is a latency period for development of malignant mesothelioma of 35–40 years after initial exposure (61). Affected patients are usually in the sixth to eighth decades of life, and males are more frequently affected than females by a ratio of approximately 4:1 (62).

Patients typically present with insidious onset of symptoms, often occurring 6–8 months prior to the diagnosis. Patients often complain of chest pain but also may have dyspnea, cough, and weight loss.

Imaging of the Pleura

Histologically, mesotheliomas are usually divided into three categories: epithelioid, sarcomatoid, and biphasic (mixed). The epithelioid variety is most common and may be difficult to distinguish histologically from metastases to the pleura (63). On gross inspection, the tumor involves the parietal pleura more extensively than the visceral layer, often forming sheetlike coalescent tumor masses that may encase the lung and extend into interlobar fissures. The prognosis of malignant mesothelioma is poor, with a median survival of approximately 10 months. Selected patients may undergo extrapleural pneumonectomy, a radical procedure associated with significant morbidity and mortality (64).

The characteristic radiographic feature of mesothelioma is unilateral diffuse, irregular, and nodular pleural thickening with or without an associated pleural effusion. Associated asbestos-related pleural disease (e.g., pleural plaques) occurs in 20–25% of cases. Mediastinal shift towards the involved hemithorax as a result of tumor encasement and volume loss may be identified. Alternatively, massive tumor bulk and large pleural effusions may produce contralateral shift of the mediastinum. Pleural effusion may obscure tumor masses and be the sole or predominant radiographic finding (Fig. 18).

CT better characterizes tumor extent and morphology and may demonstrate focal or diffuse pleural masses, nodular pleural thickening, and fissural involvement. Involvement is typically circumferential with involvement of the mediastinal pleura. The cross-sectional imaging features of malignant mesothelioma are often indistinguishable from metastatic involvement of the pleura (65,66). Invasion of the chest wall, mediastinum, and diaphragm may be

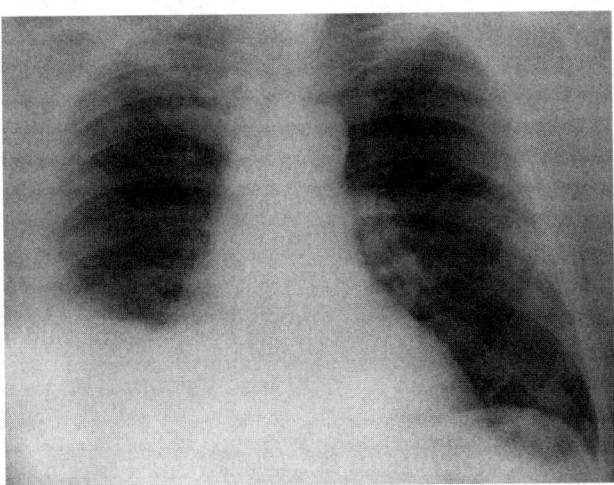

Figure 18 Mesothelioma: PA radiograph. A large right pleural effusion obscures the right lower hemithorax and its underlying involvement by malignant mesothelioma.

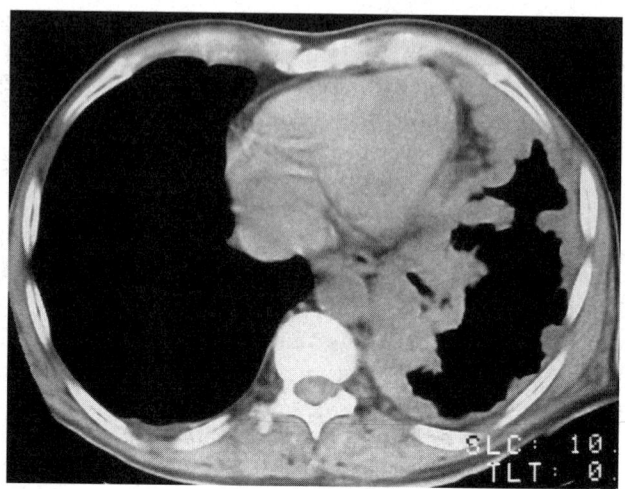

Figure 19 Mesothelioma: CT demonstrates extensive nodular pleural thickening, which circumferentially involves the left hemithorax and extends into the medial and lateral aspects of the interlobar fissure anteriorly.

demonstrated by CT, but early invasion is often not apparent or may be underestimated (Fig. 19).

MR imaging may better characterize the invasive features of mesothelioma. Tumor typically manifests as minimally increased signal on T1-weighted images and moderately increased signal on T2-weighted images. The multiplanar capabilities of MR may allow better detection and visualization of chest wall, mediastinal, and diaphragmatic extension of tumor and help predict resectability (67) (Fig. 20). Diffuse superficial spread of mesothelioma throughout the pleural space may be difficult to detect by any of the above modalities.

B. Metastases

Pleural metastases are the most common form of neoplastic involvement of the pleura. Most metastases are adenocarcinomas, typically arising from primary sites in the lung, breast, ovary, and stomach. Lymphomas may also involve the pleura. Metastatic tumor usually involves both the visceral and parietal pleura and often produces malignant pleural effusion (9).

On CT, metastases may manifest as marked thickening and nodularity of the pleura, usually with an associated pleural effusion. In some cases the effusion

---

Figure 20 Mesothelioma: (a) sagittal MR demonstrates a large mesothelioma posteriorly that does not appear to invade the chest wall or hemidiaphragm; (b) coronal MR of a different patient shows extensive circumferential nodular pleural masses involving the entire right hemithorax and extending into the minor interlobar fissure.

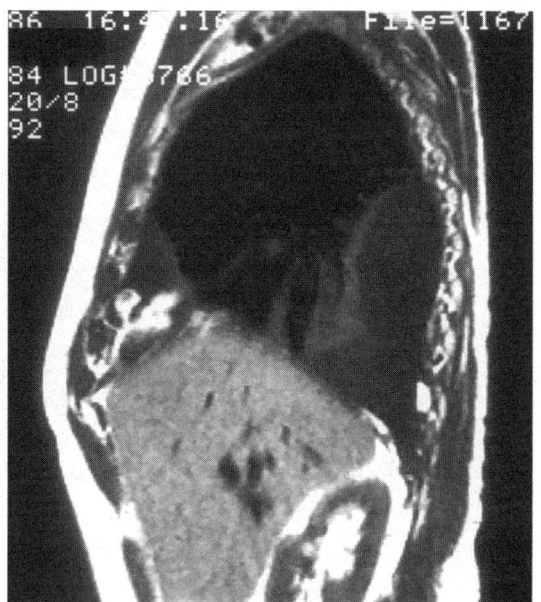

(a)

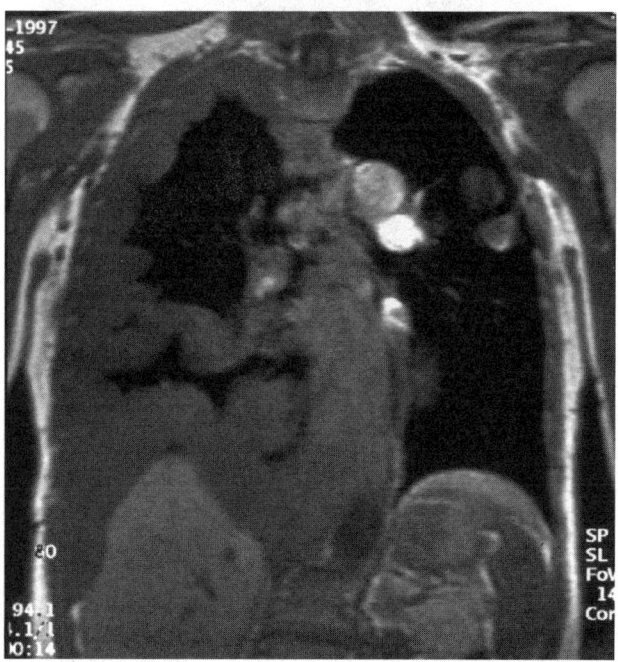

(b)

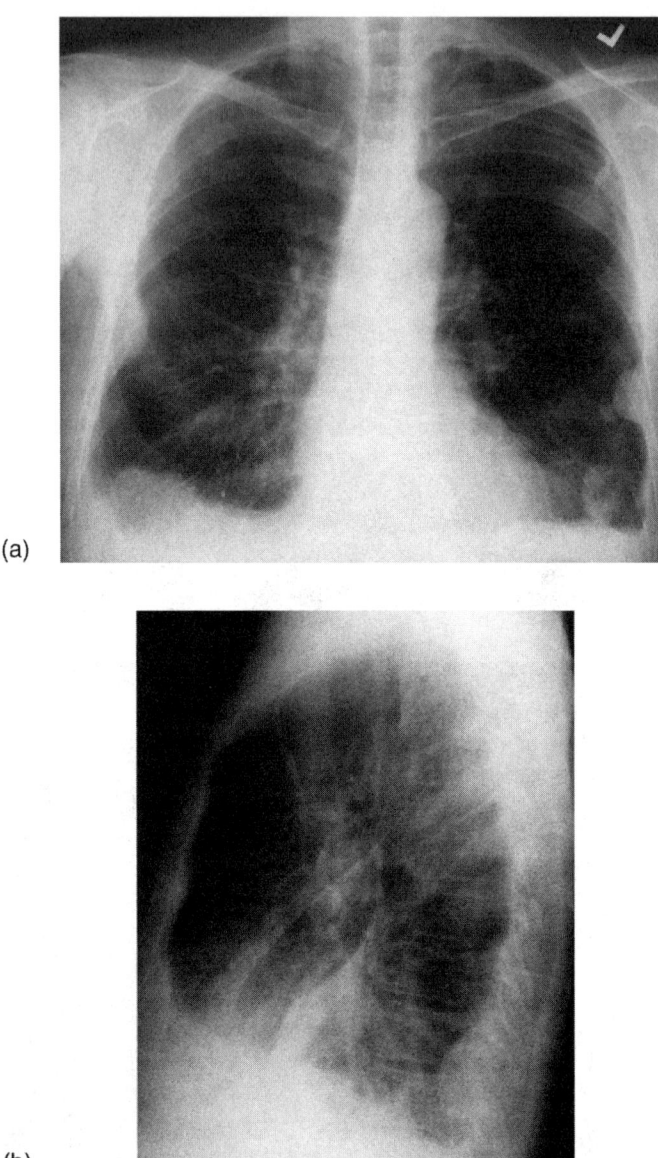

Figure 21 Pleural metastases (renal cell carcinoma): (a,b) PA and lateral radiographs demonstrate multiple areas of nodular pleural thickening that are >1 cm and appear circumferential within the left hemithorax. Involvement of the mediastinal pleura is apparent in the medial aspect of the apical portion of the left hemithorax on the PA view.

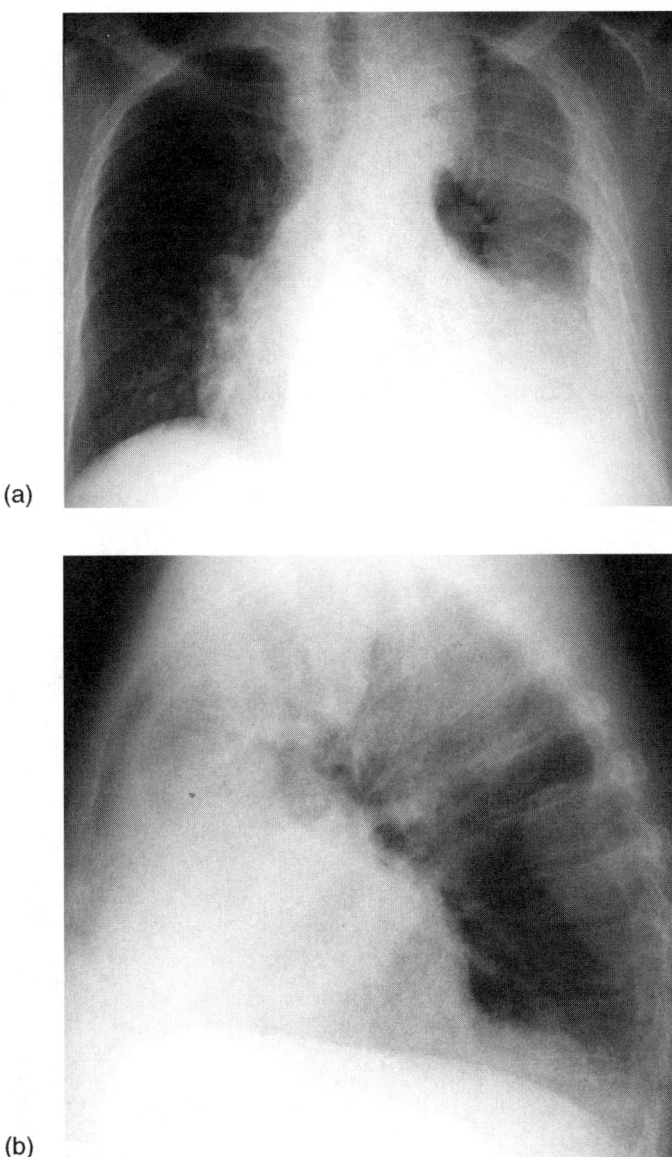

Figure 22 Pleural metastases (lymphoma): (a,b) PA and lateral radiographs demonstrate large, contiguous pleural masses in the left hemithorax with marked nodularity and extensive circumferential involvement; (c) CT demonstrates the pleural configuration of the masses with involvement of the mediastinal pleura and invasion of adjacent mediastinal structures.

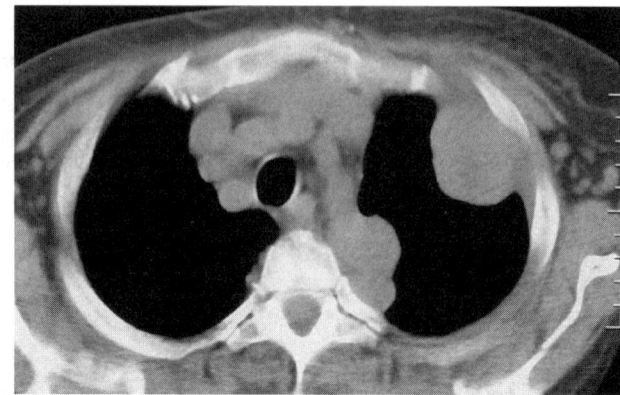

(c)

Figure 22 Continued.

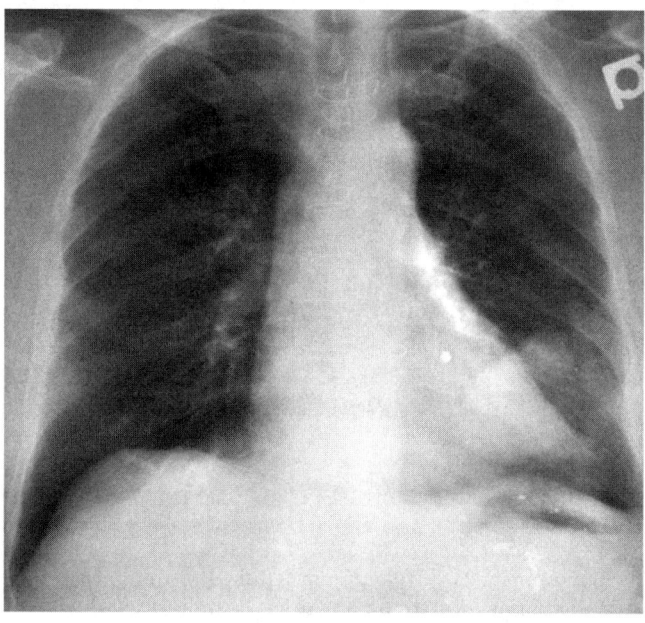

(a)

Figure 23 Thoracic splenosis: (a,b) PA and lateral radiographs demonstrate multiple opacities from gunshot wound to the left lower chest. A posterior pleural opacity in the lower left hemithorax has incomplete margins on the lateral view, suggesting its extraparenchymal location; (c) CT shows two adjacent pleural masses posterolaterally in the lower left hemithorax. The diagnosis was confirmed by radionuclide scanning using ^{99m}Tc sulfur colloid (not shown).

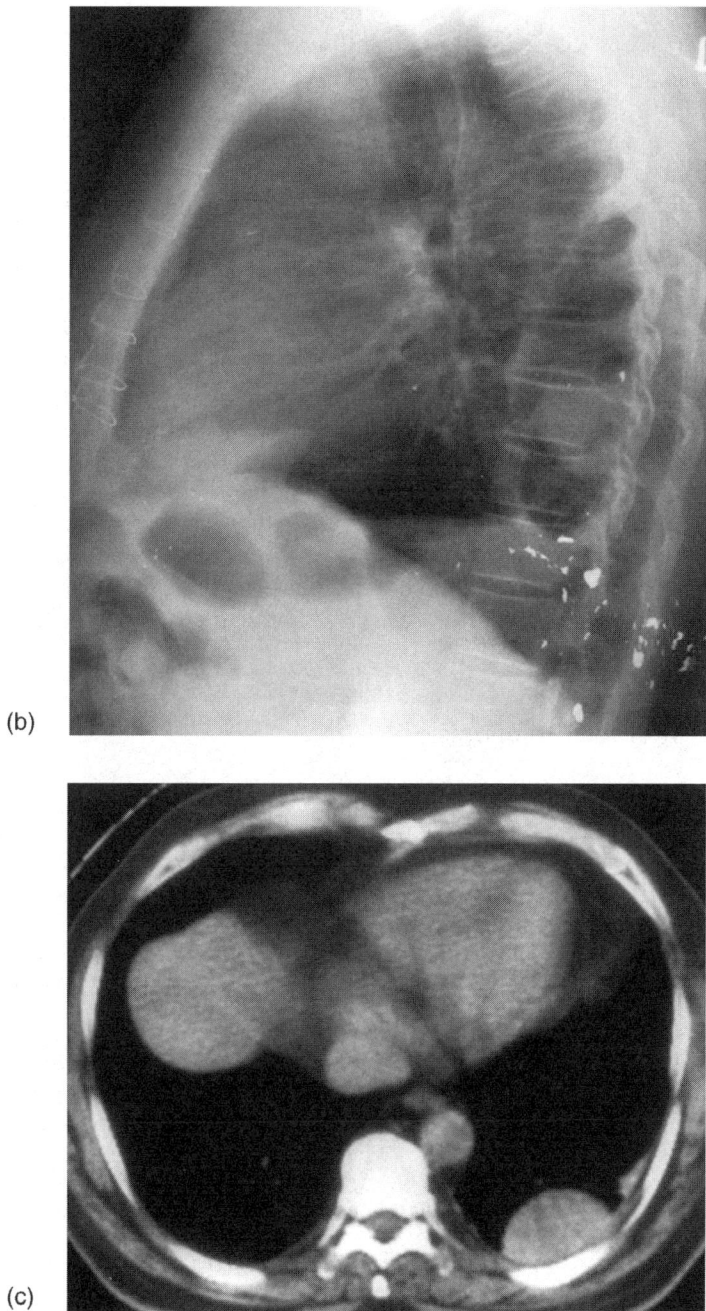

Figure 23 Continued.

may be large and tumor foci may be difficult to identify. Metastases may mimic malignant mesothelioma, and the two entities cannot be reliably distinguished by cross-sectional imaging (58) (Figs. 21, 22).

Finally, certain tumors such as malignant thymoma may produce focal seeding of the pleura. This is usually manifest on CT scanning as localized focal pleural nodules, which may be bilateral or unilateral.

The differentiation of malignant from benign pleural thickening provides a challenge for the radiologist. There is overlap of the radiological manifestations of benign and malignant pleural processes. Leung et al. (57) in a study of 74 consecutive patients with proven diffuse pleural disease demonstrated that CT can play a major role in providing the distinction. Features that were helpful in distinguishing malignant from benign pleural disease included (a) circumferential pleural thickening, (b) nodular pleural thickening > 1 cm in thickness, and (c) mediastinal pleural involvement, all of which occurred more consistently with malignant lesions. These features may be seen in mesothelioma and metastatic pleural disease but are unusual in benign pleural disease. The presence of pleural calcification is also suggestive of a benign process. In the study by Leung et al. (57), calcification was seen in 6 of 35 patients with benign pleural thickening and in only 3 of 39 patients with malignant pleural disease. Although calcified pleural plaques may be seen in cases of mesothelioma, they are uncommon.

VI. Thoracic Splenosis

Thoracic splenosis is a rare pathological entity that may mimic pleural neoplasia. Affected patients have a history of thoracoabdominal trauma that ruptures and fragments the spleen. Splenic fragments may implant and grow on the adjacent peritoneal surfaces. With concomitant penetrating trauma to the diaphragm, splenic fragments may implant and grow along pleural surfaces in the lower aspect of the left hemithorax and manifest as multifocal pleural masses ranging in size from 3 to 7 cm (Fig. 23). The diagnosis may be confirmed by radionuclide scans using ^{99m}Tc sulfur colloid (68).

References

1. Light RW, MacGregor MI, Luchsinger PC, Ball WC Jr. Pleural effusions: the diagnostic separation of transudates and exudates. Ann Intern Med 1972; 77:507–513.
2. Raasch BN, Carsky EW, Lane EJ, O'Callaghan JP, Heitzman ER. Pictorial essay: pleural effusion; explanation of some typical experiences. AJR 1982; 139:899–904.
3. Heitzman ER. The Lung: Radiologic-Pathologic Correlations. 2d ed. St. Louis: Mosby, 1984.
4. Oestreich AE, Haley C. Pleural effusion: the thorn sign. Chest 1981; 79:365–366.
5. Moskowitz H, Platt RT, Schachar R, Mellins H. Roentgen visualization of minute

pleural effusion: an experimental study to determine the minimum amount of pleural fluid visible on a radiograph. Radiology 1973; 109:33–35.
6. McLoud TC, Flowers CD. Imaging the pleura: sonography CT and MR imaging. AJR 1991; 156:1145–1153.
7. Yang PC, Luh KT, Chang DB, Wu HD, Yu CJ, Kuo SH. Value of sonography in determining the nature of pleural effusion: analysis of 320 cases. AJR 1992; 159: 29–33.
8. Friedman RL. Infrapulmonary pleural effusions. Am J Roentgenol Radium Ther Nucl Med 1954; 71:613–623.
9. Fraser RS, Muller NL, Colman N, Pare' PD. Diagnosis of Diseases of the Chest. 4th ed. Philadelphia: WB Saunders, 1999:2737–2840.
10. Naidich DP, Zerhouni EA, Siegelman SS. Pleura and chest wall. In: Naidich DP, Zerhouni EA, Siegelman SS, eds. Computed Tomography and Magnetic Resonance Imaging of the Thorax. 2d ed. New York: Raven-Lippincott, 1991:407–471.
11. Stark DD, Federle MP, Goodman PC, Podrasky AE, Webb WR. Differentiating lung abscess and empyema: radiography and computed tomography. AJR 1983; 141:163–167.
12. McLoud TC. The pleura and chest wall. In: Haaga JR, Lanzieri CF, Sartoris DJ, Zerhouni Ea, eds. Computed Tomography and Magnetic Resonance Imaging of the Whole Body. St. Louis: Mosby, 1994:772–787.
13. Dwyer RA. The displaced crus: a sign for distinguishing between pleural fluid and ascites on computed tomography. J Comput Assist Tomogr 1978; 2:598–599.
14. Griffin DJ, Gross BH, McCrackenn S, Glazer GM. Observation on CT differentiation of pleural and peritoneal fluid. J Comput Assist Tomogr 1984; 8:24–28.
15. Halvorsen RA, Fedyshin PJ, Korobkin M, Foster WL Jr, Thompson WM. Ascites or pleural effusion? CT differentiation: four useful criteria. RadioGraphics 1986; 6:135–149.
16. Chiles C, Ravin CE. Radiographic recognition of pneumothorax in the intensive care unit. Crit Care Med 1986; 14:677–680.
17. Schwartz DA. New developments in asbestos-related pleural disease. Chest 1991; 99:191–198.
18. Muller NL. Imaging the pleura. Radiology 1993; 186:297–309.
19. McLoud TC. Asbestos-related diseases: the role of imaging techniques. Postgrad Radiol 1989; 9:65–74.
20. Hillerdal G. Pleural plaques in a health survey material: frequency, development and exposure to asbestos. Scand J Respir Dis 1978; 59:257–261.
21. Rockoff SD, Kagan E, Schwartz A, Kriebel D, Hix W, Rohatgi P. Visceral pleural thickening in asbestos exposure: the occurrence and implications of thickened interlobar fissures. J Thorac Imaging 1987; 2:58–66.
22. Gefter WB, Conant EF. Issues and controversies in the plain-film diagnosis of asbestos-related disorders in the chest. J Thorac Imaging 1988; 3:11–28.
23. Fisher MS. Asymmetric changes in asbestos-related disease. J Can Assoc Radiol 1985; 36:110–112.
24. Withers BF, Ducatman AM, Yang WN. Roentgenographic evidence for predominant left-sided location of unilateral pleural plaques. Chest 1984; 95:1262–1264.
25. Sargent EN, Boswell WD, Ralls PW, Markovitz A. Pleural plaques: a signpost of asbestos chest inhalation. Semin Roentgenol 1977; 12:287–297.
26. Anton HC. Multiple pleural plaques, Part III. BJ Radiol 1968; 41:341–348.

27. Sargent EN, Gordonson J, Jacobson G, Birnbaum W, Shaub M. Bilateral pleural thickening: a manifestation of asbestos exposure. AJR 1978; 131:579–585.
28. Greene R, Boggin C, Jantsch H. Asbestos-related pleural thickening: effect of threshold criteria on interpretation. Radiology 1984; 152:569–573.
29. International Labour Office. Guidelines for the Use of the ILO International Classification of Radiographics of Pneumoconioses, Revised Edition. International Labour Office Occupational Safety and Health Series, No. 22 (revised 1980). Geneva, Switzerland: International Labour Office, 1980.
30. Schwartz DA, Fuortes LJ, Galvin JR, Burmeister LF, Schmidt LE, Leistikow BN, LaMarte FP, Merchant JA. Asbestos-induced pleural fibrosis and impaired lung function. Am Rev Respir Dis 1990; 141:321–325.
31. Wain SL, Roggli VL, Foster WL. Parietal pleural plaques, asbestos bodies, and neoplasia: a clinical, pathologic, and roentgenographic correlation of 25 consecutive cases. Chest 1984; 86:707–713.
32. Hourihane DO, Lessog L, Richardson PC. Hyaline and calcified pleural plaques as an index of exposure to asbestos: a study of radiological and pathological features of 100 cases with a consideration of epidemiology. Br Med J 1977; 1:1069–1074.
33. Sargent EN, Boswell WD Jr, Ralls PW, Markovitz A. Subpleural fat pads in patients exposed to asbestos: distinction from non-calcified pleural plaques. Radiology 1984; 152:273–277.
34. Proto AV. Conventional chest radiographs: anatomic understanding of newer observations. Radiology 1992; 183:593–603.
35. Kreel L. Computed tomography in the evaluation of pulmonary asbestosis. Acta Radiol 1976; 17:405–412.
36. Kreel L. Computed tomography of the lung and pleura. Semin Roentgenol 1978; 131:213–225.
37. Theros EG, Feigin DS. Pleural tumors and pulmonary tumors: differential diagnosis. Semin Roentgenol 1977; 12:239–247.
38. England DM, Hockholzer L, McCarthy MJ. Localized benign and malignant fibrous tumors of the pleura: a clinicopathologic review of 223 cases. Am J Surg Pathol 1989; 13:640–658.
39. Briselle M, Mark EJ, Duhersin GR. Solitary fibrous tumors of the pleura: eight new cases and review of 360 cases in the literature. Cancer 1981; 47:2678–2689.
40. Soulen MC, Greco-Hunt VT, Templeton P. Cases from A^3CR^2, migratory chest mass. Invest Radiol 1990; 25:209–211.
41. Dedrick CG, McLoud TC, Shepard JO, Shipley RT. Computed tomography of localized pleural mesothelioma. AJR 1985; 144:275–280.
42. Mendelson DS, Meary E, Bay JN, Pigeau I, Kirschner PA. Localized fibrous pleural mesothelioma: CT findings. Clin Imaging 1991; 15:105–108.
43. Desser TS. Solitary fibrous tumor of the pleura. J Thoracic Imag 1998; 13:27–35.
44. Buxton RC, Tan CS, Kline NM, Cuasay NS, Shor MJ, Spigos DG. Atypical transmural thoracic lipoma. CT diagnosis. J Comput Assist Tomogr 1988; 12:196–198.
45. Epler GR, McLoud TC, Munn CS, Colby TV. Pleural lipoma: diagnosis by computed tomography. Chest 1986; 90:265–268.
46. Evans AR, Wolstenholte RJ, Shettan SP, Yogish H. Primary pleural liposarcoma. Thorax 1985; 40:554–555.
47. Munk PC, Muller NL. Pleural liposarcoma: CT diagnosis. J Comput Assist Tomogr 1988; 12:709–710.

48. Chalaoui J, Sylvestre J, Dussault RG, Pinsky M, Palayew MJ. Thoracic fatty lesions, some usual and unusual appearances. J Can Assoc Radiol 1980; 32:197–201.
49. Yeh HC, Gordon A, Kirschner PA, Cohen BA. Computed tomography and sonography of thymolipoma. AJR 1983; 140:1131–1133.
50. Biondetti PR, Fiore D, Perrin B, Ravasini R. Infiltrative angiolipoma of the thoracoabdominal wall. J Comput Assist Tomogr 1982; 6:847.
51. Mendez G, Isilkoff MB, Isilkoff SK, Sinner WN. Fatty tumors of the thorax demonstrated by lung CT. AJR 1979; 133:207–212.
52. Piehler J, Pairolere PC, Weiland LH, O'Brien PC. Bronchogenic carcinoma with chest wall invasion: factors affecting survival following en bloc resection. Ann Thorac Surg 1986; 34:684–687.
53. Quint Le, Francis IT, Wahl RL, Gross BH, Glazer GM. Pre-operative staging of non-small cell carcinoma of the lung: imaging methods. AJR 1995; 164:1349–1354.
54. Shirakawa T, Fukuda K, Miyamoto Y, Tanabe H, Tada S. Parietal pleural invasion of lung masses: evaluation with CT performed during deep inspiration and expiration. Radiology 1994; 192:809–814.
55. Padovani B, Mouroux J, Seksik L, Chanalet S, Sedat J, Rotomondo C, Richelme H, Serres JJ. Chest wall invasion by bronchogenic carcinoma: evaluation by MR imaging. Radiology 1993; 198:32–37.
56. McLoud TC, Woods BO, Carrington CB, Epler GR, Gaensler EA. Diffuse pleural thickening in an asbestos exposed population: prevalence and causes. AJR 1985; 144:9–18.
57. Leung AN, Muller NL, Miller RR. CT in differential diagnosis of diffuse pleural disease. AJR 1990; 154:487–492.
58. Friedman AC, Fiel SB, Redeiki PD, Lev-Toaff AS. Computed tomography of benign pleural and pulmonary parenchymal abnormalities related to asbestos exposure. Semin Ultrasound CT MR 1990; 11:393–408.
59. McLoud TC. The use of CT in the examination of asbestos-exposed persons. Radiology 1988; 169:862–863.
60. Rusch VW, Piantadaosi S, Holmes EC. The role of exrapleural pneumonectomy in malignant pleural mesothelioma. J Thorac Cardiovasc Surg 1991; 102:1–9.
61. Selikoff IJ, Hammond EC, Seidman H. Latency of asbestos disease among insulation workers in the United States and Canada. Cancer 1980; 46:2736–2740.
62. Pisani RJ, Colby TV, Williams DE. Malignant mesothelioma of the pleura. Mayo Clin Proc 1988; 63:1234–1244.
63. Roggi VL, Sanfilippo F, Shelburne JD. Mesothelioma. In: Roggli VL, Greenberg SD, Pratt PC, eds. Pathology of Asbestos-Associated Diseases. Boston: Little, Brown, 1992:109–153.
64. Aisner J. Current approach to malignant mesothelioma of the pleura. Chest 1995; 107:332S–344S.
65. Wechsler RJ, Rao VM, Steiner RM. The radiology of thoracic malignant mesothelioma. Crit Rev Diagn Imaging 1983; 20:283–310.
66. Kawashima A, Libshitz HI. Malignant pleural mesothelioma: CT manifestations in 50 cases. AJR 1990; 155:965–969.
67. Miller BH, Rosado-de-Christenson ML, Mason AC, Fleming MV, White CS, Krasna MJ. Malignant pleural mesothelioma: radiologic-pathologic correlation. Radiographics 1996; 16:613–644.
68. Normand J-P, Rioux M, Dumont M, Bouchard G, Letourneau L. Thoracic splenosis after blunt trauma: frequency and imaging findings. AJR 1993; 161:739–741.

7

The Role of Ultrasonography in the Evaluation of Pleural Diseases

OK HWA KIM and KYUNG JOO PARK
Ajou University Medical Center
Suwon, South Korea

I. Introduction

Patients with chest lesions have been considered poor candidates for ultrasonographic examination because air-filled lungs and bony structures are not good media to transmit ultrasound (US) beams. With the rapid advances of transducer design, signal processing, and Doppler technology, great improvement has been achieved in imaging quality of sonography. The pleura, a relatively superficial structure, is easily accessible to sonography and has been examined by US since its early development (1–5). Since US gained recognition as a highly useful tool in the evaluation of pleural lesions, its role has expanded in imaging as well as in therapeutic goals, particularly in pleural fluid collection.

Pathological processes that involve the pleura, either directly from isolated pleural disease or indirectly from neighboring pulmonary lesions, manifest as pleural fluid collections, which is one of the main causes of increased opacity in the hemithorax seen on chest radiography. US is ideal for imaging with this radiological finding, which can also be due to other causes, such as pulmonary consolidation or masses. US easily identifies the cause of the opaque chest on radiography by their acoustic properties and avoids unnecessary invasive procedures (6–9).

US can also be used to provide imaging guidance for pleural drainage procedures (10). With US one can determine the depth of the fluid collection and decide on the safest manner to approach for draining fluid. Sonography-guided thoracentesis or catheter drainage of pleural fluid is a safe, well-tolerated procedure with a high success rate.

Pleural tumors can be detected and diagnosed with sonography. In patients with pleural origin tumors, either primary or metastatic, pleural implants may hide behind pleural fluid collections and go unnoticed on chest radiography. Sonography can be useful in finding pleural masses and indicating the origin of the pleural collection. In these patients, guided biopsy by real-time sonographic monitoring increases the chances of obtaining tissue.

The purpose of this chapter is to summarize the sonographic features of pleural diseases as well as the role of sonography in the therapeutic work-up of pleural pathology. We describe the technique of pleural sonography, the characteristic US appearances of pleural effusion, pneumothorax, and pleural tumors, and give an overview of US-guided diagnostic and therapeutic procedures.

II. Technique of Pleural Ultrasonography

The optimal frequency of the transducer for pleural US varies with the age of the patient. Young children are best imaged with a high-resolution 5–10 MHz linear-array transducer; adolescents and adults may require 2–4 or 4–7 MHz sector or linear-array transducer (6,11,12). Either a linear or a curved array probe gives a broad view of the near field when used to image through intercostal approach and excellent visualization of the pleura/lung interface is obtained with the transducer sweeping along the intercostal spaces. A sector probe is useful for imaging the diaphragmatic pleura by subxiphoid and transdiaphragmatic approaches with liver or spleen as the acoustic window (7,8,11,12).

Every patient undergoes routine frontal or lateral chest radiography before US. US is performed in the sitting, supine, prone, or decubitus position, with the presumed location of the lesion based on the radiographic findings. In the sitting position the dorsal and lateral costal pleura are visualized, whereas the supine position is preferred for visualizing the ventral costal pleura (7). Images are obtained in the transverse, longitudinal, and inclined transverse or longitudinal planes to maximize demonstration of the pleural lesion. Bedridden and intensive care patients are examined by turning them to the oblique position in the bed.

III. Normal Pleura and Artifacts of Pleural Ultrasonography

The normal pleura is composed of two membranes comprising the opposed visceral and parietal layers, which are seen as a highly echogenic curvilinear structure (Fig. 1a). Between these two layers there are small hypoechoic inhomogeneities. It is not always possible to visualize sonographically both layers

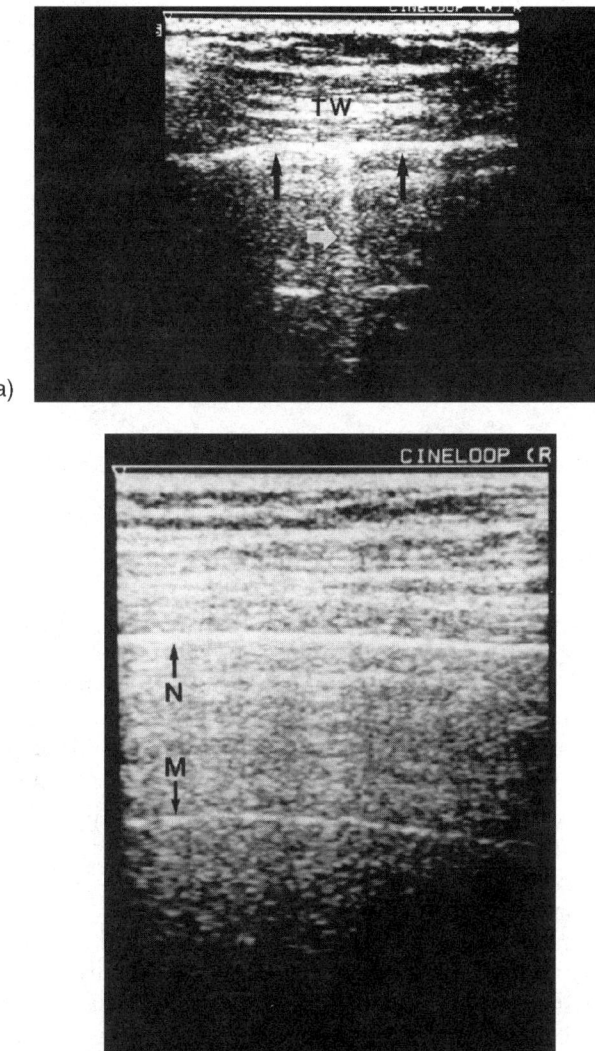

Figure 1 Sonographic normal pleura and artifacts. (a) Normal pleura and comet-tail artifact. Linear transverse US scan shows highly echogenic band of normal pleura opposed parietal and visceral pleura and interface reflection of aerated lung (arrows), which can be distinguished from the thoracic wall (TW). A vertical reverberation echo, comet-tail artifact (white arrow) evoked at the boundary between the visceral pleural and the ventilated lung is also seen. (b) Mirror artifact. Linear transverse US scan shows two echogenic bands, one is normal pleura (N) and the other one is a mirror image (M) of normal pleura in the lung. Duplication of structures outside the pleural space is projected into the lung due to total reflection of sound waves at the lung surface.

and the hypoechoic space between them (7). The echogenic visceral pleura line moves during respiratory excursions. This has been termed the "lung sliding" sign (13). Sometimes the parietal pleura is accompanied by a thin hypoechoic layer and nodular hypoechoic spreading, which represents subpleural fat (7).

At the interphase between the pleura and the ventilated lung tissue, intensive band-like reverberation echoes (comet-tail artifacts) are seen during the breathing movements (14–16) (Fig. 1a). This artifact can be evoked only at the boundary between the visceral pleura and ventilated pulmonary alveoli. Mirror artifacts are commonly seen as duplication of structures external to the pleura projected over the lung because of total reflection of the sound waves at the pleural surface when the US beam strikes the lung surface at certain angles (Fig. 1b).

IV. Pleural Effusion

The conventional chest radiographic findings of pleural fluid collections are variable and depend on the amount and age of the fluid collection. These findings range from complete opacification of the hemithorax to less striking but puzzling areas of increased opacity, especially in patients with loculated empyema or associated peripheral pulmonary lesions (6). The patient with a completely opaque hemithorax is an ideal candidate of sonography for differentiation of massive pleural effusion from pleural or lung masses. The presence of pleural fluid may not be identified with chest radiographs when there is extensive pulmonary consolidation or collapse (17,18). If there is any doubt whether a pleural effusion exists, US allows easy distinction of pleural fluid from increased opacity due to pulmonary parenchymal lesion (Fig. 2).

On US imaging through an intercostal approach, pleural fluid between the parietal and visceral pleura is demarcated with a sharp echogenic line delineating the visceral pleura and lung. Posterior sonic enhancement is absent because the underlying lung usually contains air (7). When scanning through the subxiphoid or transdiaphragmatic approach, the fluid collection is seen behind the liver and just above the diaphragm (19,20). On this view, there are sonographic signs of pleural fluid that help to distinguish it from ascites: the crus sign and *the bare area sign*. The crus sign results from displacement of the diaphragmatic crus away from the spine due to interposition of fluid between the diaphragm and the vertebral column. *The bare area sign* represents fluid collection in the bare area, the posterior part of the right lower lobe of the liver (Fig. 3). All fluid accumulation in this area is necessarily located in the pleural space because the bare area is directly attached to the diaphragm without the covering layer of the peritoneum and peritoneal fluid cannot extend behind this area. Sonography can also demonstrate subpulmonic effusion in patients with an apparently elevated hemidiaphragm on plain chest radiographs (Fig. 4), which is particularly useful to detect hemothorax in trauma patients, accurate, and significantly faster than supine and decubitus portable chest radiography (21,22).

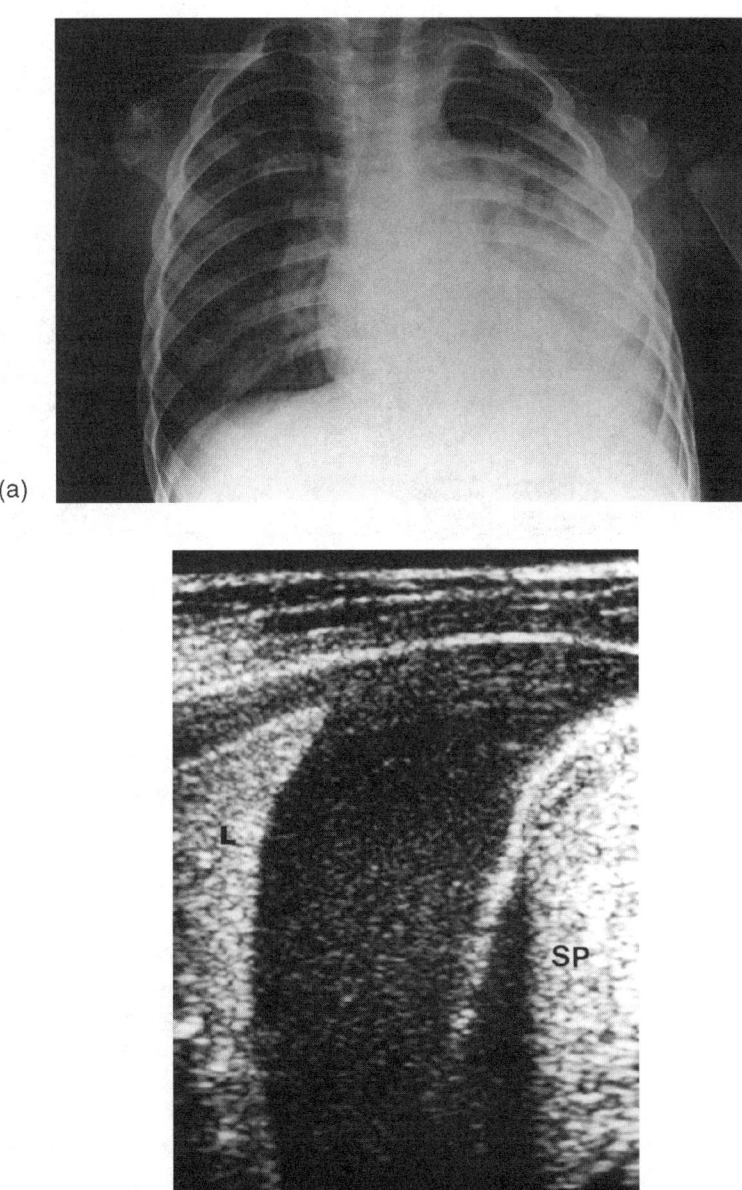

Figure 2 Sonographic distinction of pleural fluid from pneumonia. (a) Chest radiograph shows an ill-defined area of increased opacity in the left lower lobe. (b) Linear longitudinal US scan through the intercostal space at the left lower lobe shows a large amount of subpulmonic hypoechoic effusion between the echogenic area of lower lobe pneumonic consolidation (L) and the spleen (SP). (From Ref. 6.)

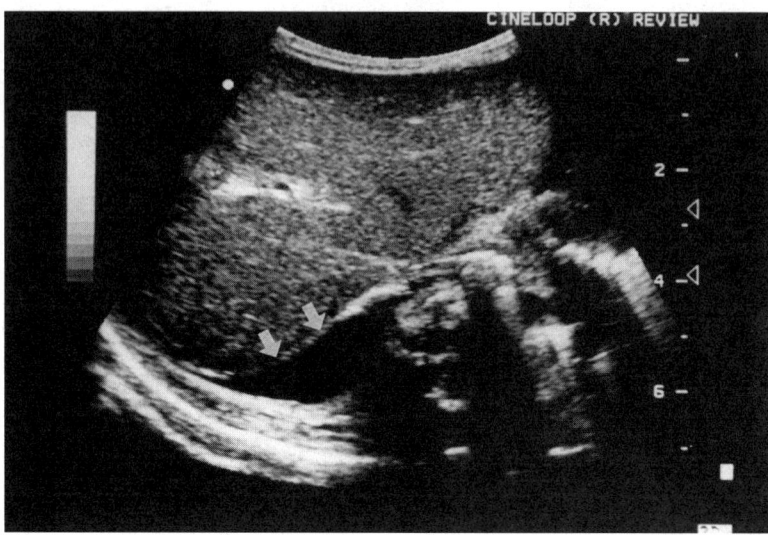

Figure 3 Pleural effusion in the bare area. Sector transdiaphragmatic approach through the liver shows pleural effusion extending behind the right posterior portion of the liver (bare area) (arrows).

At US, pleural fluid may be characterized as a simple or complicated nature of the fluid. Yang et al. (23) assessed the value of sonography in determining the nature of pleural effusions of various causes. A simple effusion appears as clear anechoic or cloudy hypoechoic fluid that may be transudates or exudates. Transudates are almost always echo-free, whereas about half of the exudates are echogenic (24). Most exudative pleural effusion is of infectious origin, which is known as parapneumonic effusion or empyema. Hypoechoic and echogenic fluid may contain diffusely distributed swirling or floating echogenicities that reflecting particles in the fluid, e.g., cells, protein, fibrin, or blood (7) (Fig. 5). Homogeneous echogenic effusions may be due to hemorrhagic effusion or empyema.

As exudative fluid collections organize, mobile, linear structures of fibrin bands or to-and-fro motion of septa, which are typical for inflammatory effusions, tend to occur (Fig. 6). This complicated effusion appears as septated or multiloculated, hypoechoic fluid. In some empyemas, the septa are so profuse that they produce a honeycomb appearance (Fig. 7). The septated or multiloculated nature of pleural fluid may not be visible with computed tomography (CT). The lung could be captured by inflammation and may not slide up and down during the respiratory cycle and no clear demarcation is visualized between the lung and pleural components (23). Sonographic findings of thickening of the parietal and visceral pleura and associated parenchymal lesions in the lung are most likely indicative of empyemas.

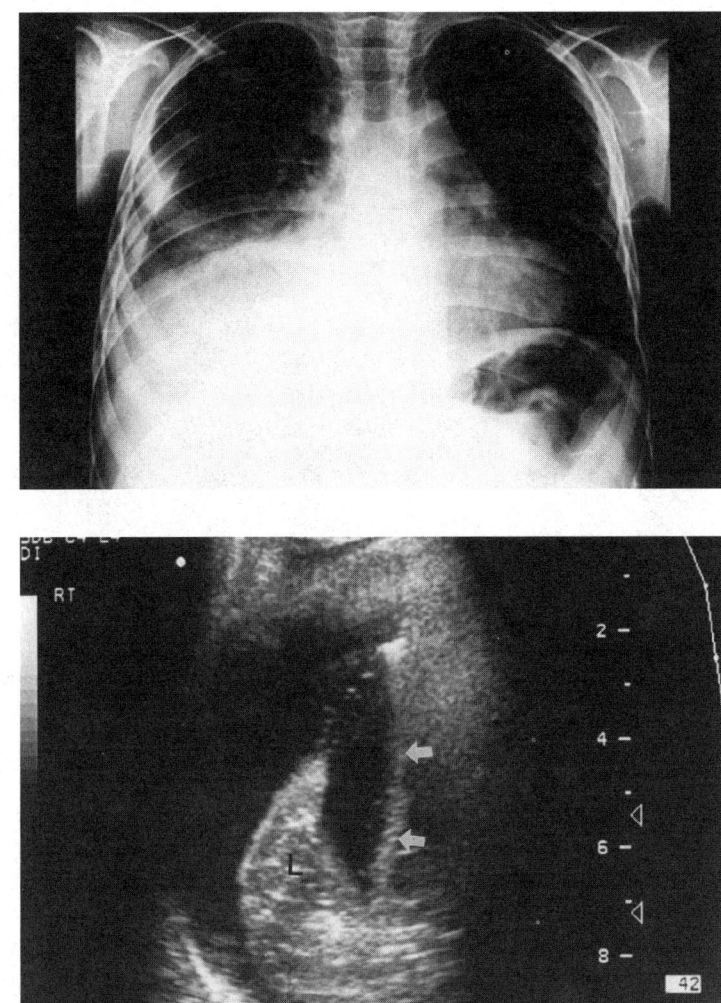

Figure 4 Elevated hemidiaphragm due to extensive subpulmonic pleural effusion. (a) Chest radiograph shows the elevated right hemidiaphragm associated with pleural effusion along the major fissure. (b) Sector oblique longitudinal US scan shows extensive pleural effusion in the subpulmonic and lateral pleural space with collapse of the right lower lobe (L). The right hemidiaphragm (arrows) is not elevated but everted due to subpulmonic effusion.

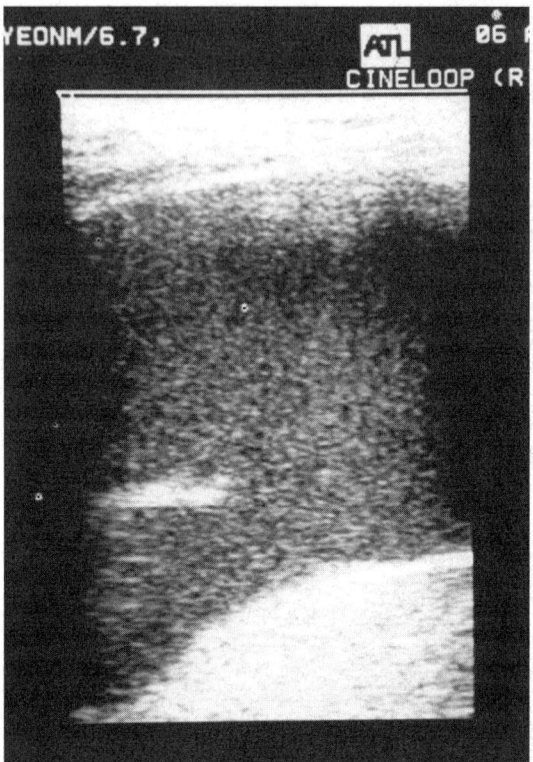

Figure 5 Homogeneously echogenic effusion in empyema. Linear transverse US scan demonstrates echogenic free fluid that reflecting floating particles.

With advance of pleural fluid organization, extensive pleural thickening or fibrothorax may ensue. This appears as echogenic, solid-appearing pleural plaque with or without some loculation of fluid (Fig. 8). Honeycomb pattern of fluid collection and pleural plaque are predictive of significant difficulties with thoracentesis. US performed with a high-resolution transducer is sensitive in demonstrating the internal derangement about the nature of pleural changes and provides detailed information to determine the planning of therapeutic approaches (6).

Septated fluids caused by fibrous strands are mainly observed in infected exudative fluid, but also in malignant effusion (25,26), and may very rarely be found in patients with tuberculous pleurisy (27) and more often in asbestosis (28). In these latter benign cases, pleural nodularities may be observed over the pleural surface on thoracoscopic studies. These nodules are characterized by small, white-gray nodules, which have a low diagnostic yield in confirming those small nodules on sonography, even on CT. Although sonographic evidence of pleural nodules is a specific finding in patients with a malignant

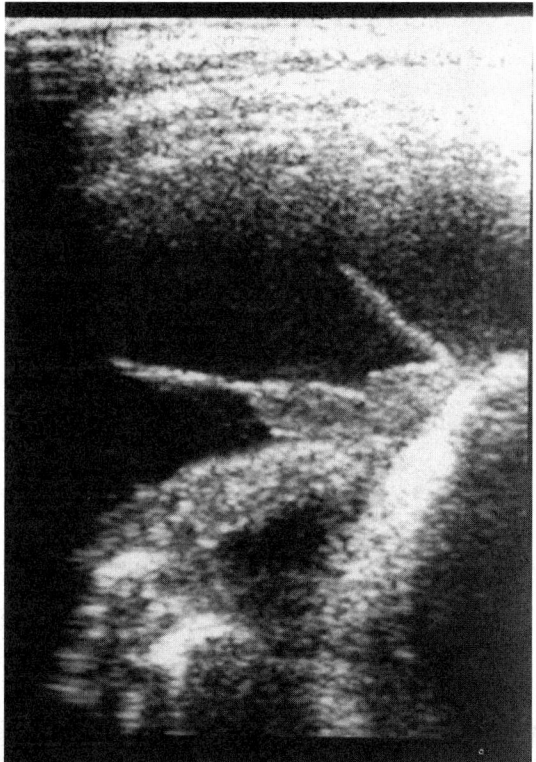

Figure 6 Fibrin bands in empyema. Linear transverse scan shows to-and-fro motion of echogenic bands within the anechoic pleural fluid. (From Ref. 6.)

effusion, sonographic differentiation between benign and malignant pleural fluid is possible only if solid nodular structures are visible (24,26). US detection of large, confluent pleural masses greater than 1 cm is indicative of malignant effusion (25) (Fig. 9).

As pleural scars and thickening appear as echogenic rind of pleural plaque, the discrimination between echogenic pleural fluid and solid pleural thickening may be difficult. It is important to determine by the nature of pleural changes whether thoracentesis is feasible. Characterization of pleural changes with US is very informative in guiding thoracentesis. Useful features in distinguishing fluid and solid thickening are changes in the shape of the fluid when the fluid shifts in response to a change in patient position or respiration, as well as demonstration of echogenic floating debris (6,18,29). Both exudates and hemorrhage may demonstrate floating echogenic debris. Wu et al. (30) described a "fluid color" sign, which is a color signal that appears within the fluid collection in the pleural space. The moving debris within the effusion may scatter the sound and produce color Doppler signals. In their study of 76

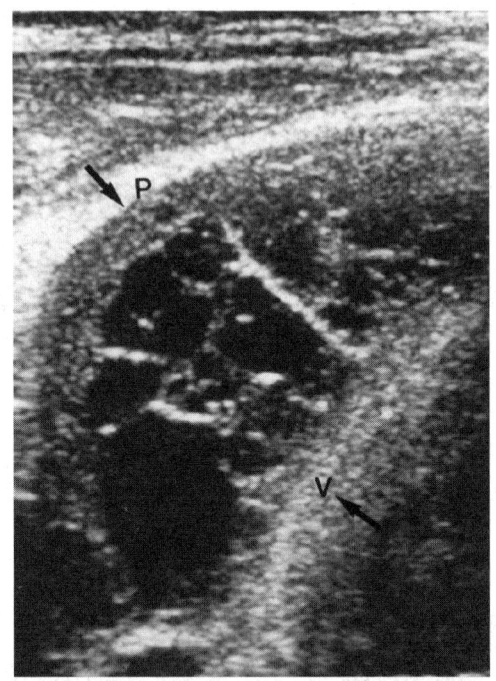

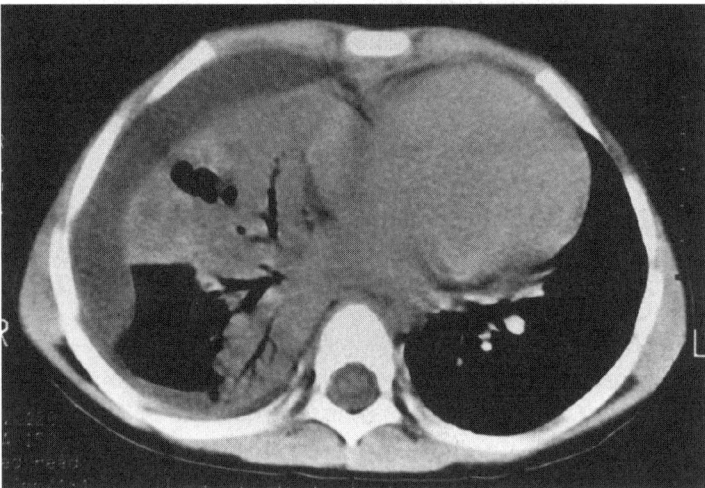

Figure 7 Complicated pleural effusion with multiple loculi. (a) The pleural space is filled with profusely septated fluid, which has a honeycomb appearance. Extensive thickening of the parietal (P) and visceral (V) pleura encircles the septated fluid. (b) CT scan in the same patient on the same day shows a rind of hypoattenuating pleural effusion. The multiloculated nature of the effusion is not visualized on CT.

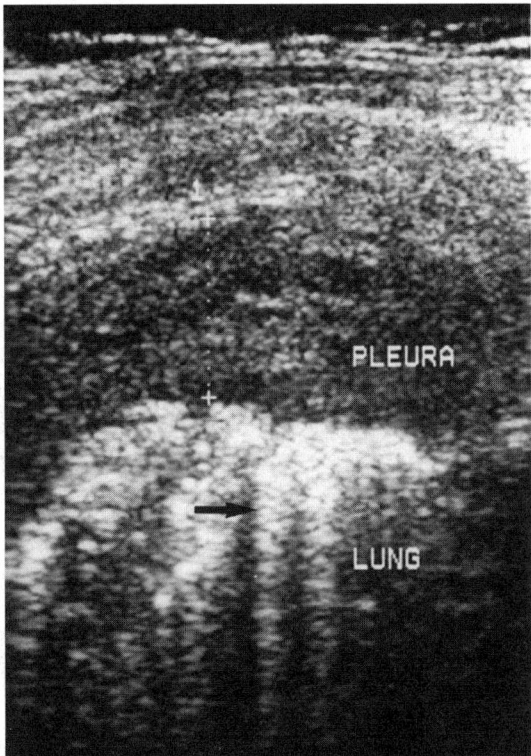

Figure 8 Adhesive fibrotic pleural thickening in the advanced empyema. Linear transverse US scan shows thick, echogenic plaque filling the pleural space (PLEURA). Comet-tail reverberation echoes (arrows) are seen at the boundary of thickened visceral pleura and the aerated lung. (From Ref. 6.)

patients, the fluid color sign had a sensitivity of 89.2% and specificity of 100% in discriminating pleural fluid from pleural thickening.

Pleural thickening may occur diffusely. According to Leung et al. (28), parietal pleural thickening of more than 1 cm on CT was specific for malignancy in 94%. In benign exudative effusions, associated pleural thickening is usually of less than 1 cm and combined mostly with a lung parenchymal change. Akhan et al. (27) reported thickening of the pleura in one third of their patients with nonmalignant pleural effusions, especially tuberculous effusions. In almost all cases, thickness was less than 1 cm and decreased with treatment within 6 months. Therefore, pleural thickening of more than 1 cm should arouse a high suspicion of malignancy (25).

Several studies have been performed to measure the volume of pleural effusion by means of sonography. Lorenz et al. (31) used a planimetric method that is measurement of the square dimensions of effusion in various longitu-

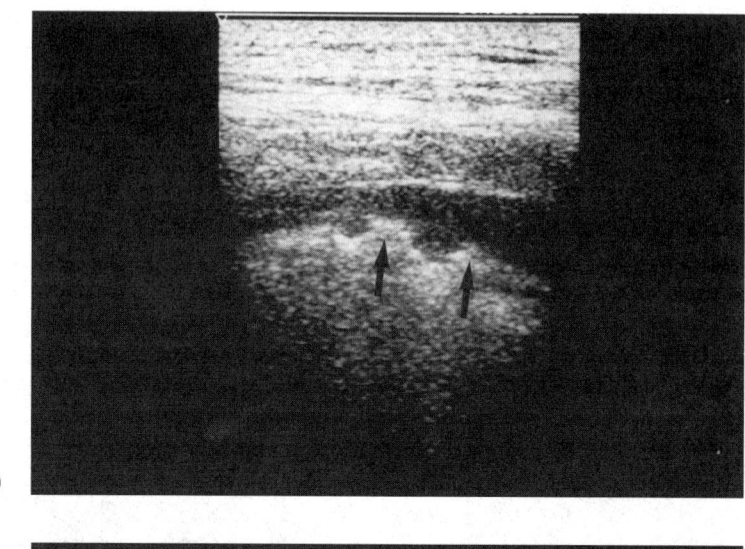

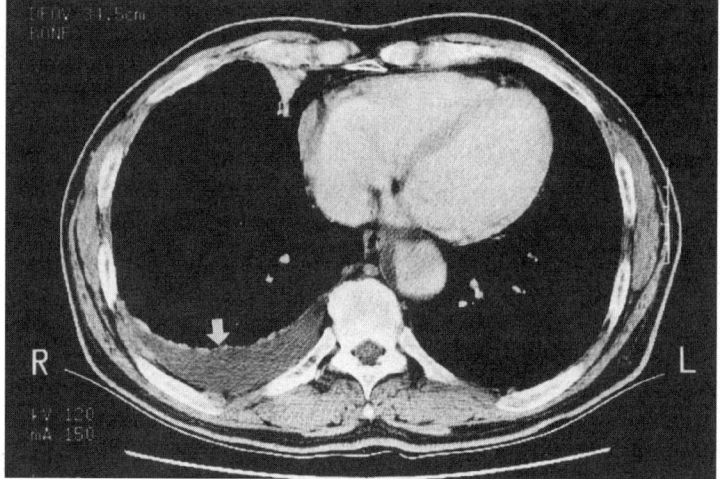

Figure 9 Pleural nodules in malignant pleural effusion. (a) Linear transverse US scan shows nodular appearance of the visceral pleura (arrows), which is well delineated by hypoechoic pleural effusion. Biopsy showed metastatic squamous cell carcinoma of the pleura. (b) CT scan in a same patient shows hypoattenuating pleural effusion with irregularity of the visceral pleura (arrow).

dinal and transverse sections. In planimetry of the effusion, planes were scanned in longitudinal sections at six positions, and the mean value was multiplied by the chest circumference and by an empirical correlation factor of 0.89. Using this procedure, the effusion volume could be calculated with a statistical variability of less than 10%. Eibenberger et al. (32) measured the maximum thickness of the pleural fluid layer with lateral decubitus radiography and supine sonography. With sonographic measurement, an effusion width of 20 mm had a mean volume of 380 mL ± 130 (standard deviation), while one of 40 mm had a mean volume of 1000 mL ± 330. Those values were compared with actual effusion volumes determined by means of complete drainage. Sonographic measurements correlated significantly better with actual effusion volume than did radiographic measurements.

V. Pleural Tumors

Benign pleural neoplasms, such as fibromas, lipomas, neurogenic tumors, and chondromas, are rounded, sharply marginated masses of high or mixed echogenicity. Localized fibrous tumor of pleura, a relatively uncommon neoplasm, appears as well-circumscribed and non-calcified hyperechoic soft tissue masses forming an obtuse angle with the chest wall (14,15). Malignant mesotheliomas are usually visualized as diffuse irregular thickenings of the pleura, including localized nodules. Large pleural effusions occur frequently together with mesotheliomas (7).

Metastases constitute the overwhelming majority of malignant neoplasms involving the pleura. Metastatic disease to the pleura often causes large pleural effusions that are probably due to impaired lymphatic drainage (19). In some patients pleural fluid is so profuse that it may mask the tumoral masses on chest radiography. Most pleural metastases are too small to be detected. However, metastases larger than 5 mm in diameter on the parietal or diaphragmatic pleura can be detected by sonography. These nodules are round, oval, broad-based, echogenic or moderately echogenic, and well delineated against effusion (Figs. 9, 10).

Sonography is useful in the evaluation of parietal pleural invasion of peripheral lung tumors and an easy and safe method for guiding pleural biopsy of either pleural masses or processes that cause diffuse pleural thickening (33). Real-time sonography can easily exclude parietal pleural invasion of bronchogenic carcinoma by assessing mobility of the tumor during breathing. If the tumor is sonographically fixed during breathing and disruption of the pleural band of reflections is present, neoplastic infiltration of parietal pleura should be highly suspected. However, a fixed peripheral pulmonary tumor with disruption of the pleura cannot confidently be diagnosed as being invasive because associated desmoplastia and inflammation can simulate tumor extension into the adjacent pleura (34). In a study by Suzuki et al. (33), who compared the usefulness of sonography and CT in this respect on 120 patients, sonography

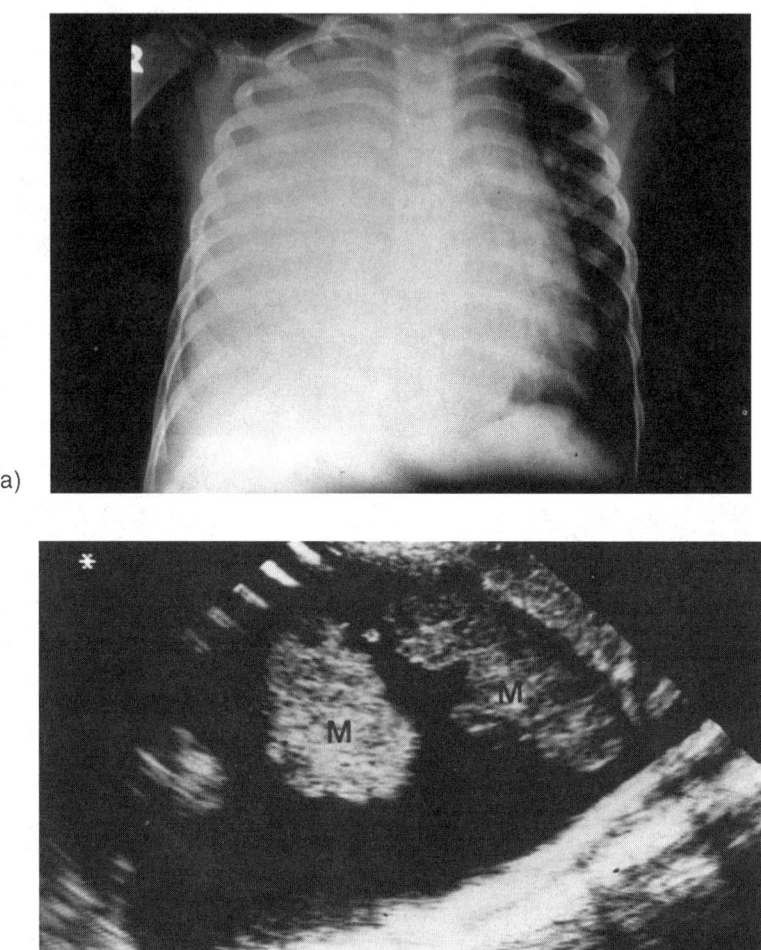

Figure 10 Opaque hemithorax due to massive pleural effusion caused by pleural metastasis. (a) Chest radiograph shows complete opacification of the right hemithorax. (b) Sector longitudinal US scan shows a massive anechoic effusion containing large echogenic masses (M), which were metastasis from Wilms tumor. (From Ref. 6.)

revealed a sensitivity of 100% (CT 68%), a specificity of 98% (CT 66%), and an accuracy of 98% (CT 67%).

For the further evaluation of pleural masses seen on plain radiographs, either sonography or CT can be used. CT has a distinct advantage in the evaluation of pleural diseases in that it can easily evaluate all parts of the pleura including the mediastinal pleura, and thus provide accurate information about the extent of disease and better detect involvement of adjacent structures and pleural-based parenchymal pulmonary lesions. Wernecke (15) recommended that CT be the first method of choice in the assessment of diffuse pleural disease and stated that it generally is also superior to sonography in the assessment of focal disease.

VI. Pneumothorax

The normal pleura/lung interface is identified by virtue of respiratory motion (sliding sign) at real-time scanning and by the detection of comet-tail artifacts at the interface. Wernecke et al. (16) reported that pneumothorax could be diagnosed by sonography on the basis of these findings. The observations were subsequently confirmed by Lichtenstein and Menu (13) and Targhetta et al. (35,36). However, a very small amount of air in the pleural space prevents sonographic visualization of visceral pleural movements and comet-tail artifacts.

Although early studies demonstrated accurate pneumothorax detection with sonography, Sistrom et al. (37) reported relatively poor performance of sonography. They blindly compared taped thoracic ultrasound examinations of patients with variable-sized pneumothoraces to determine the efficacy of real-time sonography for the detection and estimation of the volume of pneumothorax. They concluded that real-time sonography is useful to localize known pneumothorax but cannot be used to exclude the diagnosis. Sonography has a significant false-positive rate and is of no use in estimating the volume of a pneumothorax.

Recently, Goodman et al. (38) used CT as a gold standard to compare sonography and erect chest radiographs in detecting pneumothorax after CT-guided lung biopsy. They reported that sonography was more sensitive than erect chest radiography. Modest pneumothorax could be inferred by the ultrasound sign of "partial lung sliding," consisting of visualization of lung sliding in a portion of the scanning window with adjacent absence of sliding noted in the same window. As the volume of pneumothorax increased, they noted a progressive loss of movement of lung sliding from the anterior window, to the lateral thorax, and finally to the posterior window.

VII. Ultrasonography-Guided Thoracentesis and Catheter Drainage

It is clear that sonography has important implications in the management of pleural effusion because of its ability to characterize the internal composition of pleural fluid. Diagnostic thoracentesis can be performed safely at the bedside without imaging guidance if the effusion is reasonably large, extending over several rib spaces on the chest radiograph. When the effusion is smaller than this, associated with underlying pulmonary collapse, or is loculated, aspiration becomes a difficult task. One of the main difficulties for clinicians performing unguided pleural aspiration is correctly identifying the level of the hemidiaphragm, thereby avoiding inadvertent infradiaphragmatic puncture of either liver or spleen. If diaphragmatic elevation is suspected on the chest radiograph, ultrasound should be performed (39).

There is still a great deal of controversy around the clinical management of empyema (40). Two main treatment approaches are used: nonoperative, in which patients are treated with antibiotics alone or combined with thoracentesis or tube drainage thoracotomy, and operative, where the good of treatment is to evacuate infected debris and reexpand the lung. Sonography is used for guidance of therapeutic thoracentesis and tube drainage of parapneumonic effusions or empyemas. Sonography clearly shows the extent of fluid collection and, therefore, is an ideal guide for thoracentesis. Furthermore, it is also an excellent modality as a guide to aspiration and drainage of pleural fluid (10,41). Urokinase instillation through the catheter can facilitate the drainage of thoracic empyema. Park et al. (42) used sonography to predict the effectiveness of urokinase in the treatment of loculated pleural effusion and found that urokinase instillation was not effective in patients whose pleural fluid had a honeycomb septation pattern on sonographic scans or whose parietal pleura was more than 5 mm thick on CT scans. Pleurodesis can be performed through sonographically placed small-bore catheters (7–15 Fr) for recurrent malignant pleural effusions or recurrent pneumothoraces with success rates comparable to those seen with large-bore, surgically placed catheters (43–45).

The sonography-guided technique has been shown to be a safe, well-tolerated procedure for obtaining fluid from the pleural space with a high success rate (46–49). However, sonography-guided thoracentesis is not always successful. Typical errors are misinterpretation of hypoechoic or anechoic lesions as fluid collection. Coagulated blood may be anechoic, whereas some tumors such as lymphomas, hamartomas, and neurogenic tumors could be very low echogenic (7).

Pneumothorax, the most common complication of pleural taps, is exceedingly rare when the procedure is performed under sonographic control. Pneumothorax rates for guided thoracentesis have been reported at 2–3%, with approximately half of these needing treatment (47–49). This compares favorably with unguided diagnostic thoracentesis rates of 9–13%. In addition, guided aspiration reduces the failure rate of aspiration from 10 to 3% (41,47) and avoids the complications associated with an elevated diaphragm. The placement of large (24–28 F) drains without imaging guidance is associated with a relatively high failure rate. One of the major reasons for this is malpositioning of the tube, and complications including laceration of the diaphragm, spleen, and liver can be avoided by ultrasound- or CT-guided drainage using catheters of 8–14 Fr (39).

Sonographically guided aspiration can be attempted either in the radiology department or at the patient's bedside using a portable machine. The latter is particularly valuable for patients in the intensive care unit. In some centers ultrasound is performed to confirm the presence of fluid and identify the best site for aspiration, which is then marked with the measurement of depth for the needle to penetrate and the patient returned to the ward for pleural aspiration by the referring clinician (39). It is particularly helpful for critically ill patients when tedious radiographic study is not possible and safe thoracentesis is mandatory.

VIII. Ultrasonography-Guided Pleural Biopsy

Although thoracentesis or closed pleural biopsy can often establish the diagnosis of pleural malignancy, those methods may not provide enough diagnostic material to confirm the presence of malignancy. Unguided pleural biopsy using Cope or Abram needle is safely performed only when the amount of pleural effusion or pneumothorax is sufficient. When the pleural disease may be focally involved, real-time US is useful in guiding pleural biopsy of focal or diffuse pleural lesions, particularly when pleural fluid is absent or minimal. Sonography clearly shows thickened pleura or pleural tumors, and the passage of biopsy needles can be monitored. Sonography guidance of the needle biopsy can increase the chances of obtaining tissue with significant pathological changes (50).

Ruffie et al. (51) reported that percutaneous needle biopsy produced sufficient tissue to diagnose malignant pleural mesothelioma in only about one third of their cases. Thus, very often it was necessary to perform open surgical biopsy. Chang et al. (52) compared non-guided biopsy with Abrams biopsy needle and with sonography-guided pleural biopsy with a Tru-cut needle in patients with malignant pleural disease. Cut needle biopsy findings were positive for malignant disease in 7 of 10 patients, but only 4 of 9 patients had positive biopsy findings at nonguided Abrams biopsy.

By using imaging guidance, the accuracy of biopsy has been remarkably increased (53–58). There are some reports in which both CT and sonography were used as guidance in cutting-needle biopsy of malignant pleural effusion (57). The overall accuracy of a correct histological diagnosis of malignant and benign pleural diseases was 91% in cutting-needle biopsy and 78% of sensitivity in fine needle aspiration. The cutting-needle biopsy was more sensitive than fine needle aspiration overall. Heilo et al. (59) reported that sonography-guided core-needle biopsy had a sensitivity of 77%, specificity of 88%, accuracy of 80%, positive predictive value of 100%, and negative predictive value of 57%. There were no serious complications. Adams and Gleeson (53) reported that image-guided fine needle aspiration results were suggestive but not diagnostic for mesothelioma in 5 of 12 patients with mesothelioma with a sensitivity of 50%. Compared with cutting-needle biopsy, fine needle aspiration is less sensitive in establishing the diagnosis of mesothelioma. Sonography-guided core-needle biopsy of possible malignant pleural mesothelioma may become the method of choice owing to its high accuracy and ease of performance. In conclusion, ultrasonography-guided pleural biopsy is a readily available, generally quick and safe procedure with which to establish the diagnosis of pleural malignancy.

References

1. Joyner CR Jr, Herman RJ, Reid JM. Reflected ultrasound in the detection and localization of pleural effusion. JAMA 1967; 200:129–132.
2. Doust BD, Baum JK, Maklad NF, Doust VL. Ultrasonic evaluation of pleural opacities. Radiology 1975; 114:134–140.
3. Hirsch JH, Rogers JV, Mack LA. Real-time sonography of pleural opacities. AJR Am J Roentgenol 1981; 136:297–301.
4. Lipscomb DJ, Flower CDR, Hadfield JW. Ultrasound of the pleura: an assessment of its clinical value. Clin Radiol 1981; 32:289–290.
5. Miller JH, Reid BS, Kemberling CR. Water-path ultrasound of chest disease in childhood. Radiology 1984; 152:401–408.
6. Kim OH, Kim WS, Kim MJ, Jung JY, Suh JH. US in the diagnosis of pediatric chest diseases. RadioGraphics 2000; 20:653–671.
7. Mathis G. Thorax sonography—part I: chest wall and pleura. Ultrasound Med Biol 1997; 23:1131–1139.
8. McLoud TC, Flower CDR. Imaging the pleura: sonography, CT, and MR imaging. AJR Am J Roentgenol 1991; 156:1145–1153.
9. Müller NL. Imaging of the pleura. Radiology 1993; 186:297–309.
10. Yang PC. Ultrasound-guided transthoracic biopsy of the chest. Radiol Clin North Am 2000; 38:323–343.
11. Ben-Ami TE, O'Dpmpvam KC, Yousefzadeh DK. Sonography of the chest in children. Radiol Clin North Am 1993; 31:517–531.
12. Herman TE, McAlister WH, Siegel MJ. Chest. In: Siegel MJ, ed. Pediatric Sonography. 2d ed. New York: Raven, 1995:139–155.
13. Lichtenstein DA, Menu Y. A bedside ultrasound ruling out pneumothorax in the critically ill. Lung sliding. Chest 1995; 108:1345–1348.
14. Wernecke K. Sonographic features of pleural disease. AJR Am J Roentgenol 1997; 168:1061–1066.
15. Wernecke K. Ultrasound study of the pleura. Eur Radiol 2000; 10:1515–1523.
16. Wernecke K, Galanski M, Peter PE. Pneumothorax: evaluation by ultrasound—preliminary results. J Thorac Imaging 1987; 2:76–78.
17. Rosenberg ER. Ultrasound in the assessment of pleural densities. Chest 1983; 84:283–285.
18. Yu CJ, Yang PC, Yang DB, Luh KT. Diagnostic and therapeutic use of chest sonography: value in critically ill patients. AJR Am J Roentgenol 1992; 159:695–701.
19. Enriquez G, Serres X. Ultrasound of the pediatric lung parenchyma and pleura. In: Brunelle F, Strife JL, eds. Syllabus: 4th International Pediatric Radiology Postgraduate Course, Paris, May 28–29, 2001. Milan: Springer, IPR, 2001:132–136.

20. Seibert JJ, Glasier CM, Leithiser RE. The pediatric chest. In: Rumack CM, Wilson SR, Charboneau JW, eds. Diagnostic Ultrasound. 2d ed. St.Louis: Mosby-Year Book, 1998:1617–1644.
21. Ma OJ, Mateer JR. Trauma ultrasound examination versus chest radiography in the detection of hemothorax. Ann Emerg Med 1997; 29:312–315.
22. Sisley AC, Rozycki GS, Ballard RB, Namias N, Salomone JP, Feliciano DV. Rapid detection of traumatic effusion using surgeon-performed ultrasonography. J Trauma 1998; 44:291–296.
23. Yang PC, Luh KT, Chang DB, Wu HD, Yu CJ, Kuo SH. Value of sonography in determining the nature of pleural effusion: analysis of 320 cases. AJR Am J Roentgenol 1992; 159:29–33.
24. Reuß J. Sonographic imaging of the pleura: nearly 30 years experience. Eur J Ultrasound 1996; 3:125–139.
25. Görg C, Restrepo I, Schwerk WB. Sonography of malignant pleural effusion. Eur Radiol 1997; 7:1195–1198.
26. Görg C, Schwerk WB, Goerg K, Walters E. Pleural effusion: an "acoustic window" for sonography of pleural metastases. J Clin Ultrasound 1991; 19:93–97.
27. Akhan O, Demirkazik FB, Özmen MN, Balkanci F. Tuberculous pleural effusions: ultrasonic diagnosis. J Clin Ultrasound 1992; 20:461–465.
28. Leung AN, Müller NL, Miller RR. CT in differential diagnosis of diffuse pleural disease. AJR Am J Roentgenol 1990; 154:487–492.
29. Lomas DG, Padley SG, Flower CD. The sonographic appearances of pleural fluid. Br J Radiol 1993; 66:619–624.
30. Wu RG, Yang PC, Kuo SH, Luh KT. "Fluid color" sign: a useful indicator for discrimination between pleural thickening and pleural effusion. J Ultrasound Med 1995; 14:767–769.
31. Lorenz J, Börner N, Nikolaus HP. Volumetry of pleural effusions by chest ultrasound. Ultraschall Med 1988; 9:212–215.
32. Eibenberger KL, Dock WI, Ammann ME, Dorffner R, Hormann MF, Grabenwoger F. Quantification of pleural effusions: sonography versus radiography. Radiology 1994; 191:681–684.
33. Suzuki N, Saitoh T, Kitamura S. Tumor invasion of the chest wall in lung cancer: diagnosis with US. Radiology 1993; 187:39–42.
34. Baron RL, Levih RG, Sagel SS. Computed tomography in the preoperative evaluation of bronchogenic carcinoma. Radiology 1982; 145:727–732.
35. Targhetta R, Bourgeois JM, Chavagneux R, Marty-Double C, Balmes P. Ultrasonographic approach to diagnosing hydropneumothorax. Chest 1992; 101:931–934.
36. Targhetta R, Bourgeois JM, Chavagneux R, Coste E, Amy D, Balmes P, Pourcelot L. Ultrasonic signs of pneumothorax: preliminary work. J Clin Ultrasound 1993; 21:245–250.
37. Sistrom CL, Reiheld CT, Gay SB, Wallace KK. Detection and estimation of the volume of pneumothorax using real-time sonography: efficacy determined by receiver operating characteristic analysis. AJR Am J Roentgenol 1996; 166:317–321.
38. Goodman TR, Traill ZC, Philips AJ, et al. Ultrasound detection of pneumothorax. Clin Radiol 1999; 54:736–739.
39. Patel MC, Flower CDR. Radiology in the management of pleural disease. Eur Radiol 1997; 7:1454–1462.
40. Ramnath RR, Heller RM, Ben-Ami T, Miller MA, Campbell P, Neblett WW III, Holcomb GW, Hernanz-Schulman M. Implications of early sonographic evalua-

tion of parapneumonic effusions in children with pneumonia. Pediatrics 1998; 101:68–71.
41. O'Moore PV, Mueller PR, Simeone JF, Saini S, Butch RJ, Hahn PF, Steiner E, Stark DD, Ferrucci JT Jr. Sonographic guidance in diagnostic and therapeutic interventions in the pleural space. AJR Am J Roentgenol 1987; 149:1–5.
42. Park CS, Chung WM, Lim MK, Cho CH, Suh CH, Chung WK. Transcatheter instillation of urokinase into loculated pleural effusion: analysis of treatment effect. AJR Am J Roentgenol 1996; 167:649–652.
43. Morrison MC, Mueller PR, Lee MJ, Saini S, Brink JA, Dawson SL, Cortell ED, Hahn PF. Sclerotherapy of malignant pleural effusion through sonographically placed small-bore catheters. AJR Am J Roentgenol 1992; 158:41–43.
44. Parker LA, Charnock GC, Delany DJ. Small bore catheter drainage and sclerotherapy for malignant pleural effusions. Cancer 1989; 64:1218–1221.
45. Seaton KG, Patz EF Jr, Goodman PC. Palliative treatment of malignant pleural effusions: value of small-bore catheter thoracostomy and doxycycline sclerotherapy. AJR Am J Roentgenol 1995; 164:589–591.
46. Harnsberger HR, Lee TG, Mukuno DH. Rapid, inexpensive real time directed thoracentesis. Radiology 1983; 146:545–546.
47. Seneff MG, Corwin RW, Gold LH. Complications associated with thoracentesis. Chest 1986; 90:97–100.
48. Collins TR, Sahn SA. Thoracentesis: clinical value, complications, technical problems, and patient experience. Chest 1987; 91:817–822.
49. Silverman SG, Saini S, Mueller PR. Pleural intervention: indications, techniques, and clinical applications. Radiol Clin North Am 1989; 27:1257–1266.
50. Yang PC, Kuo SH, Luh KT. Ultrasonography and ultrasound guided needle biopsy of chest diseases: indications, techniques, diagnostic yields and complications. J Med Ultrasound 1993; 2:53–63.
51. Ruffie P, Feld R, Minkin S, Cormier Y, Boutan-Laroze A, Ginsberg R, Ayoub J, Shepherd FA, Evans WK, Figueredo A, et al. Diffuse malignant mesothelioma of the pleura in Ontario and Quebec: a retrospective study of 332 patients. J Clin Oncol 1989; 7:1157–1168.
52. Chang DB, Yang PC, Luh KT, Kuo SH, Yu CJ. Ultrasound-guided pleural biopsy with Tru-cut needle. Chest 1991; 100:1328–1333.
53. Adams RF, Gleeson FV. Percutaneous image-guided cutting-needle biopsy of the pleura in the presence of a suspected malignant pleural effusion. Radiology 2001; 219:510–514.
54. Rusch VW. Diagnosis and treatment of pleural mesothelioma. Semin Surg Oncol 1990; 6:279–285.
55. Heilo A. US-guided transthoracic biopsy. Eur J Ultrasound 1996; 3:141–151.
56. Scott EM, Marshall TJ, Flower CDR, Stewart S. Diffuse pleural thickening: percutaneous CT-guided cutting needle biopsy. Radiology 1995; 194:867–870.
57. Metintas M, Ozdemir N, Isiksoy S, Kaya T, Ekici M, Erginel S, Harmanci E, Erdinc P, Ulgey N, Alatas F. CT-guided pleural needle biopsy in the diagnosis of malignant mesothelioma. J Comput Assist Tomogr 1995; 19:370–374.
58. Mueller PR, Saini S, Simeone JF, Silverman SG, Morris E, Hahn PF, Forman BH, McLoud TC, Shepard JO, Ferrucci JT Jr. Image-guided pleural biopsies: indication, technique, and results in 23 patients. Radiology 1988; 169:1–4.
59. Heilo A, Stenwig AE, Solheim ØP. Malignant pleural mesothelioma: US-guided histologic core-needle biopsy. Radiology 1999; 211:657–659.

8

Pleural Thoracentesis and Biopsy

ANDREAS H. DIACON and CHRIS T. BOLLIGER

University of Stellenbosch
and Tygerberg Hospital
Capetown, South Africa

I. Introduction

Diagnostic thoracentesis has been performed for more than 150 years and remains the first step to take in the evaluation of a pleural effusion of unknown origin (1). Thoracentesis can be combined with closed needle pleural biopsy, a procedure first described in 1955 and refined thereafter (2). The analysis of pleural fluid offers the opportunity to diagnose the underlying disease directly, or provides valuable information for narrowing the spectrum of possible causes. Moreover, pleural fluid findings may precipitate immediate therapeutic steps in parapneumonic effusions or empyema. Closed needle biopsy, although less often practiced nowadays, is of importance in tuberculosis (tb) pleurisy, and pleural malignancy. Diagnostic thoracentesis as well as closed needle biopsy are simple and straightforward procedures, and severe complications are rare. This chapter will discuss the technique, indications and contraindications, yield, complications and limitations of each method. Slight overlap with other chapters may occur where diagnostic yields are dealt with, and the reader is kindly asked to consult the relevant chapters for in-depth information about specific diseases.

II. Indications, Contraindications

A. Diagnostic Thoracentesis

Diagnostic pleurocentesis to obtain up to 50 mL of pleural fluid is indicated in almost all patients with pleural effusion of unknown origin. If a pleural effusion can be explained by a known medical condition with a high degree of certainty, a watchful waiting strategy may be endorsed. The same is true for expected transudative effusions, since their diagnostic value is limited. In all instances where an exudative effusion is likely, analysis of a pleural effusion offers an excellent opportunity to diagnose the underlying disease. In a series of 129 consecutive patients, a definitive diagnosis could be made in 18% of cases with pleural fluid analysis, and a presumptive diagnosis in up to 75% of cases when correlated with clinical findings. Moreover, previously suspected diseases could be excluded in many cases (3).

With closed needle biopsy, a small piece of pleura is obtained for histological and microbiological evaluation. Because of the higher morbidity and the higher cost of needle biopsy, routine use with every thoracentesis is not generally recommended (4). Since its first description in 1955, closed needle pleural biopsy has been an important diagnostic tool in pleural effusions of unknown origin (2). Its indications have, however, been narrowed to suspected pleural malignancy and tuberculous pleurisy by the American Thoracic Society (ATS) in 1989, and the use of closed needle biopsy has decreased further in recent years (5). Since operator experience is crucial for the yield of the method, declining levels of experience may further decrease the effectiveness of the procedure (6). There is ongoing controversy about the role of closed needle biopsy in current practice due to advances in pleural fluid analysis and revived interest in thoracoscopy (4). We recommend closed needle biopsy when tuberculous pleurisy is suspected, with chemical analysis of adenosine deaminase (AdA) or gamma-interferon (IFN-γ) remaining inconclusive, or when pleural malignancy is suspected despite repeatedly negative cytology and thoracoscopy is not available.

There are no absolute contraindications to performing a diagnostic pleurocentesis. If the management of the patient is likely to be influenced by findings in the pleural fluid, a diagnostic pleurocentesis can also be done in patients with relative contraindications like bleeding diathesis and anticoagulation, while closed needle pleural biopsy is contraindicated in cases with severe coagulopathy. Caution is warranted for both procedures in patients with chest wall infections, and the risk of transferring the infection into the pleural space at the site of puncture must be individually assessed. In patients with small effusions, ultrasound assistance may be required. Mechanically ventilated patients are at increased risk for pneumothorax, but pleurocentesis can be safely done with ultrasound guidance (7). In empyema, closed needle biopsies are rarely indicated, which minimizes the risk of a subcutaneous abscess. A risk-benefit ratio based on clinical grounds should be calculated in patients with an unstable medical condition (5).

Pleural Thoracentesis and Biopsy

III. Technique

A. Positioning

It is important to take enough time to position the patient and operator for a pleural procedure, serving both the patient's comfort and the operator's need for easy access to the pleural puncture or biopsy site. Both diagnostic pleurocentesis and pleural biopsy are best performed with the patient sitting upright on the side of a bed or stretcher, facing away from the investigator, with arms crossed and resting on a bedside table. The feet should rest on a footstool. The operating height should be adjusted to accommodate the operating physician, excessive bending over should be avoided, and enough space for the necessary tools to be laid out must be provided (Fig. 1). For patients unable to sit, a puncture can be attempted in the midaxillary line with the head of the bed maximally elevated. Alternatively, a puncture can be tried with the patient

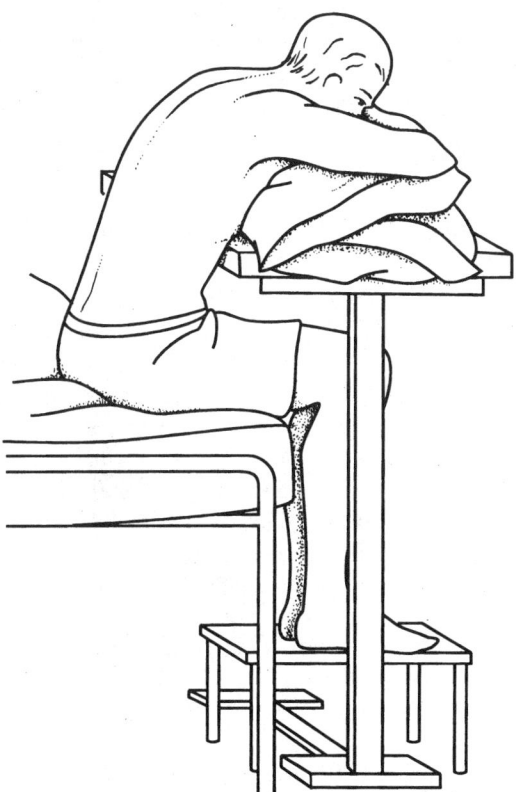

Figure 1 Optimal positioning of patient for thoracentesis.

lying in a decubitus position with the effusion side down. In both cases, soft bedding makes access to the most dependent part of the chest difficult, and the patient should be moved as far as possible to the bedside to avoid excessive bulging of the mattress into the working field.

Once a comfortable position for operator and patient is achieved, the site for the puncture must be selected. With the patient in a vertical position, the lowest part of the thorax is usually posterior and pleural fluid can accumulate where a puncture can be achieved easiest. The chest radiograph indicates an approximate location, and the definite site is selected with clinical examinations, i.e., chest percussion and tactile fremitus. In contrast to the aerated lung above the effusion, the light percussion note becomes dull over the effusion and the tactile fremitus is lost. The puncture should be attempted one intercostal space further down from where fremitus and light percussion note are lost.

Puncture site selection is key to the success of pleurocentesis. If the clinical technique described above is endorsed, most pleurocentesis attempts failing to produce fluid will be situated too low, as demonstrated in a study reviewing cases of failed thoracentesis with ultrasound (8). Factors contributing to the wrongful selection of a puncture site in this series of 26 patients were small effusion with little or no detectable fluid on sonography, blunt costo-phrenic angle on chest x-ray (CXR), pleural effusion with multiple loculations, and pulmonary consolidation simulating a large pleural effusion. In challenging situations for puncture site selection, pleural ultrasound may be considered.

Ultrasound is superior to CXR in identifying pleural fluid collections, which was proven by several studies more than a decade ago (9–14). However, a reduction in complications or dry taps has not consistently been shown, and cost-effectiveness of ultrasound for routine pleurocentesis has been questioned (12). In the early days, when ultrasound was a stationary and expensive modality, patients frequently had to be transferred for the examination, causing inconvenience and delay, and were finally punctured by a different physician in a potentially different body position than during the ultrasound examination. In recent years, considerable technical development has taken place, and the advent of affordable and transportable ultrasound units has made the technique accessible for the physician at the bedside, and on-site sonography by the physician performing the puncture is increasingly popular. A recent study using a mobile ultrasound unit showed excellent yield for obtaining pleural fluid with a very low complication rate in mechanically ventilated patients (7). Despite the lack of recent data, it seems reasonable to recommend ultrasound up front for small effusions and those with the above-mentioned risk constellations. Frequent use of ultrasound for pleural procedures promotes the understanding of how clinical findings are related to anatomical conditions and increases the level of confidence of the operator. We believe that bedside ultrasound will ultimately be incorporated into the training and practice of pulmonary physicians and that ultrasound should be used liberally whenever available (15,16).

B. Local Anesthesia and Diagnostic Thoracentesis

The spot to perform the puncture and eventually the biopsy should be chosen not too close to the spine and just above an easily palpable rib in order to avoid contact with the intercostal vessels and nerves situated right below the ribs. Local anesthesia is compulsory if pleural biopsy is planned, and of debatable value for straightforward thoracentesis. In the hand of experienced operators, the trauma of local anesthesia usually matches the one inflicted by the procedure itself if only one needle is used. Unless the patient is very anxious or the puncture is anticipated to be difficult, e.g., in very obese subjects, an experienced operator may abstain from local anesthesia for diagnostic pleurocentesis only. Since most of the action happens out of the patient's view, we find it very useful to keep up a continuous flow of information from operator to patient about the progress of the ongoing procedure.

The puncture should be done perpendicular to the skin, and a puncture pointing upwards must be avoided at all times. We always thoroughly disinfect the selected spot with a wide margin of safety with alcohol. Local anesthesia is performed in three steps: anesthesia of the skin, the rib periostium, and the pleura (Fig. 2). The skin is best punctured with a short 24G (0.55 mm) needle, and less than 1 mL of lidocaine is usually applied to create a small wheal (Fig. 2a). This needle is then replaced with a 22G (0.7 mm) needle of 4 cm length, which is inserted through the same spot. With the needle tip in the subcutaneous tissue, the skin is easily moved up and down to adjust for the rib below the planned entry site into the thorax. While moving the needle forward towards the pleural space, small amounts of lidocaine are continuously injected, slowly advancing the needle with frequent aspirations. When the rib periostium is reached, the needle is worked upwards by withdrawing the needle from the rib, moving skin and subcutanous tissue upwards with the needle inserted, and readvancing the needle, until it passes over the rib (Fig. 2b). When the pleura is finally punctured, pleural fluid should be easily aspirated (Fig. 2c). For diagnostic aspiration, the syringe is now changed and the fluid can be sampled. If a direct puncture without local anesthesia is attempted, a 22G or 21G (0.8 mm) needle attached to an empty 20 mL syringe is directly inserted under constant aspiration with the same technique as described above.

If no fluid can be aspirated with a 22G or 21G needle inserted all the way (4 cm), the needle is either too short, too far advanced, or there is no pleural fluid at the attempted site. The needle should be slowly withdrawn under constant aspiration, because a very small rim of effusion can be missed when inserting the needle. If the patient is very obese or muscular, the needle should be replaced by a longer needle, and the attempt should be repeated. Pleural fluid is almost never too thick to be aspirated through a 21G or 22G needle. If air is

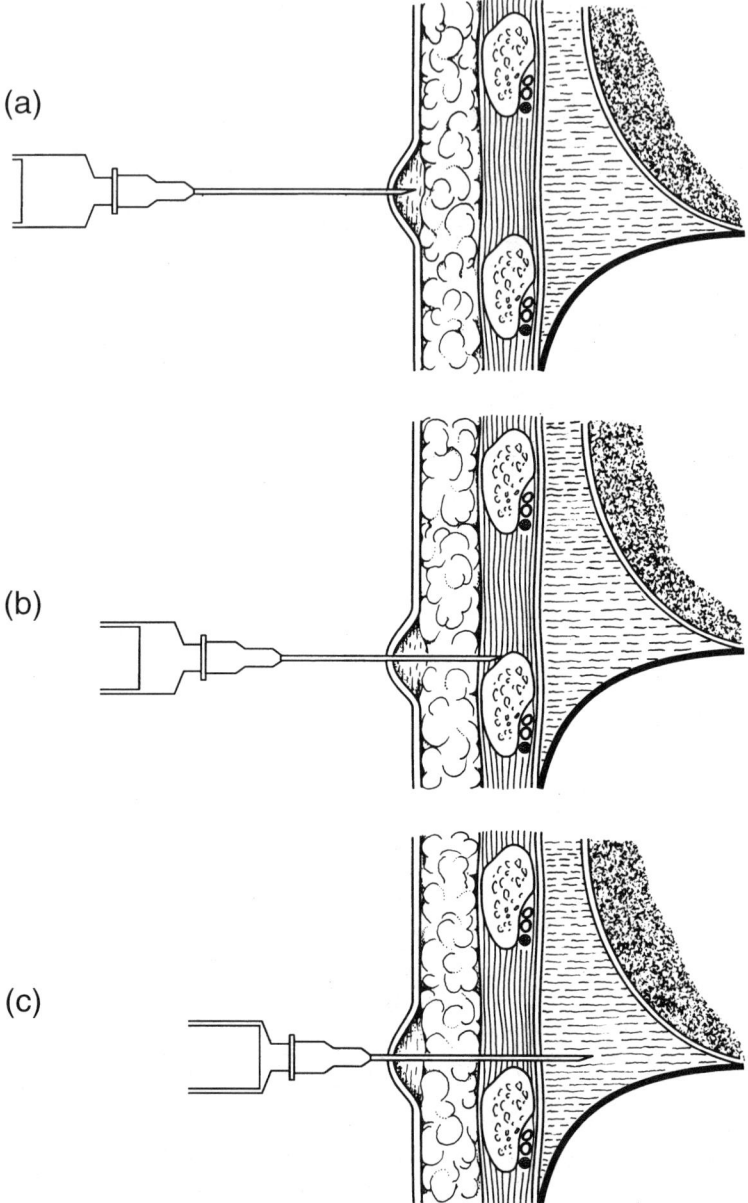

Figure 2 Performing local anesthesia for thoracentesis. Application of local anesthetic to the skin (a), to the upper edge of a rib (b), and needle positioned just above a rib within the pleural fluid (c). Note the location of the intercostal neurovascular structures under the rib.

aspirated, the puncture is probably too high and should be repeated one interspace lower, and if no air is aspirated, the puncture was probably too low and should be repeated one interspace higher. If the presence of pleural fluid is doubtful and the initial attempt is unsuccessful, a repetition of the puncture with ultrasound assistance should be considered.

C. Needle Types and Technique of Closed Needle Pleural Biopsy

The site for the biopsy is identified in the same way as for diagnostic pleurocentesis. Most needles for pleural biopsy allow for pleural fluid collection as well. Local anesthesia is always needed for closed needle biopsy and is performed as described above. The choice among the several types of needles in use depends on availability and operator experience.

The Abrams, Cope, and Raja needles are designed for diagnostic fluid aspiration as well as biopsy of the pleura and the immediate subpleural tissue. For safe use of these needles, a certain amount of pleural effusion is necessary. If no fluid is found on aspiration during local anesthesia, closed needle biopsy should not be attempted (17). The tru-cut needle, in contrast, is designed for core tissue biopsies of presumed pleural-based tumors or abundant pleural thickening. Pleural fluid cannot be aspirated through a tru-cut needle, and fluoroscopy or sonography is mostly used for guidance, especially when no pleural fluid is present.

Abrams Needle

The Abrams needle (Fig. 3a) was first described in 1958 as a refinement of the needle described by De Francis in 1955 (2,18). The Abrams needle consists of three parts: a blunt-tipped outer trocar with a notch, an inner cannula with a sharp cutting terminal part, and a solid inner stylet. The biopsy procedure is shown in detail in Figure 4. After a small scalpel skin incision is made, all three parts are introduced together into the pleural space with gentle pressure. Once the needle is believed to be in the pleural space, the stylet is removed and a syringe attached to the system. After opening the distal notch by rotating the inner cannula, fluid can be aspirated (Fig. 4a). To change syringes, the notch is closed so that no air can enter the pleural space. To take the biopsy, the notch must be in the open position and the knob in the outer trocar turned away from the upper rib. The needle has to be withdrawn slowly under permanent suction until the notch is hooked at the visceral pleura (Fig. 4b). In this position it should be possible to still aspirate pleural fluid through the needle, otherwise the needle is probably out of the pleural space and must be repositioned. Finally, the inner trocar is rotated into the closed position to cut off the biopsy specimen (Fig. 4c). The needle is withdrawn with the biopsy specimen contained within it. This procedure should be repeated at least four times.

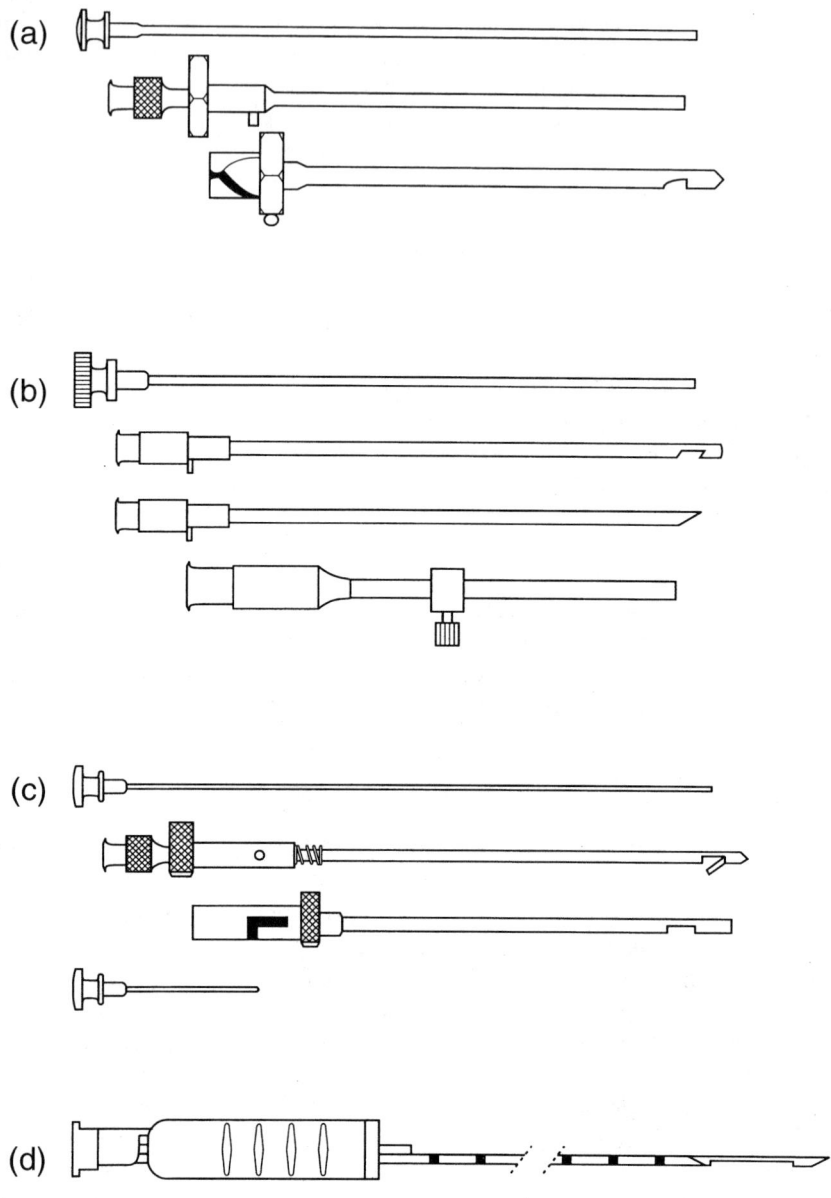

Figure 3 Different types of needles used for pleural biopsy: (a) Abrams needle; (b) Cope needle; (c) Raja needle; (d) tru-cut needle in open (top) and closed position (bottom).

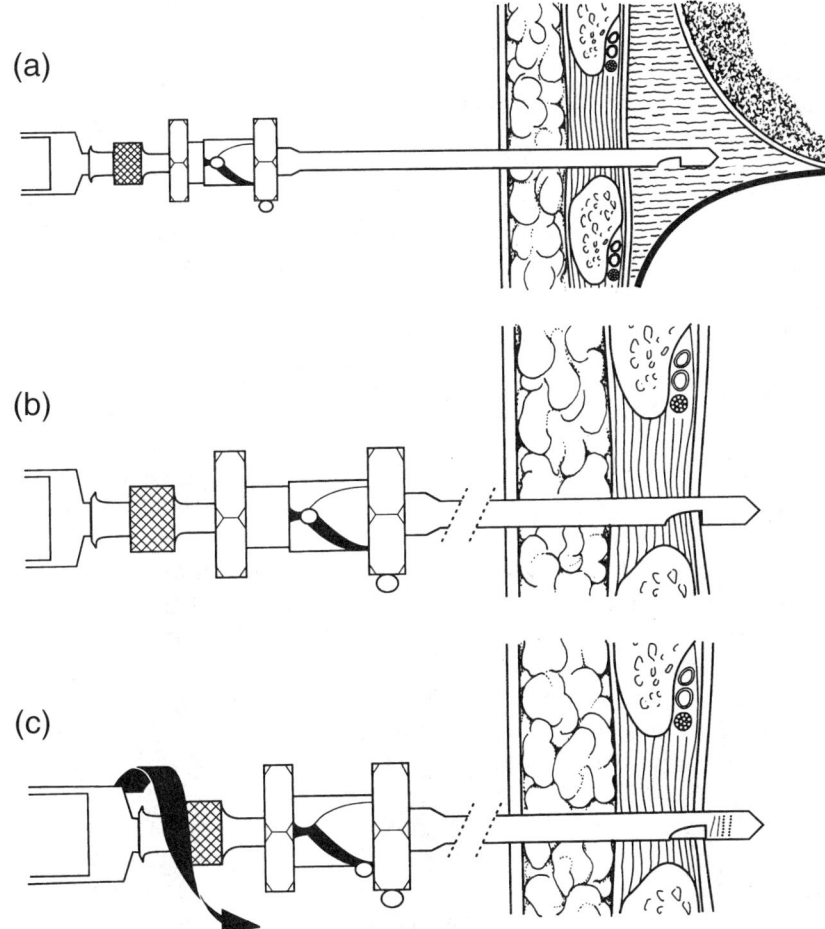

Figure 4 Pleural biopsy with Abrams needle. After introduction into the pleural space, the needle tip with the distal notch open allows for easy aspiration of fluid (a). For the biopsy, the visceral pleura is hooked with the notch (b) and by closure of the notch the biopsy material is sheared off and transferred into the needle tip (c), from where it can be harvested. Note the location of the intercostal neurovascular structures and that the knob on the outer trocar pinpoints the position of the cutting edge inside the thorax.

Cope Needle

The Cope needle (Fig. 3b) was first described in 1958 (19). The Cope needle consists of four parts: a large, sharp-tipped outer cannula, an inner trocar with a hooked notch and a blunt tip, a simple hollow trocar, and a solid inner stylet. After the skin incision, the outer cannula is introduced into the pleural space with the hollow trocar and the stylet in place. Fluid can be aspirated with a syringe attached to the outer cannula after the trocar and the stylet are removed.

The inner stylet and cannula can also directly be replaced by the blunt-tipped biopsy trocar with a syringe attached to it. To take a biopsy, the apparatus is withdrawn with the notch directed inferiorly until it hooks at the parietal pleura. The biopsy is taken by advancing the outer sharp cannula toward the pleural space in a gyrating motion. The specimen is then removed with the hooked cannula. This procedure can be repeated until the required number of biopsies is obtained. When using this needle, it is important to occlude the trocar with a syringe, stopcock, or the operator's thumb whenever the cannulas are changed to prevent a pneumothorax by air entering the pleural space, and the patient should hold his breath at the end of a normal expiration each time. This procedure can be repeated until the required number of biopsies are obtained.

Raja Needle

The Raja needle (Fig. 3c) is a closed system similar to the Abrams needle, first described in 1989 (20). The Raja needle consists of three parts: a blunt outer cannula with a notch, an inner sharp-tipped cannula with a notch and a biopsy flap, and a solid inner stylet. After a scalpel incision, the two outer parts assembled are inserted into the pleural space connected with a syringe. After entering the pleural space, the inner cannula is slightly moved back until the two notches are in a corresponding position and the biopsy flap can deploy into the pleural space. Pleural fluid can be aspirated in this position. To take the biopsy, the flap is turned inferiorly and the needle withdrawn until the flap is hooked at the parietal pleura. The outer cannula is then withdrawn over the inner cannula, forcing the flap with the hooked specimen back into the inner cannula and closing the notch. The apparatus is then removed with the specimen. This procedure can be repeated until the required number of biopsies is obtained. Initial reports by the inventor showed very encouraging results compared to the Abrams needle (21,22). To date, the number of studies with this type of needle is still limited, and no conclusive recommendation can be given.

Abrams Needle Versus Cope Needle

In general, the rate of success with closed needle biopsy seems to be more dependent on the operator's skills than on the needle type used, and diagnostic yields are almost identical (6,23). The blunt tip of the Abrams needle makes insertion somewhat more difficult but is safer for concomitant therapeutic thoracentesis because of reduced risk of lacerating the lung. The Abrams needle also seems easier to use and is a closed system, while the Cope needle has the risk of pneumothorax from air entering the pleural space from outside if not properly handled.

Tru-Cut Needle

The tru-cut needle (Fig. 3d) is not a genuine pleural biopsy needle and is generally used to obtain core biopsies from solid tissue material. Different brands and dimensions of this needle are available. Fluid cannot be aspirated with this system, but the needle can be used for conventional pleural biopsy. The tru-cut needle consists of a sharp-tipped, cutting outer cannula and a inner needle with a sharp tip and a notch. When closed, the notch is hidden in the outer cannula, and one sharp tip is formed by the two components. To take biopsies, the two parts are inserted in the closed position into the pleural cavity or into the tumor. The inner needle is then moved forward so that the tissue to biopsy can bulge into the notch. The specimen is obtained by moving the cutting cannula forward over the inner cannula, which is fixed in its position. To harvest the specimen, the whole needle in the closed position is removed. For pleural biopsy, it is somewhat more difficult than with the other needle types to feel the distal end hooking in the pleura, and the inexperienced operator tends to take biopsies of intercostal tissue rather than of pleura. Because of the sharp tip and the large biopsies that can be obtained, the blind use of this type in dry chests without fluoroscopic or ultrasound guidance is not encouraged (17).

IV. Processing of Material

A. Pleural Fluid

For diagnostic pleurocentesis it is usually sufficient to tap off 50 mL of pleural fluid. For cytology, it may be suitable to tap off even more, because more cells may be obtained for preparation with cytospin. We carefully note color, viscosity, and smell of the fluid. Fluid pH should be measured with a blood gas machine whenever a parapneumonic effusion or malignancy is suspected. Proposed routine tests performed on the fluid are listed in Table 1.

Required amounts of fluid and the appropriate tubes for each category may vary in different hospitals. Very helpful, but seldom seen, is a kit of tubes designed for pleural fluid and with a single request form that can contain some

Table 1 Recommended Routine Tests on Pleural Fluid

Category	Amount	Specific tests
Hematology	5 mL	Total cell count and differentiation
Chemistry[a]	5 mL	LDH, protein, albumin
Serology[a]		Adenosine deaminase
Microbiology	5 mL	Gram stain
		Aerobic and anaerobic culture
		Tuberculosis stain and culture
		Fungus stain and culture
pH	2 mL	Blood gas machine
Cytology	Rest	

[a] Additional tests may be requested according to the clinical situation and the aspect of the fluid.

useful hints as to how to order the appropriate test. Since most pleural punctures are done by less experienced and notoriously overworked junior medical staff, such a kit is most welcome and certainly enhances the consistency and usefulness of the tests done. Recent serum values are helpful to interpret the pleural fluid values of certain parameters. A stepwise approach with an initial step to determine whether the fluid is a trans- or an exudate and more detailed testing done in exudates only would be ideal, but is not realistic in practice. A more in-depth approach to testing of pleural fluid can be found elsewhere in this book.

B. Processing of Closed Needle Biopsy Specimens

Biopsy specimens should be sent for histology in formalin, and at least one sample should be submitted for mycobacterial culture in saline. The ideal number of biopsies for tb-pleurisy has been determined to be four in one report, and seven or more biopsy attempts produced at least two specimens containing pleural tissue in another study (24,25). At some institutions electron microscopy is available, and tissue for workup must be submitted in a specific medium.

V. Complications

In essence, the frequency and nature of complications of closed needle biopsy are the same as with diagnostic pleurocentesis. However, lacerations of intercostal vessels are more likely to lead to serious complications due to the cutting character of the devices, and hemothorax as well as arterio-venous fistulas have been described after closed needle biopsy.

Penetration of the lung (aspiration of air) or of an infra-diaphragmatic organ (dry tap) with a thin needle as described above does not necessarily lead to complications. Dry taps are reported in 10–13% of attempts for thoracentesis (3,8,11,26). Pneumothorax is the most frequent complication occurring in 11–30% of punctures, and a chest drain is necessary in about 2% (3,12,26). A pneumothorax can occur after laceration of the lung with the tip of the instrument, causing a pulmonary air leak. Air can also inadvertently enter the pleural space during the procedure from the outside. In the latter case, the pneumothoraces tend to be small and stable, while a persistent air leak in the lung will produce an increasing pneumothorax requiring drainage. In closed needle biopsy, the Cope needle as an open system might favor air entry from outside, but pneumothorax is not reported as a significant problem (27). The incidence of pneumothorax seems to be reduced with more experienced operators and to be increased in patients with underlying COPD (28,29). In our opinion it is unnecessary to routinely obtain a CXR for exclusion of a iatrogenic pneumothorax after each procedure. We routinely repeat percussion and tactile fremitus after the procedure, or repeat the ultrasound when available on site, and check for unexplained alterations of these findings indicating a pneumothorax. Only if air was aspirated, unexplained symptoms occur, or these screening tests fail do we order a CXR. This conservative approach is endorsed by the findings of several recent studies (30–33).

Very sensitive individuals can suffer a vaso-vagal syncope during the procedure, probably triggered by emotional factors and possibly by penetration of the pleura with the needle and promoted by the sitting position of the subject. The procedure should then be immediately interrupted and the patient moved into a supine position. Infection of the pleural space, hemothorax, subdiaphragmatic hematoma, and lacerations of subdiaphragmatic organs are rare but serious adverse events. Hemothorax has occasionally been reported through laceration of an intercostal artery (34–36). Endorsing the technique described above, which avoids contact with intercostal vessels, and following a sterile approach can prevent most of these complications. Seeding of the needle tract with malignant cells is frequently observed in malignant mesothelioma and can be prevented by local irradiation (37).

The use of sonography for puncture site identification seems to reduce the rate of dry taps as well as the rate of complications. The incidence of pneumothorax was only 3% in one study employing ultrasound in 188 patients, and the number of dry taps was reduced in several studies (11,12,14). In a recent large study of 255 pleural procedures in 205 patients with mostly small effusions, a low incidence of pneumothorax was reported in connection with liberal use of ultrasound (30). The risk for complications is increased in small effusions, loculated pleural effusions, blunt costo-phrenic angles and lung consolidation (8,15). It seems therefore reasonable to recommend routine ultrasound for these risk constellations to avoid complications and increase the yield of pleural taps.

VI. Yield of Pleural Thoracentesis and Biopsy

A. Diagnostic Thoracentesis

Diagnostic thoracentesis is an extremely helpful diagnostic tool, though the yield varies with different diseases. In a prospective study of 129 consecutive diagnostic thoracenteses, a definitive diagnosis could be made in 18%. In 56% of cases, a presumptive diagnosis correlated with clinical findings was possible, while only 26% of the taps remained nondiagnostic (3). Diseases to diagnose on the grounds of pleural fluid findings only are listed in Table 2 (38). In many situations, pleural fluid analysis will reveal clues to ruling in or out specific diseases, many of which are discussed in separate chapters in this book. Since closed needle biopsy is done mainly in suspected pleural tuberculosis and malignancy, we will discuss their relative yield in these selected diseases below. Pleural malignancies and tb-pleurisy are dealt with in depth in the relevant chapters.

B. Diagnostic Thoracentesis and Closed Needle Biopsy in TB-Pleurisy

Untreated tuberculous pleurisy usually has a self-limiting course. Nevertheless, the proper identification of the disease is important, because most patients with

Table 2 Diagnoses Established by Pleural Fluid Analysis

Disease	Diagnostic characteristics
Empyema	Pus on aspiration
Malignancy	Malignant cells on cytology
Tb-pleurisy	Positive AFB stain or culture
Fungal infection	Positive stain or culture
Chylothorax	Elevated triglycerides and cholesterol
Hemothorax	Hematocrit > 50% of blood hematocrit
Rheumatoid pleurisy	Typical cytology
Lupus pleurisy	Typical cytology
Esophageal rupture	Very low pH, high amylase

untreated tb-pleurisy will develop some other form of active tuberculosis later in life (39,40). Moreover, the administration of antituberculous therapy dramatically reduces the incidence of subsequent tuberculosis (41). With the high prevalence of HIV infection, the numbers of tuberculosis cases are rising in many developing countries, and invasive procedures for the diagnosis of tuberculous pleuritis are not uniformly available and relatively expensive. A simple and cheap diagnostic tool for pleural tuberculosis in high-prevalence areas is therefore of substantial epidemiological interest.

Diagnostic Thoracentesis in TB-Pleurisy

Unfortunately, the diagnostic yield of staining and culture for mycobacteria in pleural fluid is low. Staining for acid-fast bacilli (AFB) has a sensitivity of only around 20%, and mycobacterial culture of pleural fluid is positive for mycobacteria in around 40% (42,43). These figures may be somewhat higher in HIV patients (44). Polymerase chain reaction (PCR) has shown inconsistent results on pleural fluid, and PCR is expensive and requires expert laboratory staff (45,46). The low yield of all these methods is due to the mainly immunological nature of tuberculous pleuritis, with only a small number of bacteria present in the pleural fluid.

The best studied and most widely used alternative test to date is adenosine deaminase (AdA) activity in pleural fluid (47–52). The test has some specificity problems with false positives occurring in bacterial empyemas and rheumatic effusions. With a cutoff level of 50 Units, combined with a pleural fluid cell count showing predominant lymphocytosis (> 75%), the sensitivity and specificity were 88% and 95%, respectively, in a study on 472 patients with exudative pleural effusions at our institution, which is situated in a high prevalence area for tb-pleurisy (49). In the future, commercially available tests for isoenzymes may further increase sensitivity and specificity of AdA on pleural fluid (53). IFN-γ in pleural fluid is less well studied but reported to have similar predictive values as AdA. Discrimination from rheumatoid effusions may be better than with AdA, but IFN-γ is expensive and will therefore not be widely available in high-prevalence areas for tuberculosis (54,55). It is important to remember that the prevalence of the disease influences decisively the value of these indirect tests on pleural fluid for tb-pleurisy. In low-prevalence areas with tuberculosis accounting for less than 5% of exudative effusions, even a test with high specificity would still produce an unacceptably high rate of false positives.

Closed Needle Biopsy in TB-Pleurisy

The traditional method of choice for the diagnosis of tb-pleurisy is closed needle biopsy showing granulomatous inflammation, which is virtually diagnostic for pleural tuberculosis (56). In a recent study in 248 patients, closed needle biopsy alone had a yield of about 80% alone, and when added to AFB staining and culture the overall yield was 91% (43). A slightly better overall sensitivity is achieved with thoracoscopy, where in contrast to closed needle biopsy the sampling error is reduced by visual identification of the affected pleural regions (4,57). The popularity of AdA and IFN-γ in regions with high incidence of tb-pleurisy seems to be responsible for the decreasing use of closed needle pleural biopsy. Yet, replacing pleural biopsy with AdA or IFN-γ will result in fewer cultures available for resistance testing. This drawback is debatable, since the diagnosis of tb-pleurisy with pleural biopsy relies rather on the finding of granulomatous tissue on histology than on culture positivity for mycobacteria, and the number of available cultures will only decrease by 20–30% when no pleural biopsy is taken (57). Moreover, the resistance to antituberculous drugs depends on regional factors. In our opinion, the decision whether or not to use closed needle pleural biopsy routinely is to be taken locally, based on the availability of pleural fluid tests and local prevalence of tb-pleurisy as well as resistance to antituberculous drugs.

C. Diagnostic Thoracentesis and Closed Needle Biopsy in Malignancy

Malignant pleural effusions are a frequent cause of pleural exudates, mostly from metastatic breast or lung cancer. Prognosis of patients with malignant pleural effusion is poor, and the disease is usually beyond a curable stage. While a certain delay in diagnosis in asymptomatic patients is acceptable, patients with symptomatic effusions should be diagnosed and referred for palliative treatment with pleurodesis to improve quality of life. Closed needle biopsy is not visually controlled and therefore prone to sampling errors in malignant pleural disease, which is not evenly distributed over the parietal pleura.

Malignant Pleural Effusions Due to Metastatic Malignancy

Cytological evaluation of pleural fluid is an excellent method to diagnose metastatic malignancies to the pleura. The yield of the method will vary with the tumor type, the type of technical examination (cell blocks or smears, use of additional tools like electron microscopy or immuno-histochemistry), the number of successive specimens submitted (the more submitted, the higher the percentage of positive results), and the skills of the involved cytologist. While the specificity of a positive result is high, a negative result does not exclude malignancy. Sensitivity varies in published reports from 40 to 87% (42,58–60). After submitting three large volume specimens, a yield of more than 80% may be expected (61).

In a considerable number of pleural effusions secondary to non–small-cell lung cancer (NSCLC), the pleural fluid may not contain malignant cells, and the pleural effusion is therefore not prohibitive for curative surgery (62). A method with higher sensitivity than pleural fluid cytology might be welcome in this situation in order to avoid unnecessary exploratory thoracotomies. Unfortunately, closed needle biopsy has a low yield for malignancy. In a study with 281 cases with proven pleural malignancy, closed needle biopsy had a sensitivity of only 43% (58). Increasing the number of biopsy sites as well as the biopsies taken per site does not significantly improve the yield of the method (24,63). In contrast, thoracoscopy under local or general anesthesia establishes the diagnosis of pleural malignancy in 90% of cases and offers the possibility of effective pleurodesis during the procedure (64–66). In our opinion, the role of closed needle biopsy in suspected malignancy is confined to situations where thoracoscopy is not an option and repeat cytology has failed to produce a diagnosis.

Malignant Effusions Due to Mesothelioma

In the case of mesothelioma, the diagnosis of malignancy can usually be made on cytological examination of pleural fluid. The distinction between metastatic adenocarcinoma and mesothelioma, however, is difficult, and in about 25% of cases the diagnosis of mesothelioma cannot be made on cytology alone, although various discriminating cytological or immuno-histochemical features with good sensitivity and specificity exist (67–72). In addition, the specific diagnosis of mesothelioma has forensic importance in many societies, because compensation can be claimed for mesothelioma associated with asbestos exposure. Traditional closed needle biopsy is usually not diagnostic for mesothelioma (67). Instead, a core tissue biopsy large enough is best acquired with thoracoscopy or open surgical biopsy. The yield of these methods is around 90% for mesothelioma (64,65,73).

VII. Limitations

Diagnostic pleurocentesis is a simple, straightforward, and safe procedure. The yield is limited, because only a minority of pleural effusions exhibit a pattern of biochemical, cytological, and microbiological markers distinctive enough for a definitive diagnosis. In our opinion, the potential benefit of diagnostic pleurocentesis is well balanced against the possible harm and discomfort in most situations where an exudative effusion may be expected on clinical grounds.

In contrast, the role of closed needle biopsy in undiagnosed exudative pleural effusions is controversial. The procedure adds little to the diagnostic value of serial pleurocentesis in metastatic malignant disease, and mesothelioma is more readily diagnosed on large tissue biopsies better obtained with different methods. In suspected tuberculous pleurisy, the yield of closed needle biopsy is still comparable to modern biochemical methods and offers the advantage of somewhat higher culture positivity. The usefulness of the technique depends greatly on the local availability of operator expertise. We believe that closed needle biopsy still has a strong role in undiagnosed lymphocytic effusions, especially if local operator experience is good and modern biochemical tests are not available.

Acknowledgment

We would like to thank Carol Lochner, who provided the artwork for this chapter.

References

1. Garrison FH. Introduction to the History of Medicine. Philadelphia: WB Saunders Co, 1929:632.
2. DeFrancis N, Klosk E, Albano E. Needle biopsy of the parietal pleura. NEJM 1955; 252:948–949.
3. Collins TR, Sahn SA. Thoracocentesis. Clinical value, complications, technical problems, and patient experience. Chest 1987; 91:817–822.
4. Baumann MH. Closed needle biopsy: a necessary tool? Pulmon Perspect 2000; 17:1–3.
5. Sokolowski JW Jr, Burgher LW, Jones FL Jr, Patterson JR, Selecky PA. Guidelines for thoracentesis and needle biopsy of the pleurad Position paper of the American Thoracic Society. Am Rev Respir Dis 1989; 140:257–258.
6. Walsh LJ, Macfarlane JT, Manhire AR, Sheppard M, Jones JS. Audit of pleural biopsies: an argument for a pleural biopsy service. Respir Med 1994; 88:503–505.
7. Lichtenstein D, Hulot JS, Rabiller A, Tostivint I, Meziere G. Feasibility and safety of ultrasound-aided thoracentesis in mechanically ventilated patients. Intensive Care Med 1999; 25:955–958.
8. Weingardt JP, Guico RR, Nemcek AA Jr, Li YP, Chiu ST. Ultrasound findings following failed, clinically directed thoracenteses. J Clin Ultrasound 1994; 22:419–426.
9. Brandt WE. The thorax. In: Rumack MC, Wilson SR, Charboneau JW, eds. Diagnostic Ultrasound. St. Louis: Mosby, 1988:575–597.
10. O'Moore PV, Mueller PR, Simeone JF, et al. Sonographic guidance in diagnostic and therapeutic interventions in the pleural space. AJR Am J Roentgenol 1987; 149:1–5.

11. Grogan DR, Irwin RS, Channick R, et al. Complications associated with thoracentesis. A prospective, randomized study comparing three different methods. Arch Intern Med 1990; 150:873–877.
12. Kohan JM, Poe RH, Israel RH, et al. Value of chest ultrasonography versus decubitus roentgenography for thoracentesis. Am Rev Respir Dis 1986; 133:1124–1126.
13. Lipscomb DJ, Flower CD, Hadfield JW. Ultrasound of the pleura: an assessment of its clinical value. Clin Radiol 1981; 32:289–290.
14. Raptopoulos V, Davis LM, Lee G, Umali C, Lew R, Irwin RS. Factors affecting the development of pneumothorax associated with thoracentesis. AJR Am J Roentgenol 1991; 156:917–920.
15. Diacon AH, Brutsche MH, Soler M. Accuracy of pleural puncture sites: a prospective comparison of clinical examination with ultrasound. Chest 2003; 123: 436–441.
16. Colt HG, Brewer N, Barbur E. Evaluation of patient-related and procedure-related factors contributing to pneumothorax following thoracentesis. Chest 1999; 116: 134–138.
17. Levine H, Szanto PB, Cugell DW. Tuberculous pleurisy. An acute illness. Arch Intern Med 1968; 122:329–332.
18. Abrams LD. A pleural-biopsy punch. Lancet 1958; 1:30–31.
19. Cope C. New pleural biopsy needle. JAMA 1958; 167:1107–1108.
20. Ogirala RG, Agarwal V, Aldrich TK. Raja pleural biopsy needle. A comparison with the Abrams needle in experimental pleural effusion. Am Rev Respir Dis 1989; 139:984–987.
21. O'Connor S, Yung T. A comparison of Abrams and Raja pleural biopsy needles. Aust NZ J Med 1992; 22:237–239.
22. Ogirala RG, Agarwal V, Vizioli LD, Pinsker KL, Aldrich TK. Comparison of the Raja and the Abrams pleural biopsy needles in patients with pleural effusion. Am Rev Respir Dis 1993; 147:1291–1294.
23. Morrone N, Algranti E, Barreto E. Pleural biopsy with Cope and Abrams needles. Chest 1987; 92:1050–1052.
24. Mungall IP, Cowen PN, Cooke NT, Roach TC, Cooke NJ. Multiple pleural biopsy with the Abrams needle. Thorax 1980; 35:600–602.
25. Kirsch CM, Kroe DM, Azzi RL, Jensen WA, Kagawa FT, Wehner JH. The optimal number of pleural biopsy specimens for a diagnosis of tuberculous pleurisy. Chest 1997; 112:702–706.
26. Seneff MG, Corwin RW, Gold LH, Irwin RS. Complications associated with thoracocentesis. Chest 1986; 90:97–100.
27. Poe RH, Israel RH, Utell MJ, Hall WJ, Greenblatt DW, Kallay MC. Sensitivity, specificity, and predictive values of closed pleural biopsy. Arch Intern Med 1984; 144:325–328.
28. Brandstetter RD, Karetzky M, Rastogi R, Lolis JD. Pneumothorax after thoracentesis in chronic obstructive pulmonary disease. Heart Lung 1994; 23:67–70.
29. Bartter T, Mayo PD, Pratter MR, Santarelli RJ, Leeds WM, Akers SM. Lower risk and higher yield for thoracentesis when performed by experienced operators. Chest 1993; 103:1873–1876.
30. Colt HG, Brewer N, Barbur E. Evaluation of patient-related and procedure-related factors contributing to pneumothorax following thoracentesis. Chest 1999; 116: 134–138.

31. Aleman C, Alegre J, Armadans L, et al. The value of chest roentgenography in the diagnosis of pneumothorax after thoracentesis. Am J Med 1999; 107:340–343.
32. Doyle JJ, Hnatiuk OW, Torrington KG, Slade AR, Howard RS. Necessity of routine chest roentgenography after thoracentesis. Ann Intern Med 1996; 124:816–820.
33. Petersen WG, Zimmerman R. Limited utility of chest radiograph after thoracentesis. Chest 2000; 117:1038–1042.
34. Carney M, Ravin CE. Intercostal artery laceration during thoracocentesis: increased risk in elderly patients. Chest 1979; 75:520–522.
35. Lai JH, Yan HC, Kao SJ, Lee SC, Shen CY. Intercostal arteriovenous fistula due to pleural biopsy. Thorax 1990; 45:976–978.
36. Ali J, Summer WR. Hemothorax and hyperkalemia after pleural biopsy in a 43-year-old woman on hemodialysis. Chest 1994; 106:1235–1236.
37. Boutin C, Rey F, Viallat JR. Prevention of malignant seeding after invasive diagnostic procedures in patients with pleural mesothelioma. A randomized trial of local radiotherapy. Chest 1995; 108:754–758.
38. Sahn SA. State of the art. The pleura. Am Rev Respir Dis 1988; 138:184–234.
39. Patila J. Initial tuberculous pleuritis in the Finnish Armed Forces in 1939–1945 with special reference to eventual post pleuritits tuberculosis. Acta Tuberc Scand 1954; 36(suppl):1–57.
40. Roper WH, Waring JJ. Primary serofibrinous pleural effusion in military personnel. Am Rev Respir Dis 1955; 71:616–634.
41. Berger HW, Mejia E. Tuberculous pleurisy. Chest 1973; 63:88–92.
42. Escudero Bueno C, Garcia Clemente M, Cuesta Castro B, et al. Cytologic and bacteriologic analysis of fluid and pleural biopsy specimens with Cope's needle. Study of 414 patients. Arch Intern Med 1990; 150:1190–1194.
43. Valdes L, Alvarez D, San Jose E, et al. Tuberculous pleurisy: a study of 254 patients. Arch Intern Med 1998; 158:2017–2021.
44. Heyderman RS, Makunike R, Muza T, et al. Pleural tuberculosis in Harare, Zimbabwe: the relationship between human immunodeficiency virus, CD4 lymphocyte count, granuloma formation and disseminated disease. Trop Med Int Health 1998; 3:14–20.
45. Villena V, Rebollo MJ, Aguado JM, Galan A, Lopez Encuentra A, Palenque E. Polymerase chain reaction for the diagnosis of pleural tuberculosis in immunocompromised and immunocompetent patients. Clin Infect Dis 1998; 26:212–214.
46. Querol JM, Minguez J, Garcia-Sanchez E, Farga MA, Gimeno C, Garcia-de-Lomas J. Rapid diagnosis of pleural tuberculosis by polymerase chain reaction. Am J Respir Crit Care Med 1995; 152:1977–1981.
47. Valdes L, San Jose E, Alvarez D, Valle JM. Adenosine deaminase (ADA) isoenzyme analysis in pleural effusions: diagnostic role, and relevance to the origin of increased ADA in tuberculous pleurisy. Eur Respir J 1996; 9:747–751.
48. Ferrer JS, Munoz XG, Orriols RM, Light RW, Morell FB. Evolution of idiopathic pleural effusion: a prospective, long-term follow-up study. Chest 1996; 109:1508–1513.
49. Burgess LJ, Maritz FJ, Le Roux I, Taljaard JJ. Combined use of pleural adenosine deaminase with lymphocyte/neutrophil ratio. Increased specificity for the diagnosis of tuberculous pleuritis. Chest 1996; 109:414–419.
50. Riantawan P, Chaowalit P, Wongsangiem M, Rojanaraweewong P. Diagnostic value of pleural fluid adenosine deaminase in tuberculous pleuritis with reference to HIV coinfection and a Bayesian analysis. Chest 1999; 116:97–103.

51. Burgess LJ, Maritz FJ, Le Roux I, Taljaard JJ. Use of adenosine deaminase as a diagnostic tool for tuberculous pleurisy. Thorax 1995; 50:672–674.
52. Valdes L, Alvarez D, San Jose E, et al. Value of adenosine deaminase in the diagnosis of tuberculous pleural effusions in young patients in a region of high prevalence of tuberculosis. Thorax 1995; 50:600–603.
53. Perez-Rodriguez E, Jimenez Castro D. The use of adenosine deaminase and adenosine deaminase isoenzymes in the diagnosis of tuberculous pleuritis. Curr Opin Pulm Med 2000; 6:259–266.
54. Villena V, Lopez-Encuentra A, Echave-Sustaeta J, Martin-Escribano P, Ortuno-de-Solo B, Estenoz-Alfaro J. Interferon-gamma in 388 immunocompromised and immunocompetent patients for diagnosing pleural tuberculosis. Eur Respir J 1996; 9:2635–2639.
55. Valdes L, San Jose E, Alvarez D, et al. Diagnosis of tuberculous pleurisy using the biologic parameters adenosine deaminase, lysozyme, and interferon gamma. Chest 1993; 103:458–465.
56. Light RW. Tubercolous pleural effusions. In: Light RW, ed. Pleural Diseases. Vol. 4. Baltimore: Williams & Wilkins, 2001:182–195.
57. Diacon AH, van de Wal BW, Wyser C, Smedemo JP, Bezuidenhout J, Bolliger CT, Walzl G. Diagnostic tools in tuberculous pleurisy: a direct comparative study. Eur Resp J 2003. In press.
58. Prakash UB, Reiman HM. Comparison of needle biopsy with cytologic analysis for the evaluation of pleural effusion: analysis of 414 cases. Mayo Clin Proc 1985; 60:158–164.
59. Dekker A, Bupp PA. Cytology of serous effusions. An investigation into the usefulness of cell blocks versus smears. Am J Clin Pathol 1978; 70:855–860.
60. Jarvi OH, Kunnas RJ, Laitio MT, Tyrkko JE. The accuracy and significance of cytologic cancer diagnosis of pleural effusions. (A followup study of 338 patients). Acta Cytol 1972; 16:152–158.
61. Light RW. Pleural effusions related to metastatic maligancies. In: Light RW, ed. Pleural Diseases. Vol. 4. Baltimore: Williams & Wilkins, 2001:108–134.
62. Rodriguez-Panadero F, Borderas Naranjo F, Lopez Mejias J. Pleural metastatic tumours and effusions. Frequency and pathogenic mechanisms in a post-mortem series. Eur Respir J 1989; 2:366–369.
63. Canto A, Rivas J, Saumench J, Morera R, Moya J. Points to consider when choosing a biopsy method in cases of pleurisy of unknown origin. Chest 1983; 84:176–179.
64. Hucker J, Bhatnagar NK, al-Jilaihawi AN, Forrester-Wood CP. Thoracoscopy in the diagnosis and management of recurrent pleural effusions. Ann Thorac Surg 1991; 52:1145–1147.
65. Menzies R, Charbonneau M. Thoracoscopy for the diagnosis of pleural disease. Ann Intern Med 1991; 114:271–276.
66. Diacon AH, Wyser C, Bolliger CT, et al. Prospective randomized comparison of thoracoscopic talc poudrage under local anesthesia versus bleomycin instillation for pleurodesis in malignant pleural effusions. Am J Respir Crit Care Med 2000; 162:1445–1449.
67. Law MR, Hodson ME, Turner-Warwick M. Malignant mesothelioma of the pleura: clinical aspects and symptomatic treatment. Eur J Respir Dis 1984; 65:162–168.
68. Stevens MW, Leong AS, Fazzalari NL, Dowling KD, Henderson DW. Cytopathol-

ogy of malignant mesothelioma: a stepwise logistic regression analysis. Diagn Cytopathol 1992; 8:333–341.
69. Wirth PR, Legier J, Wright GL Jr. Immunohistochemical evaluation of seven monoclonal antibodies for differentiation of pleural mesothelioma from lung adenocarcinoma. Cancer 1991; 67:655–662.
70. Frisman DM, McCarthy WF, Schleiff P, Buckner SB, Nocito JD Jr, O'Leary TJ. Immunocytochemistry in the differential diagnosis of effusions: use of logistic regression to select a panel of antibodies to distinguish adenocarcinomas from mesothelial proliferations. Mod Pathol 1993; 6:179–184.
71. Carella R, Deleonardi G, D'Errico A, et al. Immunohistochemical panels for differentiating epithelial malignant mesothelioma from lung adenocarcinoma: a study with logistic regression analysis. Am J Surg Pathol 2001; 25:43–50.
72. Brown RW, Clark GM, Tandon AK, Allred DC. Multiple-marker immunohistochemical phenotypes distinguishing malignant pleural mesothelioma from pulmonary adenocarcinoma. Hum Pathol 1993; 24:347–354.
73. Boutin C, Rey F, Gouvernet J, Viallat JR, Astoul P, Ledoray V. Thoracoscopy in pleural malignant mesothelioma: a prospective study of 188 consecutive patients. Part 2: Prognosis and staging. Cancer 1993; 72:394–404.

9

Chest Tubes

MICHAEL H. BAUMANN

University of Mississippi Medical Center
Jackson, Mississippi, U.S.A.

I. Introduction

A. History

Reportedly, Hippocrates was first to describe tube drainage of an infected pleural space (1). Continuous chest tube drainage of the pleural space incorporating an underwater seal device appears to have first occurred in the 1870s in a patient suffering empyema unresponsive to repeated aspiration (2). Extensive interest in effective methods of pleural drainage and experimentation investigating the appropriate role of these pleural drainage measures, including chest tube drainage, occurred after the 1917 postinfluenza epidemic of empyema (3). Postoperative use of chest tube drainage in thoracic surgery, including after lobectomy for suppurative lung disease, was reported in 1922 (4). However, not until the Korean War was postoperative chest tube placement standard after major thoracic surgical procedures (5). Chest tubes made of a myriad of materials in different designs and sizes have evolved since this time and have been accompanied by a host of different pleural drainage units.

B. Indications/Contraindications

Indications for chest tube (tube thoracostomy) placement are noted in Table 1 (1). Absolute contraindications do not exist, but careful consideration of the

Table 1 Indications for Chest Tube Placement

Pneumothorax
Empyema and parapneumonic effusion
Recurrent symptomatic effusion
Hemothorax
Chylothorax
Postoperatively in thoracic surgery
Bronchopleural fistula

risks and benefits of chest tube placement should occur before placing a chest tube in a patient with a coagulopathy; consideration to correction of the disorder should be given if patient stability permits (1,6). Chest tube insertion in an area of a dermatological disorder should be avoided if possible (6).

II. Chest Tube Placement Technique and Complications

Traditionally, the site of chest tube insertion has been determined by the material to be removed from the pleural space. Given that air rises to the least gravity-dependent portion of the chest, chest tube placement in the third to fifth intercostal space in the midaxillary line with the tube directed apically and anteriorly is suggested for pneumothorax. Alternately, the tube may be placed in the midclavicular line in the second intercostal space. Free-flowing fluid of any type is best drained by placing the tube in the sixth intercostal space in the midaxillary line with the tube directed inferiorly and posteriorly (1). Image-directed tube placement by computed tomography (CT) or ultrasound (US) is often used for the drainage of loculated pleural fluid.

Chest tubes traditionally have been placed by two major approaches: blunt dissection (incisional) and trocar insertion (1,6). Given concerns about damage to the underlying lung by utilizing a rigid, sharp trocar (1), many physicians prefer the blunt dissection approach. The development of chest tubes that may be placed by the Seldinger technique (guide wire placement) offers an additional alternative (7) that will also be briefly described. The reader is referred to two pictorial references outlining both techniques (6,7).

Regardless of the insertion technique, the site chosen should be thoroughly cleaned with an antiseptic solution covering an adequate area allowing alternate insertion sites if needed. Generous use of local anesthesia (lidocaine or similar) with infiltration of the adjacent tissue and tissue superior to the rib is recommended. Limiting the anesthesia and insertion area to the tissues just above the superior surface of the rib is recommended to avoid damage to the neurovascular bundle located inferior to the rib. If blunt dissection is planned, adequate anesthesia along the length of the incision site is required. Aspiration of air or fluid into the anesthetic syringe indicates entrance in the pleural space. Subsequent withdrawal of the needle to the point of absence of aspiration of either air or fluid indicates proximity to the visceral pleural surface. Liberal application of anesthetic to the visceral pleural surface is recommended.

When using the blunt dissection approach, most hospitals utilize tube thoracostomy (chest tube) trays containing instruments and other materials needed for tube placement. Selection of the type and size of chest tube is done separately. After allowing several minutes for development of adequate local anesthesia effects, make a small skin incision parallel to the superior surface of the rib with the length determined by the size of the tube being inserted. Usually, a 3–4 cm incision will suffice. Then, careful blunt dissection just above the superior rib surface is accomplished using a Kelly clamp. Entrance to the pleural space is often heralded by the appearance of pleural fluid or the sound of air entering and leaving the chest through the insertion site due to normal pleural pressure fluctuations with respiration (sucking sound). The Kelly clamp is then used to widen the tract from the skin to pleural space. The Kelly is slowly withdrawn while simultaneously inserting a finger in the tract to maintain the tract and to allow digital sweeping of the immediate visceral pleural surface to clear any adjacent adhesions. The distal end of the chest tube (end inserted into the chest) is then clamped with forceps and inserted through the tract and into the pleural space. Rotation of the forceps with the distal tip of the chest tube clamped in the forceps will facilitate placement of the tube superiorly (apically) or inferiorly. A subsequent chest radiograph is obtained to confirm placement.

The chest tube placed by blunt dissection should be sewn in place using heavy suture material mounted on a curved cutting needle. I prefer 0 silk suture. A purse string suture around the tube is suggested with a half square (surgeon's) knot left in place. The half-knot maintains tension in the purse string, thus sealing the chest tube within the pleural space. This also allows prompt closure of the wound upon tube removal and easy completion of the square knot. I keep the excess suture material in place and wrap it around the tube and tie it off, allowing additional security against tube removal. This excess suture material also allows easy completion of a square knot upon tube removal. The site may be dressed using sealing antiseptic gauze (Adaptic X xeroform gauze non-adherent dressing, Johnson and Johnson, Arlington, TX), serving to help seal the site against air leaks. Next, cut 4″ × 4″ gauze squares (cut halfway through, creating a slit within which to place the chest tube) are placed around the chest tube. Finally, after skin preparation with an adhesive substance (Benzoin Compound, tincture USP, Paddock Laboratories, Minneapolis, MN), the site is taped. The most successful tape, in my practice, has been Microfoam (3M Medical, Surgical Division, St. Paul, MN). Tape applied around the chest tube near the connection with the pleural drainage device (if used) in an umbilical/omental configuration adds security against tube removal.

Chest tubes may also be inserted using a Seldinger technique wherein a guide wire plays a central role in tube placement. This technique is core to many commercially available kits such as those made by the companies Arrow™ and Cook™. Both large- and small-bore chest tubes may be inserted by this approach. After adequate sterile cleansing of the site and local anesthesia, the pleural space is located with a sterile needle. Subsequently, a guide wire is placed through the needle into the space, with the wire directed apically (for air) or inferiorly (for fluid) depending upon the material to be drained. Subsequently, a tract dilator (several graduated dilator sizes may be used for larger tubes) is passed. The actual chest tube is then placed over the guide wire and the wire removed. The tube may then be dressed similarly to tubes placed by blunt dissection. Commercially available kits often have tube-securing devices included.

Perhaps the most frequent *complication* of chest tube placement is patient discomfort during tube placement, tube residence, or tube removal (6). Harvey and Prescott note that pain may be particularly problematic with larger tubes as compared to smaller tubes while in place; paradoxically, no difference was noted between large and small tubes during tube insertion (8). Other common complications directly related to the tube itself include misplacement of the tube during insertion, disconnection of the tube while in place, and leakage around the tube, possibly resulting in subcutaneous emphysema (6). Pneumothorax recurrence in mechanically ventilated patients may occur due to initial tube malposition. Radiographic demonstration of interlobar chest tube placement has a positive predictive value of 86% for pneumothorax recurrence. Optimally, the chest tube should parallel the chest wall and be in the anterior hemithorax in patients with a pneumothorax (9).

Few studies are available specifically addressing directly related chest tube complications. Millikan and colleagues prospectively assessed chest tube–related complications in the acute thoracic trauma setting (10). Four of 447 patients suffered a technical complication of chest tube placement by blunt dissection. These included diaphragm laceration (two patients), lung laceration (one patient), and one patient with avulsion injury to the lesser curve of the stomach, laceration to the left lobe of the liver, and left diaphragm defect. In 1249 patients (trocar and blunt dissection chest tube placements), 30 cases of empyema occurred. No deaths were directly attributed to chest tube placement.

Currently at least 60% of surveyed pulmonologists are inserting chest tubes (11). Chest tubes placed for indications including pneumothorax and pleural effusions of various causes are successfully and safely placed by pulmonologists (12). Complications associated with 126 chest tube placements included malpositioned tube (1), nonfunctional tube (10), laceration of trapped lung (1), site infection (1), and leak around the tube (1). Complications were more frequently associated with small-bore tubes (4 of 11, 36%) than large-bore tubes (10 of 115, 9%) ($p = 0.02$).

III. Specific Chest Tube–Related Questions

Common questions related to chest tube placement will be generally addressed in this section. Specific answers to these questions related to common indications for chest tube placement will be explored further in Section V.

A. What Size Chest Tube Should Be Used?

Various sizes of chest tubes are now available, increasing the options for treatment of various pleural conditions but potentially leading to selection of tube sizes inappropriate to the condition. Flow of a humid gas through a chest tube is governed by the Fanning equation:

$$v = \pi^2 r^5 P / fl$$

where v is flow, r is radius, l is length, P is pressure, and f is friction factor (13–15). Flow is further complicated by the presence of liquids of various viscosities. Obviously, the critical factor in chest tube selection is the bore (internal diameter) of the tube, and less so the tube length. Hence, selection of a chest tube must take into account what is being drained and the rate at which the material is being formed. Patients with a large bronchopleural fistula on mechanical ventilation or patients with a briskly bleeding chest lesion require a larger tube than patients with small air leaks or static pleural fluid collections.

Knowledge of flow rates through various commercially available small-bore chest tubes (catheters) is key when considering their use. Generally, use of a small-bore tube for fluid collection needs careful consideration, particularly if fluid production is brisk, given that flow rates will be more limited for fluid than that for air. Additionally, not all small-bore catheters are of equal efficacy in their ability to handle air flow (16). This problem is compounded by the use of commercial thoracentesis kits that contain drainage catheters as a source for indwelling catheters. As expected from the Fanning equation, smaller-bore catheters handle lower flow rates, with 8 F catheter rates ranging from 2.6 to 5.5 L of air per minute. Eight F thoracentesis catheters handle significantly lower flow rates than the 8 F pneumothorax catheters made by the same manufacturer. Lower flow rates with the thoracentesis catheter appear due to different proximal catheter hardware. Particularly concerning are lower air flow rates delivered by larger- (16 F, 14.8 L/min) and smaller-bore Cook™ catheters (14 F, 12.8 L/min) compared with the 14 F Arrow™ catheters (16.8 L/min). The flow rate differences of identical bore catheters possibly represent true bore differences, catheter side hole variations, and length differences. In any case, such flow differences could be clinically significant in the setting of significant pleural air leaks or pleural fluid production.

B. Should Suction Be Applied?

After placement of the chest tube, the tube may be connected to a pleural drainage unit (PDU). The option then exists to utilize suction regulated through the PDU to the pleural space. Limited information is available to provide clear guidance as to the role of suction in the various indications for chest tube placement. Notably, air and free-flowing fluid will generally drain from the chest without the need for suction. Suction becomes necessary when a compromising accumulation of air or fluid occurs due to their rate of development or due to the viscosity of fluid hampering efficient gravity drainage. See Section III.E regarding the role of suction in chest tube removal.

C. How Can Reexpansion Pulmonary Edema Be Avoided?

Reexpansion pulmonary edema may occur after the drainage of pleural air or fluid (17). The etiology and risk factors leading to the development of reexpansion pulmonary are likely multifactorial (15). Increased vascular permeability, oxygen-free radical generation, and mechanical injury have been implicated as possible causes (18–20). Young age and extent of lung collapse are noted by Matsuura and colleagues (21) to be independent risk factors for reexpansion pulmonary edema. Patients 20–39 years in age are particularly prone to edema compared with older patients (21). Duration of collapse, noted as an associated risk in earlier studies (17,22,23), was less strongly associated with the development of reexpansion pulmonary edema in Matsuura et al.'s study (21). Trapnell and Thurston (17) and Mahfood and colleagues (24) suggest that lung collapse longer than 3 days may be associated with a greater incidence of reexpansion pulmonary edema. However, Mahfood and colleagues (24) note that reexpansion edema may occur after removal of pleural air present for only a "few hours" and may be related to rapid reexpansion. Their review also notes reexpansion pulmonary edema may occur in the absence of suction and may occur in the contralateral lung. As noted by Mahfood and colleagues, the rate of reexpansion may be more critical than the amount of fluid or air removed or the degree of suction applied (24).

A question related to that regarding issues prompting concern for reexpansion pulmonary edema is how much pleural fluid should initially be removed during a diagnostic or therapeutic thoracentesis. Clinicians placing a chest tube should be aware of the issues raised by this question given that chest tube removal of fluid is governed by the same concerns. The development of excess negative pleural pressures [below -20 cm (25) or below or equal to -19 cm (26) H_2O pressure during pleural fluid drainage of 1 L or 0.5 L, respectively] should be avoided and may herald the presence of a trapped lung (25,26) and reduced success of pleural sclerosis (26). Safe pleural fluid removal may continue as long as pleural pressures do not fall below -20 cm of water pressure (25).

However, the tools to measure pleural pressure during fluid removal are cumbersome, and most clinicians do not measure pressures. The American Thoracic Society (ATS) statement on management of malignant pleural effusions (27) provides expert-based advice on pleural fluid removal without pleural pressure monitoring. Recommended is the removal of only 1–1.5 L of fluid at any one sitting provided the patient does not develop dyspnea, chest pain, or severe cough (27). Additionally, I perform all chest tube placements and thoracenteses with an oxygen saturation monitor in place and discontinue drainage for a drop in saturation of more than 3–5% that does not resolve promptly with a short halt in fluid drainage. This said, however, removal of several liters of fluid is likely safe in the patient with contralateral shift of the mediastinum (shift away from the fluid) who does not develop chest tightness, cough, or dyspnea during fluid removal. The patient without mediastinal shift or with ipsilateral mediastinal shift (shift toward the fluid) likely has a fixed mediastinum, trapped lung, or endobronchial obstruction. In those patients, the chance of a marked fall in pleural pressure is increased and pleural pressure monitoring should be used or only a small volume of fluid (<300 mL) should be removed. Reexpansion pulmonary edema can develop after rapid removal of air or pleural fluid and may not be related to the absolute level of negative pleural pressure (27).

D. Should Talc Be Used as a Pleural Sclerosant?

Talc is a successful (91%) pleural sclerosant whether applied by chest tube (slurry) or by poudrage (by thoracoscopy) for both pneumothorax and pleural effusion (28). However, controversy regarding its use has arisen, with a cogent debate recently published (29,30). Key to this debate is the reported, and undisputed, occurrence of acute respiratory failure/acute respiratory distress syndrome (ARDS) that may occur with talc poudrage or slurry (29,30). Incidence of ARDS in reports varies considerably from no events to up to 33%, including event-associated deaths, with respiratory failure not firmly related to talc dose (29). Sahn, however, emphasizes from compiled published reported talc use in 2393 cases that only 17 acute respiratory failure events are reported (0.71%) (30). The etiology of talc-associated respiratory failure is unclear. Talc contamination with bacteria may play a role, but adequate sterilization methods make this unlikely (31). Diffuse bodily distribution of talc beyond the pleural space may play a role in precipitating acute lung injury or simply be an epiphenomenon (29,30). Small talc particle size may contribute to its distribution throughout the body and in turn be related to geographic origin of the talc (32). Recent pleural disruption by pleural biopsy or other invasive procedures may promote systemic talc distribution (33). Given these concerns and available alternative pleural sclerosants, the patient should be informed of their options and associated risks before proceeding with talc pleural sclerosis. If talc is chosen, the dose is not clearly established. Doses of as little as 2 g by poudrage have been reported to be associated with ARDS (29). Alternately, a large review notes a dose by poudrage or slurry of 5 g as successful and comparatively safe (28).

E. How Should a Chest Tube Be Removed?

Once the primary purpose for placement of a chest tube has passed, tube removal should be considered promptly. Continued chest tube residence increases the risk of possible pleural space contamination and infection. One of the most important issues to consider before tube removal is whether an air leak is present. Tube removal prior to cessation of an air leak, even a small leak, can lead to the development of a tension pneumothorax.

A commonly asked question is whether to remove a chest tube at the end of inspiration or the end of expiration (34). Either approach can be advocated based upon pulmonary mechanics. At the end of inspiration, the lung is maximally expanded with the pleural space minimized. At the end of forceful expiration pleural pressure is positive compared with atmosphere minimizing the chance of air entering into the pleural space. A recent randomized trial by Bell and colleagues assessing 102 chest tube placements in 69 patients suffering blunt or penetrating thoracic trauma requiring tube placement found no difference in the occurrence of post–chest tube removal pneumothoraces by either method (end inspiration, 8% occurrence; end expiration, 6%) (34). These findings occurred regardless of the mechanism of injury prompting tube placement, presence of hemothorax, history of thoracotomy or thoracoscopy, previous lung disease, or chest tube duration. Hence, patients having resolution of pneumothorax or a small stable pneumothorax by chest radiograph, lack of an air leak while the chest tube is applied to water seal, and, as demonstrated in the current study, chest tube output of < 200 mL/day may have their chest tube removed safely by either approach (34).

Whether to place a chest tube to suction or to place a chest tube to water seal, both through a PDU, prior to removal is not clear. Several complementary studies address this question. In Davis and colleagues' (35) study, 80 patients with pneumothorax and/or hemothorax from blunt or penetrating trauma, initially placed to chest tube suction, were randomized to continued suction or placement to water seal at the time of air leak termination. Both the suction and water seal groups had a similar incidence of recurrent pneumothorax after chest tube removal. However, both the total chest tube time (72.2 vs. 92.5 hr) and the time between air leak cessation and tube removal (25.2 vs. 35.6 hr) were significantly shorter in the suction group (35). Martino and colleagues (36) assessed 205 patients with chest tubes inserted for blunt or penetrating trauma randomized after cessation of any air leak to water seal or immediate chest tube removal. There were no differences in the chest tube duration or hospital length of stay in the two groups. Although the water seal group had a higher incidence of recurrent pneumothorax after tube removal (13 vs. 9 patients, respectively; $p < 0.05$), the no water seal group required reinsertion of a chest tube more frequently than the water seal group (7 vs. 1 patient, respectively; $p < 0.05$) (36). A similar pneumothorax recurrence problem related to immediate chest tube removal after air leak cessation has been reported by Sharma and colleagues (37) in a group of patients suffering spontaneous pneumothorax. Immediate (within 6 hr of lung reexpansion) versus late (within 48 hr of lung reexpansion) tube removal resulted in a 25% recurrence of lung collapse in the immediate removal group versus no recollapse in the late removal group (37). Based upon this information, continued chest tube suction after lung reexpansion and air leak cessation for several hours may be advisable before chest tube removal. Suction may assist in the detection of small air leaks. It has also been proposed by Davis and colleagues that subclinical air leaks seal better under the influence of suction (35).

Chest Tubes

The optimal duration of suction after air leak resolution has yet to be studied. Davis and colleagues continued suction for 24 hours after resolution of the air leak (35). Alternate approaches to the removal of a chest tube, including suction discontinuation and chest tube clamping to detect occult air leaks, are addressed by the American College of Chest Physicians (ACCP) consensus statement on the management of spontaneous pneumothorax (see Sec. V.A) (38). Additional randomized controlled trials are needed to determine the optimal approach to chest tube removal, thereby limiting chest tube residence time and hospital length of stay.

IV. The Pleural Drainage Unit

Depending upon the clinical indication, once a chest tube is placed, a PDU may be attached to provide suction and/or water seal to prevent backflow of air into the pleural space. The same resistance considerations in choosing a chest tube need to be assessed for the connecting tubing and the multichambered drainage device comprising a PDU (15,39–42). Commercially available PDUs differ considerably in their flow rates and the accuracy of delivered negative pressures (41). The most recent assessment of commercial PDUs available in the United States notes that air flow rate capabilities at −20 cm H_2O pressure vary, ranging from 10.8 to 42.1 L/min. The accuracy of the measured level of suction delivered varies significantly but may be of a magnitude that is not clinically significant (41).

The recently assessed commercially available PDUs are all based upon the traditional three-chamber device (41). This device (Fig. 1) is now commercially packaged into compartmentalized, durable, convenient single units providing easy mobility and specimen collection. The three compartments, se-

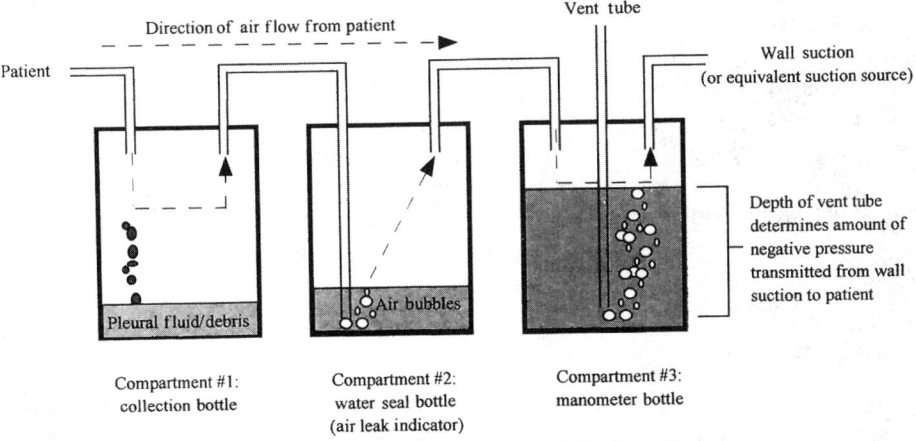

Figure 1 Three-compartment pleural drainage unit (PDU).

quentially, include: the collection bottle to trap liquid material and suspended debris (frequently with sampling ports) from the patient's pleural space while allowing any pleural air to pass through the next two compartments; the water seal bottle to prevent air flow back to the patient's pleural space and to allow detection of an air leak (bronchopleural fistula); the manometer bottle to regulate the amount of negative pressure transmitted back to the patient from the wall suction device (or equivalent suction source). The manometer bottle has an input and output tube and a central vent tube that may be raised or lowered. Adjusting the depth of the central vent tube in the chamber water determines the negative pressure transmitted from the wall suction back to the patient's pleural space (1). Most commercially available PDUs utilizing a water manometer compartment adjust the amount of negative pressure transmitted to the patient by raising and lowering the level of water in compartment number 3 instead of raising or lowering a vent tube. Commercial PDUs are now available as "wet" or "dry" devices depending upon whether they have a traditional water-based manometer (compartment 3) or a system based on a spring-loaded valve system (dry system) (41).

Simple one-way valve systems consisting of easily collapsible rubber tubing housed in a rigid plastic tube with entrance and exit ports are available and commonly contained with commercial pneumothorax kits (personal investigation). Such a device may be attached to a chest tube in lieu of the more elaborate PDU devices described above. A Heimlich valve is such a device. Caution is urged when incorporating a Heimlich valve, or similar device, particularly when a patient is sent home with the device attached to a chest tube. Clear instructions regarding device orientation (appropriate for air flow out of the chest) and maintenance are requisite to prevent complications including tension pneumothorax (43,44). A commercially available device having a self-contained needle, catheter, and one-way valve is also available (TRU-CLOSE Thoracic Vent; Davis and Geck, Wayne, NJ). A recent report of the development of a bronchopleural fistula after placement of a TRU-CLOSE highlights the necessity of a careful patient history regarding prior chest interventions leading to chest wall adhesions (45). Chest wall adhesions that may prevent lung collapse with a pneumothorax may allow perforation of the lung during placement of any device into the pleural space. The presence of viscous material such as blood should be a relative contraindication to the use of any of these alternative PDU devices for fear of device occlusion and the development of a tension pneumothorax.

V. Selected Applications

A. Pneumothorax

Current pulmonary medicine textbook and journal reviews subdivide pneumothoraces into spontaneous pneumothoraces (SP) and traumatic pneumothoraces (46,47). Spontaneous pneumothoraces occur without preceding trauma or an obvious underlying cause (15,46,47). Spontaneous pneumothoraces are categorized as primary and secondary. Primary spontaneous pneumothoraces (PSP) arise in patients without clinically obvious lung disease. Secondary spontaneous pneumothoraces (SSP) occur in patients with underlying lung disease, often chronic obstructive lung disease (15,46,47). Traumatic pneumothoraces result from direct or indirect trauma to the chest including from diagnostic or therapeutic interventions. Traumatic pneumothoraces resulting from medical interventions are termed iatrogenic pneumothoraces (47).

Spontaneous Pneumothorax

Management of SP has been quite heterogeneous (48). A limited number of randomized controlled trials addressing SP management and the myriad of therapeutic options have contributed to this heterogeneity. Recently published ACCP guidelines provide management direction (38). Patient observation, simple aspiration, chest tube placement, surgical interventions including thoracoscopy and thoracotomy for management of SP patients are outlined. Observational management is the preferred ACCP guideline approach for stable PSP patients with a small pneumothorax (< 3 cm lung collapse); some form of lung reexpansion procedure, such as chest tube placement, is recommended for a large (≥3 cm lung collapse) pneumothorax.

Chest tube placement plays a central role in the management of other SP patients in these new ACCP guidelines, while simple aspiration has a limited place. Initial placement of a chest tube and hospital admission is preferred management of an unstable patient with a large (≥3 cm lung collapse) PSP or any SSP patient with a large pneumothorax or with clinical instability. Patients with a PSP (unlikely at risk for a large air leak) suitable for chest tube placement should have their lung reexpanded using a small-bore catheter (≤14 F) or placement of a 16–22 F chest tube. Patients with a SSP, by the nature of their underlying lung disease, may be at greater risk of a large air leak or may require mechanical ventilation (38). Stable SSP patients not at great risk for a large air leak (not mechanically ventilated) who are chest tube candidates should have a 16–22 F chest tube placed; smaller tubes (≤14 F) may be acceptable in selected patients. Unstable SSP patients and SSP patients on mechanical ventilation should have a 24–28 F chest tube placed because of the risk for large air leaks (38).

Once placed, the initial management of the chest tube is quite variable (48). Limited information regarding the value of suction is available. So and Yu (49) and Minami and colleagues (50) found no clear advantage to the use of suction. The ACCP guidelines suggest attaching a chest tube to a water seal device with or without suction as acceptable in most SP patients. If the lung does not reexpand promptly, suction should then be applied. A Heimlich valve may be incorporated in selected stable SP patients in lieu of a water seal device, although the consensus of the ACCP expert group was that a water seal device is a better option in most SSP patients (38).

Once a chest tube is in place, tube-directed pleural sclerosis for pneumothorax recurrence prevention is an available option. However, in PSP patients, thoracoscopy is the preferred recurrence prevention intervention after the second pneumothorax event. Chest tube–directed pleural sclerosis is acceptable in patients with a PSP refusing surgery and for those with increased surgical risks (e.g., bleeding diathesis). Doxycycline or talc slurry is the preferred sclerosing agent (38). Recurrence prevention by thoracoscopy, after the first pneumothorax episode, is preferred in patients with a SSP. Chest tube–directed pleural sclerosis my be used in certain circumstances based on patient contraindications to surgery, management preferences, and poor prognosis of underlying disease. As with PSP, doxycycline or talc slurry is the preferred sclerosant in SSP patients (38).

Once a pneumothorax air leak has resolved and recurrence prevention issues are addressed, removal of the chest tube is considered. Tubes should be removed in a staged sequence to ensure that any air leak has resolved before tube removal. A radiograph demonstrating lung re-expansion and no clinical evidence of an air leak is necessary. Any applied suction should be discontinued as part of this assessment (38). The role of chest tube clamping to ensure the absence of small air leaks not readily detected by monitoring the pleural drainage device water seal chamber for bubbling remains controversial. The ACCP consensus group was divided regarding the utility of clamping with 47% and 59% of the group incorporating clamping as part of chest tube removal in PSP and SSP, respectively (38). Opponents of tube clamping raise concerns for the development of unnoticed lung collapse (51); supporters of clamping note that air leaks may not be obvious in the air leak indicator chamber and carefully monitored tube clamping may detect small air leaks and circumvent chest tube replacement due to an overlooked air leak (52). If clamping is incorporated, the tube should be clamped for approximately 4 hours in PSP and 5–12 hours in SSP with a subsequent chest radiograph obtained to assess for pneumothorax recurrence (38).

Traumatic Pneumothorax

Pneumothorax ranks second to rib fractures as the most common manifestation of traumatic chest injury and is noted in 40–50% of patients with chest trauma (53–55). Many of these pneumothoraces are occult (not seen on an initial chest radiograph but found by additional imaging) and may occur in up to 51% of trauma patients (55). Up to 20% of prospectively evaluated patients with chest trauma or multitrauma have an accompanying hemothorax not appreciated on initial chest radiograph but revealed by computed tomography (CT) of the chest (56). Traumatic pneumothoraces should generally be treated with placement of a chest tube (54). Chest tube placement then serves the dual purpose of evacuating both air and blood, affording the surgical team the opportunity to monitor the tempo of blood loss as a potential marker of the need for urgent operative intervention. Given the potential for the presence of both air and blood, a large-bore tube (28–36 F) is recommended. Conservative management (close observation without chest tube placement) may be successful in carefully selected patients suffering a traumatic pneumothorax, particularly those not subjected to positive pressure mechanical ventilation (57).

Iatrogenic Pneumothorax

The incidence and causes of iatrogenic pneumothorax vary considerably. The most common causes of iatrogenic pneumothorax in the Veterans Administration patient population are transthoracic needle aspiration, subclavian vein catheterization, and thoracentesis (58,59). Treatment of a patient with an iatrogenic pneumothorax is quite variable. Development of management protocols is complicated by insufficient tracking and reporting of these iatrogenic events (60). A current text recommends observation and oxygen supplementation for patients not mechanically ventilated with minimal symptoms and a limited (<15%) pneumothorax (47). If a patient has more than minimal symptoms or a larger pneumothorax (>15%), simple aspiration is recommended (47). Patients with CT evidence of emphysema sustaining a pneumothorax during needle lung biopsy more often require chest tube placement than patients without evidence of emphysema (27% with evidence vs. 9% without) (61). Given this information, initial placement of a small-bore chest tube and forgoing observation is recommended in such patients. Iatrogenic pneumothoraces secondary to positive pressure mechanical ventilation may develop tension pneumothorax and are likely to develop bronchopleural fistula (40). Such patients require placement of a larger-bore chest tube and observation is not recommended.

B. Parapneumonic Pleural Effusions and Empyema

The most appropriate therapeutic approach to a parapneumonic effusion and empyema continues to be debated. However, new ACCP guidelines provide evidence-based direction while emphasizing the limited information available to base the suggested recommendations (62). The ACCP guidelines divide patients with parapneumonic effusion and empyema into four categories reflecting increasing risk for poor outcome. Category 1 patients include those with minimal, free-flowing effusion (<10 mm on lateral decubitus) with culture, Gram stain and pleural fluid pH unknown. Category 2 patients include those with a small to moderate free-flowing effusion (>10 mm and less than half the hemithorax) with negative culture and Gram stain, and a pH of ≥ 7.20. Category 3 patients are those with a large, free-flowing effusion (half the hemithorax or greater), loculated effusion, or effusion with thickened parietal pleura. Also, a category 3 patient could simply have a positive culture or Gram stain or a pleural fluid pH of < 7.20. A category 4 patient may have category 3 characteristics as outlined but is found to have pus in the pleural space. The guidelines advise that category 1 and 2 patients may not require drainage (62) by chest tube or other means. Drainage is recommended for category 3 and 4 patients, noting that therapeutic thoracentesis or chest tube placement alone appears insufficient for most of these patients. However, the use of therapeutic thoracentesis or chest tube placement as a planned interim step before a subsequent drainage procedure may be successful in individual patients, obviating further intervention. Chest tube–directed application of fibrinolytics, video-assisted thoracoscopic surgery, and surgery are acceptable management options for category 3 and 4 patients; the statement notes that these approaches in category 3 and 4 patients are associated with the lowest mortality and need for a second intervention (62).

C. Recurrent Symptomatic Pleural Effusions

Chest tube placement with subsequent introduction of pleural sclerosing agent offers the potential opportunity to prevent the reaccumulation of a recurrent symptomatic effusion. Although perhaps more commonly considered in recurrent symptomatic malignant effusions, this therapeutic maneuver may be useful in selected benign effusions as well.

Benign Pleural Effusions

A physician may consider preventing future recurrence of a benign effusion if it recurs with significant symptoms, if the physician is comfortable with the etiological diagnosis, and no further invasive pleural diagnostic studies are planned. Generally, the patient should also be unresponsive to medical treatment of the underlying cause of the effusion. A diagnostic and therapeutic (talc poudrage) thoracoscopic approach may be taken or a chest tube may be placed with subsequent instillation of a pleural sclerosing agent. A chest tube–directed approach is often more feasible for most clinicians given its ready availability.

Chest tube–directed pleurodesis successfully prevents effusion recurrence in nonmalignant exudative and transudative effusions (63,64). Talc pleurodesis demonstrates greater success (97%) than the overall success of other unspecified sclerosing agents combined (60%) in benign effusion cases (64). Underlying diagnoses and reported success with chest tube–directed talc pleurodesis include congestive heart failure (100%), liver cirrhosis (89%), systemic lupus erythematosus (100%), chylothorax (benign causes including lymphangiolyomyomatosis) (95%), yellow nail syndrome (100%), nephrotic syndrome (100%), peritoneal dialysis (100%), and unknown underlying causes (100%) (64). Importantly, however, these effusions may be benign only in their etiology. Four of 16 patients (25%) in Glazer and colleagues' case series (one patient each with liver cirrhosis, congestive heart failure, chylothorax, and undiagnosed effusion) died of their underlying disease within 2–6 months of chest tube–directed pleural sclerosis (64).

Malignant Pleural Effusions

The recent ATS statement on the management of malignant pleural effusions provides guidance on the role of chest tubes in malignant effusions (27). This statement notes that nearly all neoplasms have been reported to involve the pleural space, with lung cancer frequently reported as the most common, accounting for approximately one third of all malignant pleural effusions. Patients most commonly present with dyspnea and symptomatic relief is the major indication for some form of palliative treatment. If a therapeutic thoracentesis provides marked symptom relief and the lung reexpands (no trapped lung or occluding endobronchial lesion) and the effusion rapidly reaccumulates with accompanying dyspnea, palliative treatment is warranted. However, if dyspnea is not relieved or the lung does not reexpand, a trapped lung or endobronchial lesion may be present and chest tube–directed sclerosis will likely fail (27).

Therapeutic options for symptomatic recurrent malignant effusions include therapeutic thoracentesis (27) that may be repeated in selected patients expected to succumb to their disease shortly. Chemical pleurodesis directed by chest tube or thoracoscopy are additional options, with the choice often dependent upon local expertise and availability of thoracoscopy. As noted with benign effusions, chest tube management may often be chosen given its generally ready availability. Talc slurry delivered by chest tube versus talc poudrage by thoracoscopy has similar success—91% in malignant effusions (27,28).

Commonly, chest tube–directed pleurodesis is performed by a large-bore tube, but similar success rates have been reported with smaller-bore tubes (8–14 F) (65,66), and this success is noted in the ATS malignant effusion statement (27). Once confirmation of lung reexpansion and fluid removal has been obtained radiographically, presclerosis narcotics and/or sedation are suggested given the pain frequently associated with sclerosis. The sclerosant, diluted in 50–100 mL of sterile saline, is introduced and the tube clamped for one hour (27). The ATS statement does not suggest patient rotation. I also do not rotate patients administered agents in *solution*, such as doxycycline, based on a study by Dryzer and colleagues demonstrating no difference in pleurodesis success for patients rotated and not rotated (67). No similar study to date has been published for talc slurry. I rotate patients administered talc slurry to effect pleural talc distribution given concerns that the talc *suspension* may settle prematurely in gravity-dependent portions of the hemithorax. The chest tube is then connected to a PDU with 20 cm of water suction until the 24-hour chest tube output is <150 mL (27).

Neither the ATS malignant effusion statement (27) nor recent texts (68) suggest waiting to proceed with sclerosis until daily chest tube output of pleural fluid reaches an arbitrary minimum. The current focus in determining when to introduce the sclerosing agent is upon the presence of successful lung reexpansion (27,68). Light (68) notes that there are no supporting data for the minimal daily fluid output goal. Success appears similar whether waiting for a minimal amount of daily fluid production or with immediate application of the sclerosing agent after lung reexpansion. Similarly, intrapleural application of an anesthetic is not recommended for pain control given no controlled studies support such a practice (68).

A myriad of sclerosing agents are available, with the ATS review specifically exploring the success of doxycycline, bleomycin, and talc. Five hundred milligrams of doxycycline in 50–100 mL of sterile saline is recommended complemented by narcotic analgesia or conscious sedation given the common complication of pain. Bleomycin is noted to be successful, but cost is the major limitation compared with doxycycline or talc. No more than 5 g of talc is suggested, and bilateral simultaneous pleurodesis with talc should be avoided (27).

In addition to palliation that may be afforded by chest tube fluid drainage and pleural sclerosis, systemic therapy should be pursued particularly in malignant effusions likely to respond to chemotherapy and may be complemented by therapeutic thoracentesis or pleurodesis. Breast cancer, small-cell lung cancer, and lymphoma tend to be chemotherapy responsive (27).

A therapeutic alternative not highlighted in the ATS statement utilizing many of the skills required for chest tube placement that can be mastered by surgeon and nonsurgeon alike is the placement of an indwelling pleural catheter (Pleurx™ catheter, Denver Biomaterials, Denver, CO) (69). This is a 15.5 F catheter with fenestrations at the pleural end and a valve on the opposing end. A wire is placed into the malignant pleural effusion using the Seldinger technique at the anterior axillary line with a 1–2 cm incision made over the wire. A 5–8 cm chest wall tunnel is created with a counterincision, and the catheter is pulled through the tunnel and out next to the wire. The catheter is then inserted over the wire and into the chest after dilation of the wire tract. The wire is then removed (69). External vacuum bottles can be used by the symptomatic patient at home to drain pleural fluid by appropriate attachment to the valve end of the catheter.

Patients underwent a 2:1 randomization to the indwelling catheter ($n = 99$) and to doxycycline pleurodesis ($n = 45$) with a median hospital stay of 1 day for the catheter group and 6.5 days for the doxycycline group ($p < 0.001$). Improvement in dyspnea and quality of life was comparable in the two groups. Twenty-one percent of the doxycycline patients and 13% of patients with the indwelling catheter had a late recurrence of their effusion or blockage of their Pleurx™ catheter after initial successful treatment ($p = 0.45$). Forty-six percent of indwelling catheter patients sent home had spontaneous pleurodesis at a median of 26.5 days (69). This approach offers an at-home management approach for patients with recurrent symptomatic malignant pleural effusions. Future study with this indwelling catheter incorporating catheter-directed pleurodesis might increase the success of this option.

D. Hemothorax

Hemothoraces may be classified as traumatic, iatrogenic, and, rarely, nontraumatic. A hemothorax is present when the pleural fluid hematocrit is ≥50%

of the peripheral blood. Given that a small amount of blood in the pleural space may appear visually significant, the hematocrit should be measured to clarify the issue in any bloody effusion (47). Drainage of a hemothorax is advisable to limit future potential complications including pleural infection (empyema) (1–5%) (70–72), retention of clotted blood in the pleural space (3%) (70), pleural effusion after chest tube removal (13%) (72), and fibrothorax (<1%) (70).

As noted in relation to traumatic pneumothorax (see above), 20% of hemothoraces in patients suffering blunt chest trauma in Trupka and colleagues' series may not be noted on routine chest radiograph but detected by chest CT (56). This study supports an earlier study finding that evaluation of the initial chest radiograph did not uncover the hemothorax in patients with blunt chest trauma in 24% of cases (73). Given the unexpected CT findings of pneumothorax in 26% of patients as well as unexpected hemothorax (20%) in Trupka's study (56), an initial CT of the chest in chest trauma patients is advised. Computed tomography of the chest more accurately predicts a residual hemothorax volume of 500 mL than chest radiographs and limits false-positive detection of fluid by chest radiographs (e.g., interpreting lung parenchymal disease as pleural blood). Such CT information has been used prospectively to indicate the need for early (within 2 days of chest tube placement) thoracoscopic intervention (74). Early diagnosis with subsequent drainage of hemothorax may limit late complications such as fibrothorax (73,74).

The finding of a hemothorax should always prompt consideration of an iatrogenic cause, particularly after thoracic surgery or after placement of a central venous or arterial catheter (47,75). A hemothorax may appear contralateral to the site of line placement (75), and contralateral radiographic findings should not dissuade consideration of a procedure-associated hemothorax. Although rare, anticoagulation should be considered as a potential cause of hemothorax, including those massive in size, usually occurring within the first week of therapy for pulmonary thromboembolism (76). Also uncommon, neoplastic pleural disease is a nontraumatic cause of hemothorax that should be considered (77).

Chest tube placement should be considered in all of these hemothorax settings. The tube allows removal of the blood from the pleural space while permitting monitoring of the tempo of blood loss that may prompt a surgical intervention. Coincidental pneumothorax in the setting of trauma may also be removed. Drainage may also help mitigate the development of subsequent pleural infection and fibrothorax (72,73). Given the viscous nature of blood, often coagulated, a large-bore tube is used (72,78). Chest tube–administered fibrinolytics appear to add little (78) and should be avoided in most cases (47). Recognition that the chest tube may not have adequately drained the space should prompt consideration of other diagnostic and therapeutic interventions, including appropriately timed thoracoscopy (79) or thoracotomy (78). Most information regarding hemothorax surgical management is found related to traumatic hemothorax; the exact timing and indications of a surgical intervention for traumatic hemothorax are variable (70,72,78). However, a recent prospective randomized trial indicates that early video-assisted thoracoscopic surgery (VATS) (within 72 hours of for retained traumatic hemothorax post-chest tube placement) compared to additional chest tube drainage decreased the total hospital length of stay, hospital cost, and duration of chest tube drainage (79).

VI. Summary

Chest tube placement is a valuable therapeutic and, at times, diagnostic tool. A myriad of chest tube devices and support equipment, including pleural drainage units, are available today. Knowledge of the appropriate use, placement, and limitations of these devices is key to the practice of chest medicine today. The few available randomized controlled trials regarding chest tube–related issues inadequately address the many aspects of chest tube management, highlighting the need for additional studies. Such studies are necessary to assist clinicians to better utilize these important tools.

References

1. Miller KS, Sahn SA. Chest tubes. Indications, technique, management and complications. Chest 1987; 91:258–264.
2. Playfair. Case of empyema treated by aspiration and subsequently by drainage: recovery. Br Med J 1875; 1:45.
3. Graham EA, Bell RD. Open pneumothorax: its relation to the treatment of empyema. Am J Med Sci 1918; 156:839–871.
4. Lilienthal H. Resection of the lung for supportive infections with a report based on 31 consecutive operative cases in which resection was done or intended. Ann Surg 1922; 75:257–320.
5. Lawrence G. Closed chest tube drainage for pleural space problems. The primary therapeutic modality. In: Problems of the Pleural Space. Vol. 28. Philadelphia: W. B. Saunders Company; 1983:13–24.
6. Silver M, Bone RC. Techniques for chest tube insertion and pleurodesis. J Crit Illness 1993; (8,631–637.
7. Bone RC. The technique of small-catheter pleural aspiration. J Crit Illness 1993; 8:827–833.
8. Harvey J, Prescott RJ. Simple aspiration versus intercostal tube drainage for spontaneous pneumothorax in patients with normal lungs. BMJ 1994; 309:1338–1339.
9. Heffner JE, McDonald J, Barbieri C. Recurrent pneumothoraces in ventilated patients despite ipsilateral chest tubes. Chest 1995; 108:1053–1058.
10. Millikan J, Moore E, Steiner E, Aragon G, Van Way C. Complications of tube thoracostomy for acute trauma. Am J Surg 1980; 140:738–741.
11. Tape TG, Blank LL, Wigton RS. Procedural skills of practicing pulmonologists. A national survey of 1,000 members of the American College of Physicians. Am J Respir Crit Care Med 1995; 151:282–287.

12. Collop NA, Kim S, Sahn SA. Analysis of tube thoracostomy performed by pulmonologists at a teaching hospital. Chest 1997; 112:709–713.
13. Swenson EW, Birath G, Ahbeck A. Resistance to air flow in bronchospirometric catheters. J Thorac Surg 1957; 33:275–281.
14. Batchelder TL, Morris KA. Critical factors in determining adequate pleural drainage in both the operated and nonoperated chest. Am Surg 1962; 28:296–302.
15. Baumann MH, Strange C. Treatment of spontaneous pneumothorax. A more aggressive approach? Chest 1997; 112:789–804.
16. Roney CW, Patel P, Petrini M, Baumann MH. Flow rates through commercially available pleural drainage catheters. Chest 2000; 118:256S.
17. Trapnell DH, Thurston JGB. Unilateral pulmonary oedema after pleural aspiration. Lancet 1970; 1:1367–1369.
18. Pavlin DJ, Nessly ML, Cheney FW. Increased pulmonary vascular permeability as a cause of re-expansion pulmonary edema. Am Rev Respir Dis 1981; 124:422–427.
19. Jackson RM, Veal CF, Alexander CB, Brannen AL, Fulmer JD. Re-expansion pulmonary edema: a potential role for free radicals in its pathogenesis. Am Rev Respir Dis 1988; 137:1165–1171.
20. Sprung CL, Loewenherz JW, Baier H, Hauser MJ. Evidence for increased permeability in reexpansion pulmonary edema. Am J Med 1981; 71:497–500.
21. Matsuura Y, Nomimura T, Murakami H, Matsushima T, Kakehashi M, Kajihara H. Clinical analysis of reexpansion pulmonary edema. Chest 1991; 100:1562–1566.
22. Waqaruddin M, Bernstein A. Re-expansion pulmonary edema. Thorax 1975; 30:54–60.
23. Sautter RD, Dreher WH, MacIndoe JH, Myers WO, Magnin GE. Fatal pulmonary edema and pneumonitis after reexpansion of chronic pneumothorax. Chest 1971; 60:399–401.
24. Mahfood S, Hix WR, Aaron BL, Blaes P, Watson DC. Reexpansion pulmonary edema. Ann Thorac Surg 1988; 45:340–345.
25. Light R, Jenkinson S, Minh V, George R. Observations on pleural fluid pressures as fluid is withdrawn during thoracentesis. Am Rev Respir Dis 1980; 121:799–804.
26. Lan R, Lo S, Chuang M, Yang C, Tsao T, Lee C. Elastance of the pleural space: a predictor for the outcome of pleurodesis in patients with malignant pleural effusions. Ann Intern Med 1997; 126:768–774.
27. Antony VB, Loddenkemper R, Astoul P, Boutin C, Goldstraw P, Hott J, Francisco Rodriguez Panadero F, Sahn SA. Management of malignant pleural effusions. Am J Respir Crit Care Med 2000; 162:1987–2001.
28. Kennedy L, Sahn SA. Talc pleurodesis for the treatment of pneumothorax and pleural effusion. Chest 1994; 106:1215–1222.
29. Light RW. Talc should not be used for pleurodesis. Am J Respir Crit Care Med 2000; 162:2024–2026.
30. Sahn SA. Talc should be used for pleurodesis. Am J Respir Crit Care 2000; 162:2023–2024.
31. Kennedy L, Vaughnan LM, Steed LL, Sahn SA. Sterilization of talc for pleurodesis: available techniques, efficacy, and cost analysis. Chest 1995; 107:1032–1034.
32. Ferrer J, Villarino MA, Tura JM, Traveria A, Light RW. Talc preparations used for pleurodesis vary markedly from one preparation to another. Chest 2001; 119:1901–1905.

33. de Campos JRM, Vargas FS, Werebe EdC, Cardoso P, Teixeira LR, Jatene FB, Light RW. Thoracoscopy talc poudrage. A 15-year experience. Chest 2001; 119:801–806.
34. Bell RL, Ovadia P, Abdullah F, Spector S, Rabinovici R. Chest tube removal: end-inspiration or end-expiration? J Trauma 2001; 50:674–677.
35. Davis JW, Mackersie RC, Hoyt DB, Garcia J. Randomized study of algorithms for discontinuing tube thoracostomy drainage. J Am Coll Surg 1994; 179:553–557.
36. Martino K, Merrit S, Boyakye K, Sernas T, Koller C, Hauser CJ, Lavery R, Livingston DH. Prospective randomized trial of thoracostomy removal algorithms. J Trauma 1999; 46:369–373.
37. Sharma TN, Agnihotri S, Jain N, Madan A, Deopura G. Intercostal tube thoracostomy in pneumothorax. Factors influencing re-expansion of the lung. Indian J Chest Dis All Sci 1988; 30:32–35.
38. Baumann MH, Strange C, Heffner JE, Light R, Kirby TJ, Klein J, Luketich JD, Panacek EA, Sahn SA. Management of spontaneous pneumothorax. An American College of Chest Physicians Delphi consensus statement. Chest 2001; 119:590–602.
39. Capps JS, Tyler M, Rusch VW, Pierson DL. Potential of chest drainage units to evacuate broncho-pleural air leaks. Chest 1985; 88:57S.
40. Baumann MH, Sahn SA. Medical management and therapy of bronchopleural fistulas in the mechanically ventilated patient. Chest 1990; 97:721–728.
41. Patel PB, Petrini M, Baumann MH. Flow rates and suction levels in commercial pleural drainage units. Am J Respir Crit Care Med 2000; 161:A400.
42. Rusch VW, Capps JS, Tyler ML, Pierson DL. The performance of four pleural drainage systems in an animal model of broncopleural fistula. Chest 1988; 93:859–863.
43. Mainini SE, Johnson FE. Tension pneumothorax complicating small-caliber chest tube insertion. Chest 1990; 97:759–760.
44. Crocker HL, Ruffin RE. Patient-induced complications of a Heimlich flutter valve. Chest 1998; 113:838–839.
45. Jones AE, Knoepp LF, Oxley DD. Bronchopleural fistula resulting from the use of a thoracic vent. A case report and review. Chest 1998; 114:1781–1784.
46. Sahn SA, Heffner JE. Spontaneous pneumothorax. N Engl J Med 2000; 342:868–874.
47. Light RW, Broaddus VC. Pneumothorax, chylothorax, hemothorax, and fibrothorax. In: Murray JF, Nadel JA, Mason RJ, Boushey HA, eds. Textbook of Respiratory Medicine. Vol. 2. 3rd ed. Philadelphia: W. B. Saunders Company, 2000:2043–2066.
48. Baumann MH, Strange C. The clinician's perspective on pneumothorax management. Chest 1997; (112,822–828.
49. So S, Yu D. Catheter drainage of spontaneous pneumothorax: suction or no suction, early or late removal? Thorax 1982; 37:46–48.
50. Minami H, Saka H, Senda K, Horio Y, Iwahara T, Nomura F, Sakai S, Shimokata K. Small caliber catheter drainage for spontaneous pneumothorax. Am J Med Sci 1992; 304:345–347.
51. Miller AC. Treatment of spontaneous pneumothorax. The clinician's perspective on pneumothorax management. Chest 1998:1423–1424.

52. Baumann MH, Strange C. Treatment of spontaneous pneumothorax. The clinicians' perspective on pneumothorax management. Chest 1998; 113:1424–1425.
53. Bridges KG, Welch G, Silver M, Schinco MA, Esposito B. CT detection of occult pneumothorax in multiple trauma patients. J Emerg Med 1993; 11:179–186.
54. Enderson BL, Abdalla R, Frame SB, Casey MT, Gould H, Maull KI. Tube thoracostomy for occult pneumothorax: a prospective randomized study of its use. J Trauma 1993; 35:726–730.
55. Wolfman NT, Myers WS, Glauser SJ, Meredith JW, Chen MYM. Validity of CT classification on management of occult pneumothorax: a prospective study. AJR 1998; 171:1317–1320.
56. Trupka A, Waydhas C, Hallfeldt K, Nast-Kolb D, Pfeifer K, Schweiberer L. Value of thoracic computed tomography in the first assessment of severely injured patients with blunt chest trauma: results of a prospective study. J Trauma 1997; 43: 405–411.
57. Johnson G. Traumatic pneumothorax: is a chest drain always necessary? J Accid Emerg Med 1996; 13:173–174.
58. Sassoon CSH, Light RW, O'Hara VS, Moritz TE. Iatrogenic pneumothorax: etiology and morbidity. Respiration 1992; 59:215–220.
59. Despars JA, Sassoon CSH, Light RW. Significance of iatrogenic pneumothoraces. Chest 1994; 105:1147–1150.
60. Berger R. Iatrogenic pneumothorax. Chest 1994; 105:980–982.
61. Cox JE, Chiles C, McManus CM, Aquino SL, Choplin RH. Transthoracic needle aspiration biopsy: variables that affect risk of pneumothorax. Radiology 1999; 212:165–168.
62. Colice GL, Curtis A, Deslaurierb, Littenberg B, Sahn S, Weinstein RA, Yusen RD. Medical and surgical treatment of parapneumonic effusions. An evidence-based guideline. Chest 2000; 118:1158–1171.
63. Sudduth CD, Sahn SA. Pleurodesis for nonmalignant pleural effusions. Recommendations. Chest 1992; 102:1855–1860.
64. Glazer M, Berkman N, Lafair JS, Kramer MR. Successful talc slurry pleurodesis in patients with nonmalignant effusions. Report of 16 cases and review of the literature. Chest 2000; 117:1404–1409.
65. Parker LA, Charnock GC, Delany DJ. Small bore catheter drainage and sclerotherapy for malignant pleural effusions. Cancer 1989; 64:1121–1218.
66. Seaton KG, Patz EF, Goodman PC. Palliative treatment of malignant pleural effusions: value of small-bore catheter thoracostomy and doxycyline sclerotherapy. AJR 1995; 164:589–591.
67. Dryzer S, Allen M, Strange C, Sahn S. A comparison of rotation and nonrotation in tetralycline pleurodesis. Chest 1993; 104:1763–1766.
68. Light RW. Pleural effusions related to metastatic malignancies. In: Light RW, ed. Pleural Diseases. 4th ed. Philadelphia: Lippincott Williams and Wilkins, 2001:108–134.
69. Putnam JB, Light RW, Rodriguez RM, Ponn R, Olak J, Pollak JS, Lee RB, Payne DK, Graeber G, Kovitz K. A randomized comparison of indwelling pleural catheter and doxycycline pleurodesis in the management of malignant pleural effusions. Cancer 1999; 86:1992–1999.
70. Beall AC, Crawford HW, DeBakey ME. Considerations in the management of acute traumatic hemothorax. J Thorac Cardiovasc Surg 1976; 52:351–360.

71. Griffith GL, Todd EP, McMillin RD, Zeok JV, Dillon ML, Utley JR, Griffen WO. Acute traumatic hemothorax. Ann Thorac Surg 1978; 26:204–207.
72. Wilson JM, Boren CH, Peterson SR, Thomas AN. Traumatic hemothorax: Is decortication necessary? J Thorac Cardiovasc Surg 1979; 77:489–495.
73. Drummond DS, Craig RH. Traumatic hemothorax: complications and management. Am Surg 1967; 33:403–408.
74. Velmahos GC, Demetriades D, Chan L, Tatevossian R, Cornwell EE, Yassa N, Murray JA, Asensio JA, Berne TV. Predicting the need for thoracoscopic evacuation of residual traumatic hemothorax: chest radiograph is insufficient. J Trauma 1999; 46:65–70.
75. Krauss D, Schmidt GA. Cardiac tamponade and contralateral hemothorax after subclavian vein catheterization. Chest 1991; 99:517–518.
76. Rostand RA, Feldman RL, Block ER. Massive hemothorax complicating heparin anticoagulation for pulmonary embolus. South Med J 1977; 70:1128–1130.
77. Berliner K. Hemorrhagic pleural effusion: an analysis of 120 cases. Ann Intern Med 1941; 14:2266–2284.
78. Parry GW, Morgan WE, Salama FD. Management of haemothorax. Ann R Coll Surg Engl 1996; 78:325–326.
79. Meyer DM, Jessen ME, Wait MW. Early evacuation of traumatic retained hemothoraces using thoracoscopy: a prospective randomized trial. Ann Thorac Surg 1997; 64:1396–1401.

10

Pleural Lavage as a Diagnostic and Research Tool

MARC NOPPEN

Free University of Brussels
and Academic Hospital AZ—VUB
Brussels, Belgium

I. Introduction

Pleural lavage (PL) is defined as an irrigation procedure of the pleural space, i.e., the instillation of a known volume of irrigation fluid (usually saline) followed by immediate aspiration. The aspirated fluid and its cellular or solute content can then be examined for diagnostic or research purposes.

As such, PL is not (yet) a universally accepted descriptive term; the procedure in itself, however, has been and still is used quite often and for various indications. The purpose of this chapter is to give a nonexhaustive overview of key papers relevant to the issue and to discuss current and future studies of PL in animal models and human pathology.

The pleural cavity is a closed space formed by a continuum of a thin serosal membrane: the pleura. The visceral pleura covers the entire surface of the lung, including the interlobar fissures; the parietal pleura covers the inner surface of the thoracic cage, mediastinum, and diaphragm. The visceral and parietal pleu-ral merge with each other at the hilum of the lung and at the pulmonary ligament (1). The pleural space contains a small amount of pleural fluid, which, in normal circumstances, maintains the necessary lubrification of the pleural surfaces enabling transmission of the forces of breathing between lung and chest wall (2).

Normal volume and cellular and solute content of pleural fluid, as well as pleural fluid dynamics, have been determined mainly in animal studies. Because of the obvious technical difficulties in retrieving atraumatically the few milliliters of fluid present in the pleural space, only a few human studies are available (3).

Pleural lavage has been used as a research tool in a number of animal studies in order to retrieve the original pleural fluid for examination of its content; in humans, PL was used in a recent paper for the determination of the volume and cellular content of normal pleural fluid (4).

In pathological processes involving the pleura, but not necessarily associated with pleural effusion (e.g., pneumothorax, asbestos-induced pleural disease), PL can be used for research purposes. Finally, PL can be used in diagnostic (staging) purposes in patients with thoracic cancers (lung, esophagus). The therapeutic use of pleural lavage, i.e., in the treatment of empyema, will not be discussed here.

II. Pleural Lavage as a Research Tool in Animals

A. Normal Pleural Fluid Volume Composition and Dynamics

Normal pleural fluid can be retrieved *directly*, e.g., using gentle aspiration after parietal pleural puncture and lung collapse (5), pleural catheterization (6), or thoracotomy (7,8) followed by fluid aspiration. The technical difficulties in performing such maneuvers (often in small animals) swiftly and atraumatically may induce significant errors and may also be responsible for the quite important within-species variations in results, e.g., on pleural fluid volumes (3). Furthermore, it is not clear whether or how the volume of liquid adherent to the lung and fissure surfaces should be included in the measurements (8,9).

Indirect approaches using PL have been performed for determining the volume of normal pleural fluid (9), the cellular content of the pleural fluid (10), and fluid dynamics (6,11). In comparing the results of normal pleural fluid volume and total cellular composition obtained by direct versus indirect (PL) retrieval, between and within species, there is some concordance. However, the disparity between various differential cell counts is unacceptably high for historical use as baseline data, and extrapolation to human pleural fluid is impossible (3). PL has also been used for the retrieval and phenotypic and functional characterization of normal pleural macrophages in rats (12).

In summary, no standardized procedure for the measurement of normal pleural fluid volumes, cellular content, and dynamics in animals is available. Direct as well as indirect (PL) methods have been used, and study results seem to a certain degree dependent on the methodology used. PL methods, however, seem technically easier to perform, especially in small-sized animals (12).

B. PL in the Study of Pathophysiological Processes in the Pleura

Animal models are widely used to study various aspects of pathological (mostly inflammatory) processes in the pleura (13). PL today seems to represent the methodology of choice, especially in small animals (e.g., various types of rodents).

In mice, for instance, PL has been used to study the cellular kinetics of inflammation in response to injection of exogenous particles such as silica or tungsten (14). In rats and hamsters, the pleural responses to inhalation of asbestos and ceramic fibers have been studied using PL techniques (15,16), and aspects of the role of various inflammatory cells in unspecific pleurisy in rats have been studied with PL (17). PL studies in mice have also been used to examine the mechanisms of eosinophilic inflammation in the pleural space (18,19).

PL is a relatively simple technique allowing for the retrieval (and examination) of the pleural fluid and its components, in normal as well as pathological situations. Especially in small laboratory animals (e.g., rodents), PL seems technically superior to direct retrieval of pleural fluid.

III. Pleural Lavage as a Research Tool in Humans

A. Normal Pleural Fluid Volume and Composition

Because of the relative inaccessibility of the pleural space, the exact volume and composition of the normal pleural fluid in humans has for long remained one of the few last secrets of human body fluid composition. Only one study, published in 1933 (20), described a direct retrieval method by intercostal puncture in healthy subjects. Pleural volume measurements varied between "a few drops of foam" up to 20 mL. Total white cell counts varied between 1700 and 6200 cells per μL; differential cell count showed 3% mesothelial cells, 53.7% cells "similar to monocytes," 10.2% lymphocytes, 3.6% granulocytes, and 29.5% "deteriorated cells of difficult classification."

Since then, only one study has addressed measurement of pleural fluid volume and cellular composition in normal humans by means of PL (4). Because of the relative invasiveness of the PL procedure, PL was performed in otherwise normal subjects who underwent elective thoracoscopic sympathectomy for essential hyperhidrosis. Lavage fluid consisted of 150 mL of prewarmed saline, which was injected under direct thoracoscopic control in the posterolateral costophrenic angle and immediately reaspirated. The effective volume of original pleural fluid was recalculated using urea as an endogenous marker; total and differential cell counts were performed using a Bürker chamber and cytospins, respectively. Expressed per kg of body mass, total pleural fluid volume (right plus left) in normal, nonsmoking humans is 0.26 ± 0.1 mL/kg. Total cell count in the original fluid was 1.716×10^3 cells/mL; differential cell count showed 75% (IR 16%) macrophages, 23% (IR 23%)

lymphocytes, 1% (IR 2%) mesothelial cells, and marginally present neutrophils and eosinophils.

PL using 500 mL of phosphate-buffered saline in patients with central bronchial tumors undergoing thoracotomy and lobe resection has been used to retrieve normal pleural macrophages for immunological characterization (21). Although performed in patients with manifest lung diseases, the pleural spaces were not directly involved.

Interestingly, using light scatter flow cytometry, pleural cell differentials seemed different from those determined by Noppen et al. (4) in normal subjects without lung disease, since 36.1 ± 24.3% "large macrophage-type" cells and 51.8 ± 22.8% "small lymphocyte-type cells" were observed. However, no cytospin preparations were made, hence direct comparison between the two studies is impossible. When compared to blood macrocytes in the same patients, pleural macrophages represented a cell type intermediate of regular CD14+ monocytes and the CD14+ CD16+ subset. Functionally, pleural macrophages were able to perform Fc-receptor1/Nmediated phagocytosis of antibody-coated sheep red blood cells to produce tumor necrosis factor, and they expressed a high constitutive IL-10 mRNA expression, which was not substantially increased by lipopolysaccharide stimulation.

PL studies of "normal" human pleural spaces have only very recently been proposed. In our opinion, PL may become an exciting new tool for the study of morphological, functional, and biochemical characteristics of normal pleural fluid and its constituents. The main disadvantage of PL in normal humans undoubtedly will be the relatively limited number of subjects with "accessible" pleural spaces. The experiences of Noppen et al. (4) and Frankenberger et al. (21) may be proof of a new theme in human pleural research.

B. PL in the Study of Pathophysiological Processes in the Pleura

The majority of pathological processes occurring in the pleural space (e.g., infectious, malignant, inflammatory) are characterized by the occurrence of associated pleural effusions. However, in a number of pathologies, pleural effusions typically are not present (e.g., spontaneous pneumothorax, some asbestos-induced pleural disorders). In these cases, PL may represent an attractive research tool in the future.

PL indeed has recently been used for the study of cellular and immunological events occurring in the pleural space of patients suffering from spontaneous pneumothorax. The presence of air in the pleural space is known to induce a pleural reaction, which is characterized by the influx of eosinophils (22). Smit et al. (23) have shown, by analyzing pleural effusions or by means of PL if no effusion was present, that an IL-5–mediated, time-dependant eosinophil influx occurs after spontaneous pneumothorax. These findings have been confirmed by others (24): in this study using exclusively PL during thoracoscopy for spontaneous pneumothorax, it was also shown that the eosinophils present in the pleural space were activated.

Further studies using PL in pneumothorax are currently being performed.

IV. Pleural Lavage as a Diagnostic Tool in Humans

A. Lung Cancer

The presence of a cytologically or histologically proven malignant effusion in lung cancer patients is associated with a poor prognosis consistent with stage IIIb disease. However, malignant cells may also be present in the pleural cavity in patients without effusions, representing localized (due to exfoliation from tumors at the pleural surface) or lymphatically disseminated disease. Various reports on pleural cavity cytology obtained by pleural lavage performed at thoracotomy before and/or after lung manipulation and resection in more than 2000 patients have been reported (25–35).

The overall incidence of positive cytologies obtained by PL at the time of thoracotomy vary between 3.7 and 46%, averaging about 15% in the larger studies. In general, positive lavage findings parallel increasing tumor stages, the presence of adenocarcinoma, and point to a significant reduction in survival and increased local recurrences. Although not universally recommended, these data suggest that all patients undergoing curative resection for non–small-cell lung cancer (especially adenocarcinoma) should undergo preresection pleural lavage for cytological evaluation in view of its significant prognostic value.

B. Esophageal Cancer

PL studies at thoracotomy before and/or after esophageal manipulation have also been performed in patients undergoing surgery for esophageal carcinoma who had no pleural effusion (36,37). Unlike the staging system in lung cancer, malignant pleural effusion is not included in the tumor node metastasis (TNM) staging system for esophageal cancer, probably due to its uncommon clinical presentation and to the fact that, from an anatomical viewpoint, the esophagus lies in the retropleural space. Nevertheless, PL studies have yielded positive cytology in 5.2–18.8 % of cases (foremost squamous cell epitheliomas) (36,37). There was no significant correlation with gender, age, clinical symptoms, histology, T or N status, TNM stage, or tumor location. The impact of positive PL cytology on prognosis or survival is unknown. Exfoliation and lymphatic spread are two plausible mechanisms to explain the etiology of positive PL cytology in esophageal cancer, considering its local invasive properties and rich lymphatic drainage.

Further studies are needed to confirm the previous rather preliminary PL results and to examine the possible impact of positive PL cytology on prognosis and survival. It is, nevertheless, conceivable that preoperative PL may become an important prognostic tool in operable esophageal carcinoma patients in the future.

V. Conclusions

PL is not a new method: it was used more than 50 years ago in research laboratories in the study of normal pleural fluid composition and pleural space physiology. Today, PL still is an excellent tool, especially in small laboratory animals such as rodents, to gain relatively uninvasive access to the content of the pleural space. In humans, PL has for the first time—and only very recently—made it possible to determine the exact volume and cellular content of normal pleural fluid. As a research tool in humans, PL has provided exciting results in the study of the pathophysiology underlying pathological processes in the pleural space that are not typically associated with pleural effusions, e.g., spontaneous pneumothorax. Finally, in daily clinical practice, preoperative PL in patients undergoing lung surgery for bronchogenic carcinoma has proven to be of significant prognostic value; preliminary data also suggest a possible role for preoperative PL in esophageal carcinoma patients.

References

1. Wang NS. Anatomy of the pleura. Clin Chest Med 1998; 19:229–240.
2. Agostoni E, Zocchi L. Mechanical coupling and liquid exchanges in the pleural space. Clin Chest Med 1998; 19:241–260.
3. Noppen M. Normal volume and cellular contents of pleural fluid. Curr Opin Pulm Med 2001; 7:180–182.
4. Noppen M, De Waele M, Li R, Vander Gucht K, D'Haese J, Gerlo E, Vincken W. Volume and cellular content of normal pleural fluid in humans examined by pleural lavage. Am J Respir Crit Care Med 2000; 162:1023–1026.
5. Sahn SA, Willcox ML, Good JT, Potts DE, Filley GF. Characteristics of normal rabbit pleural fluid: physiologic and biochemical implications. Lung 1979; 156:63–69.
6. Broaddus VC, Araya M. Liquid and protein dynamics using a new minimally invasive pleural catheter in rabbits. J Appl Physiol 1992; 72:851–857.
7. Broaddus VC, Araya M, Carlton P, Blaud RD. Developmental changes in pleural liquid protein concentration in sheep. Am Rev Respir Dis 1991; 143:38–41.
8. Miserocchi G, Agostoni E. Contents of the pleural space. J Appl Physiol 1971; 30:208–213.
9. Stewart PB, Burgen SV. The turnover of fluid in the dog's pleural cavity. J Lab Clin Med 1958; 52:212–230.
10. Stauffer JL, Potts DE, Sahn SA. Cellular content of the normal rabbit pleural space. Acta Cytol 1978; 22:570–574.
11. Wiener-Kronish JP, Albertine KH, Licko V, Staub NC. Protein egress and entry rates in pleural fluid and plasma in sheep. J Appl Physiol 1984; 56:459–463.
12. Gjomarkaj M, Pace E, Melis M, Spatafora M, Profita M, Vignola AM, Bonsig-

nore G, Toews GB. Phenotypic and functional characterization of normal rat pleural macrophages in comparison with autologous peritoneal and alveolar macrophages. Am J Respir Cell Mol Biol 1999; 20:135–142.
13. Marchi E, Broaddus VC. Mechanisms of pleural liquid formation in pleural inflammation. Curr Opin Pulm Med 1997; 3:305–309.
14. Peao MN, Ageras AP, Grande NR. Cellular kinetics of inflammation in the pleural space of mice in response to the injection of exogenous particles. Exp Lung Res 1992; 18:863–876.
15. Oberdoerster G, Ferin J, Marcello NL, Meinhold SH. Effect of intrabronchially instilled amosite on lavagable lung and pleural cells. Environm Health Perspect 1983; 51:41–48.
16. Everitt JI, Gelzleichter TR, Bermudez E, Mangum JB, Wong BA, Janszen DB, Moss OR. Comparison of pleural responses of rats and hamsters to subchronic inhalation of refractory ceramic fibers. Environm Health Perspect 1997; 105:1209–1213.
17. Nishida M, Uchikawa R, Tegoshi T, Yamada M, Matsuda S, Hyoh Y, Arizono N. Migration of neutrophils is dependent on mast cells in nonspecific pleurisy in rats. APMIS 1999; 107:929–936.
18. Bozza PT, Castro-Faria-Neto HC, Penido C, Larangeira AP, Silva PMR, Martins MA. Cordeiro RSB. IL-5 accounts for the mouse pleural eosinophil accumulation triggered by antigen but not by LPS. Immunopharmacology 1994; 27:131–136.
19. Bozza PT, Castro-Faria-Neto HC, Penido C, Larangeira AP, Silva PMR, Martins MA, das Gracas M, Henriques MO, das Santos RS. Requirements for lymphocytes and resistant macrophages in LPS-induced pleural eosinophil accumulation. J Leukoc Biol 1994; 56:151–158.
20. Yamada S. Über die Seröse Flüssigkeit in der Pleurahöhle der gesunden Menschen. Z Ges Exp Med 1933; 90:342–348.
21. Frankenberger M, Passlick B, Hofer T, Siebeck M, Maier KL, Ziegler-Heitbrock LHW. Immunological characterization of normal human pleural macrophages. Am J Respir Cell Mol Biol 2000; 23:419–426.
22. Saini JS, Lal M, Rai J. Eosinophilic pleural effusion following pneumothorax. Ind J Chest Dis 1980; 22:133–136.
23. Smit HJ, Van den Heuvel MM, Barbierato SB, Beelen RJ, Postmus PE. Analysis of pleural fluid in idiopathic spontaneous pneumothorax. Respir Med 1999; 93:262–267.
24. Noppen M, Vanderlinden E, Demanet C, De Waele M. Pleural inflammation in spontaneous pneumothorax. Am J Respir Crit Care Med 2001; 163:A957.
25. Spjut JH, Hendrix VJ, Ramirez GA, Roper CL. Carcinoma cells in pleural cavity washings. Cancer 1958; 11:1222–1225.
26. Eagan RT, Bernatz PE, Payne WS, Pairolero PC, Williams DE, Goellner JR, Piehler JM. Pleural lavage after pulmonary resection for bronchogenic carcinoma. J Thorac Cardiovasc Surg 1984; 88:1000–1003.
27. Buhr J, Berghauser KH, Morr H, Dobroschke J, Ebner HJ. Tumor cells in intraoperative pleural lavage— an indicator for poor prognosis of bronchogenic carcinoma. Cancer 1990; 65:1801–1804.
28. Okumura M, Okshima S, Kotake Y, Morino H, Kikui M, Yasumitsu T. Intraoperative pleural lavage cytology in lung cancer patients. Ann Thorac Surg 1991; 51:564–599.

29. Kondo H, Asamura H, Suemasu K, Goya T, Tsuchiya R, Naruke T, Yamagishi K, Uei Y. Prognostic significance of pleural lavage cytology immediately after thoracotomy in patients with lung cancer. J Thorac Cardiovcasc Surg 1993; 106: 1092–1097.
30. Kjellberg SI, Dresler CM, Foldberg M. Pleural cytologies in lung cancer without pleural effusions. Am Thorac Surg 1997; 64:941–944.
31. Buhr J, Berghauser KH, Gonner S, Kelm C, Burkhardt EA, Padberg WM. The prognostic significance of tumor cell detection in intra-operative pleural lavage and lung tissue cultures for patients with lung cancer. J Thorac Cardiovasc Surg 1997; 133:683–690.
32. Okada M, Tsubota N, Yoshimura M, Miyamoto Y, Maniwa Y. Role of pleural lavage cytology before resection of primary lung carcinoma. Ann Surg 1999; 229(4):579–584.
33. Vinette-Leduc D, Yazdi HM, Kalji A, Shanji F, Maziak D. Pre- and post-resection thoracic washings in non-small cell carcinoma of the lung: a cytological study of 44 patients without pleural effusion. Diagn Cytopathol 2000; 22:218–222.
34. Higashiyama M, Kodawa K, Yokouchi H, Takami K, Nakayama T, Horai T. Clinical value of pleural lavage cytological positivity in lung cancer patients without intra-operative malignant pleuritis. JJTCVS 2000; 48:611–617.
35. Higashiyama M, Doi O, Kodama K, Yokouchi H, Tateishi R, Korai T. Pleural lavage cytology immediately after thoracotomy and before closure of the thoracic cavity for lung cancer without pleural effusion and dissemination: clinicopathological and prognostic analysis. Ann Surg Oncol 1997; 4:409–415.
36. Jiao X, Zhang M, Wen Z, Krasna MJ. Pleural lavage cytology in esophageal cancer without pleural effusions: clinicopathological analysis. Eur J Cardiothor Surg 2000; 17:575–579.
37. Natsuga S, Shimada M, Nakashima S, Tokuda K, Matsumoto M, Kijima F, Baka M, Shimizu K, Tamaka S, Aikov T. Intra-operative pleural lavage in esophageal carcinoma. Ann Surg Oncol 1999; 6:305–307.

11

Medical Thoracoscopy

PHILIPPE ASTOUL

University of the Mediterranean
and Hôpital Sainte-Marguerite
Marseille, France

I. Introduction

For a long time thoracoscopy was performed to achieve pneumonolysis in patients with tuberculosis. More recently many physicians in Europe have documented the usefulness of thoracoscopy for pneumonological indications other than tuberculosis. Taking into account that the evolution of medical technologies incited physicians to seek new and potentially less invasive ways of performing diagnostic and therapeutics chest procedures, a distinction must be made between medical thoracoscopy, which may be video-assisted, and surgical thoracoscopy or video-assisted thoracoscopic surgery (VATS) (1,2).

Thoracoscopy is only slightly more invasive than a simple percutaneous pleural needle biopsy but provides infinitely more information. In all cases where a chest tube is required, it should take a pulmonologist only a few minutes to introduce an endoscope via the same incision, to inspect the pleura, to locate the adhesions, to take pleural samples, and to verify that the tube will be well positioned. In patients with primary pleural cancer, thoracoscopy is the only procedure able to give a diagnosis at the early stage of the disease, and for other pleural effusions biopsies are made under visual control with a diagnostic rate of more than 95% of patients (3).

The use of thoracoscopy has been resumed as a result of considerable progress in modern techniques:

Endoscopic telescopes have been greatly improved with extremely high optical quality despite their very small diameter (4).

Adequate instrumentation, including video camera, forceps, endoscopic scalpel, and stapler, enables the physician or surgeon to carry out interventional thoracoscopy (5).

Progress in anesthetics allows for a wide choice that ranges from local anesthesia in outpatients to general anesthesia (6,7).

Thoracoscopy, while allowing full exploration of the pleural cavity, is much less invasive and incapacitating than thoracotomy (8). Complications are uncommon and rarely occur when the procedure is performed according to appropriate recommendations.

Diagnostic or therapeutic medical thoracoscopy is performed using one or several points of entry. In addition to visual inspection of the thoracic cavity, a number of procedures can be performed. Biopsies can be collected from the pleura and, more rarely, the lung. Adherences preventing exploration can be cut. Coagulation can be performed to stop bleeding or remove small blebs or superficial bullae in patients with spontaneous pneumothorax. A pleural drain is placed at the end of the examination to ensure prompt expansion of the lung against the chest wall. If lung biopsy or pleurodesis is performed, the mean duration of drainage is 3–4 days. In simple cases involving pleurisy, the examination can be performed as an ambulatory procedure (9).

To practice thoracoscopy, a chest physician needs specific training to learn thoracic anatomy, use of instrumentation (biopsy forceps, coagulation systems, video-endoscopic equipment), and surveillance of drainage during the recovery period.

II. Equipment and Technique

A. Equipment

Thoracoscopy can be performed either in a properly equipped operating room or in an endoscopy suite. The procedure room must be equipped with a procedure table, anesthesia equipment, Mayo stands, a roller tray for instruments, diathermo-coagulation, and patient-monitoring devices.

Thoracoscopic instruments have been designed to facilitate operative procedures. Forceps, graspers, lung manipulators, cautery and cutting devices, suction/irrigation instruments, and a variety of disposable and reusable pleural trocars and cannulas are currently available (10).

A rigid thoracoscope with a cold light source is used in most cases. Optics have been considerably improved, and telescopes have greater depth of field, magnification, and arc of vision. The major equipment requierements for medical thoracoscopy are trocars, telescopes, and forceps (Fig. 1). Trocars consist of

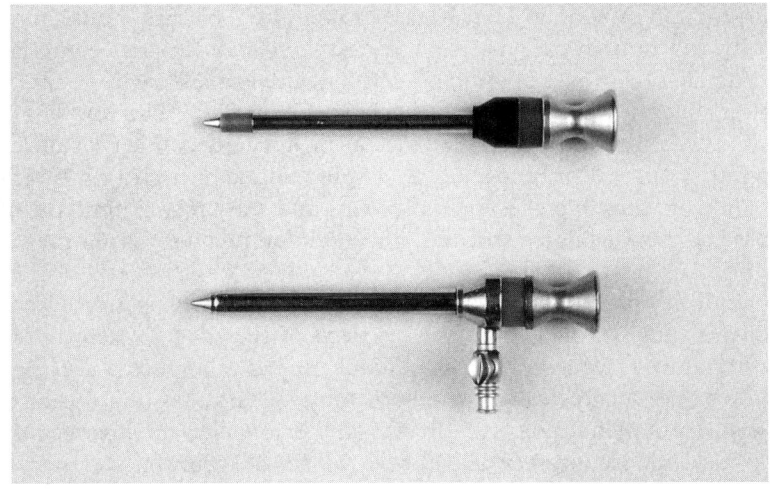

Figure 1 Major equipment for medical thoracoscopy: (a) trocars (5 and 7 mm); (b) from top to bottom—7 mm telescope (0° angle), 4 mm telescope, illuminated forceps, coagulating forceps.

an obturator and a cannula. To facilitate examination, trocars should not be too large; with a 7 mm trocar, insertion is easy, and painful, procedure-limiting pressure against the ribs is minimal. Telescopes are available with various angle of vision, including 180° (straightforward) and 50 or 90° (oblique). Illuminated forceps are ideal for biopsy of the parietal pleura under direct vision using a single point of entry. For biopsy of the diaphragmatic pleura or fibrous pleural lesions and for sampling the visceral pleura and the lung, 5 mm coagulating forceps via a 5 mm insulated trocar in a second point of entry is a more suitable device (1).

Visualization of the contents of the pleural cavity is facilitated by a videocamera that is attached to the eyepiece of the rigid telescope. The size and quality of these cameras has considerably improved in recent years, and the addition of video makes viewing, documentation, and assisting during procedures far easier than in the days of direct visualization. Newer telescopes magnify the subject being visualized (usually about 4× for a 7 mm rigid telescope), and the increased availability of couplers of varying sizes allows greater depth of field and increased field of vision without distortion to enhance visibility.

For routine patient care purposes, a single-chip videocamera, a basic single standard medical-grade monitor or other video display, and simple VHS videorecorder amply suffice. Eventually, smaller telescopes with excellent illumination and visualization capabilities may be used for microthoracoscopy (11).

Medical thoracoscopy must be carried out under sterile conditions. The thoracoscopy room should be sterilized in the same way as an operating room. The trocar, telescopes, forceps, connecting wire, fibreoptic fibers, and all other accessories are sterilized after careful cleaning (12). Calibrated talc is sterilized by autoclaving at 160°C.

B. Technique

Medical thoracoscopy is an invasive procedure that should be used only when other, more simple methods fail (13). Moreover, as with all technical procedures, appropriate training is mandatory before full competence can be achieved. The technique is very similar to chest-tube insertion by means of a trocar, the difference being that, in addition, the pleural cavity can be vizualized and biopsies can be taken from several intrapleural sites.

Anesthesia

Several modalities can be described based on the experience of the team, the local facilities, and the indications of the procedure (6,14).

Premedication

Usually meperidine, 50–100 mg, and atropine sulfate, 0.5 mg, given by intramuscular injection about 30 minutes before the procedure, are used.

Medical Thoracoscopy

Local Anesthesia

This is always recommended if the thoracoscopy procedure is to be brief in a low-risk patient whose pleural cavity is free of adhesions. Local anesthesia is also preferable to general anesthesia in high-risk patients exhibiting poor general health, compromised respiratory function, or cardiac insufficiency (15).

General Anesthesia

General anesthesia may be necessary in some cases. It is the technique of choice for procedures requiring intubation. General anesthesia may be delivered and not preclude spontaneous ventilation, which is usually recommended. This method is a relief for patient and physician alike, since it allows time for multiple biopsies, section of extensive adhesions, and electrocautery (7).

Endoscopy Procedure

The examination is performed with the patient lying on the healthy side. The entry site is generally made on the axilla midline in the third to seventh intercostal space. An absolute prerequisite for thoracoscopy is the presence of an adequate pleural space, which should be at least 6–10 cm in diameter. If not present, a pneumothorax is induced, immediately on the operating table or the day before the procedure. If extensive pleuropulmonary adhesions are present, "extended thoracoscopy" without creating a pneumothorax can be carried out, but this requires special skills and should not be undertaken without special training.

Induced Pneumothorax

A pleural trocar for making punctures, measuring 2 or 3 mm in diameter and 100 mm in length, is ideal for inducing pneumothorax. It is inserted into the pleural cavity, and by opening the trocar tap, the air is allowed to enter. The characteristic whistle of air can be heard as it passes through the trocar. As soon as the lung is in a state of equilibrium—an equal amount of air is heard entering the pleura during inhalation as leaving it during exhalation—the pleural trocar is removed and the thoracoscopy trocar is inserted (1,3).

Point of Entry

The puncture site is usually in the midaxillary zone between the third and sixth intercostal spaces because pleural adhesions are uncommon in this area. Choice of the point of entry can vary depending on the indication of the procedure. In patients with spontaneous pneumothorax, the offending leak is usually in the upper lobe so that the best location is between the third and fourth intercostal spaces. In patients with pleural effusion the fifth, sixth, or seventh intercostal space is the best site of entry. Pulmonary biopsies are facilitated by entry through the fourth/fifth intercostal space.

Examination

A procedure includes the following phases:

> Careful aspiration of secretions.
> Insufflation of air into the cavity, if necessary.
> Section of adhesions preventing inspection.
> Inspection using a lateral viewing or a direct viewing telescope. Perfect knowledge of normal and pathological endoscopic anatomy is mandatory. Biopsy can be performed with illuminated forceps through a single point of entry. When the parietal pleura is thin, specimens should be taken against the rib to avoid injuring the intercostal neurovascular bundle (1). In this regard it is noteworthy that the main danger is hemorrhage fom an intercostal vessel (16). A well-trained endoscopist can quickly create a second point of entry if he or she needs additional instrumentation to sever adhesions, take lung biopsies, coagulate bleeding vessels.
> Collection of multiple biopsy samples (wall, diaphragm, lung) for light microscopy, electronic microscopy, hormone receptor assay, mineral detection, bacteriology, tumor culture.
> Aspiration for fluid cytology.
> Talc pleurodesis, if necessary.

At the end of the procedure, a chest tube is inserted and air aspirated. The surveillance of the patient is done in the recovering room, and a control chest x-ray is required. After a diagnostic thoracoscopy for pleural effusion, the tube can be removed as soon as the lung is clinically or radiologically reexpanded against the chest wall (17,18). Sometimes the patient can be discharged the same day. After lung biopsy, tubing must be prolonged for 24–48 hours. After a therapeutic procedure, especially after talc pleurodesis, pleural drainage should be maintained until the lung is reexpanded, bubbling has stopped and the volume of fluid collected is less than 100 mL/day. This can take 2–5 days.

III. Complications and Contraindications

A. Complications

Thoracoscopy is one of the safest pneumonological examinations. In a review of 8000 cases, Viskum and Enk noted only one death (19). In this review, no mention of wound infection was found in any study, empyema occurred in only 12 of 652 cases in three studies, and hemorrhage occurred in 6 of 356 cases described in three other studies. O_2 desaturation during thoracoscopy under local anesthesia is reportedly less than 2%. The mortality rate was 0.09% for Boutin and colleagues in a series of 4300 procedures (1). In an experience of more than 6000 thoracoscopies, Loddenkemper and colleagues do not report the need for surgical intervention to stop bleeding caused by thoracoscopy (20). Reported mortality rates (<0.01%) are very low. Even several liters of fluid can be completely removed during thoracoscopy with little risk of pulmonary edema, because equilibration of pressures is provided by direct entrance of air through the cannula into the pleural space (2). If the reexpansion potential of the lung appears to be diminished, low-pressure suction should be applied. Such complication can be prevented by assessing the intrapleural pressure before the procedure (21). The most serious complication of thoracoscopy is air or gas embolism after air insufflation for artificial pneumothorax, which occurs very rarely (<0.1%), as long as necessary precautionary measures are observed. One of these recommandations is to use a double-balloon air insufflator to induce or to increase an artificial pneumothorax (1).

Although comparative studies have not been performed, it is possible that complication rates may be increased in this setting because of the increased morbidity of patients undergoing these procedures, the use of general anesthesia, and the invasive scope of procedures being performed (22).

For routine medical thoracoscopy, complications can best be prevented by observing the following rules:

1. Postpone thoracoscopy for several days if the patient is coughing.
2. Measure blood gases, monitor cardiac signs by simultaneous ECG.
3. Oxygenate the patient during thoracoscopy.
4. Avoid taking biopsy samples from the internal parts of the fissures or from the mediastinum.
5. Coagulate and ensure hemostasis if hemorrhage exceeds 20 mL.
6. Insert a chest tube (at least until the lung expands) to prevent subcutaneous emphysema.
7. Prevent local invasion in cases of malignant pleural mesothelioma, administer radiation therapy (7 Gy/day for 3 consecutive days) to the scar area (23).

B. Contraindications

Contraindications are uncommon and rarely absolute. The main limitation is the size of free pleural space. If extensive adhesions are present, an extended thoracoscopy (without first creating a pneumothorax) can be carried out, but this requires special skills and should not be undertaken without special training (24).

Several factors may make it necessary to delay thoracoscopy but are rarely prohibitive. They are cough, hypoxemia, hypocoagulability (prothrombin time <60% and/or platelet count <60,000 per mm^3) and cardiological abnormalities. The thoracoscopist must evaluate the benefit: risk ratio in each case (25).

The contraindications for pulmonary biopsy are as follows:

Mean pulmonary arterial pressure >35 mmHg
Chest x-ray with a honeycomb image of the lung or end-stage interstitial fibrosis

Suspicion of arteriovenous pulmonary aneurysm
Hydatic cyst
Vascular tumor

IV. Clinical Applications

Medical thoracoscopy is today primarily a diagnostic procedure, but it can also be applied for therapeutic purposes (12).

A. Basic Indications for Medical Thoracoscopy

Pleural Effusion

Even algorithms for investigating pleural effusion of unknown etiology typically begin with thoracentesis; diagnosis of pleural effusions is the prime indication for medical thoracoscopy (13,26). Because cytological examination is diagnostic in only 60–80% of patients with metastatic pleural involvement and in <20% of patients with mesotheliomas, thoracoscopic parietal pleural examination and biopsy present an opportunity to achieve earlier diagnosis, which is an important prognostic factor for such diseases (27).

Although the possibility of tuberculosis should not be ruled out, malignancy has been found more frequently in recent decades, and most experts agree that when the initial evaluation of a pleural effusion is nondiagnostic, especially when neoplastic disease is suspected, thoracoscopic exploration and parietal pleural biopsy should be considered (28). The diagnostic accuracy of thoracoscopy is between 90 and 100%, compared with an approximate sensitivity of 44% for closed needle pleural biopsy and 62% for fluid cytology; false negatives occur most frequently in cases of early malignant mesothelioma (29). If the patient has a malignancy and negative cytology on thoracentesis, thoracoscopy is preferred over closed needle pleural biopsy because it will establish the diagnosis in >90% of cases (30).

Metastatic Pleural Malignancies

Needle biopsies are successful in only 50% of metastatic pleural malignancies. Moreover, unlike thoracoscopy, closed pleural biopsies are of little value for localized tumors and of absolutely no use for metastatic tumors confined to the diaphragmatic, visceral, or mediastinal pleura. In fact, the success of closed techniques depends on tumor extension. The greater the extent of invasion, the more likely closed biopsy is successful and high yield is achieved only in advanced stages of diseases. This explains why centers dealing with more advanced cancer report higher success rates with needle biopsy. Similarly, pleural fluid cytology exhibits variable success. A yield of 50–60% from pleural fluid cytology is certainly a more representative figure (26).

The main advantage of thoracoscopy is its ability to achieve early diagnosis when pleural biopsy and pleural fluid cytology have failed (31,32).

In 85% of patients with malignancy, thoracoscopy reveals features suggestive of malignancy, including nodules 1–5 mm in diameter, large polypoid lesions, localized tumoral masses, rough, pale, thickened pleural surface, and hard, poorly vascularized pachypleuritis (Fig. 2). However, since appearances can be misleading, macroscopic diagnosis must always be confirmed by histology. In this regard it is important to note that some malignancies mimic nonspecific inflammation and some inflammatory lesions can look like tumors (33). Even mesotheliomas have the appearance of ordinary inflammation rather than its fairly characteristic grape-like nodular form. Histopathological findings are the only criteria for certain diagnoses.

The major stumbling block for thoracoscopy in cancer patients is cases of adherent pleura (34). The ability to obtain a biopsy depends on the practitioner's skill at dividing and cutting adhesions, and there are some cases where biopsy is impossible.

Therapeutically, fluid can be completely and immediately removed during thoracoscopy with little risk of pulmonary edema. The reexpansion of the lung can be evaluated by visual inspection. Furthermore, the extent of intrapleural tumor spread can be described. The main advantage is certainly that talc poudrage can be performed during medical thoracoscopy.

Complete evacuation of pleural fluid, maximization of lung expandability by removing adhesions, and pleurodesis by talc insufflation results in short- and long-term success rates of >90% (35). Distribution of sterile, calibrated, asbestos-free talc powder on all pleural surfaces is confirmed by thoracoscopic visualization. Following pleurodesis, low-grade fevers should be expected in up to 30% of patients, and hospitalization duration averages 4.8 days. To date, talc poudrage is considered the best conservative option for pleurodesis (36). However, survival of patients with advanced pleural carcinomatosis is often short, and the risks and benefits of thoracoscopic pleurodesis must be carefully weighed against those of repeat thoracentesis, tube thoracostomy, or bedside pleurodesis through an indwelling chest tube (37). Careful comparative studies are mandatory between these pleurodesis techniques.

Tuberculous Pleural Effusions

Tuberculosis now accounts for less than 10% of all effusions seen in Europe and the United States and a still lower percentage of all chronic cases. In 70–90 % of cases diagnosis may be achieved using specimens obtained by percutaneous needle biopsy for histology and culture in conjunction with culture of gastric contents aspirated immediately after awakening. With a second needle biopsy, definite diagnosis can be made in 95% of the cases (5).

The endoscopic appearence of tuberculosis consists of grayish-white granulomata blanketing the whole parietal and diaphragmatic pleura and, in particular, the costovertebral gutter (Fig. 3). Lesions have often lost their specific appearance by the time of thoracoscopy and mimic a simple inflammatory process, with increased vascularity, a reddish color, an important and sometimes hemorrhagic fibrinous reaction, and numerous adhesions. Thora-

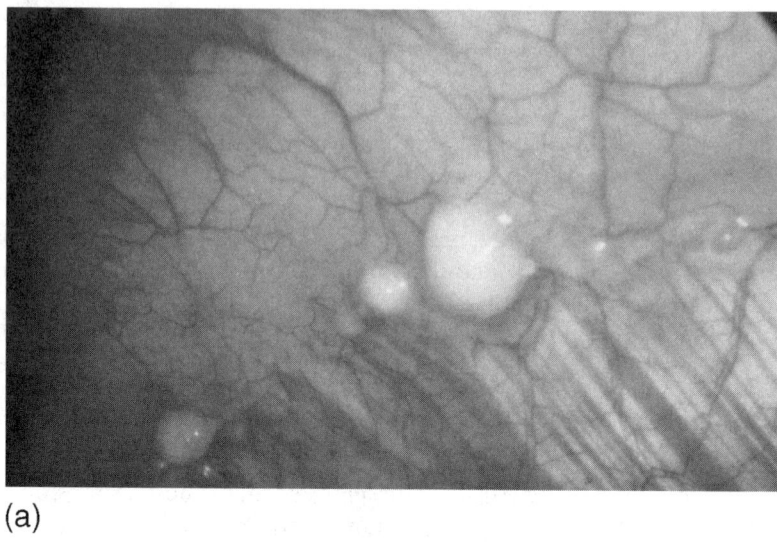

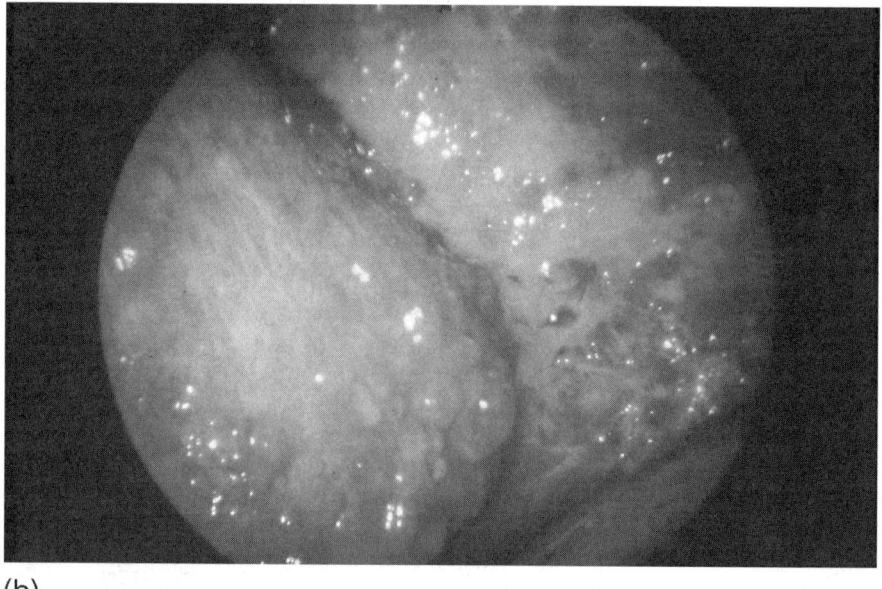

Figure 2 Metastatic pleural malignancy: (a) nodules on the parietal pleura; (b) intrapleural disseminated nodules.

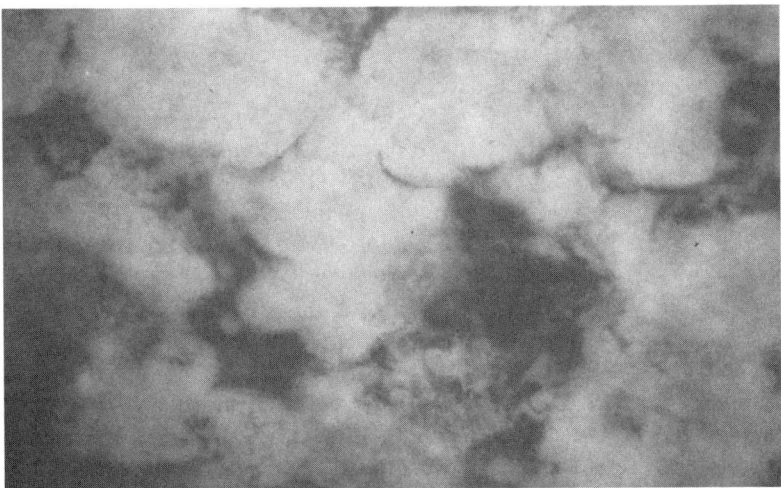

Figure 3 Pleural tuberculosis.

coscopy is usually unnecessary, therefore, to establish the diagnosis of a tuberculous effusion. A combined yield of only 6% for thoracoscopy preceded by negative thoracentesis and closed needle pleural biopsy has been reported. Thoracoscopy may be beneficial in difficult diagnostic situations, however, when lysis of adhesions is necessary or when larger amounts of tissue are warranted to assure diagnosis when drug resistance is suspected.

Therefore, thoracoscopy plays no significant role in the diagnosis of this disease, and the discovery of tuberculous granulomata on thoracoscopic biopsy sample is usually fortuitous.

Malignant Mesothelioma

Diagnosis of malignant mesothelioma depends foremost on histological findings. In the past, histologists were reluctant to advance a diagnosis without an autopsy report to bolster their findings. With the increased incidence of this disease and the availability of immunohistochemical techniques, histologists are most forthcoming, although they still hide behind the cover of a group of experts ("panel"). Obtaining biopsy samples for diagnosis of mesothelioma is one of the best indications for thoracoscopy (33,38). Endoscopy is much less invasive than thoracotomy and allows equally good tissue sampling for pathological diagnosis. By allowing direct visualization of lesions, thoracoscopy facilitates the choice of biopsy sites and correlation of staging with survival. It also allows pulmonary biopsies to document prior exposure to asbestos.

Medical diagnostic thoracoscopy is indicated in any patient without precise histopathological diagnosis in whom clinical and laboratory findings raise suspicion of mesothelioma: cardinal characteristics are age between 55 and 60 years, previous exposure to asbestos, pleural effusion or radiological images showing irregular and nodular lesions of the parietal pleura, especially in the posterior and inferior part of the costovertebral gutter.

Macroscopically the lesions range from 1–3 mm to 1 cm in diameter or even larger, depending on the stage (Fig. 4). In most patients nodules and masses are associated with parietal pleural thickening up to several millimeters. In 20% of cases nodules are small (1–5 mm in diameter). A typical aspect of mesothelioma is the "grape-like" aspect, which consists of a patch of closely spaced smooth, translucid, poorly vascularized nodules 5–10 mm in diameter with a clear or yellowish appearance. Upon biopsy these lesions may be either friable and filled with sticky fluid or hard and difficult to remove. The "grape-like" aspect is typical of mesothelioma—generally at the advanced stage—but it is not specific, since it is also encountered in patients with metastatic cancer of the pleura. Unlike benign inflammation, malignant thickness of the pleura associated with mesothelioma is hard and inelastic. When biopsy samples are taken, the cut edge is clear and there is little or no bleeding (33).

In 10–15% of all cases and in 50% of stage Ia cases, the lesions observed during thoracoscopy are macroscopically nonspecific: benign inflammation of the parietal or diaphragmatic pleura with lymphangitis in some cases. In these cases a more discrete sign is irregular thickening located mainly in the posterior and inferior region of the parietal pleura where lymphatic vessels are most numerous. The more nonspecific the lesions, the more biopsies should be taken (up to 15 or 20).

An important diagnostic finding is involvement of the visceral pleura and lung. These structures can be easily visualized during thoracoscopy. The visceral pleura is always less involved than the parietal pleura, with nodules being not only less numerous but also smaller. In many cases the visceral pleura appears macroscopically normal, but routine biopsy should be performed to confirm or exclude the diagnosis (39).

In contrast with the high sensitivity of thoracoscopy, the combined sensitivity of fluid cytology and needle biopsy was only 38.2%. The overall sensitivity of these conventional methods is poor, and most investigators prefer open surgical biopsy, which is more painful, less safe, and less cost-effective than a surgical procedure.

Other Pleural Effusions

Pleural effusions associated with lung cancer result from direct carcinomatous involvement of the pleura or are paramalignant effusions (40). Even patients in whom cytological examination of pleural fluid is negative are often found on thoracotomy to have unresectable lesions. Thoracoscopy is preferable to thoracotomy for identifying this small group of patients who could potentially benefit from a surgical resection (8). Thoracoscopy is also useful for staging both lung and esophageal cancer because it may complement cervical mediastinoscopy and allows staging of mediastinal lymphadenopathy. Ideally, diagnostic thoracoscopy and surgical resection can be performed sequentially

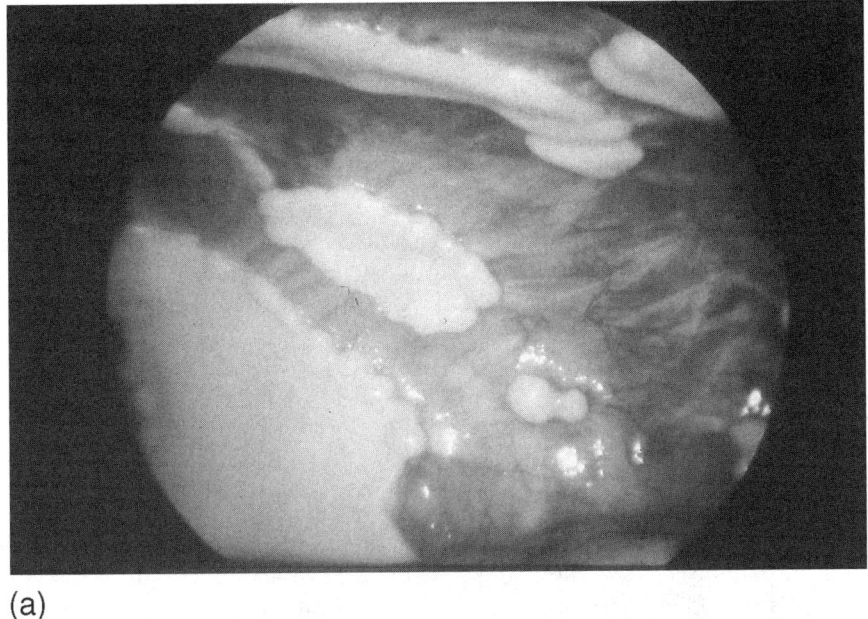

(a)

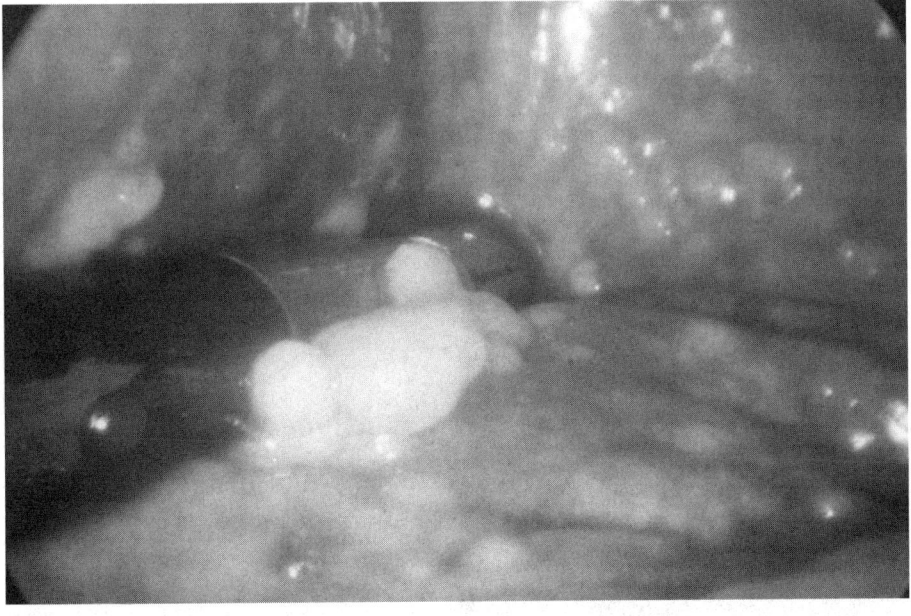

(b)

Figure 4 Malignant pleural mesothelioma (MPM): (a) early-stage disease (pleural plaques with neoplastic lymphangitis); (b) advanced-stage disease.

during the same period of general anesthesia. Although curative resections can be performed thoracoscopically, it is unlikely that this technique will replace standard open surgical approaches for lobectomy and pneumonectomy.

Recurrent pleural effusions of benign etiology are frequently caused by heart failure, cardiac surgery, nephrotic syndrome, connective tissue diseases, and other inflammatory disorders (41) (Fig. 5). Thoracoscopy may be warranted when recurrent effusions cause symptoms and are not controlled by repeated large-volume thoracentesis. Usually, pleural biopsy specimens are obtained to exclude infectious or neoplastic etiologies, and pleurodesis is performed. Results are usually excellent when talc is used, with success rates varying from to 65 to >90%.

In some selected case of recurrent pleural effusions of nonmalignant etiology, including chylothorax, pleurodesis may be induced by applying talc poudrage during medical thoracoscopy (42).

Spontaneous Pneumothorax

If a chest tube is introduced by trocar technique, it is easy to use an optic for visual inspection of the lung and the pleural cavity. Then, thoracoscopy provides an excellent alternative to repeated chest tube drainage in patients with recurrent or prolonged (usually >5 days) pneumothorax for diagnostic and therapeutic purposes (43,44). Thoracoscopic findings in patients with

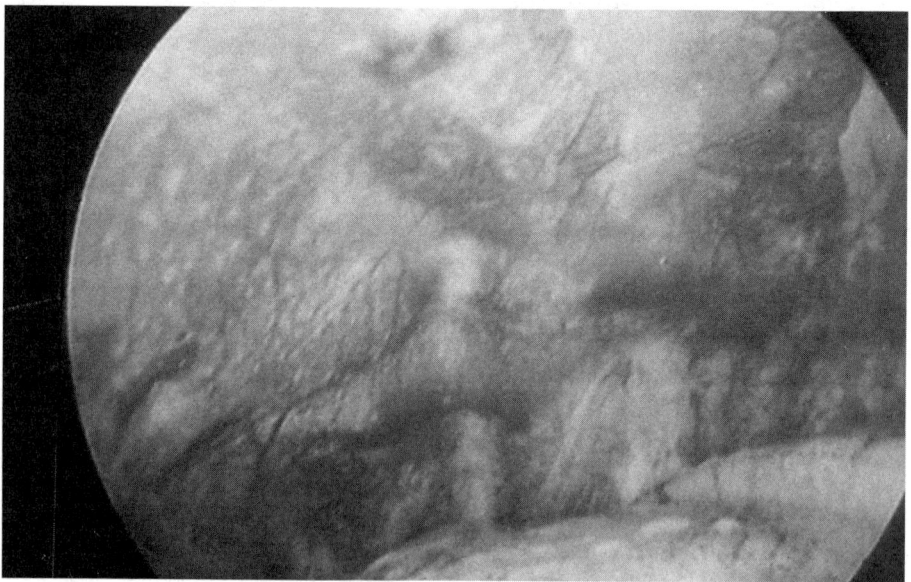

Figure 5 Endopleural sarcoidosis.

spontaneous pneumothorax include, as described by Vanderschueren, normal appearance (type 1), pleural adhesions (type 2), small blebs (<2 cm) on the visceral pleural surface (type 3), and large bullae (>2 cm) (type 4) (6,45) (Fig. 6a,b). Usually these lesions are too fine to be seen on computed tomography (CT) scans. The visibility of bullae and blebs can be enhanced if the patient performs a Valsalva maneuver or by creating positive airway pressure with the anesthesia mask during the procedure.

Lesions can be removed using electrocautery (Fig. 6c,d), argon plasma coagulation, or stapled lung resection if the skills and facilities for this technique are available, with results similar to those obtained after open thoracotomy (although the resultant pleurodesis may be somewhat less effective: recurrence rates are reportedly 5–10% vs. 1–3% after open thoracotomy). However, there is no proof to date that the endoscopic treatment of minimal lesions on the surface of the lung is required (46,47).

In case of recurrent pneumothorax, talc insufflation for pleurodesis may also be effective and is recommended by several teams. Talc poudrage achieves the best conservative treatment results, with a recurrence rate of <10% (48). However, it still remains a controversial issue due to severe secondary side effects. It seems that these complications are due to the quality of talc preparation, which must be carefully assessed (37).

Medical thoracoscopy is justified in all patients with spontaneous pneumothorax where tube drainage is indicated. This procedure offers several advantages: assessment of the underlying lesion under visual control, choice of the best treatment measures, and by severing of adhesions, if necessary, selecting the best location for chest tube placement (49,50).

B. Advanced Indications for Medical Thoracoscopy

Empyema

Medical thoracoscopy is useful in the management of early empyema (51,52). During the exudative and organizing phase of empyema, in cases with multiple loculations, thoracoscopic visualization allows debridement of fibrinous adhesions and evacuation of loculated fluid in removing the fibrinopurulent membranes by forceps to create one single pleural cavity (Fig. 7). In draining and irrigating the pleural cavity much more successfully, this procedure may shorten the length of hospital stay and avoid thoracotomy. However, this treatment should be carried out early in the course of empyema, before the adhesions become too fibrous and adherent (53).The timing of thoracoscopic intervention is critical and should be considered if the indication for a placement of a chest tube is present (54). This procedure is similar to chest tube placement that allows the creation of a single pleural cavity. The precise role for thoracoscopy instead of chest tube drainage, instillation of fibrinolytic agents, rib resection, or thoracotomy-decortication is still controversial, and prospective comparative studies have not yet been done.

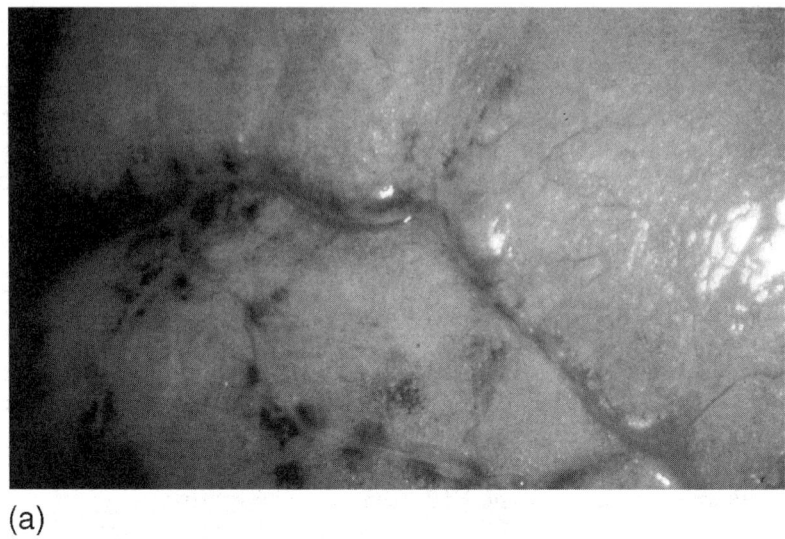

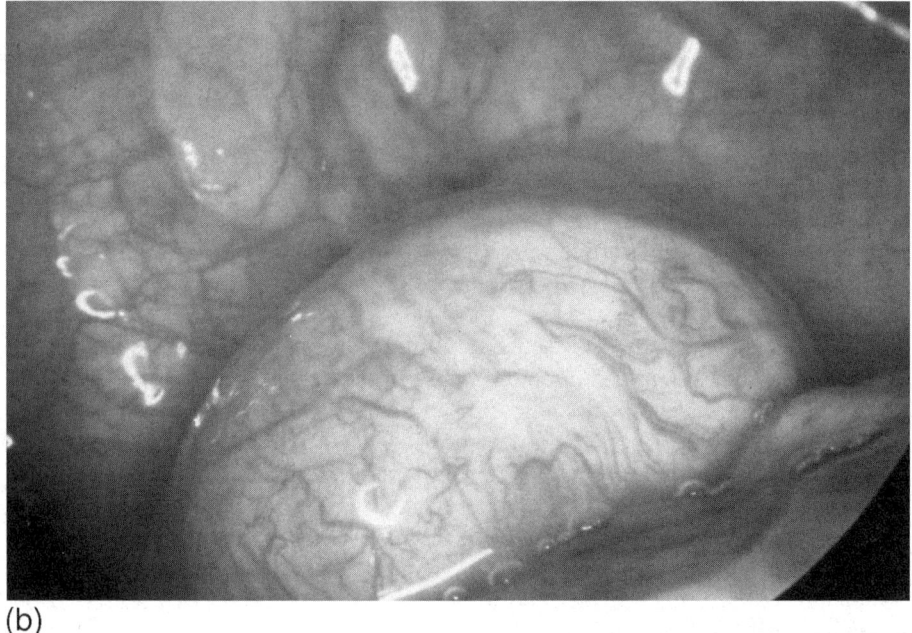

Figure 6 Pneumothorax: (a) blebs on the fissure (type III); (b) bullae (type IV); (c) coagulation of a bullae; (d) adhesiolysis with electrocautery (type II).

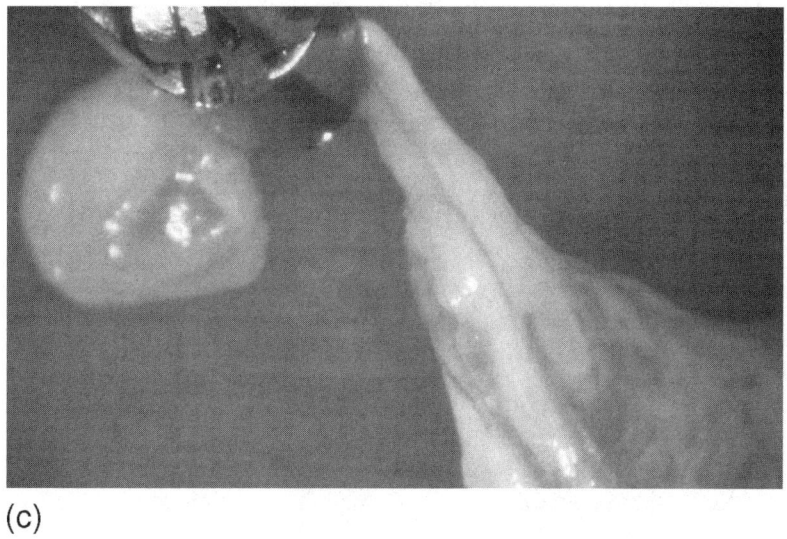

(c)

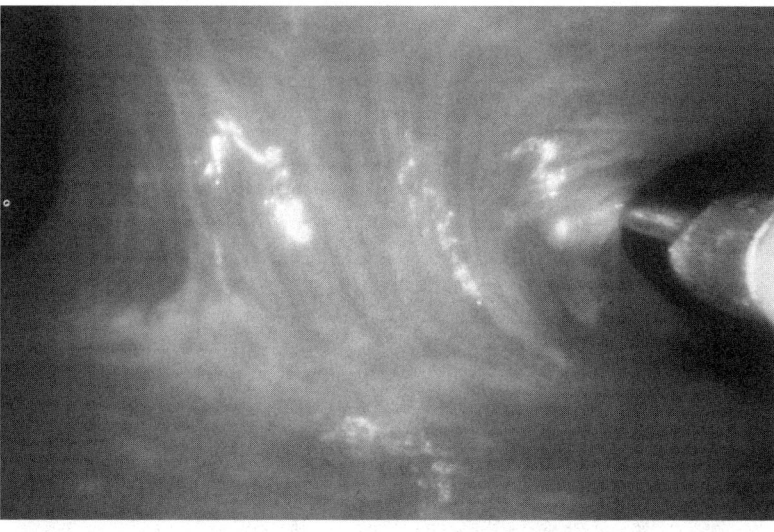

(d)

Figure 6 Continued.

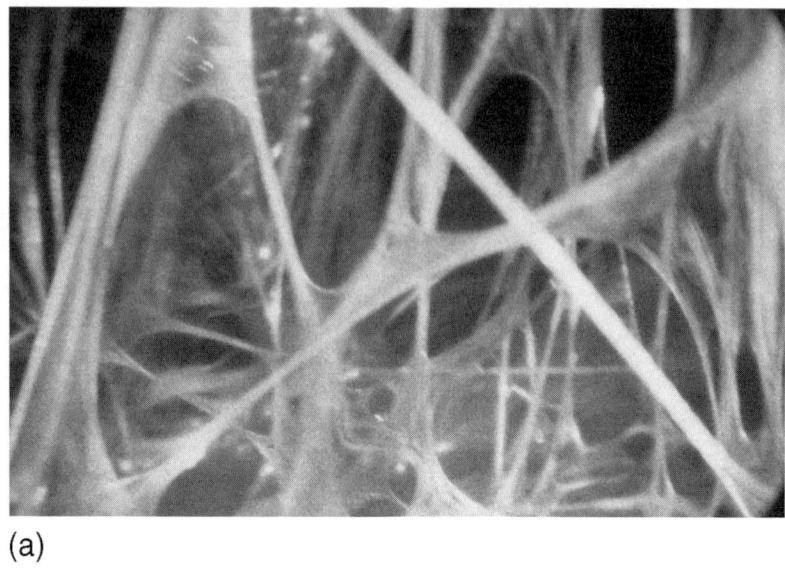

(a)

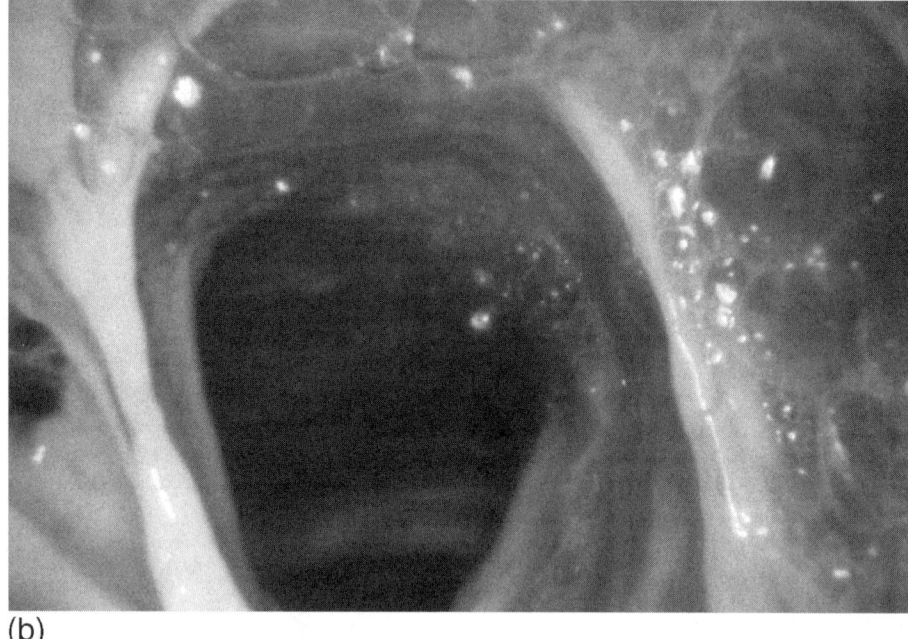

(b)

Figure 7 Empyema: (a) early-stage parapneumonic effusion; (b) endopleural purulent adhesions; (c) empyema.

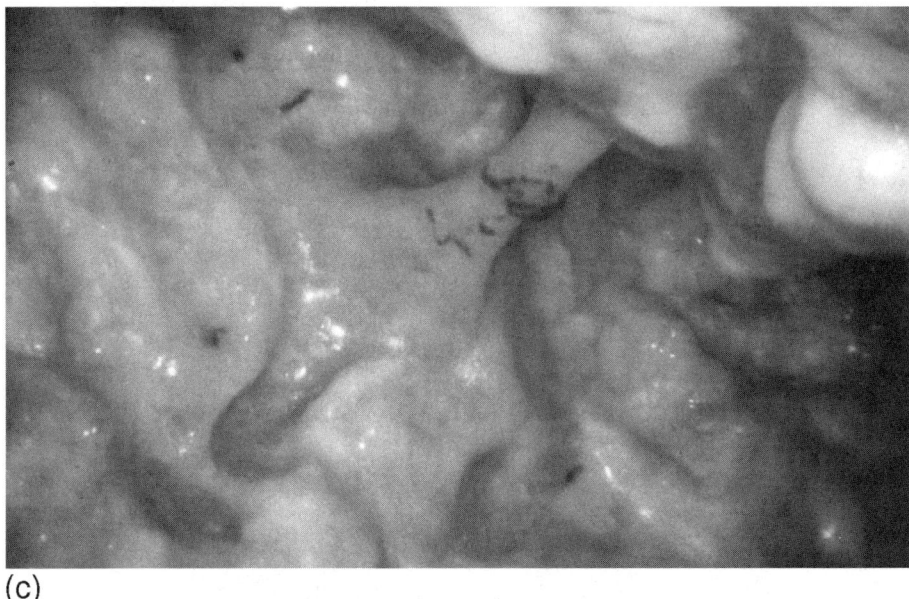
(c)

Figure 7 Continued.

Diffuse Pulmonary Diseases

Thoracoscopic lung biopsy helps establish the diagnosis of diffuse or focal interstitial lung disease and pulmonary infection, in particular when transbronchial biopsy (TBB) or bronchoalveolar lavage has failed to provide a diagnosis (55). The possibility of taking several biopsies from different sites under visual control and the lower morbidity are the most important advantages. In addition, it provides tissue for mineralogical studies of pneumoconioses and for diagnosis of pulmonary infiltrates or peripheral nodular lesions of unknown etiology.

Specimens are usually obtained using a cup biopsy forceps, which is dipped in the lung parenchyma. After lung palpation with the forceps in the closed position, the forceps is opened, the lung is grasped, and the forceps is closed while applying short pulses of diathermy coagulation (Fig. 8). In many cases patients can be discharged from the hospital in fewer than 3 days with little morbidity. Postoperative stay in an ICU is rarely necessary (56).

The diagnostic rate of diseases such as pneumoconiosis, sarcoidosis, or carcinomatous lymphangitis is very high. Frequently more than 90% of samples taken are useful for analysis. The diameter of the biopsies varies from 2.1 to 6.6 mm—much larger than TBB. Coagulation artefacts are not a major problem if coagulation time is kept to <2 seconds. The diagnostic accuracy of the technique depends on the distribution pattern of the interstitial disease, the lobular compartment involved, and the histological specificity of the disease.

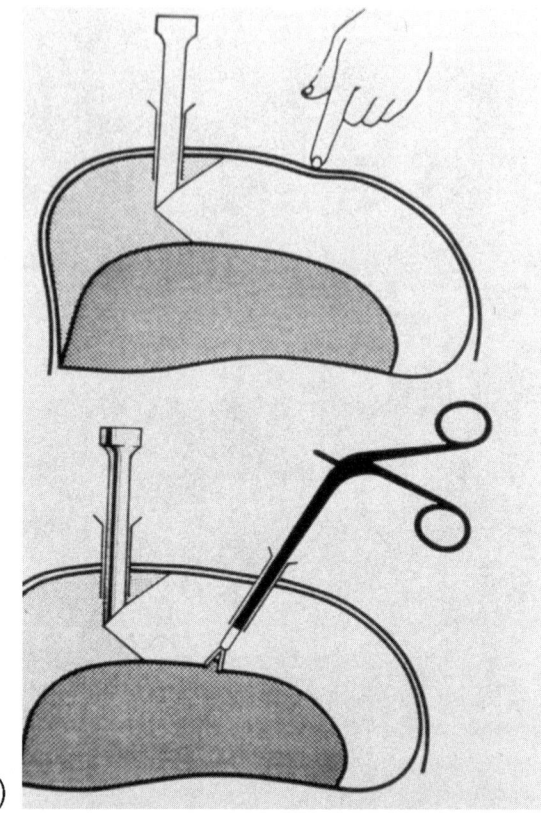

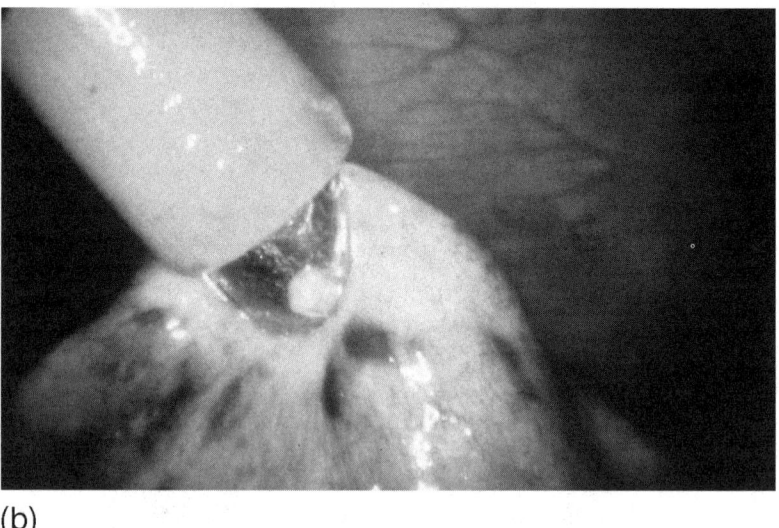

Figure 8 Lung biopsy: (a) two points of entry; (b) lung biopsy; (c) lung scar after biopsy.

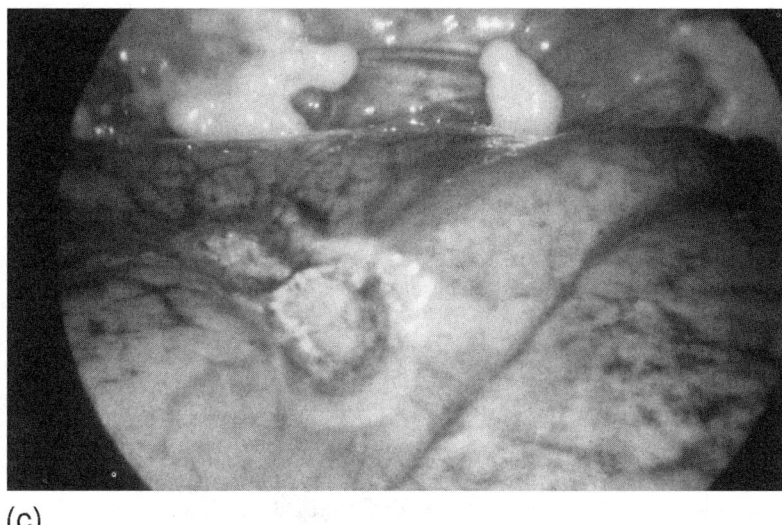

(c)

Figure 8 Continued.

Diagnoses of chonic interstitial pneumonitis of the usual or desquamative type or end-stage lung fibrosis could be made with confidence. Although the diagnosis of suspected pulmonary vasculitis or other pulmonary vascular disorders is more difficult and the technique of medical thoracoscopy less powerful in such cases, it remains useful in suspected vascular pathology, especially if there are lesions in the smaller pulmonary arterioles (57).

No major complications such as important bleeding or persistent fistula usually occur after the procedure. However, prolonged air leak is the most troublesome problem, which is not correlated with the number or size of biopsies but to the preexisting total lung capacity and static compliance. Such a complication is to be anticipated in patients with very stiff or honeycombing lungs where the use of a stapler or open lung biopsy with a suture may be a reasonable alternative. Medical thoracoscopic lung biopsy must be avoided in case of suspected major pleural adhesions, in severe pulmonary hypertension and in a very sick ventilated patients, in whom open lung biopsy carries less risk.

Thoracoscopy has prompted many practitioners to consider lung biopsy earlier in the management algorithm of patients with parenchymal disease of unclear origin, especially when bronchoscopic lung biopsies have been nondiagnostic.

Vaso-Motor Syndrome of the Upper Limb

Interruption of the upper dorsal sympathetic chain at the D2 and D3 level represents a permanent cure in patients with Raynaud's syndrome, causalgia, or essential hyperhydrosis (58). Thoracoscopic sympathectomies are performed using either electrocautery, dissection, or excision (59). Sympathectomy by medical thoracoscopy route is feasible, and this technique has been proven simple and safe with skill practicionners, with excellent short-term clinical results (60,61). Side effects and complications are minor (compensatory hyperhydrosis) or self-limiting (pain). The key problem is to prevent Horner's syndrome in avoiding the stellate ganglion with careful examination of the upper posterior part of the pleural cavity.

Exposure is usually through the anterior chest wall, and procedures can be performed bilaterally at a single setting (62,63).

Intrapleural Treatment

Intrapleural immunotherapy or chemotherapy can be administered after thoracoscopic placement of intrapleural implantable access system to treat cancer (64). Proper placement of the catheter under thoracoscopic guidance ensures that the drug is applied directly to the lesions (65,66). The subcutaneous location of the site reduces the risk of infection (67). The main indications for intrapleural therapy are malignant pleural mesothelioma as single treatment or in multimodal strategy as neoadjuvant treatment.

V. Conclusion

Potential advantages of thoracoscopy over more conventional techniques include certainty of representative tissue for diagnosis, reduced requirements for postoperative analgesia, shorter hospital stays, and a shorter duration of chest tube drainage compared with thoracotomy. The thoracoscopic approach to pleural and lung diseases has to demonstrate safety and cost-effectiveness compared with more conventional approaches. Potential adverse events including bleeding, persistent pneumothorax, intercostal nerve and vessel injury, cardiac disturbances, complications related to anesthesia, respiratory failure, wound infections, and malignant seeding of the chest wall have been reported; procedure-related mortality is rare (0.24%, comparable to that of bronchoscopic biopsy) in experienced hands.

Future directions in the field of medical thoracoscopy include developing "mini-invasive" procedures (68). One of the more exciting tasks in this field is to develop physician training and education to allow chest physicians to analyze the pleural cavity and to enhance their understanding of anatomical relationships and pleuropulmonary physiology (69).

References

1. Boutin C, Viallat JR, Aelony Y. Practical Thoracoscopy. Heidelberg: Springer-Verlag, 1991.

2. Loddenkemper R. Thoracoscopy—state of the art. Eur Respir J 1998; 11:213–221.
3. Boutin C, Astoul P. Diagnostic thoracoscopy. Clin Chest Med 1998; 19:295–309.
4. Colt HG. Thoracoscopy: window to the pleural space. Chest 1999; 116:1409–1415.
5. Loddenkemper R, Schonfeld N. Medical thoracoscopy. Curr Opin Pulm Med 1998; 4:235–238.
6. Vanderschueren RG. Thoracoscopie sous anesthésie locale. Poumon Coeur 1981; 37:21–23.
7. Plummer S, Hartley M, Vaughan RS. Anaesthesia for telescopic procedures in the thorax. Br J Anaesth 1998; 80:223–234.
8. Landreneau RJ, Mack MJ, Dowling RD, Luketich JD, Keenan RJ, Ferson PF, Hazelrigg SR. The role of thoracoscopy in lung cancer management. Chest 1998; 113(suppl 1):6S–12S.
9. Mathur PN, Astoul P, Boutin C. Medical thoracoscopy: technical details. Clin Chest Med 1995; 16:479–486.
10. Little AG. Thoracoscopy: current status. Curr Opin Pulm Med 1996; 2:315–319.
11. Yamada S, Kosaka A, Masuda M, Toyoshima M. Minimally invasive lung and pleural biopsies using 2-mm and standard thoracoscopic equipment. Jpn J Thorac Cardiovasc Surg 2000; 48:700–702.
12. Mathur P, Martin WJ. Clinical utility of thoracoscopy. Chest 1992; 4:1–4.
13. Light RW. Diagnostic principles in pleural disease. Eur Respir J 1997; 10:476–481.
14. Danby CA, Adebonojo SA, Moritz DM. Video-assisted talc pleurodesis for malignant pleural effusions utilizing local anesthesia and IV sedation. Chest 1998; 113:739–742.
15. Tschopp JM, Brutsche M, Frey JG. Treatment of complicated spontaneous pneumothorax by simple talc pleurodesis under thoracoscopy and local anaesthesia. Thorax 1997; 52:329–332.
16. DeCamp MM Jr, Jaklitsch MT, Mentzer SJ, Harpole DH Jr, Sugarbaker DJ. The safety and versatility of video-thoracoscopy: a prospective analysis of 895 consecutive cases. J Am Coll Surg 1995; 18:113–120.
17. Russo L, Wiechmann RJ, Magovern JA, Szydlowski GW, Mack MJ, Naunheim KS, Landreneau RJ. Early chest tube removal after video-assisted thoracoscopic wedge resection of the lung. Ann Thorac Surg 1998; 66:1751–1754.
18. Astoul Ph, Boutin C, Seitz B, Fico JL. Diagnostic thoracoscopy in short term hospitalisation. Acta Endo 1990; 20:79–83.
19. Viskum K, Enk B. Complications of thoracoscopy. Poumon Coeur 1981; 37:25–28.
20. Brandt HJ, Loddenkemper R, Mai J. Atlas of Diagnostic Thoracoscopy. New York: Thieme Stuttgart, 1985.
21. Lan RS, Lo SK, Chuang ML, Yang CT, Tsao TC, Lee CH. Elastance of the pleural space: a predictor for the outcome of pleurodesis in patients with malignant pleural effusion. Ann Intern Med 1997; 126:768–774.
22. Hansen M, Faurschou P, Clementsen P. Medical thoracoscopy, results and complications in 146 patients: a retrospective study. Respir Med 1998; 9:228–232.
23. Boutin C, Rey F, Viallat JR. Prevention of malignant seeding after invasive diagnostic procedures in patients with pleural mesothelioma: a randomized trial of local radiotherapy. Chest 1995; 108:754–758.
24. Janssen J, Boutin C. Extended thoracoscopy: a biopsy method to be used in case of pleural adhesions. Eur Respir J 1992; 5:763–766.
25. Colt HG. Thoracoscopy: a prospective study of safety and outcome. Chest 1995; 108:324–329.

26. Renshaw AA, Dean BR, Antman KH, Sugarbaker DJ, Cibas ES. The role of cytologic evaluation of pleural fluid in the diagnosis of malignant mesothelioma. Chest 1997; 111:106–109.
27. Colt HG. Thoracoscopic management of malignant pleural effusions. Clin Chest Med 1995; 16:505–518.
28. Rodriguez-Panadero F. Malignant pleural diseases. Monaldi Arch Chest Dis 2000; 55:17–19.
29. Boutin C, Frenay C, Astoul P. [Endoscopic diagnosis of mesothelioma]. Rev Mal Respir 1999; 16:1257–1262.
30. Wilsher ML, Veale AG. Medical thoracoscopy in the diagnosis of unexplained pleural effusion. Respirology 1998; 3:77–80.
31. McLean AN, Bicknell SR, McAlpine LG, Peacock AJ. Investigation of pleural effusion: an evaluation of the new Olympus LTF semiflexible thoracofiberscope and comparison with Abram's needle biopsy. Chest 1998; 114:150–153.
32. de Groot M, Walther G. Thoracoscopy in undiagnosed pleural effusions. S Afr Med J 1998; 88:706–711.
33. Boutin C, Rey F. Thoracoscopy in pleural mesothelioma. A prospective study of 188 consecutive patients. Part I: Diagnosis. Cancer 1993; 72:389–393.
34. Mason AC, Miller BH, Krasna MJ, White CS. Accuracy of CT for the detection of pleural adhesions: correlation with video-assisted thoracoscopic surgery. Chest 1999; 115:423–427.
35. Aelony Y, King R, Boutin C. Thoracoscopic talc poudrage pleurodesis for chronic reccurent pleural effusions. Ann Intern Med 1991; 115:778–782.
36. Aelony Y, King RR, Boutin C. Thoracoscopic talc poudrage in malignant pleural effusions: effective pleurodesis despite low pleural pH. Chest 1998; 113:1007–1012.
37. Light RW. Diseases of the pleura: the use of talc for pleurodesis. Curr Opin Pulm Med 2000; 6:255–258.
38. Canto A, Guijarro R, Arnau A, Galbis J, Martorell M, Garcia Aguado R. Video-thoracoscopy in the diagnosis and treatment of malignant pleural mesothelioma with associated pleural effusions. J Thorac Cardiovasc Surg 1997; 45:16–19.
39. Boutin C, Rey F, Gouvernet J, Viallat JR, Astoul Ph, Ledoray V. Thoracoscopy in pleural malignant mesothelioma: a prospective study of 188 patients. Part 2: prognosis and staging. Cancer 1993; 72:394–404.
40. Sahn SA. Pleural diseases related to metastatic malignancies. Eur Respir J 1997; 10:1907–1913.
41. Mouroux J, Perrin C, Venissac N, Blaive B, Richelme H. Management of pleural effusion of cirrhotic origin. Chest 1996; 109:1093–1096.
42. Mares DC, Mathur PN. Medical thoracoscopic talc pleurodesis for chylothorax due to lymphoma: a case series. Chest 1998; 114:731–735.
43. Janssen JP, Schramel FM, Sutedja TG, Cuesta MA, Postmus PE. Videothoracoscopic appearance of first and recurrent pneumothorax. Chest 1995; 108:330–334.
44. Delaunois L, el Khawand C. Medical thoracoscopy in the management of pneumothorax. Monaldi Arch Chest Dis 1998; 53:148–150.
45. Schramel FMNH. Current aspects of spontaneous pneumothorax. Eur Respir J 1997; 10:1372–1379.
46. Sahn SA, Heffner JE. Spontaneous pneumothorax. N Engl J Med 2000; 342:868–874.
47. Milanez JRC, Vargas FS, Filomeno LTB, Fernandez A, Jatene A, Light RW.

Intrapleural talc for the prevention of recurrent pneumothorax. Chest 1994; 106: 1162–1165.
48. Schramel FM, Sutedja TG, Braber JC, van Mourik JC, Postmus PE. Cost-effectiveness of video-assisted thoracoscopic surgery versus conservative treatment for first time or recurrent spontaneous pneumothorax. Eur Respir J 1996; 9:1821–1825.
49. Miller AC, Harvey JE. Guidelines for the management of spontaneous pneumothorax. Standards of Care Committee—British Thoracic Society. BMJ 1993; 307: 114–116.
50. Baumann MH, Strange C, Heffner JE, Light R, Kirby TJ, Klein J, Luketich JD, Panacek EA. Management of spontaneous pneumothorax. An American College of Chest Physicians Delphi Consensus statement. Chest 2001; 119:590–602.
51. Striffeler H, Gugger M, Im Hof V, Cerny A, Furrer M, Ris HB. Video-assisted thoracoscopic surgery for fibrinopurulent pleural empyema in 67 patients. Ann Thorac Surg 1998; 65:319–323.
52. Karmy-Jones R, Sorenson V, Horst HM, Lewis JW Jr, Rubinfeld I. Rigid thoracoscopic debridement and continuous pleural irrigation in the management of empyema. Chest 1997; 111:272–274.
53. Silen ML, Naunheim KS. Thoracoscopic approach to the management of empyema thoracis: indications and results. Chest Surg Clin North Am 1996; 6:491–499.
54. Cassina PC, Hauser M, Hillejan L, Greschuchna D, Stamatis G. Video-assisted thoracoscopy in the treatment of pleural empyema: stage-based management and outcome. J Thorac Cardiovasc Surg 1999; 117:234–238.
55. Krasna MJ, White CS, Aisner SC, Templeton PA, McLaughlin JS. The role of thoracoscopy in the diagnosis of interstitial lung disease. Ann Thorac Surg 1995; 59:348–351.
56. Ravini M, Ferraro G, Barbieri B, Colombo P, Rizzato G. Changing strategies of lung biopsies in diffuse lung diseases: the impact of video-assisted thoracoscopy. Eur Respir J 1998; 11:99–103.
57. Vansteenkiste J, Verbeken E, Thomeer M, Van Haecke P, Eeckout AV, Demedts M. Medical thoracoscopic lung biopsy in interstitial lung disease: a prospective study of biopsy quality. Eur Respir J 1999; 14:585–590.
58. Di Lorenzo N, Sica GS, Sileri P, Gaspari AL. Thoracoscopic sympathectomy for vasospastic diseases. J Soc Laparoendosc Surg 1998; 2:249–253.
59. Noppen M, Herregodts P, D'haese J, D'Haens J, Vincken W. A simplified T2-T3 thoracoscopic sympatholysis technique for the treatment of essential hyperhidrosis: short-term results in 100 patients. J Laparoendosc Surg 1996; 6:151–159.
60. Noppen M, Vincken W. Thoracoscopic sympathicolysis for essential hyperhidrosis: effects on pulmonary function. Eur Respir J 1996; 9:1660–1664.
61. Noppen M, Dendale P, Hagers Y, Herregodts P, Vincken W, D'haen J. Changes in cardiocirculatory autonomic function after thoracoscopic upper dorsal sympathicolysis for essential hyperhidrosis. J Auton Nerv Syst 1996; 60:115–120.
62. Noppen M, Dab I, D'Haese J, Meysman M, Vincken W. Thoracoscopic T2-T3 sympathicolysis for essential hyperhidrosis in childhood: effects on pulmonary function. Pediatr Pulmonol 1998; 26:264–264.
63. Noppen M, Sevens C, Gerlo E, Vincken W. Plasma catecholamine concentrations in essential hyperhidrosis and effects of thoracoscopic D2-D3 sympathicolysis. Eur J Clin Invest 1997; 27:202–205.

64. Driesen P, Boutin C, Viallat JR, Astoul PH, Vialette JP, Pasquier J. Implantable access system for prolonged intrapleural immunotherapy. Eur Respir J 1994; 7: 1889–1892.
65. Astoul Ph, Bertault-Peres P, Durand A, Catalin J, Vignal F, Boutin C. Pharmacokinetics of intrapleural recombinant interleukin-2 in immunotherapy for malignant pleural effusion. Cancer 1994; 73:308–313.
66. Monjanel-Mouterde S, Frenay C, Catalin J, Boutin C, Durand A, Astoul Ph. Pharmacokinetics of intrapleural cisplatin for the treatment of malignant pleural effusions. Oncol Rep 2000; 7:171–175.
67. Astoul Ph, Picat-Joossen D, Viallat JR, Boutin C. Intrapleural administration of interleukin-2 for the treatment of patients with malignant pleural mesothelioma. Cancer 1998; 83:2099–2104.
68. d'Alessandro AA. Microthoracoscopy at the cutting edge of thoracic surgery. J Laparoendosc Adv Surg Tech A 1997; 7:313–318.
69. Yim AP. Training in thoracoscopy in the Asia-Pacific. Int Surg 1997; 82:22–23.

12

Diagnostic Video-Assisted Thoracoscopic Surgery in Pleural Disease

GEORGE LADAS

Royal Brompton Hospital
and Imperial College School of Medicine
London, England

I. Background

Video-assisted thoracoscopic surgery (VATS), an evolution of traditional thoracoscopy, is one of the most exciting developments in thoracic surgery in the last decade. The availability of sophisticated high-quality digital imaging systems and a wide range of thoracoscopic instruments, in combination with advances in anesthetic techniques and intraoperative monitoring, facilitated its use and resulted in an ever-expanding range of indications. The minimally invasive nature of VATS makes it particularly popular for the diagnosis of pleural disease, where simpler techniques like thoracocentesis or blind pleural biopsy have failed.

II. Historic Overview

Bozzini is credited with the first endoscopic diagnostic procedure in 1806, with the use of a hollow tube illuminated by a candle to inspect the urinary bladder (1). Visualization was poor, and the discomfort felt by the patients was such that the Surgical Academy of Vienna censured his work. A major advance in the field of endoscopy came in the 1870s with the introduction of the *cystoscope* designed by Nitze in Vienna (2). This consisted of a working channel, a light source, and an optical lens, through which light was reflected. Newman in 1883 incorporated the recently invented Edison electrical bulb to further improve illumination of cystoscopes. In the early 1900s Kelling (3) developed the intracavitary technique and in 1902 performed the first laparoscopic operations in dogs. He finally reported the first laparoscopic operations in humans in 1916. Hans Christian Jacobeus, a professor of internal medicine working in a sanatorium in Sweden and a previous student of Kelling, was the first to perform a *pleuroscopy* or *thoracoscopy* in 1910. This was used to divide pleural adhesions in patients with tuberculosis to improve lung collapse following iatrogenic pneumothorax treatment (pneumolysis) (4). In 1921 Jacobeus reported his experience in using thoracoscopic procedures for the diagnosis of pleural and lung tumors (5). Thoracoscopy became a popular therapeutic procedure, with thousands of operations performed worldwide up to the early 1950s (6), when, with the introduction of antituberculous drugs, collapse treatment was abandoned. During the following 20 years, thoracoscopy evolved into a widely used diagnostic procedure for the management of pleural effusions as well as primary and metastatic pleural tumors, and several large series with more than 1000 patients each were reported (7). Interest in the procedure was renewed in the early 1970s when thoracoscopy was reintroduced as a minimally invasive diagnostic and therapeutic tool. Finally, with the introduction of modern thoracoscopic digital video imaging systems, advanced optics, and instrumentation in the early 1990s, the full potential of the technique was realized for the first time (8–10).

III. Indications

The most common indication for thoracoscopy in the diagnosis of pleural disease is the patient who presents with a pleural effusion and in whom first-line techniques like thoracocentesis and blind percutaneous pleural needle biopsy have failed to secure diagnosis, a situation occurring in as many as 20–25% of cases (11,12). A VATS pleural biopsy is particularly important when the patient has a history of malignancy at another site, previous exposure to asbestos, involvement of two serous cavities, as for example pericardial and pleural, or family history of malignancy (13). VATS allows excellent visualization of most of the visceral and parietal pleura, so that multiple targeted biopsies from suspicious areas or pleural masses can be obtained. In recurrent symptomatic pleural effusions, VATS can be used very conveniently to first confirm the presence of pleural malignancy and then provide definitive palliation during the same procedure. If the lung can still reexpand following drainage of the effusion, a talc pleurodesis is performed. If a malignant restricting cortex prevents reexpansion (trapped lung), then insertion of a pleuro-peritoneal shunt is indicated (14).

Another important indication is the assessment of pleural effusions when staging patients presenting with primary lung cancer. Metastatic involvement of the parietal pleura signals inoperability and is staged as T4 disease, stage IIIb (15).

Table 1 Etiology of Paramalignant Effusions

Proximal bronchial obstruction and atelectasis or pneumonitis
Proximal lymphatic obstruction
Systemic tumor effect (pulmonary embolism, hypoproteinemia)
Result of chemotherapy or radiotherapy

In 5% of patients with primary lung cancer and a pleural effusion, the pleura is not involved by the malignancy and the effusion does not contain malignant cells (*paramalignant effusion*) (Table 1). In patients who are otherwise operable and pleural fluid cytology from three consecutive pleural aspirations is negative, thoracoscopy is indicated. If pleural biopsies are negative for malignancy once again, then these patients are candidates for curative surgery.

The use of diagnostic thoracoscopy just for categorizing patients following the first episode of spontaneous pneumothorax has been proposed but is not widely practiced.

IV. Contraindications

Video-assisted thoracoscopy requires single lung anesthesia, so it is contraindicated in patients severely hypoxic due to concomitant chronic lung disease, who cannot tolerate collapse of the lung on the operated side intraoperatively.

Complete obliteration of the pleural space by uniform adhesions is another absolute contraindication for VATS. Patients with pleural mesothelioma often present with a pleural effusion early in the course of the disease, and VATS can be used for obtaining pleural biopsies. Later, as the disease progresses, the pleural space becomes completely obliterated by tumor encroaching on the lung, making VATS impossible. In these circumstances, we find that the easiest way of obtaining diagnostic tissue is to perform a mini (4 cm) thoracotomy and resect a short 2 cm length of a rib. This provides access to the underlying thickened parietal and visceral pleura, and generous, full-thickness biopsies can easily be obtained. A preoperative computed tomography (CT) scan of the chest is used to select the most appropriate target area. Since the pleural space is completely fused, there is no need for a chest drain to be used. The procedure still requires general anesthesia, but there is no need for single lung anesthesia. Patients are able to leave the hospital on the first postoperative day.

V. Instrumentation and Technique

The basic VATS instrumentation includes a 0° and 30° thoracoscope, a set of single or multiple use thoracoscopic ports, a camera system, a digital image amplifier, a light source, and one or two monitors (Fig. 1). There are now even

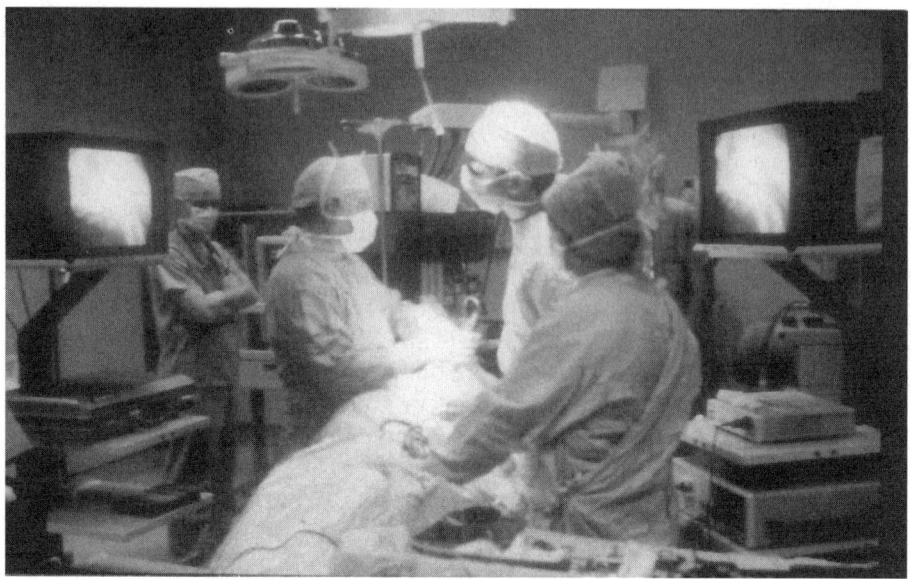

Figure 1 A video-assisted thoracoscopic procedure. The surgeon is holding the thoracoscopic camera and uses the monitor opposite for viewing. On that video rack, one can see the monitor, the digital image amplifier, and the light source (from top to bottom). A second monitor is used by the assistant.

camera systems allowing a quasi-3D image for improved operator depth-of-field perception. A wide variety of special thoracoscopic instruments is available, in disposable or multiple use form. For the purpose of diagnosis of pleural disease, a thoracoscopic biopsy forceps is required as well as combined thoracoscopic suction-diathermy catheter, for securing hemostasis. Talc insufflation can be performed with reusable insufflators loaded with medical grade iodized talc or with single-use, aerosol-type, fine-powdered talc minicontainers.

The technique of diagnostic VATS thoracoscopy for pleural disease is described in detail in Chapter 27. In principle, we use double lumen endotracheal tubes to achieve single lung anesthesia, passively collapsing the lung on the operated side. Contrary to laparoscopic procedures, CO_2 insufflation is used by only very few surgeons in thoracoscopic surgery, due to the potentially life-threatening complication of tension pneumothorax on the dependent non-operated side. We routinely use a single, 22 mm oval metal thoracoscopic port for the procedure. This will admit the standard thoracoscope in combination with one other instrument—suction diathermy, biopsy forceps, as well as the nozzle of the talc insufflator, if necessary—with ease. Pleural biopsies are sent for a frozen section to ensure diagnostic material (Fig. 2). If malignancy is confirmed and a symptomatic pleural effusion is present, we proceed to surgical palliation. If, following drainage of the effusion, the lung can reexpand using

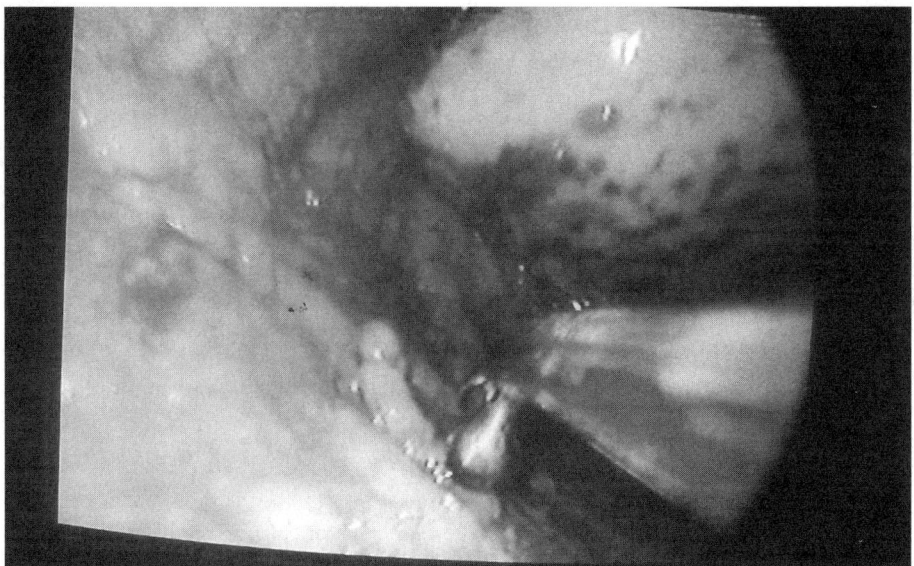

Figure 2 A view obtained during video-assisted thoracoscopy for malignant pleural effusion. The lung has been allowed to collapse using the double lumen endotracheal tube. The pleural effusion has been aspirated, and fluid specimens sent for microbiology and cytology. The ribs and intercostal spaces are clearly delineated. The parietal pleura is grossly abnormal, thickened, and uniformly covered by tumor deposits. The endoscopic biopsy forceps is used to obtain a punch biopsy of the parietal pleura, with a specimen also sent for frozen section. If malignancy is confirmed, a talc pleurodesis will follow, as the visceral pleura is relatively normal, and the lung can reexpand following drainage of the effusion.

mild (20 cmH$_2$O) intrabronchial pressures, then we perform talc pleurodesis with 8 g of iodized talc; otherwise a pleuroperitoneal shunt is used.

VI. Results

VATS thoracoscopy is successful in securing a diagnosis of pleural disease in 95–98% of cases (16,17). Talc pleurodesis for malignant pleural effusion is successful in 95% of the cases. The length of hospital stay is largely dictated by whether an additional palliative procedure was performed. The average hospital stay following VATS thoracoscopy and pleural biopsy with talc pleurodesis or insertion of pleuro-peritoneal shunt is 4 days. The procedure is technically very simple, and the morbidity and mortality due to the procedure itself is extremely low. Care is necessary, though, when operating on debilitated, frail patients with probable metastatic malignancy, as in some of them the combined physiological impact of general anesthesia and this minor procedure can at times be devastating.

References

1. Bush RB, Leonhardt H, Bush IV, et al, Dr. Bozzini's Lichtleiter. A translation of his original article (1806). Urology 1974; 3:119–123.
2. Nitze M. Eine neue Boebachtungs- und Untersuchungsmethode für Harnrohre, Harnblase, und Rektum. Wien Med Wochenschr 1879; 24:649–652.
3. Kelling G. Über Oesophagoskopie, Gastroskopie, und Koelioskopie. Münch Med Wochenschr 1902; 52:21.
4. Jacobeus HC. Possibility of the use of the cystoscope for investigation of serous cavities. Münch Med Wochenschr 1910; 57:2090–2092.
5. Jacobeus HC. The practical importance of thoracoscopy in surgery of the chest. Surg Gynecol Obstet 1921; 32:493–500.
6. Bloomberg AE. Thoracoscopy in perspective. Surg Gynecol Obstet 1978; 147:433.
7. Das K, Rothberg M. Thoracoscopic surgery: historical perspectives. Neurosurg Focus October, 2000; 9(4). Article 10.
8. Hucker J, Bhatnagar NK, Al-Jilaihawi AN, Forrester-Wood CP. Thoracoscopy in the diagnosis and management of recurrent pleural effusions. Ann Thorac Surg 1991; 52, 1145–1147.
9. Tampino-Golos I. Endoscopic thoracotomy: a new approach to thoracic surgery. AORN J 1992; 55:1167–1180.
10. Landreneau RJ, Mack MJ, Keenan RJ, Hazelrigg SR, Dowling RD, Ferson PF. Strategic planning for video-assisted thoracic surgery. Ann Thorac Surg 1993; 56:615–619.
11. Loddenkemper E. Thoracoscopy: results in non cancerous and idiopathic pleural effusions. Poumon-Coeur 1981; 37:261–264.
12. Poe RH, Israel RH, Utell MV. Sensibility, specificity and predictive values of closed pleural biopsy. Arch Intern Med 1984; 114:325.
13. Cantó A, Saumench J, Moya J. Points to consider when choosing a biopsy method in cases of pleuritis of unknown origin with special reference to thoracoscopy. In: Deslauriers J, Lacquet LK, eds. St. Louis: International Trends in General Thoracic Surgery CV Mosby, 1990:49.
14. Genc O, Petrou P, Ladas G, Goldstraw P. The long term morbidity of pleuroperitoneal shunts in the management of recurrent malignant effusions. Eur J Cardio-Thorac Surg 2000; 18:143–146.
15. Mountain CF. Revisions in the international system for staging lung cancer. Chest 1997; 111:1710–1717.
16. Menzies R, Charbonneau M. Thoracoscopy for the diagnosis of pleural disease. Ann Intern Med 1991; 114:271–276.
17. Harris RJ, Kavuru MS, Rice TA. The diagnostic and therapeutic utility of thoracoscopy: a review. Chest 1995; 108(3):828–841.

13

Therapeutic Use of Thoracoscopy for Pleural Diseases

GILBERT MASSARD

Université Louis Pasteur
and Hôpitaux Universitaires
  de Strasbourg
Strasbourg, France

PASCAL THOMAS

Sainte Marguerite University Hospital
  of Marseille
Marseille, France

I. Introduction

The therapeutic use of thoracoscopy is not a recent addition to our armamentarium (1). Illustrations in physiology textbooks from the 1950s show ports, forceps, and hooks similar to those still in use; optical interface with video transmission and the creation of endoscopic staplers and disposable instruments are the extent of new technology. For half a century, thoracoscopy has been an important adjunct to collapse therapy for tuberculosis, which was the mainstay of treatment prior to the advent of major antituberculous drugs. Thoracoscopy was used to separate pleural adhesions in order to create pneumothorax. It is therefore paradoxical that now one of the main indications for thoracoscopy is treatment of pneumothorax!

For approximately 10 years surgeons, physicians, and patients have been subjected to a campaign in favor of minimally invasive techniques. The exponential development of these techniques has reinvigorated the biomedical industry. This chapter will critically review the therapeutic use of videothoracoscopy in pleural diseases to define the optimal indications and compare to classic alternatives where available.

II. Potential Indications for Therapeutic Thoracoscopy

Use of thoracoscopy for diagnostic purposes in pleural diseases is described elsewhere in this book. We therefore concentrate here on treatment of pleural diseases and more particularly on the management of empyema and spontaneous pneumothorax.

Traditional indications also included pleurodesis for recurrent pleural effusions (in particular metastatic effusions) with talc poudrage or various other irritative substances. The sine-qua-non condition for a successsful pleurodesis in this setting is that the lung is able to reexpand and completely seal the pleural space. Therefore, it is mandatory to perform this pleurodesis at an early stage, before metastatic deposits on the visceral pleura encase the lung. It is well known that talc is both the most efficient and the least expensive material; we therefore consider that this indication does not need any further development (2).

Several single case reports describe successful management of chylothorax with thoracoscopic ligation of the thoracic duct. However, chylothorax remains a rare event, and it is impossible to estimate the proportion of patients amenable to safe thoracoscopic management, as the proportion of those managed by formal thoracotomy remains unknown. We consider this indication as—hopefully—anecdotal and will not further develop this issue (3,4).

In stable patients with traumatic hemothorax, early thoracoscopy may allow for adequate cleaning of the pleural space and thus avoid clotting; early recognition of various underlying traumatic lesions such as rupture of the diaphragm, rupture of the pericardium, and parenchymal tears will lead to adequate early management (5,6). However, many patients are either unstable, or cannot be brought to immediate thoracoscopy because of associated extrathoracic injuries; classic treatment with chest tube placement followed by thoracotomy if required by persistent bleeding still has its place.

III. Preliminary Remarks

We consider all procedures described below as surgical procedures to be undertaken only by certified thoracic surgeons. In Europe, we recommend certification by the National Colleges of Thoracic Surgeons. The latter should be progressively replaced by the recently awarded European Board of Cardiothoracic Surgery, which is promoted by the European Association for Cardiothoracic Surgery and by the European Society of Thoracic Surgeons. Any of these procedures may result in life-threatening intraoperative complications with disastrous consequences, unless a skilled thoracic surgeon may immediately converts to thoracotomy and proceeds with a classic open operation. According on intraoperative findings, extensive surgical background is required to guarantee adequate surgical decision making.

Although such procedures have been conducted under local anesthesia since their inception, it seems preferable for both the patient and surgeon to use general anesthesia. Anesthesia should be administered with double lumen intubation, or at least with use of bronchial blockers, to achieve safe single lung ventilation: the only way to allow a thorough inspection of the pleural cavity is to take the lung down by stopping its ventilation. Administration of general anesthesia will also avoid loss of precious time should a serious complication occur.

IV. Video-Assisted Thoracic Surgery Management of Empyema

At first look, treatment modalities for empyema are confusing. When comparing different publications, it appears that patient populations and diagnostic criteria differ, that classifications have not been homogenized, and that guidelines for treatment depend on the type of unit the patient has been admitted to (surgery, pulmonology, internal medicine, or intensive care). Finally, endpoints of such studies also fail to converge.

We should also clearly separate two very different entities: parapneumonic empyema and secondary empyema (Table 1). In the event of parapneumonic empyema, early surgical intervention is a valuable option. When facing secondary empyema, the individual prognosis depends on the precise cause; most often complex surgery is required in such patients. The most common cause of secondary empyema is postoperative, as happens following pneumonectomy, lobectomy, or esophageal resection. Empyema may also be associated with mediastinitis in patient with spontaneous or instrumental esophageal disruption or with necrotizing descending mediastinitis originating from a dental or tonsillar abcess. These days is rare that a subphrenic abscess is not diagnosed prior to its spreading to the pleural cavity. Finally, spinal abscesses may also drain to the pleura.

Table 1 Causes of Empyema

Primary lung infection
    Parapneumonic
    Tuberculosis
Postoperative complications
    Lobectomy
    Pneumonectomy
    Esophageal resection
Diffusion of neighboring infection
    Mediastinitis (esophageal disruption)
    Descending necrotizing mediastinitis
    Spinal abscess
    Subphrenic abscess

A. Principles of Treatment for Empyema

From a theoretical point of view, cure of empyema requires evacuation and cleaning of the pleural space and complete reexpansion of the lung. Expansion of the lung will seal the pleural space, which eventually marks healing of empyema. In modern medicine, this double goal should be reached as quickly as possible in order to reduce duration of treatment and hospital stay and duration of physical disability. The sligtht cost of treatment with use of modern tools should be counterbalanced favourably by the reduction of the global cost.

The process of parapneumonic empyema is well documented (7). The first stage is the exudative phase, when plasma with high protein content escapes towards a free pleural space. This stage is usually very short—no longer than 48 hours. The second stage is the fibrinopurulent stage, in which fibrin deposits on the visceral pleura become thicker, septae develop between the parietal and visceral pleura, and loculations appear. The duration of this stage is about 14 days. The third stage is the organizing phase. The pleural peel is well defined, and ingrowth of fibroblasts transforms the initially soft, jelly-like material into a firm envelope. We now observe progressive encasement of the lung, inhibiting spontaneous reexpansion.

B. Stage 1 Empyema: Minimally Invasive Treatment Not Required

Patients with stage 1 empyema can be successfully managed without the use of minimally invasive surgical techniques. Simple thoracentesis or, even better, tube thoracostomy may evacuate the pleural effusion and hence reexpand the lung (8). Antibiotics and physiotherapy will definitely cure the patient. Unfortunately, patients are seldom caught at this stage.

C. Stage 3 Empyema: Minimally Invasive Treatment No Longer Possible?

In patients with stage 3 empyema, external drainage cannot succeed because spontaneous reexpansion of the lung is no longer possible; in such patients, a formal decortication needs to be performed to free the surface of the lung. Most surgeons will advocate an open approach to guarantee a safe procedure (7,9,10). Such aggressive surgery ensures rapid relief from sepsis at a low mortality even in very ill patients (7): despite high sepsis or low performance status, mortality was limited to 3.9%.

However, some very skilled surgeons have reported successful decortication using video-assisted thoracic surgery (VATS). One of the teams promoting its use is the group from Krasnodar, Russia (11). In the western literature, Waller and Rengarajan recently published their initial experience (12). VATS decortication was attempted in 36 patients and succeeded in 21; conversion to thoracotomy was required in 15. Exclusive use of VATS allowed a shortening of hospital stay of 2.9 days. The authors concluded that success was significantly related to increasing operative experience.

D. Stage 2 Empyema: Minimally Invasive Treatment Optional

In patients with fibrilopurulent empyema, there are four options:

Repeated thoracentesis
External drainage
Intrapleural fibrinolysis
Minimally invasive debridement

Each of these options requires backup with antibiotic treatment and aggressive chest physiotherapy. It is now well accepted that repeated thoracentesis has a high failure rate and that early placement of a chest tube may be beneficial. The chest tube offers the possibility to proceed with intrapleural fibrinolysis if required. Most authors also agree that biochemistry is of limited use to define treatment and that computed tomography (CT) scan offers the optimal information needed to choose the suitable option (8,13–15).

Classic treatment was made with external drainage, followed by daily pleural lavages through the chest tube for 2–3 weeks. With modern health care economics and social evolution, quicker treatment options must be promoted. Fibrinolytic therapy has been used since the 1960s to accelerate detersion of fibrinous material, and its benefit has been stressed by recent scientific studies (16,17). Robinson et al. reported a primary success rate of 77%, with a mean duration of treatment of 6.8 days (16). With a slightly longer treatment time of 11 days, Bouros et al. were able to increase the primary success rate to 92% (17).

Some authors question the precise mechanism of such treatments: Is success due to effective fibrinolysis, or does increase of exudate by stimulation of the pleura help to wash out the pleural deposits (18,19)?

With the explosive development of videothoracoscopic surgery, minimally invasive debridement of empyema has been advanced. We should underline that the approach is not new; early pleural debridement with thoracotomy was recommended during the 1980s. Such an approach was at that time not easily accepted by pulmonologists or by patients (20,21). Weissberg and Refaely used classic, "optical" thoracoscopy for many years, which has been replaced by video equipment (22).

The first study reporting favorable results with VATS by Angelillo Mackinlay reported a 100% success rate, with a median duration of treatment of 4.3 days (23). These optimistic data were confirmed by Striffeler et al., who reported a primary success rate of 96% and median duration of hospital stay of 4.1 days (24).

Further comparison of treatments requires controlled trials. Medline research identified a single randomized study comparing fibrinolysis to VATS debridement, unfortunately, a relatively low cohort of patients. Nevertheless, the results strongly support early operative management (25). Chest tube time was 5.8 days in the surgical group and 9.8 days in the streptokinase group; total hospital stay was 8.7 days in the surgical group and 12.8 days in the streptokinase group. Primary success rate was 91% after surgical debridement, and 44% after fibrinolysis. Total estimated cost was $16,642 in surgical patients and $24,052 in medical patients. These data suggest that early operative management may considerably reduce the duration of treatment and favor an earlier return to occupational habits. Another advantage of surgery is that the stage of empyema may be assessed adequately and that conversion to classic decortication is feasible at once if required.

Chest physicians' opinions about these different treatment options were elicited by questionnaire at an interactive symposium of the American College of Chest Physicians (Table 2). For example, more than two thirds were in favor of immediate surgery for multiloculated empyema (26).

E. Tuberculous Empyema

At an early stage, before encasement of the lung, tuberculous empyema may be determined by simple pleural biopsy, and its treatment based on drainage and specific antituberculous therapy is most often effective. The problem is different when the diagnosis is made at the stage of pulmonary encasement. Antibiotic therapy may well halt the infectious process, but reexpansion of the lung requires formal decortication. This is usually performed by a conventional thoracotomy approach. Porkhanov and colleagues have used a technique of video-assisted decortication where the pleural pocket is entered and the visceral peel is dissected off the surface of the lung from the pleural reflexions toward the center (11). Such operations require great experience. It is quite understandable that in countries with a high prevalence of pleural tuberculosis and little money allotted to health care, a reduction in hospital stay is sought. This applies especially to the countries of the former Soviet Union.

Table 2 Physician Opinions of Optimal Treatment of Multiloculated Empyema

Type of treatment	% of Physicians in favor of treatment	Total % in favor of treatment
Medical treatment		
Bedside chest tube	8%	
Multiple CT-guided catheters	7%	
Chest tube + fibrinolysis	14%	29%
Surgical treatment		
Thoracotomy + chest tubes	22%	
Formal decortication	49%	71%

Source: Ref. 26.

F. Postpneumonectomy Empyema: A Potential Indication for Thoracoscopy?

Empyema is observed as a complication of pneumonectomy, with a reported prevalence varying from 2 to 10% in most series; risk factors for empyema are pneumonectomy for benign disease, completion pneumonectomy, intraoperative spillage from infected parenchymal cavities, and postoperative hemothorax (27,28). Classic management has consisted of either tube thoracostomy with repeated lavage or open window thoracostomy with iterative gauze packing.

Recent publications underline the contribution of VATS in the management of this complication. Thoracoscopy allows for complete debridement and removal of fibrinous deposits and septations and is followed by pleural irrigation for several days until pleural fluid cultures become sterile. Hollaus et al. reported successful management without long-term recurrence in patients followed for 204–1163 days (29).

V. VATS Management for Spontaneous Pneumothorax

Recurrent spontaneous pneumothorax is a disabling disorder, which may present either in young and otherwise healthy patients (primary pneumothorax) or as a complication of an underlying lung disease (secondary pneumothorax). Minimally invasive management has two advantages: earlier return to occupational habits for younger patients and less physiological harm due to less operative trauma in older ones. It is possible to distinguish two different philosophies of approach: the medical approach, based on chemical pleurodesis, which may be undertaken by blinded instillation or thoracoscopy (30,31), and the minimally invasive surgical approach, merely reproducing the classic surgical techniques formerly performed by open surgery.

A. Indications

Indication of chemical pleurodesis or surgical management should refer to the potential risk of recurrence. Recurrence rates after chest tube drainage of a first episode range from 10 to 21%; recurrence after a second episode is estimated close to 50% and may reach 80% following a third episode (32,33). Therefore, "classic" indications are defined as follows:

Second ipsilateral recurrence
First contralateral recurrence
Bilateral simultaneous pneumothorax
Persisting pneumothorax (air leaks beyond day 7 of tube drainage)
   spontaneous hemopneumothorax
      at-risk professions (pilots, scuba divers, etc.)

B. "Classic" Surgical Treatment

The principles of surgical management for primary spontaneous pneumothorax include (1) treatment of the apex and (2) pleurodesis. Treatment of the apex means resection of visible blebs, suture of perforations, and even blind apical resection when no obvious lesion has been identified. Pleurodesis may be performed either by pleural abrasion or by parietal pleurectomy (34,35). Pleural abrasion theoretically preserves the extrapleural space, which should be helpful in the hypothesis of a subsequent ipsilateral thoracotomy. Most authors cited a chemical abrasion of the visceral pleura by iodine or silver nitrate (36,37). These operations performed through a classic or muscle-sparing thoracotomy provided excellent results, with less than 1% recurrence (Table 3) (37–39). Pleurectomy has been credited with a slight advantage over abrasion: recurrence rate was 0.4% following pleurectomy ($n = 752$) and 2.3% after abrasion ($n = 301$) (39). Although the primum movens of spontaneous pneumothorax is a lung disorder, pleurodesis appears to be mandatory: Körner and colleagues have performed apical wedge resections without pleurodesis through thoracotomy, resulting in a recurrence rate of 5% (40). Incidence of postoperative complications has been close to 15% (Table 3), with most complications related to the patients' status (e.g., COPD) rather than to the thoracotomy itself. When separating primary and secondary pneumothorax, it appeared that significantly more complications occurred in patients with underlying lung disease: the respective rates were 26.3% for secondary pneumothorax versus 7.2% for primary pneumothorax ($p < 0.01$) (37). The main complications were hemothorax and prolonged air leaks. Postoperative hemothorax is seen more particularly following pleurectomy and occurred in 0–4% of cases. Total pleurectomy led to an increased complication rate when compared to apical pleurectomy (39). Prolonged air leaks have been observed in 5–10% of patients and were more frequent in patients with COPD (36).

Most classic series reported by European centers relate a prolonged postoperative hospital stay close to 14 days, which may be due to "cultural" reasons: chest tubes were left in place for 4–6 days as a rule, and both patients and doctors believed that thoracotomy required a hospitalization of at least 2 weeks

Table 3 Outcome Following Open Surgery for Spontaneous Pneumothorax

N	Pleurodesis	Complications (%)	Recurrence (%)	Follow-up (months)	Ref.
400	Abrasion	15	0.25	n.s.	36
107	Abrasion	14	0	27	37
278	Pleurectomy	6.5	1	84	38
233	Pleurectomy	17	0.4	56	39
120	None		5		40

for adequate recovery. Nonetheless, hospital stay was prolonged by 4 days in patients with secondary pneumothorax (37).

We should also mention a classic approach that can be considered as the precursor of minimally invasive surgery: the transaxillary minithoracotomy popularized by Becker and Munro in 1976 (41). The operation is made through an incision placed just below the axillary hairline and extended over 5–6 cm at most; the chest is entered through the 3rd intercostal space. Apical pleurectomy or abrasion is performed, and the apexes of the upper and lower lobe are carefully inspected. Blebs or bullae can be drawn to the level of the skin and stapled outside the chest. A single tube is left for 24 hours. In 1980 Deslauriers and colleagues published their experience with 362 consecutive patients (42). Four patients required reoperation for bleeding ($n = 3$) or air leak ($n = 1$), and a further 30 experienced minor complications (9.4%). Mean hospital stay was 6 days. Only 2 patients (0.4%) presented with recurrent pneumothorax.

C. Chemical Pleurodesis

Chemical pleurodesis has been promoted by chest physicians comfortable with thoracoscopy, thus prolonging the traditions of physiology. The basic principle is to create a "chemical pleuritis," scarring from which will cause dense adhesions. The most popular agents, talc, tetracycline, and silver nitrate, share the substantial advantage of low cost. Silver nitrate has lost favor over the years because its application is particularly painful and induces a major exudative reaction (30). Injectable tetracycline is no longer commercially available; besides, results with it were not satisfactory, since the recurrence rate was estimated at 16% in a series of 390 consecutive patients (43). Talc poudrage has the lowest recurrence rate of all chemical agents (2). In a comparative trial including 96 patients, recurrence rate was 36% after simple drainage, 13% following tetracycline pleurodesis, and 8% after talc poudrage (44). The reported failure rates after talc poudrage range from 10 to 15% (31,45,46) (Table 4). Half of the failures are immediate failures, prompting repeated thoracoscopy or subsequent thoracotomy (31).

In addition to a relatively high rate of failure, concerns about talc poudrage include asbestos contamination and restrictive changes of lung function. Fear of asbestos contamination can be excluded; no single case of mesothelioma occurred in a cohort of 210 patients followed for 14–40 years (47). Further,

Table 4 Success Rates with Talc Poudrage for Spontaneous Pneumothorax

No. patients	Success rate (%)	Ref.
109	87	31
200	92.7	45
356	88	46

the threat of restrictive respiratory impairment is unfounded. In a series of 75 patients followed for 22–35 years after talc poudrage, a mild restrictive impairment of lung function (mean TLC 89% of predicted) was shown (48). Spirometry showed normal values in 42 patients reviewed by Gurin et al. (31). However, most surgeons favor pleural abrasion or pleurectomy because granuloma formation is considered excessive and might offer a challenging barrier in the event of a subsequent ipsilateral thoracotomy. In contrast, patchy distribution of talc will lead to incomplete pleurodesis and require a subsequent thoracotomy to complete pleurodesis in technically critical conditions. The more recently developed fibrin glue is not an option because the recurrence rate of 25% is unacceptable (49). In addition, this type of material has a relatively high cost and entails biological risks.

In conclusion, results of chemical pleurodesis are not satisfactory; therefore, talc poudrage should be restricted to otherwise inoperable patients with secondary pneumothorax.

D. Global Results with VATS

As expected, the use of a modern approach to the pleural cavity has not yet ended the debate on pleurodesis. Most authors have merely transferred their usual technique to minimally invasive procedures, and the majority seem to favor abrasion (50–52). As previously recommended, isolated resection of blebs without pleurodesis is seldom performed (53). Other publications show that technique has evolved with growing experience; Inderbitzi and colleagues performed isolated ligation or wedge excision without pleurodesis for half of their patients and subsequently added apical pleurectomy to the procedure (32). We will discuss the results with reference to open surgery, in particular for postoperative complications and quality of long-term prevention of recurrence.

Complications

Complication rates are quite similar to those for open thoracotomy (54). In the series by Mouroux and colleagues, the total complication rate was 10% (51). When considering the cause of pneumothorax, the complication rate was 6.75% for primary pneumothorax versus 27.7% for secondary pneumothorax (51). The most frequent complication is prolonged air leak (>5 days), observed in approximately 8% of patients (32,52,55). Initial failure of pleurodesis and hemothorax require reoperation; the incidence of reoperation has been close to 5% (50).

Recurrence After Surgery

Most series suggest that at medium term (less than 3 years of follow-up), the recurrence rate ranges from 5 to 10% (Table 5) (50–57). In addition, "failure during hospitalisation treated by thoracotomy" (54) should be considered as an early recurrence. Recurrences are certainly increased when compared to thora-

Table 5 Recurrence Rates Following VATS for Spontaneous Pneumothorax

No. patients	Follow-up (months)	% Recurrence	% Lost for follow-up	Ref.
79	19.6	8.3	6.3	32
163	24.5	3.6[a]	8.5	50
100	30	3	n.s.	51
113	13.1	4.1	10	52
100	17	4	n.s.	55
109	53.2	4.6	0	56
99	29	4.8	0	57

[a] 3.6% long-term recurrence, but 4 early failures requiring reoperation by thoracotomy, which equals a total of 6% of failures.
n.s., not stated.

cotomy: in a comparison study, recurrence rate was 0.4% after thoracotomy and 6% after VATS (chi^2 = 10.635; $p < 0.01$) (54). A multicenter study by Naunheim and colleagues (52) reported a heterogeneous series of 113 patients, since pleurodesis differed: abrasion, 45%; sclerotic agents, 24%; laser, 13%; pleurectomy, 10%; none, 10%. The overall recurrence rate was 4.1%, and actuarial freedom of recurrence was estimated at 95% at 6 months. Similarly, Bertrand and colleagues (50) reported a freedom of recurrence of 95% at 42 months in a review of 163 patients. In the latter series, 3 patients had a complete recurrence requiring a second operation, and 3 had partial recurrence managed conservatively, which accounts for a recurrence rate of 3.6%. However, 4 patients were reoperated via thoracotomy for immediate failure during the initial postoperative hospital stay; when including these patients, the total rate of recurrence was 6%. A national survey in the United States reported a 7% failure rate in 1993 (58). No definitive conclusion as to recurrence rates can be drawn without a controlled trial. Also, published series probably underestimate the real recurrence rate: follow-up is short and 8.5–10% of patients are lost to follow-up (50,52). This proportion of patients lost to follow-up seems far too high for a benign disease and short-term surveillance; it is likely that patients with postoperative recurrence choose a different surgeon, as they would for failed hernia repair or recurring varicose veins.

Recurrence depends on surgical technique; compared to open surgery, it is lowest when both apical resection and pleurodesis have been performed. The importance of apical stapling has been particularly stressed by Naunheim and colleagues (52). In a univariate analysis, two factors predicted recurrence. When no bleb had been identified, the recurrence rate was 27.3% versus 0% and 2.7% when 1 or multiple blebs were seen. Apical stapling reduced recurrence rate to 1.8% versus 23% when no excision was made (52). Mouroux and colleagues (51) confirmed these data in a series of 100 consecutive patients. Overall recurrence rate was 3%; 2 out of 10 patients without apical stapling recurred (20%) versus 1 out of 87 in whom an apical lesion had been wedged (1.5%).

The importance of pleurodesis is nicely demonstrated by Inderbitzi and colleagues (32), who observed a total of 6 recurrences in 72 patients (8.3%). The results varied considerably, and appeared that combined resection of blebs and pleurodesis is the safest treatment (Table 6). In contrast, isolated ligation of bullae had a failure rate of 19.2% when including prolonged air leaks; therefore, the results did not differ from those for simple chest tube drainage. Chemical pleurodesis instead of abrasion or pleurectomy is also less successful: combination of thoracoscopic bullectomy and tetracycline pleurodesis resulted in an early failure rate of 9% (59).

Causes of Recurrence

It is not likely that learning curve alone can explain the less than optimal results of VATS. Bertrand and colleagues (50) failed to show any difference between two subsequent time periods.

Why should there be less success when the technique allows for improved visibility in comparison to a minithoracotomy? Presumably, fewer blebs are recognized and treated during VATS (50). Open surgery is usually performed with single lumen intubation, while VATS requires double lumen intubation and one lung ventilation. Single lung ventilation will deflate blebs as well as the lung, so that blebs may be missed despite careful inspection of the apex. Remaining blebs or bullae are commonly identified during reoperation after failed VATS.

A second reason might be a certain disinclination to use abrasion. With magnification, the perception of hemorrhage is exaggerated and a less than optimal abrasion may be performed. Finally, the area between the trocars remains out of view and may not be abraded adequately.

The lower degree of tissue trauma and the less intense biological reaction observed with VATS might result in less efficient pleurodesis: release of inflammatory and vasoactive mediators (C-reactive protein, prostacyclin, and thromboxane A_2) was significantly lower in VATS patients as compared to a similar sample of thoracotomy patients (60).

Table 6 Recurrence with Respect to Operative Technique

Technique	Recurrence rate	% Recurrence
Isolated ligation of bulla	3/26	11.5
Isolated wedge resection	1/14	7.1
Isolated pleurectomy	1/16	6.3
Pleurectomy + wedge	1/18	5.6

Source: Ref. 32.

Therapeutic Use of Thoracoscopy

Finally, absence of or less optimal abrasion of the visceral pleura on a deflated lung could be an important factor.

E. Potential Advantages of VATS

Improved Intraoperative Visibility

From a theoretical point of view, thoracoscopy offers a complete panoramic view of the pleural cavity and underlying lung, which cannot be achieved by a small-sized thoracotomy. This improved visualization is certainly a major advantage to the teaching surgeon, who can easily follow his trainee at each step of the operation.

Catamenial pneumothorax is a situation in which VATS should be advantageous. This variant is related either to pleural endometriosis or to diaphragmatic perforations. In the latter case, permanent cure is achieved after adequate repair of the diaphragm. VATS certainly offers an improved view of the diaphragm in comparison to a minithoracotomy (61).

Duration of Postoperative Hospital Stay and Disability

Although there have not been many randomized studies, we may anticipate that VATS allows a reduction in hospital stay of about 4 days (Table 7). However, this reduction in hospital stay is not solely explained by the new technology. In Western Europe, economic considerations and administrative pressure have had a major impact on discharge policy. Psychologically, VATS is considered as "less than surgery" by both patients and physicians, leading to earlier discharge. In former series, even axillary thoracotomy was often regarded as a reason for routine hospitalization for at least 10 days, although patients might have been fit for an earlier discharge. Further, hospital stay obviously depends on drainage time; minimally invasive techniques certainly have led to revised policies and promotion of early removal of chest tubes (Table 8) (51).

Table 7 Comparative Duration of Postoperative Hospital Stay

Country	Time in hospital (days)		Ref.
	VATS	Thoracotomy	
France	6.9	10.3	50
France	8		51
France	9.5	14	54
France	7	11.5	64
Switzerland	4.2		32
United States	4.3		52
Hong Kong	4		55

Table 8 Comparative Duration of Postoperative Chest Tube Drainage

Country	Drainage time		Ref.
	VATS	Thoracotomy	
France	6.5 days	8 days	29
France	5 days		26
France	5 days		34
France	4.4 days	5.6 days	25
Switzerland	46 hours		6
Hong Kong	2 days		30

Postoperative Pain

VATS avoids large transsections of chest wall muscles and the particularly painful spreading of ribs. Reduced surgical trauma should result in a considerable reduction of postoperative pain. Subjectively, most patients having undergone bilateral operations state that VATS is less painful. Dumont and colleagues demonstrated a significantly lower level of pain after VATS when compared to a control group operated through lateral thoracotomy: 42% of VATS patients required level 3 analgesics versus 95% in the case of formal thoracotomy (54). With a similar methodology, Hazelrigg and colleagues compared 20 and 26 patients gathered in a multicenter trial; 7.7% of VATS patients and 70% of thoracotomy patients required parenteral narcotics after 48 hours (62).

Another distressing problem in thoracic surgery is persistent pain at long term. Such pain is usually explained by intercostal nerve injury and intraoperative tension on the costo-vertebral joints due to use of rib spreaders. Bertrand and colleagues estimated that 63% of patients experienced residual chest pain following VATS for pneumothorax, which was considered minimal in 58%, moderate in 38%, and severe in 4%. Comparatively, 61% had persistent pain following lateral thoracotomy for pneumothorax, considered minimal in 65%, moderate in 33%, and severe in 2% (50). Mouroux reported a similar incidence of severe chest pain of 3% (51). Passlick and colleagues (63) reported that with a mean follow-up of 59 months, 31.7% of patients complained of chronic pain and 3.3% required daily pain medications. The incidence of chronic pain was increased following pleurectomy (47.1%) when compared to abrasion (25.6%).

These studies show that chronic pain has not been reduced by VATS. In fact, use of relatively large instruments in narrow intercostal spaces causes significant crushing injury to the intercostal nerves.

Return to Activity

Return to occupational activity has been evaluated in two series with reference to historic control groups. A first series demonstrated a return to activity within a mean of 42 days after VATS and 74 days after thoracotomy (50). In a second series comparing two groups of 16 patients, return to work was possible 1 month after VATS and 2.6 months after thoracotomy ($p < 0.002$); leisure activities were resumed at 2 months after VATS and 4 months after thoracotomy ($p < 0.0005$) (64). However, a controlled prospective study is lacking; one should not neglect a changing philosophy towards postoperative recovery between these two comparisons.

Cost-Efficiency

Cost of treatment must be taken into account because pneumothorax is a rather common problem. At first look, VATS might be less expensive owing to a shorter hospital stay. Dumont and colleagues demonstrated that hospital stay was reduced by 4.5 days when comparing VATS patients to a control group (54). The reduction in cost was estimated at $2300, whereas the increase in cost due to stapling material was estimated at $245. The shorter hospital stay should counterbalance the enhanced cost for disposable surgical materials. These conclusions are biased, because shortening of hospital stay is not the result only of a changing operative approach. Accurate cost analysis should not focus only on hospital stay, which might be the same for VATS and for open surgery with a limited thoracotomy (41,42). An objective cost analysis should also take into account the cost of video equipment. Such evaluations have been made for patients undergoing lung biopsy, which is a relatively similar operation. VATS increases the cost over minithoracotomy by $1000 when the cost of video equipment is taken into account (65). Similarly, Allen and colleagues estimated the median operating room charge to be $1970 for VATS versus $778 for thoracotomy (66). Miller and colleagues estimated the total cost to be $10400 for VATS procedures versus $6150 to $6750 for thoracotomy; they concluded that at the present time no procedure can be done more inexpensively by video-assisted thoracoscopy than by conventional open technique (67).

Hidden costs include prolonged OR time, video equipment, and disposable materials, as well as the increased cost of double lumen catheter intubation, which is mandatory for VATS. The disposables are more expensive; most anesthesiologists perform bronchoscopy to check for adequate position of the tube; induction of anesthesia takes more time. Many colleagues perform routine CT scans preoperatively to decrease the risk of missing blebs (68).

Knowing that some authors recommend VATS at the first episode, we need to further evaluate the increased cost due to expanded indications (69). Cost of recurrence should also be considered; also, the psychological impact of recurrence in operated patients is inestimable (70).

F. Controlled Studies

Only two controlled studies are available to date for this relatively frequent disease. Both conclude that there is no significant difference in early outcome between VATS and open surgery with limited incisions.

Waller and colleagues compared VATS and thoracotomy in a consecutive series of 60 patients, who were followed for a median time of 15 months. All patients were treated by bleb resection and apical pleurectomy; thoracotomy was a limited posterolateral incision carried through the auscultatory triangle. Operative time was longer by 8 minutes in the VATS group ($p < 0.01$). There was no difference in morphine consumption, in duration of drainage, or in hospital stay. However, postoperative FEV_1 was lower in the thoracotomy group (71).

Kim and colleagues compared VATS and transaxillary minithoracotomy. Operative time, amount of opioids, and duration of drainage were comparable. However, 4 of 30 patients managed with VATS did recur. The authors favor transaxillary minithoracotomy as the preferred approach owing to the lower cost and improved cosmetic result (72).

G. Should VATS Be Recommended for an Initial Episode of Pneumothorax?

The advent of VATS has certainly promoted an earlier and more aggressive approach. Obviously, most colleagues will perform an operation at the first recurrence. This seems reasonable, since spontaneous recurrence rate is certainly in excess of 50%. The definition of persistent pneumothorax has also been remastered, knowing that an air leak persisting beyond 48 hours is unlikely to seal.

We consider excessive the recommendation to operate as soon as the first episode (69). Some colleagues argue that immediate thoracoscopy under local anesthesia will select the patients at risk for recurrence when disclosing apical blebs. But there is no proven correlation between thoracoscopic findings and patterns of recurrence (44). Outside of large teaching hospitals, such a strategy is further limited by the lack of availability of experienced and skilled physicians (46). Schramel and colleagues concluded that VATS should be performed for first episodes by comparing total cost of conservative management and thoracoscopic management over two time periods (69). However, this study is biased because surgical patients of the control group underwent formal thoracotomy; when total hospitalization is taken into account, including waiting time before VATS, cost efficiency does not result.

H. Management of Recurrent Pneumothorax Following VATS Treatment

This situation is encountered in 5–10% of patients having undergone VATS pleurodesis, and it is therefore surprising that only a single study has been dedicated to this question. Most surgeons would assume that if VATS has failed at the first attempt, it would be insufficient at the second attempt as well, and they would recommend an open approach. Also, almost 50% of patients show bullae during reoperation that obviously were not identified during VATS.

Cardillo and colleagues performed 19 reoperations with VATS techniques. The conversion rate was 5.2% (1 patient). Pleurodesis was achieved with talc poudrage, and apical resection was added in 10 patients because of bullae or leak. There has been no recurrence with a mean follow-up of 32 months (73). On the basis of this experience, we conclude that an attempt at repeated VATS is justified, provided that the operating surgeon has sufficient experience.

VI. Conclusion

Minimally invasive surgery has become a major tool for the treatment of pleural diseases such as spontaneous pneumothorax and parapneumonic empyema. Shortened duration of recovery and excellent medium-term results justify an early and aggressive approach to empyema, which, like many diseases, profits from early diagnosis and treatment.

The final judgment regarding use of VATS for spontaneous pneumothorax requires some deliberation. Chemical pleurodesis should be limited to otherwise inoperable patients. VATS pleurectomy or pleural abrasion probably allows for less postoperative pain and a shorter hospital stay when compared to an open approach; however, long-term prevention of recurrent pneumothorax remains less than optimal with VATS techniques. Economic considerations might reawaken the interest of the surgical community in transaxillary minithoracotomy.

References

1. Dumarest F. La pratique du Pneumothorax Thrapeutique. Paris: Masson edit, 1945.
2. Walker-Renard PB, Vaughan ML, Sahn SA. Chemical pleurodesis for malignant pleural effusion. Ann Intern Med 1994; 120:56–64.
3. Wurnig PN, Hollaus PH, Ohtsuka T, Flege JB, Wolf RK. Thoracoscopic direct clipping of the thoracic duct for chylopericardium and chylothorax. Ann Thorac Surg 2000; 70:1662–1665.
4. Buchan KG, Hosseinpour AR, Ritchie AJ. Thoracoscopic thoracic duct ligation for traumatic chylothorax. Ann Thorac Surg 2001; 72:1366–1367.
5. Thomas P, Moutardier V, Ragni J, Giudicelli R, Fuentes P. Video-assisted repair of a ruptured right hemidiaphragm. Eur J Cardio-thorac Surg 1994; 8:157–159.
6. Lang-Lazdunski L, Mouroux J, Pons F, Grosdidier G, Martinod E, Elkaim D, Azorin J, Jancovici R. Role of videothoracoscopy in chest trauma. Ann Thorac Surg 1997; 63:327–331.
7. Le Mense GP, Strange C, Sahn SA. Empyema thoracis. Therapeutic management and outcome. Chest 1995; 107:1532–1537.
8. Sasse S, Nguyen TK, Mulligan M, Wang M, Mahutte CK, Light RW. The effects of early chest tube placement on empyema resolution. Chest 1997; 111:1679–1683.
9. Renner H, Gabor S, Pinter H, Maier A, Friehs G, Smolle-Juttner FM. Is aggressive surgery in pleural empyema justified? Eur J Cardio-thorac Surg 1998; 14:117–122.
10. Cassina PC, Hauser M, Hillejan L, Greschuchna D, Stamatis G. Video-assisted thoracoscopy in the treatment of pleural empyema: stage based management and outcome. J Thorac Cardiovasc Surg 1999; 117:234–238.

11. Porkhanov VA, Bodnia VN, Kononenko VB, Poliakov IS, Semendiaev SS. Video-assisted thoracoscopy in treatment of pleural empyema. Khirurgia (Mosk) 1999; 11:40–43.
12. Waller DA, Rengarajan A. Thoracoscopic decortication: a role for video-assisted surgery in chronic post-pneumonic pleural empyema. Ann Thorac Surg 2001; 71: 1813–1816.
13. Heffner JE, McDonald J, Barbieri C, Klein J. Management of parapneumonic effusions. An analysis of physicians practice patterns. Arch Surg 1995; 130:433–438.
14. Ashbaugh DG. Empyema thoracis. Factors influencing morbidity and mortality. Chest 1991; 99:1162–1165.
15. Poe RH, Marin MG, Israel RH, Kallay MC. Utility of pleural fluid analysis in predicting tube thoracostomy/dec parapneumonic effusions. Chest 1991; 100: 963–967.
16. Robinson LA, Moulton AL, Fleming WH, Alonso A, Galbraith TA. Intrapleural fibrinolytic treatment of multiloculated thoracic empyema. Ann Thorac Surg 1994; 57:803–813.
17. Bouros D, Schiza S, Patsourakis G, Chalkiadakis G, Panagou P, Siafakas NM. Intrapleural streptokinase versus urokinase in the treatment of complicated parapneumonic effusions: a prospective, double-blind study. Am J Respir Crit Care Med 1997; 155:291–295.
18. Strange C, Allen ML, Harley R, Lazarchik J, Sahn SA. Intrapleural streptokinase in experimental empyema. Am Rev Respir Dis 1993; 147:962–966.
19. Chin NK, Lim TK. Controlled trial of intrapleural streptokinase in the treatment of pleural empyema and complicated parapneumonic effusions. Chest 1997; 111: 275–279.
20. Van Way C, Narrod J, Hopeman A. The role of early limited thoracotomy in the treatment of empyema. J Thorac Cardiovasc Surg 1988; 96:436–439.
21. Hutter JA, Harari D, Braimbridge MV. The management of empyema thoracis by thoracoscopy and irrigation. Ann Thorac Surg 1985; 39:517–520.
22. Weissberg D, Refaely Y. Pleural empyema: 24-year experience. Ann Thorac Surg 1996; 62:1026–1029.
23. Angelillo Mackinlay TA, Lyons GA, Chimondeguy DJ, Barboza M, Piedras A, Angaramo G, Emery J. VATS debridement versus thoracotomy in the treatment of loculated postpneumonia empyema. Ann Thorac Surg 1996; 61:1626–1630.
24. Striffeler H, Gugger M, Im Hof V, Cerny A, Furrer M, Ris HB. Video-assisted thoracoscopic surgery for fibrinopurulent pleural empyema in 67 patients. Ann Thorac Surg 1998; 65:319–323.
25. Wait MA, Sharma S, Hohn J, Dal Nogare A. A randomized trial of empyema therapy. Chest 1997; 111:1548–1551.
26. Strange C, Sahn SA. The clinician's perspective on parapneumonic effusions and empyema. Chest 1993; 103:259–261.
27. Massard G, Lyons G, Wihlm JM, Fernoux P, Dumont P, Kessler R, Roeslin N, Morand G. Early and long-term results after completion pneumonectomy. Ann Thorac Surg 1995; 59:196–200.
28. Massard G, Dabbagh A, Wihlm JM, Kessler R, Barsotti P, Roeslin N, Morand G. Pneumonectomy for chronic infection is a high-risk procedure. Ann Thorac Surg 1996; 62:1033–1037.
29. Hollaus PH, Lax F, Wurnig PN, Janakiev D, Pridun NS. Videothoracoscopic

debridement of the postpneumonectomy space in empyema. Eur J Cardio-thorac Surg 1999; 16:283–286.
30. Wied U, Halkier E, Hoeier-madsen K, Plucnar B, Rasmussen E, Sparup J. Tetracycline versus silver nitrate pleurodesis in spontaneous pneumothorax. J Thorac Cardiovasc Surg 1983; 86:591.
31. Guérin JC, Champel F, Biron E, Kalb JC. Talcage pleural par thoracoscopie dans le traitement du pneumothorax. Rev Aml Resp 1985; 2:25–29.
32. Inderbitzi RGC, Leiser A, Furrer M, Althaus U. Three years experience in video-assisted thoracic surgery (VATS) for spontaneous pneumothorax. J Thorac Cardiovasc Surg 1994; 107:1410–1415.
33. Cran IR, Rumball CA. Survey of spontaneous pneumothorax in the Royal Air Force. Thorax 1967; 22:462–465.
34. Gaensler EA. Parietal pleurectomy for recurrent spontaneous pneumothorax. Surg Gynecol Obstet 1956; 102:293–308.
35. Clagett OT. The management of spontaneous pneumothorax. J Thorac Cardiovasc Surg 1968; 55:761–762.
36. Dumont P, Nebia A, Roeslin N, Massard G, Wihlm JM, Morand G. Traitement chirurgical du pneumothorax. Etude d'une srie de 400 cas. Ann Chir: Chir Thorac Cardio-vasc 1995; 49:235–240.
37. Thomas P, Le Mee F, Le Hors H, et al. Résultats du traitement chirurgical des pneumothorax persistants ou récidivants. Ann Chir: Chir Thorac Cardio-vasc 1993; 47:136–140.
38. Thévenet F, Gamondès JP, Bodzongo D, Balawi A. Pneumothorax spontané et rcidivant. Traitement chirurgical. A propos de 278 observations. Ann Chir: Chir Thorac Cardio-vasc 1992; 46:165–169.
39. Weeden D, Smith GH. Surgical experience in the management of spontaneous pneumothorax, 1972–82. Thorax 1983; 38:737–743.
40. Körner H, Andersen KS, Stangeland L, Ellingsen I, Engedal H. Surgical treatment of spontaneous pneumothorax by wedge resection without pleurodesis or pleurectomy. Eur J Cardio-thorac Surg 1996; 10:656–659.
41. Becker RM, Munro DD. Transaxillary minithoracotomy: the optimal approach for certain pulmonary and mediastinal lesions. Ann Thorac Surg 1976; 22:254–259.
42. Deslauriers J, Beaulieu M, Després JP, et al. Transaxillary pleurectomy for treatment of spontaneous pneumothorax. Ann Thorac Surg 1980; 30:569–574.
43. Olsen PS, Andersen HO. Long-term results after tetracycline pleurodesis in spontaneous pneumothorax. Ann Thorac Surg 1992; 53:1015–1017.
44. Almind M, Lange P, Viskum K. Spontaneous pneumothorax: comparison of simple drainage, talc pleurodesis, and tetracycline pleurodesis. Thorax 1989; 44: 623–627.
45. el Khawand C, Marchandise FX, Mayne A, et al. Pneumothorax spontan. Résultats du talcage sous thoracoscopie. Rev Mal Resp 1995; 12:275–281.
46. van de Brekel JA, Duurkens VA, Vanderschueren RG. Pneumothorax. Results of thoracoscopy and pleurodesis with talc poudrage and thoracotomy. Chest 1993; 103:345–347.
47. Chappel AG, Johnson A, Charles J, et al. A survey of the long term effects of talc and kaolin pleurodesis. Br J Dis Chest 1979; 73:285–288.
48. Lange P, Mortensen J, Groth S. Lung function 22–35 years after treatment of idiopathic spontaneous pneumothorax with talc poudrage or simple drainage. Thorax 1988; 43:559–561.

49. Guérin JC, Van Der Schueren RG. Traitement des pneumothorax récidivants par application de colle de fibrine sous endoscopie. Rev Mal Resp 1989; 6:443–445.
50. Bertrand PC, Regnard JF, Spaggiari L, et al. Immediate and long-term results after surgical treatment of primary spontaneous pneumothorax by VATS. Ann Thorac Surg 1996; 61:1641–1645.
51. Mouroux J, Elkaïm D, Padovani B, et al. Video-assisted thoracoscopic treatment of spontaneous pneumothorax: technique and results of one hundred cases. J Thorac Cardiovasc Surg 1996; 112:385–391.
52. Naunheim KS, Mack MJ, Hazelrigg SR, et al. Safety and efficacy of video-assisted thoracic surgical techniques for the treatment of spontaneous pneumothorax. J Thorac Cardiovasc Surg 1995; 109:1198–1204.
53. Nezu K, Kushibe K, Tojo T, Takahama M, Kitamura S. Thoracoscopic wedge resection of blebs under local anesthesia with a sedation for treatment of a spontaneous pneumothorax. Chest 1997; 111:230–235.
54. Dumont P, Diemont F, Massard G, Toumieux B, Wihlm JM, Morand G. Does a thoracoscopic approach for surgical treatment of spontaneous pneumothorax represent progress? Eur J Cardio-thorac Surg 1997; 11:27–31.
55. Yim AP, Ho JK. One hundred consecutive cases of video-assisted thoracoscopic surgery for primary spontaneous pneumothorax. Surg Endosc 1995; 9:332–336.
56. Hatz RA, Kaps MF, Meimarakis G, Loche F, Muller C, Furst H. Long-term results after video-assisted thoracoscopic surgery for first-time and recurrent spontaneous pneumothorax. Ann Thorac Surg 2000; 70:253–257.
57. Passlick B, Born C, Haussinger K, Thetter O. Efficiency of video-assisted thoracic surgery for primary and secondary spontaneous pneumothorax. Ann Thorac Surg 1998; 65:324–327.
58. Cole FH Jr., Cole FH, Khandekar A, Maxwell JM, Pate JW, Walker WA. Video-assisted thoracic surgery: primary treatment for spontaneous pneumothorax? Ann Thorac Surg 1995; 60:931–935.
59. Waterworth PD, Kallis P, Townsend ER, Fountain SW. Thoracoscopic bullectomy and tetracycline pleurodesis for the treatment of spontaneous pneumothorax. Respir Med 1995; 89:563–566.
60. Gebhard FT, Becher HP, Gerngross H, Bruckner UB. Reduced inflammatory response in minimal invasive surgery of pneumothorax. Arch Surg 1996; 131:1079–1082.
61. Kirschner PA. Porous diaphragm syndromes. Chest Surg Clin North Am 1998; 8:449–472.
62. Hazelrigg SR, Landreneau RJ, Mack M, et al. Thoracoscopic stapled resection for spontaneous pneumothorax. J Thorax Cardiovasc Surg 1993; 105:389–393.
63. Passlick B, Born C, Sienel W, Thetter O. Incidence of chronic pain after minimally invasive surgery for spontaneous pneumothorax. Eur J Cardio-thorac Surg 2001; 19:355–359.
64. Bernard A, Bélichard C, Goudet P, Lombard JN, Viard H. Pneumothorax spontané. Comparaison de la thoracoscopie et de la thoracotomie. Rev Mal Respir 1993; 10:433–436.
65. Molin LJ, Steinberg JB, Lanza LA. VATS increases costs in patients undergoing lung biopsy for interstitial lung disease. Ann Thorac Surg 1994; 58:1595–1598.
66. Allen MS, Deschamps C, Lee RE, Trastek VF, Daly RC, Pairolero PC. Video-assisted thoracoscopic stapled wedge excision for indeterminate pulmonary nodules. J Thorac Cardiovasc Surg 1993; 106:1048–1052.

67. Miller JI. The present role and future considerations of video-assisted thoracoscopy in general thoracic surgery. Ann Thorac Surg 1993; 56:804–806.
68. Warner BW, Bailey WW, Shipley RT. Value of computed tomography of the lung in the management of primary spontaneous pneumothorax. Am J Surg 1991; 162:39–42.
69. Schramel FM, Sutedja TG, Braber JC, van Mourik JC, Postmus PE. Cost-effectiveness of video-assisted thoracoscopic surgery versus conservative treatment for first time or recurrent spontaneous pneumothorax. Eur Respir J 1996; 9:1821–1825.
70. Nazari S. Psychological implications in the surgical treatment of pneumothorax. Ann Thorac Surg 1997; 63:1830.
71. Waller DA, Forty J, Morritt GN. Video-assisted thoracoscopic surgery versus thoracotomy for spontaneous pneumothorax. Ann Thorac Surg 1994; 58:372–377.
72. Kim KH, Kim HK, Han JY, Kim JT, Won YS, Choi SS. Transaxillary mini-thoracotomy versus video-assisted thoracic surgery for spontaneous pneumothorax. Ann Thorac Surg 1996; 61:1510–1512.
73. Cardillo G, Facciolo F, Regal M, Carbone L, Corzani F, Ricci A, Martelli M. Recurrences following videothoracoscopic treatment of primary spontaneous pneumothorax: the role of redo-videothoracoscopy. Eur J Cardio-thorac Surg 2001; 19:396–399.

14

Discrimination Between Transudative and Exudative Pleural Effusions

Evaluating Diagnostic Tests in the Pleural Space

JOHN E. HEFFNER

Medical University of South Carolina
Charleston, South Carolina, U.S.A.

I. Introduction

The initial step in evaluating pleural effusions of uncertain etiology is the performance of thoracentesis with the classification of pleural fluid as exudates or transudates (1). The presence of an exudative effusion presents a wide differential diagnosis of various inflammatory and malignant conditions, which usually warrants additional diagnostic testing. Conversely, the presence of a transudative effusion may limit the need for further clinical evaluation because these effusions are often attributable to clinically apparent conditions, such as congestive heart failure, cirrhosis with ascites, or nephrosis. Accurate classification of effusions, therefore, is fundamentally important in managing patients with pleural disease. This chapter will review existing approaches for discriminating between exudative and transudative effusions and critically appraise the evidence supporting the diagnostic accuracy of each approach.

II. Approaches to Diagnosis and Available Tests

Light and coworkers (2) demonstrated that the analysis of pleural fluid and serum protein and lactate dehydrogenase (LDH) discriminated between exudates and transudates with a high degree of accuracy. These observations have supported the widespread adoption of Light's criteria for identifying exudative effusions. These criteria include (1) a pleural fluid LDH of more than two-thirds the upper limits of normal for the laboratory's serum value, (2) a pleural fluid–to–serum LDH ratio of >0.6, and/or (3) a pleural fluid–to–serum protein ratio of >0.5 (1). The tests are used in parallel with an "and/or" diagnostic rule wherein a positive result for any one of the three tests indicates the presence of an exudative effusion.

During the subsequent 30 years since the report by Light and coworkers, multiple investigators have promoted the use of alternative pleural fluid tests on the basis of greater cost-effectiveness or higher diagnostic accuracy as compared with Light's (3). These alternative tests include pleural fluid–to–serum albumin ratio (4,5), pleural fluid cholesterol (6–10), pleural fluid–to–serum cholesterol ratio (4,7–10), and pleural fluid–to–serum bilirubin ratio (4,11).

The decision thresholds (cutpoints) proposed for these tests by the various study investigators are listed in Table 1. The cutpoints for several tests differ between reports because of the small sample sizes of the primary studies. Our group recently published a meta-analysis of these studies using patient-level data provided by the primary investigators (12). This report in-

Table 1 Cutoff Points Proposed for Various Pleural Fluid Tests That Discriminate Between Exudative and Transudative Effusions

Test	Reported cutoff points	Meta-analysis ROC cutoff point
Pleural fluid protein	>3 g/dL	>2.9 g/dL
Pleural fluid–to–serum protein ratio	>0.5	>0.5
Pleural fluid LDH	>2/3 of upper limits of normal	>0.45 of upper limits of normal
Pleural fluid–to–serum LDH ratio	>0.6	>0.6
Pleural fluid Cholesterol	>45 mg/dL	>45 mg/dL
	>54 mg/dL	
	>55 mg dL	
	>60 mg/dL	
Pleural fluid–to–serum cholesterol ratio	>0.3	>0.3
Albumin gradient	≤1.2 g/dL	≤1.2 g/dL
Pleural fluid–to–serum bilirubin ratio	>0.6	>0.6

ROC = receiver operating characteristic analysis.
Source: Ref. 12.

cluded 1448 patients and provides estimates of cutpoints using receiver operating characteristic analysis from the largest patient population available (Table 1).

The competition between the various tests for identifying pleural fluid exudates has led to vigorous discussions in the literature regarding the relative merits of differing approaches (3). The wealth of studies that compare pleural fluid tests and their continuing publication have generated editorial commentaries pleading for the end of efforts to unseat Light's criteria as the diagnostic gold standard; editorialists argue that Light's criteria is already highly accurate and additional attempts to improve the criteria are not worth the effort (13). Although this dialogue has not identified the ideal approach to discriminating between exudative and transudative pleural effusions, it has underscored the need to reexamine how pleural diagnostic tests should be used in clinical practice. The remainder of this chapter will review the clinical use of diagnostic tests using pleural fluid studies as the frame of reference and conclude with recommendations for estimating the likelihood of an exudative effusion.

III. Derivation and Clinical Use of Diagnostic Tests

Although most diagnostic tests dichotomize patients into categories of "condition present" and "condition absent" (14), few tests applied in everyday practice are truly dichotomous in nature and perfectly accurate in performance. Pelvic ultrasound for detecting intrauterine pregnancies near term is one example of a purely dichotomous and entirely accurate test: a fetus is either present or absent without intermediate, false-positive, or false-negative test results. Pleural tests that identify exudative effusions differ from the ideal dichotomous test in that they generate results along a continuous range of values, which require cutpoints to categorize patients into the two diagnostic groups of exudate and transudate. Effusions categorized into positive (exudate present) or negative (exudate absent) groups have different likelihoods of having the target condition, which is an exudative effusion. The extent to which effusions are correctly categorized determines the diagnostic accuracy or the "operating characteristics" of the test. Because of biological variation, tests that generate continuous values never display perfect discrimination between groups.

IV. Measures of Diagnostic Accuracy

Values for the measured diagnostic accuracy of the available pleural tests for discriminating between exudative and transudative effusions are shown in Table 2. These estimates were calculated in a meta-analysis of 1448 patients previously reported in the literature (12).

Table 2 Diagnostic Accuracy of Individual Pleural Fluid Tests for Identifying Exudative Pleural Effusions

Pleural fluid test	Sensitivity, % (95% CI)	Specificity, % (95% CI)	+PV, % (95% CI)	−PV, % (95% CI)	AUC (95% CI)
P-PF $n = 1187$	91.5 (89.3–93.7)	83.0 (77.6–88.4)	94.6 (93.8–97.1)	75.0 (69.1–80.9)	94.2 (92.6–95.9)
P-R $n = 1393$	89.5 (87.4–91.6)	90.9 (87.4–94.5)	96.9 (95.6–98.1)	73.3 (68.4–78.1)	95.4 (94.3–96.7)
LDH-PF $n = 1438$	88.0 (85.8–90.3)	81.8 (77.1–86.6)	93.9 (92.2–95.6)	68.3 (63.1–73.6)	93.3 (91.8–94.8)
LDH-R $n = 1388$	91.4 (89.4–93.3)	85.0 (80.6–89.4)	95.1 (93.5–96.6)	75.7 (70.7–80.7)	94.7 (93.4–96.0)
C-PF $n = 1348$	89.0 (86.8–91.2)	81.4 (76.6–86.2)	93.8 (92.1–95.5)	70.1 (64.8–75.3)	93.3 (91.7–94.8)
C-R $n = 1123$	92.0 (90.1–93.9)	81.4 (76.6–86.2)	94.0 (92.3–95.7)	76.3 (71.2–81.4)	94.1 (92.5–95.7)
A-G $n = 386$	86.8 (82.2–91.4)	91.8 (86.4–97.3)	95.8 (93.0–98.7)	76.3 (68.6–83.9)	94.0 (91.3–96.6)
BILI-R $n = 303$	84.3 (79.3–89.3)	61.1 (51.2–70.9)	82.3 (77.1–87.5)	64.4 (54.6–74.3)	81.3 (76.3–86.4)

P-PF = pleural fluid protein; P-R = pleural fluid–to–serum protein ratio; LDH-PF = pleural fluid LDH; LDH-R = pleural fluid to serum LDH ratio; C-PF = pleural fluid cholesterol; C-R = pleural fluid–to–serum cholesterol ratio; A-G = pleural fluid–to–serum albumin gradient; BILI-R = pleural fluid–to–serum bilirubin ratio; PV = predictive value; CI = confidence interval.
Source: Ref. 12.

A. Sensitivity and Specificity

Several measures are used to describe the performance of a test, of which sensitivity and specificity are most frequently used. Sensitivity describes the proportion of patients with the target condition (exudative effusion) who are correctly classified by a positive test result. Specificity is the proportion of patients without the target condition (a transudative rather than an exuative effusion) who have a negative test result (Fig. 1). Although clinicians favor sensitivity and specificity to describe the performance of tests they use in clinical practice, these terms actually provide only limited information as to how a positive or negative test result increases or decreases the probability that a patient has an exudative effusion (15,16). If a test has a 100% sensitivity, a *negative* test *rules out* the target condition. If a test has a 100% specificity, a *positive* test *rules* in the target condition. Other test results and lower values for sensitivity and specificity leave clinicians in varying degrees of uncertainty about the clinical meaning of the test result.

The values of sensitivity and specificity for a diagnostic test are closely interrelated, which has created confusion in the literature regarding the relative

REFERENCE STANDARD RESULT

	Exudate	Transudate	Total
Positive	a True positives	b False negatives	a+b
Negative	c False positives	d True negatives	c+d
Total	a+c	b+d	a+b+c+d

Test result (row label)

Sensitivity = a/(a+c)

Specificity = d/(b+d)

Positive predictive value = a/(a+b)

Negative predictive value = d/(c+d)

Figure 1 Two-by-two table showing how measures of test performance are calculated.

merits of Light's criteria as compared with other tests that discriminate between exudates and transudates. Light's criteria have been stated to be equal in sensitivity but lower in specificity as compared with other pleural fluid (1,17). This observation, however, results from the linkage of sensitivity with specificity rather than any unique attributes of Light's criteria. When a combination of two or more tests are used with an "and/or" rule, as is done with Light's criteria, the chance of identifying patients with the target condition of an exudtive effusion (true positives) increases, which raises the test's sensitivity. The cost of raising sensitivity includes the increased probability that patients without the target condition will be misidentified as having the condition (false-positives). Increasing the false-positive rate necessarily lowers the test's specificity (Fig. 2). Light's criteria, therefore, would be expected to have a lower sensitivity as compared with diagnostic approaches that use a single pleural

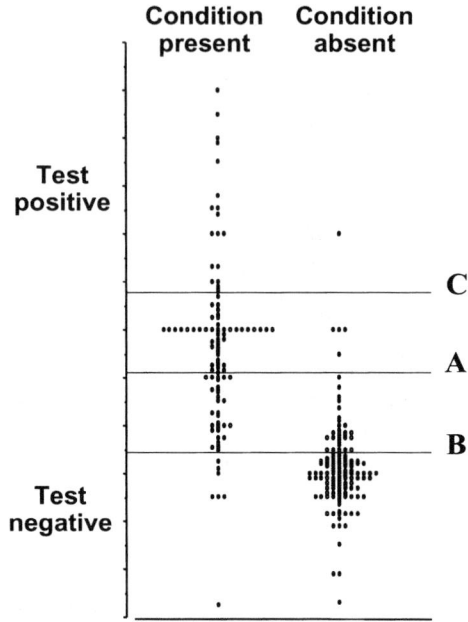

Figure 2 Interrelationship of sensitivity and specificity for tests with continuous values for test results. The graph shows the distribution of data points for patients with a condition (condition present) and without the condition (condition absent) along a continuous scale. Sensitivity and specificity were calculated using the cutpoint shown by the line at "A." If a lower cutpoint is selected ("B"), more patients with the target condition will have values above the cutpoint and will be considered to have a positive test, which will increase sensitivity. More patients without the condition, however, will also have a positive test, which will decrease specificity. Raising the cutpoint to a higher level ("C") will decrease sensitivity but increase specificity.

fluid test when the *single* test has the same operating characteristics as each of the three tests that compose Light's criteria.

The interrelationship between the sensitivity and specificity of a test or test combination is an important observation for two reasons. Multiple investigators have initiated studies with a goal of identifying tests that would have an equal sensitivity but a higher specificity than Light's criteria. Considering that each of the three component tests of Light's criteria have sensitivities greater than 90% and specificities that range from 82 to 91%, it is doubtful that a new single test could have a better performance in view of the biological variation of pleural fluid findings in patients with pleural effusions. The new test, however, might appear to have a higher specificity than Light's criteria only because the three test components of Light's criteria are combined with an "and/or" rule, which lowers the specificity of the test combination.

The interrelationship of sensitivity and specificity is also important because the lowering of specificity with the three-test combination of Light's criteria causes more patients with conditions associated with transudative effusions to be misclassified with exudative effusions (false positives) as compared with the available single test approaches. False-positive categorization as an exudate occurs most commonly with Light's criteria in patients with congestive heart failure who experience increasing concentrations of protein and LDH in their pleural space after undergoing diuresis. Such effusions have been termed "pseudoexudates" to describe their exudative classification by Light's criteria and their likely transudative origin based on the presence of congestive heart failure (18). Some investigators have recommended evaluating "pseudoexudative" effusions with follow-up tests of pleural fluid cholesterol, which is stated to have a higher specificity than Light's criteria (18). It would be expected, however, that pleural fluid cholesterol, as a single test, would have a higher specificity than the three-test combination of Light's criteria and would more likely classify these effusions correctly as transudates.

Pleural effusions misclassified by Light's criteria as exudates and described as "pseudoexudates" should be more accurately defined as false-positive test results. The confusing term "pseudoexudate" can be abandoned if physicians consider the pretest probability of an exudative effusion in their interpretation of pleural fluid tests and use likelihood ratios, which will be discussed below.

B. Positive and Negative Predictive Values

Positive and negative predictive values are more clinically useful measures of a test's diagnostic performance than sensitivity and specificity. The positive predictive value describes the proportion of patients with a positive test who have the target condition, an exudative effusion (Fig. 1). The negative predictive value describes the proportion of patients with a negative test who do not have the target condition (no exudative effusion, i.e., a transudative effusion is present). Knowledge of the positive and negative predictive values of a test allows clinicians to use the test result in estimating the probability that a patient has the target condition.

Unfortunately, predictive values present problems in clinical use because they are influenced by the prevalence of the target disorder in the tested population. We have previously reported in a meta-analysis of primary reports that 75% of patients who undergo diagnostic thoracentesis have exudative pleural effusions (12). The predictive values of pleural fluid tests listed in Table 2 are based on a 75% prevalence of exudative effusions in the tested population. If thoracentesis is performed in populations of patients with a different prevalence of exudates as compared with transudates, clinicians cannot assume that positive and negative test results signify the positive and negative predictive values listed in Table 2.

C. Likelihood Ratios

Likelihood ratios measure test performance in a manner that provides clinicians with information about the probability that a target condition exists. Likelihood ratios quantify the likelihood of a given test result in patients with a condition compared with the likelihood of the same result in patients without the condition (14,19). Likelihood ratios, however, do not depend on the prevalence of the condition in the test population as do positive and negative predictive values. They are calculated by creating multiple levels along a continuum of test results and computing the likelihood of a positive test result for each target condition within a single test result level (Table 3). Likelihood ratios, in contrast to other measures of test performance, provide information about how much a test result increases or decreases the probability that a patient has the target condition of an exudative effusion. Likelihood ratios above a value of 1 increase the likelihood that an exudate exists, and likelihood ratios below 1 decrease the probability of an exudate making a transudate more likely.

Clinicians use likelihood ratios to modulate the degree to which their pretest suspicion of an exudate is altered by a test result. To do so, physicians first estimate the pretest probability of an exudative effusion based on the patient's clinical presentation (20). For instance, a 50-year-old patient with congestive heart failure and a slowly resolving pleural effusion after diuretic therapy would be considered by most physicians to have a transudative effusion. Because the patient is also a heavy smoker, a clinician might be concerned also about an atypical presentation of a malignant effusion. The pretest suspicion remains high in this setting, however, for a transudate due to heart failure, so the pretest

Table 3 Method for Calculating Likelihood Ratios

Pleural fluid test result	Exudates, n	Transudates, n	LR
>5.0	265	2	47.25
4.6–5.0	184	2	32.80
4.1–4.5	138	3	16.40
3.6–4.0	120	18	2.38
3.1–3.5	66	23	1.02
2.6–3.0	51	35	0.52
2.1–2.5	21	42	0.18
1.6–2.0	18	88	0.07
≤1.5	12	99	0.04
Total	875	312	

Likelihood ratios (LRs) are calculated by separating patients into multiple levels grouped by strata of test results and by target conditions (exudates and transudates). Likelihood ratios are then derived by the proportion of total exudates within a strata divided by the total transudates within the same strata. For instance, the LR for effusions with a pleural fluid protein >5.0 g is (265/875)/(2/312) = 47.25. These values are shown for example purposes only; actual LRs for pleural fluid tests are presently being developed.

probability of an exudate might be estimated to be only 10%. This pretest probability can be transformed to pretest odds by the following equation: pretest odds = pretest probability/(1.00 − pretest probability), which, in this example, would be 0.11 (i.e., 0.10/(1.00 − 0.10)).

Posttest odds can be calculated by multiplying pretest odds by the likelihood ratio of the test result. For this example, the first pleural fluid test result obtained by the clinician was a pleural fluid-to-serum protein ratio of 0.6. By Light's criteria, even without knowledge of the results of the other two components of Light's criteria, the effusion would be classified as an exudate. Because the clinician might remain convinced that heart failure undergoing diuresis was the cause of the effusion, the patient would be tempted to classify the effusion as a "pseudoexudate."

Likelihood ratios, however, provide a more accurate classification of the effusion that does not require post hoc "second guessing" of the test result by naming it a "pseudoexudate." Referring to a source of likelihood ratios for different pleural fluid tests, the clinician would find that the likelihood ratio for a pleural fluid-to-serum protein ratio test result of 0.6 might be 1.34. This value indicates that a test result of 0.6 increases the pretest odds of an exudate by a factor of 1.34. This low value for the likelihood ratio would be expected because the test result of 0.6 is only slightly higher than the cutoff point (0.5) for protein ratios when these tests are used in the traditional dichotomous manner of Light's criteria (Table 1). The pretest odds of 0.11 is multiplied by 1.34 to give the posttest odds of 0.15. Because clinicians find probabilities more easily interpretable, the posttest probability can be calculated by the following equation: posttest odds/(posttest odds + 1.00). This equation computes a posttest probability of an exudative effusion of 0.13 or 13%. Since the probability of an exudate is only 13%, the clinician would conclude that the patient most likely (87% likelihood) has a transudate. Even though the test was "positive" for an exudate by traditional Light's criteria, the borderline positive result did not raise the clinician's pretest estimation of the probability of an exudate sufficiently to alter the diagnosis of a transudative effusion due to congestive heart failure.

Likelihood ratios progressively increase or decrease the further a test result is above or below the cutoff point used to determine a "positive" or "negative" test result. Test results near the cutoff point result in likelihood ratios close to 1, which do not alter the pretest probability of the target condition. Extremely high or low results generated by test results far beyond the cutoff points produce extremely high or low likelihood ratios, which have a large effect in changing the pretest probability of disease. Likelihood ratios, therefore, provide the clinician with more information regarding the meaning of a test result as compared with strategies that bin both borderline and extreme test results into dichotomous categories of "condition present" (exudate) and "condition absent" (transudate) (12,19,20). To demonstrate the value of this added information for the previous example, now consider that the pleural fluid-to-serum protein ratio had an extreme test result that was much higher than 0.6 and was associated with a likelihood ratio of 45. Repeating the same calculations with this new likelihood ratio calculates a posttest probability of an exudative effusion of 83% (posttest odds = 0.15 × 45 = 4.95; posttest probability = 4.95/(1 + 4.95) = 0.83). With this second laboratory result, the clinician would diagnose an exudate and initiate further evaluation for a malignancy. In both examples, the pleural fluid test was "positive" for an exudate by Light's criteria, but only the extremely high value established the presence of an exudate when evaluated by likelihood ratios. Use of likelihood ratios avoid the coinage of confusing terms, such as "pseudoexudate," which really describe the clinician's discomfort with a test result that does not fit the clinical picture.

Likelihood ratios from different tests can be combined in a serial manner to increase diagnostic certainty. In the instance of Light's criteria, results of each of the three test components have likelihood ratios that can be used to calculated posttest odds in a serial manner (Table 4).

Unfortunately, likelihood ratios have not yet been published for the tests that discriminate between exudative and transudative effusions. Our group is generating data to calculate likelihood ratios, which will be published in the near future.

Table 4 Use of Likelihood Ratios to Calculate Posttest Probability Using Results of Three Tests that Measure Protein and Lactate Dehydrogenase (LDH) in Blood and Pleural Fluid Samples

---

Pleural fluid results
  Pleural fluid–to–serum protein ratio = 0.46
  Pleural fluid LDH (fraction of lab normal) = 0.63
  Pleural fluid–to–serum LDH ratio = 0.72
Calculation of posttest probability
  Pretest probability of an exudate = 25%
  Pretest odds = pretest probability/(1.00−pretest probability) = 0.25/(1.00 − 0.25) = 0.33
  Pleural fluid protein ratio likelihood ratio (LR) = 0.50
  Posttest odds$_1$ = pretest odds × LR = 0.33 × 0.50 = 0.17
  Pleural fluid LDH likelihood ratio = 2.05
  Posttest odds$_2$ = 0.17 × 2.05 = 0.35
  Pleural fluid LDH ratio likelihood ratio = 1.25
  Posttest odds$_3$ = 0.35 × 1.25 = 0.44
  Posttest probability of an exudate = posttest probability/(1.00 + posttest probability) = 0.44/(1.00 + 0.44) = 0.31 = 31%

The patient has the test results shown under "Pleural fluid results," which by Light's criteria would be categorized as an exudate. The clinician estimated the patient's pretest probability of having an exudate to be 25%. The pretest probability is converted to a pretest odds, which is multiplied serially by LRs for each test result. Likelihood ratios would be obtained from a source for LRs. The final posttest odds (posttest odds$_3$) is then converted to a posttest probability.

V. Diagnostic Performance of Pleural Fluid Tests

Light's criteria used with dichotomous cutpoints as a parallel "and/or" rule provide sufficient accuracy for most clinical purposes. Clinicians should recognize, however, that a proportion of patients evaluated by these criteria will be misclassified. Test results that establish the presence of a transudative or exudative effusion are "probabilistic" statements and do not exclude, for instance, that a patient with a transudative effusion does not have an underlying malignant effusion (21). Results from these tests always need to be evaluated in the context of the clinical circumstances related to the individual patient undergoing evaluation.

One criticism of Light's criteria is that they contain three test components, two of which are highly correlated. A general principle for using multiple diagnostic tests with "and/or" rules states that individual tests should not have a high correlation with another test in the diagnostic strategy. Otherwise, the tests would demonstrate "multicollinearity" and would not be expected to perform well in a diagnostic model because each would examine patients for the same clinical factor (22). In Light's criteria, pleural fluid LDH and the pleural fluid-to-serum LDH ratio both incorporate the results of pleural fluid LDH and demonstrate a high degree of correlation (Pearson coefficient of correlation = 0.84) (12). We have previously suggested that an "abbreviated Light's criteria" using only two test components of pleural fluid-to-serum protein ratio and either pleural fluid LDH or pleural fluid-to-serum LDH ratio simplifies pleural fluid analysis and does not decrease specificity to the degree observed with the three-test combination of Light's criteria (12).

In comparing Light's criteria with other pleural fluid tests, most investigators have compared sensitivities and specificities between the different tests and testing strategies without calculating the confidence intervals for the reported values of sensitivity and specificity. Also, differences between testing strategies are usually reported using hypothesis-testing statistics, such as Chi square, which are not designed to compare the operating characteristics between different diagnostic tests.

A recent meta-analysis combined patient-level data from existing studies to calculate confidence intervals for the measures of performance for different pleural fluid tests and compared tests using receiver operating characteristics analysis (12). Receiver operating characteristics analysis is a method for comparing the performance of tests across the entire range of test results and for selecting test result cutpoints (23,24). The results of this analysis demonstrated that most of the tests that have been studied to diagnose exudative pleural effusions have similar operating characteristics, with the exception of the pleural fluid-to-serum bilirubin ratio. The other available tests have overlapping confidence intervals for sensitivity, specificity, and positive and negative predictive values (Table 2). Also, the areas under the ROC curves (AUC), a measure of test performance, were not statistically significant between tests (Table

2). These findings indicate that pleural fluid tests for discriminating between exudative and transudative effusions have similar utility in clinical practice. Differences shown in primary studies between various tests probably result from small sample sizes and unique clinical factors within the studied patients rather than intrinsic differences between tests or testing strategies. This conclusion complements the biological rationale for these tests, which is based on the influx of large molecules from the vasculature into the pleural space in conditions associated with exudative pleural effusions.

Tradition, however, supports the ongoing use of Light's criteria, because these criteria are well accepted into routine clinical practice. The "abbreviated" Light's criteria, however, simplify patient evaluation and do not result in any loss of diagnostic accuracy. Light's criteria also provide an advantage of a high sensitivity—albeit at the cost of a lower specificity—by virtue of having multiple test components. This strategy supports the clinician's goal of erring on the side of not overlooking patients with exudative effusions (high sensitivity to avoid false-negative test results) because of the important clinical implications of having an exudate.

Some rationale exists, however, for the use of test combinations other than Light's criteria that do not require serum test results. We have previously suggested that diagnostic approaches that use a two-test combination of pleural fluid LDH and pleural fluid cholesterol or a three-test combination of pleural fluid protein, pleural fluid LDH, and pleural fluid cholesterol in an "and/or" rule perform as well as Light's criteria but do not require the results of a blood test. Cutoff points for these tests are shown in Table 1.

VI. Limitations of Pleural Fluid Tests

Although extensively studied, the major weaknesses of all pleural fluid tests relate to the difficulties in designing rigorous studies to define the tests' operating characteristics. No gold standard test exists to establish the benchmark categorization of study populations into groups of exudative and transudative effusions. Consequently, various clinical studies (lung scans, echocardiographic examinations, pleural biopsies) are performed on patients to establish the underlying disease (e.g., heart failure, lung cancer, pulmonary embolism). Once the underlying condition is diagnosed, effusions are categorized as the type (exudate or transudate) that is typically associated with the underlying condition. Considering that many patients with heart failure undergoing diuresis may have exudative effusions and some patients with pleural malignancies may have transudative effusions by Light's criteria, the "gold standard" may misclassify numerous patients.

Other limitations of existing studies pertain to deficiencies in study design. Although standards for evaluating diagnostic tests are well described (15,19,25–36), these standards have been poorly applied to most studies that examine the diagnostic accuracy of pleural fluid tests (12,37,38). Until more rigorous studies are available, the existing data remain the best available (12), which requires clinicians to blend their clinical impressions with test results.

VII. Conclusions

Pleural tests do not absolutely establish the nature of a pleural effusion with certainty. Discrimination between an exudate and a transudate is a "point of departure" for evaluation of a pleural effusion and should be considered a probabilistic statement. Clinicians should consider their level of confidence in making such probabilistic statements to determine the need for additional testing and the appropriateness of therapeutic interventions. Most of the available pleural fluid tests have similar operating characteristics. If the patient's clinical features do not match the test results, clinicians should pursue alternative diagnoses and recall that pleural fluid tests only alter the pretest probability of a diagnosis given the clinical information that the clinician already has at hand (35).

References

1. Light RW. Pleural Disease. Baltimore: Williams & Wilkins, 1995.
2. Light RW, MacGregor I, Luchsinger PC, Ball WC. Pleural effusion: the diagnostic separation of transudates and exudates. Ann Intern Med 1972; 77:507–513.
3. Antony VB, Holm KA. Testing the waters. Differentiating transudates from exudates. Chest 1995; 108:1191–1192.
4. Burgess L, Maritz FJ, Taljaard JJF. Comparative analysis of the biochemical parameters used to distinguish between pleural transudates and exudates. Chest 1995; 107:1604–1609.
5. Roth BJ, O'Meara TF, Cragun WH. The serum-effusion albumin gradient in the evaluation of pleural effusions. Chest 1990; 98:546–549.
6. Costa M, Quiroga T, Cruz E. Measurement of pleural fluid cholesterol and lactate dehydrogenase. A simple and accurate set of indicators for separating exudates from transudates. Chest 1995; 108:1260–1263.
7. Hamm H, Brohan U, Bohmer R, Missmahl H-P. Cholesterol in pleural effusions. A diagnostic aid. Chest 1987; 92:296–302.
8. Romero S, Candela A, Martín C, Hernández L, Trigo C, Gil J. Evaluation of different criteria for the separation of pleural transudates from exudates. Chest 1993; 104:399–404.
9. Suay VG, Moragón EM, Viedma EC, Tordera MP, Fábregas ML, Aldás JS. Pleural cholesterol in differentiating transudates and exudates. A prospective study of 232 cases. Respiration 1995; 62:57–63.
10. Valdés L, Pose A, Suàrez J, Gonzalez-Juanatey JR, Sarandeses A, San José E, Dobaña JMA, Salgueiro M, Suàrez JRR. Cholesterol: a useful parameter for distinguishing between pleural exudates and transudates. Chest 1991; 99:1097–1102.
11. Meisel S, Shamiss A, Thaler M, Nussinovitch N, Rosenthal T. Pleural fluid to serum bilirubin concentration ratio for the separation of transudates and exudates. Chest 1990; 98:141–144.

12. Heffner JE, Brown LK, Barbieri C. Diagnostic value of tests that discriminate between exudative and transudative pleural effusions. Chest 1997; 111:970–979.
13. Bartter T, Santarelli RJ, Pratter MR. Transudate vs exudate: genug! Chest 1996; 109:1419–1421.
14. Sox HC Jr, Blatt MA, Higgins MC, Marton KI. Medical Decision Making. Boston: Butterworths, 1988.
15. Sheps SB, Schechter MT. The assessment of diagnostic tests: a survey of current medical research. JAMA 1984; 252:2418–2422.
16. Riegelman RK, Hirsch RP. Studying a Study and Testing a Test. How to Read the Health Science Literature. Boston: Little, Brown and Co, 1996.
17. Romero S, Martinez A, Hernandez L, Fernandez C, Espasa A, Candela A, Martin C. Light's criteria revisited: consistency and comparison with new proposed alternative criteria for separating pleural transudates from exudates. Respiration 2000; 67:18–23.
18. Chakko SC, Caldwell SH, Sforza PP. Treatment of congestive heart failure. Its effect on pleural fluid chemistry. Chest 1989; 95:798–802.
19. Jaeschke R, Guyatt G, Sackett D. Users' guides to the medical literature. III. How to use an article about a diagnostic test. JAMA 1994; 271:703–707.
20. Sackett DL, Straus SE, Richardson WS, Rosenberg W, Haynes RB. Evidence-Based Medicine. How to Practice and Teach EBM. Edinburgh: Churchill Livingstone, 2000.
21. Ashchi M, Golish J, Eng P, O'Donovan P. Transudative malignant pleural effusions: prevalence and mechanisms. South Med J 1998; 91:23–26.
22. Katz MH. Multivariable Analysis. A Practical Guide for Clinicians. Cambridge: University Press, 1999.
23. Hanley JA, McNeil BJ. The meaning and use of the area under the receiving operating characteristic (ROC) curve. Radiology 1982; 143:29–36.
24. Hanley JA. Receiver operating characteristic (ROC) methodolgy: the state of the art. Crit Rev Diagn Imag 1989; 29:307–335.
25. Ransohoff DF, Feinstein AR. Problems of spectrum and bias in evaluating the efficacy of diagnostic tests. N Engl J Med 1978; 299:926–930.
26. Nierenberg AA, Feinstein AR. How to evaluate a diagnostic marker test: lessons from the rise and fall of dexamethasone suppression test. JAMA 1988; 259:1699–1702.
27. Fineberg HV, Hiatt HH. Evaluation of medical practices: the case for technology assessment. N Engl J Med 1979; 301:1086–1091.
28. Becker DM, Philbrick JT, Abbitt PL. Real-time ultrasonography for the diagnosis of lower extremity deep venous thrombosis: the wave of the future? Arch Intern Med 1989; 149:1731–1734.
29. Cooper LS, Chalmers TC, McCally M, Berrier J, Sacks HS. The poor quality of early evaluations of magnetic resonance imaging. JAMA 1988; 259:3277–3280.
30. Kent DL, Haynor DR, Longstreth WT, Larson EB. The clinical efficacy of magnetic resonance imaging in neuroimaging. Ann Intern Med 1994; 120:856–871.
31. Greenes RA, Begg CB. Assessment of diagnostic technologies: methodology for unbiased estimation from samples of selectively verified patients. Invest Radiol 1985; 20:751–757.
32. Bates AS, Margolis PA, Evans AT. Verification bias in pediatric studies evaluating diagnostic tests. J Pediatr 1993; 122:585–590.

33. Arroll B, Schechter MT, Sheps SB. The assessment of diagnostic tests: a comparison of medical literature in 1982 and 1985. J Gen Intern Med 1988; 3:443–447.
34. Guyatt GH, Tugwell PX, Feeny DH, Haynes RB, Drummond M. A framework for clinical evaluation of diagnostic technologies. Can Med Assoc J 1986; 134:587–594.
35. Begg CB. Biases in the assessment of diagnostic tests. Stat Med 1987; 6:411–423.
36. Kent DL, Larson EB. Disease, level of impact, and quality of research methods: three dimensions of clinical efficacy assessment applied to magnetic resonance imaging. Invest Radiol 1992; 27:245–254.
37. Heffner JE, Feinstein D, Barbieri C. Methodologic standards for diagnostic test research in pulmonary medicine. Chest 1998; 114:877–885.
38. Heffner JE. Evaluating diagnostic tests in the pleural space. Differentiating transudates from exudates as a model. Clin Chest Med 1998; 19:277–293.

15

Differentiating Between Benign and Malignant Pleural Effusions

D. KEITH PAYNE and MICHAEL W. OWENS

Louisiana State University Health Sciences Center
Shreveport, Louisiana, U.S.A.

I. Introduction

The vast majority of pleural effusions in the United States, as in many parts of the world, are caused by congestive heart failure, pulmonary infections, malignancy, and pulmonary embolism. These are common disease processes, especially in older populations. Therefore, distinguishing benign from malignant pleural effusions is a common challenge in the practice of chest medicine and is of wide interest to many physicians and their patients. The intent of this chapter is to summarize methods, both proven and experimental, for achieving this goal. For the purposes of this discussion, we define malignant effusion in a broad sense to include any pleural effusion associated with malignancy by cytology, pleural biopsy, or autopsy as well as those effusions associated with a known malignancy with no other explanation for their formation, even in the absence of positive fluid cytology, pleural biopsy, or autopsy (some authors prefer to call these paramalignant effusions). Benign effusions are pleural effusions arising from all other disease processes.

II. Clinical Manifestations of Benign and Malignant Pleural Effusion

The history and physical examination may provide clues that assist in distinguishing benign from malignant pleural effusions. Although many patients may be asymptomatic or have minimal symptoms, pain, cough, and shortness of breath are the most common symptoms of patients with clinically significant pleural effusions (1). While symptoms alone do not have sufficient positive or negative predictive value to accurately distinguish between benign and malignant effusions, in selected patient populations they may be especially helpful. Marel et al. studied 171 patients referred to a pulmonary specialty clinic for evaluation of pleural effusion (2). Among this relatively small and somewhat biased population sample (63% had effusions due to malignancy), patients with malignant effusions were more likely to report the occurrence of severe dyspnea as well as dull chest pain compared to patients with effusions of benign etiology. A history of exposure to carcinogens at work as well as a personal history of cancer was significantly more common in patients with malignant effusions. Patients with benign effusions reported a significantly increased incidence of pleuritic type chest pain as well as an increased incidence of fever. Finally, the age of the patient is a consideration in providing clues to the etiology of the pleural effusion. Malignant effusions are much more common in older patients (greater than age 60) than in younger individuals.

The physical examination may also be helpful, if not diagnostic. For instance, patients with pleural effusions accompanied by elevated neck veins, cardiomegaly, and peripheral edema may be suspected to have congestive heart failure. Subcutaneous nodules and joint disease may indicate the presence of a rheumatoid effusion. A breast mass or the presence of hard, fixed nodes may indicate carcinoma.

III. Diagnostic Approaches

A. Imaging Techniques

Following the initial evaluation of the patient, imaging tests are frequently used to confirm the presence of pleural effusion. Several complementary imaging modalities are now available to assess the pleural space. Although seldom diagnostic, certain findings are very suggestive of a malignant cause for the effusions.

Chest Radiograph

The chest radiograph (CXR) is frequently the initial imaging test to be ordered and is the usual method by which a suspected pleural effusion is confirmed. Certain patterns on the CXR can be helpful in distinguishing benign from malignant effusions. If the pleural effusion is accompanied by an ipsilateral chest mass, then bronchogenic carcinoma may be suspected (1). If an entire hemithorax is occupied by pleural effusion, a massive effusion is said to be present. This finding strongly suggests a malignant etiology for the effusion, accounting for 31 of 46 (67%) cases in one series of patients with massive pleural effusion (3). The presence of bilateral pleural effusions with a normal heart size was found to predict malignancy as the cause in 50% of the 78 patients in an earlier study (4). Other diagnoses among this group of patients included nephrotic syndrome, lupus, hepatic hydrothorax, constrictive pericarditis, and esophageal rupture. Pleural effusions accompanied by mediastinal node involvement frequently signal the presence of a malignant etiology, particularly lymphoma (5). Unfortunately, the chest radiograph can easily miss mediastinal adenopathy, even when present (6).

Computed Tomography

Computed tomography (CT) is more sensitive than CXR in detecting a variety of lung and mediastinal masses, which, when associated with pleural effusions suggest a malignant origin. CT may also be useful in distinguishing malignant from benign pleural disease. Hierholzer et al. studied 42 patients referred for evaluation of pleural disease (7). CT findings most suggestive of malignant disease were infiltration of the chest wall and diaphragm, irregular and nodular pleural thickening, circumferential pleural thickening, and mediastinal pleural involvement. These findings were predictive of malignancy with a sensitivity of 93% and specificity of 87%. Pleural calcification suggested a benign cause of pleural disease with a sensitivity of 33% and specificity of 96%. An earlier study reported similar findings using CT to distinguish malignant from benign pleural disease, albeit with a somewhat lower sensitivity and specificity of 72% and 83%, respectively (8).

Magnetic Resonance Imaging

There is some evidence to suggest that magnetic resonance imaging (MRI) may be useful in distinguishing between exudative or hemorrhagic effusions and transudative effusions (9,10). Another small study of 34 patients found that malignant pleural lesions always displayed a high signal intensity on proton density-weighted and T2-weighted images, making them hyperintense in relation to intercostal muscles (11). Benign pleural lesions were isointense or hypointense. At the present time, however, the main usefulness of MRI appears to be as a complementary imaging study to better assess the extent of chest wall and diaphragmatic involvement by pleural tumor. Carlsen et al. found that MRI was more sensitive in detecting chest wall and pleural sites of disease in lymphoma patients compared to CT (12). In a retrospective study of 42 patients, Hierholzer et al. actually found MRI to be superior to CT in differentiating between benign and malignant pleural disease with a sensitivity of 100%

and specificity of 93% (7). CT was more sensitive in detecting pleural calcification and bone destruction.

Positron Emission Tomography

The role of positron emission tomography (PET) in the evaluation of benign and malignant pleural disease continues to evolve as additional studies are published. Early results from small studies appear promising, especially in the evaluation of mesothelioma. Carretta et al. investigated 14 patients presenting to their institution with pleural effusion, pleural masses, or pleural thickening (13). A histological diagnosis of malignancy was obtained in 13 of the 14 patients (most had malignant mesothelioma). PET correctly identified 12 of the 13 patients with malignant pleural disease as well as the patient with benign pleural disease. A false-negative result was obtained in one patient with epithelial mesothelioma. An overall accuracy of 92% was reported. Benard et al. investigated 28 consecutive patients presenting with pleural disease from suspected mesothelioma (14). Malignant disease was proven in 24 of the 28 (22 being mesothelioma). PET correctly predicted malignant disease in 22 of the 24 patients and predicted benign pleural disease in 3 of the remaining 4 patients. In this study, PET had a 92% sensitivity, a 75% specificity, and an accuracy of 89%. Gerbaudo et al. reported similar results in a group of 15 patients, 11 of whom had malignant mesotheliomas (15). Erasmus et al. studied 25 patients with non–small-cell lung cancer and a pleural effusion on CT scan (16). Of these 25 patients, 22 were proved to have malignant pleural disease by thoracentesis or pleural biopsy. In this nonmesothelioma study, PET was reported to have a sensitivity of 95%, a specificity of 67%, and an overall accuracy of 92% for predicting pleural metastases.

B. Diagnostic Thoracentesis

Cytology

The diagnosis of a malignant pleural effusion is most commonly made by the cytological analysis of pleural fluid obtained at thoracentesis. The diagnostic utility of cytological examination of pleural fluid is influenced by a number of factors including the type and extent of the tumor, how many samples are submitted, the skill of the cytologist, and the presence of other paramalignant diseases.

The percentage of patients in which cytology can establish the diagnosis of malignant pleural effusions ranges from 40 to 87% (17–19). The degree of usefulness of the cytological examination of pleural fluid varies with the type of malignancy being examined, being greatest with adenocarcinoma. It is significantly less with squamous cell carcinoma, sarcoma, and mesothelioma. Pleural fluid cytologies are positive in diffuse histiocytic lymphoma approximately 75% of the time, but only 25% of the time with Hodgkin's lymphoma (20).

Paramalignant pleural effusions may develop in conditions associated with cancer, but without direct involvement of the pleura. Cytologically negative pleural effusions can be caused by low oncotic pressure due to hypoproteinemia, pulmonary emboli, post-obstructive pneumonia, and blockage of major lymphatic vessels due to central tumors, such as lymphoma and squamous cell carcinoma (21).

Biochemical Parameters

Malignant pleural effusions almost always have exudative characteristics (22). Approximately 1–5% of the time, malignant effusions may be transudates, although alternative explanations may be present in a number of these patients (23,24).

An elevation in the pleural fluid amylase level in patients where esophageal rupture and acute pancreatitis are not expected suggests carcinoma, particularly adenocarcinoma (25). Lymphoma, ovarian cancer, and pancreatic cancer can also be associated with high pleural fluid amylase levels (26,27).

Recently, pleural fluid adenosine deaminase (ADA) has been proposed as both a sensitive and specific marker for the presence of tuberculous pleuritis. Ocana et al. studied 221 patients with pleuroperitoneal effusions and found that all patients with pleural ADA levels above 70 U/L had tuberculosis while no patient with an ADA level below 40 U/L had tuberculous pleuritis (28). In areas with a high incidence of tuberculosis, ADA cutoff levels of 47–50 U/L have been found to be approximately 90% sensitive and specific for the diagnosis of tuberculous pleuritis in patients with a lymphocytic predominant pleural effusion (29–31).

A pleural fluid pH less than 7.30 is seen in about one third of malignant pleural effusions (32). It is not diagnostic of a malignant effusion, but limits the possibilities to a handful of diagnoses that include it. Malignant pleural effusions with a lower pH are more likely to have a positive pleural fluid cytology (33).

Matrix metalloproteinases constitute a family of endopepetidases that degrade and turnover extracellular matrix proteins. They are produced by mesothelial cells and have been measured in a variety of pleural effusions. A study by Eickelberg et al. demonstrated that interstitial collagenase, gelatinase A, and TIMP-1 are found in pleural fluid of all causes (34). Gelatinase B was expressed in exudates, but not in transudates. The ratio of gelatinase B to gelatinase A was found to be highest in pleural effusions of paramalignant origin.

The diagnostic value of pleural fluid levels of interleukin-1-alpha (IL-1-α), interleukin-6 (IL-6), and tumor necrosis factor in determining the etiology of pleural effusions has been recently examined (35). IL-6 was demonstrated to be the only cytokine that differed significantly among the three types of exudates examined (malignant, parapneumonic, tuberculous). IL-6 levels were significantly lower in malignant effusions compared to parapneumonic and tuberculous effusions. There were no significant differences in TNF and IL-1-a between the three groups.

Immunohistochemical Stains

To perform immunohistochemistry studies, tissue samples or cytological preparations are incubated with an antibody and then counterstained with a specific antibody tagged with alkaline phosphatase or similar agent. The diagnostic utility of immunohistochemistry in the diagnosis of malignant pleural effusions secondary to adenocarcinoma, mesothelioma, and lymphoma has been established (36,37). These techniques have little value in the diagnosis of pleural effusions due to squamous cell carcinoma and small-cell carcinoma.

The best markers for the diagnosis of adenocarcinoma are carcinoembryonic antigen (CEA), Leu-M1, B72.3, Ber-EP4, and BG-8 (38). The best markers for mesothelioma are calretinin and cytokeratin 5/6 (39). Calretinin and cytokeratin 5/6 cannot separate mesothelioma cells from benign mesothelial cells. A panel of these antibodies can be used to separate adenocarcinoma from mesothelioma (37). If the specimen studied is positive for all three (CEA, B72.3, and Leu-M1), the specificity for adenocarcinoma is 100% with a sensitivity of 70%. If the specimen is negative for all three, the specificity is 99% for mesothelioma.

Oncogenes and DNA/RNA Analysis

In general, oncogene analysis is of limited value in giving a definitive diagnosis because of a low sensitivity and specificity. The p53 oncogene was not detected in benign effusions in a study by Zoppi et al., but it was found in only one third of the malignant effusions (40). The CMYC oncogene was found in both malignant and benign effusions (41). The CHARAS oncogene was detectable in the vast majority of malignant effusions, but was also found in over one third of benign effusions (42).

Flow cytometry is a technique used to quantitate nuclear DNA levels. It is useful in the evaluation of lymphocytic pleural effusions in which lymphoma is a diagnostic possibility. Otherwise, flow cytometry has little diagnostic utility in the differentiation of benign and malignant effusions because a large number of malignant effusions do not have aneuploidy and a significant number of benign effusions do (43–45).

Quantitative competitive reverse transcription/polymerase chain reaction techniques were used to detect aberrant mucin genes in pleural effusions (46). The authors examined three mucin genes (MUC1, MUC2, and MUC5AC) in patients with pleural effusions secondary to a variety of etiologies. The expression ratios of MUC1 and MUC5AC were significantly higher in malignant compared to benign pleural effusions. The combination of MUC1 and MUC5AC had a sensitivity of 86.1%, specificity of 91.5%, positive predictive value of 93.3%, and a negative predictive value of 82.7%.

The use of the competitive reverse transcription-polymerase chain reaction technique to analyze cells in pleural effusions for a specific CD44 variant RNA, CD44v8-10, was recently examined (47). The authors used the assay to determine the relative expression of CD44v8-10 with CD44v10, which is predominantly expressed in leukocytes. Ratios of CD44v8-10/CD44v10 greater than 1.0 were able to detect the presence of exfoliated cancer cells with a sensitivity of 76% and a specificity of 94%. The ratios of CD44v8-10/CD44v10 were consistently low in a variety of benign conditions, including inflammatory processes.

Tumor Markers

A variety of tumor markers have been studied to establish their utility in the diagnosis of malignancies involving the pleural space. Overall, the ability of tumor markers to discriminate between benign and malignant pleural effusions is poor.

A number of studies have examined the use of CEA in the diagnosis of malignant pleural effusions. In general, an elevated CEA level is suggestive of malignancy but not diagnostic. Previous studies have found that patients with pleural fluid CEA levels above 10–12 ng/mL have a malignancy about 35–50% of the time (48,49). Tamura et al. found that no patients with a benign effusion had a CEA level above this (49). However, an occasional benign effusion with a CEA level above 100 ng/mL was seen in another study (50).

Vascular endothelial growth factor (VEGF) is a cytokine that increases vascular permeability and is an important angiogenic factor for malignant tumors. Many malignant pleural effusions appear to have especially high levels of VEGF. Cheng et al. measured VEGF levels in a group of 70 patients with pleural effusion and found that the highest median levels occurred in malignant effusions and the lowest median levels were found in transudative effusions (51). Inflammatory diseases of the pleura yielded intermediate values for VEGF. Significant overlap in VEGF levels between the groups was found to limit the clinical usefulness of the test in separating benign from malignant conditions. Setting very high cutoff values for pleural fluid VEGF levels as well as measuring other key cytokines in pleural fluid such as tumor necrosis factor alpha (TNF-α) may improve diagnostic utility of VEGF measurements (52).

The carbohydrate antigens (CA) 15-3, 19-9, and 72-4 have significant overlap between benign and malignant effusions (53,54). Cytokeratin 19 (CYFRA 21-1) is found in cytoskeleton intermediate filaments of epithelium. It tends to be overexpressed in carcinomas and mesotheliomas, reaching levels above 100 ng/mL approximately 60% of the time (55). However, there is a substantial overlap between effusions due to benign and malignant etiologies. Enolase, a glycolytic enzyme found in neuroendocrine tumors, and squamous cell carcinoma antigen have been studied and found to have little utility in the diagnosis of malignant effusions secondary to small cell carcinoma and squamous cell carcinoma, respectively (53,56).

Hyaluronate concentrations above 1 mg/mL, as measured by the HPLC technique, were able to identify 37% of mesotheliomas in one study (57). None of the effusions due to causes other than mesothelioma had hyaluronate concentrations above 0.8 mg/mL. Other studies have been unable to demonstrate that hyaluronate concentrations can discriminate between pleural effusions due to adenocarcinoma or mesothelioma (58,59).

C. Closed Pleural Biopsy

Needle biopsy of the pleura historically has been useful for the diagnosis of tuberculosis or malignancy in the setting of an exudative lymphocytic pleural effusion of unknown etiology. In areas with a high incidence of tuberculosis, pleural biopsy may show caseous granulomas in 80% of cases and pleural tissue cultures may be positive in 12% (60). Closed pleural biopsy is less sensitive than pleural fluid cytology in diagnosing malignant pleural effusion with a reported diagnostic yield of 40–75% (61–64). If cytology is negative, the addition of closed pleural biopsy can be expected to yield a diagnosis of malignancy in only 7–12% of patients (64,65). Lack of involvement of the costal parietal pleura by tumor cells, especially early in the course of disease, as well as the blind nature of the sampling procedure along with operator inexperience likely contribute to the relatively low yield of this test (66).

D. Medical Thoracoscopy

Medical thoracoscopy for diagnostic purposes has a number of advantages to recommend it over both blind pleural biopsy and surgical biopsy of the pleural. It can be performed safely in properly equipped endoscopy suites in spontaneously breathing patients using local anesthesia or conscious sedation and is considerable less expensive than a surgical approach (67). Visual inspection of the pleural space permits much more accurate biopsy compared to blind needle biopsy in the diagnosis of pleural effusion of unknown etiology. In skilled hands a diagnostic sensitivity of approximately 95% can be obtained in malignant effusions (68,69). Tuberculous involvement of the pleural space can also be diagnosed with a sensitivity of over 90% (67).

E. Surgical Biopsy

Surgical biopsy procedures are usually reserved for those few cases in which the cause of pleural effusion remains unknown after less invasive diagnostic methods. Video-assisted thoracic surgery (VATS) is considerably more involved than medical thoracoscopy (66). It is usually performed in the operating room arena using general anesthesia and single lung ventilation. Multiple incisional ports may be used to facilitate viewing of the pleural space and for the introduction of special instrumentation. If the patient cannot tolerate single lung ventilation or if complications are encountered, such as the presence of widespread pleural adhesions, the surgeon may elect to convert to an open pleural biopsy procedure. Even after surgical biopsy procedures it is possible that a diagnosis for the etiology of the pleural effusion may not be obtained even after years of close clinical follow-up (70).

IV. Summary

Cytology and pleural tissue histology remain the most accepted means to differentiate benign from malignant pleural effusions. The history and physical examination may provide useful clues that direct the clinician in the workup of the effusion. Imaging studies provide an invaluable adjunct for further diagnostic efforts. Although a plethora of biochemical and genetic tests are being investigated, at the present time none are sensitive and specific enough to be diagnostic of a malignant pleural effusion. In general, the clinician should proceed from the least invasive tests that promise the best diagnostic yield, such as thoracentesis with simple pleural fluid chemistries and cytology, to more invasive sampling of the pleura. Operator expertise and institutional resources and policy are important determinants of which invasive test will be used. If a careful, systematic approach is applied with appropriate use of minimally invasive and surgical procedures, fewer than 10% of pleural effusions should remain undiagnosed (66,68).

References

1. Light RW. Pleural Diseases. Philadelphia: Lippincott Williams and Wilkins, 2001: 42–43.
2. Marel M, Stastny B, Melinova L, Svandova E, Light R. Diagnosis of pleural effusions. Experience with clinical studies, 1986 to 1990. Chest 1995; 107:1598–1603.
3. Maher G, Berger H. Massive pleural effusion: malignant and nonmalignant causes in 46 patients. Am Rev Respir Dis 1972; 105:458–460.
4. Rabin CB, Coleman NS. Bilateral effusions and significance in association with a heart of normal size. J Mt Sinai Hosp 1957; 24:45–53.
5. Bruneau R, Rubin P. The management of pleural effusions and chylothorax in lymphoma. Radiology 1965; 85:1085–1092.
6. Celikoglu F, Teirstein A, Krellenstein D, Strauchen J. Pleural effusion in non-Hodgkin's lymphoma. Chest 1992; 101:1357–1360.
7. Hierholzer J, Luo L, Bittner RC, Stroszczynski C, Schroder RJ, Schoenfeld N, Dorow P, Loddenkemper R, Grassot A. MRI and CT in the differential diagnosis of pleural disease. Chest 2000; 118:604–609.
8. Leung AN, Muller NL, Miller RR. CT in differential diagnosis of diffuse pleural disease. Am J Radiol 1990; 154:487–492.
9. Shiono T, Yoshikawa K, Takenaka E, Hisamatsu K. MR imaging of pleural and peritoneal effusion. Radiat Med 1993; 11:123–126.
10. Davis SD, Henschke CI, Yankelevitz DF, Cahill PT, Yi Y. MR imaging of pleural effusions. J Comput Assist Tomogr 1990; 14:192–198.
11. Falaschi F, Battolla L, Mascalchi M, Cioni R, Zampa V, Lencioni R, Antonelli A, Bartolozzi C. Usefulness of MR signal intensity in distinguishing benign from malignant pleural disease. AJR Am J Roentgenol 1996; 166:963–968.
12. Carlsen SE, Bergin CJ, Hoppe RT. MR imaging to detect chest wall and pleural involvement in patients with lymphoma: effect on radiation therapy planning. AJR Am J Roentgenol 1993; 160:1191–1195.

13. Carretta A, Landoni C, Melloni G, Ceresoli GL, Compierchio A, Fazio F, Zannini P. 18-FDG positron emission tomography in the evaluation of malignant pleural diseases—a pilot study. Eur J Cardiothorac Surg 2000; 17:377–383.
14. Benard F, Sterman D, Smith R, Kaiser L, Albelda S, Alavi A. Metabolic imaging of malignant pleural mesothelioma with fluorodeoxyglucose positron emission tomography. Chest 1998; 114:713–722.
15. Gerbaudo VH, Sugarbaker DJ, Britz-Cunningham S, Carli MFD, Mauceri C, Treves ST. Assessment of malignant pleural mesothelioma with (18)F-FDG dual-head gamma-camera coincidence imaging: comparison with histopathology. J Nucl Med 2002; 43:1144–1149.
16. Erasmus JJ, McAdams HP, Rossi SE, Goodman PC, Coleman RE, Patz EF. FDG PET of pleural effusions in patients with non-small cell lung cancer. AmJ Radiol 2000; 175:245–249.
17. Bueno CE, Clemente G, Castro BC. Cytologic and bacteriologic analysis of fluid and pleural biopsy specimens with Cope's needle. Arch Intern Med 1990; 150:1190–1194.
18. Grunze H. The comparative diagnostic accuracy, efficiency and specificity of cytologic techniques used in the diagnosis of malignant neoplasm in serous effusions of the pleural and pericardial cavities. Acta Cytol 1964; 8:150–164.
19. Jarvi OH, Kunnas RJ, Laitio MT. The accuracy and significance of cytologic cancer diagnosis of pleural effusions. Acta Cytol 1972; 16:152–157.
20. Melamed MR. The cytological presentation of malignant lymphomas and related diseases in effusions. Cancer 1963; 16:413–431.
21. Naylor B, Schmidt RW. The case for exfoliative cytology of serous effusions. Lancet 1964; 1:711–712.
22. Light RW, MacGregor MI, Luchsinger PC, Ball WC. Pleural effusions: the separation of transudates and exudates. Ann Intern Med 1972; 77:507–513.
23. Ashchi M, Golish J, Eng P, O'Donovan P. Transudative malignant pleural effusions: prevalence and mechanisms. South Med J 1998; 91:23–26.
24. Assi Z, Caruso J, Herndon J, Patz E Jr. Cytologically proved malignant pleural effusions: distribution of transudates and exudates. Chest 1998; 113:1302–1304.
25. Kramer MR, Saldana MJ, Cepro RJ, Pitchenik AE. High amylase in neoplasm-related effusion. Ann Intern Med 1989; 10:567–569.
26. Cramer SF, Bruns DE. Amylase-producing ovarian neoplasm with pseudo-Meigs' syndrome and elevated pleural fluid amylase: case report and ultrastructure. Cancer 1979; 44:1715–1721.
27. Joseph J, Viney S, Beck P, Strange C, Sahn S, Basran G. A prospective study of amylase-rich pleural effusions with special reference to amylase isoenzyme analysis. Chest 1992; 102:1455–1459.
28. Ocana I, Martinez-Vazquez JM, Segura RM, Fernandez-De-Sevilla T, Capdevila JA. Adenosine deaminase in pleural fluids. Test for diagnosis of tuberculous pleural effusion. Chest 1983; 84:51–53.
29. Burgess LJ, Maritz FJ, Le Roux I, Taljaard JJ. Use of adenosine deaminase as a diagnostic tool for tuberculous pleurisy. Thorax 1995; 50:672–674.
30. Valdes L, San Jose E, Alvarez D, Sarandeses A, Pose A, Chomon B, Alvarez-Dobano JM, Salgueiro M, Rodriguez J, Suarez R. Diagnosis of tuberculous pleurisy using the biologic parameters adenosine deaminase, lysozyme, and interferon gamma. Chest 1993; 103:458–465.
31. Valdes L, Alvarez D, San Jose E, Juanatey JR, Pose A, Valle JM, Salgueiro M,

Suarez JR. Value of adenosine deaminase in the diagnosis of tuberculous pleural effusions in young patients in a region of high prevalence of tuberculosis. Thorax 1995; 50:600–603.
32. Sahn SA, Good JT. Pleural fluid pH in malignant effusions. Diagnostic, prognostic, and therapeutic implications. Ann Intern Med 1988; 1988:345–349.
33. Rodriguez-Pandero F, Lopez-Mejias L. Low glucose and pH levels in malignant pleural effusions. Diagnostic significance and prognostic value in respect to pleurodesis. Am Rev Respir Dis 1989; 139:663–667.
34. Eickelberg O, Sommerfeld CO, Wyser C, Tamm M, Reichenberger F, Bardin PG, Soler M, Roth M, Perruchoud AP. MMP and TIMP expression pattern in pleural effusions of different origins. Am J Respir Crit Care Med 1997; 156:1987–1992.
35. Xirouchaki N, Tzanakis N, Bouros D, Kyriakou D, Karkavitsas N, Alexandrakis M, Siafakas NM. Diagnostic value of interleukin-1{alpha}, interleukin-6, and tumor necrosis factor in pleural effusions. Chest 2002; 121:815–820.
36. Guzman J, Bross KJ, Costabel U. Malignant lymphoma in pleural effusions: an immunocytochemical cell surface analysis. Diagn Cytopathol 1991; 7:113–118.
37. Brown RW, Clark GM, Tandon AK. Multiple-marker immunohistochemical phenotypes distinguishing malignant pleural mesothelioma from pulmonary adenocarcinoma. Hum Pathol 1993; 24:347–354.
38. Ordonez NG. The immunohistochemical diagnosis of epithelial mesothelioma. Hum Pathol 1999; 30:313–323.
39. Barberis MC, Faleri M, Veronese S. Calretinin. A selective marker of normal and neoplastic mesothelial cells in serous effusions. Acta Cytol 1997; 41:1757–1761.
40. Zoppi JA, Pellicer EM. Diagnostic value of p53 protein in the study of serous effusions. Acta Cytol 1995; 39:721–724.
41. Tawfik MS, Coleman DV. C-myc expression in exfoliated cells in serous effusions. Cytopathology 1991; 2:83–92.
42. Athanassiadou PP, Veneti SZ, Kyrkou KA. Detection of c-Ha-ras oncogene expression in pleural and peritoneal smear effusions by in situ hybridization. Cancer Detect Prev 1993; 17:585–590.
43. Pinto MM. DNA analysis of malignant effusions. Comparison with cytologic diagnosis and carcinoembryonic antigen content. Anal Quant Cytol Histol 1992; 14:222–226.
44. Rodriguez de Castro F, Molero T, Acosta O. Value of DNA analysis in addition to cytological testing in the diagnosis of malignant pleural effusions. Thorax 1994; 49:692–694.
45. Rijken A, Dekker A, Taylor S. Diagnostic value of DNA analysis in effusions by flow cytometry and image analysis. A prospective study on 102 patients as compared with cytologic examination. Am J Clin Pathol 1991; 95:6–12.
46. Yu C-J, Shew J-Y, Liaw Y-S, Kuo S-H, Luh K-T, Yang P-C. Application of mucin quantitative competitive reverse transcription polymerase chain reaction in assisting the diagnosis of malignant pleural effusion. Am J Respir Crit Care Med 2001; 164:1312–1318.
47. Okamoto I, Morisaki T, Sasaki J, Miyake H, Matsumoto M, Suga M, Ando M, Saya H. Molecular detection of cancer cells by competitive reverse transcription-polymerase chain reaction analysis of specific CD44 variant RNAs. J Natl Cancer Inst 1998; 90:307–315.
48. Loewenstein MS, Rittgers RA, Feinerman AE, Kupchik HZ, Marcel BR, Koff RS,

Zamcheck N. Carcinoembryonic antigen levels in benign and malignant pleural effusions. Ann Intern Med 1978; 88:631–634.
49. Tamura S, Nishigaki T, Moriwaki Y, Fujioka H, Nakano T, Fujii J, Yamamoto T, Nabeshima K, Hada T, Higashino K. Tumor markers in pleural effusion diagnosis. Cancer 1988; 61:298–302.
50. Garcia-Pachon E, Padilla-Navas I, Dosda MD, Miralles-Llopis A. Elevated level of carcinoembryonic antigen in nonmalignant pleural effusions. Chest 1997; 111: 643–647.
51. Cheng D, Rodriguez RM, Perkett EA, Rogers J, Bienvenu G, Lappalainen U, Light RW. Vascular endothelial growth factor in pleural fluid. Chest 1999; 116: 760–765.
52. Momi H, Matsuyama W, Inoue K, Kawabata M, Arimura K, Fukunaga H, Osame M. Vascular endothelial growth factor and proinflammatory cytokines in pleural effusions. Respir Med 2002; 96:817–822.
53. Miedouge M, Rouzaud P, Salama G, Pujazon MC, Vincent C, Mauduyt MA, Reyre J, Carles P, Serre G. Evaluation of seven tumour markers in pleural fluid for the diagnosis of malignant effusions. Br J Cancer 1999; 81:1059–1065.
54. Villena V, Lopez-Encuentra A, Echave-Sustaeta J, Martin-Escribano P, Ortuno-de-Solo B, Estenoz-Alfaro J. Diagnostic value of CA 72-4, carcinoembryonic antigen, CA 15-3, and CA 19-9 assay in pleural fluid. A study of 207 patients. Cancer 1996; 78:736–740.
55. Salama G, Miedouge M, Rouzaud P, Mauduyt MA, Pujazon MC, Vincent C, Carles P, Serre G. Evaluation of pleural CYFRA 21-1 and carcinoembryonic antigen in the diagnosis of malignant pleural effusions. Br J Cancer 1998; 77:472–476.
56. San M, Jose E, Alvarez D, Valdes L, Sarandeses A, Valle JM, Penela P. Utility of tumour markers in the diagnosis of neoplastic pleural effusion. Clin Chim Acta 1997; 265:193–205.
57. Rasmussen KN, Faber V. Hyaluronic acid in 247 pleural fluids. Scand J Respir Dis 1967; 48:366–371.
58. Pettersson T, Froseth B, Riska H, Klockars M. Concentration of hyaluronic acid in pleural fluid as a diagnostic aid for malignant mesothelioma. Chest 1988; 94:1037–1039.
59. Hillerdal G, Lindqvist U, Engstrom-Laurent A. Hyaluronan in pleural effusions and in serum. Cancer 1991; 67:2410–2414.
60. Valdes L, Alvarez D, San Jose E, Penela P, Valle JM, Garcia-Pazos JM, Suarez J, Pose A. Tuberculous pleurisy: a study of 254 patients. Arch Intern Med 1998; 158: 2017–2021.
61. Escudero BC, Garcia CM, Cuesta CB, et al. Cytological and bacteriologic analysis of fluid and pleural biopsy specimens with Cope's needle. Arch Intern Med 1990; 150:1190–1194.
62. Poe RH, Israel RH, Utell MJ, Hall WJ, Greenblatt DW, Kallay MC. Sensitivity, specificity, and predictive values of closed pleural biopsy. Arch Intern Med 1984; 144:325–328.
63. Starr RL, Sherman ME. The value of multiple preparations in the diagnosis of malignant pleural effusions. A cost-benefit analysis. Acta Cytol 1991; 35:533–537.
64. Prakash UB, Reiman HM. Comparison of needle biopsy with cytologic analysis for the evaluation of pleural effusion: analysis of 414 cases. Mayo Clin Proc 1985; 60:158–164.
65. Loddenkemper R, Grosser H, Gabler A, Mai J, Preussler H, Brandt HJ. Prospective evaluation of biopsy methods in the diagnosis of malignant pleural effusions:

intrapatient comparison between pleural fluid cytology, blind needle biopsy and thoracoscopy. Am Rev Respir Dis 1983; 127(suppl 4):114.
66. Antony VB, Loddenkemper R, Astoul P, Boutin C, Goldstraw P, Hott J, Rodriguez Panadero F, Sahn SA. Management of malignant pleural effusions. Am J Respir Crit Care Med 2000; 162:1987–2001.
67. Boutin C, Astoul P. Diagnostic thoracoscopy. Clin Chest Med 1998; 19:295–309.
68. Boutin C, Viallat JR, Cargnino P, Farisse P. Thoracoscopy in malignant pleural effusions. Am Rev Respir Dis 1981; 124:588–592.
69. Loddenkemper R. Thoracoscopy—state of the art. Eur Respir J 1998; 11:213–221.
70. Ryan CJ, Rodgers RF, Unni KK, Hepper NG. The outcome of patients with pleural effusion of indeterminate cause at thoracotomy. Mayo Clin Proc 1981; 56:145–149.

16

Clinical Evaluation of the Patient with a Pleural Effusion

STEVEN A. SAHN

Medical University of South Carolina
Charleston, South Carolina, U.S.A.

I. Introduction

The clinical recognition of a pleural effusion, either on physical examination or radiologically, as a marker of an abnormal physiological state has resulted in greater formation than removal of pleural fluid. Disease in virtually any organ system can be the cause of a pleural effusion (1). In the approach to the patient with a pleural effusion, the clinician must be cognizant that not only can disease in the thorax be causative, but disease of organs juxtaposed to the diaphragm, such as the liver or spleen, can as well. Furthermore, systemic diseases, such as systemic lupus erythematosus and rheumatoid arthritis, may involve the pleura, as can diseases of the lymphatic system, such as yellow nail syndrome. Therefore, the evaluation of a pleural effusion must begin with a complete history and physical examination and follow with pertinent laboratory tests to formulate a prethoracentesis diagnosis.

II. Value of Pleural Fluid Analysis

It is important to recognize that pleural fluid analysis alone will establish a definitive diagnosis in only a minority of patients; the number of definitive diagnoses will vary with the population being evaluated. In a prospective study of 129 patients with pleural effusion, thoracenteses provided a definitive diagnosis in only 18% of patients and a presumptive diagnosis in 55% of patients (2). In the remaining 27% of patients, the pleural fluid findings were not helpful diagnostically, as the values were compatible with two or more clinical possibilities; however, in a number of these patients, the findings were useful in excluding possible diagnoses, such as empyema. Therefore, history and physical examination, radiological evaluation, and ancillary blood tests are crucial in establishing a pretest diagnosis; pleural fluid analysis is a valuable test that usually does not provide a definitive diagnosis but can provide a secure clinical diagnosis if there is a thoughtful prethoracentesis evaluation.

Diagnoses that can be "established definitively" by pleural fluid analysis include malignancy, complicated parapneumonic effusion, empyema, lupus pleuritis, chylothorax, urinothorax, hemothorax, peritoneal dialysis, chronic rheumatoid pleurisy, esophageal rupture, extravascular migration of a central venous catheter, rupture of an amebic liver abscess, and a duro-pleural fistula (1,3).

III. Symptoms with Pleural Effusions

The patient may present with (e.g., lupus pleuritis) (4) or without (e.g., BAPE) (5) symptoms related to the pleural effusion. Patients without underlying cardiopulmonary disease who develop a small effusion may be asymptomatic and the effusion discovered by routine chest radiograph. When patients with a pleural effusion are symptomatic, dyspnea and chest pain are the most common findings. Dyspnea may be caused by a large or massive pleural effusion in a patient with normal lungs, a moderate effusion with underlying lung disease, and a small effusion with severe lung disease. A large pleural effusion causes ipsilateral mediastinal shift, depression of the ipsilateral diaphragm, outward movement of the ipsilateral chest wall, and lung compression when there is no endobronchial lesion or fixed mediastinum. The breathlessness perceived by patients with a large to massive pleural effusion is due to its effect on the previously mentioned structures with input by neurogenic receptors from the lung and chest wall (6). Small to moderate effusions tend to cause lung displacement rather than lung compression and generally have minimal to no effect on pulmonary function (7). Chest pain with splinting and atelectasis or a primary parenchymal process from infection or malignancy may be the major cause of dyspnea in patients with a small to moderate pleural effusion.

Patients with a pleural effusion may present with pleuritic chest pain, which is associated with pleural inflammation (8). The pain with pleurisy will vary with the degree of pleural inflammation. Pleuritic chest pain has been described as having a stitch in the side, stabbing or shooting. The pain may be exacerbated by deep inspiration, cough, or sneeze. Any maneuver that results in chest wall splinting, such as manual pressure over the chest wall, will minimize the pain.

However, it should be noted that a splinting maneuver will not differentiate other causes of pleuritic-like chest pain, such as rib fractures, from inflammation of the pleura itself.

With inflammation of the costal pleura, the pain is located directly over the site of pleural involvement, often with associated tenderness on pressure; cutaneous hypersensitivity and abdominal pain are absent. When the lateral anterior and parts of the posterior diaphragmatic pleura are inflamed, the perceived pain covers a more diffuse area including the lower thorax, back, and abdomen; this pain, typically accompanied by cutaneous hyperesthesia, is exacerbated by pressure and muscle rigidity. Inflammation of the central portion of the diaphragmatic pleural does not elicit pain in the immediate area but results in referred pain to the ipsilateral posterior neck, shoulder, and trapezius muscle; the pain is associated with tenderness, hyperesthesia, hyperalgesia, and muscle spasm. The referred pain from central diaphragmatic inflammation occurs because the majority of the sensory fibers of the phrenic nerve enter at the C4 level of the spinal cord, the usual entry point of sensation from the shoulder (8).

The primary symptoms of a pleural effusion, chest pain and dyspnea, are nonspecific; therefore, further history is important in limiting the differential diagnosis prior to pleural fluid analysis. Features such as loss of consciousness in an alcoholic who presents with fever suggests that the effusion is an anaerobic empyema. The acute onset of dyspnea in an individual who sustained a recent leg fracture that required a cast suggests that the effusion is caused by a pulmonary embolism. Pleural effusion from asbestos exposure should be suspected in a man who was a shipyard worker for the past 20 years. A patient who sustained a myocardial infarction 2 weeks previously and presents with fever, dyspnea, and pleuritic chest pain may have the post–cardiac injury syndrome. Esophageal rupture should be considered in the patient who provides a history of severe retching and upper abdominal or lower chest pain. A known diagnosis of systemic lupus erythematosus or a history of taking procainamide should raise the possibility of lupus pleuritis. A history of sarcoidosis, rheumatoid disease, or chronic dialysis (uremic pleural effusion, tuberculous pleurisy) should alert the clinician to the possible cause of the pleural effusion. Although the number of drugs that are associated with pleural disease is substantially less than those that are purported to cause parenchymal disease, pleural disease should always be a consideration in the patient who presents with a drug-induced pleural effusion. Drugs that have been associated with a pleural effusion in more than a single case report include bromocriptine, cyclophosphamide, dantrolene, nitrofurantoin, mitomycin, practolol, procarbazine, methotrexate, mesalamine, and isotretinoin (9).

IV. Physical Examination

Pleural fluid separates the lung from the chest wall and interferes with sound transmission. The physical signs of a pleural effusion will vary depending upon the volume of pleural fluid and the degree of lung compression. The examination will also be affected by the status of the underlying lung and the patency of the bronchial tree.

A small amount of pleural fluid (approximately 250–300 cc) will be difficult to detect on physical examination (10). When approximately 500 cc of fluid is present, the following physical findings typically are present: (1) dullness to percussion; (2) decreased fremitus; and (3) normal vesicular breath sounds, possibly of lower intensity than on the normal side. When the effusion volume exceeds 1000 cc, there usually is (1) mild bulging and an absence of inspiratory retraction of the lower intercostal spaces, (2) decreased expansion of the ipsilateral chest wall, (3) dullness to percussion to the level of the scapula and possibly to the axilla, (4) decreased or absent fremitus at the posterior base and laterally, (5) decreased broncho-vesicular breath sounds at the upper level of the effusion, and (6) egophony at the upper level of the effusion. If there is more marked lung compression, auscultation may reveal bronchial breath sounds (10).

With a massive pleural effusion, physical examination will show (1) bulging of the intercostal spaces, (2) virtual absence of chest wall expansion, (3) a dull percussion note over the entire hemithorax, (4) absent breath sounds over the majority of the chest with possible broncho-vesicular or bronchial breath sounds at the uppermost portion of the effusion, (5) egophony at the upper level of the effusion, and (6) palpation of the liver or spleen due to significant diaphragmatic depression (10).

With transudative pleural effusions, the prethoracentesis history and physical examination should increase the likelihood of a presumptive diagnosis. Patients with congestive heart failure typically relate symptoms of orthopnea and paroxysmal nocturnal dyspnea and have a gallop rhythm and bibasilar fine crackles, usually associated with increased jugular venous pressure. Patients with hepatic hydrothorax show the stigmata of cirrhosis and have clinical ascites. Those with nephrotic syndrome and a pleural effusion generally have anasarca. Patients who develop atelectatic effusions are those who are postoperative, are in an intensive care unit, or have upper abdominal or lower chest pain.

V. Laboratory Tests

A. Peripheral Leukocyte Count

The finding of peripheral leukocytosis with a left shift with an associated pleural effusion suggests a bacterial infection, most commonly from pneumonia; however, other diagnoses to consider include subphrenic abscess, esophageal rupture, hepatic or splenic abscess, or severe inflammation as with pancreatitis. Leukopenia with a pleural effusion may be seen with systemic lupus erythematosus, viral pleurisy, severe pneumonia with sepsis, or pneumonia in an HIV-positive patient.

B. Chest Radiograph

Finding an isolated pleural effusion or associated findings on chest radiograph may narrow the differential diagnosis prior to pleural fluid analysis (1). When the only abnormality on the chest radiograph is a pleural effusion, the clinician should consider infectious causes, such as tuberculous pleurisy or viral pleurisy, in addition to a small bacterial pneumonia. Connective tissue diseases, such as rheumatoid pleurisy and lupus pleuritis, should be considered in the appropriate clinical setting. Metastatic carcinoma, non-Hodgkin's lymphoma, and leukemia can present as a solitary pleural effusion. Other diseases where a pleural effusion is the only radiographic abnormality include benign asbestos pleural effusion (BAPE), pulmonary embolism, drug-induced pleural disease, yellow nail syndrome, hypothyroidism, uremic pleuritis, chylothorax, and constrictive pericarditis. When the effusion is massive and causes contralateral mediastinal shift, the most likely diagnosis is carcinoma, usually a nonlung primary (11). When there is no contralateral shift, lung cancer (12) and malignant mesothelioma (13) are most likely.

A pleural effusion as the only radiographic abnormality may also be associated with disease below the diaphragm. This radiographic finding is seen with transudates from hepatic hydrothorax, nephrotic syndrome, urinothorax, and peritoneal dialysis and exudates from acute pancreatitis and pancreatic pseudocyst, Meigs' syndrome, chylous ascites, subphrenic abscess, hepatic abscess, and splenic abscess or infarction (1).

When a patient has bilateral effusions on chest radiograph, the effusion is most likely a transudate and, therefore, is seen with congestive heart failure, nephrotic syndrome, hypoalbuminemia, peritoneal dialysis, and constrictive pericarditis. Bilateral exudative effusions can occur with malignancy, usually an extra-lung primary or lymphoma, lupus pleuritis, and yellow nail syndrome (14).

In patients whose chest radiograph shows a pleural effusion with interstitial lung disease, the differential diagnosis includes congestive heart failure, rheumatoid disease, asbestos-induced pleuropulmonary disease, lymphangitic carcinomatosis, lymphangioleiomyomatosis (LAM), viral and mycoplasma pneumonia, Waldenström's macroglobulinemia, sarcoidosis, and *Pneumocystis carinii* pneumonia.

Pleural effusions associated with pulmonary nodules suggest metastatic cancer, Wegener's granulomatosis, rheumatoid disease, septic pulmonary emboli, sarcoidosis, and tularemia.

C. Pleural Fluid Analysis

Virtually all patients with a newly discovered pleural effusion should have a thoracentesis performed to aid in diagnosis and management. Exceptions would be a secure clinical diagnosis, such as typical congestive heart failure, and a very small volume of pleural fluid, as with viral pleurisy. Observation may be warranted in the above situations; however, if the clinical situation worsens, a thoracentesis should be performed promptly. Only 30–50 cc of pleural fluid is needed for complete pleural fluid analysis. An effusion that layers on a lateral decubitus radiograph of at least 10 mm from the inside of the chest wall to the fluid line is generally safe to sample by thoracentesis if the physical examination is confirmatory. Thoracentesis with ultrasound guidance should be used with a very small or loculated effusion that is not clearly localized by examination.

Observation of Pleural Fluid

Some diagnoses can be established immediately at the bedside by visual examination of the fluid (Table 1). For example, if pus is aspirated from the pleural space, the diagnosis of empyema is established and, if the pus has a putrid odor, anaerobic organisms are causative. A chylothorax can be suspected if there is milky fluid; however, this appearance could also be due to empyema or a cholesterol effusion. Centrifugation of the specimen will be helpful, for if the supernatant remains turbid, a lipid effusion (either chylothorax or cholesterol

Table 1 Observations of Pleural Fluid Helpful in Diagnosis

	Suggested diagnosis
Color of fluid	
Pale yellow (straw)	Transudate, some exudates
Red (bloody)	Malignancy, BAPE, PCIS, or pulmonary infarction in absence of trauma
White (milky)	Chylothorax or cholesterol effusion
Brown	Long-standing bloody effusion; amebic liver abscess
Black	*Aspergillus*
Yellow-green	Rheumatoid pleurisy
Color of enteral tube feeding or central venous line infusate	Feeding tube has entered pleural space; extravascular catheter migration
Character of fluid	
Pus	Empyema
Viscous	Mesothelioma
Debris	Rheumatoid pleurisy
Turbid	Inflammatory exudate of lipid effusion
Anchovy paste	Amebic liver abscess
Odor of fluid	
Putrid	Anaerobic empyema
Ammonia	Urinothorax

effusion) is likely; if the supernatant clears, the turbidity is caused by a large number of leukocytes. With a bloody effusion, if the pleural fluid hematocrit is >40–50% of the blood hematocrit, a diagnosis of hemothorax can be established that requires different management than a hemorrhagic effusion (usual PF hematocrit <5%). Brownish, anchovy-paste fluid is virtually diagnostic of an amebic liver abscess that has ruptured through the diaphragm into the right pleural space (15). If the pleural effusion is the color of the enteral feeding or central venous line infusate, the diagnosis that the feeding tube has entered the pleural space (16) and the vascular catheter has migrated out of the vessel (17), respectively, is confirmed. A fluid that appears to contain debris is characteristic of rheumatoid pleurisy (18), and a clear yellow fluid that has the smell of ammonia diagnoses a urinothorax (19).

Transudate Versus Exudate

The determination of whether an effusion is a transudate or an exudate is an important diagnostic step in pleural fluid analysis. Because the clinical diagnosis of a transudative effusion is relatively straightforward based on the clinical presentation, the patient typically does not require an extensive diagnostic evaluation (Table 2). In contrast, finding an exudative pleural effusion presents

Table 2 Causes of Transudative Pleural Effusions

Diagnosis	Comment
Congestive heart failure	Acute diuresis can increase PF protein and LDH concentrations
Cirrhosis	Rare without clinical ascites
Nephrotic syndrome	Typically small and bilateral; unilateral, larger effusion may be due to pulmonary embolism
Peritoneal dialysis	Large right effusion develops within 48 hours of initiating dialysis
Hypoalbuminemia	Edema fluid rarely isolated to pleural space; small bilateral effusions
Urinothorax	Unilateral effusion caused by ipsilateral obstructive uropathy
Atelectasis	Small effusion caused by increased intrapleural negative pressure; common in ICU patients
Constrictive pericarditis	Bilateral effusions with normal heart size
Trapped lung	Unilateral effusion from remote inflammatory process
Superior vena caval obstruction	Due to acute systemic venous hypertension or acute obstruction of lymphatics
Duropleural fistula	CSF in pleural space

a much larger number of possibilities and may be diagnostically problematic, requiring a multiplicity of tests (Table 3).

Exudative effusions, caused predominantly by neoplastic or inflammatory processes or impaired lymphatic pleural space drainage, are characterized by the presence of higher concentrations of large molecular weight proteins than transudative effusions, the by-product of hydrostatic and oncotic pressure imbalances. While an early approach to detecting exudates was the measurement of pleural fluid specific gravity, pleural fluid protein later replaced this measurement. However, pleural fluid protein concentration alone has insufficient sensitivity as a screening strategy. Light and colleagues (20) reported the use of pleural fluid protein and LDH values compared to serum values in a combination test. Light's criteria "established" the presence of an exudate if one or more of three criteria were satisfied. A modification of these three criteria are as

Table 3 Causes of Exudative Pleural Effusions

Infectious	*Malignancy*	*Connective tissue disease*
Bacterial pneumonia	Carcinoma	Lupus pleuritis
Tuberculous pleurisy	Lymphoma	Rheumatoid pleurisy
Fungal disease	Mesothelioma	Mixed connective
Atypical pneumonias	Leukemia	tissue disease
Nocardia, actinomyces	Chylothorax	Churg-Strauss syndrome
Subphrenic abscess		Wegener's granulomatosis
Hepatic abscess	*Other inflammatory*	Familial Mediterranean
Splenic abscess	Pancreatitis	fever
Hepatitis	BAPE	
Spontaneous esophageal	Pulmonary infarction	*Endocrine dysfunction*
rupture	Radiation therapy	Hypothyroidism
Parasites	Uremic pleurisy	Ovarian hyperstimulation
		syndrome
Iatrogenic	Sarcoidosis	
Drug-induced	Post–cardiac injury	*Lymphatic abnormalities*
Esophageal perforation	syndrome	Malignancy
Esophageal sclerotherapy	Hemothorax	Yellow nail syndrome
Central venous catheter	ARDS	Lymphangiomyomatosis
misplacement/migration		(chylothorax)
Enteral feeding tube in	*Increased negative*	Lymphangiectasis
pleural space	*intrapleural pressure*	
	Atelectasis	*Movement of fluid from*
	Trapped lung	*abdomen to pleural space*
	Cholesterol effusion	Acute pancreatitis
		Pancreatic pseudocyst
		Meigs' syndrome
		Carcinoma
		Chylous ascites
		Urinothorax

follows: (1) a pleural fluid–to–serum protein ratio of >0.5; (2) a pleural fluid–to–serum lactate dehydrogenase (LDH) ratio of >0.6; and (3) a pleural fluid LDH concentration > 0.67 of the upper limits of normal for a laboratory's serum LDH value. Heffner and coworkers (21), using pooled data from several primary investigators, reported that Light's criteria had a sensitivity of 98% and a specificity of 74% in identifying an exudative effusion. They also reported results from a meta-analysis of over 1400 patients that decision thresholds, determined by receiver operating characteristic (ROC) analysis for separation of transudates and exudates, had a similar cut points for pleural fluid to serum protein ratio of >0.5 and LDH (>0.67, the upper limits of normal of serum) (21). In a ROC analysis of 200 consecutive patients, Joseph and colleagues (22) found that a PF LDH value of >0.82 of the upper limits of normal of the serum LDH value had excellent discriminative value. They also noted that, because pleural fluid LDH concentration is not influenced by the serum LDH concentration, there is no basis for using the pleural fluid–to–serum LDH ratio in the diagnostic separation of transudative or exudative pleural effusions. Other investigators have suggested the use of pleural fluid cholesterol as a discriminating test between transudates and exudates and that pleural fluid cholesterol has a lower sensitivity but higher specificity compared with Light's criteria (23–25). It has been suggested, therefore, that pleural fluid cholesterol can be used as a confirmatory test for patients who have a condition usually associated with a transudate, such as congestive heart failure, but have an exudate by Light's criteria. Clinicians should understand that pleural fluid values simply enhance or diminish their pretest probability that the fluid is an exudative effusion. The degree of the clinician's clinical suspicion, whether high or low, should not be affected by a borderline test result.

Total Protein and LDH Concentrations

The total protein concentrations may help with clinical diagnosis in certain situations. For example, tuberculous pleural effusions virtually always have a total protein concentration of >4.0 g/dL, while protein concentrations show a wide range in parapneumonic effusions and carcinomatous and lymphomatous pleural effusions (20). When a total protein concentration of 7.0–8.0 g/dL is detected, Waldenström's macroglobulinemia (26) and multiple myeloma (27) should be considered. Several features about the pleural fluid LDH may also help in the diagnostic evaluation of a pleural effusion. When pleural fluid LDH value is in the usual exudative range but the total protein measurement falls in the typical transudative range, malignancy (20), parapneumonic effusions (20), and *P. carinii* pneumonia should be considered (28). With an upper limit of normal of the serum LDH of 200 IU/L, finding a pleural fluid LDH concentration of >1000 IU/L, the differential diagnosis usually narrows to a complicated parapneumonic effusion or empyema (29,30), rheumatoid pleurisy (31), or pleural paragonimiasis (32); an LDH value of >1000 IU/L is less often observed with malignancy and rarely with tuberculous pleurisy (20).

Most transudates have nucleated cell counts of <1000 per μL, while most exudates are have >1000 nucleated cell counts per μL (1,33). The total pleural fluid nucleated cell count is rarely diagnostic; however, counts of >50,000 per μL are usually seen only in complicated parapneumonic effusions and empyema but can occasionally occur in acute pancreatitis and pulmonary infarction (1,33). Pleural fluid nucleated cell counts of >10,000 per μL are only found in parapneumonic effusions and may occasionally be found with pulmonary infarction, acute pancreatitis, malignancy, tuberculosis, post–cardiac injury syndrome, and lupus pleuritis (1,34). Chronic exudates typified by tuberculous pleurisy and malignancy usually have nucleated cell counts of <5,000 per μL (35,36). It should be remembered that, when pus is aspirated from the pleural space, the nucleated cell count may be less than anticipated, even as low as a few hundred neutrophils, because the remainder of the neutrophils have undergone autolysis because of the harsh environment of low pH and low oxygen tension. Pus, a yellowish-white, creamy, thick, opaque fluid has its appearance because of cellular debris, fibrin, and coagulated pleural fluid.

The timing of thoracentesis in relation to acute pleural injury determines the predominant cellular population. The acute response to pleural injury attracts neutrophils to the pleural space (37). Interleukin-8 (IL-8) is one of the major chemotaxins for neutrophils in the pleural space (38,39). It has been demonstrated that absolute neutrophil counts are correlated with IL-8 levels, with the highest IL-8 levels being found with purulent effusions (39). When the acute injury ceases over the next few days, mononuclear cells move into the pleural space from the peripheral blood and become the predominant cell (40). In chronic effusions, the lymphocyte predominates. Therefore, in diseases in which the patient presents shortly after the onset of symptoms, such as bacterial pneumonia, pulmonary embolism with infarction, and acute pancreatitis, neutrophils predominate. In diseases with a more insidious onset, such as malignancy and tuberculous pleurisy, the predominant cell is the lymphocyte.

The finding of >80% lymphocytes limits the possibilities of the exudative pleural effusion (3) (Table 4). The most common of these diagnoses is tuberculous pleurisy (41). Other causes include lymphoma (41), yellow nail syndrome (42), chronic rheumatoid pleurisy (36,43), sarcoidosis (44), trapped lung (45), chylothorax (46), and acute lung rejection (47). All of the above-mentioned diagnoses can occur when the lymphocyte population is <80%; however, the lymphocyte percentage is rarely <50%. In contrast to lymphoma, only about 60% of patients with carcinomatous pleurisy have lymphocyte populations of >50–70% (41). An undiagnosed lymphocytic-predominant exudative effusion is the most appropriate indication for percutaneous pleural biopsy, and the most sensitive diagnostic procedure in tuberculous pleurisy (48,49). Lymphoma, carcinoma, sarcoidosis, and occasionally rheumatoid pleurisy may be diagnosed by percutaneous pleural biopsy.

Pleural fluid eosinophilia (PFE) is defined as a pleural fluid eosinophil count of >10% of the total nucleated cell count (Table 5). IL-5 appears to be an important chemotactic factor attracting bone marrow–produced eosinophils

Table 4 Pleural Fluid Lymphocyte Predominant (>80%) Exudates

Disease	Comment
Tuberculous pleurisy	Most common cause of lymphocyte predominant exudate; usually 90–95% lymphocytes
Chylothorax	2000–20,000 lymphocytes/µL; lymphoma most common cause
Lymphoma	Often 100% of nucleated cells are lymphocytes; diagnostic yield on cytology or pleural biopsy higher with non-Hodgkin's lymphoma
Yellow nail syndrome	A cause of effusion present for months to years
Rheumatoid pleurisy (chronic)	Usually associated with trapped lung
Sarcoidosis	Usually > 90% lymphocytes
Acute lung rejection	New or increased effusion 2–6 weeks after transplant

into the pleural space (50). In patients who require thoracotomy for spontaneous pneumothorax, eosinophilic pleuritis is commonly encountered (51). While eosinophils appear to move rapidly into the pleural space following pneumothorax, following hemothorax eosinophils tend not to appear for 7–14 days (52). Interestingly, PFE is associated with peripheral blood eosinophilia following trauma that does not resolve until no pleural fluid remains (53). BAPE is a

Table 5 Pleural Fluid Eosinophila

Disease	Comment
Pneumothorax	Common cause of PFE
Hemothorax	May take 1–2 weeks for PFE
BAPE	30% incidence; up to 50% eosinophils
Pulmonary embolism	Associated with radiographic infarction and hemorrhagic effusion
Previous thoracentesis	Usually due to pneumothorax
Parasitic disease	Paragonimiasis, hydatid disease, amebiasis, ascariasis
Fungal disease	Histoplasmosis, coccidioidomycosis
Drug-induced	Dantrolene, bromocriptine, nitrofurantoin
Lymphoma	Hodgkin's disease
Carcinoma	Prevalence of PFE the same in malignant and nonmalignant effusions
Churg-Strauss syndrome	PFE is usual finding
Tuberculous pleurisy	Rare

PFE = PF eosinophils/total nucleated PF cells >10%.

common cause of PFE, occurring in 30–50% of patients, with eosinophil percentages reaching 50% (54,55); often these effusions are hemorrhagic. The most common cause of PFE is air or blood in the pleural space (52,56); therefore, pneumothorax, hemothorax, benign asbestos pleural effusion, pulmonary embolism with infarction, and carcinoma are known causes of pleural fluid eosinophilia. Two recent studies found that the prevalence of PFE was the same in malignant and non-malignant effusions (57,58). Other causes of PFE include parasitic disease, fungal pleurisy, drug-induced pleurisy, Churg-Strauss syndrome, and lymphoma. Tuberculous pleurisy is a rare cause of pleural fluid eosinophilia.

Pleural fluid macrophages, which have their origin in the blood monocyte (40), are not of diagnostic value. Mesothelial cells are exfoliated into normal pleural fluid in small numbers. While mesothelial cells are common in transudative effusions and some exudates, they are rare in tuberculous pleurisy, probably due to the extensive pleural involvement not permitting mesothelial cell shedding into the pleural space (41,59). This same phenomenon is observed with inflammatory processes, such as empyema, chemical pleurodesis, rheumatoid pleurisy, and chronic malignant effusions.

A large number of plasma cells in pleural fluid suggests multiple myeloma with pleural involvement (27). A small number of plasma cells in serous fluid is nondiagnostic and has been observed in a number of nonmalignant diseases.

Pleural Fluid Glucose and pH

A pleural fluid glucose or pH should be measured on all exudative pleural effusions because (1) it can narrow the differential diagnosis (60–62), (2) with a parapneumonic effusion, it provides information helpful management strategies (29,30,63–65), and (3) in malignant pleural effusions, it provides information relating to extent of pleural involvement with tumor, ease of diagnosis, prognosis, and management (66–70). A low pleural fluid glucose is defined as a glucose concentration of <60 mg/dL with a normal serum glucose or a pleural fluid/serum glucose ratio of <0.5. A low pleural fluid pH is defined as a pH value of <7.30 with a normal blood pH. Normal pleural fluid has a pH of approximately 7.60 (71), transudates have a pH ranging from 7.45 to 7.55, and most exudates have a pH ranging from 7.30 to 7.45 (1,60,62). Therefore, finding a pleural effusion with a pH of <7.30 signifies a substantial accumulation of hydrogen ions in the pleural space. There is a direct relationship between pleural fluid pH and glucose; if the pleural fluid pH is low, the glucose is low, and when the pH is normal, the glucose is normal (60,61,65). This correlation suggests that the pathophysiological processes responsible for this biochemical phenomenon are interrelated. The mechanism of the low pH and glucose in parapneumonic empyema and esophageal rupture is an increased rate of glucose utilization by neutrophil phagocytosis and bacteria metabolism with the accumulation of the end-products of glycolysis, CO_2, and lactic acid, causing the pH to fall (72). In contrast, in malignant pleural effusions (73) and rheumatoid pleural effusions

(74,75), the mechanism of low pH and glucose is related to an abnormal pleural membrane rather than increased pleural fluid metabolism. The abnormally thickened pleural membrane in rheumatoid pleurisy and malignancy creates a barrier to glucose entry into the pleural space and a barrier to the efflux of CO_2 and lactic acid, causing the glucose and pH to fall. The mechanism in tuberculous and lupus pleuritis has not been extensively studied but probably represents a combination of the above-mentioned mechanisms.

Table 6 shows the usual pleural fluid pH and glucose as well as the ranges and incidence in the six diagnoses associated with a low pleural fluid pH and glucose. The lowest pHs are found in parapneumonic empyema (29,30,62,65) and esophageal rupture (76), both of which can produce an anaerobic empyema. Glucoses of zero are found only in rheumatoid pleural effusions (61,74) and empyemas (61). In malignancy, tuberculous pleurisy, and lupus pleuritis, the pH and glucose values tend to higher than with the aforementioned diagnoses (60–62). Pleural fluid pH should always be measured in a radiometer system.

Pleural Fluid Amylase

The finding of an amylase-rich pleural effusion, defined as a pleural fluid amylase in excess of the upper limits of normal for serum amylase or a pleural fluid/serum amylase of >1.0, signifies that the exudative effusion is either due to pancreatic disease (77–80), malignancy (79,81,82), or esophageal rupture (83–85). A pleural fluid high in amylase can be observed with acute or chronic pancreatitis, the latter associated with pseudocyst formation and a fistulous tract into the mediastinum or pleural space. Rare causes of an amylase-rich effusion include pneumonia, ruptured ectopic pregnancy, hydronephrosis, and cirrhosis (79). Several mechanisms are responsible for the formation of a pancreatic pleural effusion and include direct contact of the pancreatic enzymes with the diaphragmatic pleura, movement of ascitic fluid into the pleural space through trans-

Table 6 Diagnoses Associated with Pleural Fluid Acidosis (pH <7.30) and Low Glucose Concentration (<60 mg/dL or PF/S <0.5)

Diagnosis	pH Range (incidence)	Glucose range concentration (mg/dL)
Complicated parapneumonic effusion/empyema	5.50–7.29 (~100%)	0–40
Esophageal rupture	5.50–7.00 (~100% by 48 hr)	20–59
Rheumatoid pleurisy	6.80–7.10 (80%)	0–30
Malignancy	6.95–7.29 (33%)	30–59
Tuberculous pleurisy	7.00–7.29 (20%)	30–59
Lupus pleuritis	7.00–7.29 (20%)	30–59

diaphragmatic defects (86,87), movement of fluid through a fistulous tract between a pseudocyst and the pleural space (80), and retroperitoneal movement into the mediastinum creating mediastinitis and eventual rupture into the pleural cavity (88,89). Pleural fluid amylase increases in concentration because of impaired lymphatic pleural space drainage; this mechanism in combination with more rapid clearance of amylase by the kidney is the explanation for the pleural fluid/serum amylase ratio being >1.0.

The pleural fluid amylase may be normal in the early phase of pancreatitis but increases over time (77). In chronic pancreatitis, the pleural fluid amylase is always elevated and may reach extremely high levels, often >100,000 IU/L (81). Serum amylase may be elevated due to back-effusion from the pleural space or may be normal (90).

Approximately 10–14% of patients with a malignant pleural effusion present with an increased pleural fluid amylase concentration (77,79,82,91). Isoenzyme analysis of these amylase-rich malignant pleural effusions demonstrate that most of the amylase is of the salivary type (77,79,82). The most common malignancy causing a salivary amylase–rich pleural effusion is adenocarcinoma of the lung, with adenocarcinoma of the ovary being the next most frequent (79,82). Other types of lung cancer, as well as lymphoma and leukemia, have also been associated with a salivary-like amylase–rich pleural effusion (79,82). Clinically, the finding of a salivary isoamylase–rich effusion makes it highly likely that the effusion is due to malignancy in the absence of esophageal rupture. Statistically, the tumor is most likely to be an adenocarcinoma of the lung and not mesothelioma, as the latter tumor has not been reported to be associated with a high salivary amylase level.

Adenosine Deaminase

Adenosine deaminase (ADA), an enzyme important in the degradation of purines, is required for lymphoid cell differentiation and is involved in monocyte-macrophage maturation. Pleural fluid/serum ADA ratios of >1 have been observed in tuberculous pleurisy, rheumatoid pleurisy, and empyema, while other exudates have similar ADA levels in pleural fluid and serum (92). Furthermore, effusions from patients with tuberculous pleurisy, rheumatoid pleurisy, and empyema have higher ADA activity than other exudates and congestive heart failure. Pleural fluid ADA levels above 70 U/L are highly suggestive of tuberculous pleuritis, while levels below 40 U/L make the diagnosis unlikely (93,94). However, patients with rheumatoid pleuritis may have pleural fluid ADA levels exceeding 70 U/L (95), and high levels have also been found in empyema, lymphoma, and leukemia (96). Recent data suggest that the determination of ADA isoenzymes enhances the diagnostic utility of ADA activity. In tuberculous effusions, ADA2 probably reflecting monocyte/macrophage origin is responsible for increased ADA content in contrast to ADA1, which originates from lymphocyte or neutrophil turnover, and causes the increased ADA in parapneumonic effusions (97).

Cytological Examination

Pleural fluid cytological examination has a positive diagnostic yield in 40–90% of patients with pleural malignancy (98,99). An important reason for the variability in diagnostic yield is that the effusion may be paramalignant (100). Paramalignant effusions are effusions associated with malignancy but are not due to pleural involvement with tumor. These effusions are due to local effects of the tumor (obstructive atelectasis or pneumonia and impaired lymphatic drainage of the pleural space), systemic effects (pulmonary embolism), and results of therapy (radiation). Other explanations for the variability in cytological diagnosis are tumor type, high positivity with adenocarcinoma and low with Hodgkin's disease (101), the number of specimens submitted (yields tend to increase with additional specimens due to exfoliation of fresher cells), and the interest and expertise of the cytopathologist (102).

Many serous samples have the tendency to clot, making cytological examination problematic. Pleural fluid should be placed immediately into sterile containers with an anticoagulant; heparin (200 units) is a satisfactory anticoagulant for up to 20 mL of pleural fluid. Although it is preferable to examine the pleural fluid cells immediately, delay of up to 24 hours generally is not deleterious provided there is no bacterial contamination. The cells in bloody fluid tend to show more rapid deterioration than those in serous fluids (103). The volume of pleural fluid submitted for cytological evaluation is probably not critical, as a few milliliters will have a diagnostic value similar to 1000 mL.

References

1. Sahn SA. The pleura. Am Rev Respir Dis 1988; 138:184–234.
2. Collins TR, Sahn SA. Thoracentesis: complications, patient experience and diagnostic value. Chest 1987; 91:811–817.
3. Sahn SA. Diagnostic value of pleural fluid analysis. Clin Chest Med 1995; 16: 269–278.
4. Good JT Jr, King TE, Antony VB, Sahn SA. Lupus pleuritis: clinical features in pleural fluid characteristics with special reference to pleural fluid anti-nuclear antibodies. Chest 1983; 84:714–718.
5. Epler GR, McLoud TC, Gaensler EA. Prevalence and incidence of benign asbestos pleural effusion in a working population. JAMA 1982; 247:617–622.
6. Estenne M, Yernault JC, De Troyer A. Mechanism of relief of dyspnea after thoracentesis in patients with large pleural effusions. Am J Med 1983; 74:813–819.
7. Anthonisen NR, Martin RR. Regional lung function in pleural effusion. Am Rev Respir Dis 1977; 116:201–207.
8. Sahn SA, Heffner JE. Approach to the patient with pleurisy. In: Kelley WN, ed. Textbook of Internal Medicine. 2d ed. Philadelphia: JB Lippincott Co, 1991: 1887–1890.
9. Morelock SY, Sahn SA. Drugs and the pleura. Chest 1999; 116:212–221.
10. Hopkins HU. Principles and Methods of Physical Diagnosis. 3rd ed. Philadelphia: W.B. Saunders, 1965:202 230.

11. Maher GG, Berger HW. Massive pleural effusions: malignant and non-malignant causes in 46 patients. Am Rev Respir Dis 1972; 105:458–460.
12. Liberson M. Diagnostic significance of the mediastinal profile in massive unilateral pleural effusions. Am Rev Respir Dis 1963; 88:176–180.
13. Heller RM, Janower ML, Weber AL. The radiological manifestations of malignant pleural mesothelioma. Am J Roentgenol 1970; 108:53–59.
14. Rabin CB, Blackman NS. Bilateral pleural effusion. Its significance in association with a heart of normal size. J Mt Sinai Hosp 1957; 24:45–53.
15. Roberts PP. Parasitic infections of the pleural space. Semin Respir Infect 1988; 3:362–382.
16. Miller KS, Tomlinson JR, Sahn SA. Pleuropulmonary complications of enteral tube feedings. Two reports, review of the literature, and recommendations. Chest 1985; 88:230–233.
17. Ellis LM, Vogel SB, Copeland EM. Central venous catheter vascular erosions. Diagnosis and clinical course. Ann Surg 1989; 209:475–478.
18. Nosanchuk JS, Naylor B. A unique cytologic picture in pleural fluid from patients with rheumatoid arthritis. Am J Clin Pathol 1968; 50:330–335.
19. Stark DD, Shanes JG, Baron RL, Roach DD. Biochemical features of urinothorax. Arch Intern Med 1982; 42:1509–1511.
20. Light RW, MacGregor MI, Luchinger PC, Ball WC. Pleural effusions: the diagnostic separation of transudates and exudates. Ann Intern Med 1972; 77:507–513.
21. Heffner JE, Brown LK, Barbieri C. Diagnostic value of tests that discriminate between exudative and transudative pleural effusions. Chest 1997; 111:970–979.
22. Joseph J, Badrinath P, Basran G, Sahn SA. Is the pleural fluid transudate or exudate? A revisit of the diagnostic criteria. Thorax 2001; 56:867–870.
23. Hamm H, Brohan U, Bohmer R, Missmahl HP. Cholesterol in pleural effusions: a diagnostic aid. Chest 1987; 92:296–302.
24. Costa M, Quiroga T, Cruz E. Measurement of pleural fluid cholesterol and lactate dehydrogenase. A simple and accurate set of indicators for separating exudates from transudates. Chest 1995; 108:1260–1263.
25. Gil Suay V, Martinez Moragon E, Cases Viedma E, Perpina Tordera M, Leon Fabregas M, Sanchis Aldas J. Pleural cholesterol in differentiating transudates and exudates. A prospective study of 232 cases. Respiration 1995; 62:57–63.
26. Winterbauer RH, Riggins RCK, Griesman FA, Bauermeister DE. Pleuropulmonary manifestations of Waldenstrom's macroglobulinemia. Chest 1974; 66:368–375.
27. Rodriguez JN, Pereira A, Martinez JC, Conde J, Pujol E. Pleural effusion in multiple myeloma. Chest 1994; 105:622–624.
28. Horwitz ML, Schiff M, Samuels J, Russo R, Schnader J. *Pneumocystis carinii* pleural effusion. Pathogenesis and pleural fluid analysis. Am Rev Respir Dis 1993; 148:232–234.
29. Light RW, Girard WM, Jenkinson SG, George RB. Parapneumonic effusions. Am J Med 1980; 69:507–511.
30. Potts DE, Levin DC, Sahn SA. Pleural fluid pH in parapneumonic effusions. Chest 1976; 70:328–331.
31. Pettersson T, Klockars M, Helmstrom PE. Chemical and immunological features of pleural effusions: comparison between rheumatoid arthritis and other diseases. Thorax 1982; 37:354–361.

32. Johnson JR, Falk A, Iber C, Davies S. Paragonimiasis in the United States. A report of nine cases in Hmong immigrants. Chest 1982; 82:168–171.
33. Light RW, Erozan YS, Ball WC Jr. Cells in pleural fluid: their value and differential diagnosis. Arch Intern Med 1973; 132:854–860.
34. Light RW. Pleural Diseases. 3rd ed. Baltimore: Williams & Wilkins, 1995:36–74.
35. Berger HW, Mejia E. Tuberculous pleurisy. Chest 1973; 63:88–92.
36. Pettersson T, Riska H. Diagnostic value of total and differential leukocyte counts in pleural effusions. Acta Med Scand 1981; 210:129–135.
37. Antony VB, Repine JE, Sahn SA. Experimental models of inflammation in the pleural space. In: Chretein J, Bignon N, Hirsch A, eds. The Pleura in Health and Disease. New York: Marcel Dekker, 1985:253–266.
38. Antony VB, Godbey SW, Kunkel SL, Hott JW, Hartman D, Burdick MD, Strieter M. Recruitment of inflammatory cells to the pleural space. Chemotactic cytokines, IL-8, and monocyte chemotactic peptide-1 in human pleural fluids. J Immunol 1993; 151:7216–7223.
39. Broaddus VC, Hebert CA, Vitangcol RV, Hoeffel JM, Bernstein MS, Boylan AM. Interleukin-8 as a major neutrophil chemotactic factor in the pleural liquid of patients with empyema. Am Rev Respir Dis 1992; 146:825–830.
40. Antony VB, Sahn SA, Antony AC, Repine JE. Bacillus Calmette-Guerin-stimulated neutrophils release chemotaxins for monocytes in rabbit pleural spaces and in vitro. J Clin Invest 1985; 76:1514–1521.
41. Yam LT. Diagnostic significance of lymphocytes in pleural effusion. Ann Intern Med 1967; 66:972–982.
42. Nordkild P, Kromann-Andersen H, Struve-Christiansen E. Yellow nail syndrome—the triad of yellow nails, lymphedema, and pleural effusion. Acta Med Scand 1986; 219:221–227.
43. Sahn SA, Kaplan RL, Maulitz RM, Good JT Jr. Rheumatoid pleurisy. Observation on the development of low pleural fluid pH and glucose levels. Arch Intern Med 1980; 140:1237–1238.
44. Nicholls AJ, Friend JAR, Legge JS. Sarcoid pleural effusions: three cases and review of the literature. Thorax 1980; 35:277–281.
45. Doelken P, Sahn SA. Trapped lung. Sem Respir Crit Care Med 2001; 22:631–635.
46. Yoffey JM, Cortice FC. Lymphatics, Lymph, and Lymphoid Tissue. Cambridge: Harvard University Press, 1956:323–390.
47. Judson MA, Handy JR, Sahn SA. Pleural effusion from acute lung rejection. Chest 1997; 111:1128–1130.
48. Scharer L, McClemant JH. Isolation of tubercle bacilli from needle biopsy specimens of parietal pleura. Am Rev Respir Dis 1968; 97:466–468.
49. Levine H, Metzger W, Lacera D, Kay L. Diagnosis of tuberculous pleurisy by culture of pleural biopsy specimen. Arch Intern Med 1970; 126:269–271.
50. Nakamura Y, Ozaki T, Yanagawa H, Yasuoka A, Ogura T. Eosinophil colony-stimulating factor induced by administration of interleukin-2 into the pleural cavity of patients with malignant pleurisy. Am Rev Respir Cell Mol Biol 1990; 3:230–291.
51. Askin FB, McCann BG, Kuhn C. Reactive eosinophilic pleuritis. Arch Pathol Lab Med 1997; 101:187–191.
52. Spriggs AI, Boddington MM. The Cytology of Effusions. 2d ed. New York: Grune & Stratton, 1986.

53. Maltais F, Laberge F, Cormier Y. Blood hypereosinophilia in the course of post-traumatic pleural effusion. Chest 1990; 98:348–351.
54. Mattson S-B. Monosymptomatic exudative pleurisy in persons exposed to asbestos dust. Scand J Respir Dis 1975; 56:263–272.
55. Hillerdal G, Ozesmi M. Benign asbestos pleural effusion: 73 exudates in 60 patients. Eur J Respir Dis 1987; 71:113–121.
56. Adelman M, Albelda SM, Gottlieb J, Haponik EF. Diagnostic utility of pleural fluid eosinophilia. Am J Med 1984; 77:915–920.
57. Rubins JB, Rubins HB. Etiology and prognostic significance of eosinophilic pleural effusions. A prospective study. Chest 1996; 110:1271.
58. Martinez-Garcia MA, Cases-Viedma E, Cordero-Rodriguez PJ, Hidalgo-Ramirez, Perpina-Tordera M, Sanchis-Moret F, Sanchis-Aidas JL. Diagnostic utility of eosinophils in the pleural fluid. Eur Respir J 2000; 15:166–169.
59. Hurwitz S, Leiman G, Shapiro C. Mesothelial cells in pleural fluid: TB or not TB? South African Med J 1980; 57:937–939.
60. Sahn SA. Pleural fluid pH in the normal state and in diseases affecting the pleural space. In: Chretien J, Bignon N, Hirsch A, eds. The Pleura in Health and Disease. New York: Marcel Dekker, 1985:253–266.
61. Sahn SA. Pathogenesis and clinical features of diseases associated with a low pleural fluid glucose. In: Chretien J, Bignon N, Hirsch A, eds. The Pleura in Health and Disease. New York: Marcel Dekker, 1985:267–285.
62. Good JT Jr, Taryle DA, Maulitz RM, Kaplan RL, Sahn SA. The diagnostic value of pleural fluid pH. Chest 1980; 78:55–59.
63. Heffner JE, Brown LK, Barbieri C, DeLeo JM. Pleural fluid chemical analysis in parapneumonic effusions. A meta-analysis. Am J Respir Crit Care Med 1995; 151:1700–1708.
64. Colice GL, Curtis A, Deslauriers J, Heffner JE, Light R, Littenberg B, Sahn SA, Weinstein RA, Yusen RD. Medical and surgical treatment of parapneumonic effusions. Chest 2000; 118:1158–1171.
65. Potts DE, Taryle DA, Sahn SA. The glucose-pH relationship in parapneumonic effusions. Arch Intern Med 1978; 138:1378–1380.
66. Sahn SA, Good JT Jr. Pleural fluid pH in malignant effusions. Diagnostic, prognostic and therapeutic implications. Ann Intern Med 1988; 108:345–349.
67. Rodriguez-Panadero F, Lopez-Mejias J. Low glucose and pH levels in malignant pleural effusions. Diagnostic significance and prognostic value in respect to pleurodesis. Am Rev Respir Dis 1989; 139:663–667.
68. Rodriguez-Panadero F, Lopez-Mejias J. Survival time of patients with pleural metastatic carcinoma predicted by glucose and pH studies. Chest 1989; 95:320–324.
69. Heffner JE, Nietert PJ, Barbieri C. Pleural fluid pH as a predictor of survival for patients with malignant pleural effusions. Chest 2000; 117:79–86.
70. Heffner JE, Nietert PJ, Barbieri C. Pleural fluid pH as a predictor of pleurodesis failure. Chest 2000; 117:87–95.
71. Sahn SA, Wilkox ML, Good JT Jr, Potts DE, Filley GF. Characteristics of normal rabbit pleural fluid: physiologic and biochemical implications. Lung 1979; 156:63–69.
72. Sahn SA, Reller LB, Taryle DA, Antony VB, Good JT Jr. The contribution of leukocytes and bacteria to the low pH of empyema fluid. Am Rev Respir Dis 1983; 128:811–815.

73. Good JT Jr, Taryle DA, Sahn SA. The pathogenesis of low glucose, low pH malignant effusions. Am Rev Respir Dis 1985; 131:737–741.
74. Carr DT, McGuckin WF. Pleural fluid glucose. Am Rev Respir Dis 1968; 97:302–305.
75. Taryle DA, Good JT Jr, Sahn SA. Acid generation by pleural fluid: possible role in the determination of pleural fluid pH. J Lab Clin Med 1979; 93:1041–1046.
76. Good JT Jr, Antony VB, Reller RB, Molitz RM, Sahn SA. The pathogenesis of the low pleural fluid pH in esophageal rupture. Am Rev Respir Dis 1983; 127:702–704.
77. Light RW, Ball WC. Glucose and amylase in pleural effusions. JAMA 1973; 225:257–260.
78. Kaye MD. Pleuropulmonary complications of pancreatitis. Thorax 1968; 23:297–306.
79. Joseph J, Viney S, Beck P, Strange C, Sahn SA, Basran GS. A prospective study of amylase-rich pleural effusion with special reference to amylase isoenzyme analysis. Chest 1992; 102:1455–1459.
80. Rockey DC, Cello JP. Pancreaticopleural fistula: a report of 7 cases and review of the literature. Medicine 1990; 69:332–344.
81. Ende N. Studies of amylase activity in pleural effusions and ascites. Cancer 1960; 13:283–287.
82. Kramer MR, Sepero RJ, Pitchenik AE. High amylase in neoplasm-related pleural effusions. Ann Intern Med 1989; 110:567–569.
83. Abbott OA, Mansour KA, Logan WD Jr, Hatcher CR Jr, Symbas PN. Atraumatic so-called "spontaneous" rupture of the esophagus. A review of 47 personal cases with comments on a new method of surgical therapy. J Thorac Cardiovasc Surg 1970; 59:67–83.
84. Sherr HP, Light RW, Merson MH, Wolf RO, Taylor LL, Hendrix TR. Origin of pleural fluid amylase in esophageal rupture. Ann Intern Med 1972; 76:985–986.
85. Maulitz RM, Good JT Jr, Kaplan RL, et al. The pleuropulmonary consequence of esophageal rupture: an experimental model. Am Rev Respir Dis 1979; 120:363–367.
86. Perry TT. Role of lymphatic vessels in the transmission of lipase in disseminated pancreatic lymphatic necrosis. Arch Pathol 1947; 43:456–465.
87. Dumont AE, Doubilet H, Mulholand JH. Lymphatic pathways of pancreatic secretion in man. Ann Surg 1960; 153:403–409.
88. Camaro JL. Chronic pancreatic ascites in pancreatic pleural effusions. Gastroenterology 1978; 74:134–140.
89. Tombroff M, Loick A, Dekoster JP, Englehorn L, Govarerts JP. Pleural effusions with pancreatico-pleural fistula. Br Med J 1973; 1:330–331.
90. Lueng AKC. Pancreatic pleural effusion with normal serum amylase levels. J Royal Soc Med 1985; 78:698.
91. Buckler H, Honeybourne D. Raised pleural fluid amylase level as an aid in the diagnosis of adenocarcinoma of the lung. Br J Clin Pract 1984; 38:359–361, 371.
92. Pettersson T, Kaarina O, Weber TH. Adenosine deaminase in the diagnosis of pleural effusions. Acta Med Scand 1984; 215:299–304.
93. Ocana I, Martinez-Vazquez JM, Segura RM, Fernandez-De-Sevilla T, Capdevila JA. Adenosine deaminase in pleural fluids. Test for diagnosis of tuberculous pleural effusion. Chest 1983; 84:51–53.
94. Fontan Bueso J, Verea Hernando H, Garcia-Buela JP, Dominguez Juncal L,

Martin Egana MT, Montero Martinez MZ. Diagnostic value of simultaneous determination of pleural adenosine deaminase and pleural lysozyme/serum lysozyme ratio pleural effusions. Chest 1988; 93:303–307.
95. Ocana I, Ribera E, Martinez-Vazquez JM, Ruiz I, Bejarano E, Pigrau C, Pahissa A. Adenosine deaminase activity in rheumatoid pleural effusion. Ann Rheum Dis 1988; 47:394–397.
96. Ungerer JP, Grobler SM. Molecular forms of adenosine deaminase in pleural effusions. Enzyme 1988; 40:7–13.
97. Ungerer JP, Oosthuizen HM, Retief JH, Bissbort SH. Significance of adenosine deaminase activity and its isoenzymes in tuberculous effusions. Chest 1994; 106:33–37.
98. Grunze H. The comparative diagnostic accuracy, efficacy, and specificity of cytologic techniques used in the diagnosis of malignant neoplasm and serous effusions of the pleuroperitoneal cavities. Acta Cytol 1964; 8:150–164.
99. Jarvi OH, Kunnas RJ, Laitio MT, Tyrkko JES. The accuracy and significance of cytologic cancer diagnosis of pleural effusions. Acta Cytol 1972; 16:152–157.
100. Sahn SA. Malignant pleural effusions. Semin Respir Med 1987; 9:43–53.
101. Naylor B, Schmidt RW. The case for exfoliate cytology of serous effusions. Lancet 1964; 1:711–712.
102. Melamed MR. The cytological presentation of malignant lymphomas and related diseases and effusions. Cancer 1963; 16:413–431.
103. Johnson WD. The cytological diagnosis of cancer in serous effusions. Acta Cytol 1966; 10:161–172.

17

Transudative Pleural Effusions

PAULA CARVALHO

University of Washington
Seattle, Washington
and VA Medical Center
Boise, Idaho, U.S.A.

I. Introduction

Pleural fluid accumulation occurs as a consequence of several physiological factors that influence pleural fluid formation or absorption. Pleural effusions develop whenever the rate of pleural fluid accumulation in the pleural space exceeds the rate of reabsorption. Pleural effusions are generally classified as exudative or transudative (1). The following criteria are used to characterize transudative pleural effusions:

1. The ratio of the pleural fluid to the serum protein level is less than 0.5.
2. The ratio of the pleural fluid to the serum LDH level is less than 0.6.
3. The absolute level of the pleural fluid LDH level is less than 200 IU/L.

Light et al. determined that any pleural effusion that meets all of the above criteria is classified as a transudate (2,3). In general, transudative pleural effusions signify that the pleural membranes are normal.

Transudation of liquid across the capillary membrane occurs due to an increase in transcapillary hydrostatic pressure and/or a decrease in intracapillary oncotic pressure. The most common cause of transudative pleural effusions is an increase in pulmonary capillary hydrostatic pressure, which occurs with congestive heart failure. In this situation, edema fluid filters through the visceral pleura and into the pleural space (4–6). Other transudates, such as those associated with atelectasis, develop due to a localized decrease in intrapleural pressure that assists fluid filtration in the pleural space. Transudative effusions also form in patients with hypoalbuminemia due to cirrhosis or nephrotic syndrome because the plasma oncotic pressure is reduced (7). In this case, the hydrostatic pressures within the pleural capillaries may be normal, but the oncotic pressure gradient is decreased. Some transudates develop due to a decrease in fluid exit rate from the pleural space, such as in superior vena cava obstruction. In hepatic hydrothorax and peritoneal dialysis, transudative effusions form due to migration of fluid along a pressure gradient from the peritoneal space, through macroscopic or microscopic diaphragmatic defects, and into the pleural space. Lymphatic obstruction may also lead to pleural fluid formation, which may be transudative or exudative in nature (8).

II. Causes of Transudative Pleural Effusions

A. Congestive Heart Failure

Congestive heart failure accounts for approximately 90% of all transudates (9). Although pleural effusions associated with congestive heart failure can appear at any age, they are more frequently present in patients who are middle-aged and older (10,11). The majority of patients with decompensated congestive heart failure will have a pleural effusion. Logue and colleagues (12) reported an incidence of 58% in patients with left ventricular failure, whereas an autopsy series by Race et al. (13) reported a 72% incidence of pleural effusion with volumes exceeding 250 mL.

Pleural effusions associated with congestive heart failure are most often bilateral, with an incidence of 88% in the autopsy series of 250 patients reported by Race and colleagues (13). Race and coworkers also measured the volume of pleural fluid and found a mean value of 1084 mL in the right pleural space and 913 mL in the left, possibly due to the difference in size of the pleural cavities. In the same study, 35 patients had unilateral effusion, but concurrent pulmonary emboli or pneumonia were present in approximately half of these. It is important to note, however, that further evaluation is merited in patients who have bilateral pleural effusions without cardiomegaly. In one series of 78 patients reported by Rabin et al. (14), only 4% had effusions due to congestive heart failure (Table 1).

In patients with unilateral effusion, right-sided effusions tend to be present in twice as many patients as left-sided effusions (12,13,15,16). The right-sided predilection of pleural effusions in patients with heart failure, though, was disputed by Peterman and Speicher (17). In a review of 55 records of patients with congestive heart failure and documented transudative pleural effusion, 19 patients had equal bilateral effusions, whereas 18 had predominantly right-sided

Table 1 Etiology of Transudative Pleural Effusions

Congestive heart failure
Hepatic hydrothorax
Nephrotic syndrome
Peritoneal dialysis
Fontan operation
Urinothorax
Superior vena caval obstruction
Atelectasis
Misplaced central line
Pericardial disease[a]
Myxedema[a]
Pulmonary emboli[a]
Malignancy[a]
Sarcoid[a]
Amyloidosis[a]

---
[a] Effusion may be transudative or exudative.

and 17 had predominantly left-sided effusions. In patients with left pleural effusions, congestive heart failure associated with pericardial disease is more common (16,18).

Pleural effusions can occur with biventricular failure, as well as with separate left and right heart failure, and the mechanisms may be multifactorial. In a dog model, Mellins et al. (19) found that biventricular decompensation predisposed to pleural effusions. In this study, they elevated systemic and pulmonary venous pressures (well above physiological values) separately or together and studied the rate of pleural fluid accumulation with each condition. They determined that a much larger amount of pleural fluid formed with the condition of systemic venous hypertension than with left atrial hypertension and, under these extreme conditions, found that that lymphatic flow was unable to provide effective drainage of the pleural cavity. There have been other studies, however, indicating that the transudative effusions caused by congestive heart failure originate from the capillary circulation of the lungs and form as a result of leakage of edema fluid from the pulmonary interstitium across the visceral pleura and into the pleural space (4–6,8).

In a model using sheep lungs isolated in situ, Broaddus et al. (5) found that volume loading resulted in an increase in fluid transudation across the lung and into the pleural space. The protein concentration in the resultant pleural effusion was the same as that in the lung lymph and in the interstitial lung edema. The total volume of pleural fluid comprised approximately 25% of all edema formed in the lung. In a study by Allen et al. (4) utilizing an intact sheep model of high-pressure pulmonary edema, left atrial hypertension resulted in pleural fluid formation, but only after pulmonary edema had developed. Accordingly, patients with congestive heart failure are more likely to have a pleural effusion if pulmonary edema is present (20).

The diagnosis of pleural effusion due to heart failure is generally made clinically, as these patients will manifest features such as dyspnea, orthopnea, peripheral edema, distended neck veins, nocturia, and an S3 ventricular gallop. The heart is almost always enlarged on chest x-ray, although the effusion can obscure the true degree of cardiomegaly (14). Sometimes pleural fluid localizes into an interlobar fissure, mainly in the right horizontal fissure, and may have the radiographic appearance of a mass (21), which disappears after treatment of heart failure and resorption of the pleural fluid (22).

Once a pleural effusion is suspected of being associated with congestive heart failure, the initial decision is whether or not to perform thoracentesis. It is recommended that thoracentesis be performed in patients with heart failure and a pleural effusion in cases when the effusion is unilateral or when bilateral effusions differ in size and when cardiomegaly is absent (23). Additionally, thoracentesis should always be performed if fever or other manifestations of infection are present, if pleuritic pain is present, or if malignancy is suspected. If the above features are not present, then thoracentesis can be deferred and performed only if the effusion does not respond to treatment of heart failure. Treatment of patients with congestive heart failure includes diuresis, afterload reduction, and inotropes as appropriate. Once congestive heart failure is compensated, pleural effusions generally resolve. Transudative effusions tend to have low total protein concentrations, on the order of <2.9 g/dL. However, acute diuresis in congestive heart failure can elevate protein levels into the exudative range. Accordingly, the pleural fluid in patients with congestive heart failure meets exudative criteria in approximately 20% of cases (24). Therefore, when a pleural effusion meets exudative criteria in a patient with a clinically suspected transudate, the difference between the serum and pleural fluid albumin levels can be measured to further assist in the differentiation. Burgess et al. (24) found that if this difference exceeds 1.2 g/dL, then the effusion is likely to be due a transudative effusion due to heart failure.

In patients with marked dyspnea, removal of pleural fluid by thoracentesis may improve breathing, although the degree of dyspnea does not necessarily correlate with the size of the effusion (25). In some cases, however, pleural effusions may persist despite optimal management of congestive heart failure. If dyspnea is relieved by therapeutic thoracentesis, consideration should be given to pleurodesis (26), although this may not be effective in all cases. Some patients with congestive heart failure and pleural effusions who have undergone pleurodesis, pleural fluid has not reaccumulated, but accumulation of fluid has occurred in other body cavities (27). For this reason pleurodesis should be used only as a last option in patients with congestive heart failure and intractable pleural effusions.

B. Pericardial Disease

Plum et al. (28) reviewed 35 patients with constrictive pericarditis and found a 60% incidence of pleural effusion. In a series of 124 patients, Weiss and Spodick (18) found that 35 (28%) had a pleural effusion. Of these, 21 (60%) were left-sided, 2 (5%) were right-sided, and the remaining 12 (35%) were bilateral.

Although there is a high incidence of pleural effusion associated with pericardial disease, the mechanism responsible for the accumulation of pleural fluid is not clear. The pleural effusion is thought to form because of congestive heart failure. If sufficiently severe, liver involvement may also occur, with subsequent development of hypoproteinemia, which may further contribute to the formation of pleural fluid (29). The elevation of pulmonary and systemic capillary pressures due to constrictive pericardial disease is thought to be the mechanism responsible for formation of transudative effusions. This phenomenon, however, does not explain the predominance of unilateral, rather than bilateral effusions in patients with inflammatory pericardial disease. Effusions accompanying inflammatory pericardial disease are predominantly left-sided, therefore, it is likely that extension of the inflammatory process to the adjacent pleura accounts for the development of pleural effusion (18).

C. Hepatic Hydrothorax

A transudative pleural effusion occurs in patients with hepatic cirrhosis with a frequency of approximately 6% (30,31). In an autopsy study of 600 cases, 1% of all pleural effusions was attributed to cirrhosis, and the frequency of pleural effusions increased with more advanced stages of cirrhosis (32). The majority of patients with hepatic hydrothorax have ascites, although pleural effusions have been reported in patients with clinically undetected ascites (33) as well as in patients with no evidence of ascites at autopsy (34). In these patients with hepatic hydrothorax in the absence of ascites, it is presumed that the ascitic fluid moves almost entirely to the pleural space due to pressure gradients (35).

There are no lymphatic connections between the peritoneal and pleural spaces (36). Therefore, the accepted mechanism for the development of hepatic hydrothorax in a patient with cirrhosis and ascites is thought to be the movement of ascitic fluid from the peritoneal to the pleural cavity through diaphragmatic defects (37). Other factors, such as azygos vein hypertension and hypoalbuminemia, are thought to be secondary (38). There is a significant amount of evidence for the presence and function of diaphragmatic defects. These have been identified in patients by intraperitoneal injection of ^{99m}Tc sulfur colloid followed by gamma scanning (39) or by methylene blue injected into the peritoneal cavity (40). Injection of ^{99m}Tc albumin aggregates into the peritoneal or pleural cavities in a patient with cirrhosis and LeVeen shunt showed that the flow of fluid is unidirectional from the abdomen to the pleural space (35). Lieberman and colleagues (41) introduced 0.5–1 L of air into the peritoneal cavity of five patients with cirrhosis, ascites, and pleural effusion. All patients developed a pneumothorax within 48 hours. Diaphragmatic defects have also been identified at thoracoscopy (42) or at autopsy (30,34,41) in patients with ascites and pleural effusion. It has been suggested, therefore, that diaphragmatic defects may be the result of diaphragmatic blebs that stretched and ruptured due to increased abdominal pressure (43). These blebs were likely formed from evagination of the peritoneum through a congenital diaphragmatic defect; the pressure of the ascites then separated the collagen fibers of the diaphragm leading to the evagination of the serosa into the thoracic cavity (30). Postmortem microscopic examination of the diaphragm has shown separation of the collagen bundles, producing a defect lined with a single layer of mesothelial cells which is continuous with the peritoneal and pleural linings (34).

The pleural effusions associated with cirrhosis and ascites can be quite large and occupy the entire hemithorax and can rapidly reaccumulate (44), as the diaphragmatic defects previously discussed allow fluid movement from the peritoneal cavity to the pleural space until the until the pleural and peritoneal pressures are equivalent. The right diaphragmatic system is larger and more developed than the left, which may explain the predominance of right-sided effusions (approximately 2/3) in patients with hepatic hydrothorax (40). Bilateral effusions are present in 16% of patients, and left-sided effusions account for another 16% (31,41). The pleural fluid protein concentration is low, and is most frequently consistent with a transudate. Exudative (45) or bloody (46) effusions are rare. In rare cases, the pleural fluid in hepatic hydrothorax can become secondarily infected either by hematogenous or contiguous spread of organisms, and empyema may develop (47,48).

Large transudative pleural effusions have also been reported in patients following liver transplant (49). These effusions were more common on the right side, developed 3–7 days after transplant, and were not associated with cardiopulmonary disease. Some patients developed transient ascites before detection of pleural fluid in the immediate postoperative period. The mechanism responsible for the accumulation of pleural fluid was presumed to be related to the subdiaphragmatic dissection performed during surgery (49).

In order to diagnose hepatic hydrothorax, paracentesis and thoracentesis should be done to confirm that the ascites and pleural fluid are both transudative. The pleural fluid protein concentration, as previously mentioned, is low, but is usually higher than that in the ascites fluid (41). An elevated polymorphonuclear cell count (>500 cells/μL) may suggest the presence of infection and the diagnosis of spontaneous bacterial pleuritis in conjunction with, or in the absence of, spontaneous bacterial peritonitis needs to be considered (47,48).

Management of hepatic hydrothorax should address treatment of ascites with diuresis, low sodium intake, and proper nutrition. The pleural pressures in patients with transudative pleural effusions resulting from ascites are higher than those in patients with other transudative effusions (50). Evacuation of pleural fluid should be avoided unless severe dyspnea is present due to a large pleural effusion, because it can further increase hypoproteinemia and tends to rapidly reaccumulate if ascites is present (44). Of note, when tube thoracostomy is performed, the volume of ascites can rapidly decrease and lead to hypovolemia with hemodynamic compromise (44), and, therefore, patients should be carefully monitored if thoracentesis is performed.

If conservative measures with dietary modification and diuresis are not effective, a transjugular intrahepatic portal-systemic shunt (TIPS) should be considered, as this may effectively manage hepatic hydrothorax in many, although not all, patients. Gordon and colleagues (51) reported a series of 24 patients with refractory hepatic hydrothorax treated with a TIPS procedure and found that 5 (21%) developed worsening hepatic function and died within 45 days. These patients who do not respond to TIPS are likely best treated with liver transplant.

For those patients who are not candidates for TIPS or liver transplant, surgical closure of the diaphragmatic defects followed by talc insufflation should be considered, as reported by Mouroux and colleagues (42). Pleurodesis via tube thoracostomy can also be considered, with careful attention to potential hemodynamic compromise from pleural fluid shifts, using intrapleural doxycycline or talc (23). In most cases, pleurodesis with a sclerosing agent can be performed without damaging the bowel (35). In patients with hepatic hydrothorax, the insertion of a peritoneo-jugular shunt is not effective due to the fact that the pleural pressure is lower than the central venous pressure (23).

D. Nephrotic Syndrome

Nephrotic syndrome is characterized by proteinuria, edema, and hypoproteinemia and is associated with a high incidence of pleural effusion (52,53). In a series of 52 patients with nephrotic syndrome, 21% had pleural effusions. These effusions were generally bilateral and frequently in a subpulmonic location (52). In nephrotic syndrome, pleural effusions have a low protein concentration, and fluid accumulates in the pleural space because of a decreased albumin concentration in plasma (usually <25 g/L) and, therefore, a decreased plasma oncotic pressure. Also, hydrostatic pressure may be increased in nephrotic syndrome due to hypervolemia from sodium retention, which can further assist with pleural fluid formation (54).

Patients with nephrotic syndrome and pleural effusion should undergo both a diagnostic thoracentesis and evaluation for pulmonary embolism, since the incidence of thromboembolic disease is high and pleural effusions due to pulmonary embolism can be both transudative or exudative. In one series of 36 patients with nephrotic syndrome, 22% had pulmonary emboli (53).

Management of pleural effusion associated with the nephrotic syndrome should focus on increasing the level of serum protein by decreasing renal protein loss. Repetitive thoracenteses should not be performed because, despite its low protein concentration, hypoproteinemia can be aggravated. In patients with respiratory symptoms due to recurrence of effusion, pleurodesis should be considered (55).

E. Peritoneal Dialysis

Acute hydrothorax associated with peritoneal dialysis was first described by Edwards and Unger in 1967 (56) and, shortly thereafter, by Holm et al. in 1971 (57). In a study by Nomoto et al. (58), 1.6% of 3195 patients receiving continuous ambulatory peritoneal dialysis developed a pleural effusion as a result of the dialysate moving from the peritoneal to the pleural cavity through diaphragmatic defects. In this series, the effusion developed within 30 days of initiation of dialysis in 50% of patients, but 18% had been receiving dialysis for over a year prior to development of effusion. The effusions resemble the dialysate but are characterized by a glucose level intermediate between that of the dialysate and the serum, a protein level below 10 g/L, and a low LDH level. The dialysate moves from the peritoneal to the pleural space through diaphragmatic defects. These defects have been identified by injection of methylene blue (59), air (41), or radiolabeled albumin (60) in the peritoneal cavity and observing their passage into the pleural space. The microscopic defects in the diaphragm may rupture due to the large volume of peritoneal dialysate with prolonged dwelling time and increased intra-abdominal pressure. In some patients, the diaphragmatic defects could not be identified, and pleural effusion was postulated to be due to hemodynamic disturbances (61,62). To minimize pleural effusion, it has been suggested that a smaller volume of dialysate be used during each cycle and the patient remain in a sitting or upright position (63). Although the communication closes spontaneously in many patients, thoracotomy for repair of the diaphragmatic defects or pleurodesis can be used (64). Alternatively, thoracoscopic closure of the diaphragmatic defects followed by pleurodesis may be warranted (65).

F. The Fontan Procedure

The Fontan operation is performed for the purpose of bypassing the right ventricle in the case of tricuspid atresia or a univentricular heart. An anastomosis is created between the pulmonary artery and the right atrium, superior or inferior vena cavae, thus directly bypassing the right ventricle. A transudative pleural effusion occurs frequently after surgery, particularly in patients who have a large number of aortopulmonary collateral vessels (66). Pleural effusion can be treated with insertion of a pleuroperitoneal shunt (67) or chemical pleurodesis. In some patients, a surgical fenestration to create a right-to-left shunt is needed (68).

G. Myxedema

Pleural effusions associated with thyroid disease may be exudative or transudative (69). When associated with a pericardial effusion in patients with myxedema, however, effusions are more often transudates. In a series of 25 patients with myxedema and pericardial effusion compiled by Smolar and colleagues (70), 13 (52%) had a concurrent pleural effusion. Effusions can range from small to moderate in size, may be unilateral or bilateral (71), and may be due to increased pleural capillary permeability (72). Although some patients with myxedema have concurrent congestive heart failure, treatment with diuretics and inotropic agents is not useful for resolution of pleural effusion (29). In contrast, thyroid hormone replacement is an effective treatment and results in the disappearance of pleural effusion in these patients.

H. Pulmonary Embolism

Pleural effusions occur in approximately 30–50% of patients with pulmonary emboli (73,74). In many series, however, less than 5% of pleural effusions are attributed to pulmonary embolism (75). It is likely that this discrepancy exists because the diagnosis of pulmonary embolism is not considered in many patients with pleural effusion. The value of pleural fluid analysis in pulmonary thromboembolic disease, however, is limited because the pleural fluid findings are nonspecific. When a paraembolic effusion is present, it is transudative in 25% of patients (76). Transudative effusions are thought to form because of decreased intrapleural pressure or because of increased central venous pressures resulting from obstruction of pulmonary vessels with a consequent elevation of central venous pressure (76). The treatment for a patient with a transudative paraembolic pleural effusion addresses the underlying condition, specifically the treatment of thromboembolic disease with anticoagulation or, if indicated, with thrombolytic therapy.

I. Urinothorax

Urinothorax has been described in patients with hydronephrosis (77), renal calculi (78), blunt trauma (79), and surgical procedures, such as placement of a percutaneous nephrostomy catheter (80). In patients with urinary tract obstruction, the effusions were ipsilateral to the site of obstruction (77,81). Once the urinary tract obstruction is corrected, pleural fluid rapidly disappears (82). In some patients with disruption to the urinary tract, therefore, such as hydronephrosis or ureteral fistula, urine may track up through the retroperitoneum and produce an effusion with low concentrations of protein and glucose, as well as a low pH (54). Although this appears to be the case in most patients with urinothorax, one patient had a pleural fluid concentration of urea nitrogen similar to that of serum, and the effusion was not characteristic of urine, but was instead a transudate due to impaired drainage from the descending transdiaphragmatic lymphatics (83). Retroperitoneal urinomas can extend into the thorax through lymphatic drainage of extravasated urine (77) or by dissection through the peritoneum and movement into the pleural space (82). This clinical finding should be recognized, because it can be present in patients with urinary tract obstruction resulting from a malignant tumor (84).

If urinothorax is suspected, measurement of pleural fluid creatinine (82) or urea (79,84) may be diagnostic. In patients without obstructive uropathy and otherwise normal renal function, the concentration of creatinine in pleural fluid does not exceed that of serum (83). However, with urinothorax, the concentration of creatinine and urea are both higher in pleural fluid than in serum (85,86). Also, radioactive iodine (^{131}I) used to perform nephrograms can show an accumulation of fluid in the pleural space (82). The treatment of urinothorax is generally aimed at correcting the source of urinary tract obstruction, as these effusions then tend to rapidly resolve.

J. Other Causes of Transudative Pleural Effusion

Sarcoidosis

The incidence of pleural effusion with sarcoid is low, on the order of 1–7% (87,88), and is only rarely transudative. The pathogenesis of pleural effusion in patients with sarcoidosis is vascular or lymphatic obstruction (89) or direct pleural involvement (90). The effusions are usually small and unilateral (generally right-sided) in approximately two thirds of cases, although massive effusions have been reported. Javaheri and Hales (89) reported a massive pleural effusion associated with obstruction of the innominate vein. The pleural effusion associated with sarcoidosis may resolve spontaneously in approximately 50% of patients (91) and usually responds well to treatment with corticosteroids (88).

Amyloidosis

Primary amyloidosis of the pleura is rare, although amyloid tumors of the lung and upper respiratory tract have been reported (92,93). Pleural amyloidosis is associated with transudative pleural effusions, but it is thought that these may be related to concurrent congestive heart failure due to myocardial amyloid infiltration (54).

Superior Vena Cava Obstruction

Obstruction of the superior vena cava is a rare cause of pleural effusion (94) and is often iatrogenic, following insertion of central venous or pulmonary arterial catheters (95). It has previously been suggested by Dhande and colleagues (96) that 2-chloroethanol or ethylene oxide residues from gas sterilization of Silastic tubes enhanced thrombosis of the vena cava due to fibrin deposition on the catheters, a finding not present on autoclaved catheters. In patients with obstruction of the superior vena cava by tumor, increased systemic venous pressure can impair resorption of pleural fluid from the parietal pleura. In 30% of cases, fluid collects in the pleural space when the absorptive capacity of the pleural surfaces is overcome (97). With superior vena caval obstruction, the increase in systemic venous pressure leads to increased water filtration from the parietal pleural capillaries, which may impede lymphatic drainage. However, there is evidence to suggest that the site of obstruction is important for pleural fluid formation. For example, in a dog model, ligation of the superior vena cava above the azygous vein did not produce pleural effusions, suggesting that obstruction of both vessels is necessary for the occurrence of pleural effusion (98).

Iatrogenic Effects of Intravascular Catheters

If a transudative pleural effusion develops shortly after a central line is placed, it is important to exclude the possibility that this is an iatrogenic effusion due to a catheter placed improperly in the pleural space or that the effusion has resulted from intravascular obstruction secondary to thrombosis. Pleural effusions are usually unilateral and can appear early, within hours after the placement of an intravascular catheter, or as a late manifestation of superior vena cava perforation (99), obstruction, or migration (96). Although perforation of a large vessel generally produces a hemothorax, in the absence of significant bleeding the effusion may be a transudate with glucose and electrolyte compositions similar to the infusing fluid (54).

Atelectasis

Lobar or segmental atelectasis or fibrosis of the visceral pleura produces a localized decrease in intrapleural pressure that promotes the filtration of fluid into the pleural space, thus leading to formation of pleural effusions. These effusions that develop as a result of lowered intrapleural pressure tend to be transudative and are known as "effusions ex vacuo." Pleural effusions developed in approximately 5% of patients treated with pneumothorax for tuberculosis as the intrapleural pressure became increasingly more negative (-20 cmH$_2$O or lower). This lowering of intrapleural pressure led to increased fluid filtration through pleural capillaries into the pleural space (100). This mechanism was thought to be responsible for the rapid reaccumulation of pleural fluid following thoracentesis in patients with idiopathic pleurisy (presumably tuberculous) whose lungs were encased in a fibrous peel, as reported by Stead and coworkers (101).

Malignancy

The major mechanisms by which tumors produce transudative effusions is by obstruction of mediastinal lymph nodes, which collect the lymphatic drainage from the pleura, and obstruction of lymphatic channels, such as the stomas connecting the pleural cavity and the lymphatics in the parietal pleura (102–105). Additionally, as previously discussed, obstruction of the superior vena cava by tumor can lead to formation of a pleural effusion due to increased systemic venous pressure and consequent impairment in fluid absorption (97).

III. Management of Transudative Pleural Effusions

The basis of management of transudative pleural effusions is the treatment of the underlying condition (106). This generally results in rapid resolution of the effusion as the primary process that results in accumulation of fluid in the pleural space is controlled or no longer active. In some patients, the pleural effusion may be quite large and lead to lung compression and consequent dyspnea. In these patients, a therapeutic thoracentesis should be performed, removing 500–1000 mL, in order to alleviate symptoms. Dyspnea diminishes after thoracentesis, presumably because the thoracic muscles are allowed to operate at a more advantageous position on their length-tension curve after the reduction of thoracic volume (107). Repetitive thoracenteses should be avoided, however, because these may lead to protein depletion. In those patients that continue to be symptomatic due to recurrent pleural effusion despite the management of the underlying condition, pleurodesis can be considered. Pleurodesis has been performed successfully in patients with transudative pleural effusions resulting from hepatic cirrhosis (108), congestive heart failure (26), and the nephrotic syndrome (55). In patients with nephrotic syndrome and pleural effusion, however, management of the underlying condition should include evaluation for pulmonary embolism, since the incidence of thromboembolic disease is high in these patients (53).

References

1. Antony VB. Drawing the line: differentiating transudates from exudates. Respiration 2002; 69:198.
2. Light RW, MacGregor MI, Luchsinger PC, Ball WC. Pleural effusions: the diagnostic separation of transudates and exudates. Ann Intern Med 1972; 77:507–513.
3. Light RW. Useful tests on the pleural fluid in the management of patients with pleural effusions. Curr Opin Pulm Med 1999; 5:245–249.
4. Allen S, Gabel J, Drake R. Left atrial hypertension causes pleural effusion formation in unanesthetized sheep. Am J Physiol 1989; 257:H690–H692.
5. Broaddus VC, Wiener-Kronish JP, Staub NC. Clearance of lung edema into the pleural space of volume-loaded anesthetized sheep. J Appl Physiol 1990; 68:2623–2630.
6. Wiener-Kronish JP, Broaddus VC. Interrelationship of pleural and pulmonary interstitial liquid. Annu Rev Physiol 1993; 55:209–226.
7. Black LF. The pleural space and pleural fluid. Mayo Clin Proc 1972; 47:493–506.
8. Broaddus VC, Light RW. What is the origin of transudates and exudates? Chest 1992; 102:658–659.
9. Light RW. Approach to the patient. Pleural Diseases. 3rd ed. Baltimore: Williams and Wilkins, 1995:75–82.
10. Sahn SA. The differential diagnosis of pleural effusions. Wes J Med 1982; 137:99–109.
11. Sah SH, Leichthling M, Bass HE. The significance of pleural effusion in patients past the age of fifty. N Engl J Med 1952; 246:927–928.
12. Logue RB, Rogers JV Jr, Gay BB Jr. Subtle roentgenographic signs of left heart failure. Am Heart J 1963; 65:464–473.
13. Race GA, Scheifley CH, Edwards JE. Hydrothorax in congestive heart failure. Am J Med 1957; 22:83–89.

14. Rabin CB, Blackman NS. Bilateral pleural effusion: its significance in association with a heart of normal size. J Mt Sinai Hosp 1957; 24:45–53.
15. McPeak EM, Levine SA. The preponderance of right hydrothorax in congestive heart failure. Ann Intern Med 1946; 25:916–927.
16. Weiss JM, Spodick DH. Brief reports: laterality of pleural effusions in chronic congestive heart failure. Am J Cardiol 1984; 53:951.
17. Peterman TA, Speicher CE. Evaluating pleural effusions: a two-stage laboratory approach. JAMA 1984; 252:1051–1053.
18. Weiss JM, Spodick DH. Association of left pleural effusion with pericardial disease. N Engl J Med 1983; 308:696–697.
19. Mellins RB, Levine OR, Fishman AP. Effect of systemic and pulmonary venous hypertension on pleural and pericardial fluid accumulation. J Appl Physiol 1970; 29:564–569.
20. Wiener-Kronish JP, Matthay MA, Callen PW. Relationship of pleural effusions to pulmonary hemodynamics in patients with congestive heart failure. Am Rev Respir Dis 1985; 132:1253–1256.
21. Laufer ST. Interlobar effusion associated with heart disease. Nova Scotia Med Bull 1965; 25:299–304.
22. Millard CE. Vanishing or phantom tumor of the lung: Localized interlobar effusion in congestive heart failure. Chest 1971; 59:675–677.
23. Light RW, Broaddus VC. Pleural effusion. In: Murray JF, Nadel JA, Mason RJ, Boushey HA Jr, eds. Textbook of Respiratory Medicine. Philadelphia: WB Saunders Co, 2000:2013–2041.
24. Burgess LJ, Maritz FJ, Taljaard JJ. Comparative analysis of the biochemical parameters used to distinguish between pleural transudates and exudates. Chest 1995; 107:1604–1609.
25. Vladutiu AO. Cardiac failure with pleural effusion. Pleural Effusion. New York: Futura Publishing Co Inc, 1986:173–174.
26. Spicer AJ, Fisher JA. Recurring pleural effusion in congestive heart failure treated by pleurodesis. J Irish Med Assoc 1969; 62:177–178.
27. Davidoff D, Naparstek Y, Eliakim M. The use of pleurodesis for intractable pleural effusion due to congestive heart failure. Postgrad Med 1983; 59:330–331.
28. Plum GE, Brower AJ, Clagett OT. Chronic constrictive pericarditis: roentgenologic findings in 35 surgically proved cases. Proc Mayo Clin 1957; 32:555–556.
29. Vladutiu AO. Miscellaneous causes of pleural effusion. Pleural Effusion. New York: Futura Publishing Co Inc, 1986:293–294.
30. Lieberman FL, Peters RL. Cirrhotic hydrothorax. Further evidence that an acquired diaphragmatic defect is at fault. Arch Intern Med 1970; 125:114–117.
31. Johnson RF, Loo RV. Hepatic hydrothorax: Studies to determine the source of the fluid and report of thirteen cases. Ann Intern Med 1964; 61:385–401.
32. McKay DG, Sparling HS Jr, Robbins SC. Cirrhosis of liver with massive hydrothorax. Arch Intern Med 1947; 79:501–509.
33. Faiyaz U, Goyal PC. Unilateral pleural effusion without ascites in liver cirrhosis. Postgrad Med 1983; 74:309–315.
34. Singer JA, Kaplan MM, Katz RL. Cirrhotic pleural effusion in the absence of ascites. Gastroenterology 1977; 73:575–577.
35. Crawford KL, McDougall IR. Prediction of satisfactory response to pleural sclerosis using radiopharmaceuticals. Study in a patient with cirrhotic hydrothorax and LeVeen shunt. Arch Intern Med 1982; 142:194–196.

36. Broaddus VC, Light RW. Disorders of the pleura: general principles and diagnostic approach. In: Murray JF, Nadel JA, Mason RJ, Boushey HA Jr, eds. Textbook of Respiratory Medicine. Philadelphia: WB Saunders C, 2000:1995–2012.
37. Kirschner PA. Porous diaphragm syndromes. Chest Surg Clin North Am 1998; 8:449–472.
38. Vladutiu AO. Liver diseases with pleural effusion. Pleural Effusion. New York: Futura Publishing Co Inc, 1986:273–276.
39. Frazer IH, Lichtenstein M, Andrews JT. Pleuroperitoneal effusion without ascites. Med J Aust 1983; 2:520–521.
40. Llaneza PP, Salt WB II. Unilateral pleural effusion without clinical ascites in Laennec's cirrhosis. Dig Dis Sci 1985; 30:88–89.
41. Lieberman FL, Hidemura R, Peters RL. Pathogenesis and treatment of hydrothorax complicating cirrhosis with ascites. Ann Intern Med 1966; 64:341–351.
42. Mouroux J, Perrin C, Venissac N. Management of pleural effusion of cirrhotic origin. Chest 1996; 109:1093–1096.
43. Crofts NF. Pneumothorax complicating therapeutic pneumoperitoneum. Thorax 1954; 9:226–228.
44. Frothingham JR. Cirrhosis of the liver complicated by persistent right hydrothorax and ascites. N Engl J Med 1942; 226:679–682.
45. Hartz RS, Bomalaski J, LoCicero J III. Pleural ascites without abdominal fluid: surgical considerations. J Thorac Cardiovasc Surg 1984; 87:141–146.
46. Mirouze D, Juttner HU, Reynolds TB. Left pleural effusion in patients with chronic liver disease and ascites. Dig Dis Sci 1981; 26:984–988.
47. Flaum MA. Spontaneous bacterial empyema in cirrhosis. Gastroenterology 1976; 70:416–417.
48. Xiol X, Castellvi JM, Guardiola J. Spontaneous bacterial empyema in cirrhotic patients: a prospective study. Hepatology 1996; 23:719–723.
49. Olutola PS, Hutton L, Wall WJ. Pleural effusion following liver transplantation. Radiology 1985; 157:594.
50. Light RW, Jenkinson SG, Minh V. Observations on pleural pressures as fluid is withdrawn during thoracentesis. Am Rev Respir Dis 1980; 121:799–804.
51. Gordon FD, Anastopoulos HT, Crenshaw W. The successful treatment of symptomatic, refractory hepatic hydrothorax with transjugular intrahepatic portosystemic shunt. Hepatology 1997; 25:1366–1369.
52. Cavina G, Vichi G. Radiological aspects of pleural effusions in medical nephropathy in children. Ann Radiol Diagn 1958; 31:163–202.
53. Llach F, Arieff AI, Massry SG. Renal vein thrombosis and nephritic syndrome: a prospective study of 36 adult patients. Ann Intern Med 1975; 83:8–14.
54. Kinasewitz GT. Transudative pleural effusions. Eur Respir J 1997; 10:714–718.
55. Jenkins PG, Shelp WD. Recurrent pleural transudate in the nephrotic syndrome: a new approach to treatment. JAMA 1974; 230:587–588.
56. Edwards SR, Unger AM. Acute hydrothorax—a new complication of peritoneal dialysis. JAMA 1967; 199:853–855.
57. Holm J, Lieden B, Lindqvist B. Unilateral pleural effusion—a rare complication of peritoneal dialysis. Scand J Urol Nephrol 1971; 5:84–85.
58. Nomoto Y, Suga T, Nakajima K. Acute hydrothorax in continuous ambulatory peritoneal dialysis. A collaborative study of 161 centers. Am J Nephrol 1989; 9:363–367.

59. O'Connor JR, Rutland M. Demonstration of pleuro-peritoneal communication with radionuclide imaging in a CAPD patient. Peritoneal Dialysis Bull 1981; 1:153–154.
60. Spadaro JJ, Thakur V, Nolph KD. Technetium-99m-labeled macroaggregated albumin in demonstration of trans-diaphragmatic leakage of dialysate in peritoneal dialysis. Am J Nephrol 1982; 2:36–38.
61. Kuehnel E. Massive pleural effusion secondary to CAPD [abstr]. Kidney Int 1981; 19:152.
62. Nassberger L. Left-sided pleural effusion secondary to continuous ambulatory peritoneal dialysis. Acta Med Scand 1982; 211:219–220.
63. Grefberg N, Danielson BG, Benson L. Right-sided hydrothorax complicating peritoneal dialysis. Nephron 1983; 34:130–134.
64. Posen GA, Sachs HJ. Treatment of recurrent pleural effusions in dialysis patients by talc insufflation. Am Soc Artif Intern Organs 1979; 8:75.
65. DiBisceglie M, Paladini P, Voltolini L. Videothoracoscopic obliteration of pleuroperitoneal fistula in continuous peritoneal dialysis. Ann Thorac Surg 1996; 62:1509–1510.
66. Spicer RL, Uzark KC, Moore JW. Aortopulmonary collateral vessels and prolonged pleural effusions after modified Fontan procedures. Am Heart J 1996; 131:1164–1168.
67. Sade RM, Wiles HB. Pleuroperitoneal shunt for persistent pleural drainage after Fontan procedure. J Thorac Cardiovasc Surg 1990; 100:621–623.
68. Rychik J, Rome JJ, Jacobs ML. Late surgical fenestration for complications after the Fontan procedure. Circulation 1997; 96:33–36.
69. Gottehrer A, Roa J, Stanford GG. Hypothyroidism and pleural effusions. Chest 1990; 98:1130–1132.
70. Smolar EN, Rubin JE, Avramides A. Cardiac tamponade in primary myxedema and review of the literature. Am J Med Sci 1976; 272:345–352.
71. Brown SD, Brashear RE, Schnute RB. Pleural effusion in a young woman with myxedema. Arch Intern Med 1983; 143:1458–1459.
72. Naye RL. Capillary and venous lesions in myxedema. Lab Invest 1963; 12:465–470.
73. Bynum LJ, Wilson JE III. Radiographic features of pleural effusions in pulmonary embolism. Am Rev Respir Dis 1978; 117:829–834.
74. Dalen JE, Haffajee CI, Alpert JS. Pulmonary embolism, pulmonary hemorrhage and pulmonary infarction. N Engl J Med 1977; 296:1431–1435.
75. Story DD, Dines DE, Coles DT. Pleural effusion: A diagnostic dilemma. JAMA 1976; 236:2183–2186.
76. Bynum LJ, Wilson JE III. Characteristics of pleural effusions associated with pulmonary embolism. Arch Intern Med 1976; 136:159–162.
77. Corriere JN Jr, Miller WT, Murphy JJ. Hydronephrosis as a cause of pleural effusion. Radiology 1968; 90:79–84.
78. Laforet EG, Kornitzer GD. Nephrogenic pleural effusion. J Urol 1977; 117:118–119.
79. Lahiri SK, Alkhafaji AH, Brown AL. Urinothorax following blunt trauma to the kidney. J Trauma 1978; 18:608–610.
80. Barek LB, Cigtay OS. Urinothorax: An unusual cause of pleural effusion. Br J Radiol 1975; 48:685–686.
81. Belis J, Milam DF. Pleural effusion secondary to ureteral obstruction. Urology 1979; 14:27–29.

82. Baron RL, Stark DD, McClennan BL. Intrathoracic extension of retroperitoneal urine collections. AJR 1981; 137:37–41.
83. Leung FW, Williams AJ, Guze PA. Lymphatic obstruction: a possible explanation for left-sided pleural effusions associated with splenic hematomas. AJR 1982; 138:182.
84. Stark DD, Shanes JG, Baron RL. Biochemical features of urinothorax. Arch Intern Med 1982; 142:1509–1511.
85. Friedland GW, Axman MM, Love TL. Neonatal urinothorax associated with posterior urethral valves. Br J Radiol 1971; 44:471–474.
86. Kamble RT, Bhat SP, Joshi JM. Urinothorax: a case report. Indian J Chest Dis Allied Sci 2000; 42:189–190.
87. Chusid EL, Siltzbach LE. Sarcoidosis of the pleura. Ann Intern Med 1974; 81:190–194.
88. Nicholls AJ, Friend JAR, Legge JS. Sarcoid pleural effusion: three cases and review of the literature. Thorax 1980; 35:277–281.
89. Javaheri S, Hales CA. Sarcoidosis: a cause of innominate vein obstruction and massive pleural effusion. Lung 1980; 157:81–83.
90. Everett ED, Iverholt EL. Sarcoidosis and pleural effusion. Military Med 1968; 133:731–733.
91. Sharma OP. Sarcoidosis: unusual pulmonary manifestations. Postgrad Med 1977; 61:67–73.
92. Bonfils-Roberts E, Marx AJ, Neaton TF. Primary amyloidosis of the respiratory tract. Ann Thorac Surg 1975; 19:313–318.
93. Michaels L, Hyams VJ. Amyloid in localized deposits and plasmacytomas of the respiratory tract. J Pathol (Lond) 1979; 128:29–38.
94. Hussey HH, Katz S, Yates WM. The superior vena cava syndrome: report of thirty-five cases. Am Heart J 1946; 31:1–26.
95. Good JT Jr, Moore JB, Fowler AA. Superior vena cava syndrome as a cause of pleural effusion. Am Rev Respir Dis 1982; 125:246–247.
96. Dhande V, Kattwinkel J, Alford B. Recurrent bilateral pleural effusions secondary to superior vena cava obstruction as a complication of central venous catheterization. Pediatrics 1983; 72:109–113.
97. Chahinian AP, Pajak TF, Holland JF, Norton L, Ambinder RM, Mandel EM. Diffuse malignant mesothelioma. Prospective evaluation of 69 patients. Ann Intern Med 1982; 96:746–755.
98. Carlson HA. Obstruction of the superior vena cava: an experimental study. Arch Surg 1934; 29:669–677.
99. Criado A, Mena A, Figueredo R. Late perforation of superior vena cava and effusion caused by central venous catheter. Anaesth Intens Care 1981; 9:286–288.
100. Farber JE, Lincoln NS. The unexpandable lung. Am Rev Tuberc 1939; 40:704–709.
101. Stead WW, Eichenholz A, Stauss HK. Operative and pathologic findings in twenty-four patients with syndrome of idiopathic pleurisy with effusion, presumably tuberculous. Am Rev Tuberc 1955; 71:473–502.
102. Wang ND. The preformed stomas connecting the pleural cavity and the lymphatics in the parietal pleura. Am Rev Respir Dis 1975; 111:12–20.
103. Meyer PC. Metastatic carcinoma of the pleura. Thorax 1966; 21:437–443.
104. Fernandez C, Martin C, Aranda I, Romero S. Malignant transient pleural transudate: a sign of early lymphatic tumoral obstruction. Respiration 2000; 67:333–336.

105. Aschi M, Golish J, Eng P, O'Donovan P. Transudative malignant pleural effusions: prevalence and mechanisms. South Med J 1998; 91:23–26.
106. Light RW. Pleural effusion. N Engl J Med 2002; 346:1971–1977.
107. Estenne M, Yernault JC, DeTroyer A. Mechanism of relief of dyspnea after thoracocentesis in patients with large pleural effusions. Am J Med 1983; 74:813–819.
108. Falchuk KR, Jacoby I, Colucci WS. Tetracycline-induced pleural symphysis for recurrent hydrothorax complicating cirrhosis. Gastroenterology 1977; 72:319–321.

18

Interventional Radiology of Pleural Disease

JOHNY A. VERSCHAKELEN

University Hospitals, Gasthuisberg
Leuven, Belgium

I. Introduction

Percutaneous nonoperative procedures were first reported in the late 1800s. Leyden (1) was probably the first to perform a transthoracic needle biopsy to confirm the presence of a pulmonary infection. The lack of small-caliber needles, causing a high rate of complications, and the difficulties pathologists had making a diagnosis from small samples or smears were responsible for the fact that these percutaneous diagnostic procedures did not experience widespread use until the 1960s. At that time Dahlgren and Nordenström (2) introduced small-gauge needles, reducing the rate of pneumothorax, popularizing the technique of transthoracic fine needle sampling of the chest. At the same time, the first report on the use of fluoroscopy during transthoracic needle biopsy was published (3). Not until the late 1970s, however, did imaging-guided percutaneous insertion of drainage catheters in fluid collections of the lung and pleura become a routine procedure (4). Fluoroscopy was initially the method of choice, but now many imaging techniques, including ultrasound (US), computed tomography (CT), and magnetic resonance (MR), are used to guide interventional procedures.

II. Imaging Guidance Modalities

A. Fluoroscopy

Uni- or biplanar fluoroscopy was the first imaging technique used to guide percutaneous pleural interventions. The technique is widely available, allows real-time control of the procedure, and gives an overview of the thorax. In addition, the technique is familiar to most investigators (5). However, fluoroscopy is not suitable for every lesion. Small lesions may be difficult or impossible to identify. Some lesions may be superimposed on or not separable from normal thoracic structures. Another important limitation is that biopsy or drainage using fluoroscopic guidance may not be advisable if the lesion is adjacent to major cardiovascular structures, such as the aorta (6).

B. Ultrasonography

Ultrasound is well suited for interventional procedures in the pleura (7,8). Because of the development of high-resolution, high-frequency probes with special biopsy ports, ultrasonographically guided biopsy of small pleural lesions has become possible (9–12). Ultrasonography is particularly indicated to guide percutaneous aspiration and catheter drainage of a pleural fluid or air collection, even in small amounts (13–21) (Fig. 1). Advantages of this technique include real-time visualization during needle placement, absence of ionizing radiation, and, in the case of biopsy of a mass, the ability to target nonnecrotic portions for sampling (10,22). In addition, US is a safe and convenient method of guiding interventional procedures at the bedside of the patient and obviates the need to transport patients on life support devices to the radiology department (23). A disadvantage is that sonography is limited by attenuation of the beam as it transverses air-filled lung or pleura.

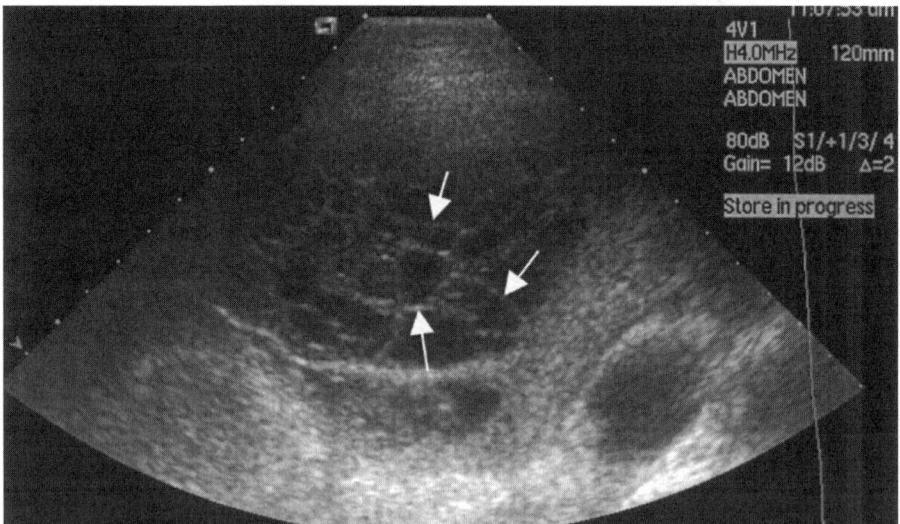

Figure 1 Ultrasonography is particularly indicated to guide percutaneous aspiration and catheter drainage of a pleural fluid collection. This technique is especially helpful to ensure accurate placement of the tube in the presence of septations (arrows).

C. Computed Tomography

A major advantage of CT over fluoroscopy is its axial format and its exquisite anatomical detail (6,13,16,17,24). It is particularly useful for sampling lesions visible in only a single radiographic projection or when great imaging detail is required for the interventional procedure. The administration of intravenous contrast can be mandatory for the identification of tissue necrosis, fluid content, and identification of normal and abnormal vascular structures. CT allows for determination of an optimal cutaneous entry point for the biopsy needle or for tube placement. Disadvantages of CT-guided interventional procedures include lack of real-time visualization, greater patient discomfort lying on the CT table, and greater expense than with fluoroscopically guided biopsies. A disadvantage compared to US is the fact that this technique also requires ionizing radiation. According to a study of Ghaye et al. (25), spiral CT had no advantages over sequential CT because this technique reduces neither procedure time nor the rate of complications. Also, pathological results did not differ compared with sequential CT, and total irradiation dose was higher with spiral scanning. However, the recent introduction of CT continuous imaging, also called real-time CT and CT fluoroscopy, has improved the ease of performing interventional thoracic procedures because it allows real-time visualization of the lesion and of the progression of the needle or tube. In this way the diagnostic accuracy can be improved and the duration of the procedure can be shortened (26–29). Compared with conventional spiral CT, there is also a markedly decreased patient radiation dose (30).

D. Magnetic Resonance

Although MR is often used for guidance of interventional procedures, little experience has been gained in thoracic or pleural interventions (31,32). This technique combines the absence of ionizing radiation with good anatomical detail and has become possible with the introduction of nonferromagnetic MR-compatible biopsy needles (33,34). Major disadvantages include, however, high cost, limited availability, the length of the procedure, and the lack of real-time control.

III. Percutaneous Drainage of Thoracic Fluid and Air Collections

A. Parapneumonic Effusion and Empyema

Imaging plays an important part in the investigation and management of pleural fluid collection. The choice of treatment depends on the fluid characteristics (i.e., transudate vs. exudate). In general, a transudate or simple parapneumonic effusion responds to antibiotic therapy, while most drainage catheter placements are reserved for exudative effusions—either infectious, inflammatory, or neoplastic (35). Chest radiographs are the first-line investigation, and most pleural effusions are clearly visible. In large pleural collections, needle aspiration and drainage are often possible without imaging control.

Although chest radiographs and fluoroscopy (36) are used successfully to guide percutaneous catheter drainage of pleural effusion, both US and CT are more sensitive than chest radiographs for the detection and localization of pleural fluid, and both can be used to differentiate between transudates and exudates (37,38). Anechoic collections may be either exudates or transudates, but the presence of homogeneous internal echos and/or septations indicates an exudate. Multiple septa not only indicate exudates, but also predict difficulties with aspiration. Ultrasound guidance can in these cases ensure accurate placement of the drain (Fig. 1). Septa are seldom detectable on CT (15,36,38,39).

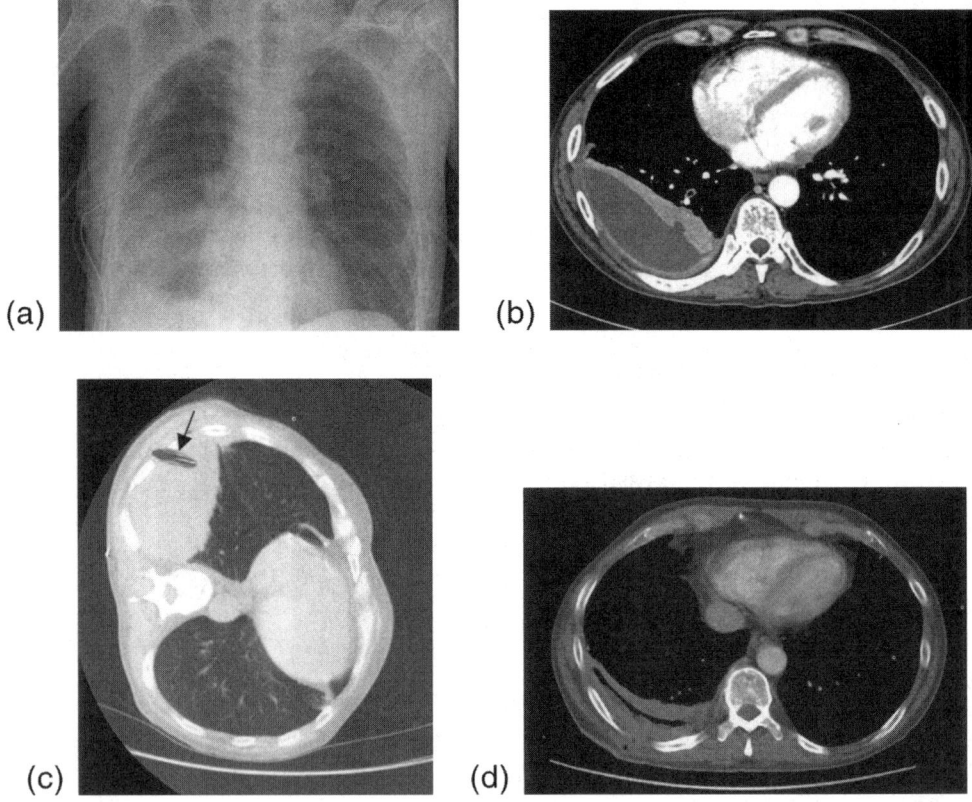

Figure 2 Chest x-ray and CT are valuable imaging modalities to locate the drain after a non-guided drainage of empyema. In this patient, chest x-ray (a) suggested and CT (b) confirmed incorrect placement of the thoracostomy tube. Under CT guidance a new tube was placed (c) and treatment was successful. A follow-up CT (d) shows an important reduction in the amount of pleural fluid but also demonstrates the presence of extensive pleural thickening.

However, this latter technique is valuable to assess the underlying lung, mediastinum, chest wall, and subdiaphragmatic regions. It is especially useful in characterizing complex pleural and parenchymal disease and is used to guide drainage of collections that are difficult to access by way of an intercostal approach (e.g., paramediastinal collections). The presence of fibrin strand septations and loculations is an indication for the installation of fibrinolytic agents, and again tube placement is facilitated when ultrasound is used to guide the procedure (40–42).

Drainage via thoracostomy, thoracocentesis, and antibiotics is standard therapeutic procedure for empyema (43–45). When these fail, excision of a rib for open drainage and open thoracostomy are more invasive alternatives. Failure of the thoracostomy tube is very often the result of a poorly positioned or nonfunctioning tube (46–48). Incorrect tube placement is not only responsible for inadequate drainage but can also produce complications such as pain, hypotension, subcutaneous emphysema, leakage, chylothorax, and bleeding (47,48). Large surgical studies have demonstrated the limitations of nonguided thoracostomy drainage of empyema (43,45) (Fig. 2). One report shows a 10% cure rate (43), while another shows a mortality rate of 5% (45). Van Sonnenberg et al. (17) used CT and US to locate and drain empyemas in 17 patients, most of whom had failed to improve with conventional chest tube drainage due to a poorly positioned tube. Fifteen patients (88.2%) were treated successfully, averting surgery or further drainage. In four patients the radiological procedure provided additional diagnostic information: two were found to have a bronchopleural fistula, in one patient a communication between the empyema and the esophagus was seen, and in one patient the empyema was communicating with a subphrenic abscess.

CT has also been used successfully to follow patients who underwent percutaneous catheter drainage for empyema (24) (Fig. 2). Up to 4 weeks after the removal of the catheter(s), CT scan demonstrated extensive pleural thickening in all of the 10 patients who entered the study. This pleural peel had decreased at 8 and 12 weeks; the pleura was essentially normal in 4 patients, demonstrated only a small area of plaque-like thickening in 4 patients, and was mildly thickened in 2 patients. Serial CT can be helpful to determine the necessity of decortication.

B. Malignant Pleural Disease and Pleural Effusions

Lung and breast carcinomas together with lymphoma are the most common causes of malignant pleural effusion (49). The majority of these pleural effusions require tube drainage with sclerosis to prevent recurrence. Imaging-guided drainage and chemical pleurodesis have become a well-accepted procedure for the management of malignant effusions (50). In addition, Davies et al. suggested that intrapleural streptokinase might be useful in the drainage of malignant multiloculated pleural effusions in patients who fail to drain adequately with a standard chest tube (51). In most cases ultrasonography is used to guide catheter placement (52). This technique is also be used to guide transthoracic needle biopsy of pleural masses (7,12,53). Real-time ultrasound visualization allows accurate needle placement, shorter procedure time, and performance in debilitated and less cooperative patients (54). CT, on the other hand, is the method of choice for guiding biopsy of small pleural masses or for biopsy in those parts of the pleura that are hidden behind bone or aerated lung tissue (Fig. 3). In a series of 33 patients with diffuse or focal pleural thickening, pleural effusion, and suspected pleural malignancy, percutaneous CT- or US-guided cutting-needle biopsy revealed a sensitivity of 88%, a specificity of 100%, and an accuracy of 91% for the correct diagnosis of malignant disease including mesothelioma (55). This is much better than pleural biopsies performed without imaging guidance, where sensitivity varies from 48 to 56% for the detection of malignant pleural disease (56–58) and from 21 to 43% for the detection of malignant mesothelioma (59,60).

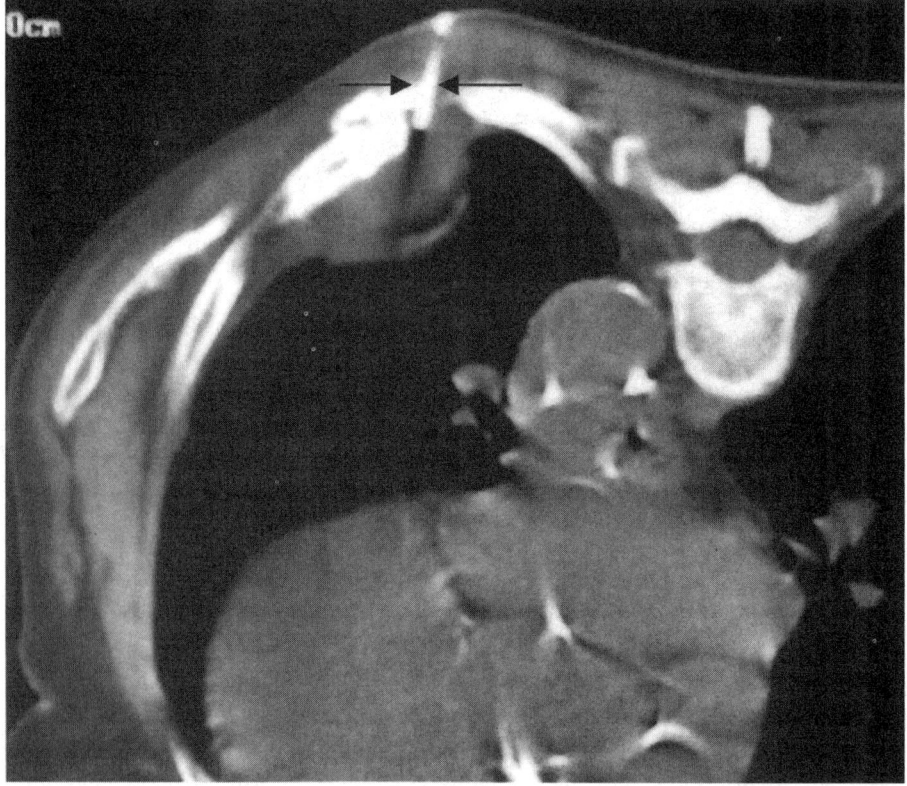

Figure 3 CT is the method of choice for guiding biopsy (arrows) of pleural masses that are hidden behind bone or aerated lung tissue.

C. Pneumothorax

Pneumothorax can be either spontaneous or posttraumatic in origin. Common causes of traumatic pneumothorax include chest trauma, central venous catheter placement, transbronchial biopsy and transthoracic biopsy, or drainage procedures (61–63). Small or stable pneumothoraces in asymptomatic patients are usually observed. Drainage is performed for large or symptomatic air collections. Large air collections can be treated without imaging guidance. Fluoroscopy can be used to guide catheter placement, although CT is more often used when the pneumothorax occurred during a CT-guided interventional procedure. CT is also helpful in accessing loculated collections (64).

IV. Imaging of Complications

The most common complications of transthoracic needle biopsy of lung lesions are pneumothorax and pulmonary hemorrhage ranging from 5 to 30% (9,65,66). These numbers are much smaller for pleural interventions since lung tissue is normally not punctured. Factors associated with higher incidence of pneumothorax include small pleural lesions, the presence of obstructive airways disease and emphysema, intractable coughing, increased duration of the procedure, and cavitary lesions.

Pulmonary hemorrhage is rare, but bleeding in the chest wall can occur when a vein or artery is damaged during the procedure. Special care should be taken to avoid intercostal and internal mammary vessels. The administration of intravenous contrast can be necessary to locate the internal mammary vessels on CT prior to the interventional procedure.

V. Video-Assisted Thoracic Surgery

Video-assisted thoracic surgery (VATS) has become a very useful diagnostic and therapeutic tool in the management of lung, pleural, and mediastinal disease (67). In the pleura it has become the preferred surgical technique for pleural drainage, lyses of adhesions, decortication, and directed pleurodesis (67,68). Thoracoscopic biopsy has a sensitivity of approximately 91–98% in the detection of malignant pleural disease, including mesothelioma (69,70). Preoperative imaging, especially CT, is very important to assess location and extent of disease and to have an idea about the nature of the lesion(s). Since the anatomical relationships of the pleura and the pleural lesions remain relatively undisturbed during the procedure, imaging guidance or imaging-guided location of the lesion is rarely necessary. This is different for lung lesions that are often not visible during the VATS procedure. Three methods of preoperative image–guided location for VATS using CT guidance have been described: skin marking, transpleural staining, and wire placement (71–76). These procedures can help the surgeon to locate the pulmonary lesion but are performed less and less frequently as the experience with thoracoscopy increases (68).

References

1. Leyden OO. Über infectiöse Pneumonie. Dtsch Med Wochenschr 1883; 9:52–55.
2. Dahlgren S, Nordenström B. Needle Transthoracic Biopsy. Stockholm: Almquist and Wiksell, 1966.
3. Hattori S, Matsuda M, Sugiyama T. Cytologic diagnosis of early lung cancer: brushing methods under x-ray television fluoroscopy. Dis Chest 1964; 45:129–135.
4. Vainrub D, Husher DM, Guinn GA, Young EJ, Septimus EJ, Travis LL. Percutaneous drainage of lung abscess. Am Rev Respir Dis 1978; 117:153–157.
5. Klein JS, Zarka M. Transthoracic needle biopsy: an overview. J Thorac Imaging 1997; 12:232–249.
6. vanSonnenberg E, Casola G, Ho M, Neff CC, Varney RR, Wittich GR, Christensen R, Friedman PJ. Difficult thoracic lesions: CT-guided biopsy experience in 150 cases. Radiology 1988; 167:457–461.
7. Heilo A, Stenwig AE, Solheim OP. Malignant pleural mesothelioma: US-guided histologic core-needle biopsy. Radiology 1999; 211:657–659.
8. Heilo A. Tumors in the mediastinum: US-guided histologic core-needle biopsy. Radiology 1993; 189:143–146.
9. Ikezoe J, Morimoto S, Kozuka T. Sonographically guided needle biopsy of thoracic lesions. Semin Intervent Radiol 1991; 8:15–22.
10. Pan JF, Yang PC, Chang DB, Lee YC, Kuo SH, Luh KT. Needle aspiration biopsy of malignant lung masses with necrotic centers. Improved sensitivity with ultrasound guidance. Chest 1993; 103:1452–1456.
11. Yang PC, Chang DB, Yu CJ, Lee YC, Wu HD, Kuo SH, Luh KT. Ultrasound-guided core biopsy of thoracic tumors. Am Rev Respir Dis 1992; 146:763–767.
12. Yang PC. Ultrasound-guided transthoracic biopsy of peripheral lung, pleural, and chest-wall lesions. J Thorac Imaging 1997; 12:272–284.
13. Casola G, vanSonnenberg E, Keightley A, Ho M, Withers C, Lee AS. Pneumothorax: radiologic treatment with small catheters. Radiology 1988; 166:89–91.
14. Hunnam GR, Flower CDR. Radiologically-guided percutaneous catheter drainage of empyemas. Clin Radiol 1988; 39:121–126.
15. Merriam MA, Cronan JJ, Dorfman GDS, Lambiase RE, Haas RA. Radiographically guided percutaneous catheter drainage of pleural fluid collections. AJR 1988; 151:1113–1116.
16. Silverman SG, Mueller PR, Saini S, Hahn PF, Simeone JF, Forman BH, Steiner E, Ferrucci JT. Thoracic empyema: management with image-guided catheter drainage. Radiology 1988; 169:5–9.
17. van Sonnenberg E, Nakamoto SK, Mueller PR, Casola G, Neff CC, Friedman PJ, Ferrucci JT Jr, Simeone JF. CT- and ultrasound-guided catheter drainage of empyemas after chest-tube failure. Radiology 1984; 151:349–353.
18. Parker LA, Melton JW, Delany DJ, Yakaskas BC. Percutaneous small bore catheter drainage in the management of lung abscesses. Chest 1987; 92:213–218.
19. O'Moore PV, Mueller PR, Simeone JF, Saini S, Butch RJ, Hahn PF, Steiner E, Stark DD, Ferrucci JT. Sonographic guidance in diagnostic and therapeutic interventions in the pleural space. AJR 1987; 149:1–5.

20. Cummin ARC, Wright NL, Joseph AE. Suction drainage: a new approach to the treatment of empyema. Thorax 1991; 46:259–260.
21. Morrison MC, Mueller PR, Lee MJ, Saini S, Brink JA, Dawson SL, Cortell ED, Hahn PF. Sclerotherapy of malignant pleural effusion through sonographically placed small-bore catheters. AJR 1992; 158:41–43.
22. Klein JS, Zarka MA. Transthoracic needle biopsy. Radiol Clin North Am 2000; 38: 235–266.
23. Yu CJ, Yang PC, Chang DB, Luh KT. Diagnostic and therapeutic use of chest sonography: value in critically ill patients. AJR 1992; 159:695–701.
24. Neff CC, vanSonnenberg E, Lawson DW, Patton AS. CT follow-up of empyemas: pleural peels resolve after percutaneous catheter drainage. Radiology 1990; 176: 195–197.
25. Ghaye B, Dondelinger RF, Dewe W. Percutaneous CT-guided lung biopsy: sequential versus spiral scanning. A randomized prospective study. Eur Radiol 1999; 9:1317–1320.
26. White CS, Meyer CA, Templeton PA. CT fluoroscopy for thoracic interventional procedures. Radiol Clin North Am 2000; 38:303–322.
27. Sheafor DH, Paulson EK, Kliewer MA, DeLong DM, Nelson RC. Comparison of sonographic and CT guidance techniques: does CT fluoroscopy decrease procedure time? AJR 2000; 174:939–942.
28. Ernst RD, Kim HS, Kawashima A, Middlebrook MR, Sandler CM. Near real-time CT fluoroscopy using computer automated scan technology in nonvascular interventional procedures. AJR 2000; 174:319–321.
29. Daly B, Templeton PA. Real-time CT fluoroscopy: evolution of an interventional tool. Radiology 1999; 211:309–315.
30. Carlson SK, Bender CE, Classic KL, Zink FE, Quam JP, Ward EM, Oberg AL. Benefits and safety of CT fluoroscopy in interventional radiologic procedures. Radiology 2001; 219:515–520.
31. Adam G, Neuerburg J, Bucker A, Glowinski A, Vorwerk D, Stargardt A, Van Vaals JJ, Gunther RW. Interventional magnetic resonance. Initial clinical experience with a 1.5-tesla magnetic resonance system combined with c-arm fluoroscopy. Invest Radiol 1997; 32:191–197.
32. Buecker A, Adam G, Neuerburg JM, Glowinski A, van Vaals JJ, Guenther RW. MR-guided biopsy using a T2-weighted single-shot zoom imaging sequence (local look technique). J Magn Reson Imaging 1998; 8:955–959.
33. Langen H-J, Kugel H, Grewe S, Gindele A, Landwehr P, Fischbach R. MR-guided biopsy using respiratory-triggered high-resolution T2-weighted sequences. AJR 2000; 174:834–836.
34. Lufkin R, Teresi L, Hanafee W. New needle for MR-guided aspiration cytology of the head and neck. AJR 1987; 149:380–382.
35. Light RW. Parapneumonic effusions and empyema. Clin Chest Med 1985; 6: 55–62.
36. Westcott JL. Percutaneous catheter drainage of pleural effusion and empyema. AJR 1985; 144:1189–1193.
37. Yang PC, Luh KT, Chang DB, Wu HD, Yu CJ, Kuo SH. Value of sonography in determining the nature of pleural effusion: analysis of 320 cases. AJR 1992; 159: 29–33.
38. Aquino SL, Webb WR, Gushiken BJ. Pleural exudates and transudates diagnosis with contrast enhanced CT. Radiology 1994; 192:803–808.

39. Light RW. Management of parapneumonic effusions (editorial; comment). Chest 1991; 100:892–893.
40. Moulton JS, Benkert RE, Weisiger KH, Chambers JA. Treatment of complicated pleural fluid collections with image-guided drainage and intracavitary urokinase. Chest 1995; 108:1252–1259.
41. Taylor RF, Rubens MB, Pearson MC, Barnes NC. Intrapleural streptokinase in the management of empyema. Thorax 1994; 49:856–859.
42. Chin NK, Lim TK. Controlled trial of intrapleural streptokinase in the treatment of pleural empyema and complicated parapneumonic effusions. Chest 1997; 111: 275–279.
43. Davis WC, Johnson LF. Adult thoracic empyema revisited. Am Surg 1978; 44: 362–368.
44. Ibarra-Pérez C, Selman-Lama M. Diagnosis and treatment of amebic "empyema". Report of eighty-eight cases. Am J Surg 1977; 134:283–287.
45. Sherman MM, Subramanian V, Berger RL. Management of thoracic empyema. Am J Surg 1977; 133:474–478.
46. Milfeld DJ, Mattox KL, Beall AC Jr. Early evacuation of clotted hemothorax. Am J Surg 1978; 136:686–692.
47. Maurer JR, Friedman PJ, Wing VW. Thoracostomy tube in an interlobar fissure: radiologic recognition of a potential problem. AJR 1982; 139:1155–1161.
48. Webb WR, LaBerge J. Major fissure tube placement. Letter to the editor. AJR 1983; 140:1039.
49. Anderson CB, Philpott GW, Ferguson TB. The treatment of malignant pleural effusions. Cancer 1974; 33:916–922.
50. Marom EM, Patz EF Jr, Erasmus JJ, McAdams HP, Goodman PC, Herndon JE. Malignant pleural effusions: treatment with small-bore-catheter thoracostomy and talc pleurodesis. Radiology 1999; 210:277–281.
51. Davies CWH, Traill ZC, Gleeson FV, Davies RJO. Intrapleural streptokinase in the management of malignant multiloculated pleural effusions. Chest 1999; 115:729–733.
52. Goff BA, Mueller PR, Muntz HG, Rice LW. Small chest-tube drainage followed by bleomycin sclerosis for malignant pleural effusions. Obstet Gynecol 1993; 81: 993–996.
53. Gleeson F, Lomas DJ, Flower CDR, Stewart S. Powered cutting needle biopsy of the pleura and chest wall. Clin Radiol 1990; 41:199–200.
54. Sheth S, Hamper UM, Stanley DB, Wheeler JH, Smith PA. US guidance for thoracic biopsy: a valuable alternative to CT. Radiology 1999; 210:721–726.
55. Adams RF, Gleeson FV. Percutaneous image-guided cutting-needle biopsy of the pleura in the presence of a suspected malignant effusion. Radiology 2001; 219:510–514.
56. vonHoff DD, Li Volsi V. Diagnostic reliability of needle biopsy of the parietal pleura: a review of 272 biopsies. Am J Clin Pathol 1975; 64:200–203.
57. Poe RH, Israel RH, Utell MJ, Hall MJ, Greenblatt DW, Kallay MC. Sensitivity, specificity, and predictive values of closed pleural biopsy. Arch Intern Med 1984; 144:325–328.
58. Dalyer WR, Eggleston JC, Erozan YS. Efficacy of pleural needle biopsy and pleural fluid cytopathology in the diagnosis of malignant neoplasm involving the pleura. Chest 1975; 67:536–539.
59. Ruffie P, Feld R, Minkin S, Cormier Y, Boutan-Laroze A, Ginsberg R, Ayoub J,

Sheperd FA, Evans WK, Figueredo A. Diffuse malignant mesothelioma of the pleura in Ontario and Quebec: a retrospective study of 332 patients. J Clin Oncol 1989; 7:1157–1168.
60. Achatzy R, Beba W, Ritschler R, Worn H, Wahlers B, Macha HN, Morgan JA. The diagnosis, therapy and prognosis of diffuse malignant mesothelioma. Eur J Cardiothorac Surg 1989; 3:445–448.
61. Conces DJ Jr, Tarver RD, Gray WC, Pearcy EA. Treatment of pneumothoraces utilizing small caliber chest tubes. Chest 1988; 94:55–57.
62. Martin T, Fontana G, Olak J, Ferguson M. Use of a pleural catheter for the management of simple pneumothorax. Chest 1996; 110:1169–1172.
63. Minami H, Saka H, Senda K, Horio Y, Iwahara T, Nomura F, Sakai S, Shimokata K. Small caliber catheter drainage for spontaneous pneumothorax. Am J Med Sci 1992; 304:345–347.
64. Klein JS. Interventional techniques in the thorax. Clin Chest Med 1999; 20:805–826.
65. Protopapas Z, White CS, Miller BH. Transthoracic needle biopsy practices: results of a nationwide survey. Radiology 1996; 201(P):270.
66. Westcott JL. Direct percutaneous needle aspiration of localized pulmonary lesions: results in 422 patients. Radiology 1980; 137:31–35.
67. Spirn PW, Shah RM, Steiner RM, Greenfield AL, Salazar AM, Liu J-B. Image-guided localization for video-assisted thoracic surgery. J Thorac Imaging 1997; 12:285–292.
68. Kaiser LR, Shrager JB. Video-assisted thoracic surgery: the current state of the art. AJR 1995; 165:1111–1117.
69. Boutin C, Rey F. Thoracoscopy in malignant mesothelioma: a prospective study of 188 consecutive patients. I. Diagnosis. Cancer 1993; 72:389–404.
70. Menzies R, Charbonneau M. Thoracoscopy for the diagnosis of pleural disease. Ann Intern Med 1991; 114:271–276.
71. Shah RM, Spirn PW, Salazar AM. Localization of peripheral pulmonary nodules for thorascopic excision: value of CT-guided wire placement. AJR 1993; 161:279–283.
72. Mack MJ, Gordon MJ, Postma TW. Percutaneous localization of pulmonary nodules for thoracoscopic lung resection. Ann Thorac Surg 1992; 53:1123–1124.
73. Lenglinger FX, Schwarz CD, Artman W. Localization of pulmonary nodules before thoracoscopic surgery: value of percutaneous staining with methylene blue. AJR 1994; 163:297–300.
74. Plumkett MB, Peterson MS, Landrenau RJ, Ferson PF, Posner MC. Peripheral pulmonary nodules: preoperative percutaneous needle localization with CT guidance. Radiology 1992; 185:274–276.
75. Templeton PA, Krasna M. Localization of pulmonary nodules for thoracoscopic resection: use of needle/wire breast-biopsy system. AJR 1993; 160:761–762.
76. Gossot D, Miaux Y, Guermazi A. The hook-wire technique for localization of pulmonary nodules during thoracoscopic resection. Chest 1994; 105:1467–1469.

19

Drug-Induced Pleural Diseases

PHILIPPE CAMUS

University of Bourgogne Medical School
and University Medical Center le Bocage
Dijon, France

I. Introduction

In the past few decades drugs and radiation therapy, in addition to medical and surgical procedures, have become a significant cause of pleural involvement (1–8). This chapter is devoted to drug- and radiation-induced pleural disease, whereas iatrogenic and procedure-induced pleural involvement is considered separately (see Chapter 45). Being cognizant of iatrogenic pleural disease enables earlier diagnosis and may prevent unnecessary search for the cause of pleural effusion or thickening.

Drug- and radiation-induced pleural involvement is in the form of uni- or bilateral effusion(s), hemothorax, pneumothorax, chylothorax, pleural thickening, or acute chest pain. Clinically, pleural disease develops in isolation, concomitant with involvement of the pericardium (serositis, polyserositis), or with systemic symptoms and positive antinuclear antibodies (ANA) in drug-induced lupus. Patients with iatrogenic pleural involvement present with dyspnea as the combined result of pleural effusion or thickening, chest pain, compression of the contralateral lung, blood loss, pericardial tamponade/constriction, and, sometimes, parenchymal involvement. Patients with massive effusion (especially if bilateral) or tension pneumothorax present with acute respiratory distress, and this requires expeditious management.

In patients with drug-induced pleural effusion, restrictive pulmonary physiology is usually present, but the diffusing capacity for carbon monoxide is often normal or increased, except in patients with associated parenchymal involvement. High-resolution computed tomography (HRCT) and thoracic echography are more sensitive in the detection of pleural effusion than is the plain chest radiograph, particularly in ICU patients in whom only the frontal chest radiograph is generally available.

General mechanisms at the origin of iatrogenic pleural involvement include increased pleural fluid output due to pleural inflammation, decreased pleural fluid clearance (e.g., in chylothorax), and/or exaggerated pleural fibrogenesis (e.g., with the use of ergolines, amiodarone, or cyclophosphamide).

Pleural effusions resulting from medical procedures (e.g., transesophageal echography, insertion of a central venous line), self-inflicted pleural laceration, empyema in patients on long-term immunosuppression, drug-induced left ventricular or renal failure, and fluid overload are not considered in this chapter.

II. Diagnostic Criteria

The sources of information used to evaluate the drug-relatedness of pleural involvement include review articles (1–8)—particularly the recent article and detailed table of drugs that produce pleural disease by Morelock and Sahn (7)—and electronic databases (9), including Pneumotox® (10). Five main criteria should be evaluated.

There should be a history of exposure to drug(s). About 70 different drugs can produce pleural involvement (10) (Table 1). This is fewer than the number of drugs implicated in causing parenchymal lung involvement. History taking should include approved and over-the-counter drugs, dietary supplements, and illicit drugs that can produce pleural involvement. Drugs of a therapeutic class may all produce similar adverse pleural effects, suggesting a common cytopathic mechanism. Examples of this include pleural effusion and thickening in patients exposed to ergolines or to certain β-blockers. Drug-induced pleural involvement develops after variable periods of treatment, ranging from a few days (e.g., nitrofurantoin) to several years (e.g., ergolines). Rarely, pleural involvement is noted after termination of treatment with the drug or physical agents (e.g., cyclophosphamide, radiation therapy).

The clinical, imaging, and pathological pattern of pleural involvement should conform to earlier observations with the drug (1–8). Interestingly, drugs tend to occasion a reproducible pattern of pleural involvement. For instance, dantrolene produces eosinophilic pleural or pleuropericardial effusions, whereas ergolines produce pleural thickening, and hydralazine occasions the lupus syndrome.

Other drugs should be ruled out as causative. This is particularly important if pleural involvement is known to occur in the course of the background disease for which the suspected drug was given (e.g., rheumatoid arthritis or inflammatory bowel disease under treatment with sulfasalazine or left ventricular failure in patients on amiodarone). Prior exposure to asbestos should also be examined, as this probably increases the risk of developing adverse pleural reactions from ergot drugs (11).

Improvement should follow discontinuation of the drug. Drug therapy withdrawal is generally followed by sustained improvement of pleural abnormalities and of pulmonary functions in patients with pleural involvement of recent onset. Patients with drug-induced pleural thickening improve more slowly (over months to years), and some degree of pleural thickening often persists indefinitely. Follow-up of the erythrocyte sedimentation rate (ESR), or of ANA levels after drug discontinuation is useful to the extent that the values were elevated at the time of diagnosis. Corticosteroids or nonsteroidal antiinflammatory drugs are used in patients with severe symptoms, or if drug withdrawal does not translate into beneficial effect. The effects of these drugs remain difficult to evaluate.

Pleural involvement should recur following reexposure to the drug. Rechallenge of patients with drug-induced pleuritis has been performed in a few patients, leading to recurrence of pleural symptoms, and this confirmed the drug etiology (12). However, rechallenge is generally avoided because it may take months for pleural symptoms to recur. Rechallenge of patients with drug-induced pleural thickening and fibrosis is generally considered unethical, as the pleural changes are largely irreversible, and this increases the risk to the patient. The "acute chest pain syndrome," which sometimes develops during treatments with bleomycin or methotrexate, may not recur following reinstitution of treatment (13).

Additional features useful to the diagnosis include:

Involvement of other serosal surfaces such as the pericardium (14–17) or, rarely, the peritoneum (18)

Involvement of the retroperitoneum (19), mediastinum (20), or heart valves (21)

Eosinophilia in pleural fluid, blood, or broncho-alveolar lavage (BAL) fluid

Elevated titers of circulating ANA or antineutrophil cytoplasmic autoantibodies (ANCA), which suggests a drug-induced autoimmune condition

High titers of ANA or of LE cells in the pleural fluid, which are strongly associated with drug-induced lupus pleuritis

As regards pleural complications of radiation therapy, patients may develop pleural involvement up to many years after exposure, and there is an inverse relationship between time to onset after exposure to radiation and the likelihood of spontaneous improvement.

III. Drug-Induced Pleural Involvement

A. Drug-Induced Lone Pleural Effusion

Drugs causing pleural involvement and the corresponding clinical features and incidence estimates are shown in Table 1. Among these drugs, clozapine, dantrolene, gliclazide, isotretinoin, mesalazine, nitrofurantoin, propylthiouracil, sulfasalazine, and valproate occasion a distinctive pattern of eosino-

Table 1 Drugs Producing Pleural Disease

Drug	Lone pleural effusion	Pleural effusion and pulmonary infiltrates[a]	Eosinophilic pleural effusion[b]	Pleural thickening[c]	Lupus pleuritis/ effusion[d]	Acute chest pain	Hemothorax	Pneumothorax
Acebutolol	*							
ACE inhibitors		*			**			
Acyclovir		**			*			
Amiodarone	*	**		*	*			
Anticoagulants (oral)							**	
BCG therapy (in urinary bladder)	*							
Bleomycin	*	*				*		*
Bromocriptine	*			**				
Cabergoline	*			**				
Carbamazepine					**			
Camustine (BCNU)								*
Clomifen	***							
Clozapine	*		*					
Cyclophosphamide	*			**				
Dapsone	*							
Dantrolene			**					
Dextran	**							
Dihydroergocistine	*			**				
Dihydroergocryptine	*			**				
Dihydroergotamine	*			**				
Docetaxel	*			**				
Ergotamine	*							
Ethchlorvynol		*						
Fenfluramine/dexfenfluramine		*						
Glicazide	*		*					
Gonadotropins		*						
G(M)-CSF								

Drug							
Heparin						*	
Hydralazine/dihydralazine	*						
Interleukin 2	**		***				
Isoniazid			*				
Isotretinoin					*		
Itraconazole	*		*				
Leuprorelin							
Lisuride							
Mesalazine	*		*				
Mesulergine	*						
Methotrexate	**		**		***	**	
Methyldopa			*				
Methysergide	***	**					
Minocycline	*	*					
Minoxidil				*			
Nevirapine					*		
Nicergoline	*	**					
Nitrofurantoin	*				**	*	
Oxprenolol	*						
Penicillamine	*						
Pergolide							
Phenytoin					*		
Pindolol	*						
Practolol			***			***	
Praziquantel				*			
Procainamide				*			
Procarbazine	*					*	
Propylthiouracil							
Quinidine	*		***				
Radiation	**		**			*	*
Retinoic acid (ATRA)	**						

Table 1 Continued

Drug	Lone pleural effusion	Pleural effusion and pulmonary infiltrates[a]	Eosinophilic pleural effusion[b]	Pleural thickening[c]	Lupus pleuritis/effusion[d]	Acute chest pain	Hemothorax	Pneumothorax
Simvastin		*			*			
Sulfamides-sulfonamides-sulfasalazine	*	**			**			
Trimipramine			*					
Troglitazone	**							
l-Tryptophan (recalled)	*	***	*					
Valproate			*					
Vitamins B$_5$			*					

[a] Pleural effusion in association with infiltrative lung disease or pulmonary edema.
[b] Eosinophilic pleural or pleuropericardial effusion.
[c] Pleural thickening: pleural effusion, usually exudative, may predate or occur in association with pleural thickening.
[d] Lupus pleuritis: i.e., the association of pleural effusion or thickening and systemic symptoms (e.g., fever, rash, arthralgias) in the context of positive antinuclear antibodies (drugs that occasion the lupus syndrome do not all cause lupus pleuritis or pleural effusion).
The number of asterisks is an estimate of incidence from * rare to *** common.

philic pleural effusion, with or without associated pericardial effusion (10). Eosinophilia is generally present in the blood, BAL, or pleural tissue, concomitant with eosinophilia in the pleural fluid. In patients with bilateral effusions, eosinophilia was present on both sides. Rechallenge with the drug has caused recurrence of symptoms in some patients.

In addition to causing eosinophilic pleural effusion, clozapine, isotretinoin, mesalazine, and sulfasalazine can also occasion the syndrome of parenchymal infiltrates with eosinophilia (10).

The development of lone pleural effusion druring treatments with amiodarone is unusual, whereas it is frequently observed in patients with amiodarone pneumonitis. On imaging, a free-flowing effusion is present, often accompanied by some degree of pleural thickening. Bilateral exudates developed in one patient placed on high-dose amiodarone (1600 mg daily, followed by 1200 mg), and the effusions subsided after drug withdrawal (22). In another patient, a large bilateral serosanguineous effusion preceded the onset of amiodarone pneumonitis (23). Generally, the pleural fluid in amiodarone-induced pleural effusion is an exudate, with a range of protein concentration of 2.8–5.5 g/dL (7) and a lymphocyte (24) or lymphocyte and neutrophil predominance (22). In one patient with bilateral effusions, the right and left pleural fluid had the same characteristics (22). Foam cells resembling those found in the BAL fluid were evidenced on cytological examination of the pleural fluid in one case (23). On histology, there is pleural thickening, and foamy macrophages can be found in pleural tissue (22). Pericardial effusion was present in some patients as an associated feature (25,26). Amiodarone rarely causes the drug-associated lupus. (27) (see below). Patients generally improved upon discontinuance of amiodarone. An important differential diagnosis is left ventricular failure, which can also produce an exudate (28).

Ergoline drugs can produce a free-flowing pleural effusion. The effusion occurs in isolation or is associated with pleural thickening (see below). Patients with a history of prior exposure to asbestos are at a greater risk of developing pleural complications during treatments with ergolines (11). Imaging studies indicate uni- or bilateral, moderate or abundant effusion. Pleural thickening and rounded pulmonary atelectasis (i.e., the folded lung) are frequently present in association. The predominant side of involvement can change with time. Analysis of the pleural fluid typically shows a lymphocyte-predominant (up to 99%) exudate (7). However, pleural eosinophilia, a serosanguineous exudate, and a transudate have also been reported (29–31). Ergot-induced effusions usually resolve with stoppage of the drug.

Approximately 3% of patients with acute nitrofurantoin lung present with bilateral pleural effusions of small or moderate volume heralded by acute chest pain (32). Chest pain and effusions quickly recur upon reexposure to the agent (33).

Following drug withdrawal, the overall prognosis of drug-induced lone pleural effusion is good (Fig 1). Persistence of the effusion or sequellae are infrequent.

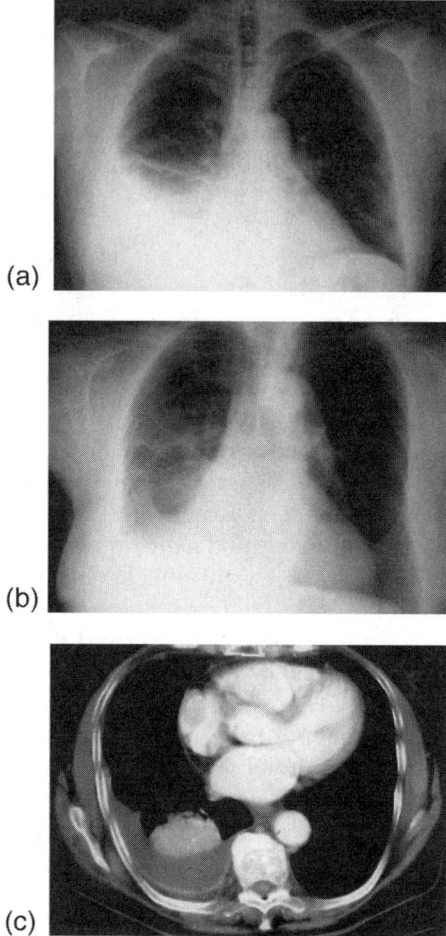

Figure 1 (a) Pleural effusion developed in a patient chronically exposed to dihydralazine. There were elevated fevers and high neutrophil counts in blood. Antinuclear antibodies were negative. The patient was seen after failure of several courses of antibiotics given empirically for presumed pleuropulmonary infection. Withdrawal of the drug was quickly followed by improvement of symptoms, and the pleural effusion disappeared over a few weeks. There was no relapse. (b) Pleural effusion developed insidiously in a patient exposed to an ergoline drug. (c) The CT scan showed pleural thickening and rounded atelectasis of the lung, in addition to the expected changes of free-flowing effusion. The effusion resolved slowly following stoppage of the drug.

B. Drug-Induced Pleural Thickening

Drug-induced pleural thickening is a slowly progressive disease characterized by chest pain, dyspnea, and increased pleural thickness on imaging with frequent areas of rounded atelectasis of the lung. Pleural calcifications are typically absent, except if there was prior exposure to asbestos. The impact upon pulmonary functions may be substantial in terms of restriction. Pleural abnormalities typically diminish after drug therapy withdrawal.

Amiodarone

Imaging studies commonly indicate smooth-edged pleural thickening in patients with amiodarone pneumonitis (34), (Fig. 2). The thickening predominates in the area where the pulmonary infiltrates are densest. Clinically, pleuritic chest pain and a friction rub may be present. The parenchymal opacities of amiodarone pneumonitis often demonstrate high attenuation on HRCT and similar changes in the liver or spleen, when present, help relate the changes on imaging with exposure to amiodarone (35). Upon drug discontinuation, some degree of pleural thickening may persist after resolution of the pulmonary opacities.

Ergolines

Ergoline drugs commonly produce fibrotic conditions with possible involvement of the pleura(e), pericardium, retroperitoneum (36), and, sometimes, cardiac valves (21), (Fig. 3). When pleural fibrosis develops, it is rarely associated with the other fibrosing syndromes seen as a result of ergoline use.

Historically, methysergide was the first ergot recognized to cause pleural fibrosis in patients who were receiving the drug for migraine (37). Similarly, bromocriptine in patients with Parkinson's disease and the newer ergolines cabergoline, dihydroergotamine, dihydrocryptine, dihydrocristine, ergonovine, ergotamine, lisuride, nicergoline, and pergolide can also occasion pleural thickening or effusion (36). The incidence is 2–4% of the treated population and is greater in patients previously exposed to asbestos (11). The onset is insidious, after months or years of treatment, and patients are often diagnosed after a long period of disabling chest or systemic symptoms (38). Symptoms include chest pain (mild to acute), dyspnea, a nonproductive cough, and slight fever. Clinical examination shows chest dullness, muffled breath sounds, and a pleural friction rub, which may be perceived by the patient. Associated manifestations include pericardial effusion, tamponade or constriction, or endomyocardial fibrosis. The ESR is generally increased (36), and ANA are negative. Imaging studies indicate bilateral symmetrical or asymmetrical involvement in the form of an increase in thickness of the pleura laterally and basally, and sometimes loculated effusions. Lung shrinkage and foci of rounded atelectasis en face the areas of increased pleural thickness are common associated findings (36). The pleural involvement is rarely apical or unilateral. Transudative or exudative pleural effusion may be present as an associated

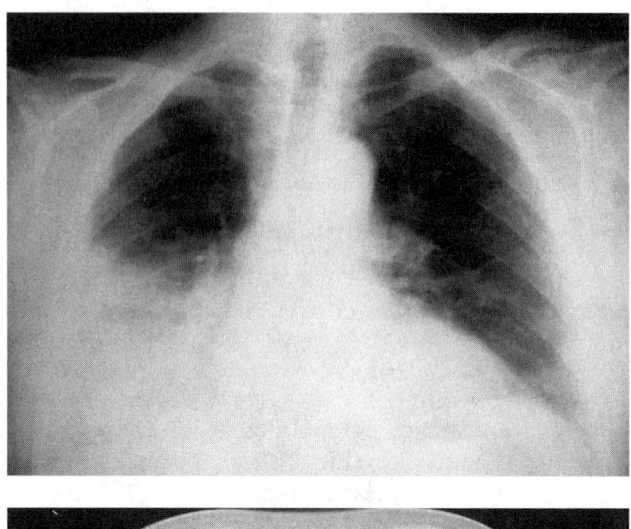

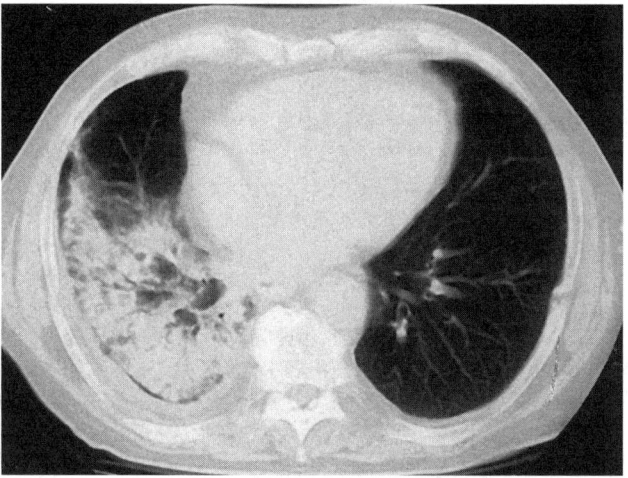

Figure 2 The CT scan of patients with amiodarone pneumonitis often displays smooth-edged pleural thickening, en face the area(s) of parenchymal involvement. In general, the CT scan is more sensitive than the chest radiograph in the detection of drug-induced pleural changes. (From Refs. 154,155.)

Figure 3 Suggestive pleural thickening induced by long-term exposure to ergolines (e.g., bromocriptine, ergotamine, lisuride, methysergide). The chest radiograph shows pleural thickening in addition to bilateral rounded atelectasis. The pleural thickening is better visualized on CT, and no calcifications are usually found, except in patients with prior exposure to asbestos, a potentiating factor for ergot-induced pleural changes (11). Ergoline-induced pleural thickening is responsible for significant loss of lung volume. Cessation of exposure to the drug is usually followed by rapid improvement of chest symptoms, whereas the improvement of imaging and of pulmonary physiology is usually lagging behind and incomplete (36).

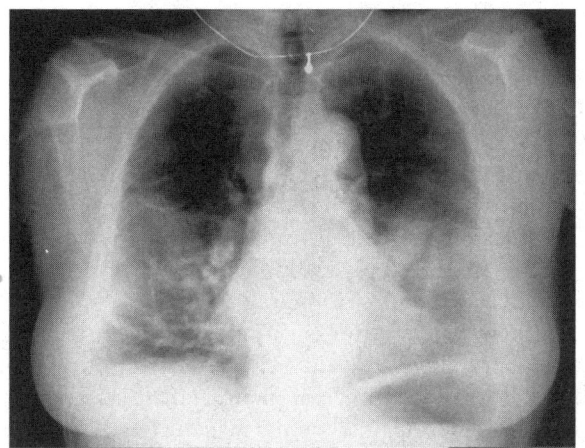
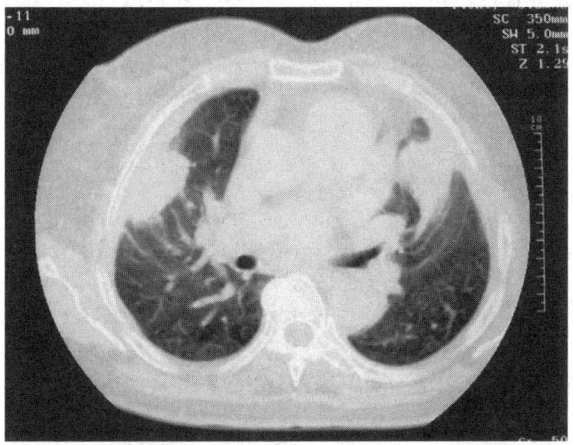
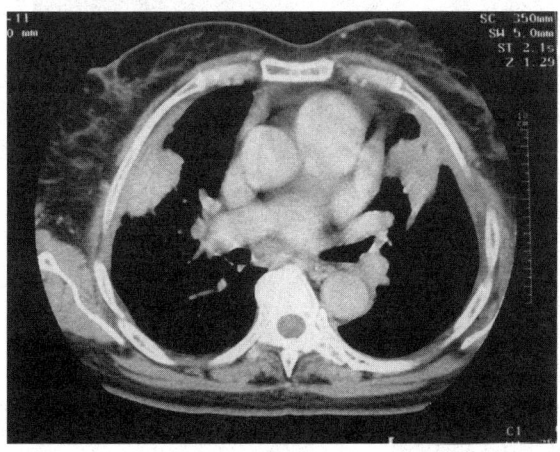

feature. An unexpectedly rapid increase in pleural thickening in a patient with prior exposure to asbestos during treatment with ergolines should alert to the possibility of the drug condition.

Restrictive pulmonary functions are present with vital capacity reduced to less than 50% of predicted in some patients, but the diffusing capacity is preserved. Peripheral edema and ascites were present in some patients will severely restrictive physiology. On thoracoscopy, the parietal or, less often, the visceral pleura is thickened in the form of a whitish peel encasing the lung (36,39). Biopsy of the abnormal pleura indicates bland pleural fibrosis (36) and sometimes perivascular inflammatory aggregates (40).

Most patients improve after stoppage of drug treatment. Systemic symptoms abate in a few days, and the ESR returns to normal in a few weeks. This is followed by the disappearance of pleural effusions, if present, and by the slow diminution of the pleural thickening, which may require several months or years to be complete (36). In patients with marked pleural thickening, the pleural thickness may never completely normalize (36). Steroids do not seem to accelerate recovery of the pleural abnormalities (41). Surgical decortication was used in the past but has no current role. Rechallenge with the same or another ergoline is discouraged, as this is followed by recurrence (12).

Cyclophosphamide

The peculiar features of late pleuropulmonary toxicity from cyclophosphamide are a pattern of pleural fibrosis, which involves the upper and lateral aspect of the pleura bilaterally, in addition to more typical changes of pulmonary fibrosis (42). Narrowing of the anteroposterior diameter of the thorax is seen in children with cyclophosphamide toxicity as they grow up, and this occasions severe restrictive physiology and respiratory failure.

Practolol

The β-blocker practolol was introduced in the 1970s in the United Kingdom. After months of treatment, and even after withdrawal of the drug, some patients developed bilateral basilar pleural thickening with or without effusion and rarely elevated ANA titers (43). Some patients also developed ocular inflammation or fibrosis, Lapeyronie's disease, or peritoneal fibrosis, which persisted upon drug therapy withdrawal. Practolol was recalled in 1976. Oxprenolol was once suspected of producing pleural abnormalities similar to those of practolol (44), but the drug was eventually exonerated (45).

C. Drug-Induced Pneumothorax

Pneumothorax can develop in patients with rheumatoid nodules, primary or metastatic lung tumors (e.g., germ cell tumor, sarcoma), or lymphoma, as they undergo treatment with cytotoxic chemotherapy. The air leak is thought to result from the necrosis of subpleurally located masses, leading to communication between the bronchial tree and the pleural space (46).

Pneumothorax with or without pneumomediastinum can develop in patients with drug-induced pneumonitis (47) or fibrosis (48). A few patients have died from the complication (49).

Pneumothorax and pneumomediastinum have been described as a complication of bronchiolitis obliterans in bone marrow transplantees (50).

D. Hemothorax

The pleura is a relatively rare site of hemorrhage in patients on chronic oral anticoagulants who have received fibrinolytic agents or heparin (51–53). Patients with a history of recent thoracic trauma, including cardiopulmonary resuscitation or pulmonary embolism and infarction, are at risk (51,53–55). In patients with pulmonary embolism, bleeding in the pleura can occur early on the side of the initial clinical symptoms, which suggests intrapleural rupture of a hemorrhagic pulmonary infarct (51,54). Less often, the hemothorax develops later and may not be on the side of the initial symptoms, which is consistent with bleeding from the pleural membrane (51).

Hemothorax often occurs as the only bleeding complication of anticoagulation, and coagulation studies are misleading, as they are within an acceptable therapeutic range in 60% of patients (51). Hemothorax has also been reported after the administration of ticlopidine and aspirin (55). Cessation of anticoagulation therapy and prompt evacuation of the pleural space are recommended.

Patients with thoracic endometriosis and pulmonary endometrial implants can develop symptoms synchronous with menses. These include recurrent hemoptysis, pleuritic chest pain, pneumothorax, hemothorax, and hemopneumothorax. The hemothorax can follow the administration of leuprorelin (56).

Hemothorax has also been reported as a complication of thrombocytopenia in patients receiving myeloablative chemotherapy (57).

E. Pleuritic Chest Pain

Moderate chest pain is a common symptom in patients with drug-induced pleural effusion or thickening, and in those with drug-induced lupus.

Intense chest pain and an audible friction rub has been described in patients with drug-induced pneumonitis or organizing pneumonia due to nitrofurantoin, (58), furazolidone (14), carbamazepine (59), and minocycline (60) (Fig. 4).

A few drugs cause severe pleuritic chest pain, often without demonstrable pleural or pulmonary involvement, and this can create significant diagnostic problems for the practitioner. In a series of 210 patients who received 3130 courses of high-dose methotrexate, marked chest pain interpreted as "chemical pleuritis" developed in 18 (incidence = 8.5%) (61). The sudden onset of chest pain occurred after the third or fourth treatment course and lasted between 3

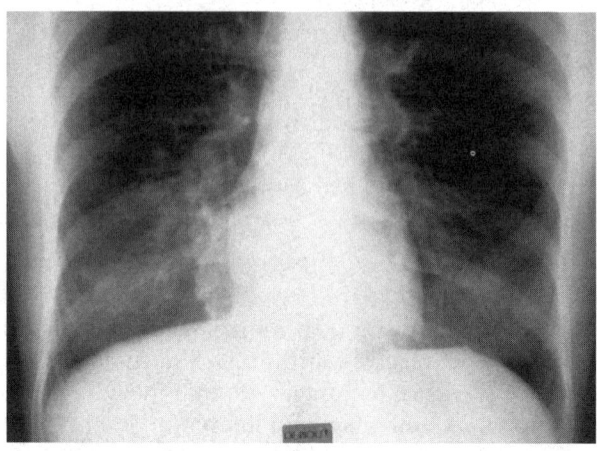

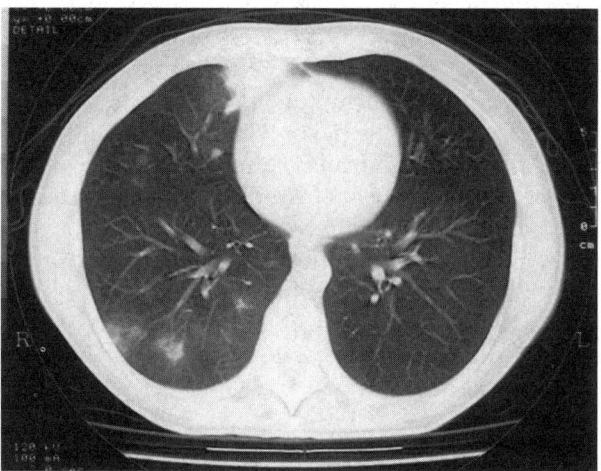

Figure 4 A few drugs, especially the chemotherapeutic agents cyclophosphamide or methotrexate when administered IV, produce excruciating pleuritic pain. On imaging, there are usually no to minimal changes in the lung or pleura. Patients with drug-induced parenchymal reactions may present with acute chest pain, especially if the parenchymal changes are subpleural. This young woman developed an acute chest syndrome and scattered pulmonary opacities while being treated with a statin drug. The clinical and imaging picture relapsed after the patient was given another statin, suggesting a drug class effect.

and 5 days. Roentgenographic examination of the chest revealed thickening of the intralobar pleura most prominent on the right side, with pleural effusion in about a third of patients (62). The outcome was good (61).

Severe chest pain suggesting acute cardiac or pulmonary events was also observed after administration of bleomycin, and incidence of the syndrome was 2.8% of patients on the drug (13). The pain was sudden in onset and described either as substernal pressure or pleuritic in character. Electrocardiographic changes suggestive of pericarditis were found in two cases. Radiographic evidence of a small pleural effusion was seen in one patient. The syndrome was self-limited or relieved with analgesics. Discontinuation of bleomycin was not necessary, although improvement was seen when the infusions were stopped. Further courses of bleomycin did not lead to recurrent episodes in most patients and are therefore not contraindicated.

The administration of dihydro-5-azacytidine to oncology patients occasioned similar symptoms (63).

Accoring to Pelz et al. (64), acute chest pain developed in 1.6% of patients who underwent occlusion of brain arteriovenous malformation(s) with liquid acrylate glue (iso-butyl-2-cyanoacrylate, or *n*-butyl-2-cyanoacrylate). The symptoms are linked to glue emboli within the pulmonary circulation, and develop within 48 hours of glue injection. Patients were treated conservatively and recovered spontaneously.

F. Pleural Effusion in the Context of Drug-Induced Pneumonitis

Pleural effusions are relatively common in patients with drug-induced pneumonitis. For instance, the incidence is about 10% in patients with methotrexate lung (65), with the effusion sometimes noted a few days after the peak of the symptoms of the infiltrative lung disease (Fig. 5a). Similarly, pleural effusion containing eosinophils may develop in patients with drug-induced eosinophilic pneumonia (Fig. 5b, c). In some cases the infiltrative lung disease and pleural effusion recured upon reexposure of the patient to the causative agent (33,66–68).

Pleural effusion is a rare occurrence in patients with gold lung, with an overall incidence of effusion and thickening of 2.9% (69). One patient presented with a lymphocyte-predominant exudate while receiving gold, and the pleural biopsy revealed nonspecific inflammation (70).

Pleural effusion was present in two of five patients with mitomycin pneumonitis in one series (71), but the fluid characteristics were not described.

In acute nitrofurantoin lung, pleural effusions were evidenced in 16% of patients, and the volume of pleural effusion ranged from simple blunting of the costophrenic angles to moderate (72). Rechallenge of one patient occasioned recurrence of blood eosinophilia and of the pleural effusion, but the pleural fluid was not examined (73). The prevalence of pleural effusion in patients with subacute or chronic nitrofurantoin lung is less (6%) than in the acute form of the disease (32).

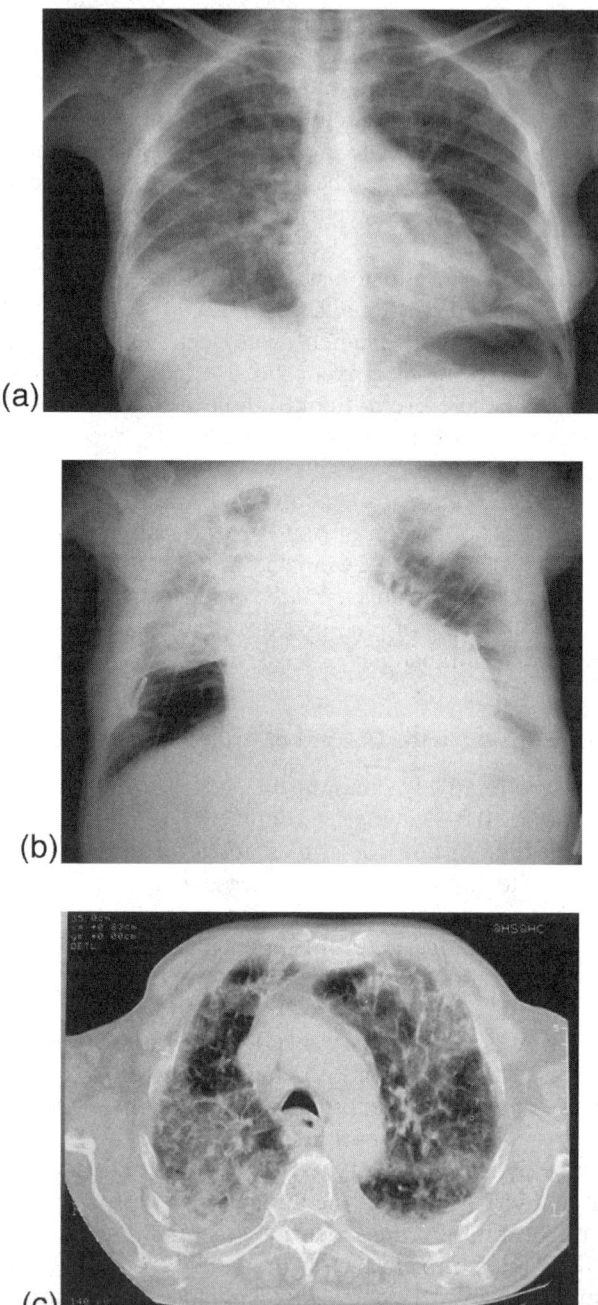

Figure 5 Pleural effusions occasionally accompany infiltrative lung disease due to (a) methotexate or (b,c) drug-induced eosinophilic pneumonias. (From Ref. 74.)

Pleural effusion, with or without chest pain, has been reported in several patients with eosinophilic pneumonia due to angiotensin-converting enzyme (ACE) inhibitors (74), diflunisal (75), fenfluramine (67), minocycline (76), nevirapine (77), tosulofloxacin (78), trypophan, Chinese herbs (79), and certain health foods (80).

An exudative pleural effusion, often unilateral and of moderate volume, develops in up to a third of patients with amiodarone pneumonitis (81).

Peripheral opacities and lung shrinkage have been reported on in patients exposed to bleomycin. Although the reaction has been called "bleomycin pleuropneumonitis," a true effusion is unusual (82,83) (Fig. 6).

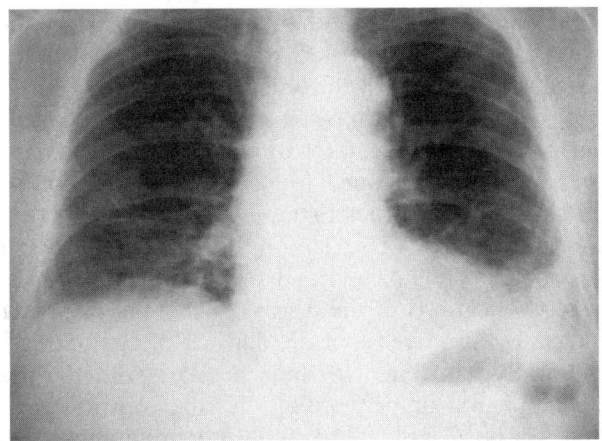

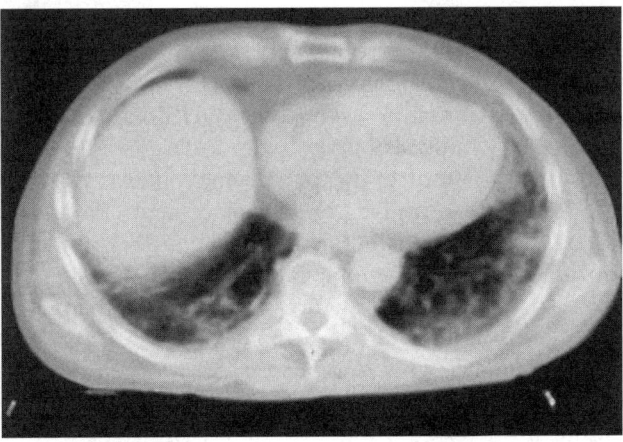

Figure 6 Bibasilar shrinking is a common feature of bleomycin pleuro-pulmonary toxicity (13,82,83,156). Clinically, patients present with dyspnea and, sometimes, intense chest pain. Parenchymal infiltrates and pleural thickening (presumably due to fibrinous pleural thickening) can be seen on imaging.

Pleural effusion does not generally occur in association with drug-induced pulmonary fibrosis.

G. Pleural Effusions Associated with Drug-Induced Increase in Pulmonary Permeability

Pleural effusions have been reported on chest radiograph in a few patients with severe drug-induced pulmonary edema or adult respiratory distress syndrome (ARDS) secondary to the administration of granulocyte-monocyte colony-stimulating factor (GM-CSF) (84), high-dose cytosine arabinoside (85), gemcitabine (86), or ethchlorvynol (87). Postmortem studies indicate extensive fibrinous pleural exudates suggestive of capillary leak (85).

Pleural effusion is rare in patients with drug-induced pulmonary edema. For instance, when all cases of hydrochlorothiazide- and aspirin-induced pulmonary edema are considered, pleural effusion was present in only one patient (88).

About 5% of women with β_2-agonist–induced pulmonary edema (a disease specific to the pregnant state) develop pleural effusion (89). In one case, the pleural effusion developed following resolution of the pulmonary opacities (90). Pleural fluid characteristics are unknown.

All-*trans*-retinoic acid (ATRA) promotes the maturation of promyelocytic cells in promyelocytic leukemia and reduces the likelihood and intensity of hemorrhagic complications of the disease. The administration of ATRA is followed 2–21 days by an increase in the number of circulating myeloid cells, and this is temporally associated in some patients with the development of weight gain, fever, pleural or pericardial effusion, pleuritic chest pain, lower extremity edema, dyspnea, pulmonary infiltrates, pulmonary edema or hemorrhage, or an ARDS picture (91). The syndrome is named the retinoic acid or ATRA syndrome. Pleural or pleuroperocardial effusion is present on imaging in most if not all patients (91). Prophylactic administration of corticosteroids has decreased the incidence of the syndrome (92).

The ovarian hyperstimulation syndrome (OHSS) is a distinctive condition observed in women of childbearing age who undergo induction of ovulation with clomifen or other gonadotropins. In a few patients, a syndrome of vascular leak occurs after ovulation and embryo replacement. Patients present with basilar atelectasis, pleural effusion(s), often of large volume, ascites, renal failure, and thromboembolic phenomena (93). A fraction of patients develop pulmonary edema or an ARDS picture. In a few women, massive pleural effusion developed in isolation. The pleural fluid is typically an exudate [pleural proteins 4.0–5.3 g/L (94)], with low lactate dehydorgenase (LDH) and cell counts suggesting increased permeability of the pleural membrane. Abdominal ultrasound can aid in determining the size and severity of ascites and pleural effusion and demonstrates the cystically enlarged ovaries. Thoracentesis and evacuation of the pleural fluid is recommended (95). In one patient with compressive pleural effusion, 10 L of pleural fluid were removed (96).

Pulmonary edema and pleural effusions have been observed in patients with pulmonary hypertension or venoocclusive disease following treatments with calcium channel blockers or prostacyclin (97,98). Pleural fluid characteristics are unknown.

Certain classic [e.g., cytosine arabinoside (99)] or novel chemotherapeutic agents (100), interleukin-2 (101)), and lymphokine-activated killer cells (101) can produce a dose-dependent vascular leak syndrome. The syndrome is associated with radiographically detectable pleural effusions in 3–50% of patients (102,103).

Patients with acute leukemia and high blast counts can develop acute respiratory failure and pleural effusions shortly after initiation of chemotherapy. In the two reported patients, the pleural fluid was an exudate with very high LDH levels (1787 and 3652 IU/L, respectively), which contained blast cells (104).

H. Pleural Involvement in Drug-Induced Systemic Conditions

Drug-Induced Systemic Lupus Erythematosus

Drug-induced lupus was first described in 1945 in a patient treated with sulfadiazine (105). Many cases of drug-induced lupus were reported in the 1950s, when hydralazine became available for the treatment of systemic hypertension (106). Hydralazine produces fever, arthralgias, and serositis, along with high titers of circulating ANA (Fig. 7). It was estimated that after 4 years of treatment, 80–100% of patients developed ANA and 30–50% eventually developed symtoms of lupus (107). At the time, the clustering of cases of drug-induced lupus produced a measurable increase in prevalence, compared to idiopathic lupus (108).

Later, isoniazid and procainamide were also recognized to cause the syndrome, and the latter drug is still considered the most potent lupus-inducing drug. Over the years, the drug lupus was described during treatments with about 50 chemically-unrelated drugs such as amiodarone, ACE inhibitors, anticonvulsants, β-blockers (mainly acebutolol), carbamazepine, chlorpromazine, oral contraceptives, recombinant cytokines or antibodies, dihydralazine, mesalazine, methyldopa, minocycline, nitrofurantoin, propylthiouracil, statins, sulfasalazine, and ticlopidine (10). Although hydralazine and procainamide are now less in use, cases of the drug-induced lupus are still regularly observed in clinical practice (109).

The overall prevalence of drug-induced lupus is 0.8 per 100,000 population, and it is estimated that drugs cause approximately 30% of all cases of lupus. Minocycline increases the risk of developing lupus 8.5-fold (109). Generally, drugs induce a form of lupus that is clinically (milder course, absence of flares, rare kidney or neurological involvement, frequent reversal upon discontinuance of drug therapy, equal distribution in men and women as opposed to the 90% female predominance in idiopathic lupus), and biologically (anti-double-strand

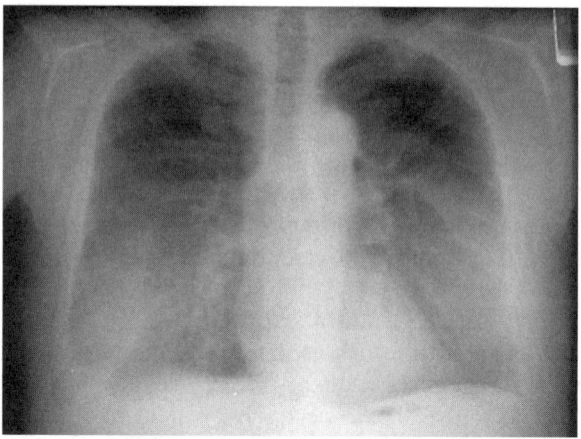

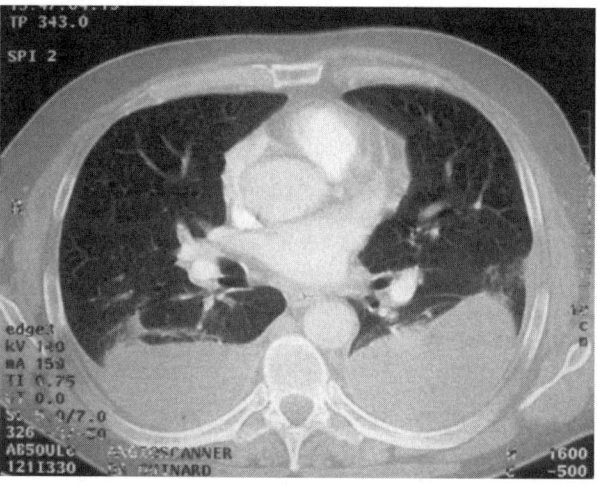

Figure 7 Bilateral free-flowing exudative effusions developed in a patient with fluoxetine-induced lupus erythematosus. In drug-induced lupus, there are usually high titers of antinuclear antibodies in blood, and even more so in the pleural fluid. Systemic symptoms or manifestations are often present in association with the pleural changes. Stoppage of the lupus-inducing drug generally leads to disappearance of the pleural effusion(s), as was the case in this patient.

DNA antibodies distinctly unusual, normal complement levels) dissimilar to the idiopathic lupus (110).

Risk factors for the development of drug-induced lupus are drug- and patient-related and include:

> The type of drug (e.g., arylamine and hydrazine drugs are potent lupus-inducing agents).

The degree of exposure (i.e., dose and duration of treatment) to the drug.

The acetylator phenotype. Patients with the slow hydralazine acetylator phenotype produce more oxidative and unconjugated metabolites, have a higher liability to disease, and develop lupus-related symptoms earlier than do rapid acetylators. Patients with the rapid acetylator phenotype metabolize hydralazine into conjugated metabolites, which have less potency as regards the induction of lupus (111).

Genetic and ethnic background. Relatives of patients with drug-induced lupus are more prone to the development of idiopathic autoimmune conditions, and drug-induced lupus develops more often in whites than it does in dark-skinned people.

Onset of the disease is progressive after months or years into treatment, with chest pain, cough, dyspnea, arthralgias, fever, skin changes, and other systemic symptoms. Approximately half the patients with drug-induced lupus present with pleuritis or pleural effusion, and up to a third present with pericardial effusion (112). Pleural fibrosis resembling that caused by ergolines occurs rarely. As the disease develops insidiously, the diagnosis is often established late.

Circulating antinuclear and antihistone antibodies are nearly always present in patients with drug-induced lupus if appropriate techniques are employed. There is no relationship between ANA levels and the likelihood of developing lupus or the type or severity of symptoms. Some patients with drug-induced lupus lacked ANA, and only antihistone antibodies were present (113). Antihistone antibodies are not specific for the drug etiology and have different specificities depending on the causative drug [H2A, H2B, or H2A-H2B-complex in procainamide-induced lupus, and H3 and H4 in hydralazine-induced lupus, respectively (114)]. Anti-DNA antibodies have been described only in a few patients with in acebutolol-, hydralazine-, penicillamine-, and procainamide-induced lupus. Hypocomplementemia and antimyeloperoxidase antibodies are also unusual findings (115). The lupus anticoagulant and anti-phospholipid antibodies were present in a few patients (115) and may associate with thromboembolic phenomena (116). The diagnosis of drug-induced lupus is complex in patients who have elevated ANA titers from their background disease. Examples of this include the association of pleural effusion and elevated ANA titers in patients with ulcerative colitis, rheumatoid arthritis, or tuberculosis while being treated with mesalazine, penicillamine, or isoniazide, respectively. In such cases, the time course of pleural involvement and of ANA upon drug therapy withdrawal will aid in determining if the condition was drug-related. Rare patients with drug-induced lupus presented with peripheral eosinophilia as an associated feature (117).

As in idiopathic lupus, the pleural fluid is an exudate (118). Cells counts range from 230 to 55,000 cells/μL (118,119), percentage of neutrophils from 10 to 100% (7,118), and pleural levels of LDH between 200 and 550 IU/L. The presence of elevated titers of ANA in the pleural fluid is a useful marker of the disease (120,121). Eleven out of 13 patients (2 drug-induced) with lupus pleuritis had pleural fluid ANA ≥ 1:160, and in 9 the pleural fluid-to-serum ANA ratio was greater than unity (118). Antinuclear antibodies are specifically present in the pleural tissue of patients with drug-induced lupus pleuritis, as opposed to pleural effusions of other causes (122). Antinuclear antibodies are also found in the pericardial fluid of patients with pericardial effusion (107).

Treatment is mainly discontinuation of the drug, and corticosteroid therapy is recommended for severe reactions. Upon stoppage of drug therapy, all symptoms diminish within a few days or weeks (109). This is followed by the more gradual decrease of circulating ANA. In a fraction of patients, ANA and/or symptoms persist for longer periods of time (109). Rechallenge of the patient with the drug leads to recurrence of symptoms within shorter periods of time (109). Patients who develop subclinical ANA during treatments with drugs known to induce lupus need simple follow-up; the drug does not need to be discontinued unless an alternate treatment choice is available or symptoms develop (123).

l-Tryptophan

In the past, ethylene-bis-tryptophan, a contaminant formed during the manufacturing process of *l*-tryptophan in one plant, was associated with epidemics of a systemic eosinophilic disease coined the "eosinophilia-myalgia syndrome." Affected patients presented with the insidious or rapid onset of constitutional symptoms, myalgias, skin changes, fasciitis, and neurological and cardiac involvement. Respiratory involvement included pulmonary infiltrates, pulmonary hypertension, or acute respiratory failure. Small-to-moderate bilateral pleural effusions were present in approximately 1/6 of patients who presented with eosinophilic pulmonary infiltrates (124). There were no sequellae, as opposed to the persistence or progression of blood eosinophilia, skin or neurological changes, or pulmonary hypertension in a fraction of the affected population (125).

Drug-Induced Vasculitides

Bilateral pleural effusions were present in a patient with montelukast-induced Churg-Strauss syndrome (126). The pleural fluid was an eosinophilic exudate (proteins 4.3 g/L) containing 152 IU/L of LDH.

A patient developed hypersensitivity vasculitis, pulmonary infiltrates, and pleural effusion while being treated with propylthiouracil for Graves' disease (127). The pleural fluid was a transudate (total proteins 1.6 g/dL), containing 64 white cells per μL, and the LDH level was 235 IU/L. The pleuropulmonary manifestations improved upon drug therapy withdrawal and institution of corticosteroids.

Pleural effusion was not a feature of the drug rash and eosinophilia systemic syndrome (DRESS) caused by carbamazepine (128) but has been observed in a case of DRESS caused by nevirapine (77).

Pleural exudate containing 48% mononucleated cells and 666 IU/L of LDH developed in conjunction with the sulfone syndrome (a constellation of symptoms including fever, malaise, hepatitis, dermatitis, hemolytic anemia, and pancreatitis) in an adolescent during treatment of *acne vulgaris* with dapsone (129).

IV. Pleural Involvement Following Chest Radiation Therapy

A. Early Effusions

Pleural effusion (typically unilateral, on the irradiated side) can develop early (2–6 months) after radiation therapy to the chest for breast or lung carcinoma (130), less commonly after mantle field radiation therapy for Hodgkin's disease or lymphoma. Formerly, pleural effusion developed in approximately 10% of women irradiated for breast carcinoma, and in nearly all of them, radiation pneumonitis was also present (131,132). The incidence of post-irradiation pleural effusion has now decreased (133). Early radiation-induced effusions are usually of moderate volume and may be associated with chest pain. Imaging studies may indicate a tent-like apperance of the effusion, especially when there is associated retraction of the upper lung segments.

The pleural fluid is an exudate containing reactive mesothelial cells (134). Early radiation-induced effusions generally follow an indolent course and rarely give rise to marked symptoms. Steroids and nonsteroidal anti-inflammatory drugs are required to control symptoms in some cases.

Pleural effusion is not a feature of radiation-induced organizing pneumonia, a syndrome of migrating parenchymal opacities that develops after breast radiation therapy (135).

B. Late Radiation-Induced Effusions

Pleural effusions can develop late to very late after mediastinal or mantle field irradiation. The pleural fluid has the characteristics of an exudate, with neutrophils, lymphocytes, and a few eosinophils. Since late radiation–induced effusions often develop in areas of the chest remote from the radiation beam, factors other than direct pleural injury are thought to play a role. Mechanisms in addition to direct pleural damage include hemodynamic factors (e.g., pericardial effusion, thickening or constriction, myocardial fibrosis) and/or altered mediastinal lymph flow dynamics (136). Sometimes the effusion is massive or recurrent, requiring pleurodesis (137), or is associated with pleural or pleuropericardial thickening and causes severe cardiorespiratory dysfunction (Fig. 8).

C. Chylothorax

Chylothorax can develop in patients with a remote history of radiation therapy to the chest [up to 23 years in one case (138)] (Fig. 9). The milky appearance of the pleural fluid suggests the diagnosis, and this is confirmed by

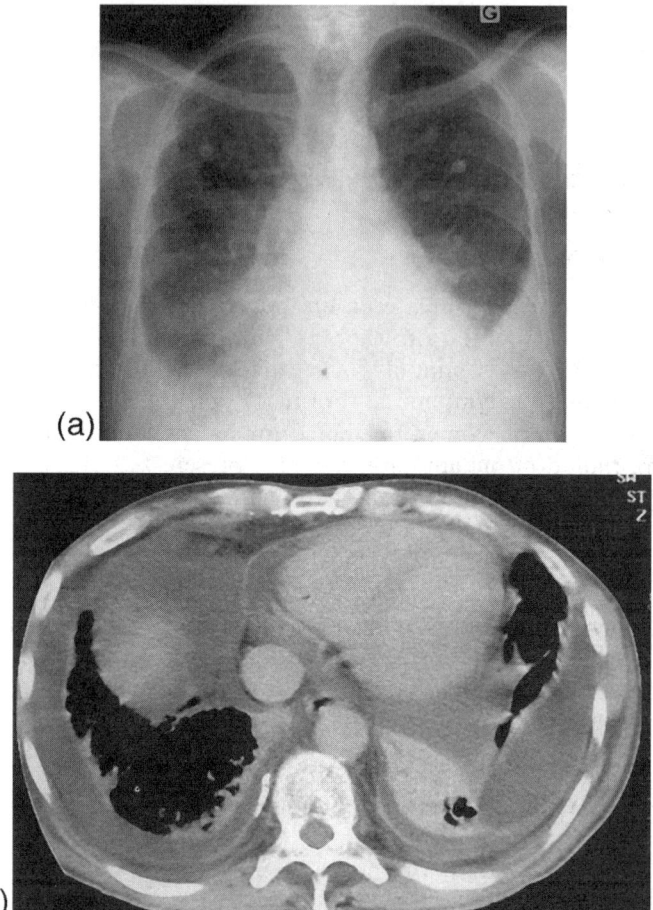

Figure 8 (a) Radiation therapy to the chest can produce cardiac changes (e.g., myocardial fibrosis, valvular stenosis or regurgitation, and thickening of coronary arteries) in addition to pleural and pericardial effusion/thickening. The combination of these changes severely impacts on lung functions. Bilateral exudative pleural effusions and pericardial effusion developed in this 60-year-old patient 35 years after he was given radiation therapy to the chest for Hodgkin's disease. He died from intractable cardiorespiratory failure, despite long-term mechanical ventilation via a tracheostomy. (b) Note the pleural calcification.

the finding of elevated levels of triglycerides and chylomicrons in the pleural fluid. Sometimes the interface between the lipid and aqueous phase is spontaneously visible on CT examination of the chest (139). Radiation-related chylothorax is thought to result from hindered lymph flow secondary to mediastinal fibrosis, less often from a tear in the thoracic duct (140). Chylous ascites may be present in association with the chylothorax. Chylous effusions

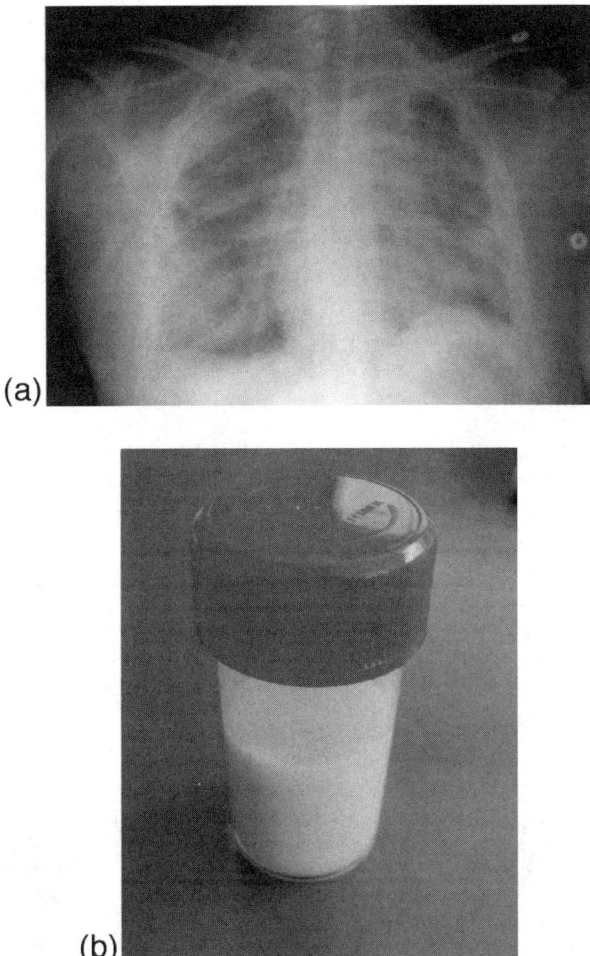

Figure 9 (a) Chylous effusions can develop after radiation therapy to the chest (157–160). (b) Inspection of the pleural fluid is diagnostic. The accumulation of lymph is thought to result in part from radiation-induced mediastinal fibrosis.

can be controlled by total parenteral nutrition followed by a low-fat diet. In rare cases in which a tear and leak could be evidenced on the thoracic duct, surgical repair was followed by control of the effusion (140).

D. Pleural Thickening

Pleural thickening is a common finding on imaging in patients with prior radiation therapy to the chest (141). In a series of 39 patients with breast cancer or various intrathoracic malignancies, pleural thickening was evidenced in 9 on conventional chest radiographs and in 15 on HRCT (142) (Fig. 10).

After mantle-field or supraclavicular and cervical radiation therapy, the localization of pleural fibrosis is typically in the apices or in paravertebral regions and may occasion severe volume loss (Fig. 11). A slight amount of pleural fluid is sometimes present as an associated feature. The impact of these changes in terms of volume restriction is variable, but is usually modest in patients treated with recent irradiation thechniques.

Pleural thickening is also observed in women who received tangential radiation therapy for the treatment of breast carcinoma. The thickening occurs in areas where the radiation dose was highest (143).

E. Pneumothorax

Pneumothorax occasionally develops late after radiation therapy to the chest or mediastinum (144) and is usually ipsilateral to the side of irradiation. It is probably related to underlying fibrosis of the irradiated lung. Patients may recover spontaneously, or exsufflation may be required.

F. Pleural Tumors

Patients can develop mesothelioma (145) or other malignant pleural tumors (146) late after chest radiation therapy. The cause-and-effect relationship remains under investigation (147).

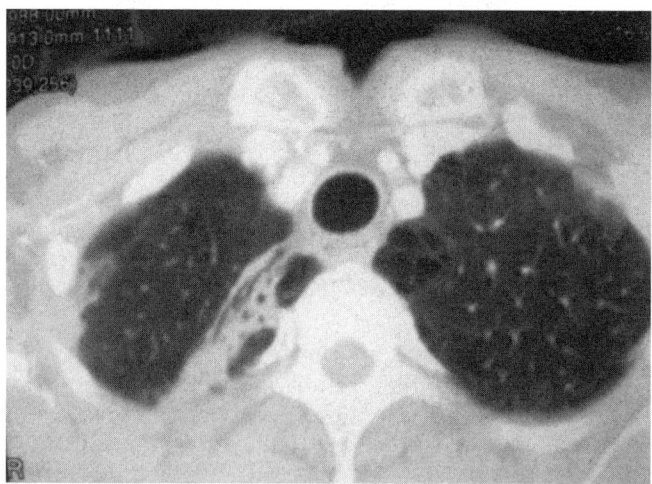

Figure 10 The pleural thickening in patients with a history of radiation therapy to the breast is often diagnosed easily when the characteristic distribution of the pleuropulmonary changes along the radiation port (oblique in the present case) is present on imaging.

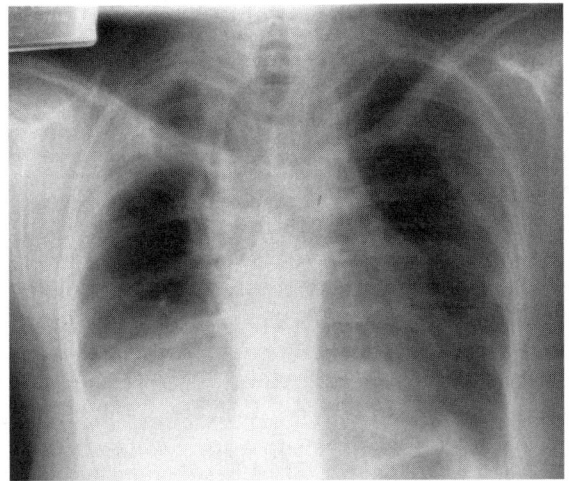

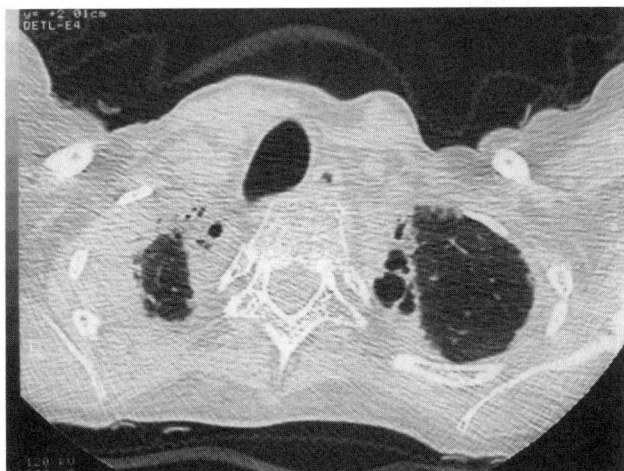

Figure 11 Thoracic changes induced by mantle radiation therapy have a predilection to localize in the superior lung sulci and in the paramediastinal regions of the lung. This results in a Y-shaped pattern of pleuro-pulmonary and mediastinal fibrosis. This 27-year-old woman had received radiation therapy as part of treatment of Hodgkin's disease in childhood and presented with severe restrictive respiratory insufficiency.

V. Complications of Intrapleural Delivery of Drugs

Intrapleural instillation of talc, bleomycin, cisplatin, and etoposide was followed by the rapid development of pulmonary edema or an ARDS picture (148–150).

VI. Pleural Disease in Drug Abusers

Drug abusers whose peripheral veins are sclerosed following the long-term administration of illicit drugs turn to other sites such as the internal jugular or the subclavian vein. The procedure is usually performed by a comrade in the street, under the name "pocket shot." During the procedure the pleura can be lacerated with resultant pneumothorax. In a series of 12 drug abusers with various complications resulting from supra- or subclavicular drug injection, 6 presented with unilateral pneumothorax and one with bilateral tension pneumothorax (151). In a large urban community, 113 pneumothorax episodes were diagnosed in 84 drug abusers, representing an alarming 21.5% rate of all causes of pneumothorax (152). In that study, 9 patients developed bilateral lung collapse, probably as the consequence of bilateral attempts at injecting the drug, and 11 patients developed recurrence. In one drug abuser, pneumothorax developed 3 months after breakage of a needle into the jugular vein (153).

Repeated Valsalva maneuvers used to increase the "high" experienced during the inhalation of cocaine or marijuana may cause pneumothorax and pneumomediastinum (5).

VII. Conclusion

Among manmade pleural diseases, those induced by drugs and radiation are common enough to warrant careful examination of the drug history in any patient with pleural effusion, hemothorax, pleural thickening, pneumothorax, or the lupus syndrome. Simple cessation of exposure to the agent will often translate into durable improvement of the pleural condition. A regularly updated list of drugs causing pleural disease is available on the Internet (10).

Acknowledgments

The invaluable help of Adeline Metchedjin and Pascal Foucher is gratefully acknowledged.

References

1. Rosenow ECI. Drug-induced bronchopulmonary pleural disease. J Allergy Clin Immunol 1987; 80:780–787.

2. Miller KS. Drug-induced pleural disease. Semin Respir Med 1987; 9:86–97.
3. Sahn SA. The pleura. Am Rev Respir Dis 1988; 138:184–234.
4. Byrd RP, Morris CJ, Roy TM. Drug-induced pleural effusions. J Kentucky Med Assoc 1991; 89:71–73.
5. Miller WTJ. Pleural and mediastinal disorders related to drug use. Semin Roentgenol 1995; 30:35–48.
6. Antony VB. Drug–induced pleural disease. Clin Chest Med 1998; 19:331–340.
7. Morelock SY, Sahn SA. Drugs and the pleura. Chest 1999; 116:212–221.
8. Ben-Noun LL. Drug-induced respiratory disorders. Incidence, prevention and management. Drug Safety 2000; 23:145–164.
9. Ebbert JO, Dupras DM, Erwin PJ. Searching the medical literature using PubMed: a tutorial. Mayo Clin Proc 2003; 78:87–91.
10. http://www.pneumotox.com: Pneumotox® Website: 1997. Producers: P Foucher - Ph. Camus: Last update: July, 2003.
11. De Vuyst P, Pfitzenmeyer P, Camus P. Asbestos, ergot drugs and the pleura. Eur Respir J 1997; 10:2695–2698.
12. Tornling G, Unge G, Axelsonn G, Noring L, Granerus AK. Pleuropulmonary reactions in patients on bromocriptine treatment. Eur J Respir Dis 1986; 68:35–38.
13. White DA, Schwartzberg LS, Kris MG, Bosl GJ. Acute chest pain syndrome during bleomycin infusions. Cancer 1987; 59:1582–1585.
14. Cortez LM, Pankey GA. Acute pulmonary hypersensitivity to furazolidone. Am Rev Respir Dis 1972; 105:823–826.
15. Petusevsky ML, Faling LJ, Rocklin RE, Snider GL, Merliss AD, Moses JM, Dorman SA. Pleuropericardial reaction to treatment with dantrolene. JAMA 1979; 242:2772–2774.
16. Webb DB, Whale RJ. Pleuropericardial effusion associated with minoxidil administration. Postgr Med J 1982; 58:319–320.
17. Debourdeau PM, Djezzar S, Estival JLF, Zammit CM, Richard RC, Catstot AC. Life-threatening eosinophilic pleuropericardial effusion related to vitamins B5 and H. Ann Pharmacother 2001; 35:424–426.
18. Marshall AJ, Baddeley H, Barritt DW, Davies JD, Lee REJ, Low-Beer TS, Read AE. Practolol peritonitis. Q J Med 1977; 46:135–149.
19. Shaunak S, Wilkins A, Pilling JB, Dick DJ. Pericardial, retroperitoneal, and pleural fibrosis induced by pergolide. J Neurol Neurosurg Psychiatry 1999; 66: 79–81.
20. Klisnick A, Fourcade J, Ruivard M, Baud O, Souweine B, Boyer L, Deteix P. Combined idiopathic retroperitoneal and mediastinal fibrosis with pericardial involvement. Clin Nephrol 1999; 52:51–55.
21. Pritchett AM, Morrison JF, Edwards WD, Schaff HV, Connolly HM, Espinosa RE. Valvular heart disease in patients taking pergolide. Mayo Clin Proc 2002; 77:1280–1286.
22. Gonzalez-Rothi RJ, Hannan SE, Hood I, Franzini DA. Amiodarone pulmonary toxicity presenting as bilateral exudative pleural effusion. Chest 1987; 92:179–182.
23. Stein B, Zaatari GS, Pine JR. Amiodarone pulmonary toxicity. Clinical, cytologic and ultrastructural findings. Acta Cytol 1987; 31:357–361.
24. Akoun G, Milleron BJ, Badaro DM, Mayaud CM, Lioté HA. Pleural T-lymphocyte subsets in amiodarone-associated pleuropneumonitis. Chest 1989; 95:596–597.
25. Clarke B, Ward DE, Honey M. Pneumonitis with pleural and pericardial effusion and neuropathy during amiodarone therapy. Int J Cardiol 1985; 8:81–88.

26. Stäubli M, Zimmermann A, Bircher J. Amiodarone-induced vasculitis and polyserositis. Postgr Med J 1985; 61:245–247.
27. Sheikhzadeh A, Schafer U, Schnabel A. Drug-induced lupus erythematosus by amiodarone. Arch Intern Med 2002; 162:834–836.
28. Gotsman I, Fridlender Z, Meirovitz A, Dratva D, Muszkat M. The evaluation of pleural effusions in patients with heart failure. Am J Med 2001; 111:375–378.
29. Dunn JM, Sloan H. Pleural effusion and fibrosis secondary to Sansert administration. Ann Thorac Surg 1973; 15:295–298.
30. Ibsen KK, Lindeneg O. Ergotaminbehandling og pleuritis. Ugeskr Laeger 1979; 141:860.
31. Diot E, Diot P, Le Roll A, Jonville AP, Lasfargues G, Lemarié E, Lavandier M, Guilmot JL. Epanchements pleuraux induits par la bromocriptine. Rev Mal Respir 1990; 7:175–177.
32. Holmberg L, Boman G. Pulmonary reactions to nitrofurantoin. 447 cases reported to the Swedish Adverse Drug Reaction Committe 1966–1976. Eur J Respir Dis 1981; 62:180–189.
33. Bayliff CD, Sobiera CJ, Paterson NAM. Nitrofurantoin induced acute pneumonitis. A review of three cases. Can J Hosp Pharm 1997; 50:247.
34. Standertskjöld-Nordenstam CG, Wandtke JC, Hood WJJ, Zugibe FT, Butler L. Amiodarone pulmonary toxicity. Chest radiography and CT in asymptomatic patients. Chest 1985; 88:143–145.
35. Kuhlman JE, Teigen C, Ren H, Hurban RH, Hutchins GM, Fishman EK. Amiodarone pulmonary toxicity: CT findings in symptomatic patients. Radiology 1990; 177:121–125.
36. Pfitzenmeyer P, Foucher P, Dennewald G, Chevalon B, Debieuvre D, Bensa P, Piard F, Camus P. Pleuropulmonary changes induced by ergoline drugs. Eur Respir J 1996; 9:1013–1019.
37. Graham RG. Cardiac and pulmonary fibrosis during methysergide therapy for headache. Am J Med Sci 1967; 254:1–12.
38. Varsano S, Gershman M, Hamaoui E. Pergolide-induced dyspnea, bilateral pleural effusion and peripheral edema. Respiration 2000; 67:580–582.
39. Danoff SK, Grasso ME, Terry PB, Flynn JA. Pleuropulmonary disease due to pergolide use for restless legs syndrome. Chest 2001; 120:313–316.
40. Messiaen T, Lefebvre C, Weynand B, Pieters T. Epanchement pleural et importants oedèmes des membres inférieurs induits par la bromocriptine. Rev Med Interne (Paris) 1996; 17:680–683.
41. Robert M, Derbaudrenghien JP, Blampain JP, Lamy F, Meyer P. Fibrotic processes associated with long-term ergotamine therapy. N Engl J Med 1984; 311:601.
42. Malik SW, Myers JL, DeRemee RA, Specks U. Lung toxicity associated with cyclophosphamide use. Two distinct patterns. Am J Respir Crit Care Med 1996; 154:1851–1856.
43. Lombard JN, Bonnotte B, Maynadié M, Foucher P, Reybet-Degat O, Jeannin L, Camus P. Celiprolol pneumonitis. Eur Respir J 1993; 9:588–591.
44. Page RL. Progressive pleural thickening during oxprenolol therapy. Br J Dis Chest 1979; 73:195–199.
45. Page RL. Pleural thickening-oxprenolol exonerated. Br J Dis Chest 1979; 73:319.
46. Lote K, Dahl O, Vigander T. Pneumothorax during combination chemotherapy. Cancer 1981; 47:1743–1745.

47. Rantala H, Kirvelä O, Anttolainen I. Nitrofurantoin lung in a child. Lancet 1979; ii:799–800.
48. Wilson KS, Brigden ML, Alexander S, worth A. Fatal pneumothorax in "BCNU lung." Med Pediatr Oncol 1982; 10:195–199.
49. Leeser JE, Carr D. Fatal pneumothorax following bleomycin and other cytotoxic drugs. Cancer Treat Rep 1985; 69:344–345.
50. Kumar S, Tefferi A. Spontaneous pneumomediastinum and subcutaneous emphysema complicating bronchiolitis obliterans after allogeneic bone marrow transplantation—case report and review of literature. Ann Hematol 2001; 80:430–435.
51. Rostand RA, Feldman RL, Block ER. Massive hemothorax complicating heparin anticoagulation for pulmonary embolus. South Med J 1977; 70:1128–1130.
52. Robinson NMK, Thomas MR, Jewitt DE. Spontaneous haemothorax as a complication of anti-coagulation following coronary angioplasty. Respir Med 1995; 89:629–630.
53. Cafri C, Gilutz H, Ilia R, Abu-ful A, Battler A. Unusual bleeding complications of thrombolytic therapy after cardiopulmonary resuscitation. Three case reports. Angiology 1997; 48:925–928.
54. Simon HB, Dagett WM, DeSanctis RW. Hemothorax as a complication of anticoagulant therapy in the presence of pulmonary infarction. JAMA 1969; 208:1830–1834.
55. Quinn MW, Dillard TA. Delayed traumatic hemothorax on ticlopidine. Chest 1999; 116:257–260.
56. Margolis MT, Thoen LD, Mercer LJ, Keith LG. Hemothorax after Lupron therapy of a patient with pleural endometriosis—a case report and literature review. Int J Fertil 1996; 41:53–55.
57. Kuhlman JE, Singha NK. Complex disease of the pleural space: radiographic and CT evaluation. RadioGraphics 1997; 17:63–79.
58. Boggess KA, Benedetti TJ, Raghu G. Nitrofurantoin-induced pulmonary toxicity during pregnancy: a report of a case and review of the literature. Obstet Gynecol Surv 1996; 51:367–370.
59. Barreiro B, Manresa F, Valldeperas J. Carbamazepine and the lung. Eur Respir J 1990; 3:930–931.
60. Sitbon O, Bidel N, Dussopt C, Azarian R, Braud ML, Lebargy F, Fourme T, Piard F, Camus P. Minocycline pneumonitis and eosinophilia: a report on 8 patients. Arch Intern Med 1994; 154:1633–1640.
61. Urban C, Nirenberg A, Caparros B, Anac S, Cacavio A, Rosen G. Chemical pleuritis as the cause of acute chest pain following high-dose methotrexate treatment. Cancer 1983; 51:34–37.
62. Walden PAM, Mitchell-Heggs PF, Coppin C, Dent J, Bagshawe KD. Pleurisy and methotrexate treatment. Br Med J 1977; ii:967.
63. Curt GA, Kelley JA, Fine RL, Huguenin PN, Roth JS, Batist G, Jenkins J, Collins JM. A phase I and pharmacokinetic study of dihydro-5-azacytidine (NSC 264880). Cancer Res 1985; 45:3359–3363.
64. Pelz DM, Lownie SP, Fox AJ, Hutton LC. Symptomatic pulmonary complications from liquid acrylate embolization of brain arteriovenous malformations. Am J Neuroradiol 1995; 16:19–26.
65. Massin F, Coudert B, Marot JP, Foucher P, Camus P, Jeannin L. La pneumopathie du méthotrexate. Rev Mal Respir 1990; 7:5–15.

66. Brander L, Selroos O. Pulmonary reaction to nitrofurantoin. Acta Med Scand 1969; 185:215–220.
67. Braun D, Tréchot P, Netter P, Danloy V, Anthoine D, Vaillant G. Recurrent interstitial pneumonitis and dexfenfluramine. Chest 1993; 103:1927.
68. Melloni B, Vergnenègre A, Bonnaud F, Antonini MT, Gaillard S, Touraine F, Germouty J. Pneumopathie induite par le pirindopril. Rev Mal Respir 1994; 11:308–311.
69. Tomioka H, King TEJ. Gold-induced pulmonary disease: clinical features, outcome, and differentiation from rheumatoid lung disease. Am J Respir Crit Care Med 1997; 155:1011–1020.
70. Baethge BA, Wolf RE. Gold-induced pneumonitis. J La State Med Soc 1988; 140:37–39.
71. Gunstream SR, Seidenfeld JJ, Sobonys RE, McMahon LJ. Mitomycin-associated lung disease. Cancer Treat Rep 1983; 67:301–304.
72. Müller U, Abbühl K, Bissig J, Baumgartner H, Mühlberger F, Scherrer M, Hoigné R. Überempfindlichkeitsreaktionen der Lunge auf Nitrofurantoin. Schweiz Med Wochenschr 1970; 100:2206–2212.
73. Israel HL, Diamond P. Recurrent pulmonary infiltration and pleural effusion due to nitrofurantoin sensitivity. N Engl J Med 1962; 266:1024–1026.
74. Benzaquen-Forner H, Dournovo P, Tandjaoui-Lambiotte H, Sullerot A, Mahé C, Bonnin A, Camus P, Valeyre D. Pneumopathie hypoxémiante sous traitement par IEC. Rev Mal Respir 1998; 15:804–810.
75. Rich MW, Thomas RA. A case of eosinophilic pneumonia and vasculitis induced by diflunisal. Chest 1997; 111:1767–1769.
76. Toyoshima M, Sato A, Hayakawa H, Taniguchi M, Imokawa S, Chida K. A clinical study of minocycline-induced pneumonitis. Intern Med 1996; 35:176–179.
77. Bourezane Y, Salard D, Hoen B, Vandel S, Drobacheff C, Laurent R. DRESS (drug rash with eosinophilia and systemic symptoms) syndrome associated with nevirapine therapy. Clin Infect Dis 1998; 27:1321–1322.
78. Kimura N, Miyazaki E, Matsuno O, Abe Y, Tsuda T. Drug-induced pneumonitis with eosinophilic infiltration due to tosufloxacin tosilate. Nippon Kokyuki Gakkai Zasshi 1998; 36:618–622.
79. Yamawaki I, Katsura H, Taira M, Kadoriku C, Hashimoto I, Chiyotani A, Kondo M, Tamaoki J, Nagai A, Konno K. Six patients with pneumonitis related to blended Chinese traditional medicines. Nihon Kyobu Shikkan Gakkai Zasshi 1996; 34:1331–1336.
80. Nakanishi M, Okamura S, Demura Y, Ishizaki T, Miyamori I, Itoh H. Acute eosinophilic pneumonia with positive response to smoking challenge test, suggesting the involvement of health food. Nihon Kokyuki Gakkai Zasshi 2001; 39:357–362.
81. Siniakowicz RM, Narula D, Suster B, Steinberg JS. Diagnosis of amiodarone pulmonary toxicity with high-resolution computerized tomographic scan. J Cardiovasc Electrophysiol 2001; 12:431–436.
82. Golding RP, van Zanten TEG, Vermorken JB. Bleomycin pleuropneumonitis. Br J Radiol 1982; 55:672–674.
83. Rimmer MJ, Dixon AK, Flower CDR, Sikora K. Bleomycin lung: computed tomographic observations. Br J Radiol 1985; 58:1041–1045.
84. Lei KIK, Leung WT, Johnson PJ. Serious pulmonary complications in patients receiving recombinant granulocyte colony-stimulating factor during BACOP

chemotherapy for agressive non-Hodgkin's lymphoma. Br J Cancer 1994; 70: 1009–1013.
85. Andersson BS, Luna BS, Yee C, Hui KK, Keating MJ, McCreadie KB. Fatal pulmonary failure complicating high-dose cytosine arabinoside therapy in acute leukemia. Cancer 1990; 65:1079–1084.
86. Rosado MF, Kett DH, Schein RMH, Baraona FJ, Shridar KS. Severe pulmonary toxicity in a patient treated with gemcitabine. Am J Clin Oncol 2002; 25:31–33.
87. Miller KS, Sahn SA. Bilateral exudative pleural effusions following intravenous ethchlorvynol administration. Chest 1989; 95:464–465.
88. Reed CR, Glauser FL. Drug-induced non cardiogenic pulmonary edema. Chest 1991; 100:1120–1124.
89. Pisani RJ, Rosenow ECI. Pulmonary edema associated with tocolytic therapy. Ann Intern Med 1989; 110:714–718.
90. Milos M, Aberle DR, Parkinson BT, Batra P, Brown K. Maternal pulmonary edema complicating beta-adrenergic therapy of preterm labor. Am J Roentgenol 1988; 151:917–918.
91. Frankel SR, Eardley A, Lauwers G, Weiss M, Warrell RP Jr. The "retinoic acid syndrome" in acute promyelocytic leukemia. Ann Intern Med 1992; 117:292–296.
92. Wiley JS, Firkin FC. Reduction of pulmonary toxicity by prednisolone prophylaxis during all-trans retinoic acid treatment of acute promyelocytic leukemia. Leukemia 1995; 9:774–778.
93. Rogé P, Erny R. Ovarian hyperstimulation syndrome in medically assisted reproduction. Rev Fr Gynecol Obstet 1994; 89:495–501.
94. Man A, Schwarz Y, Greif J. Pleural effusion as a presenting symptom of ovarian hyperstimulation syndrome. Eur Respir J 1997; 10:2425–2426.
95. Roden S, Juvin K, Homasson JP, Israel-Biet D. An uncommon etiology of isolated pleural effusion. The ovarian hyperstimulation syndrome. Chest 2000; 118:256–258.
96. Thomas F, Kalfon P, Niculescu M. Acute respiratory failure, lactic acidosis, and shock associated with a compressive isolated right pleural effusion following ovarian hyperstimulation syndrome. Am J Med 2003; 114:165–166.
97. Chaouat A, Kessler R, Weitzenblum E. Pulmonary oedema and pleural effusion in two patients with primary pulmonary hypertension treated with calcium channel blockers. Heart 1996; 75:383.
98. Gugnani MK, Pierson C, Vanderheide R, Girgis RE. Pulmonary edema complicating prostacyclin therapy in pulmonary hypertension associated with scleroderma—a case of pulmonary capillary hemangiomatosis. Arthr Rheum 2000; 43:699–703.
99. Tham RTOTA, Peters WG, de Bruine FT, Willemze R. Pulmonary complications of cytosine-arabinoside therapy: radiographic findings. Am J Roentgenol 1987; 149:23–27.
100. Pavlidis N, Hanauske AR, Gamucci T, Smyth J, Lehnert M, te Velde A, Lan J, Verweij J. A randomized phase II study with two schedules of the novel indoloquinone EO9 in non-small-cell lung cancer: a study of the EORTC early clinical studies group (ECSG). Ann Oncol 1996; 7:529–531.
101. Villani F, Galimberti M, Rizzi M, Manzi R. Pulmonary toxicity of recombinant interleukin-2 plus lymphokine-activated killer cell therapy. Eur Respir J 1993; 6:828–833.

102. Lee RE, Lotze MT, Skibber JM, Tucker E, Bonow RO, Ognibene FP, Carrasquillo JA, Shelhamer JH, Parrillo JE, Rosenberg SA. Cardiorespiratory effects of immunotherapy with interleukin-2. J Clin Oncol 1989; 7:7–20.
103. Saxon RR, Klein JS, Bar MH, Blanc P, Gamsu G, Webb WR, Aronson FR. Pathogenesis of pulmonary edema during interleukin-2 therapy: correlation of chest radiographic and clinical findings in 54 patients. Am J Roentgenol 1991; 156:281–285.
104. Myers TJ, Cole SR, Klatsky AU, Hild DH. Respiratory failure due to pulmonary leukostasis following chemotherapy of acute nonlymphocytic leukemia. Cancer 1983; 51:1808–1813.
105. Hoffman BJ. Sensitivity of sulfadiazine resembling acute disseminated lupus erythematosus. Arch Dermatol Syph 1945; 51:190–192.
106. Dustan HP, Taylor RD, Corcoran AC, Page IH. Rheumatic and febrile syndrome during prolonged hydralazine treatment. JAMA 1954; 154:23–29.
107. Goldberg MJ, Husain M, Wajszczuk WJ, Rubenfire M. Procainamide-induced lupus erythematosus pericarditis encountered during coronary bypass surgery. Am J Med 1980; 69:159–162.
108. Siegel M, Lee SL, Peress NS. The epidemiology of drug-induced systemic lupus erythematosus. Arthr Rheum 1967; 10:407–415.
109. Gordon MM, Porter D. Minocycline induced lupus: case series in the west of Scotland. J Rheumatol 2001; 28:1004–1006.
110. Cohen MG, Prowse MV. Drug-induced rheumatic syndromes. Diagnosis, clinical features and management. Med Toxicol 1989; 4:199–218.
111. Hofstra AH. Metabolism of hydralazine: relevance to drug-induced lupus. Drug Metab Rev 1994; 26:485–505.
112. Siddiqui MA, Khan IA. Isoniazid-induced lupus erythematosus presenting with cardiac tamponade. Am J Ther 2002; 9:163–165.
113. Carter JD, Valeriano-Marcet J, Kanik KS, Vasey FB. Antinuclear antibody-negative, drug-induced lupus caused by lisinopril. South Med J 2001; 94:1122–1123.
114. Portanova JP, Arndt RE, Tan EM, Kotzin BL. Anti-histone antibodies in idiopathic and drug-induced lupus recognize distinct intrahistone regions. J Immunol 1987; 138:446–451.
115. Pape L, Strehlau J, Latta K, Ehrich JH, Offner G. Drug-induced lupus as a cause of relapsing inflammatory disease after renal transplantation. Pediatr Transplant 2002; 6:337–339.
116. Asherson RA, Zulman J, Hugues GRV. Pulmonary thromboembolism associated with procainamide-induced lupus syndrome and anticardiolipin antibodies. Ann Rheum Dis 1989; 48:232–235.
117. Khosla R, Butman AN, Hammer DF. Simvastatin-induced lupus erythematosus. South Med J 1998; 91:873–874.
118. Good JTJ, King TE, Antony VB, Sahn SA. Lupus pleuritis: clinical features and pleural fluid characteristics with special reference to pleural fluid antibody titers. Chest 1983; 84:714–718.
119. Smith PR, Nacht RI. Drug-induced lupus pleuritis mimicking pleural space infection. Chest 1992; 101:268–269.
120. Kaplan AI, Zakher F, Sabin S. Drug-induced lupus erythematosus with in vivo lupus erythematosus cells in pleural fluid. Chest 1978; 73:875–876.
121. Hiraoka K, Nagata N, Kawajiri T, Suzuki K, Kurokawa S, Kido M, Sakamoto

N. Paradoxical pleural response to antituberculous chemotherapy and isoniazid-induced lupus. Review and report of two cases. Respiration 1998; 65:152–155.
122. Chandrasekhar AJ, Robinson J, Barr L. Antibody deposition in the pleura: a finding in drug-induced lupus. J Allergy Clin Immunol 1978; 61:399–402.
123. Rubin RL, Nusinow SR, Johnson AD, Rubenson DS, Curd JG, Tan EM. Serologic changes during induction of lupus-like disease by procainamide. Am J Med 1986; 80:999–1002.
124. Campagna AC, Blanc PD, Criswell LA, Clarke D, Sack KE, Gold WM, Golden JA. Pulmonary manifestations of the eosinophilia-myalgia syndrome associated with tryptophan ingestion. Chest 1992; 101:1274–1281.
125. Pincus T. Eosinophilia-myalgia syndrome: patient status 2-4 years after onset. J Rheumatol 1996; 23(suppl 46):19–24.
126. Villena V, Hidalgo R, Sotelo MT, Martin-Escribano P. Montelukast and Churg-Strauss syndrome. Eur Respir J 2000; 15:626.
127. Stankus SJ, Johnson NT. Propylthiouracil-induced hypersensitivity vasculitis presenting as respiratory failure. Chest 1992; 102:1595–1596.
128. de Vriese ASP, Philippe J, Van Renterghem DM, De Cuyper CA, Hindryckx PHF, Matthys EGJ, Louagie A. Carbamazepine hypersensitivity syndrome: report of 4 cases and review of the literature. Medicine (Balt) 1995; 74:144–150.
129. Corp CC, Ghishan FK. The sulfone syndrome complicated by pancreatitis and pleural effusion in an adolescent receiving dapsone for treatment of acne vulgaris. J Pediatr Gastroenterol Nutr 1998; 26:103–105.
130. Braun SR, doPico GA, Olson CE, Caldwell W. Low-dose radiation pneumonitis. Cancer 1975; 35:1322–1324.
131. Bachman AL, Macken K. Pleural effusions following supervoltage radiation for breast carcinoma. Radiology 1959; 72:699–709.
132. Gross NJ. Pulmonary effects of radiation therapy. Ann Intern Med 1977; 86: 81–92.
133. Polansky SM, Ravin CE, Prosnitz LR. Pulmonary changes after primary irradiation for early breast carcinoma. Am J Roentgenol 1980; 134:101–105.
134. Fentanes de Torres E, Guevara E. Pleuritis by radiation. Acta Cytol 1981; 25: 427–429.
135. Crestani B, Valeyre D, Roden S, Wallaert B, Dalphin JC, Cordier JF. Bronchiolitis obliterans organizing pneumonia syndrome primed by radiation therapy to the breast. Am J Respir Crit Care Med 1998; 158:1929–1935.
136. Whitcomb ME, Schwarz MI. Pleural effusion complicating intensive mediastinal radiation therapy. Am Rev Respir Dis 1971; 103:100–107.
137. Rodriguez-Garcia JL, Fraile G, Moreno MA, Sanchez-Corral JA, Penalver R. Recurrent massive pleural effusion as a late complication of radiotherapy in Hodgkin's disease. Chest 1991; 100:1165–1166.
138. McWilliams A, Gabbay E. Chylothorax occurring 23 year post-irradiation: literature review and management strategies. Respirology 2000; 5:301–303.
139. Bishop PC, Elwood PC. Chylous effusion in Hodgkin's disease. N Engl J Med 1998; 339:1515.
140. Zoetmulder F, Rutgers E, Baas P. Thoracoscopic ligation of a thoracic duct leakage. Chest 1994; 106:1233–1234.
141. Logan PM. Thoracic manifestations of external beam radiotherapy. Am J Roentgenol 1998; 171:569–577.
142. Bell J, McGivern D, Bullimore J, Hill J, Davies ER, Goddard P. Diagnostic imaging of post-irradiation changes in the chest. Clin Radiol 1988; 39:109–119.

143. Srinivasan G, Kurtz DW, Lichter AS. Pleural-based changes on chest x-ray after irradiation for primary breast cancer: correlation with findings on computerized tomography. Int J Radiat Oncol Biol Phys 1983; 9:1567–1570.
144. Epstein DM, Littman P, Gefter WB, Miller WT, Raney RBJ. Radiation-induced pneumothorax. Med Ped Oncol 1983; 11:122–124.
145. Melato M, Rizzardi C. Malignant pleural mesothelioma following chemotherapy for breast cancer. Anticancer Res 2001; 21:3093–3096.
146. Henley JD, Loehrer PJ, Ulbright TM. Deciduoid mesothelioma of the pleura after radiation therapy for Hodgkin's disease presenting as a mediastinal mass. Am J Surg Pathol 2001; 25:547–548.
147. Neugut AI, Ahsan H, Antman KH. Incidence of malignant pleural mesothelioma after thoracic radiotherapy. Cancer 1997; 80:948–950.
148. Rinaldo JE, Owens GR, Rogers RM. Adult respiratory distress syndrome following intrapleural instillation of talc. J Thorac Cardiovasc Surg 1983; 85:523–526.
149. Audu PB, Sing RF, Mette SA, Fallahnejhad M. Fatal diffuse alveolar injury following use of intrapleural bleomycin. Chest 1993; 103:1638.
150. Tohda Y, Iwanaga T, Takada M, Yana T, Kawahara M, Negoro S, Okishio K, Kudoh S, Fukuoa M, Furuse K. Intrapleural administration of cisplatin and etoposide to treat malignant pleural effusions in patients with non-small cell lung cancer. Chemotherapy 1999; 45:197–204.
151. Lewis JWJ, Groux N, Elliott JPJ, Jara FM, Obeid FN, Magilligan DJJ. Complications of attempted central venous injections performed by drug abusers. Chest 1980; 78:613–617.
152. Douglass RE, Levison MA. Pneumothorax in drug abusers. An urban epidemic? Am Surg 1986; 52:377–380.
153. Reinmuth N, Forster R, Scheld HH. From the neck to the lung: pneumothorax caused by a lost needle. Eur J Cardiothorac Surg 1995; 9:216–217.
154. Mason JW. Amiodarone pulmonary toxicity and Professor Hounsfield. J Cardiovasc Electrophysiol 2001; 12:437–438.
155. Rossi SE, Erasmus JJ, McAdams P, Sporn TA, Goodman PC. Pulmonary drug toxicity: radiologic and pathologic manifestations. RadioGraphics 2000; 5:1245–1259.
156. Kuhlman JE. The role of chest computed tomography in the diagnosis of drug-related reactions. J Thorac Imaging 1991; 6:52–61.
157. Neelakandan B, Neelakandhan KS. Delayed chylothorax after irradiation. Ann Thorac Surg 1996; 61:277.
158. Perrin C, Mouroux J, Tamisier R, Vandenbos F, Dumon MC, Blaive B. Un chylothorax d'origine particulière: la fibrose médiastino-pulmonaire post-radique. Presse Med 1996; 25:259.
159. Promisloff RA, Hogue DJ. Chylothorax: the result of previous radiation therapy? J Am Osteopath Assoc 1997; 97:164–166.
160. Lee YC, Tribe AE, Musk AW. Chylothorax from radiation-induced mediastinal fibrosis. Aust NZ J Med 1998; 28:667–668.

20

Parapneumonic Pleural Effusions and Empyema

DEMOSTHENES BOUROS

Demokritos University of Thrace
Medical School
and University Hospital of Alexandroupolis
Alexandroupolis, Greece

**MARIA PLATAKI
and SOPHIA E. SCHIZA**

University Hospital of Heraklion
Heraklion, Crete, Greece

I. Introduction

Parapneumonic pleural effusions (PPE) present a frequently difficult diagnostic and therapeutic challenge in clinical practice because of their heterogeneity. Their spectrum ranges from a small pleural effusion that does not require specific therapy to multiloculated pleural empyema with pleural fibrosis, trapped lung, systemic sepsis, respiratory failure, and metastatic infection. Today the physician is warranted to play an increasing role in the timely and modern management, with new available techniques, of the patients with PPE and pleural empyema (1).

This chapter reviews the epidemiological factors that influence their clinical course, the existing classification systems for PPE, and the current diagnostic and therapeutic options and offers guidelines for treating the various stages of PPE and PE.

II. Definitions

Infectious pleural effusions are usually of parapneumonic origin; however, they may also have other causes, such as surgery, trauma, or esophageal perforation

Table 1 Causes of Bacterial Empyema

Pulmonary infection
  Bacterial pneumonia
  Lung abscess
  Bronchiectasis
  Septic pulmonary emboli
Postoperative
  Thoracic surgery
  Cardiac surgery
  Esophageal surgery
Trauma
Mediastinitis
  Esophageal perforation
  Dental abscess
  Epiglottitis
Abdominal infection
  Subdiaphragmatic abscess
  Peritonitis
Spontaneous pneumothorax
Thoracentesis
Sepsis
Complicating rheumatoid pleurisy
Miscellaneous or unknown

(see Table 1). Any pleural effusion associated with bacterial pneumonia, lung abscess, or bronchiectasis is a parapneumonic effusion. An effusion is called an empyema when the concentration of leukocytes becomes macroscopically evident as a thick, highly viscous, whitish-yellow, opaque, and turbid fluid (pus). It consists of fibrin, cellular debris, and living or dead bacteria. There is no consensus on the white blood cell (WBC) count or the biochemistry for an empyema. The extent of the definition of empyema in a nonpurulent fluid with only the presence of a positive Gram stain or culture is not widely accepted (2).

Uncomplicated (simple) PPEs are usually small, not loculated, and not infected. Most often they resolve spontaneously under antibiotic treatment. Complicated PPEs are usually associated with pleural invasion of the infectious agent and require at least drainage and possibly further interventions. A loculated PPE is a non–free-flowing pleural effusion. A multiloculated PPE is a pleural effusion with more than one loculus (3).

III. Epidemiology

The annual incidence of bacterial pneumonia is estimated to be 2–4 million in the United States, with approximately 20% of patients requiring hospitalization (3). It is estimated that 40–60% of patients with pneumonia develop PPE (4), which is associated with an increased morbidity and mortality, despite the advent of potent antibiotics. Infection is the second leading cause of a pleural effusion after congestive heart failure in developed countries (3). Pleural infection caused by an underlying pneumonia is the most common cause of empyema and accounts for 70% of reported empyemas (2). Pleural empyemas occur in 5–10% of patients with PPE and seem to affect more frequently the elderly and debilitated and hospitalized patients with community acquired pneumonia and men more than women (male-to-female ratio 1.8:1) (2). An important cause of PPE is the delayed diagnosis and initiation of proper antibiotic treatment or effective tube drainage in the course of a bacterial pneumonia.

Comorbidities include preexisting pulmonary diseases, such as bronchiectasis, chronic obstructive pulmonary disease (COPD), lung cancer, malignancy, previous tuberculosis (post-tuberculous bronchiectasis), rheumatoid pleuropulmonary disease (drug immunosuppression, rupture of subpleural necrobiotic nodules, increased risk of infection because of impaired neutrophil function and altered bacterial clearance by a chemically inflamed pleura and low pleural fluid pH and glucose), acquired immunodeficiency syndrome (AIDS), and diabetes (5–10). Clinical factors that predict the presence of anaerobic pneumonia include poor dental hygiene, sedative drug use, alcoholism, seizures, mental retardation, and gastroesophageal reflux (6).

The majority of non-PPE and empyemas are iatrogenic either after thoracic surgery (about 20% of all causes of empyemas) or after thoracic surgical procedures. Trauma and esophageal perforation account for 5% each, while thoracentesis is responsible for almost 2% of all causes of empyemas (Table 1). Rare causes of empyema include secondary pulmonary infarctions (11), post-obstructive pneumonitis because of foreign body aspiration (12) and extension of head and neck infection from dental abscesses (more common in the preantibiotic era) (13).

The role of the pathogen in the underlying pneumonia and the likelihood of the patient to develop PPE is not clear since there are no comparative studies from a single institution. A cases series has shown that *Mycoplasma pneumoniae* (20%) (14) is less likely than *Streptococcus pneumoniae* (40–57%) to cause PPE (15). It is unusual for a loculation of a PPE or progress to empyema to occur after initiation of appropriate antibiotic therapy. Small patient series indicate that patients with pneumonia caused by gram-positive, gram-negative, or anaerobic bacteria have a 50% incidence of parapneumonic effusions when examined with decubitus chest radiographs (5).

Morbidity and mortality is higher in patients with PPE than in patients with pneumonia alone. Mortality from pleural empyema ranges from 5 to 30% (16). The mortality rate for immunocompromised patients can be as high as 40% (4).

In terms of the economic impact of PPE, little information is available. Patients with PPE or pleural empyema often have protracted duration of hospitalization. In a review of case series the mean hospital stay for patients with empyema ranged from 12.3 to 56.8 days and the mortality rates ranged from 0 to 51%. (17) It was found, in an NIH-sponsored study (18) that the presence of bilateral pleural effusions at the time of hospital admission is independently correlated with an increase in early (<7 days) and late (<30 days) mortality rates [total relative risk 2.8, 95% confidence interval (CI) 1.4–5.8). It is speculated that congestive heart failure as a comorbid condition played an additional role in the outcome.

IV. Pathophysiology

When a patient develops pneumonia, the pleura responds to the presence of microbes with a vigorous inflammatory response. The rate of pleural fluid formation, consisting of an exudate of WBC and proteins, is increased. The increase is mainly due to lung interstitial fluid, and secondary to Increased permeability of the capillaries in the pleurae. When the amount of pleural fluid entering the pleural space exceeds the capacity of the pleural lymphatics to reabsorb the fluid, a pleural effusion develops. Initially, the pleural fluid has a normal glucose and pH and the lactate dehydrogenase (LDH) level and the WBC count are low (3). Mesothelial cells are actively phagocytic, initiating inflammatory response when activated by the presence of bacteria, releasing a battery of chemokines (C-X-C group), cytokines (IL-1, IL-6, IL-8, TNF-α), oxidants, and proteases (19).

In some patients the process progresses with bacteria invading the pleural fluid. Consequently, the pleural fluid glucose and pH become progressively lower, the LDH progressively higher, and the fluid increasingly more viscid. In addition, sheets of fibrin form loculi of fluid and cover the visceral pleura, which prevents the underlying lung from reexpanding if the fluid is removed. The process is reversible with the institution of proper antibiotic therapy during the early exudative phase. The evolution of a simple PPE to an empyema represents a continuous progression from a small amount of freeflowing, noninfected pleural fluid to a large amount of frank pus, which is multiloculated and is associated with thick visceral pleura. In accordance, a PPE can be divided into four stages (Table 2), which are not sharply defined but gradually merge together.

A. The Pleuritis Sicca Stage

In this stage the inflammatory process of the lung extends to the visceral pleura, causing a local reaction. This leads to audible pleural rub and pleuritic chest pain, originating from the sensitive innervation of the adjacent parietal pleura. A significant number of patients with pneumonia report pleuritic chest pain without developing a pleural effusion (1,20), suggesting that the involvement of the pleura may be limited to this stage in many cases of pneumonia.

Table 2 Pathophysiological Phases of Evolution of Parapneumonic Pleural Effusions and Empyema

1. Pleuritis sicca phase
    Pleural rub and pleuritic chest pain without pleural effusion
    Involvement of the pleura may be limited to this stage
2. Exudative phase
    Thin, free-flowing fluid
    Normal pleural fluid leukocytes, pH, LDH, glucose
3. Fibrinopurulent phase
    Increased viscosity of pleural fluid
    Fibrin deposition
    Bacteria may be present
    Increased leukocytes and LDH (>500 IU)
    Decreased pH (<7.2), glucose (<60 mg/dL)
4. Organizing phase
    Purulent fluid
    Increased leukocytes and LDH (>1000 IU)
    Decreased pH (<7.0), glucose (<40 mg/dL)
    Pleural peel

B. The Exudative Stage

The parapneumonic effusion that occurs in the initial hours tends to be small in volume and is a sterile, neutrophil predominant exudate. The ongoing inflammatory process leads to a mediator-induced increase of the permeability of local tissue and of regional capillaries. The following accumulation of fluid in the pleural space is probably the combined result of the influx of pulmonary interstitial fluid (21) and of a local microvascular exudate. This stage is the capillary leak or exudative stage. Typically, the pleural fluid is usually clear and sterile, the pH is >7.30, the glucose is >60 mg/dL, and the LDH is <500 U/L (1–3,22,23). Patients in this first stage can be treated successfully with antibiotics without the need for pleural space drainage.

C. The Fibropurulent Stage

If the pneumonia progresses, bacteria continue to multiply in the lung with invasion and persistence in the pleural space, while endothelial injury becomes more prominent with worsening pulmonary edema and increased pleural fluid formation. The pleural fluid in this bacterial invasion/fibrinopurulent stage is characterized by an increased number of polymorphonuclear cells (PMNs), by the effect of the major chemotactic factor interleukin-8 (IL-8), by a fall in pleural fluid pH and glucose, and by an increase in pleural fluid LDH (19). The pleural fluid/serum glucose ratio decreases to <0.5, with an absolute concentration of usually <40 mg/dL because of the increased rate of glycolysis from

PMN phagocytosis and bacterial metabolism (1–3). As the end products of glucose metabolism, CO_2 and lactic acid accumulate in the pleural space and the pH falls (<7.2). The LDH increases (>1000 U/L), because of PMN lysis. The pleural fluid becomes clottable as procoagulants from the blood move into the pleural space in conjunction with a loss of pleural space fibrinolytic activity from mesothelial injury (20,24–28). Fibrin and collagen are deposited in a continuous sheet, covering the visceral and parietal pleura, and compartmentalize the pleural fluid into loculations by bridging the two pleural surfaces, making drainage increasingly difficult. In addition, pleural thickening limits lung expansion with deposition on the visceral pleura. Pleural fluid volume may increase further because of blockage of the parietal pleural stoma by fibrin and collagen and mesothelial swelling (25–28). Early in this stage antibiotics alone may be effective, but later, pleural space drainage is usually required (29,30).

D. The Organizational/Empyema Stage

According to Hippocrates, "Pleurisy that does not clear up in fourteen days, results in empyema" (31). Indeed, without treatment, this stage ensues over the next few weeks, characterized by the invasion of fibroblasts, leading to the transformation of intrapleural fibrin membranes into a thick and nonelastic pleural "peel," forming a single or multiple loculations. As a consequence, impairment of pleural fluid drainage and inhibition of lung expansion occurs. Functionally, gas exchange can be severely impaired on the side of the organizing empyema ("trapped lung"). Empyema fluid is a thick, purulent coagulum, which may not be adequately drained by tube thoracostomy. Pus is characterized by the coagulability of pleural fluid, the abundance of cellular debris, and increased fibrin and collagen deposition. Untreated empyema rarely resolves spontaneously. It may drain through the chest wall (empyema necessitatis) or into the lung (bronchopleural fistula) or may format lung abscess. Patients with empyema always require drainage for resolution of pleural sepsis.

V. Classification of Parapneumonic Effusion and Empyema

Numerous classification schemes (20,22,23,32–34) have been proposed to categorize the entire spectrum of PPE (Table 3). One common classification divides PPE into the following three categories:

1. Uncomplicated parapneumonic effusion. This corresponds to the exudative stage of a PPE. It is characterized by an exudative, predominantly neutrophilic effusion that occurs when the lung interstitial fluid increases during pneumonia. It resolves with the resolution of the pneumonia. No drainage is needed.

Table 3 Classification Schemes for Patients with Parapneumonic Pleural Effusion and Empyema and Key Characteristics

Early	STAGE →		Late	Ref.
Exudative	Fibrinopurulent		Organizing	32
Nonloculated	Loculated		Empyema	33
Uncomplicated/nonloculated	Complicated/loculated		Empyema	34
Uncomplicated	Complicated		Empyema	35
Nonsignificant Typical Borderline	Simple Complex	Simple E	Complex E	36
Category 1 A0 + Bx + Cx	Category 2 A1 + Bo + Co	Category 3 A2 or B1 or C1	Category 4 B2	37

See Table 5 for details. E = empyema.

2. Complicated parapneumonic effusion. This corresponds to the fibrinopurulent stage of a PPE. Complicated effusions occur when there is persistent bacterial invasion of the pleural space. Bacterial invasion typically leads to an increased number of neutrophils and the development of pleural fluid acidosis, which results from anaerobic utilization of glucose by the neutrophils and bacteria. In addition, lysis of neutrophils increases the LDH concentration in the pleural fluid to values often in excess of 1000 IU/L. Complicated parapneumonic effusions are often sterile because bacteria can be cleared rapidly from the pleural space (4). This occurs despite the deposition of a dense layer of fibrin on both the visceral and parietal pleurae that can lead to pleural loculation (4).

3. Thoracic empyema. This corresponds to the organizational/empyema stage of a PPE. It is characterized by bacterial organisms seen on Gram stain or by the aspiration of pus on thoracentesis. A positive culture is not required for diagnosis. A negative bacterial culture may be due to anaerobic organisms, which are difficult to culture, sampling after antibiotic treatment, and aspiration adjacent to an infected loculus of infection. Table 4 shows the biochemical characteristics of a para-

Table 4 Biochemical Characteristics of the Stages of Parapneumonic Pleural Effusions and Empyema

Parameter	Uncomplicated	Undetermined	Complicated
pH	>7.3	7.3–7.1	<7.1
Glucose (mg/dL)	>60	60–40	<40
LDH (IU)	<500	<1000	>1000

pneumonic effusion. Cases with borderline biochemical parameters on pleural fluid analysis characterize an undetermined PPE and need close follow-up. Table 5 presents a practical classification scheme introduced by Light.

The American College of Chest Physicians has developed a new classification system for PPE/PE (34), which is based upon the radiological characteristics of the effusion, the pleural fluid bacteriology, and the pleural fluid chemistry (Table 6). The key aspects are the characteristics that indicate that the patient has a moderate to high risk of a poor outcome without drainage. Radiological characteristics associated with a poor prognosis are an effusion that occupies >50% of the hemithorax, is loculated, or (paradoxically) is associated with thickened parietal pleura. However, pleural thickening is not related to the requirement for surgery (35). Bacteriological criteria associated with a poor

Table 5 Classification, Characteristics and Treatment Scheme of Parapneumonic Pleural Effusion and Empyema

Category of PPE/PE	Characteristics/treatment
Class 1 Nonsignificant	<10 mm thick on decubitus radiograph No thoracentesis indicated
Class 2 Typical PPE	>10 mm thick Glucose >40 mg/dL, pH >7.2, Gram stain and culture negative; antibiotics alone
Class 3 Borderline complicated PPE	7.0 < pH < 7.2 or LDH > 500, and glucose >40 mg/dL Gram stain and culture negative Antibiotics plus serial thoracentesis
Class 4 Simple complicated PPE	pH <7.0 or glucose <40 mg/dL, or Gram stain or culture positive Not loculated, not frank pus Tube thoracostomy plus antibiotics
Class 5 Complex complicated PPE	pH <7.0 or glucose <40 mg/dL, or Gram stain or culture positive Multiloculated Tube thoracostomy plus thrombolytics Thoracoscopy if above ineffective
Class 6 Simple empyema	Frank pus present Single locule or free flowing Tube thoracostomy plus thrombolytics ± decortication
Class 7 Complex empyema	Frank pus present Multiple locules Tube thoracostomy plus thrombolytics Usually require thoracoscopy or decortication

Source: Modified from Ref. 33.

Table 6 Classification Scheme of Risk for Poor Outcome in Patients with Parapneumonic Pleural Effusion and Empyema and Drainage Recommendations

Pleural space anatomy		Pleural fluid bacteriology		Pleural fluid chemistry	Category	Risk of poor outcome	Drainage
A0 Minimal, free-flowing effusion (<10 mm on lateral decubitus)	and	Bx culture and Gram stain results unknown	and	Cx pH unknown	1	Very low	No
A1 Small to moderate free-flowing effusion (<10 mm and <1/2 hemithorax)	and	B0 negative culture and Gram stain	and	C0 pH >7.20	2	Low	No
A2 Large, free-flowing effusion (≥1/2 hemithorax), loculated effusion, or effusion with thickened parietal pleura	or	B1 positive culture and Gram stain	or	C1 pH <7.20	3	Moderate	Yes
		B2 pus			4	High	Yes

Source: Ref. 34.

prognosis are a positive culture and/or Gram stain or the presence of pus. The pleural fluid chemistry criterion associated with a poor prognosis is a pleural fluid pH of 7.20. Alternative pleural fluid chemistry criteria are a pleural fluid glucose <60 mL/dL or a pleural fluid LDH more than three times the upper limit of normal serum levels.

VI. Etiology of PPE/PE

The bacteriology of PPE/PE is related to that of the pneumonic infection. Before the advent of modern antibiotics, the most common pleural infections occurred with streptococcal and staphylococcal species. Current series of empyemas support the continuing role of these organisms while documenting the emergence of anaerobes and gram-negative organisms as common pathogens. The reported spectra depend on the patient populations studied by various investigators. Animal models suggest that infection with a mixed bacterial flora containing aerobes and anaerobes is more likely to produce an empyema than a single organism infection (36,37). Anaerobic bacteria have been cultured in 36–76% of empyemas (38,39). According to many series (38–45) the majority of culture-positive effusions are due to aerobic organisms, while up to 15% are caused exclusively by anaerobic bacteria. This high incidence probably results from the indolent nature of these pneumonias, which permits pleural penetration of bacteria before antibiotics are instituted. The most frequent anaerobic isolates are *Bacteroides* species and *Peptostreptococcus*. Empyemas, particularly if they are multiloculated, may harbor multiple bacteria (29).

The remainder are usually due to a mixture of aerobic and anaerobic organisms. Streptococci (mostly *S. pneumoniae*) and staphylococci (mostly *S. aureus*) usually dominate gram-positive isolates, while *Escherichia coli*, *Klebsiella* species, *Pseudomonas* species, and *Haemophilus influenzae* are the most common gram-negative isolates (18,29). Particularly *E. coli* and anaerobic organisms are often found in combination with other organisms. Reports on viral, fungal (most frequently *Aspergillus*), and parasitic pleural infections are rare, although the incidence and awareness is increasing (46). Readers wanting further details are referred to a review article (46).

VII. Clinical Picture

The clinical presentation of patients with pneumonia with or without PPE is usually very much alike, with no significant differences between these two groups of patients regarding WBC count and occurrence of pleuritic chest pain (20). The clinical picture depends mainly on whether the pneumonia is caused by aerobic or anaerobic bacteria. Patients with aerobic bacterial pneumonia usually suffer from an acute-onset fever, while anaerobic infections tend to present as a more subacute or chronic condition with longer duration of symptoms and weight loss (47). Anaerobic pleuropulmonary infections often follow aspiration of oral or gastric contents. These patients usually have poor oral hygiene (*fetor ex ore!*) with anaerobic colonization of the oropharynx and often suffer from conditions that predispose to aspiration like seizures, syncopes, or alcoholism. Alcoholism has been found to be associated in 29% (4) to 40% (41) of the cases. Leukocytosis (> 20.000/mL) and anemia are common findings in the majority of patients (47).

In general, patients who have a longer history of symptoms before seeking medical attention or have received insufficient treatment are more likely to have complicated PPE/PE (29). Among gram-positive pneumonias, *S. pneumoniae* is even today responsible for most PPE. Among the gram-negative pneumonias, those caused by *E. Coli* are more frequently related with complicated PPE (3). PPE are more common in anaerobic pneumonia, while some of them have no concomitant parenchymal infiltration (3).

The finding of a purulent effusion without pneumonia may represent a postpneumonic empyema in which the pulmonary infiltrates have already resolved. However, pleural empyemas are not necessarily caused by pneumonias (Table 1). The majority of nonpneumonic empyemas are of iatrogenic origin, most commonly as a complication of a pneumonectomy or other thoracic surgical procedures.

VIII. Diagnosis

Physicians should be alert for PPE in any patient with pulmonary infection who has a pleural effusion on presentation. Symptoms and signs of PPE—fever, pleurodynia, cough, and dyspnea—merge with those of underlying pneumonia. Up to 10% of patients with PPE and empyema are relatively asymptomatic, while 60–80% have underlying comorbidities (40,45). Prompt thoracentesis is recommended before antibiotics are administered to improve the diagnostic yield of pleural fluid culture. A diagnostic thoracentesis should usually be performed when clinical findings and/or imaging techniques suggest the presence of a significant pleural effusion. Smaller effusions can safely be reached, e.g. by ultrasound guidance. Very small (<10 mm), difficult-to-reach effusions may be observed only.

A foul-smelling pleural fluid suggests the presence of anaerobic bacteria (47). Only 60% of anaerobic empyemas have feculent odor (47,48). Since not all PPE have an acute presentation, and caution should be exercised for the possibility of PPE in all patients with a pleural effusion.

IX. Imaging Techniques

Radiology is central in the evaluation and proper management of PPE. Conventional radiographs, including decubitus films, and newer imaging techniques, including contrast enhanced computed tomography (CT) scans and real-time ultrasound, provide more detailed morphological information in terms of size and nature of the effusion, but they do not obviate the need for a thoracentesis or other invasive diagnostic procedures (29,49).

A. Chest Radiograph

A chest radiograph showing a pleural-based opacity that has an abnormal contour or does not flow freely on lateral decubitus views first suggests the presence of a complicated PPE/PE. Conventional chest radiographs usually show a pulmonary infiltrate with ipsilateral pleural fluid. A lateral chest radiograph is particularly useful to detect blunting of the posterior costophrenic angle (Fig. 1). Accumulation of >200 mL of pleural fluid usually blunts the lateral costophrenic angle, although up to 500 mL may be present without blunting or other radiographic abnormalities (50). A meniscus sign is seen in nonloculated pleural effusions in excess of 500 mL. The lateral decubitus film can detect pleural effusion as small as 5 mL (51) and is used in the decision making of a thoracentesis (3). A lateral decubitus radiograph with the diseased lung up is also useful since it allows for a better evaluation of the presence of pleural fluid loculi and the extent of pneumonia. Supine radiographs have a sensitivity and specificity of about 70% compared with lateral decubitus films in demonstrating a pleural effusion (52). Increased opacity in the hemithorax without obscuration of the vascular markings, blunting of the costophrenic angle or apical cap indicate a pleural effusion in a supine radiograph (53). Interlobular loculation of pleural fluid is referred to as pseudotumor and has an oval shape and longitudinal orientation. The presence of consolidated or atelectatic lower lobe can obscure the silhouette of the diaphragm, concealing a PPE, and may require additional imaging examination by ultrasound or CT scan for detection (53,54).

B. Ultrasound

Ultrasonography (US) is a good method to confirm or rule out a pleural effusion in cases where chest radiographs are inconclusive. Also, it is the method of choice to guide a thoracentesis or place a chest tube. It is especially useful for small effusions and in other difficult circumstances, which require precise targeting, for instance, loculated effusions. A distinct advantage of ultrasound is the ability to study the patient at the bedside. In patients with minimal pleural abnormalities on conventional radiographs, ultrasound can detect small amounts of pleural fluid and reliably distinguishes small effusions from pleural thickening (55). When decubitus views fail to show layering of pleural fluid, sonography can significantly increase the diagnostic yield from thoracentesis.

Pleural collections as seen on sonography are characterized as echo-free, complex septated, complex nonseptated, and homogeneously echogenic (56). Transudates are always anechoic, but exudates may also be anechoic. Effusions

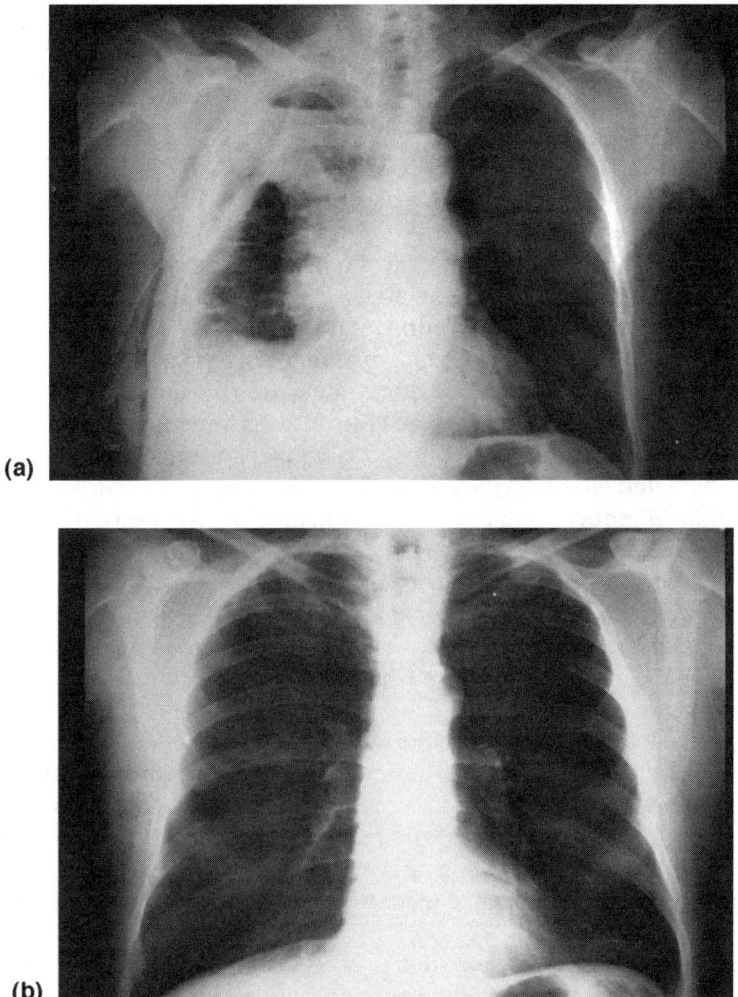

Figure 1 A posteroanterior chest radiograph of a patient with extensive multiloculated parapneumonic pleural effusion on the right before (a) and after treatment with intrapleural urokinase instillation for 5 days (b).

are usually exudates when they are septated or show a complex or homogeneously echogenic pattern. Dense echogenic patterns are most often associated with hemorrhagic effusions or empyemas (57). The real-time evaluation of the movement of pleural collections appears to be a more useful indicator of successful thoracentesis than the echogenicity of the collection. However, the use of ultrasound guidance has been shown to be the single most significant factor in reducing the incidence of pneumothorax after thoracentesis (58). Sonographic evaluation is more accurate in estimating pleural fluid volume than a decubitus radiograph (59), while it was found to expedite patient management in 49% of cases by either clarifying the nature of the pleural collection or identifying the most appropriate sites for thoracentesis (60).

C. Computed Tomography

Although diagnosis can be facilitated by thoracentesis under ultrasound guidance, optimal management requires a chest CT scan with contrast, which enhances the pleural surface and assists in delineating pleural fluid loculi (Fig. 2). CT scan may show pleural abnormalities at an earlier stage than other imaging modalities. Its useful in distinguishing pleural from parenchymal abnormalities, in detecting pleural fluid loculation in the mediastinal pleura, where ultrasound is usually negative (18), in determining the precise location and extent of pleural disease, and in occasionally providing information for the specific characterization of pleural fluid. It also may detect airway or parenchymal abnormalities (such as endobronchial obstruction), the extent of underlying pneumonia and its features (necrotizing pneumonia), or the presence of lung abscesses. Furthermore, chest CT can assess the position of chest tubes and give evidence for the presence of bronchopleural fistula or gas-forming organisms. Contrast-enhanced chest CT aids in better outlining of the thick inflammatory pleura in empyema. However, it cannot differentiate inflammatory from malignant disease (61). Pleural thickening and thickening of extrapleural fat did not correlate with clinical stages or outcome (62). A chest CT scan performed after the intravenous administration of iodinated contrast that shows parietal and visceral pleural enhancement, thickening of the extrapleural subcostal tissues, and increased attenuation of the extrapleural fat is highly suggestive of an empyema (49,63). The combination of fluid between the enhancing thickened pleural layers has been termed the split pleura sign of empyema.

Mediastinal lymphadenopathy is a common finding (36%) in PPE/PE (64,65). Multiple sites may be involved, and node diameters may reach 2 cm. CT may also be used for image-guided drainage and monitoring response to closed drainage or intrapleural fibrinolytic therapy.

D. Magnetic Resonance Imaging

The role of magnetic resonance imaging (MRI) in the clinical evaluation of pleural infection is limited. Although MRI is able to show pleural fluid collections, it is severely limited in assessing lung parenchyma (49).

Sagittal T1-weighted MR images allow a detailed analysis of the layers of the chest wall and their possible infiltration by inflammatory or malignant processes. Uncomplicated parapneumonic effusions do not seem to induce visible changes of the chest wall, whereas malignant effusions are frequently asso-

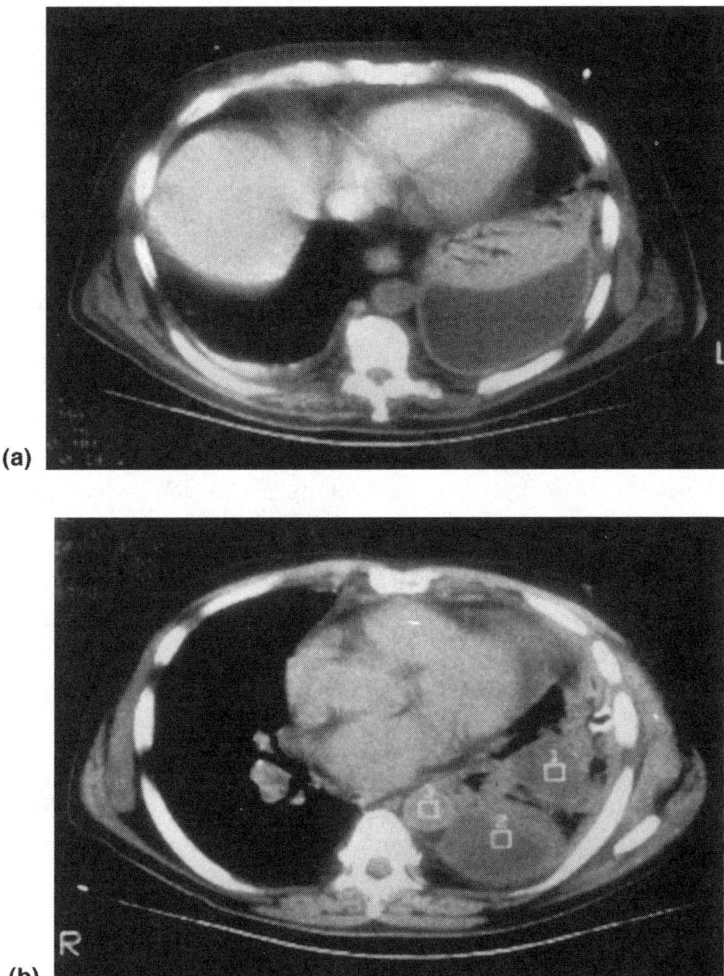

Figure 2 Chest computed tomographies showing a single loculus of pleural empyema (a) on the left, and a multiloculated parapneumonic pleural effusion on the left hemithorax (b).

ciated with alterations of the peripleural fat layer and the innermost intercostal muscles (66,67). While these findings were interpreted as helpful in the differential diagnosis of benign and malignant effusions, it remains doubtful that complicated effusions and empyemas show infiltration of the chest wall similar to malignant disease. The use of MRI in the routine differentiation of transudates from exudates is not practical or cost-effective at the present time (68,69).

X. Pleural Fluid Analysis

All suspected PPE should undergo a thoracentesis, unless they are very small (Table 5). The pleural fluid should be sent to microbiology lab for Gram stain and bacterial culture, WBC count and differential, and to biochemistry for determination of glucose, LDH, and pH.

A. Pleural Fluid Chemistry

Parapneumonic pleural effusions are exudates and are identified by application of Light's criteria (70) and/or the cholesterol level (71) and measuring the pleural fluid protein and LDH levels. If the pH is determined, it must be done with the same care as is an arterial pH level. The fluid should be collected in a heparinized syringe and placed in ice for its transfer to the blood gas laboratory. pH meters and dip sticks do not provide sufficiently accurate pH measurements (3). In the case of frank empyema, a pH measurement is not useful, as the purulent material is at risk of filling the membrane of the arterial blood gas machine.

Several pleural fluid parameters have been described to assess the severity and to predict the future course of a PPE. Patients with complicated PPE/PE tend to have a lower pleural fluid pH and glucose level and a higher LDH activity (1,72–76). The glucose concentration correlates directly with the pH (76). The cause for pleural fluid acidosis and low glucose levels is the local metabolic activity of inflammatory cells and bacteria (77). The superiority of the pH over glucose or LDH measurements in PPE/PE has been confirmed in a metaanalysis of seven studies using receiver operating characteristic (ROC) statistical techniques (78). The decision threshold to identify complicated effusions ranged between pH 7.21 and 7.29. A pleural pH in this range appeared to represent the threshold for consideration of drainage of a complicated PPE. It should be noted, however, that other diseases are associated with pleural fluid acidosis, including malignancy, tuberculosis, rheumatoid pleurisy, and lupus pleuritis.

It may suffice to measure the pH alone, but it must be emphasized that there are still not enough large-scale studies that have firmly established the predictive and discriminative power of this parameter. Further, pH measurements are only valid when performed properly, which means (1) collection and transport under strict anaerobic conditions, and (2) immediate measurement in a calibrated blood gas machine. It should also be kept in mind that the pleural fluid pH may not be useful in patients with systemic pH alterations (72) and in infections due to *Proteus* species, which can induce a local metabolic alkalosis due to ammonia production (79). Also, in loculated pleural effusions it is possible to find pleural fluid with different macroscopic characteristics and pH values.

There is general clinical consensus that pleural fluid pH is the most important chemical parameter to predict the further course of a PPE/PE, and various recommendations have been made for the best cut-off point to distinguish complicated from uncomplicated cases (1,3,80,81). In a recently published consensus statement of the American College of Chest Physicians (34), a pH of <7.20 is recommended as one of the parameters that predict poor outcome and should lead to chest tube drainage (see Table 2).

B. Pleural Fluid Cytology

PPE/PE are polymorphonuclear dominated effusions. Any other finding suggests another diagnosis (e.g., predominance of lymphocytes in an exudate is most often associated with tuberculosis or malignancy). The finding of food particles in the pleural fluid suggests the presence of esophageal-pleural fistula (82).

C. Bacteriology

Bacteriological studies should include a Gram stain and aerobic and anaerobic cultures. Delayed thoracentesis results in prolonged hospitalization (78,83). Pleural fluid cultures should be repeated if there is any alteration in the expected clinical status and radiological appearance, because new pathogens may be introduced in the pleural cavity via thoracentesis needles, percutaneous catheters, intercostal tubes, or open thoracotomies.

XI. Differential Diagnosis

Fever, pulmonary infiltrates, and a pleural effusion are not invariably due to pneumonia or to a complication of some surgical procedure. Pulmonary embolism is a common disorder, and paraembolic effusions occur in about 25–50% of the cases (84). The effusions may become infected and will then require treatment identical to complicated PPE. Other disorders that should be considered include tuberculosis, lupus erythematosus and other autoimmune disorders, acute pancreatitis and other diseases of the gastrointestinal-tract, and drug-induced pleuropulmonary disease. The turbid or milky aspect of empyemas may sometimes resemble the aspect of a chylothorax or pseudochylothorax.

XII. Treatment Strategy

The therapeutic options for a PPE depend on the particular type or stage of parapneumonic effusion. The best therapeutic approach for PPE and PE remains controversial (1,3,4,84–86). The development of new options for treatment further complicates decision making. There are only few prospective, randomized trials to guide intervention. A survey conducted at the 1991 American College of Chest Physicians (ACCP) Annual Scientific Assembly in order to record their personal management preferences reported heterogeneous approaches to management (87). The British Thoracic Society Research Committee conducted the first prospective multicenter study to document the present-day clinical course and management of empyema, which reported a great diversity in treatment approaches and outcomes of PPE and PE (6). Recently, the Health and Sciences Policy Committee (HSP) of the ACCP recognized the variability in clinical practice and convened a panel of experts in this field to develop a clinical practice guideline on the medical and surgical treatment of PPE (34). The rationale for effective management is to identify the pathophysiological stage and intervene quickly and appropriately to prevent progression to empyema.

Uncomplicated parapneumonic effusions resolve with antibiotics alone. Complicated parapneumonic effusions have a variable response to appropriate antibiotic therapy alone. Although some patients can be managed solely with antibiotics (18), there is a bias that early pleural fluid drainage of all loculi of fluid speeds clinical recovery and hospital discharge. Until clinical trials demonstrate the safety of alternative therapies, these patients are normally treated as though they have thoracic empyema. Thoracic empyema should be sterilized with appropriate antibiotics; at least 4–6 weeks of therapy are required, and a longer course may be necessary unless there is prompt resolution of fever and leukocytosis. Complete pleural fluid drainage with large bore chest tube is sine qua non and evidenced by minimal chest tube output (< 50 mL/24 h) and US or CT documentation that no residual loculations persist. Obliteration of the empyema cavity by adequate lung expansion is also important (18).

When a patient with pneumonia is first evaluated, one should attempt first to determine whether a pleural effusion is present. A lateral radiograph should be obtained to screen. If both diaphragms cannot be seen throughout their entirety on the lateral chest radiograph, bilateral decubitus chest radiographs, chest CT scan, or US should be obtained. The amount of free pleural fluid can be estimated by measuring on the lateral chest radiograph the distance between the inside of the chest wall and the outside of the lung. If the thickness of the pleural fluid is >10 mm, thoracentesis should be performed. One should perform the thoracentesis as soon as the pleural effusion is recognized because a free-flowing, easily treated PPE can progress to a multiloculated PPE within a day (35,84).

It is important to realize that not all PPE and not all complicated PPE are the same. The classification outlined in Tables 3, 5, and 6 was developed to assist the practicing physician in the initial care of patients with parapneumonic effusions. A practical management plan is shown in Figure 3.

If the thickness of the pleural fluid is <10 mm, the effusion is nonsignificant and no thoracentesis is indicated (3,84). If it appears from the standard radiographs that the patient has a loculated pleural effusion, this possibility should be evaluated with ultrasound. When a patient has a PPE of >10 mm in thickness on the decubitus radiograph, a thoracentesis should be performed to determine the category of the effusion. It is reasonable to perform a therapeutic rather than a diagnostic thoracentesis (18,33,35). If the fluid is removed com-

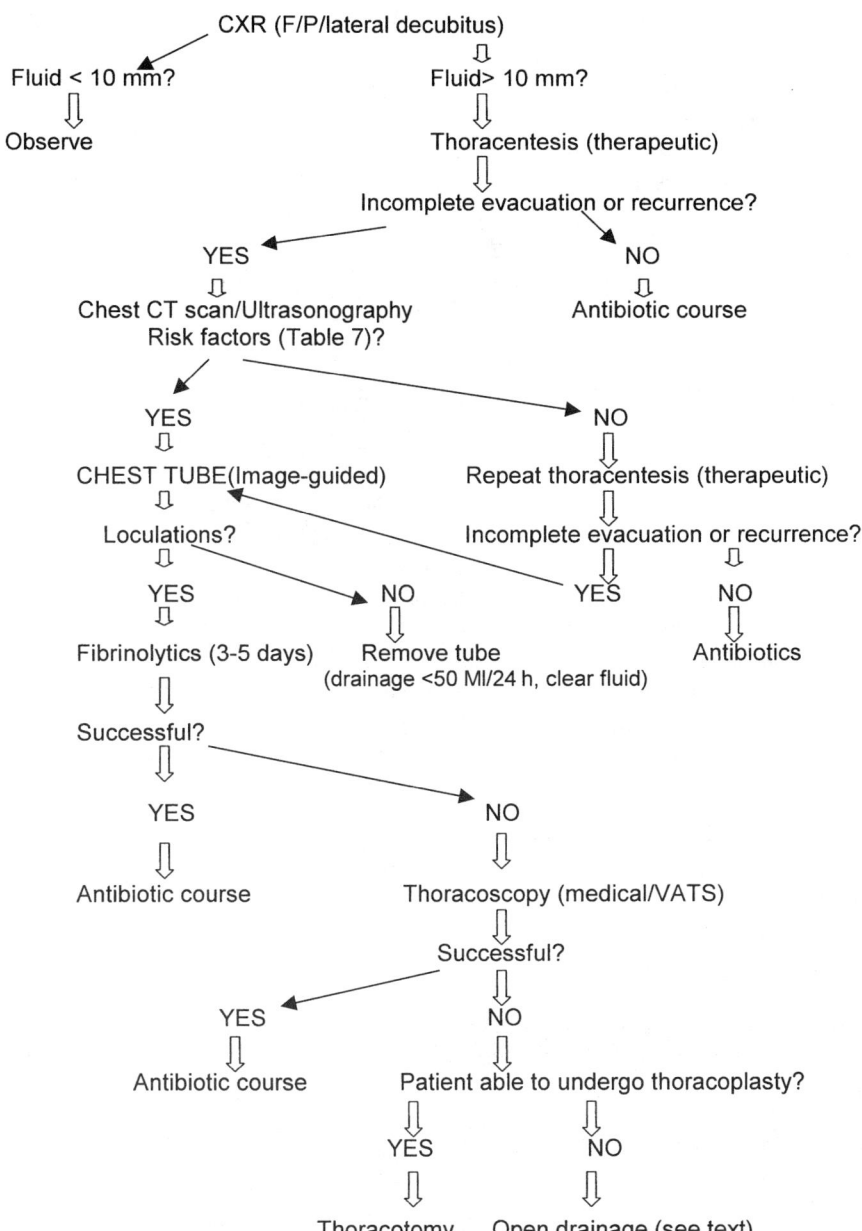

Figure 3 Management algorithm for patients with parapneumonic pleural effusion and empyema.

pletely with the therapeutic thoracentesis and does not reaccumulate, no additional therapy is needed.

If the therapeutic thoracentesis removes all the pleural fluid and the fluid recurs, the next step is guided by the initial pleural fluid findings (3). If none of the poor prognostic indicators are present (Table 7), a repeat thoracentesis should be considered if the size of effusion is progressively increasing, while no invasive procedures are indicated if the patient is doing well clinically or the effusion is small. If any of the poor prognostic indicators were present at the initial thoracentesis, a small 8–13 French chest tube should be inserted into the pleural space. The chest tube is removed if the drainage is <50 mL/24 h. If the pleural fluid cannot be removed completely with a small chest tube, it is probably loculated. If the pleural fluid is loculated and if any of the poor prognostic factors listed in Table 7 are present, efforts should be made to break down the loculations in order to obtain complete drainage of the pleural space. Loculations can be broken down either chemically with intrapleural instillation of fibrinolytics or mechanically by thoracoscopy. If one selects intrapleural fibrinolytics, thoracoscopy should be performed if the fibrinolytics are not successful within 3–5 days. If the lung does not expand at thoracoscopy, one should proceed to decortication unless the patient is too debilitated. In such a case open drainage should be considered (Fig. 3). The primary mistake in the management of patients with complicated PPE/PE is that one progresses from one therapy to another too slowly. A definitive procedure should be done within 10–14 days after the patient is initially seen (3).

Table 7 Risk Predictors in Parapneumonic Effusions, Indicating the Need for Chest Tube Drainage and/or Further Invasive Procedures

Clinical signs
  Prolonged symptoms
  Comorbidity
  Failure to respond to antibiotics
  Pathogen (anaerobic, virulent pathogen)
Imaging signs
  Large effusion ($\geq 1/2$ hemithorax)
  Loculations (single or multiple, large)
  Air-fluid level
  Pleural thickening
  Complex sonographic pattern
Pleural fluid signs
  Macroscopic signs (turbid fluid or frank pus, odorous)
  Low pleural fluid pH (<7.20)
  Low pleural fluid glucose (<40 mg/dL)
  High pleural fluid LDH (>1000 IU)
  Positive pleural fluid Gram stain/culture

XIII. Methods for Treatment of PPE/PE

Today there are various medical and surgical methods for the treatment of PPE/PE (Table 8).

A. Medical Methods

A number of medical methods are available for the treatment of pleural space infection. The choice of therapy depends in part upon whether the PPE/PE is loculated.

Antibiotic Therapy

Antibiotic therapy is indicated for all patients with PPE and PE. Early institution of appropriate antibiotic therapy may prevent the development of PPE and clear small effusions before they become complicated.

The antibiotic selection depends primarily on whether the pneumonia is community or hospital acquired and not on the presence or absence of a PPE. Thus, initial treatment should follow the existing guidelines for treatment of community or hospital-acquired pneumonia (4,88), but with the following in mind: antibiotics that exhibit satisfactory penetration into the pleural fluid include the penicillins, cephalosporins, aztreonam, clindamycin, and ciprofloxacin (3,89). The concentrations of parenterally administered aminoglycosides, particularly gentamicin, were found to be substantially lower in empyema pus than in sterile pleural fluid (see Chapter 50) (89,90).

The recommended empiric treatment for a patient with community-acquired pneumonia that is not severe is a β-lactam-β-lactamase inhibitor with or without a macrolide (4). Alternatively, the newer generation fluoroquinolones,

Table 8 Methods for Treatment of Parapneumonic Effusions and Pleural Empyema

---
Medical
   Antibiotics
   Daily thoracentesis
   Tube thoracostomy (standard chest tube)
   Image-guided percutaneous catheter insertion
   Intrapleural fibrinolytic debridement
   Succion drainage
   Medical thoracoscopy
Surgical
   Video-assisted thoracoscopic surgery (VATS)
   Standard thoracotomy
   Open drainage

such as moxifloxacin and levofloxacin, can be used. The recommended treatment for severe community-acquired pneumonia is a macrolide or a new generation fluoroquinolone plus cefotaxime, ceftriaxone, or a β-lactam-β-lactamase inhibitor (4). Enteric gram-negative bacilli, or *S. aureus* with or without oral anaerobes frequently causes pneumonia acquired in institutions such as nursing homes or hospitals. If methicillin-resistant S. aureus infection is suspected, vancomycin should be administered. If gram-negative infection is suspected, the patient should be treated with a third-generation cephalosporin or a β-lactam-β-lactamase inhibitor plus an aminoglycoside.

Given the high incidence of anaerobic infection in empyema and the difficulty in isolating anaerobes in many clinical laboratories, most clinicians cover for anaerobes, even if cultures are negative. Options for empiric therapy, which also covers anaerobic organisms, include penicillin, metronidazole, clindamycin, extended spectrum penicillins (such as ticarcillin, piperacillin, ampicillin-sulbactam, or piperacillin-tazobactam), or imipenem.

There is still debate over the use of intrapleural antibiotics. Several studies have reported positive results, but none of them included a randomized control group (91,92).

Repeat Thoracentesis

Repeat therapeutic thoracentesis is the least invasive technique to treat PPE and PE. Nowadays it is used rarely as a mode of treatment. There is lack of controlled randomized trials to evaluate its efficacy. In the few reported nonrandomized series the success rate ranged widely from 25 to 94%, and the mortality from 0 to 25%, probably due to variability in the PPE stage (85,87,92–95). Repeat thoracentesis should be performed in cases where pleural fluid recurs or when the PPE is undetermined (Table 5, Figure 3).

Storm et al. (92) in a retrospective study of 94 patients with PPE or PE compared patients who were treated with daily thoracentesis, saline rinse, systemic antibiotics, and in some patients local antibiotics in the medical ward and patients with tube drainage and systemic antibiotics in the surgical ward. The thoracentesis group had a lower frequency of complications and a shorter duration of hospital stay than the tube drainage group. The overall mortality was 8.5% with no difference between the two groups. The outcome, however, could be due to inclusion of more severe cases in the surgical group (92).

Standard Chest Tubes

In many centers even today relatively large (26F–28F) chest tubes are usually used to drain PPE, especially PE. The success rate ranges from 6 to 76% (mean 50%) (1,6,85,86,92,93,96–104). Their failure to drain PPE is usually due to misplacement, malfunctioning, or loculation of the pleural fluid. In a study by Huang et al. loculation and PPE leukocyte count $> 6.400/\mu L$ were independent predicting factors of poor outcome of tube thoracostomy drainage (103). The chest tube is removed when the daily drainage is < 50 mL/24 h and the fluid is clear and yellow. Complications include hemorrhage, pneumothorax, subcutaneous emphysema, or pain. The mortality ranges from 0 to 24% (mean 9.5%) (1,3,4,6,85,86,92,93,96–104).

Image-Guided Transcutaneous Catheters

Today image-guided transcutaneous catheter (IGTC) insertion is used increasingly as they are more comfortable for pleural drainage. Interventional radiologists or pneumonologists can easily and safely use IGTC under US or CT scan guidance. Their size ranges between 8 and 14F (Malecot or pigtail). Their success rate ranges from 0 to 94% (mean 70%) (1,3,104–112). These wide differences are due to patient selection. IGTC drainage is successful if instituted early in the course of the disease process. They are indicated for small, inaccessible or multiloculated effusions, are not suitable for PE, and work better in free or single loculated effusion. They can also be used for fibrinolytic instillation. No major complications have been noted.

Intrapleural Instillation of Fibrinolytics

Intrapleural instillation of fibrinolytic agents (streptokinase or urokinase) has been shown, in a number of studies, to be an effective and safe mode of treatment in complicated PPE and PE, minimizing the need for surgical intervention.

Technique of Instillation

The optimum dose, frequency, and duration of instillation of fibrinolytics into the pleural space have not been determined. The most commonly used dose of streptokinase (SK) is 250,000 IU and that of urokinase (UK) 100,000 (50,000–450,000 IU). The drug is usually diluted in 100 mL of normal saline. Dwell time varies from 2 to 4 hours, the duration of treatment from 3 to 5 days, and the chest tube size from 10 to 40 F. Duration of treatment is based on the presence of residual pleural fluid as determined by repeat chest radiograph, US, and/or CT scan.

Success Rate

The mean success rate in the published uncontrolled series of streptokinase is about 85% (range 38–100%) (Fig. 4) and that of urokinase 88% (range 63–100%) (113) (Fig. 5).

Six controlled and/or randomized trials of the use of intrapleural fibrinolytics have been reported (Table 9). Bouros et al. (114) compared the efficacy and safety of SK and UK in the treatment of PPE. Fifty consecutive patients were randomly allocated to receive either SK (250000 IU in 100 mL normal saline solution) or UK (100000 IU in 100 mL normal saline) through tube thoracostomy in a double-blinded fashion. All patients had inadequate drainage (<70 mL/24 h) through a chest tube before fibrinolytic treatment. Pleural fluid drainage significantly increased with fibrinolytic therapy, and the increase in pleural fluid drainage was similar for patients treated with UK and SK. Most

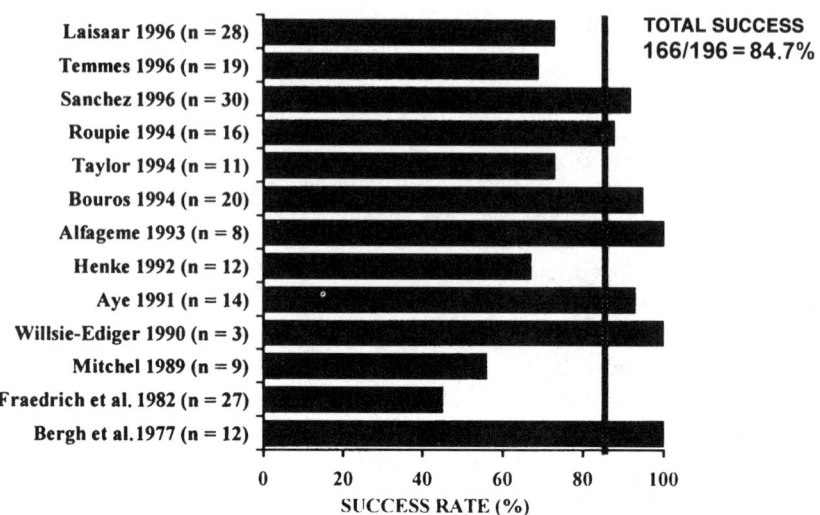

Figure 4 Reported case series (1977–1996) of the success rate of the streptokinase intrapleural instillation in patients with parapneumonic pleural effusion and empyema.

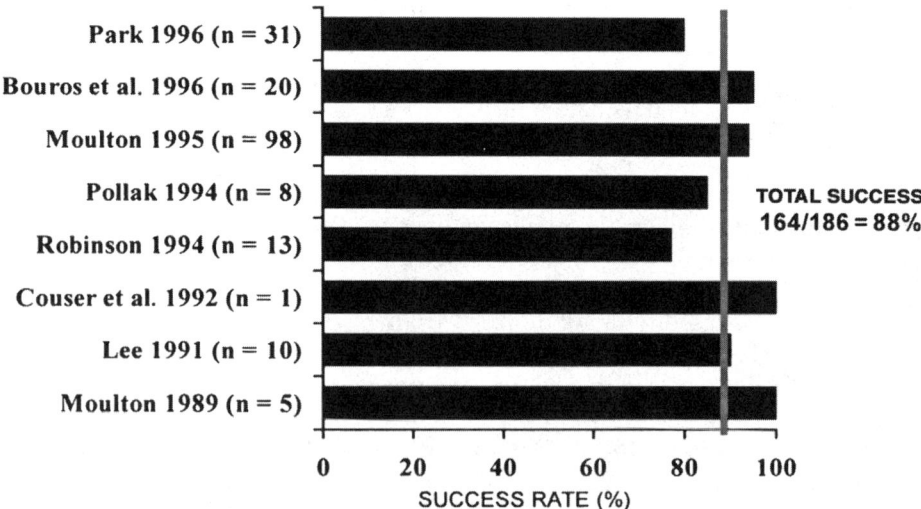

Figure 5 Reported case series (1989–1996) of the success rate of the urokinase intrapleural instillation in patients with parapneumonic pleural effusion and empyema.

Table 9 Success Rate in the Published Controlled Studies of Fibrinolytics in Parapneumonic Effusions and Pleural Empyema

SK n (%)	UK n (%)	CT + NS n (%)	VATS n (%)	CT n (%)	Ref.
23/25 (92)	23/25 (92)				114
12 (100)		3/12 (25)			100
4/9 (44)			10/11 (91)		115
16/23 (70)				19/29 (66)	98
	13/15 (86.5)	4/16 (25)			116
	25 (60)	24 (29)			117

CT = chest tube; SK = streptokinase; UK = urokinase; NS = normal saline; VATS = video-assisted thoracoscopic surgery.

patients in both treatment groups had marked clinical improvement with fibrinolytic therapy. UK was suggested as the fibrinolytic of choice due to the lower incidence of drug-related adverse events and its only slightly higher cost (114).

In another randomized, prospective, controlled trial, Davies et al. (100) compared the efficacy of SK (250000 IU in 20 mL of saline with a 2-hour dwell time daily for 3 days) with normal saline flushes in 24 patients. Patients who received SK had greater daily and total pleural fluid drainage as well as more evidence of chest radiographic improvement at discharge. Three patients in the tube thoracostomy control group required a second intervention to effectively drain versus none in the fibrinolytic group. There were no significant differences between the two treatment groups in hospital length of stay, time to defervescence, and time to normalization of WBC (100).

Wait et al. (115) compared the results after fibrinolytic therapy with video-assisted thoracoscopic surgery (VATS) in the management of PPE. Twenty patients were randomly allocated to receive either SK (250000 IU in 100 mL normal saline solution) administered daily for 3 days through tube thoracostomy or immediate VATS. They found that the VATS group had a significantly higher treatment success rate than the fibrinolytic group. The hospital length of stay and duration of chest tube drainage were significantly shorter in the VATS group (115).

Chin and Lim (98), in a controlled, nonrandomized trial, analyzed the treatment responses of PPE to either tube thoracostomy or fibrinolytics. A historical control group, studied from 1990 to 1992, of 29 patients was treated with tube thoracostomy and a second one of 23 patients, evaluated from 1992 to 1995, was given SK (250000 IU in 100 mL normal saline solution) daily through tube thoracostomy. Decortication was done in 17% and the overall mortality rate was 15%. There were no differences between the two groups in time to defervescence, days of chest tube drainage, and hospital stay, although the fibrinolytic group did have a greater amount of total pleural fluid drainage. The death rate was lower for the group treated with fibrinolytics but the need for a second intervention to drain the pleural space was similar for the two treatment groups (98).

Bouros et al. (116) in a randomized, controlled double-blind trial compared UK (15 patients) to tube thoracostomy (16 patients) in managing PPE. No patients died in this series, but the fibrinolytic group needed a second intervention to manage the PPE less often (2 of 15, or 13.5%) than the group receiving normal saline (12 of 16, or 75%). From this study it was suggested that UK is effective in the treatment of loculated pleural effusions through the lysis of pleural adhesions and not through the volume effect (116). Tuncozgur et al. in a recent randomized, controlled study confirmed the data of our own study (117).

At the present time there is an ongoing multicenter study in the United Kingdom comparing streptokinase with normal saline. It is estimated to have 400 patients upon its completion and is expected to definitely determine the degree of efficacy of fibrinolytics in PPE.

Monitoring for Efficacy and Adverse Reactions

Fibrinolytic agents are most effective if used early in the evolution of PPE before significant collagen is deposited in the pleural space (early in the fibrinopurulent stage) (1). Factors to consider in evaluating whether or not intrapleural instillation of fibrinolytics is effective include an assessment of clinical response. Preposition for clinical response is the installation via a patent, properly placed chest tube. Its use should be started early if after chest tube placement inadequate evacuation of pleural fluid is noted radiographically with no clinical improvement. Measurement of pleural fluid drainage, WBC count, chest radiographs, and US and/or CT could be used to monitor treatment efficacy.

In the face of fever persistence or pleural sepsis, a markedly elevated WBC with left sift, or unresponsiveness of the pleural process to drainage, the clinician should reevaluate whether or not alternative therapy should be employed. In this situation further invasive intervention, such as thoracoscopy, is indicated (1,3, 113,114,116,118).

Initial use of nonpurified solutions of SK and streptodornase had as a result frequent febrile reactions, general malaise, and leukocytosis. Newer preparations cause fewer allergic reactions. The most frequently observed adverse reaction is fever (0–20%), which in rare cases can be severe (1,113,118).

Anaphylactic intravenous reactions to -UK have been rarely reported, which were usually mild. Only one possible case of ventricular fibrillation following IPUK has been reported in a patient with pleural empyema (119). A case of acute hypoxemic respiratory failure following intrapleural instillation of both SK and UK 24 hours apart for hemothorax has been described (120).

Intrapleural fibrinolytic treatment does not seem to have a measurable effect on systemic coagulation parameters (121). A case of major hemorrhage following intrapleural instillation SK in a dose of 500,000 IU, which is higher than the usual, has been reported (122) in a patient who was also taking carbenicillin and prophylactic heparin.

Although intravenous use of SK can potentially lead to antistreptokinase antibodies in the blood, which may lead to an allergic reaction if SK is readministered later (after an acute myocardial infarction), this has not been systematically studied in intrapleural instillation. It is possible that these antibodies may cause allergic reactions or neutralization in a further treatment with SK (122,123). Furthermore, its use is contraindicated in patients with recent streptococcal infection. Contraindications for intrapleural administration of fibrinolytics are not well known. However, caution should be exercised in certain situations (Table 10).

Timing of Decision for Additional Therapy

Failure of the pleural infection to resolve, both clinically and radiologically, within 3–5 days with the use of intrapleural fibrinolytics is considered as an indication for further intervention (1,118). Clinicians should be aware that patients with clinical improvement but with remaining radiographic pleural shadowing may have pleural peels that will resolve in a period of weeks (3).

In a recent study Bouros et al. (124) reported that in 20 consecutive patients with complicated PPE/PE, intrapleural urokinase instillation failed to achieve complete drainage. This was achieved by applying VATS in 17 patients (85%). In the other three (15%) patients the VATS procedure had to be con-

Table 10 Contraindications for Intrapleural Fibrinolytic Use

Absolute contraindications
  History of allergic reaction to the agent
  History of hemorrhagic stroke
  Cranial surgery or head trauma within 14 days
  Bronchopleural fistula
  Trauma or surgery within 48 h
Relative contraindications
  Major thoracic or abdominal surgery within 7–14 days
  Biopsy or invasive procedure in a location inaccessible to external compression within 7–14 days
  Coagulation defects
  Cerebrovascular accident (nonhemorrhagic)
  Previous streptokinase thrombolysis
  Streptococcal infection (?)

Source: Adapted from Ref. 118.

verted to open thoracotomy due to a thickened visceral pleural peel. Therefore, in PPE patients who have failed to resolve with initial treatment with fibrinolytics, VATS could be the next procedure of choice.

Suction Drainage

Cummin et al. used strong suction (-100 mmHg) with the catheter directed, under US guidance, into most parts of the infected cavity, permitting removal of septations and drainage of pus (125). However, others have not applied this technique up to now.

B. Surgical Methods

The various surgical methods used for patients with more advanced stages of PPE and PE are shown in Table 8 and discussed briefly in this chapter. For more details, see other chapters in this book.

Thoracoscopy

Today thoracoscopy (medical or surgical), conventional or video-assisted, for the breakdown of adhesions is considered as the procedure of choice and a major innovation when tube thoracostomy plus intrapleural thrombolytic therapy fails (124). Medical thoracoscopy is performed under local anesthesia in the bronchoscopy suite (126). It is easy to learn and should be applied increasingly by pulmonologists. In one series the success rate was 75% (127).

Video-assisted thoracic surgery is being used increasingly (128–137). However, it needs one lung ventilation, general anesthesia, expertise, availability, and is not suitable for chronic PE (success rate <50%). The conversion rate to thoracotomy ranges from 10 to 30% according to patient selection. In five retrospective studies and one prospective study, a mean success rate of 82% in a total of 212 patients has been reported (1,128–133) (Fig. 6).

Open Thoracotomy

With open thoracotomy the patient is submitted to debridement or decortication. The decision to proceed to open thoracotomy usually follows the failure of less invasive methods to control pleural sepsis. Decortication is a major thoracic operation that is not indicated for markedly debilitated patients (1,3). Decortication in the acute phase of a PPE is performed in order to control pleural sepsis and not for pleural thickening. Pleural fibrosis usually begins to resolve once the pleural infection is controlled. Late decortication (>6 months) is indicated for persistent pleural thickening that leads to reduced pulmonary function and restrictive pulmonary function tests. Success and mortality rates range from 87 to 100% (mean 93.4%) and 0 to 9% (mean 2.5%), respectively (3,138–140). Comparative studies between VATS and thoracotomy showed similar rates of success, but VATS offered substantial advantages in terms of resolution of the disease, hospital stay, and cosmesis (128,140).

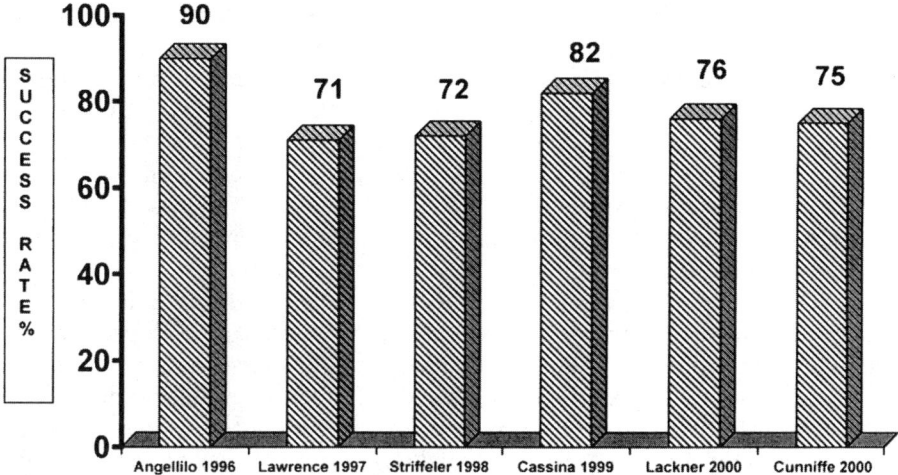

Figure 6 Success rate of video-assisted thoracoscopic surgery (VATS) in patients with parapneumonic effusions in six published series during the period 1995–2000. Mean success rate 78%. (Adapted from Ref. 1.)

Open Drainage

Open drainage is an alternative to decortication in patients who are markedly debilitated. It involves rib resection and insertion of large-bore tubes to permit open drainage at the inferior border of the PE cavity. Daily irrigation with a mild antiseptic solution is necessary, while a colostomy bag can be used for drainage collection. In order for open drainage to be performed, fusion of the two pleural layers is required to avoid lung collapse. Early open drainage of pleural fluid before the fusion of the two pleural layers can lead to increased mortality, as happened during the Word War I (3). With this technique the patient is freed from the closed drainage system. A more complicated procedure is the Eloesser technique. A skin and muscle flap creates a skin-lined fistula, providing drainage without chest tubes. The time of healing, howeverm, is lengthy (usually 6 months) (3,29).

XIV. Summary

PPE/PE are frequent complications of bacterial pneumonia and one of the oldest known diseases. Even today PPE/PE continue to be a significant medical problem, with high mortality in cases of late intervention. Their clinical presentation may vary from small, uncomplicated effusions to severe multiloculated empyemas. It is critical to assess the individual severity and risk of a PPE using imaging techniques and early thoracentesis with pleural fluid analysis and bacteriology. Imaging techniques identify the size and the loculations of an effusion and may help to identify empyemas. There is widespread clinical consensus that the pleural fluid pH is the best chemical parameter to assess a PPE. A pH of <7.20 usually predicts a more complicated course. A positive Gram stain and/or culture of the pleural fluid, a low glucose (<40 mg/dL), a high LDH (>100 IU), large effusions (≥1/2 hemithorax), loculations, and the presence of frank pus are further important markers of severity and indications for chest tube drainage. These risk factors are associated with a complicated course. Small nonloculated effusions have a high probability of spontaneous resolution under appropriate antibiotic therapy and should be observed.

There are no general guidelines for the management of PPE/PE. The appropriate therapeutic approach should be individualized for each patient. The stage of the pneumonia and the PPE is critical to the outcome. Early detection and institution of adequate therapy are essential for the resolution of PPE/PE (141). The evolution from one stage to the other could progress quickly and an aggressive therapeutic modality is needed if less invasive techniques fail ("the sun should never set on a PPE").

The pulmonologist should play a pivotal role, becoming increasingly active by the introduction of newer trends (intrapleural fibrinolytics, medical thoracoscopy, imaging-guided transcutaneous catheters) for the treatment of PPE. The application of these newer modalities protects patients from surgical intervention and its associated risks. These methods have been found to be efficient in the hands of experts in specialized centers. However, methodological weaknesses in the existing literature and lack of controlled, randomized trials relevant to the management of PPE do not permit the formulation of practical guidelines.

References

1. Bouros D, Hamm H. Infectious pleural effusions. Eur Respir Mon 2002; 22:204–218.
2. Strange C, Sahn SA. The definitions and epidemiology of pleural space infection. Semin Respir Infect 1999; 14:3–8.
3. Light RW. Pleural Diseases. 4th ed. Philadelphia: Lippincott Williams & Wilkins, 2001.
4. Niederman MS, Mandell LA, Anzueto A, Bass JB, Broughton WA, Campbell GD, Dean N, File T, Fine MJ, Gross PA, Martinez F, Marrie TJ, Plouffe JF, Ramirez J, Sarosi GA, Torres A, Wilson R, Yu VL. Guidelines for the management of adults with community-acquired pneumonia. Diagnosis, assessment of severity, antimicrobial therapy, and prevention. Am J Respir Crit Care Med 2001; 163:1730–1754.
5. Jerng JS, Hsueh PR, Teng LJ, Lee LN, Yang PC, Luh KT. Empyema thoracic and lung abscess caused by viridans streptococci. Am J Respir Crit Care Med 1997; 156:1508–1514.
6. Ferguson AD, Prescott RJ, Selkon JB, Watson D, Swinburn CR. The clinical course and management of thoracic empyema. QJM 1996; 89:285–289.
7. Chin NK, Lim TK. Treatment of complicated parapneumonic effusions and pleu-

ral empyema: a four-year prospective study. Singapore Med J 1996; 37:631–635.
8. Densai GA, Mugala DD. Management of empyema thoracis at Lusaka Zambia. Br J Surg 1992; 79:537–538.
9. Hassan I, Mabogunje 0. Adult empyema in Zaria, Nigeria. East African Med J 1992; 69:97–100.
10. Weissberg D, Refaely Y. Pleural empyema: 24-year experience. Ann Thorac Surg 1996; 62:1026–1029.
11. Bashir Y, Benson MK. Necrotizing pneumonia and empyema due to *Clostridium perfringens* complicating pulmonary embolus. Thorax 1990; 45:72–73.
12. Baethge GA, Eggerstedt JM, Olash FA. Group F streptococcal empyema from aspiration of a grass inflorescence. Ann Thorac Surg 1990; 49:319–320.
13. Zachariades N, Mezitis M, Stavrinidis P, Konsolaki-Agouridaki E. Mediastinitis, thoracic empyema, and pericarditis as complications of a dental abscess: report of a case. Oral Maxillofac Surg 1988; 46:493–495.
14. Fine NL, Smith LR, Sheedy PF. Frequency of pleural effusions in mycoplasma and viral pneumonias. N Engl J Med 1970; 283:790–793.
15. Taryle DA, Potts DE, Sahn SA. The incidence and clinical correlates of parapneumonic effusions in pneumococcal pneumonia. Chest 1978; 74:170–173.
16. Sasse SA. Parapneumonic effusions and empyema. Curr Opin Pulm Med 1996; 2:520–526.
17. Hasley PB, Albaum MN, Li YH, Fuhrman CR, Britton CA, Marrie TJ, Singer DE, Coley CM, Kapoor WN, Fine MJ. Do pulmonary radiographic findings at presentation predict mortality in patients with community-acquired pneumonia? Arch Intern Med 1996; 156:2206–2212.
18. Strange C, Sahn SA. Management of parapneumonic pleural effusions and empyema. Infect Dis Clin North Am 1991; 5:539–559.
19. Antony VB, Mohammed KA. Pathophysiology of pleural infections. Semin Respir Infect 1999; 14:9–17.
20. Light RW, Girard WM, Jenkinson SG, George RB. Parapneumonic effusions. Am J Med 1980; 69:507–512.
21. Wiener-Kronish JP, Sakuma T, Kudoh I, Pittet JF, Frank D, Dobbs L, Vasil ML, Matthay MA. Alveolar epithelial injury and pleural empyema in acute P aeruginosa pneumonia in anesthetized rabbits. J Appl Physiol 1993; 75:1661–1669.
22. Potts DE, Levin DC, Sahn SA. Pleural fluid pH in parapneumonic effusions. Chest 1976; 70:328–331.
23. Potts DE, Taryle DA, Sahn SA. The glucose-pH relationship in parapneumonic effusions. Arch Intern Med 1978; 138:1378–1380.
24. Antony VB, Hadley KJ, Sahn SA. Mechanisms of pleural fibrosis in empyema: pleural macrophage-mediated inhibition of fibroblast proliferation. Chest 1989; 95S:230–231.
25. Sahn SA, Taryle DA, Good JT Jr. Experimental empyema: time course and pathogenesis of pleural fluid acidosis and low pleural fluid glucose. Am Rev Respir Dis 1979; 120:355–361.
26. Broaddus VC, Hebert CA, Vitangcol RV, Hoeffel JM, Bernstein MS, Boylan AM. Interleukin-8 is a major neutrophil chemotactic factor in pleural liquid of patients with empyema. Am Rev Respir Dis 1992; 146:825–830.
27. Sahn SA, Reller LB, Taryle DA, Antony VB, Good JT Jr. The contribution of

leukocytes and bacteria to the low pH of empyema fluid. Am Rev Respir Dis 1983; 128:811–815.
28. Idell S, Girard W, Koenig KB, McLarty J, Fair DS. Abnormalities of pathways of fibrin turnover in the human pleural space. Am Rev Respir Dis 1991; 144:187–194.
29. Hamm H, Light RW. Parapneumonic effusion and empyema. Eur Respir J 1997; 10:1150–1156.
30. Light RW, MacGregor M, Ball WCj, Luchsinger PC. Diagnostic significance of pleural fluid pH and pCO_2. Chest 1973; 64:591–596.
31. Hippocrates. Aphorisms. In: Jones WHS, trans, eds. Hippocrates Works. Vol. II. Cambridge, MA: Harvard University Press, 1967; Aphorisms No. VII, 87.
32. Andrews NC, Parker EF, Shaw RR. Management of nontuberculous empyema. Am Rev Respir Dis 1962; 85:935–936.
33. Light RW. A new classification of parapneumonic effusions and empyema. Chest 1995; 108:299–301.
34. Colice GL, Curtis A, Deslauriers J, Heffner J, Light R, Littenberg B, Sahn S, Weinstein RA, Yusen RD. Medical and surgical treatment of parapneumonic effusions. Chest 2000; 18:1158–1171.
35. Light RW. The management of parapneumonic effusions and empyema. Pneumon 2002; 15:127–132.
36. Bhattacharyya N, Umland El, Kosloske AM. A bacteriologic basis for the evolution and severity of empyema. J Pediatr Surg 1994; 29:667.
37. Strange C. Pathogenesis and management of parapneumonic effusions and empyema. UpToDate 2002, March 2.
38. Brook I, Frazier EH. Aerobic and anaerobic microbiology of empyema: A retrospective review in two military hospitals. Chest 1993; 103:1502.
39. Bartlett JG, Gorbach SL, Thadepalli H, Finegold SM. Bacteriology of empyema. Lancet 1974; 1:338.
40. Alfagame I, Munoz F, Pena N, Umbria S. Empyema of the thorax in adults. Etiology, microbiologic findings, and management. Chest 1993; 103:839–843.
41. LeMense GP, Strange C, Sahn SA. Empyema thoracis—therapeutic management and outcome. Chest 1995; 107:1532–1537.
42. Yeh TJ, Hall DP, Ellison RG. Empyema thoracis: a review of 110 cases. Am Rev Respir Dis 1963; 88:785–790.
43. Snider GL, Saleh SS. Empyema of the thorax in adults: review of 105 cases. Chest 1968; 54:12–17.
44. Smith JA, Mullerworth MH, Westlake GW, Tatoulis J. Empyema thoracis: 14-year experience in a teaching center. Ann Thorac Surg 1991; 51:39–42.
45. Kelly JW, Morris MJ. Empyema thoracis: medical aspects of evaluation and treatment. South Med J 1994; 87:1103–1110.
46. Everts RJ, Reller LB. Pleural space infections: microbiology and antimicrobial therapy. Semin Respir Infect 1999; 14:18–30.
47. Bartlett JG, Finegold SM. Anaerobic infections of the lung and pleural space. Am Rev Respir Dis 1974; 110:56–77.
48. Bartlett JG. Anaerobic bacterial infections of the lung. Chest 1987; 91:901–909.
49. Levin DL, Klein JS. Imaging techniques for pleural space infections. Semin Respir Infect 1999; 14:31–38.
50. Blackmore CC, Black WC, Dallas RV, et al. Pleural fluid volume estimation: a chest radiograph prediction rule. Acad Radiol 1996; 3:103–109.

51. Moskowitz H, Platt RT, Schachar R, Mellins H. Roentgen visualization of minute pleural effusion. Radiology 1973; 109:33–35.
52. Ruskin JA, Gurney JW, Thorsen MK, Goodman LR. Detection of pleural effusion on supine chest radiographs. AJR 1987; 146:681–683.
53. Muller NL. Imaging of the pleura. Radiology 1993; 186:297–309.
54. McLoud TC, Flower CDR. Imaging the pleura: sonography, CT, and MR imaging. AJR Am J Roentgenol 1991; 156:1145–1153.
55. Pugatch RD, Spirn PW. Radiology of the pleura. Clin Chest Med 1985; 6:17–32.
56. Hirsh JH, Rogers JV, Mack LA. Real-time sonography of pleural opacities. AJR 1981; 136:297–301.
57. Yang PC, Luh KT, Chang DB, Wu HD, Yu CJ, Kuo SH. Value of sonography in determining the nature of pleural effusion: analysis of 320 cases. AJR 1992; 159:29–33.
58. Raptopoulos V, Davis LM, Lee G, Umali C, Lew R, Irwin RS. Factors affecting the development of pneumothorax associated with thoracentesis. AJR 1991; 156:917–920.
59. Eibenberger KL, Dock WI, Ammann ME, Dorffner R, Hormann MF, Grabenwoger F. Quantification of pleural effusions: sonography vs. radiography. Radiology 1994; 191:681–684.
60. Lipscomb DJ, Flower CDR, Hadfield JW. Ultrasound of the pleura: an assessment of its clinical utility. Clin Radiol 1981; 32:289–290.
61. Aquino SL, Webb WR, Gushiken BJ. Pleural exudates and transudates: diagnosis with contrast-enhanced CT. Radiology 1994; 192:803–808.
62. Kearney SE, Davies CW, Davies RJ, Gleeson FV. Computed tomography and ultrasound in parapneumonic effusions and empyema. Clin Radiol 2000; 55:542–547.
63. Arenas-Jimenez J, Alonso-Charterina S, Sanchez-Paya J, Fernandez-Latorre F, Gil-Sanchez S, Lloret-Llorens M. Evaluation of CT findings for diagnosis of pleural effusions. Eur Radiol 2000; 10:681–690.
64. Haramati LB, Alterman DD, White CS, Kerr AS. Intrathoracic lymphadenopathy in patients with empyema. J Comput Assist Tomogr 1997; 21:608–611.
65. Kearney SE, Davies CW, Tattersall DJ, Gleeson FV. The characteristics and significance of thoracic lymphadenopathy in parapneumonic effusion and empyema. Br J Radiol 2000; 73:583–587.
66. Bittner RC, Schnoy N, Schönfeld N, Grassot A, Loddenkemper R, Lode H, Kaiser D, Krumhaar D, Felix R. High-resolution magnetic resonance tomography (HR-MRT) of the pleura and thoracic wall: normal findings and pathological findings. Rofo Fortschr Geb Röntgenstr Neuen Bildgeb Verfahr 1995; 162:296–303.
67. Davis SD, Henschke CI, Yankelevitz DF, Cahill PT, Yi Y. MR imaging of pleural effusions. J Comput Assist Tomogr 1990; 14:192–198.
68. Himelman RB, Kallen PW. The prognostic value of loculations in parapneumonic pleural effusions. Chest 1986; 90:852–856.
69. Frola C, Cantoni S, Turtulici I, Leoni C, Loria F, Gaeta M, Derchi LE. Transudative vs. exudative pleural effusions: differentiation using Gd-DTPA enhanced MRI. Eur Radiol 1997; 7:860–864.
70. Light RW, Macgregor MI, Luchsinger PC, Ball WC Jr. Pleural effusions: the diagnostic separation of transudates and exudates. Ann Intern Med 1972; 77:507–513.

71. Hamm H, Brohan U, Bohmer R, Missmahl HP. Cholesterol in pleural effusions. A diagnostic aid. Chest 1987; 92:296–302.
72. Light RW, MacGregor M, Ball WCj, Luchsinger PC. Diagnostic significance of pleural fluid pH and pCO2. Chest 1973; 64:591–596.
73. Potts DE, Levin DC, Sahn SA. Pleural fluid pH in parapneumonic effusions. Chest 1976; 70:328–331.
74. Poe RH, Marin MG, Israel RH, Kallay MC. Utility of pleural fluid analysis in predicting tube thoracostomy/decortication in parapneumonic effusions. Chest 1991; 100:963–967.
75. Good JT, Taryle DA, Maulitz RM, Kaplan RL, Sahn SA. The diagnostic value of pleural fluid pH. Chest 1980; 78:55–59.
76. Potts DE, Taryle DA, Sahn SA. The glucose-pH relationship in parapneumonic effusions. Arch Intern Med 1978; 138:1378–1380.
77. Sahn SA, Reller LB, Taryle DA, Antony VB, Good JT. The contribution of leucocytes and bacteria to the low pH of empyema fluid. Am Rev Respir Dis 1983; 128:811–815.
78. Heffner JE, Brown LK, Barbieri C, DeLeo JM. Pleural fluid chemical analysis in parapneumonic effusions. Am J Respir Crit Care Med 1995; 151:1700–1708.
79. Pine JR, Hollmann JL. Elevated pleural fluid pH in *Proteus mirabilis* empyema. Chest 1983; 84:109–111.
80. Sahn SA. Management of complicated parapneumonic effusions. Am Rev Respir Dis 1993; 148:813–817.
81. Light RW, Rodriguez RM. Management of parapneumonic effusions. Clin Chest Med 1998; 19:373–382.
82. Massard G, Wihlm JM. Early complications. Esophagopleural fistula. Chest Surg Clin North Am 1999; 9:617–631.
83. Chu MW, Dewar LR, Burgess JJ, Busse EG. Empyema thoracis: lack of awareness results in a prolonged clinical course. Can J Surg 2001; 44:284–288.
84. Sahn SA. State of the art. The pleura. Am Rev Respir Dis 1988; 138:184–234.
85. Lemmer JH, Botham MJ, Orringer MB. Modern management of adult thoracic empyema. J Thorac Cardiovasc Surg 1985; 90:849–885.
86. Mandal AK, Thadepalli H. Treatment of spontaneous bacterial empyema thoracis. J Thorac Cardiovasc Surg 1987; 94:414–418.
87. Strange C, Sahn SA. The clinician's perspective on parapneumonic effusions and empyema. Chest 1993; 103:259–261.
88. Campbell GD, Niederman MS, Broughton WA, Craven DE, Fein AM, Fink MP, Gleeson K, Hornick DB, Lynch JP, Mandell LA, Mason CM, Torres A, Wunderink RG. Hospital-acquired pneumonia in adults: diagnosis, assessment of severity, initial antimicrobial therapy, and preventive strategies. Am J Respir Crit Care Med 1995; 153:1711–1725.
89. Teixeira LR, Sasse SA, Villarino MA, Nguyen T, Mulligan ME, Light RW. Antibiotic levels in empyemic pleural fluid. Chest 2000; 117:1734–1739.
90. Thys JP, Vanderhoeft P, Herchuelz A, Bergmann P, Yourassowsky E. Penetration of aminoglycosides in uninfected pleural exudates and in pleural empyemas. Chest 1988; 93:530–532.
91. Rosenfeldt FL, McGibney D, Braimbridge MV, Watson DA. Comparison between irrigation and conventional treatment for empyema and pneumonectomy space infection. Thorax 1981; 36:272–277.
92. Storm HK, Krasnik M, Bang K, Frimodt-Moller N. Treatment of pleural em-

pyema secondary to pneumonia: thoracentesis regimen versus tube drainage. Thorax 1992; 47:821–824.
93. Benfield GF. Recent trends in empyema thoracis. Br J Dis Chest 1981; 75:358–366.
94. Vianna NJ. Nontuberculous bacterial empyema in patients with and without underlying disease. JAMA 1971; 215:69–75.
95. Wehr CJ, Adkins RB Jr. Empyema thoracis: a ten-year experience. South Med J 1986; 79:171–176.
96. Ali I, Unruh H. Management of empyema thoracis. Ann Thorac Surg 1990; 50:355–359.
97. Berger HA, Morganroth ML. Immediate drainage is not required for all patients with complicated parapneumonic effusion. Chest 1990; 97:731–735.
98. Chin NK, Lim TK. Controlled trial of intrapleural streptokinase in the treatment of pleural empyema and complicated parapneumonic effusion. Chest 1997; 111:275–279.
99. Cohn LH, Blaisdell EW. Surgical treatment of nontuberculous empyema. Arch Surg 1970; 100:376–381.
100. Davies RJO, Traill ZC, Gleeson FV. Randomised controlled trial of intrapleural streptokinase in community acquired pleural infection. Thorax 1997; 52:416–421.
101. Hoover EL, Hsu HK, Webb H, Toporoff B, Minnard E, Cunningham JN. The surgical management of empyema thoracis in substance abuse patients: a 5-year experience. Ann Thorac Surg 1988; 46:563–566.
102. Roupie E, Bouabdallah K, Delclaux C, Brun-Buisson C, Lemaire F, Vasile N, Brochard L. Intrapleural administration of streptokinase in complicated purulent pleural effusion: a CT-guided strategy. Intensive Care Med 1996; 22:1351–1353.
103. Huang HC, Chang HY, Chen CW, Lee CH, Hsiue TR. Predicting factors for outcome of tube thoracostomy in complicated parapneumonic effusion for empyema. Chest 1999; 115:751–756.
104. Thourani VH, Brady KM, Mansour KA, Miller Jl Jr, Lee RB. Evaluation of treatment modalities for thoracic empyema: a cost-effectiveness analysis. Ann Thorac Surg 1998; 66:1121–1127.
105. Westcott JL. Percutaneous catheter drainage of pleural effusion and empyema. Am J Roentgenol 1985; 144:1189–1193.
106. Merriam MA, Cronan JJ, Dorfman GS, Lambiase RE, Haas RA. Radiographically guided percutaneous catheter drainage of pleural fluid collections. Am J Roentgenol 1988; 151:1113–1116.
107. Silverman SG, Mueller PR, Saini S, Hahn PF, Simeone JF, Forman BH, Steiner E, Ferrucci JT. Thoracic empyema: management with image-guided catheter drainage. Radiology 1988; 169:5–9.
108. VanSonnenberg E, Nakamoto SK, Mueller PR, Casola G, Neff CC, Friedman PJ, Ferrucci JT Jr, Simeone JF. CT- and ultrasound-guided catheter drainage of empyemas after chest-tube failure. Radiology 1984; 151:349–353.
109. Moulton JS, Benkert RE, Weisiger KH, Chambers JA. Treatment of complicated pleural fluid collections with image-guided drainage and intracavitary urokinase. Chest 1995; 108:1252–1259.
110. Shankar S, Gulati M, Kang M, Gupta S, Suri S. Image-guided percutaneous drainage of thoracic empyema: can sonography predict the outcome? Eur Radiol 2000; 10:495–499.

111. Ulmer JL, Choplin RH, Reed JC. Image-guided catheter drainage of the infected pleural space. J Thorac Imaging 1991; 6:65–73.
112. Maier A, Domej W, Anegg U, Woltsche M, Fell B, Pinter H, Smolle-Juttner FM. Computed tomography or ultrasonically guided pigtail catheter drainage in multiloculated pleural empyema: a recommended procedure? Respirology 2000; 5:119–124.
113. Bouros D, Schiza S, Siafakas N. Fibrinolytics in the treatment of parapneumonic effusions. Monaldi Arch Chest Dis 1999; 54:558–563.
114. Bouros D, Schiza S, Patsourakis G, Chalkiadakis G, Panagou P, Siafakas NM. Intrapleural streptokinase versus urokinase in the treatment of complicated parapneumonic effusions. A prospective, double-blind study. Am J Respir Crit Care Med 1997; 155:291–295.
115. Wait MA, Sharma S, Hohn J, Dal Nogare A. A randomized trial of empyema therapy. Chest 1997; 111:1548–1551.
116. Bouros D, Schiza S, Tzanakis N, Chalkiadakis G, Drositis J, Siafakas N. Intrapleural Urokinase versus normal saline in the treatment of complicated parapneumonic effusions and empyema. Am J Respir Crit Care Med 1999; 159:37–42.
117. Tuncozgur B, Ustunsoy H, Sivrikoz MC, Dikensoy 0, Topal M, Sanli M, Elbeyli L. Intrapleural urokinase in the management of parapneumonic empyema: a randomised controlled trial. J Clin Pract 2001; 55:658–660.
118. Bouros D, Schiza S, Siafakas N. Utility of fibrinolytic agents for draining intrapleural infection. Semin Respir Infect 1999; 14:39–47.
119. Alfageme I, Vazquez R. Ventricular fibrillation after intrapleural UK. Intensive Care Med 1997; 23:352.
120. Frye MD, Jarratt M, Sahn SA. Acute hypoxemic respiratory failure following intrapleural thrombolytic therapy for hemothorax. Chest 1994; 105:1595–1596.
121. Berglin F, Ekroth R, Teger-Nilsson A, et al. Intrapleural instillation of streptokinase effects on systemic fibrinolysis. Thorac Cardiovasc Surg 1981; 11:265–268.
122. Godley P1, Bell RC. Major hemorrhage following administration of intrapleural streptokinase. Chest 1984; 86:486–487.
123. Lee HS. How safe is the readministration of streptokinase? Drug Saf 1995; 13:76–80.
124. Bouros D, Antoniou KM, Chalkiadakis G, Drositis J, Petrakis I, Siafakas N. The role of video-assisted thoracoscopic surgery in the treatment of parapneumonic empyema after the failure of fibrinolytics. Surg Endosc 2002; 16:151–154.
125. Cummin AR, Wright NL, Joseph AE. Suction drainage: a new approach to the treatment of empyema. Thorax 1991; 46:259–260.
126. Loddenkemper R. Thoracoscopy—state of the art. Eur Respir J 1998; 11:213–221.
127. Soler M, Wyser C, Bolliger T, Perruchoud AP. Treatment of early parapneumonic empyema by medical thoracoscopy. Schweiz Med Wochenschr 1997; 127:1748–1753.
128. Angelillo Mackinlay TA, Lyons GA, Chimondeguy DJ, Piedras MA, Angaramo G, Emery J. VATS debridement versus thoracotomy in the treatment of loculated postpneumonia empyema. Ann Thorac Surg 1996; 61:1626–1630.
129. Lawrence DR, Ohri SK, Moxon RE, Townsend ER, Fountain SW. Thoracoscopic debridement of empyema thoracis. Ann Thorac Surg 1997; 64:1448–1450.
130. Striffleler H, Gugger M, Im Hof V, Cerny A, Furrer M, Ris HB. Video-assisted

thoracoscopic surgery for fibrinopurulent pleural empyema in 67 patients. Ann Thorac Surg 1998; 65:319–323.
131. Cassina PC, Hauser M, Hillejan L, Greschuchna D, Stamatis G. Video-assisted thoracoscopy in the treatment of pleural empyema: stage-based management and outcome. J Thorac Cardiovasc Surg 1999; 117:234–238.
132. Lackner RP, Hughes R, Anderson LA, Sammut PH, Thompson A. Video-assisted evacuation of empyema is the preferred procedure for the management of pleural space infections. Am J Surg 2000; 179:27–30.
133. Cunniffe MG, Maguire D, McAnena OJ, Johnston S, Gilmartin JJ. Video-assisted thoracoscopic surgery in the management of loculated empyema. Surg Endosc 2000; 14:175–178.
134. Hornick P, Townsend ER, Clark D, Fountain SW. Videothoracoscopy in the treatment of early empyema: an initial experience. ann Royal Coll Surg Eng 1996; 78:45–48.
135. Sendt W, Forster E, Hau T. Early thoracoscopic debridement and drainage as definite treatment for pleural empyema. Eur J Surg 1995; 161:73–623.
136. Waller DA, Rengarajan A. Thoracoscopic decortication: a role for video-assisted surgery in chronic postpneumonic pleural empyema. Ann Thorac Surg 2000; 71:1813–1816.
137. Silen ML, Naunheim KS. Thoracoscopic approach to the management of empyema thoracis. Indications and results. Chest Surg Clin North Am 1996; 6:491–499.
138. Mayo P. Early thoracotomy and decortication for nontuberculous empyema in adults with and without underlying disease. A twenty-five year review. Am Surg 1985; 51:230–236.
139. Muskett A, Burton NA, Karwande SV, Collins MP. Management of refractory empyema with early decortication. Am J Surg 1988; 156:529–532.
140. Mackinlay TAA, Lyons GA, Chimondeguy DJ, Piefreas MAB, Angaramo G, Emery J. VATS debridement versus thoracotomy in the treatment of loculated postpneumonia empyema. Ann Thorac Surg 1996; 61:1626–1630.
141. Chu MW, Dewar LR, Burgess JJ, Busse EG. Empyema thoracis: lack of awareness results in a prolonged clinical course. Can J Surg 2001; 44:284–288.

21

Postsurgical Pleural Infection

JOSEPH A. LoCICERO III

The University of South Alabama
Mobile, Alabama, U.S.A.

I. Postoperative Changes in the Pleura

An operation performed either by the standard open technique or by minimally invasive or thoracoscopic technique disrupts the natural bond between the lung and the pleura. The pleural surface is exposed to the atmosphere, which initiates an inflammatory response that affects its normal functions.

At the site of violation of the pleura, the well-established process of wound healing begins. As in the peritoneum, the ultimate outcome is the formation of adhesions between the pleural wound and any tissue adjacent to it. The usual tissue at the pleural wound is the lung. Reoperation on the same hemithorax will demonstrate adherence of the lung or, in some cases, the diaphragm or pericardial fat to the pleural wound. These adhesions are formed early but are mature within 4–6 weeks of the operation. Such adhesions lead to compartmentalization of the pleural cavity.

Where the air contacts intact pleura, it becomes edematous within 3 hours, showing thickening under the microscope (1). Over the ensuing hours, the pleura appears thickened to as much as 10 times its normal size. Within 2–3 weeks, the pleura shrinks back to normal thickness. By 6 weeks, it is indistinguishable from intact, unviolated pleura.

These changes suggest that, early after an operation, the pleura cannot function normally. Clinically, the pleura exudes excessive fluid that it cannot reabsorb. This process continues for days to weeks following operation as evidenced by the amount of drainage into the chest drainage system. This exudative fluid sometimes becomes trapped and loculated either from the incisional adhesions or secondary to solidification of the proteinaceous material. When infection does not occur, these loculated areas slowly resolve.

II. Residual Space Following Surgical Intervention

A. Etiology

Pleural apposition of tissue against the pleura is the most important principle in the prevention of postoperative infection. "No space, no problem" is the surgeon's mantra. As noted above, spaces may occur secondary to loculation of areas that become isolated from the chest tubes. These spaces may contain only air but often contain pleural fluid exuded by the altered postoperative pleural surface. Spaces that contain air usually are formed when an area of lung with an air leak becomes isolated from the chest tubes placed at the time of the operation. In this scenario, a space develops immediately following the operation. If the space can be eliminated within the first few hours, no problem will develop. The longer a space exists, the higher the chance that the space will become loculated. Usually, if the space persists beyond the third postoperative day, it will become loculated and chronic.

B. Natural History

Few surgeons write about the postoperative space today. One must go back nearly a half century to find thoughtful investigations into the evolution of the persistent pleural space (2–5). These authors describe what is now known as classic postoperative natural compensatory mechanisms. For a pneumonectomy, the body tries to compensate for the space voided by the absence of the lung. The body accomplishes this through four mechanisms. The first mechanism is the movement of the mediastinum toward the operated side. The mediastinum is freely mobile and has low compliance compared to the remaining lung (6). In some cases it can move far enough to compromise venous return to the heart. The second mechanism is the elevation of the hemidiaphragm. On the right this is limited by the liver, which is attached to the undersurface of the dome of the diaphragm. In some cases, surgeons have tried to accentuate this mechanism by crushing the phrenic nerve and/or producing an artificial pneumoperitoneum. The third mechanism is diminution in the size of the interspaces. Without the lung and its natural residual volume of alveolar air, there is unopposed contraction of the intercostal muscles causing the outer contour of the hemithorax to contract in size. These three mechanisms reduce the space to less than the residual volume of the single lung that was removed. However, these mechanisms cannot reduce the space to zero, so the final mechanism is exudation of fluid by the pleura, obliterating the remaining space.

When there is residual lung tissue in the hemithorax, the mechanisms of space elimination are similar but include expansion of the lung. In fact, there can be compensatory overexpansion of the remaining lung tissue (7). Although there is no increase in alveolar units, this mechanism allows the remaining lung to expand beyond its normal elastic recoil. Complete expansion of the lung will often obliterate the residual space. In some cases, the remaining lung is insufficient to fill the entire hemithorax. Sometimes the lung does not expand for the reasons listed above and loculations develop. If a loculated space remains uncontaminated and there is no persistent air leak, the area of loculation will fill with exudative fluid but will resolve over time. A space with a continued air leak will remain with little fluid accumulation.

C. Prevention and Management

The best approach is early elimination of any space and air leak in the operated chest. The only exception is a pneumonectomy. In this case, the prevention of a bronchopleural fistula is most important. The surgeon should attempt to seal any air leaks from the remaining lung. This can be accomplished through stapling, suturing, or application of fibrin or synthetic sealants. In the uncomplicated operation, every effort should be directed toward expansion of any remaining lung tissue. If one ascertains that the lung cannot fill the space, maneuvers should be used to decrease the size of the hemithorax. The pulmonary ligament should be released and the lung freed at the hilus so that it can elevate into the apex, which is the most common site of non-expansion.

If the lung does not expand into the apex, a pleural tent should be considered. This is a maneuver involving release of the pleura from the upper half of the chest, leaving the mediastinal pleura attached. This pedicled patch is folded down over the apex of the lung and sewn onto the lung. This effectively makes the space an extrapleural space that acts like a space that is outside of the chest.

Finally, the chest tubes should be placed strategically to effectively drain any air or fluid that collects in the hemithorax. Usually this is accomplished with one anterior tube placed near the apex or near any air leak from the lung and one posterior tube placed in the most dependent portion of the chest that will drain any accumulating fluid.

When a loculation of air or fluid develops, aggressive management of the chest tubes should be initiated. Tubes should be stripped to keep them patent, and consideration should be given to increasing the suction on the drainage system. If the space is large and does not communicate with the current tubes, consideration should be given to placement of another tube directly into the area. Again, if the space is small and there is no air leak, it should resolve spontaneously.

III. Development of Space Infection

A. Etiology

It is rare for an infection to develop if there is no residual space or continued air leak. Occasionally, following operation for pulmonary or pleural infection, residual infectious agents remain. If the chest tubes are removed too soon before the draining fluid has diminished back to baseline, accumulating fluid may become contaminated with bacteria that could develop into a new infection.

When a loculated space develops in an uninfected patient, it will resolve unless there is a source of continued contamination. The most common problem is contamination from a chest tube that remains in the chest to evacuate a continued air leak. After several days, skin contaminants enter through the chest tube portal and colonize the space. If there is no space, even with a persistent air leak, it is unusual to develop a space infection.

B. Bacteriology

Little is written about the usual bacteria involved in such infections. A study in the early 1980s compared patients receiving penicillin versus no antibiotic for perioperative prophylaxis (8). The prophylactic penicillin regimen had no effect on the incidence of empyema or lower respiratory tract infections. *Staphylococcus aureus* and *Haemophilus influenzae* were identified as the major pathogens in postoperative infections. Penicillin significantly reduced the incidence of *S. aureus* in spite of resistance to penicillin in most isolated strains, while the frequency of *H. influenzae* was similar in the two treatment groups. Colonization with Enterobacteriaceae and *Pseudomonas aeruginosa* was pronounced in the penicillin group.

Another, much later study from Italy looked at more modern antibiotic prophylaxis using and aztreonam (9). In patients undergoing routine lung cancer operations, one group received no antibiotics while the other group received antibiotic prophylaxis for the operation and continued the antibiotics until the drains were removed. In the placebo group, empyema was due to gram-positive bacteria, while in the prophylaxis group, infection was due to gram-negative bacteria.

IV. Management of Postoperative Pleural Infection

A. Postresection (Less Than Pneumonectomy) Space Infection

Postoperative spaces, even those that are infected, have been traditionally treated with a great deal of conservatism. Walter Barker (10), drawing on a lifetime of surgical experience, stated the following in 1996:

> It is emphasized that a decision for or against surgical intervention in the management of residual spaces, irrespective of cause, will not be required for several months after their occurrence in most cases. The stresses associated with the

critical period of disability occasioned by a prolonged air leak, even if not voluminous, may preclude premature surgical intervention. The indications for initial surgical resection and the diseases for which it was required often are sufficiently debilitating to the patient to produce a protracted period of convalescence, necessitating prolonged observation before a decision for aggressive surgical therapy is mandated or indicated. In our experience, these pleural spaces are not a major threat to the health of the patient. In many cases, the concern over them and the fear that more egregious postoperative problems will ensue have resulted in premature and overzealous treatment that may lead to iatrogenic complications. If, instead, they are left alone and followed with judicious observation based on appropriate clinical, physiologic, and radiologic criteria, a more favorable outcome will result. Haste in arriving at a decision to intervene surgically therefore is not warranted.

These principles still endure, albeit with more sophisticated imaging techniques and less invasive interventional options. During the postoperative period, any patient who develops a persistent loculated space should be monitored for symptoms and signs of the development of infection. If the patient shows signs of sepsis, all the usual sources of infection should be checked. If signs point to the operated chest as the septic source, a CT of the chest will help to define the number, size, and location of any areas of loculation. This study can also help to define if the chest tubes are in communication with these collections. Any likely areas that could be a source should be evaluated by thoracentesis, Gram stain, and culture. Depending on location, ultrasound-guided aspiration may be the easiest procedure. For large collections, chest tube drainage is most appropriate. However, it is often simpler to tap the fluid during the CT evaluation. If a collection is suspicious for infection, a CT-guided catheter may be placed. These are especially useful for posterior pockets that are difficult to place a large chest tube into, either because of the paraspinous muscles or because the patient will be uncomfortable with such a sizable drain in the back. These tubes rarely need to be placed on closed suction drainage because these pockets are isolated by the mechanisms described above and the lung does not pull away further from the chest wall. Initiation of appropriate antibiotics should be concomitant with the drainage of the space. Since it is difficult to predict the organism, broad-spectrum antibiotics such as piperacillin/tazobactam or the combination of vancomycin and ceftriaxone should be chosen.

To enhance the drainage of the space, instillation of streptokinase can be beneficial (11). Aliquots of 250,000 units of streptokinase in 100 mL normal saline are instilled into the pleural cavity and the tube clamped for 4 hours and then drained. Suction may be used but often is of little additional benefit. This may be repeated daily for up to 2 weeks. Irrigation of the space with plain saline may be as effective. The drainage tube should be left in place until the drainage decreases and the space contracts. If a bronchopleural fistula is associated with the space, the drainage tube should be left in place until the air leak stops as well.

For larger cavities that are resistant to these techniques, open drainage should be considered. A local rib resection to open the cavity will allow an adequate opening to irrigate and pack the space. In a soft tissue abscess, incision and drainage allows the cavity to collapse. In the chest, the rigid chest wall does not allow the cavity to collapse. Opening of the cavity permits these large cavities to heal quicker. If there is a catheter in the space, the surgeon can follow the catheter into the space resection at the rib just above or below the drainage tube. If there is no catheter in the space, ultrasound works well to mark the space. This can be accomplished in the Radiology suite or in the operating room at the time of open drainage.

Two types of open drainage are utilized today. They differ in the type of skin incision employed. In the Eloesser procedure, the surgeon makes a "U" incision. After rib removal, the flap is sewn into the upper end of the cavity. In the modified Shede thoracoplasty, the surgeon makes a linear incision, removing sections of two ribs. All edges of the skin are sewn into the cavity to cover the ends of the ribs and completely marsupialize the cavity. In both, the cavity is irrigated and packed daily, permitting inside-out healing.

B. Postpneumonectomy Space Infection

Postpneumonectomy space infections are almost always associated with a bronchopleural fistula. Drainage is of utmost importance to prevent contamination of the contralateral lung. Initial drainage is best accomplished with a tube thoracostomy. The next step is bronchoscopy to assess the bronchial stump. If one exists, it must be closed before definitive management of the space infection can be accomplished. Methods of bronchial stump closure are beyond the scope of this treatise.

The space must be clean in order to establish closure. A new approach is to explore and debride the hemithorax with the thoracoscope (12). This has been successful in initial management of the space. Eventually, the space must be obliterated. The time-honored Clagett procedure involves making the cavity as clean as possible and then filling the space with an antibiotic solution and closing all openings in the chest wall. This technique has, at best, a 50% success rate unless combined with a muscle flap to manage the bronchopleural fistula (13).

For large spaces or those that fail more conservative therapies, autogenous material transferred into the cavity has become the standard. Omentum works well, especially on the left side (14). The latissimus dorsi, pectoralis, and the serratus anterior muscles work equally well to close the space (15,16).

References

1. LoCicero J, Frederiksen JW, Hartz RS, Michaelis LL. Pulmonary procedures assisted by optosurgical and electrosurgical devices: comparison of damage potential. Lasers Surg Med 1987; 7:263–272.
2. Wareham EE, Barber H, McGoey JS. The persistent pleural spaces following partial pulmonary resection. J Thorac Surg 1956; 31:593–599.
3. Bell JW. Management of the postresection space in tuberculosis. Role of pre and postresection thoracoplasty. J Thorac Surg 1956; 32:580–585.

4. Silver AW, Espinos EE, Byron FW. The fate of postresection spaces. Ann Thorac Surg 1966; 2:311–316.
5. Barker WL, Langston HT, Noffah P. Postresectional thoracic spaces. Ann Thorac Surg 1966; 2:229–310.
6. Van de Woestijne KP, Trop D, Clement J. Influence of the mediastinum on the measurement of esophageal pressure and lung compliance in man. Pflugers Arch 1971; 323:323–241.
7. Arnup ME, Greville HW, Oppenheimer L, Mink SN, Anthonisen NR. Dynamic lung function in dogs with compensatory lung growth. J Appl Physiol 1984; 57:1569–1576.
8. Frimodt-Moller N, Ostri P, Pedersen IK, Poulsen SR. Antibiotic prophylaxis in pulmonary surgery: a double-blind study of penicillin versus placebo. Ann Surg 1982; 195:444–450.
9. Ratto GB, Fantino G, Tassara E, Angelini M, Spessa E, Parodi A. Long-term antimicrobial prophylaxis in lung cancer surgery: correlation between microbiological findings and empyema development. Lung Cancer 1994; 11:345–352.
10. Barker WL. Natural history of residual air spaces after pulmonary resection. Chest Surg Clin North Am 1996, 530–613.
11. Taylor RF, Rubens MB, Pearson MC, Barnes NC. Intrapleural streptokinase in the management of empyema. Thorax 1994; 49:856–859.
12. Podbielski FJ, Halldorsson AO, Vigneswaran WT. Video-assisted thoracoscopic management of post-pneumonectomy empyema. JSLS 1997; 1:255–258.
13. Deschamps C, Allen MS, Miller DL, Nichols FC III, Pairolero PC. Management of postpneumonectomy empyema and bronchopleural fistula. Semin Thorac Cardiovasc Surg 2001; 13(1):3–19.
14. Levashev YN, Akopov AL, Mosin IV. The possibilities of greater omentum usage in thoracic surgery. Eur J Cardiothorac Surg 1999; 15:465–468.
15. Widmer MK, Krueger T, Lardinois D, Banic A, Ris HB. A comparative evaluation of intrathoracic latissimus dorsi and serratus anterior muscle transposition. Eur J Cardiothorac Surg 2000; 18(4):435–439.
16. Nomori H, Horio H, Hasegawa T, Suemasu K. Intrathoracic transposition of a pectoralis major and pectoralis minor muscle flap for empyema in patients previously subjected to posterolateral thoracotomy. Surg Today 2001; 31(4):295–299.

22

Surgical Management of Empyema

DEAN M. DONAHUE and DOUGLAS J. MATHISEN

Harvard Medical School
and Massachusetts General Hospital
Boston, Massachusetts, U.S.A.

I. Introduction

Empyema thoracis occurs when bacteria enter the sterile pleural space and overwhelm the normal pleural defense mechanisms. The most common mode of entry for these bacteria is transpleural migration following pneumonia. Bacteria may also enter the pleural space following a thoracic surgical procedure or after the development of a bronchopleural fistula. Empyema can result from extension of a subphrenic abscess or through esophageal rupture. Identifying and correcting the etiology of the empyema is critical to successful treatment.

The management of empyema is based on the surgical principle that *pus needs to be drained and empty space needs to be obliterated*. Treatment must begin immediately by adequately draining the pleural space. Depending upon the patient's presentation, this can be done through thoracentesis, closed tube drainage, or by opening the pleural space surgically. Once drainage is established, two issues must be addressed. First is the presence or absence of a bronchopleural fistula (BPF), and second is the existence of a residual pleural space. A BPF can occur peripherally from a necrotizing pneumonia, or centrally with the dehiscence of a post-resection bronchial closure. Either type may heal spontaneously following drainage and debridement of the pleural space, but more commonly a well-timed operative repair is required. Any residual pleural space after drainage must be addressed. One option for obliterating the space is filling it with viable tissue, such as the underlying lung following decortication, or with a transposed flap of muscle or omentum. Alternatively, collapsing the chest wall with a thoracoplasty can eliminate this space.

II. Empyema Without BPF

A. Etiology

Pneumonia with parapneumonic effusion remains the most common etiology for empyema. In the pre-antibiotic era approximately 10% of patients with pneumonia developed empyema with *Streptococcus pneumoniae* being the predominant organism in two thirds of all cases (1). With the advent of antibiotics, Staphylococcus species became more prevalent. More recently, penicillin-resistant Staphylococcus, Gram-negative bacteria, and anaerobic organisms are increasing in incidence (2).

The second most common etiology for empyema is infection following a thoracic surgical procedure. This most frequently occurs after pneumonectomy and is associated with a BPF from dehiscence of the bronchial closure in up to 80% of cases. However, it can occur following any thoracic surgical procedure with or without a pulmonary resection. Empyema following pulmonary resection is more complex because it is frequently associated with a BPF, and the residual space resulting from the resection will need to be addressed. Empyema may also occur following esophageal injury or anastamotic leak. Bacterial migration across the diaphragm can result in empyema from intraperitoneal infections.

B. Pathophysiology of Parapneumonic Effusion

To determine both the timing and the extent of surgical intervention for parapneumonic pleural space infections, a thorough understanding of its pathophysiology is necessary. A pleural space infection due to pneumonia is a continuum of three stages: exudative (Stage I), fibrinopurulent (Stage II), and organizing (Stage III). The stage at presentation correlates with the length of time between the onset of the pneumonia and the initiation of antibiotic therapy.

The first stage begins as an exudative effusion. The infected lung parenchyma will develop a vascular endothelial injury mediated by migrating neutrophils. This vascular injury results in fluid leaking into the pleural space that is initially sterile. With progressive injury pleural fluid production exceeds the lymphatic drainage capacity, particularly when deposited fibrin obstructs the pleural lymphatic channels. The fluid is initially free flowing and turbid with a pH >7.30, a glucose >60 and LDH <500 IU/l. These early parapneumonic effusions occur to some degree in up to 50–60 percent of cases; however, most resolve with early initiation of appropriate antibiotic therapy.

If the pneumonia remains untreated, bacteria will enter the pleural space and the empyema progresses to the fibrinopurulent stage. Additional fibrin is deposited to act as scaffolding for white blood cell (WBC) migration. These WBC's utilize glucose and produce lactate and carbon dioxide, resulting in a low glucose and pH in the pleural fluid. A high LDH results from cell death and lysis. Clinically this second stage is characterized by purulent fluid with progressive loculations.

Unchecked, this progresses on to the sequelae of chronic inflammation with collagen deposition and organization. This organizing stage of an empyema results in an inelastic "peel" of collagen encasing the lung and chest wall, thus preventing their expansion. An empyema will rarely spontaneously resolve. If untreated it will drain out of the chest wall (empyema necessitatis) or into the lung, creating a BPF.

C. Diagnosis

Empyema in the absence of BPF typically presents as an extension of the symptoms of the underlying pneumonia. Patients most commonly present with symptoms of dyspnea, fever, cough, and chest pain (3). The duration of symptoms prior to initiating antibiotic treatment will correlate with the degree of pleural space contamination and severity of the symptoms. Bacterial invasion typically occurs several days after the formation of a pleural exudate.

A thoracentesis draining as much of the pleural fluid as possible is the initial step in evaluation and treatment. Pleural fluid characteristics, as outlined in the preceding section, will stage the empyema and help in the initial decision on the need for chest tube drainage (Table 1).

D. Treatment of Empyema Without BPF

Understanding the stages of empyema formation helps guide surgical therapy. Following thoracentesis, an early exudative stage with a small residual effusion can be observed if effective antibiotic treatment is followed by immediate clinical improvement with resolution of the effusion and expansion of the lung. The dilemma facing the clinician in the exudative phase is whether antibiotics alone are appropriate, or should the pleural space be drained with a chest tube. There are several clinical, radiographic and pleural fluid features that suggest the need for pleural space drainage (Table 1). Early tube drainage is indicated for an effusion in a patient with pneumonia caused by a virulent organism such as an anaerobic organism or group A β-hemolytic streptococcus. Evidence of loculations on radiographic studies such as pleural thickening or enhancement, or debris in the pleural space is an indication for tube placement. Patients who fail to improve clinically soon after the initiation of appropriate antibiotic therapy should undergo tube drainage.

Table 1 Indicators for Tube Drainage of Parapneumonic Effusion

Clinical
  1. Duration of pneumonia symptoms prior to initiation of antibiotic therapy
  2. Lack of clinical improvement with proper antibiotic
  3. Pneumonia due to virulent pathogen
Radiographic
  1. Chest x-ray
    a. Size of effusion
    b. Presence of air-fluid level
  2. Computerized tomography
    a. Presence of loculations
    b. Pleural thickening or enhancement on contrast scans
  3. Ultrasonography
    a. Presence of loculations or debris
Pleural fluid
  1. WBC >25,000 cells/mL
  2. Organisms seen on Gram stain or a positive culture
  3. pH <7.30
  4. Glucose <50% serum level
  5. LDH >1000 IU/L

Chest tube drainage often suffices in treating the exudative or early fibrinopurulent stage of parapneumonic effusion and empyema. This is because the low-viscosity fluid is easily drained and the lung is able to expand and fill the pleural space. In patients who present later in the course, the fibrinopurulent debris may not be able to be drained through a closed tube system. The options that exist in this scenario include instillation of a fibrinolytic agent through the chest tube, video-assisted thoracoscopy (VATS) for debridement, or open drainage with rib resection.

A minimally invasive approach with VATS is particularly helpful in the fibrinopurulent or early organizing stage when tube placement has failed to expand the lung. Two or three 1–2 centimeter incisions are required for this procedure. This has the advantage of allowing a complete inspection of the pleural space with debridement and disruption of loculated collections. An early non-fibrous peel can be decorticated allowing re-expansion of the lung. Several series of VATS management of parapneumonic empyema have been reported (4,5). The likelihood of success depends upon the stage of empyema at operation. Recently, Cassina and associates reported a prospective series of 45 patients with nontuberculous empyema who had failed initial management with chest tube drainage plus fibrinolytic therapy and antibiotics (6). None of the patients had undergone prior thoracotomy or pulmonary resection. Persistent fever and chest pain was present in 60 percent of patients, and 47 percent continued to have bacteria in the empyema fluid in spite of antibiotics. All patients underwent VATS debridement, which successfully treated the empyema in 82 percent of patients. In the remaining 8 patients (18%) the underlying lung did not re-expand. This necessitated a thoracotomy and decortication in 7 patients. Two of these patients required lung resection because of destroyed parenchyma with peripheral bronchopleural fistula. One patient was managed with open thoracostomy. Full re-expansion of the lung, which is critical to the success of the VATS approach needs to be confirmed with the thoracoscope at the end of the procedure.

An alternative to a VATS approach is to convert a closed tube thoracostomy to open drainage. This involves resecting a short segment of rib, leaving the wound open around a large bore tube for both drainage and irrigation. However, if this is done too early in the course of empyema formation, an open pneumothorax will be created. To ensure that the lung will not collapse with open drainage, the patient's chest tube is disconnected from the drainage system and left open to air. If the patient's clinical condition and chest x-ray is unchanged, then open drainage can be performed. An extension of this procedure is an open thoracostomy using the techniques first described by Eloesser (7), and later modified by Symbas and associates (8). This "Eloesser flap" typically involves resecting a 4–6 cm. segment of two ribs near a dependent portion of the empyema cavity. The skin is then sutured to the parietal pleura, creating a window for irrigation or gauze dressing changes.

Following drainage of the pleural space, if the lung does not expand to fill the cavity, the surgeon can either attempt lytic therapy or proceed to a thoracotomy for a decortication. A full discussion on the role of fibrinolytic therapy is beyond the scope of this chapter, but it is more successful when used in the earlier stages (9,10). In the later stage of empyema formation, collagen is deposited and organizes into a fibrothorax. This inhibits both lung and chest wall expansion resulting in restrictive physiology (11). Decortication of the lung involves removing the constricting layer from the parietal and visceral pleural surfaces, allowing the lung and chest wall to re-expand. The ease of freeing the entrapped lung depends upon the extent of fibrosis that has occurred over time. Preventing the development of fibrothorax is the basis for early and aggressive intervention in the management of pleural space infection. Before a decortication is performed, the quality of the underlying lung must be assessed. If the lung is densely consolidated, it may not expand. This will create the undesirable situation of a persistent pleural space with parenchymal air leaks.

The technique of decortication involves peeling the constricting rind off of the lung, chest wall, and diaphragm. This can be attempted with a VATS approach in the fibroproliferative or early organizing phase. With organized fibrosis, a posterolateral thoracotomy is usually required. An anesthetic technique allowing single lung ventilation should be used; however, stripping the peel from the surface of the lung is frequently aided by intermittent positive pressure ventilation of the underlying lung. This helps delineate the fibrous peel from the lung tissue. Once the lung is fully expanded, the pleural space is drained with two or three chest tubes. If the underlying lung does not fill the remaining pleural space, further techniques are needed to fill the pleural space and to prevent recurrence. These techniques will be discussed later in this chapter.

III. Empyema with BPF

A. Etiology

The development of a communication between the bronchial tree and the pleural space provides access for bacteria to enter and develop an empyema. BPF can occur with the dehiscence of a bronchial closure following pulmonary resection. It can also develop from lung parenchyma following either necrotizing pneumonia or a spontaneous pneumothorax with a prolonged air leak.

Understanding and identifying the risk factors for postoperative bronchial dehiscence (Table 2) prior to resection allows for adjustment of operative strategy to prevent this complication. The most significant predictor for BPF in our own series of 256 consecutive pneumonectomy patients was the need for postoperative mechanical ventilation (12). The presence of residual infection within the pleural space such as a patient with preoperative suppurative lung or pleural disease increases the risk of a postoperative empyema. All attempts should be made to control the infection preoperatively with adequate antibiotic therapy or drainage.

Several factors related to the technical aspects of the surgical resection can increase the risk of bronchial dehiscence. Patients undergoing a right pneumonectomy have been found to have a higher risk, as have patients with prior

Table 2 Risk Factors for Postpneumonectomy Bronchopleural Fistula and Empyema

Preexisting suppurative lung or pleural disease
    Postobstructive pneumonia
    Bronchiectasis
    Empyema
Systemic factors
    Age >70 years
    Corticosteroid therapy
    Malnutrition
Associated treatment
    Radiation therapy
    Postoperative mechanical ventilation
Operative considerations
    Completion pneumonectomy
    Right pneumonectomy
    Mediastinal lymph node dissection
    Carcinoma at bronchial margin
    Bronchial devascularization

lung surgery that requires a completion pneumonectomy. Patients undergoing a mediastinal lymph node dissection or procedures that disrupt the bronchial blood supply are also at greater risk. The presence of carcinoma at the bronchial resection margin increases the possibility of fistula formation. Other groups at risk include patients with preoperative radiation therapy or systemic conditions such as malnutrition or corticosteroid therapy.

B. Clinical Presentation

Empyema from a peripheral BPF presents with the typical signs of empyema such as fever, dyspnea, cough, and chest pain. In addition there will be radiographic evidence of an intrapleural air-fluid level.

Fistula formation from bronchial closure dehiscence following pneumonectomy occurs within the first week after surgery in one half of cases. During this time a fistula is identified clinically by the production of thin watery sputum, or by a fall in the pleural cavity fluid level seen on an upright chest radiograph. The fistula causes varying degrees of respiratory distress depending upon the extent that the pleural fluid contaminates the remaining lung.

Delayed fistula formation and empyema has a more insidious presentation with chest pain, dyspnea, fatigue, cough, and weight loss. These symptoms can occur following any major thoracic surgical procedure, but they will worsen rather than improve in a patient with a BPF. Diagnosis is facilitated by having a high index of suspicion, particularly in patients with risk factors for the development of a bronchopleural fistula and empyema (Table 2).

C. Initial Management

The potentially life-threatening nature of postpneumonectomy BPF requires immediate diagnostic and therapeutic maneuvers. Routine chest radiography is mandatory to evaluate the fluid level within the pneumonectomy space as well as the condition of the remaining lung. In the absence of a bronchopleural fistula, a postpneumonectomy empyema may have an unremarkable chest radiograph. The clinical suspicion of a postpneumonectomy empyema or BPF mandates an immediate bronchoscopy to evaluate the bronchial closure. If the diagnosis remains uncertain, a CT scan of the chest should be performed. This may localize areas within the pleural space to guide a diagnostic thoracentesis. In rare cases a ventilation scan with xenon 133 can be obtained to look for ventilation into the empty pleural cavity.

In a patient with obvious clinical or radiographic features of BPF, immediate therapy is indicated to protect the remaining lung from contamination. The patient is positioned with the pneumonectomy space in a dependent position to minimize the amount of pleural fluid draining into the contralateral lung. A tube thoracostomy is performed above the level of the thoracotomy incision as the hemidiaphragm frequently rises to this level postoperatively. Immediate tube drainage is also the appropriate initial measure in BPF following pulmonary resection other than a pneumonectomy.

D. Closure of BPF

Successful management of a BPF depends upon the correct timing and technique of closure. The optimal time to close a BPF can be a difficult decision. It is determined by the presence of pleural space contamination and the patients overall condition including the existence of risk factors for BPF that may be corrected prior to repair.

Repair should be considered in an early postoperative fistula that is identified immediately after it develops. This requires a pleural space free from contamination and a patient that was clinically well. Our group has reported successfully resuturing the bronchus and tissue flap coverage up to one month after pneumonectomy (12). Each of these cases was closed without recurrence or empyema formation. Critical to the success of a fistula closure is further resection of the anterior bronchial wall. This allows the membranous wall flap to be sutured to the anterior wall without tension. Equally as important is a completely clean pleural cavity with no sign of any purulence.

Immediate closure of a postoperative fistula should be avoided if there is any pleural space contamination. It should also be avoided if the patient is at high risk for recurrence of the BPF if that risk factor can be corrected. In these instances an urgently placed tube thoracostomy is frequently present. This is converted to an open thoracostomy with an Eloesser flap (8). Gauze dressings are then applied and changed once or twice daily depending upon the degree of pleural contamination. This will debride the pleural space and allow for the formation of granulation tissue. This large wound creates a metabolic demand on the patient, and their nutritional status needs to be optimized and closely followed. Systemic antibiotic therapy is a critical component in the control of the initial sepsis. Once the pleural space begins to clear with dressing changes, the antibiotics can be discontinued.

By controlling the pleural sepsis, a small BPF may heal by secondary intention in up to one third of cases (13). When this fails to occur, direct operative repair is required. Repair should only be considered when the pleural space is clean and lined with healthy granulation tissue.

Operative repair is typically approached through the initial thoracotomy incision. The bronchial stump is identified in the mediastinum and debrided back to viable tissue. A tension-free closure is accomplished by resecting a segment of anterior cartilaginous wall as previously described. It is our preference (12) as well as that of other groups (14–17) to reinforce the BPF closure with tissue flap transfer techniques detailed in the following section. This technique results in successful closure in at least 75% of cases.

IV. Management of the Pleural Space

Definitive management of the pleural space in an empyema depends upon the presence or absence of a BPF. Regardless of the existence of a fistula, if there is a residual pleural space it will need to be obliterated. The options available are filling the space with either an antibiotic solution or with viable tissue, or collapsing it with thoracoplasty. A combination of these procedures may be required.

Once the pleural space contamination is cleared with drainage and irrigation or dressing changes, some small, early fistulae may spontaneously close. In the absence of a BPF, or following fistula closure, the technique described by Clagett and colleagues may be used to treat the residual pleural space (18). This involves filling the pleural space with an antibiotic solution and closing the soft tissue over the thoracostomy in a watertight fashion. The choice of antibiotic is adjusted to the cultured flora of the pleural space. Successful treatment was reported by Stafford and Clagett in up to 88 percent of cases (19). If a recurrent empyema develops, it is likely due to residual pleural space infection or an unsuspected BPF. This can be treated by re-establishing drainage followed by pleural irrigation or dressing changes. The identical procedure can be repeated with a similar success rate to the initial attempt. This technique has a low morbidity and is a reasonable choice in the initial attempt to close a clean pleural space.

Transposing healthy tissue into the pleural space is also an important component to both re-enforcing the closure of a BPF and filling space. A variety of muscle flaps exist with varying bulk and axis of rotation (Table 3). These can be selected based on the need to fill a specific area in the hemithorax. The flaps can be brought into the pleural space through the primary chest incision, but more frequently require a separate rib resection to create a window of entry. This window needs to be placed properly to minimize tension and kinking of the vascular pedicle, which would compromise the viability of the tissue flap.

The latissimus dorsi is an excellent muscle flap because of its proximity and size. It is our preferred muscle flap for intrathoracic procedures; however, it is frequently divided in patients who have had a prior thoracotomy. If this muscle is intact, it is harvested by raising tissue flaps over the muscle exposing its entire surface. Electrocautery is then used to divide the distal origin. If additional length is needed, the tendinous insertion to the humerus is divided,

Table 3 Tissue Flaps Commonly Used for Filling the Pleural Space

Tissue	Arterial supply
Muscle	
Latissimus dorsi	Thoracodorsal
Serratus anterior	Lateral thoracic
Pectoralis major	Thoracoacromial
Rectus abdominus	Superior epigastric
Omentum	Right gastroepiploic

avoiding the adjacent thoracodorsal artery. This muscle is brought into the chest by resecting a segment of the second or third rib. The serratus anterior muscle also has the advantage of proximity, and is useful in the upper half of the hemithorax. This is mobilized by raising it off of its origin along the chest wall. Some of the insertion to the scapula may need to be divided to increase the mobility of the flap.

Other tissue available includes the pectoralis major muscle. It is large and is particularly useful for upper anterior cavities. The rectus abdominis may be used for lower thoracic spaces, but a modified transverse rectus abdominis myocutaneous (TRAM) flap with a deepithelialized pedicle has been used successfully up to the apex of the chest (17).

The omentum is an excellent treatment option, particularly in cases associated with a BPF. The pliable omentum will conform to the mediastinal contour and has the angiogenic property ideal for covering a fistula repair (20). We find it particularly useful in patients with prior high-dose radiation therapy (21). The omentum is first mobilized off of the transverse colon. The gastroepiploic branches along the greater curvature are divided as the omentum is removed from the stomach. The flap is based on the right gastroepiploic artery and brought into the hemithorax substernally or through a small opening created in the peripheral hemidiaphragm.

An alternative means of obliterating the pleural space is the technique of thoracoplasty. This involves a series of subperiosteal rib resections allowing the soft tissues of the chest wall to collapse into the pleural space (22). The extent of thoracoplasty varies with the size of the cavity that needs to be ablated. It can be used alone, or in conjunction with tissue transposition. This procedure can be applied to the treatment of any pleural space problem including cavitary or drug resistant tuberculosis, but in order to preserve chest wall integrity our first preference is to fill the pleural space with muscle or omentum.

V. Conclusion

The two most common etiologies for empyema are parapneumonic and postoperative. Therapy can be distilled down to two principles: complete drainage of the pleural cavity and obliteration of any residual pleural space. The management of a parapneumonic effusion depends upon many factors—most importantly the duration of symptoms prior to antibiotic therapy. A diagnostic thoracentesis is strongly encouraged, and we would favor an aggressive approach to drainage. A residual pleural space following drainage can be treated with lytic therapy early in the patient's course. Failure to improve clinically, persistent loculations, or incomplete lung reexpansion is an indication for decortication. This can be attempted with a minimally invasive VATS, but if unsuccessful, a thoracotomy is mandated.

In cases of empyema where there is insufficient lung tissue present to fill the pleural space, treatment begins with open drainage to clear the pleural space infection. If present, a reinforced closure of a BPF is performed. The timing of this repair is critical. It depends upon adequately clearing the pleural space contamination and correcting any underlying causative factors. Any residual pleural space can then be closed with a Claggett procedure, filled with tissue flap transfer, or obliterated with a thoracoplasty.

References

1. Ehler AA. Non-tuberculous thoracic empyema: a collective review of the literature from 1934 to 1939. Int Abstr Surg 1941; 72:17.
2. Brook I, Frazier EH. Aerobic and anaerobic microbiology of empyema. A retrospective review in two military hospitals. Chest 1993; 103:1502.
3. Varkey B, Rose HD, Kutty CP, Politis J. Empyema thoracis during a ten-year period. Analysis of 72 cases and comparison to a previous study (1952 to 1967). Arch Intern Med 1981; 141:1771.
4. Angelillo Mackinlay T, Lyons G, Chimondeguy D, Piedras MA, Angaramo G, Emery J. VATS Debridement versus thoracotomy in the treatment of loculated postpneumonia empyema. Ann Thorac Surg 1996; 61:1626–1630.
5. Weissberg D, Refaely Y. Pleural empyema: 24-year experience. Ann Thorac Surg 1991; 62:1026–1029.
6. Cassina P, Hauser M, Hillejan L, Greschuchna D, Stamatis G. Video-assisted thoracoscopy in the treatment of pleural empyema: stage-based management and outcome. J Thorac Cardiovasc Surg 1999; 117:234–238.
7. Eloesser L. An operation for tuberculous empyema. Surg Gynecol Obstet 1935; 60:1096.
8. Symbas PN, Nugent JT, Abbott OA, Logan WD Jr, Hatcher CR Jr. Non-tuberculous pleural empyema in adults. The role of a modified Eloesser procedure in its management. Ann Thorac Surg 1971; 12:69–78.
9. Jerejes-Sanches C, Ramirez-Rivera A, Elizalde JJ, Delgado R, Cicero R, Ibarra-Perez C, Arroliga AC, Padua A, Portales A, Villareal A, Perez-Romo A. Intapleural fibrinolysis with streptokinase as an adjunctive treatment in hemothorax and empyema: a multicenter trial. Chest 1996; 109:1514–1519.
10. Chin NK, Lim TK. Controlled trial of intrapleural streptokinase in the treatment of pleural empyema and complicated parapneumonic effusions. Chest 1997; 111: 275–279.
11. Liu CT, Cellerino A, Baldi S, Huang NQ, Tian YL, Rapellino M, Oliaro, Scappaticci E, Obert R, Coni F, et al. Pulmonary function in patients with pleural effusion of varying magnitude and fibrothorax. Panminerva Med 1991; 33:86–92.
12. Wright C, Wain J, Mathisen D, Grillo H. Postpneumonectomy bronchopleural fistula after sutured bronchial closure: incidence, risk factors, and management. J Thorac Cardiovasc Surg 1996; 112:1367–1371.
13. Wain JC. Management of late postpneumonectomy empyema and bronchopleural fistula. Chest 1996; 6:529–541.
14. Miller JI, Mansour KA, Nahai F, Jurkiewicz MJ, Hatcher CR Jr. Single-stage complete muscle flap closure of the post pneumonectomy empyema space. A new method and possible solution to a disturbing complication. Ann Thorac Surg 1984; 38:227.

15. Regnard J, Alifano M, Puyo P, Fares E, Magdeleinat P, Levasseur P. Open window thoracostomy followed by intrathoracic flap transposition in the treatment of empyema complicating pulmonary resection. J Thorac Cardiovasc Surg 2000; 120: 270–275.
16. Francel T, Lee G, Mackinnon S, Patterson G. Treatment of long-standing thoracostoma and bronchopleural fistula without pulmonary resection in high risk patients. Plastic Reconstruct Surg 1997; 99:1046–1053.
17. Serletti J, Feins R, Carras A, Losee JE, Kpjmstpme DW, Herrera H, Hicks GL Jr. Obliteration of empyema tract with de-epithelialized unipedicle transverse rectus abdominis myocutaneous flap. J Thorac Cardiovasc Surg 1996; 112:631–636.
18. Clagett OT, Geraci JE. A procedure for the management of post pneumonectomy empyema. J Thorac Cardiovasc Surg 1963; 45:141.
19. Stafford EG, Clagett OT. Postpneumonectomy empyema: neomycin instillation and definitive closure. J Thorac Cardiovasc Surg 1972; 63:771.
20. Goldsmith H, Griffith A, Kupferman A, Catsimpoolas N. Lipid angiogenic factor from omentum. JAMA 1984; 252:2034.
21. Mathisen DJ, Grillo HC, Vlahakes G, Daggett W. The omentum in the management of complicated cardiothoracic problems. J Thorac Cardiovasc Surg 1988; 95:677–684.
22. Barker WL. Thoracoplasty. Chest Surg Clin North Am 1994; 4:593.

23

Malignant Pleural Effusions

STEVEN A. SAHN

Medical University of South Carolina
Charleston, South Carolina, U.S.A.

I. Introduction

Malignant pleural effusions (MPE) are a common consequence of malignancy and result in substantial morbidity for those inflicted. With the virtual epidemic of lung cancer and breast cancer, both in the United States and worldwide, clinicians will face the challenge of managing patients with malignant pleural effusions, as the aforementioned cancers are the most common cause of these effusions. For example, in the United States there are approximately 160,000 deaths due to lung cancer and 44,000 deaths due to breast cancer annually (1). Based on the reported incidence of malignant pleural effusions in lung cancer (8–15%) and breast cancer (2–12%), clinicians in the United States can expect to care for approximately 75,000 patients a year with malignant pleural effusions due to lung cancer and 30,000 patients annually with breast cancer (1). With the estimated incidence of malignant pleural effusion in lymphoma of 7% and the contribution from nonlung primaries, more than 150,000 cases of malignant pleural effusions are diagnosed in the United States annually (1).

The primary goal of palliation in these patients is relief of breathlessness. Decisions relating to palliation should be determined only after global evaluation of the patient and should not be based on a single factor. In this chapter, I will discuss the pathogenesis, clinical manifestations, radiographic features, diagnostic techniques, prognosis, and management of patients with malignant pleural effusions.

II. Pathogenesis of Metastasis and Effusions

Autopsy studies report several mechanisms for pleural metastases, including pulmonary vascular invasion with tumor emboli to the visceral pleural surface (the major mechanism in lung cancer) with subsequent seeding of the parietal pleura, direct tumor invasion (lung and breast cancer), hematogenous metastases to the parietal pleura from extrapulmonary primaries, and lymphatic involvement (2–5).

The mechanisms of pleural metastasis have not been clearly defined. However, it is clear that for tumor to metastasize to a distant site, such as the pleura, a succession of events needs to occur. If these sequential processes ensue, the pleura will be seeded by tumor cells and independent growth of the tumor will occur. These processes—adhesion, migration, propagation, and angiogenesis—appear to be mediated by the interaction of mesothelial and neoplastic cells (6,7). Initially, the primary malignant cell must detach from the core tumor. Second, the malignant cell must adhere to and penetrate through the wall of the blood vessel. Third, migration must occur from the vasculature to the pleural surface. Lastly, for the potentiation of local growth and spread of the tumor, autocrine growth factors need to be operative and angiogenesis needs to be induced. Several systems may influence the remodeling with the stroma of neoplasms and growth of the tumor in the pleural space. Both the procoagulant and fibrinolytic systems (8,9) and the urokinase—urokinase receptor systems have been linked to the invasiveness of malignant mesothelioma cells and may be operative in other malignancies (10,11).

Tumors may produce specific growth, permeability, and adhesion—related factors. Vascular endothelial growth factor (VEGF), an important angiogenic factor, results in both new vessel formation and an alteration of mesothelial permeability (12). In addition, interleukin-8 (IL-8) functions as a growth factor for both malignant melanoma and mesothelial cells (13). The present evidence suggests that an interaction between the malignant cell, the mesothelial cell, and their extracellular matrix prevents the host from controlling the malignant cells and the independent growth and function of these cells on the pleura.

Malignant pleural effusions (malignant cells identified in pleural fluid or pleural tissue) are probably formed by several mechanisms, including increased capillary permeability, impaired lymphatic drainage from the pleural space, thoracic duct rupture, and pericardial involvement.

At times a patient has a known malignancy and a pleural effusion that does not demonstrate malignant cells in pleural fluid or pleural tissue; these effusions are termed "paramalignant" and are not the direct result of pleural involvement

Table 1 Paramalignant Pleural Effusions

Cause	Comments
Local effects of tumor	
Lymphatic obstruction	Important mechanism for pleural fluid accumulation
Bronchial obstruction with pneumonia	Parapneumonic effusion; does not exclude operability in lung cancer
Bronchial obstruction with atelectasis	Transudate; does not exclude operability in lung cancer
Trapped lung	Exudate; due to extensive tumor/fibrosis of visceral pleura with capillary link
Chylothorax	Disruption of thoracic duct; non-Hodgkin's lymphoma most common cause
Superior vena cava syndrome	Transudate; due to increased systemic venous pressure
Malignant pericardial effusion	Transudative effusion due to increased pulmonary and systemic venous pressures
Systemic effects of tumor	
Pulmonary embolism	Hypercoagulable state; adenocarcinoma
Hypoalbuminemia	Serum albumin < 1.5 g/dL; associated with anasarca
Complications of therapy	
Radiation therapy	
Early	Pleuritis 6 weeks to 6 months after radiation completed; loculated exudative effusion
Late	Fibrosis of mediastinum Constrictive pericarditis Vena caval obstruction
Chemotherapy	
Methotrexate	Pleuritis or effusion; ± blood eosinophilia
Procarbazine	Blood eosinophilia; fever and chills
Cyclophosphamide	Pleuropericarditis
Mitomycin/bleomycin	Associated with interstitial disease

Source: Adapted from Ref. 14.

with tumor but related to the primary tumor (14) (Table 1). Examples of paramalignant effusions include endobronchial obstruction with pneumonia and parapneumonic effusion or a transudative effusion from atelectasis, a transudative effusion from low oncotic pressure from severe malnutrition, and chylothorax from thoracic duct obstruction. Radiation and chemotherapy can also be causative. At times, a pleural effusion may develop that is unrelated to the malignancy, such as from congestive heart failure. Therefore, it is important to establish the cause of the effusion; as it will relate to prognosis (see below).

III. Clinical Features

Breathlessness is the most common presenting symptom in patients with malignant pleural effusions, occurring in more than half of the patients (4). Because malignant pleural effusions represent an advanced stage of the malignancy, patients may also have systemic manifestations, such as malaise, anorexia, and weight loss (4) (Table 2). The pathogenesis of dyspnea from a large pleural effusion has not been clearly defined, but it appears that several factors may be operative, including decreased chest wall compliance, contralateral mediastinal shift, decreased ipsilateral lung volume, and reflex stimulation from the chest wall and lung parenchyma (15).

While dull, aching chest pain is common in malignant mesothelioma (16), it is relatively uncommon in the patient with lung cancer (4). In contrast, the patient with malignant pleural effusion and hemoptysis suggests that the underlying malignancy is bronchogenic cancer and not mesothelioma or an extralung primary. A known history of malignancy is an important historical finding, as is occupational exposure, particularly asbestos, which should increase the suspicion for lung cancer or mesothelioma.

Since most patients presenting with a malignant pleural effusion have a moderate volume of fluid in the pleural space, the typical physical findings of a pleural effusion are present (4). Lymphadenopathy and cachexia is seen in less than half the patients at presentation (Table 2).

A malignant pleural effusion should be the primary consideration when an older individual (in the sixth or seventh decade) presents with a unilateral effusion or bilateral pleural effusions with a normal heart size and the insidious onset of dyspnea or a patient with a known malignancy develops a pleural effusion.

Table 2 Clinical Manifestations of Patients with Carcinomatous Pleural Effusions on Admission to Hospital ($n = 96$)

Symptoms	Patients No.	%	Physical findings	Patients No.	%
Dyspnea	55	57	Pleural effusion	88	92
Cough	41	43	Cachexia	35	37
Weight loss	31	32	Adenopathy	20	21
Chest pain	25	26	Fever	9	9
Malaise	21	22	Chest wall tenderness	4	4
Anorexia	14	15	Clubbing	2	2
Fever	8	8	Pleural rub	2	2
Chills	5	5	Cyanosis	2	2
Asymptomatic	22	23			

Source: Ref. 4.

IV. Radiological Findings

At presentation, patients with metastatic carcinoma to the pleura typically have >1,000 cc of fluid in the pleural space (4). While small effusions (estimated <500 cc) are seen in about 10% of these patients, an additional 10% present with a massive pleural effusion, which involves the entire hemithorax (4). In the majority of patients who present with a massive pleural effusion, malignancy is the most likely diagnosis (17), this volume of fluid typically results in contralateral mediastinal shift, diaphragm depression, and outward movement of the chest wall (Fig. 1). The tumor responsible for this radiographic finding is usually from an extrapulmonic primary (18). However, when there is an absence of contralateral mediastinal shift with an apparent large pleural effusion, lung cancer involving the ipsilateral mainstem bronchus should be suspected (18) (Fig. 2). Other causes of the absence of contralateral mediastinal shift include malignant mesothelioma, fixation of the mediastinum due to malignant lymph nodes, or rarely marked tumor infiltration of the parenchyma.

The presence of bilateral pleural effusions with a heart of normal size makes malignancy a possible diagnosis, usually the result of an extrapulmonic primary (19) (Fig. 3). However, transudative effusions from nephrotic syndrome, hypoalbuminemia, hepatic hydrothorax, and constrictive pericarditis

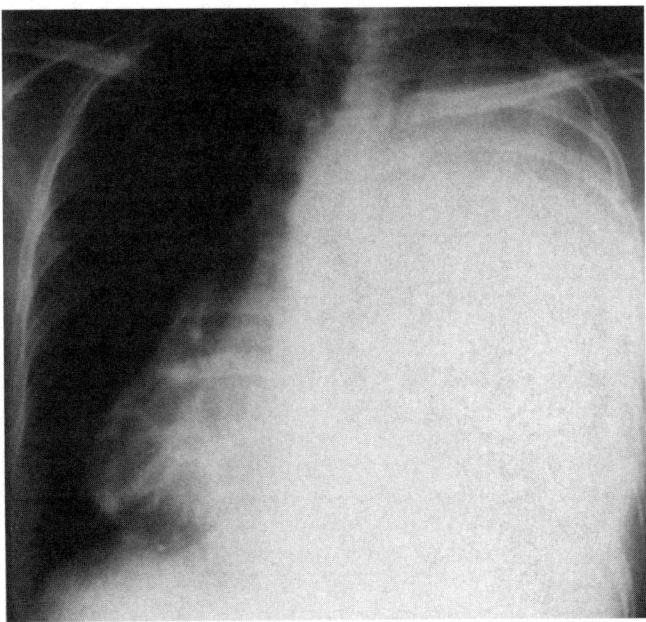

Figure 1 Posteroanterior chest radiograph of a woman with cervical carcinoma metastatic to the left pleura and mediastinum resulting in a massive pleural effusion with contralateral mediastinal shift. (From Ref. 128.)

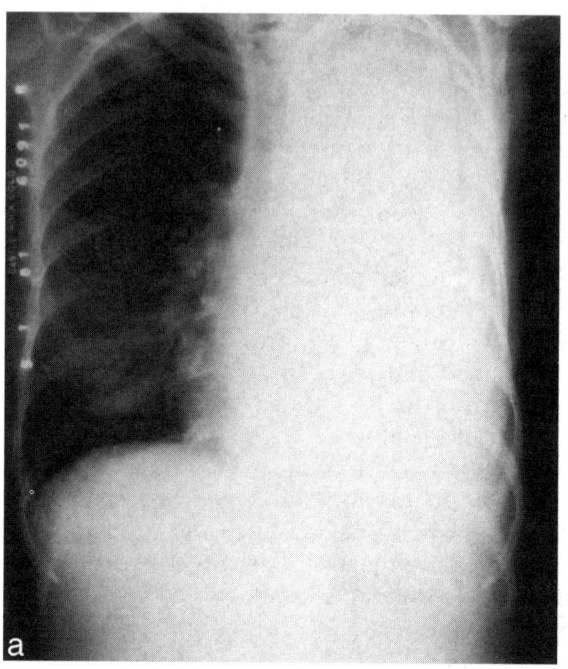

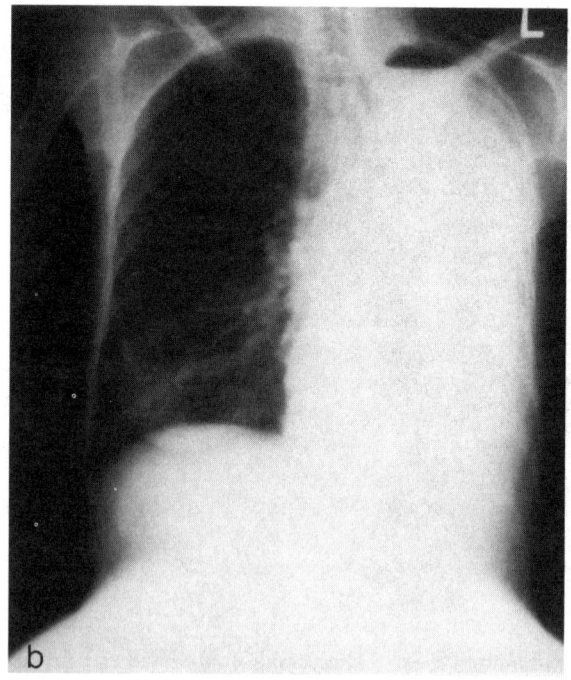

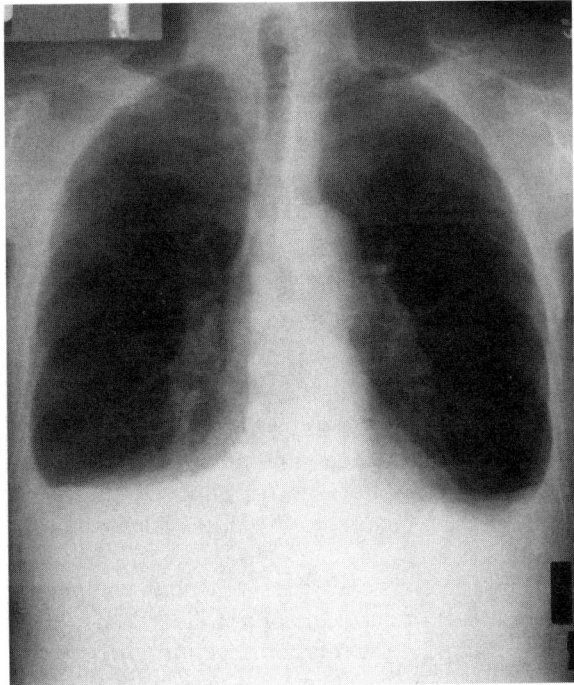

Figure 3 Posteroanterior chest radiograph of an elderly man with prostate cancer metastatic to mediastinum and pleura. Note bilateral effusions with a normal heart size.

and exudative effusions from lupus pleuritis and yellow nail syndrome can also cause the aforementioned radiographic findings. While patients with lung cancer and lymphoma often show other radiographic abnormalities in addition to the effusion, patients with extrathoracic primary malignancies usually present with a pleural effusion as the only radiographic abnormality.

Computerized tomography of the chest may be helpful in the evaluation of patients with a malignant effusion by demonstrating mediastinal lymph node involvement, parenchymal disease, and airway involvement that cannot be detected on standard chest radiograph (20). In addition, CT scan can identify

---

Figure 2 (a) Posteroanterior chest radiograph of a woman with small-cell lung cancer with total obstruction of the left mainstem bronchus. There is complete opacification of the left hemithorax with minimal ipsilateral mediastinal shift. (b) Posteroanterior chest radiograph following thoracentesis with resultant accentuation of ipsilateral mediastinal shift due to the increased intrapleural negative pressure from removal of pleural fluid in the setting of complete lung collapse. (From Ref. 129.)

pleural abnormalities and distant metastases. If pleural plaques are noted, lung cancer and malignant mesothelioma need to be considered. Magnetic resonance imaging (MRI) may be helpful in evaluating chest wall involvement (21). Positron emission tomography (PET scanning) may be helpful in evaluating the extent of pleural involvement in malignant mesothelioma (22).

V. Diagnosis

A. Pleural Fluid Analysis

Virtually all patients with an undiagnosed pleural effusion should undergo a diagnostic thoracentesis. Thirty to 50 cc of pleural fluid is necessary for diagnostic studies. Malignant pleural effusions can be serous, hemorrhagic, or grossly bloody. Nucleated cell count is typically low, generally <3000/µL, composed mainly of lymphocytes, macrophages, and mesothelial cells (4). About half the time in carcinomatous pleural effusions, lymphocytes range from 50 to 70% of the nucleated cells and are typically >80% of the nucleated cells in lymphomatous effusions (23).

The pleural fluid is a classic exudate (4,24) but, on rare occasions, can be transudative, if the patient has a concomitant disease such as congestive heart failure, atelectasis from endobronchial obstruction, or is in the early phase of lymphatic obstruction (4,24,25). The absolute LDH value usually satisfies exudative criteria when compared to the upper limits of normal of the serum (either 0.45,(26) 0.67,(24) or 0.80(27)). The pleural fluid-protein serum ratio may be <0.5 in some malignant pleural effusions, while the LDH criterion is virtually always in the exudative range.

The presence of pleural fluid eosinophilia should not dissuade the clinician from pursuing the diagnosis of malignancy. Two investigations have demonstrated that the prevalence of malignancy is similar in both eosinophilic and non—eosinophilic effusions (28,29).

A low pleural fluid pH (<7.30) and a low pleural fluid glucose (<60 mg/dL) with a normal serum glucose or a PF/serum glucose ratio of <0.5 is a marker of advanced disease in the pleural space with increased tumor burden. These biochemical findings are associated with a decreased survival, a higher sensitivity of diagnosis by initial cytologic examination and pleural biopsy, and less successful pleurodesis than those patients with a pH >7.30 and glucose >60 mg/dl (30–33).

Ten to 14% of patients with malignant pleural effusions have an increased amylase concentration (34). Isoenzyme analysis demonstrates that the amylase is composed predominantly of the salivary type (34,35). Adenocarcinoma of the lung is the most common cause of a salivary amylase—rich pleural effusion with adenocarcinoma of the ovary being next most frequent. A high salivary amylase content has been found in tumor tissue. Clinically, the finding of an elevated pleural fluid salivary amylase, in the absence of esophageal rupture, virtually establishes the diagnosis of a malignant pleural effusion.

B. Cytology

Pleural fluid cytology is the least invasive method for diagnosing malignant pleural effusion. With improvement in cytological techniques and appropriate specimen handling, exfoliative cytology is diagnostic in 60 to 90% of patients with the sensitivity depending on the extent of pleural involvement and the primary malignancy (36–40); most malignant effusions are due to adenocarcinomas. However, it is problematic to determine the true sensitivity and specificity of malignancy in pleural fluid. The only "gold standard" would be a post–mortem following thoracentesis (41). While some investigators recommend the routine use of cell blocks plus cytology smears (42,43), others have shown that the routine use of cell blocks is not cost effective (41). It appears that the volume of fluid submitted to the cytology laboratory does not effect the diagnostic yield.

C. Pleural Biopsy

Percutaneous pleural biopsy is a blind sampling procedure whose sensitivity varies between 40 and 75% (39,40,44–46), depending on the extent of parietal pleural involvement, number and adequacy of biopsies obtained, and the experience of the operator. A reason for a low yield of percutaneous biopsy in early metastatic disease to the pleura is that the initial lesions tend to be established on the mediastinal and diaphragmatic pleura with progression cephalad along the costal parietal pleura (47).

D. Thoracoscopy

In a sequential study of pleural fluid cytology, percutaneous pleural biopsy, and medical thoracoscopy in 208 consecutive patients, the diagnostic sensitivity of malignancy was 62%, 44%, and 95%, respectively (40). Similar results have been reported by others (48).

Medical thoracoscopy and video—assisted thoracic surgery (VATS) are clearly the most sensitive diagnostic procedures and approach 100% with experienced operators. Even in the early stages of pleural involvement, the yield with thoracoscopy can be high with a thorough examination by a skilled thoracoscopist. The reasons for false negative thoracoscopies include operator inexperience (48), incomplete examination due to pleural adhesions (48,49), and insufficient and non–representative tissue samples.

Medical thoracoscopy, primarily a diagnostic procedure, can be performed using local anesthesia with conscious sedation in an endoscopy suite using non-disposable rigid instruments, making it less invasive and costly than VATS. In contrast, (VATS) requires general anesthesia and single lung ventilation. A more extensive procedure can be done with VATS than medical thoracoscopy and treatment is often combined with diagnosis. Substantial adhesions, which may prevent thoracoscopy, can be suspected by the chest radiograph or ultrasonography. When extensive adhesions are initially appreciated at the time of VATS, the surgeon can convert to an open procedure.

Adhesions most commonly result from repeated thoracenteses or previous pleurodesis attempts (49).

E. Other Studies

With relatively low sensitivity and specificity, immunohistochemical staining with monoclonal antibodies to tumor markers and chromosomal analysis are not reliable for diagnosis. There are circumstances, however, where these tests may be useful, such as chromosomal analysis (50) in lymphomatous and leukemic effusions and flow cytometry (51) with identification of DNA aneuploidy for detection of a false negative with initial cytologic screen. Tumor markers, such as CEA, LEU-1, and mucin may be helpful in differentiating adenocarcinomas from mesothelioma (52–54).

VI. Management

The major indication for palliative treatment in patients with a malignant pleural effusion is relief of dyspnea. The degree of dyspnea is dependent, not only on the volume of pleural fluid, but also the underlying condition of the lungs and pleura. When palliation is considered, in addition to the patient's degree of breathlessness, their general health, functional status, and expected survival need to be assessed.

A. Therapeutic Thoracentesis

Therapeutic thoracentesis should be performed in virtually all dyspneic patients with a malignant pleural effusion to determine its effect on breathlessness and the rate and degree of recurrence. However, some clinicians choose to proceed directly to chest tube drainage and chemical pleurodesis or thoracoscopy with talc poudrage in dyspneic patients with large pleural effusions and contralateral mediastinal shift. Rapid recurrence of the effusion following therapeutic thoracentesis dictates the need for immediate treatment, while stabilization with relief of dyspnea may warrant observation. When dyspnea is not relieved by thoracentesis, other causes of breathlessness should be considered, such as lymphangitic carcinomatosis, atelectasis, tumor embolism, and thromboembolism.

Therapeutic thoracentesis may be the sole therapeutic option in patients with far-advanced disease, poor performance status, tumors associated with a poor survival, and very low pleural fluid pH. These patients can be treated with periodic outpatient thoracenteses rather than hospitalization for more invasive procedures that are associated with morbidity and higher costs.

The volume of fluid that can be removed safely from the pleural space is unknown. Monitoring of the pleural fluid pressure during thoracentesis would be optimal. If the pressure does not decrease to < -20 cmH$_2$O with removal of several hundred cc, fluid removal usually can be continued safely (55). As most clinicians do not measure pleural fluid pressure, it is recommended to remove no more than one and a half liters of fluid at a single sitting, if the patient does not develop dyspnea, chest pain, or severe cough. After six or eight hours with the patient improved, removal of several liters of fluid probably is safe in the setting of contralateral mediastinal shift on chest radiograph. It must be remembered that neither the patient nor operator may be aware of a precipitous decrease in pleural pressure. In patients with ipsilateral mediastinal or no shift with a large effusion, the likelihood of a precipitous decrease in pleural pressure is increased, and either the pressure should be monitored during thoracentesis or a small volume of fluid should be removed. Furthermore, in the patient with ipsilateral mediastinal shift, it is unlikely that thoracentesis will result in significant relief of breathlessness, as there likely is either mainstem bronchial occlusion or trapped lung. Reexpansion pulmonary edema can occur after rapid removal of either air or fluid from the pleural space and may not be related to the absolute level of negative pleural pressure. The mechanism of pulmonary edema is believed to be increased capillary permeability with the injury related to mechanical forces causing vascular stretching during reexpansion (56) or to ischemia–reperfusion.

B. Trapped Lung

In the setting of malignancy, a trapped lung occurs when a large tumor burden or tumor–induced fibrosis prevents partial or complete lung expansion to the chest wall. In the area where the lung cannot expand, a space *in vacuo* is created, which increases the pleural interstitial/pleural space pressure gradient, resulting in fluid movement from the interstitium into the pleural space to reach a volume of fluid that results in a new steady state of formation and resorption of fluid (57–59). If fluid is withdrawn from the space, the same volume will recur rapidly within 48 to 72 hours. A trapped lung can be suggested by any of the following criteria in the absence of endobronchial obstruction: (1) failure of the lung to expand completely after most of the fluid has been removed by therapeutic thoracentesis, as demonstrated by chest radiograph; (2) an initial pleural fluid pressure of <-5 cmH_2O (60); (3) a decrease in pleural fluid pressure to <-20 cmH_2O after one liter of fluid is removed (55,61); or (4) a pleural space elastance (ELpl) of >19 cmH_2O when removing 500 cc of fluid (62). In a prospective cohort study of 65 patients with malignant pleural effusion, eleven (79%) of 14 patients with ELpl >19 cmH_2O had trapped lung; while only 3 (6%) of 51 patients with ELpl of <19 cmH_2O had trapped lung ($p<0.001$). Furthermore, none of the 14 patients with ELpl of >19 cmH_2O and none of the 14 patients with trapped lung had successful pleurodesis. In contrast, 42 (98%) of 43 patients with ELpl <19 cmH_2O who did not have a trapped lung had successful pleurodesis with bleomycin. It is futile to perform a therapeutic thoracentesis or to attempt pleurodesis in patients who have extensive trapped lung. However, there are patients with trapped lung due to malignancy who show relief of dyspnea with thoracentesis or pleuroperitoneal shunt. These patients do not have a classic trapped lung; in these patients, the fluid in the pleural space represents a combination of fluid produced by the malignancy plus lung entrapment (59). The fluid is exudative due to malignancy and by removing the fluid produced by the malignancy, there is some relief. In classic trapped lung, the transudative fluid forms on a hydrostatic basis only and there is no other mechanism for fluid formation; these patients do not have relief of dyspnea with fluid removal (59).

C. Chemotherapy and Radiation

Malignant pleural effusions that are likely to respond favorably to chemotherapy include those from small-cell lung cancer (63), breast carcinoma (64–66), lymphoma, prostate cancer, ovarian cancer, germ cell tumor, and thyroid cancer. All other malignant pleural effusions are unlikely to be controlled by chemotherapy alone. In lymphomatous chylothorax, mediastinal radiation (67) may be effective and pleuroperitoneal shunt (68) may be helpful in failed therapy, as it can recirculate chyle. When chemotherapy is unavailable, contraindicated, or has become ineffective, local therapy such as pleurodesis should be considered.

D. Pleurodesis

Chemical pleurodesis is an accepted palliative treatment for patients with recurrent, symptomatic pleural effusions. A number of chemical agents have been used for pleurodesis; however, adequate assessment of the effectiveness of these agents has been problematic because 1) reported series have evaluated small numbers of patients, 2) different pleurodesis techniques have been employed, 3) different criteria for success have been used, and 4) patients have been followed for varying time periods. In addition, there have been limited studies of direct comparisons between agents under similar conditions in similar patient populations. In addition, very few studies have prospectively evaluated adverse effects.

Walker–Renard and colleagues (69) analyzed 1,168 patients who received chemical pleurodesis as reported in the English language literature from 1966 through 1992. They found a complete response rate of 64% (752 of 1,168), defined as no recurrence of the effusion determined by clinical examination or chest radiograph. They found talc to be the most effective agent with a complete response rate of 93% with *Corynebacterium parvum* being successful in 76%, doxycycline in 72%, tetracycline in 67%, and bleomycin in 54% (Table 3). The most common reported adverse effects with all agents in 1,140 patients were chest pain (23%) and fever (19%) with the incidence varying between agents (69) (Table 4). Talc was found to be superior to both bleomycin and tetracycline in comparative studies of pleurodesis success (70–72).

Talc Pleurodesis

On literature review, when analyzed by method of administration, pleurodesis by poudrage (418 of 461) and slurry (168 of 185) had similar success rates of 91% (73). In a small series of 57 patients randomized to receive 5 gm of either

Table 3 Success Rates of Commonly Used Agents for Pleurodesis in Malignant Pleural Effusions

Chemical agent	Patients (n)	Complete success[a] (n)	Complete success (%)	Dose
Talc	165	153	93	2.5–10 g
Corynebacterium parvum	169	129	76	3.5–14 mg
Doxycycline	60	43	72	500 mg (often multiple doses)
Tetracycline	359	240	67	500 mg–20 mg/kg
Bleomycin	199	108	54	15–240 units

[a] Complete success = absence of reaccumulation of effusion (CXR or clinical).
Source: Adapted from Ref. 69.

talc slurry through a chest tube or talc poudrage with thoracoscopy, no difference in recurrence was found between the two methods (74). A recently completed large, randomized multicenter trial by the North American Cooperative Oncology Groups comparing the effectiveness of talc poudrage and talc slurry found no difference in efficacy.

The most common adverse effects of talc pleurodesis are fever (16%) and chest pain (7%) (69). When fever occurs following talc pleurodesis, its typical onset is 4 to 12 hours following the procedure with a duration of up to 72 hours (73). It is rare for the fever to exceed 102.4°. Empyema has been reported with talc slurry in 0–11% of cases and with talc poudrage in 0–3% of patients (73). Cardiovascular events such as arrythmias, cardiac arrest, chest pain, myocardial infarction, and hypotension have been documented, but it is unclear whether these complications are the result of the procedure itself, are related to talc per se, or the patient's underlying disease (73).

Table 4 Incidence of Chest Pain and Fever with Chemical Pleurodesis

Chemical agent	Patients (n)	Chest pain (%)	Fever (%)
Talc	131	7	16
Corynebacterium parvum	169	43	59
Doxycycline	60	40	31
Tetracycline	359	14	10
Bleomycin	199	28	24

Source: Adapted from Ref. 69.

There has been recent concern about acute respiratory failure following talc pleurodesis. In a review of the English language literature from 1958 through 2001 in an attempt to determine the incidence and causality of acute respiratory failure following talc pleurodesis, I found 3,064 patients with malignant pleural effusions, 1,009 with pneumothorax, and 178 patients with nonmalignant effusions treated with either talc slurry or talc poudrage (73–89). There were 43 patients who developed acute respiratory failure, 41 (1.3%) occurred in patients with malignant effusions, 2 (0.2%) patients with pneumothorax, and none with nonmalignant effusion. Therefore, of the 4,252 patients who received talc poudrage and slurry pleurodeses, there was a 1% incidence of acute respiratory failure reported. After careful reading of these manuscripts, it was my opinion that, approximately half of the reported cases of acute respiratory failure either provided no information that allowed determination of the cause of the acute respiratory failure, occurred in severely compromised patients (severe underlying COPD, widespread tumor involving the lung and mediastinum) (75), or received excess narcotics (75). In the most recent report from de Campos and colleagues (82) of 614 patients who received talc pleurodesis, 7 (1.5%) of 457 patients with malignant pleural effusions developed acute respiratory failure; 2 of these patients had received multiple pulmonary and pleural biopsies prior to poudrage, one patient had lymphoma of the mediastinum and bilateral chylothoraces and had bilateral talc poudrage, and the other 4 patients were described as having "very limited pulmonary reserve". None of the 108 patients with nonmalignant effusions or 49 patients with pneumothorax developed respiratory failure post talc pleurodesis (82).

In a retrospective review of complications of talc pleurodesis from 1993 to 1997 with 78 patients who had 89 pleurodeses, a number of respiratory complications were noted (81). The predominant method was talc slurry, which was used in 70 patients. Five grams of talc was used in 85 of the pleurodeses. Seven patients were reported with ARDS who had 8 pleurodesis procedures. One of the patients with AIDS and *Pneumocystis carinii* pneumonia–induced pneumothorax had bilateral simultaneous talc pleurodeses preceded by a pleural abrasion. The other 6 patients all had malignant pleural effusions; 2 had pleural abrasion prior to talc poudrage while the other 4 had only talc slurry pleurodesis. Therefore, it would have been more appropriate for the authors to state that with 89 pleurodeses, 4 patients developed ARDS, which may have been solely related to talc.

Possible causes for acute respiratory failure following talc pleurodesis include a systemic inflammatory syndrome (SIRS) or ARDS from talc, reexpansion pulmonary edema, excess premedication, severe comorbid disease, terminal malignancy, sepsis from unsterile talc or poor chest tube technique, and excess talc (high-dose or bilateral sequential pleurodesis). If talc is the culprit, it may be due to very small particle size (<30 mm) (90), a contaminant, or endotoxin (91).

Long-term studies have not shown development of mesothelioma with the use of asbestos-free talc (92–94). In a short-term follow-up of patients receiving talc poudrage for pneumothorax, no difference in lung function was found when compared to patients who received a thoracotomy without talc poudrage (95,96). Twenty-two to 35 years following talc poudrage for pneumothorax, total lung capacity was 89% of predicted in 46 patients compared to 97% of predicted for 29 patients treated with tube thoracostomy alone (93). Although a minimal reduction in total lung capacity was found following talc poudrage, as well as pleural thickening observed on chest radiograph, these changes were clinically unimportant. None of the 46 patients who received talc poudrage developed mesothelioma over the similar time of follow-up (93). Although a link has been found between talc and cancer in those who mine and process talc (97), the association has been attributed to asbestos exposure, which is commonly found with talc, rather than with talc per se. In a group of patients who received talc pleurodesis for pneumothorax and had long-term follow-up, there was no increased incidence of lung cancer (92).

At present, with the data available on talc pleurodesis, I have reached the following conclusions:

1. Poudrage and slurry are effective for treating malignant pleural effusions, nonmalignant effusions, and pneumothoraces.
2. Poudrage and slurry appear to be equally effective in the management of malignant pleural effusions.
3. Long-term (up to 35 years) safety has been documented.
4. Acute respiratory failure has been reported in approximately 1% of over 4,200 patients, virtually all of whom had malignant pleural effusions.
5. In approximately half of the patients with acute respiratory failure, factors other than talc could be implicated.
6. In approximately half of the reported cases of talc-associated respiratory failure, other predisposing factors were present, such as prior pleural abrasions or biopsies, bilateral pleurodeses were done, or the patient had severe underlying pulmonary disease.
7. Talc-induced acute respiratory failure could be caused by contaminants in the talc, endotoxin, non–sterile talc, or small particle size.

To virtually eliminate the possibility of talc-induced acute respiratory failure, the sterility of talc should be assured, the majority of talc particles should be >30 microns in diameter, the absence of endotoxin should be documented, no more than 3 g of talc should be used, pleural abrasion and multiple biopsies should be avoided prior to pleurodesis, and pleurodesis should not be attempted in terminal patients or those with marginal lung function.

Pleural Fluid pH and Glucose

Approximately a third of patients on presentation with a malignant pleural effusion have a low pleural fluid pH (<7.30) and a glucose (<60 mg/dl) (30). These patients have more pleural tumor than those with normal pH and glucose effusions. Pleural fluid pH and glucose are low in patients with far-advanced disease of the pleural space primarily because the end-products of glucose metabolisms (CO_2 and lactic acid) have a decreased rate of efflux from the pleural space and subsequently high pleural fluid values because tumor has created a barrier to removal through the pleural membrane (98). There is a direct correlation between pleural fluid pH and survival with those patients with lower pH having a decreased survival (30–33,99). Those with a lower pleural fluid pH also have less success with pleurodesis (30–33). However, a meta-analysis of 417 patients with malignant pleural effusion from multiple investigators from North America and Europe was found that even in the lowest pH (6.70–7.26) quartile, 45% of these patients were still alive at 3 months (99). Furthermore, in the same low pH quartile, only 35% failed chemical pleurodesis (100). Therefore, the clinician should not use pleural fluid pH as a single factor, but in conjunction with other variables, when deciding whether pleurodesis should be offered to the patient.

Technique of Pleurodesis

Proper technique is critical for successful pleurodesis. Several issues relating to pleurodesis technique have been controversial. These include chest tube size, pain control, patient rotation, dwell time, and timing of instillation of the pleurodesis agent and chest tube removal. Twelve studies with a combined 245 patients have been published on the response of small-bore (7–16 F) catheters with chemical pleurodesis (101–112). Fifty-five of the patients had pleurodesis with talc slurry, 50 with doxycycline, 94 with bleomycin, and 46 with tetracycline. Talc had the best success rate of 88%, followed by doxycycline at 80%, bleomycin at 75%, and tetracycline at 75%. The overall success rate (complete or partial) of the 245 patients who had chemical pleurodesis using small-bore catheters was 78%. Small-bore catheters are as effective as standard chest tubes for pleurodesis and are associated with less patient morbidity.

In my experience, the administration of 2 to 3 mg of intravenous morphine and 2 to 3 mg of intravenous midazolam provides excellent pain control and an amnestic response, respectively, for pleurodesis. These drugs should be administered 5–10 mins prior to the instillation of the pleurodesis agent. If pain does occur, it is generally immediate and short-lived.

We previously have demonstrated that radiolabeled tetracycline dispersed immediately and completely throughout the pleural space when instilled through a chest tube (113). In a follow-up to the distribution study, we randomized patients who received tetracycline pleurodesis either to rotation or nonrotation following instillation (114). There was no difference found in pleurodesis success suggesting that it was not necessary to rotate patients when using a soluble agent such as tetracycline. However, with the use of talc slurry, my current recommendation is that rotation should be performed over a one-hour period, moving the patient through right and left lateral decubitus positions, head of the bed at 45° to 60°, Trendelenburg, and supine because dispersion may not be as complete with a slurry as with a soluble agent.

Since the mesothelial cell initiates the inflammatory cascade that leads to a fibrotic response and mesothelial cell injury occurs virtually instantaneously after contact with the chemical agent (115), a one hour (possibly 2 hours) dwell time would appear to be adequate, as the two pleural surfaces should be juxtaposed as soon as possible.

The dogma has been perpetuated over time that the chemical agent should be instilled into the pleural space when the lung is fully expanded on chest radiograph and there is <150 cc of daily drainage through the chest tube. The "standard of care" also suggests that the chest tube be removed when there is <100 to 150 cc of drainage over 24 hours. In a small, randomized study of 25 patients with malignant pleural effusions evaluating timely instillation and chest tube drainage, 15 patients were randomized to standard chest tube drainage and 10 patients to short-term chest tube drainage (116). Patients in the standard group had the chest tube in place until there was lung reexpansion on chest radiograph and the volume of fluid drained from the pleural space was <100 mL for 24 hours before 1,500 mg of tetracycline was instilled. The chest tube was removed when the amount of fluid drained was <150 mL for 24 hours after the tetracycline was administered. In the 10 patients in the short-term group, the same dose of tetracycline was instilled as soon as the chest radiograph showed lung reexpansion and the effusion was drained, which was usually within 24 hours, regardless of the volume of chest tube drainage; the chest tube was removed the day after instillation of tetracycline. Pleurodesis success was 80% in each group, but the duration of chest tube drainage was significantly shorter (median 2 days, range 2–9 days) in the short-term chest tube group compared with the standard group (median 7 days, range 3–19 days), ($p < 0.01$). This small, randomized study suggests that, as soon as the lung is fully expanded on chest radiograph with an absence or minimal volume of fluid, the pleurodesis agent should be instilled, regardless of the volume of drainage through the chest tube. The chest tube should be removed the following day regardless of drainage. The use of this technique could substantially shorten the patient's hospital stay or could be done as an outpatient, both minimizing cost. However, if the postpleurodesis chest tube drainage is >250–300 cc for 24 hours, the chest tube should not be removed as success would be unlikely; pleurodesis should be repeated if the lung is expanded.

Recommendations for Pleurodesis

Factors that should be considered before recommending pleurodesis to a patient with a malignant effusion include their response to therapeutic thoracentesis, general health, performance status, expected survival, pleural space anatomy by chest radiograph or chest CT, pleural space elastance, primary malignancy, and pleural fluid pH. Absolute contraindications to pleurodesis include absence of relief of dyspnea with therapeutic thoracentesis, extensive trapped lung, or mainstem bronchial occlusion. Relative contraindications to pleurodesis include a terminal patient, widespread metastatic disease, poor performance status, active air leak, low pleural fluid pH, severe underlying disease, and following extensive pleural abrasion or multiple biopsies.

E. Short-Term Chest Tube Drainage

Five studies have evaluated the response of short-term (3–12 days) chest tube drainage for recurrent malignant pleural effusion (117–121). The range of reported successful pleurodeses in these 5 series was 0% to 77%. Of the total 126 patients who were treated with standard chest tube drainage without a pleurodesis agent, 78 (62%) patients had successful treatment of their malignant pleural effusions. Although the response rate seems high, in several of the article the observation period was not clearly defined. Furthermore, if a chest tube is placed in these patients and the lung expands with drainage, a pleurodesis agent should be instilled if there is no contraindication.

F. Chronic Indwelling Catheters

Two studies with chronic indwelling catheters have shown that these 15.5 F catheters are effective in the relief of dyspnea, safe, as successful as pleurodesis with doxycycline or talc, and less costly than chemical pleurodesis. In a multicenter prospective trial, 144 patients were randomized in a 2:1 distribution to chronic indwelling silastic catheter (n = 99) or chest tube drainage with doxycycline pleurodesis (n = 45) (122). Relief of dyspnea was the same in both groups after initial treatment and at 90 days and improved from baseline. Patients with the indwelling catheter had significantly fewer hospital days. No patient in the catheter group had symptomatic recurrence compared to 27% of patients who received doxycycline pleurodesis. Pleurodesis success was not different between the indwelling catheter group and the doxycycline group, both being low at 18% and 28%, respectively. Putnam and colleagues (123) retrospectively reviewed 100 consecutive indwelling pleural catheter patients, 60 treated as outpatients and 40 as inpatients, and compared them to 68 consecutive inpatients treated with chest tube drainage and doxycycline or talc pleurodesis who were treated for malignant pleural effusions. The median survival was 3.4 months and did not differ significantly between treatment groups. No deaths occurred in the chronic indwelling catheter group, and 81 (81%) of the 100 patients had no complications. The other 19 patients had complications that included removal of the malfunctioning catheter and an infected pleural space. Those treated with the indwelling catheter as outpatients, as expected, had significantly lower costs than those treated with the catheter as inpatients or those treated with chest tube pleurodesis as inpatients. Chronic indwelling catheters should be considered for patients with lung entrapment who cannot undergo or who have failed pleurodesis.

G. Pleuroperitoneal Shunting

Pleuroperitoneal shunt has been used in patients who have failed chemical pleurodesis, chemotherapy, or radiation therapy, or have a trapped lung or malignant chylothorax. Petrou and colleagues (79) reported their 10-year experience with patients who were referred for surgical palliation of malignant pleural effusion. One hundred thirty-four patients (74%) had previous treatment, which included thoracentesis, tube thoracostomy, pleurodesis, and pleurectomy. One hundred seventeen patients demonstrated full lung expansion at thoracoscopy or mini-thoracotomy and underwent talc pleurodesis; the remaining 63 patients had trapped lung and received a pleuroperitoneal shunt, which resulted in palliation in 98% of patients. Nine shunt occlusions occurred from several days to 2.5 months and were found to be infected. The occluded shunts were replaced in 4, revised in 2, and removed with open drainage in 3. There were no intraoperative deaths. Pleuroperitoneal shunting can provide effective palliation in patients with a trapped lung and chylothorax (68,124) or others who have failed pleurodesis.

H. Parietal Pleurectomy

Parietal pleurectomy offers definitive treatment for patients with malignant pleural effusions but carries a high morbidity and mortality that is not justified in patients with a poor prognosis. Martini and coworkers (125) reported their results in 106 patients treated by pleurectomy for malignant pleural effusions. Sixteen (19%) of 83 patients were alive 2 years following pleurectomy with a survival range of 2 to 6 years. The primary postoperative complication was prolonged air leak in those that required decortication for trapped lung. The overall 30-day postoperative mortality was 10%. Fry and Khandekar (126) performed parietal pleurectomy in 24 patients who did not respond to standard treatment for malignant pleural effusion using axillary thoracotomy. Three (13%) patients died in the postoperative period. In the remaining 21 patients, satisfactory control of their malignant pleural effusion was obtained with survival of 2–30 months (average 10.6). Waller and colleagues (127) reported the use of VATS pleurectomy in 19 patients with malignant pleural effusions (13 mesothelioma and 6 metastatic adenocarcinoma). All patients were successfully extubated in the operating room without the need for mechanical ventilation and were discharged from the hospital with a median postoperative stay of 5 days (range 2–20). There were no postoperative deaths; 6 patients died of their underlying disease 4 to 17 months following surgery. Of the remaining 13 patients, two developed recurrent effusions. Because of its significant morbidity and mortality, parietal pleurectomy should be reserved for patients who have failed chemical pleurodesis, have a trapped lung, or if the malignant pleural effusion is found at the time of thoracotomy for resection of an intrathoracic tumor. The procedure should not be offered to patients who have a poor performance status and an expected survival of <6 months.

The goal of improving the quality of life of our patients is particularly germane in the setting of malignant pleural effusions where relief of breathlessness remains the primary objective. The least invasive, morbid and costly therapy should be recommended for patients who have a limited survival. Hospitalization should be minimized so that cost can be contained and the patient not removed from their family. Success of the initial procedure is important, as repeat procedures are associated with additional hospitalization, patient discomfort, and added expense. Therefore, the selection of patients for palliation and the specific procedure to be utilized needs to be chosen carefully, based on multiple factors, such as their general health, performance status, expected survival and others. The clinician currently cannot rely on prospective, randomized, controlled trials that will help in these important therapeutic decisions. Prospective studies are needed that will evaluate the course of small, symptomatic, malignant pleural effusions, assess the potential of intrapleural immune modulators, compare ambulatory and hospital-based management, and study the issue of talc–associated respiratory failure.

VII. Prognosis

In a combined series of 417 patients with malignant pleural effusions from 9 investigators in the United States and Europe, lung cancer represented 43% and breast cancer 18% of the primary malignancies (99). Eighty percent were alive at one month, 54% at 3 months, 31% at 6 months, and 13% at one year. Lung cancer ($n = 146$) patients had a median survival of 3 months, GI cancers ($n = 18$) 2.3 months, and ovarian cancer ($n = 9$) 3.6 months. Those with breast cancer ($n = 60$) had a median survival of 5 months, mesothelioma ($n = 29$) 6 months, and lymphoma ($n = 7$) 9 months.

VIII. Conclusion

Malignant pleural effusions are a common consequence of the primary tumor that cause substantial morbidity for the patient. There are approximately 150,000 new cases of malignant pleural effusions diagnosed in the United States annually, with lung cancer and breast cancer being the most common cause. Pleural metastases occur through pulmonary vascular invasion and embolization to the visceral pleural surface, direct invasion from lung and breast cancer, hematogenous metastases, and lymphatic involvement. Breathlessness, the most common presenting symptom, occurs in more than half of the patients. Bilateral pleural effusions with a normal heart size, a massive pleural effusion, and a large pleural effusion without contralateral mediastinal shift are suggestive of a malignant etiology. Malignant pleural effusions can be serous, hemorrhagic, or grossly bloody exudates with a low number of nucleated cells that commonly are lymphocyte predominant. The prevalence of malignancy is similar in both eosinophilic as well as noneosinophilic pleural effusions. A pleural fluid pH <7.30 and a glucose <60 mg/dl are found in a third of patients who present with a malignant pleural effusion and are associated with ease of diagnosis and decreased survival. Ten to 14% of patients with malignant effusions have an increased salivary amylase effusion, the most common cause of which being adenocarcinoma of the lung. Pleural fluid cytology is the least invasive method for diagnosis with a sensitivity of 60–90%. Percutaneous pleural biopsy has a sensitivity of 40–75%. The diagnostic sensitivity of the aforementioned procedures increases with the extent of pleural involvement. Thoracoscopy is clearly the most sensitive diagnostic procedure approaching 100% with experienced operators. The major indication for palliative treatment for patients with a malignant effusion is relief of dyspnea. Therapeutic thoracentesis would be the therapeutic option in patients with far-advanced disease, poor performance status, a tumor associated with poor survival, and very low pleural fluid pH. Malignant effusions from small cell lung cancer, breast cancer, and lymphoma are likely to have a favorable response to chemotherapy. Mediastinal radiation may be effective for treating lymphomatous chylothorax. Chemical pleurodesis is an accepted palliative treatment for patients with recurrent, symptomatic pleural effusions. Talc, either as a poudrage or slurry, has been shown to be the most effective pleurodesis agent, with less success with doxycycline and bleomycin. The most common adverse effects of all pleurodesis agents are chest pain and fever. The incidence of acute respiratory failure associated with talc pleurodesis is approximately 1%. In about half of the patients reported with acute talc-associated respiratory failure, factors other than talc could be implicated. It would be unlikely for talc-induced acute respiratory failure to occur if the sterility of talc was assured, the majority of talc particles were >30 microns in diameter, endotoxin was not present, no more than 3 gm of talc were used, pleural abrasion was not done prior to the procedure, simultaneous bilateral pleurodeses were not attempted, and pleurodesis was not performed in terminal patients or those with marginal lung function. Factors that need to be considered prior to recommending pleurodesis include the response to therapeutic thoracentesis, general health, performance status, expected survival, pleural space anatomy, pleural space elastance, primary malignancy, and pleural fluid pH. Absolute contraindications to pleurodesis include absence of relief of dyspnea with therapeutic thoracentesis, extensive trapped lung, or mainstem bronchial occlusion. Therapies that can be considered if patients are not candidates for or have failed chemical pleurodesis include indwelling catheters and pleuroperitoneal shunts. The least invasive, morbid and costly therapy should be recommended for patients who have a limited survival outlook.

References

1. Antony VB, Loddenkemper R, Astoul P, Boutin C, Goldstraw P, Hott J, Rodriguez-Panadero F, Sahn SA. Management of malignant pleural effusions. Am J Respir Crit Care Med 2000; 162:1987–2001.
2. Rodriguez-Panadero F, Borderas-Naranjo F, Lopez-Mejias J. Pleural metastatic tumours and effusions. Frequency and pathogenic mechanisms in a post-mortem series. Eur J Respir Dis 1989; 2:366–369.
3. Meyer PC. Metastatic carcinoma of the pleura. Thorax 1966; 21:437–443.

4. Chernow B, Sahn SA. Carcinomatous involvement of the pleura. An analysis of 96 cases. Am J Med 1977; 63:695–702.
5. Kolin A, Koutoulakis T. Invasion of pulmonary arteries by bronchial carcinomas. Hum Pathol 1987; 18:1165–1171.
6. Jiang W. In vitro models of cancer invasion and metastasis: recent developments. Eur J Surg Oncol 1994; 20:493–499.
7. Zetter B. Adhesion molecules in tumor metastasis. Semin Cancer Biol 1993; 4:219–229.
8. Shetty S, Kumar A, Johnson A, Idell S. Expression of the urokinase-type plasminogen activator receptor in human malignant mesothelial cells: role in tumor cell mitogenesis and proteolysis. Am J Physiol Lung Cell Mol Physiol 1995; 12:L972–L982.
9. Idell S, Pueblitz S, Emri S, Gungen Y, Gray L, Kumar A, Holiday D, Koenig KB, Johnson AR. Regulation of fibrin deposition by malignant mesothelioma. Am J Pathol 1995; 147:1318–1329.
10. Shetty S, Idell S. A urokinase receptor MRNA binding protein–MRNA interaction regulates receptor expression and function in human pleural mesothelioma cells. Arch Biochem Biophys 1998; 35:265–279.
11. Shetty S, Idell S. Post-transcriptional regulation of urokinase receptor gene expression in human lung carcinoma and malignant mesothelioma cells in vitro. Mol Cell Biochem 1999; 199:189–200.
12. Hott KW, Yu L, Antony VB. Role of VEGF in the formation of malignant pleural effusions. Am J Respir Crit Care Med 1999; 159:A212.
13. Galffy G, Mohammed KA, Ward MJ, Dowling PA, Antony VB. Interleukin 8—an autocrine growth factor for malignant mesothelioma. Am Cancer Res 1999; 59:367–371.
14. Sahn SA. Malignant pleural effusions. In: Light RW, ed. Pleural Diseases. Philadelphia: WB Saunders, 1985:113–125.
15. Estienne M, Yeranult JC, DeTroyer A. Mechanism of relief of dyspnea after thoracentesis in patients with large pleural effusions. Am J Med 1983; 74:813–819.
16. Tammilehto L, Maasilita P, Kostianen S, Appelqvist P, Holsti LR, Mattson K. Diagnosis and prognostic factors in malignant pleural mesothelioma: a retrospective analysis of 65 patients. Respiration 1992; 52:129–135.
17. Maher GG, Berger HW. Massive pleural effusions: malignant and non-malignant causes in 46 patients. Am Rev Respir Dis 1972; 105:458–460.
18. Liberson M. Diagnostic significance of the mediastinal profile in massive unilateral pleural effusions. Am Rev Respir Dis 1963; 88:176–180.
19. Rabin CB, Blackman NS. Bilateral pleural effusion. Its significance in association with a heart of normal size. J Mt Sinai Hosp 1957; 24:45–53.
20. O'Donovan PB, Eng P. Pleural changes in malignant pleural effusions: appearance on computed tomography. Cleve Clin J Med 1994; 61:127–131.
21. Bittner RC, Felix R. Magnetic resonance (MR) imaging of the chest: state-of-the-art. Eur Respir J 1998; 11:1392–1404.
22. Benard F, Sterman D, Smith RJ, Kaiser LR, Albelda SM, Alavi A. Metabolic imaging of malignant pleural mesothelioma with fluorodeoxyglucose positron emission tomography. Chest 1998; 144:713–722.
23. Yam LT. Diagnostic significance of lymphocytes in pleural effusions. Ann Intern Med 1967; 66:972–982.
24. Light RW, MacGregor MI, Luchsinger PC, Hall WC. Pleural effusions: the

diagnostic separation of transudates and exudates. Ann Intern Med 1972; 77: 507–513.
25. Fernandes C, Martin C, Aranda R, Romero S. Malignant transient pleural transudate: a sign of early lymphatic tumoral obstruction. Respiration 2000; 67:333–336.
26. Heffner JE, Brown LK, Barbieri CA. Diagnostic value of tests that discriminate between exudative and transudative pleural effusions. Chest 1997; 111:970–980.
27. Joseph J, Badrinath P, Basran G, Sahn SA. Is the pleural fluid transudate or exudate? A revisit of the diagnostic criteria. Thorax 2001; 56:867–870.
28. Rubins JB, Rubins HB. Etiology and prognostic significance of eosinophilic pleural effusions: a prospective study. Chest 1996; 11:1271–1274.
29. Martinez-Garcia MA, Cases-Viedma E, Cordero-Rodrigues PJ, Hidalgo-Ramirez M, Perpina-Tordera M, Sanchis-Moret F, Sanchis-Aldas JL. Diagnostic utility of eosinophils in the pleural fluid. Eur Respir J 2000; 15:166–169.
30. Sahn SA, Good JT Jr. Pleural fluid pH in malignant effusions: diagnostic, prognostic, and therapeutic implications. Ann Intern Med 1988; 108:345–349.
31. Sanchez-Armengol A, Rodriguez-Panadero F. Survival and talc pleurodesis in metastatic pleural carcinoma, revisited. Chest 1993; 104:1482–1485.
32. Rodriguez-Panadero F, Lopez-Mejias L. Low glucose and pH levels in malignant effusions: diagnostic significance and prognostic value in respect to pleurodesis. Am Rev Respir Dis 1989; 139:663–667.
33. Rodriguez-Panadero F, Lopez-Mejias L. Survival time of patients with pleural metastatic carcinoma predicted by glucose and pH studies. Chest 1989; 95:320–324.
34. Kramer MR, Saldana MJ, Cepro RJ, Pitchenik AE. High amylase in neoplasm-related pleural effusions. Ann Intern Med 1989; 10:567–569.
35. Joseph J, Viney S, Beck P, Strange C, Sahn S, Basran GS. A prospective study of amylase-rich pleural effusions with special reference to amylase isoenzyme analysis. Chest 1992; 102:1455–1459.
36. Johnston WW. The malignant pleural effusion: a review of cytopathological diagnoses of 584 specimens from 472 consecutive patients. Cancer 1985; 56:905–909.
37. Hsu C. Cytologic detection of malignancy in pleural effusion: a review of 5,255 samples from 3,811 patients. Diagn Cytopathol 1987; 3:8–12.
38. Molangraft FL, Fooijs GP. The interval between the diagnosis of malignancy and the development of effusions, with reference to the role of cytologic diagnosis. Acta Cytol 1988; 32:183–187.
39. Starr RL, Sherman ME. The value of multiple preparations in the diagnosis of malignant pleural effusions. Acta Cytol 1991; 35:533–537.
40. Loddenkemper R, Grosser H, Gabler A, Mai J, Preussler H, Brandt HJ. Prospective evaluation of biopsy methods in the diagnosis of malignant pleural effusions: intra-patient comparison between pleural fluid cytology, blind needle biopsy, and thoracoscopy. Am Rev Respir Dis 1983; 127(suppl 4):S114.
41. Jonasson JG, Ducatman BS, Wang HH. The cell block for body cavity fluids: Do the results justify the cost? Mod Pathol 1990; 3:667–670.
42. Dekker A, Bupp PA. Cytology of serous effusions: an investigation into the usefulness of cell blocks versus smears. Am J Clin Pathol 1978; 70:855–860.
43. Irani DR, Underwood RD, Johnson EH, Greenberg D. Malignant pleural effusions. A clinical cytopathologic study. Arch Intern Med 1987; 147:1133–1136.
44. Prakash UBS, Reiman HM. Comparison of needle biopsy with cytologic analysis

for the evaluation of pleural effusions: analysis of 414 cases. Mayo Clin Proc 1985; 60:158–164.
45. Poe RH, Israel RH, Utell MJ, Hall WJ, Greenblatt DW, Kallen MC. Sensitivity, specificity, and predictive values of closed pleural biopsy. Arch Intern Med 1984; 144:325–328.
46. Escudero BC, Garcia CM, Cuesta CB, Molinos ML, Rodriguez RS, Gonsalez PA, Martinez Glez-Rio J. Cytological and bacteriologic analysis of fluid and pleural biopsy specimens with Cope's needle. Arch Intern Med 1990; 150:1190–1194.
47. Canto A, Rivis J, Saumench J, Morera R, Moy J. Points to consider when choosing a biopsy method in cases of pleurisy of unknown origin. Chest 1983; 83:176–179.
48. Boutin C, Viallat JR, Cargaino P, Farisse P. Thoracoscopy in malignant pleural effusions. Am Rev Respir Dis 1981; 124:588–592.
49. Loddenkemper R, Boutin C. Thoracoscopy: diagnostic and therapeutic indications. Eur Respir J 1993; 6:1544–1555.
50. Mentintas M, Ozdemir N, Solak M, Artan S, Ozdemir M, Basaran N, Ekici M, Erginel S. Chromosome analysis in pleural effusions: efficiency of this method in the diagnosis of pleural effusions. Respiration 1994; 61:330–335.
51. Rijken A, Dekker A, Taylor S, Hoffman P, Blank M, Krause J. Diagnostic value of DNA analysis in effusions by post-cytometry and image analysis. Am J Clin Pathol 1991; 95:6–12.
52. Sheibani K, Esteban J, Bailey A, Battifora H, Wiess L. Immunopathologic and molecular studies as an aid in the diagnosis of malignant mesothelioma. Hum Pathol 1992; 23:107–116.
53. Shield PW, Callan JJ, Devine PL. Markers for metastatic adenocarcinoma in serous effusion specimens. Diagn Cytol 1994; 11:237–245.
54. Mezger J, Stotzer O, Schilli G, Bauer S, Wilmanns W. Identification of carcinomas cells in acidic and pleural fluid: comparison of 4 panepithelial antigens with carcinoembryonic antigen. Acta Cytol 1992; 36:758–781.
55. Light RW, Stansbury DW, Brown SE. The relationship between pleural pressures and changes in pulmonary function after therapeutic thoracentesis. Am Rev Respir Dis 1986; 133:658–661.
56. Sprung CL, Loewenherz JW, Baier H, Hauser JM. Evidence of increased permeability in re-expansion pulmonary edema. Am J Med 1981; 71:497–500.
57. Black LF. The pleural space and pleural fluid. Mayo Clin Proc 1972; 47:493–506.
58. Lai-Fook SJ. Mechanics of the pleural space: fundamental concepts. Lung 1987; 165:249–267.
59. Doelken P, Sahn SA. Trapped lung. Semin Respir Crit Care Med 2001; 22:631–635.
60. Villena V, Lopez-Encuentra A, Pozo F, De-Pablo A, Martin-Escribano P. Measurement of pleural pressure during therapeutic thoracentesis. Am J Respir Crit Care Med 2000; 162:1534–1538.
61. Light RW, Jenkinson SG, Minh V-D, George RB. Observations on pleural fluid pressures as fluid is withdrawn during thoracentesis. Am Rev Respir Dis 1980; 121:799–804.
62. Lan R, Singh KL, Chuang M, Yang C-T, Tsao TC-Y, Lee C-H. Elastance of the pleural space: a predictor for the outcome of pleurodesis in patients with malignant effusion. Ann Intern Med 1997; 126:768–774.

63. Livingston RV, McCracken JD, Trauth CJ, Chen T. Isolated pleural effusion in small cell lung cancer: favorable prognosis. Chest 1982; 81:208–210.
64. Fentiman IS, Reubens RD, Hayward JL. Control of pleural effusions in a patient with breast cancer. Cancer 1983; 52:737–739.
65. Lees AW, Hoy W. Management of pleural effusions in breast cancer. Chest 1979; 75:51–53.
66. Poe RH, Qazi R, Israel RH, Wichs CM, Reubins JM. Survival of patients with pleural involvement by breast carcinoma. Am J Clin Oncol 1983; 6:523–527.
67. Xaubet A, Diumenjo MC, Masin A, Montserrat E, Estopa R, Llebaria C, Austi A, Rozman C. Characteristics and prognostic value of pleural effusions in non-Hodgkin's lymphomas. Eur J Respir Dis 1985; 6:135–140.
68. Murphy MC, Newman BM, Rodgers BM. Pleuroperitoneal shunts in the management of persistent chylothorax. Ann Thorac Surg 1989; 48:195–200.
69. Walker-Renard PB, Vaughan LM, Sahn SA. Chemical pleurodesis for malignant pleural effusions. Ann Intern Med 1994; 120:56–64.
70. Hamed H, Fentiman IS, Chaudary MA, Reubens DS. Comparison of intracavitary bleomycin and talc for control of pleural effusions secondary to carcinoma of the breast. Br J Surg 1989; 76:1266–1267.
71. Hartman DL, Gaither JM, Kesler MA, Mylet DM, Brown JW, Mathur PN. Comparison of insufflated talc under thoracoscopic guidance with standard tetracycline and bleomycin pleurodesis for control of malignant pleural effusions. J Thorac Cariovasc Surg 1993; 105:743–748.
72. Fentiman IS, Reubens RD, Hayward JL. A comparison of intracavitary talc and tetracycline for the control of pleural effusions secondary to breast cancer. Eur J Cancer Clin Oncol 1986; 22:1079–1081.
73. Kennedy L, Sahn SA. Talc pleurodesis for the treatment of pneumothorax and pleural effusion. Chest 1994; 106:1215–1222.
74. Yim AP, Chan AT, Lee TW, Wan IY, Ho JK. Thoracoscopic talc insufflation versus talc slurry for symptomatic malignant pleural effusions. Ann Thorac Surg 1996; 62:1655–1658.
75. Kennedy L, Rusch VW, Strange C, Ginsberg RJ, Sahn SA. Pleurodesis using talc slurry. Chest 1994; 106:342–346.
76. Sahn SA. Talc should be used for pleurodesis. Am J Respir Crit Care Med 2001; 62:2024–2025.
77. Viallat J-R, Rey F, Astoul P, Boutin C. Thoracoscopic talc poudrage pleurodesis for malignant effusions. A review of 360 cases. Chest 1996; 110:1387–1393.
78. Campos JR, Werebe EC, Vargas FS, Jatene FB, Light RW. Respiratory failure due to insufflated talc. Lancet 1997; 349:251–252.
79. Petrou M, Kaplan D, Goldstraw P. Management of recurrent malignant pleural effusions. The complementary role of talc pleurodesis and pleuroperitoneal shunting. Cancer 1995; 75:801–805.
80. Weissberg D, Ben-Zeev I. Talc pleurodesis: experience with 360 patients. J Thorac Cardiovasc Surg 1993; 106:689–695.
81. Rehse DH, Aye RW, Florence MG. Respiratory failure following talc pleurodesis. Am J Surg 1999; 177:437–440.
82. de Campos JRM, Vargas FS, de Campos Werebe E, Cardoso P, Teixeira LR, Jatene FB, Light RW. Thoracoscopy talc poudrage. A 15-year experience. Chest 2001; 119:801–806.
83. Glazer MM, Berkman N, Lafair JS, Kramer MR. Successful talc slurry

pleurodesis in patients with non-malignant pleural effusion. Report of 16 cases and review of the literature. Chest 2000; 117:1404–1409.
84. Sudduth CD, Sahn SA. Pleurodesis for nonmalignant pleural effusions; recommendations. Chest 1992; 102:1855–1860.
85. Cardillo G, Facciolo F, Guinti R, Gasparri R, Lopergolo M, Orsetti R, Martelli M. Videothoracoscopic treatment of primary spontaneous pneumothorax: a six year experience. Ann Thorac Surg 2000; 69:357–362.
86. Mares DC, Mathur PN. Medical thoracoscopic talc pleurodesis for chylothorax due to lymphoma. Chest 1998; 114:731–735.
87. Rinaldo JE, Owens GR, Rodgers RM. Adult respiratory distress syndrome following intrapleural instillation of talc. J Thorac Cardiovasc Surg 1983; 85:523–526.
88. Bouchama A, Chastre J, Gaudichet A, Soler P, Gibert C. Acute pneumonitis with bilateral pleural effusion after talc pleurodesis. Chest 1984; 86:795–797.
89. Lineau C, Le Coz A, Quinquenel ML, Le Tulzo Y, Kernec J, Delaval P. Acute respiratory insufficiency after pleural talcage of pneumothorax. Apropos of a case. Rev Pneumol Clin 1993; 49:153–155.
90. Ferrer J, Villarino MA, Tura JM, Traveria J, Light RW. Comparison of size and composition of nine different talcs. Its relevance for pleurodesis. Am J Respir Crit Care Med 1998; 157A:A66.
91. Shaffer JP, Allen JN, Prior RB. Detection of endotoxin in talc preparations used for pleurodesis. Chest 2000; 118:130.
92. Chappell AG, Johnson A, Charles WJ, Seal RME, Berry G, Nicholson D. A survey of the long-term effects of talc in kaolin pleurodesis. Br J Dis Chest 1979; 73:285–288.
93. Lange P, Mortensen J, Groth S. Lung function 22–25 years after treatment of idiopathic spontaneous pneumothorax with talc poudrage with simple drainage. Thorax 1988; 43:559–561.
94. Viskum K, Lange P, Mortensen J. Long-term sequelae after talc. Pneumonolige 1989; 43:105–106.
95. Paul JS, Geatiee EJ, Blades B. Lung function studies in poudrage treatment of recurrent spontaneous pneumothorax. J Thorac Surg 1951; 22:52–61.
96. Knowles JH, Storey CF. Effects of talc poudrage on pulmonary function. J Thorac Surg 1957; 340:250–256.
97. Kleinfeld M, Messite J, Kooyman O, Zaki MH. Mortality among talc miners and millers in New York State. Arch Environ Health 1967; 14:663–667.
98. Good JT Jr, Taryle DA, Sahn SA. The pathogenesis of low glucose, low pH malignant effusions. Am Rev Respir Dis 1985; 131:737–741.
99. Heffner JE, Nietert PJ, Barbieri C. Pleural fluid pH as a predictor of survival of patients with malignant pleural effusions. Chest 2000; 117:79–86.
100. Heffner JE, Nietert PJ, Barbieri C. Pleural fluid pH as a predictor of pleurodesis failure. Chest 2000; 117:87–95.
101. Walsh FW, Alberts M, Solomon DA, Goldman AL. Malignant pleural effusions: pleurodesis using small-bore catheter. So Med J 1989; 82:963–972.
102. Parker LA, Charnock GC, Delany DJ. Small-bore catheter drainage and sclerotherapy for malignant effusions. Cancer 1989; 64:1218–1221.
103. Morrison MC, Mueller PR, Lee MJ, Saini S, Brink JA, Dawson SL. Sclerotherapy of malignant pleural effusion through sonographically placed small-bore catheters. AJR 1992; 158:41–43.

104. Goff BA, Mueller PR, Muntz HG, Rice LW. Small chest-tube drainage followed by bleomycin sclerosis from malignant pleural effusions. Obstet Gynecol 1993; 84:993–996.
105. Seaton KG, Patz EF Jr, Goodman PC. Palliative treatment of malignant pleural effusions: value of small-bore catheter thoracostomy and doxycycline sclerotherapy. AJR 1995; 164:589–591.
106. Patz EF Jr, McAdams HP, Goodman PC, Blackwell S. Ambulatory sclerotherapy for malignant pleural effusions. Radiology 1996; 199:133–135.
107. Hsu WH, Chiang CD, Chen CY, Kwan PC, Hsu JY. Ultrasound-guided small-bore Elecath tube insertion for the rapid sclerotherapy of malignant pleural effusion. Jpn J Clin Oncol 1998; 28:187–191.
108. Patz EF Jr, McAdams HP, Erasmus JJ, Goodman PC, Culhane DK, Gilkeson RC, Herndon J. Sclerotherapy for malignant pleural effusions. A prospective randomized trial of bleomycin versus doxycycline with small-bore catheter drainage. Chest 1998; 113:1305–1311.
109. Thompson RL, Yau JC, Donnelly RF, Gowan DJ, Matzinger FR. Pleurodesis with iodized talc for malignant effusions using pigtail catheters. Ann Pharmacother 1998; 32:739–742.
110. Marom EM, Patz EF Jr, Erasmus JJ, McAdams HP, Goodman PC, Herndon JE. Malignant pleural effusions. Treatment with small-bore-catheter thoracostomy and talc pleurodesis. Radiology 1992; 210:277–281.
111. Bloom AI, Wilson MW, Kerlan RK Jr, Gordon RL, LaBerge JM. Talc pleurodesis through small-bore percutaneous tubes. Cardiovasc Interv Radiol 1999; 22:433–438.
112. Saffran L, Ost DE, Fein AM, Schiff MJ. Outpatient pleurodesis of malignant pleural effusions using a small-bore pigtail catheter. Chest 2000; 118:417–421.
113. Lorch BG, Gordon L, Wooten S, Cooper JF, Strange C, Sahn SA. The effect of patient positioning on the distribution of tetracycline of pleural space during pleurodesis. Chest 1988; 93:527–529.
114. Dryzer S, Allen ML, Strange C, Sahn SA. A comparison of rotation and non-rotation in tetracycline pleurodesis. Chest 1993; 104:1763–1766.
115. van den Heuvel MM, Smit HJ, Barbierato SB, Havenith CE, Beelen RH, Postmus PE. Talc-induced inflammation in the pleural cavity. Eur Respir J 1998; 12:1419–1423.
116. Villaneuva AG, Gray AW Jr, Shahian DM, Williamson WA, Beamis JF Jr. Efficacy of short-term versus long-term tube thoracostomy drainage of tetracycline pleurodesis in the treatment of malignant pleural effusions. Thorax 1994; 49:23–25.
117. Lambert CJ, Shah HH, Urshel HC Jr, Paulson DL. Treatment of malignant pleural effusions by closed trocar tube drainage. Ann Thorac Surg 1967; 3:1–5.
118. Anderson CB, Philpott GW, Ferguson TB. The treatment of malignant pleural effusions. Cancer 1974; 33:916–922.
119. Izbicki R, Weyhing BT III, Baker L, Caoili EM, Vaitkevicius VK. Pleural effusion in cancer patients. A prospective randomized study of pleural drainage with the addition of radioactive phosphorus to the pleural space versus pleural drainage alone. Cancer 1975; 36:1511–1518.
120. Sorensen PG, Svendsen TL, Enk B. Treatment of malignant pleural effusion with drainage with and without instillation of talc. Eur J Respir Dis 1984; 65:131–135.
121. Groth G, Gatzemeier U, Haussigen K, Heckmayr M, Magnussen H, Neuhauss

R, Pavel JV. Intrapleural palliative treatment of malignant pleural effusion with mitoxantrone versus placebo (pleural tube alone). Ann Oncol 1991; 2:213–215.
122. Putnam JB Jr, Light RW, Rodrigues RM, Ponn R, Olak J, Pollak JS, Lee RB, Payne DK, Graeber G, Kovitz KL. A randomized comparison of indwelling pleural catheter and doxycycline pleurodesis in the management of malignant pleural effusions. Cancer 1999; 86:1992–1999.
123. Putnam JB Jr, Walsh GL, Swisher SG, Roth JA, Suell DM, Vaporciyan AA, Smythe WR, Merriman KW, DeFord LL. Outpatient management of malignant pleural effusion by chronic indwelling pleural catheter. Ann Thorac Surg 2000; 69:369–375.
124. Rheuban KS, Kron IL, Carpenter MA, Gutgesell HP, Rodgers BM. Pleuroperitoneal shunts for refractory chylothorax after operation for congenital disease. Ann Thorac Surg 1992; 53:85–87.
125. Martini N, Bains M, Beattie EJ Jr. Indications for pleurectomy in malignant effusions. Chest 1975; 35:734–738.
126. Fry WA, Khandekar JD. Parietal pleurectomy for malignant pleural effusion. Ann Thorac Oncol 1995; 2:160–164.
127. Waller DA, Morritt GN, Forty J. Video-assisted thoracoscopic pleurectomy in the management of malignant pleural effusion. Chest 1995; 107:1454–1456.

24

Pleural Effusion in Lung Carcinoma

MARIOS E. FROUDARAKIS

University of Crete Medical School
and University Hospital of Heraklion
Heraklion, Crete, Greece

PIERRE FOURNEL

University Hospital of Saint-Etienne
Saint-Etienne, France

I. Introduction

Carcinoma of the lung is the most common cause of malignant pleural effusion. The incidence of pleural effusion due to lung carcinoma was reported in 641 cases out of 1783 patients (36%), while the second most common cause was breast carcinoma in 449 cases (25%) (1). The incidence of pleural effusion in patients with lung carcinoma ranges between 7% (280 of 4000 cases) (2) and 23% (5,888 of 25,464 cases) (3). All histological types of bronchogenic carcinomas are likely to present pleural effusion (3). However, the most frequent histological type seems to be adenocarcinoma, in about 40% of the cases, as it is more likely to arise in the periphery next to the pleura, which may be invaded by the tumor. The second most common tumor is small-cell lung carcinoma, a tumor with highly invasive potential, accounting for about 25% of the cases (3,4).

Pleural effusion is mostly diagnosed by a simple chest radiograph and/or computed tomography (CT). In lung cancer, its presence is associated with advanced stage disease and therefore with poor prognosis (5). However in some cases, pleural effusion is due to postobstructive pneumonia or atelectasis, venous obstruction by tumor compression, or lymphatic obstruction by mediastinal lymph nodes, and is not associated with direct pleural involvement (6). In the case of negative pleural cytology, medical or surgical video-assisted thoracoscopy (VATS) must be performed in order to evaluate the extension of the disease and prove the possible malignant infiltration of the pleura (7).

439

II. Pathogenesis

The occurrence of pleural effusion in malignancy is mainly due to an obstacle of lymphatic drainage from the pleural space, such as pleural thickening by widespread carcinomatosis, obstruction caused by infiltration of mediastinal lymph nodes, or obstruction caused by tumor emboli (4,8,9). Local response with inflammatory reaction to tumors next to the pleura might play an important role in pleural effusion development by increasing capillary permeability (10). These mechanisms explain the existence of lymphocyte predominance in malignant pleural effusion, although their role is still unclear. Some authors believe that T lymphocytes have an important role in host-versus-tumor local defense in malignant pleural effusions (11).

Pathogenetic mechanisms of pleural effusion due to lung carcinoma have been reported in postmortem studies (4,8). Most of the patients have both parietal and visceral pleura infiltration. It has been shown that invasion of parietal pleura is due to neoplastic spread across the pleural cavity from visceral pleural sites along pleural adhesions that are preformed or secondary to the malignant process. Also, parietal pleura is invaded by the attachment of exfoliated cells from the visceral pleura. Visceral pleura might be invaded primarily by pulmonary arterial invasion and embolization (4,8).

When the tumor infiltrates blood vessels directly and/or occludes venules, a bloody pleural effusion may occur. Another mechanism of hemorrhagic pleural effusion might be capillary dilatation due to vasoactive substances (8,9). Bilateral pleural metastases from lung carcinoma are due to hematogenous spread to the contralateral hemithorax secondary to the presence of liver metastases (8). Non-malignant pleural effusions (paramalignant) may occur due to bronchial obstruction causing atelectasis or pneumonia with parapneumonic effusion, due to mechanical, obstruction without malignant cell infiltration of lymphatics or blood vessels. Lung carcinoma is also frequently associated with heart failure, as both bronchogenic carcinoma and heart disease have the same terrain of occurrence. The same finding is observed in patients associating bronchogenic carcinoma with hepatic insufficiency. Cases also report the association of pulmonary embolism and pneumothorax (12) in patients with bronchogenic carcinoma.

III. Diagnostic Approach

Pleural effusion in patients with lung carcinoma may be present in two situations: as a presenting syndrome revealing, during the work up an unknown previously lung carcinoma, or as a pleural effusion in the evolution of a known carcinoma. The diagnostic approach, although basically the same, must be specific to each case according to the patient's prognosis relies on.

In the first case, a pleural effusion is discovered after the patient consults his physician for worsening progressively dyspnea, dry cough, lateral thoracic pain, or hemoptysis. General symptoms may be associated, such as fever, weight loss, loss of appetite and restriction of the daily activity (13–15). About 25% of patients are totally asymptomatic, and pleural effusion is discovered after a routine chest radiograph (15,16). Typically on physical examination a pleural syndrome is confirmed by chest radiograph, which shows the extent of the pleural effusion (13–15).

Pleural effusion may be free-flowing or loculated (17). The chest radiograph may also show the cause of the pleural effusion, such as peripheral lesion in contact with the thoracic wall, central lesion with atelectasis, or obstructive pneumonia (Fig. 1) (18,19). It also provides useful information about associated findings, such as pericardial effusion, air in the pleural space, and mediastinal lymph node enlargement (17–19). In 15% of cases, chest radiograph is negative because of the location of the tumor (in the pleural effusion and/or cardiac, and/or diaphragmatic shadows, endobronchial). A profile chest radiograph must be performed in order to help diagnosis (17).

Spontaneous pneumothorax may be a rare manifestation of lung cancer. It has been estimated that air in the pleural space occurs in 1% of patients with lung cancer (12,20,21). Also, lung cancer causes only about 0.05% of cases of

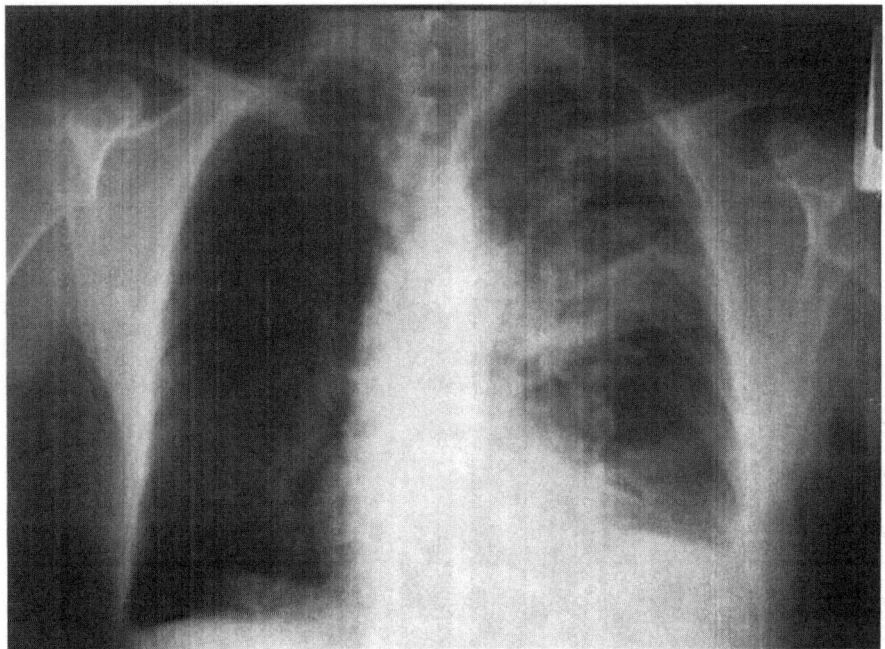

Figure 1 Chest radiograph showing pleural effusion with ventilation defects of the upper and lower lobes due to central (hilar) obstruction.

pneumothorax (20). Pneumothorax may develop as a complication of bronchopleural fistula du to both pleural and bronchial infiltration from the tumor, of peripheral necrotizing tumor invading the pleura, or of obstructive hyperinflation due to central obstruction (20,21). In most cases pneumothorax occurs when lung cancer is at an advanced stage (21).

Pleural extension must also be assessed by chest (5,22). Chest CT is sensitive in recognizing pleural effusion (Fig. 2), but cannot identify its possible malignant nature (22,23). However, some patterns may indicate malignancy, such as a thickness of the pleura >1 cm, indicating pleural carcinomatosis (24). Controversy exists as to whether CT is useful in identifying associated findings missed by the standard chest radiograph, such as a peripheral nodule and/or mass infiltrating the thoracic wall, the diaphragm, or the mediastinum (23,25,26), as soft tissue swelling may be due to inflammation and/or fibrosis rather than direct infiltration (27). It seems that focal chest pain is more accurate than chest CT in predicting chest wall invasion (28). However, the presence of these findings may be indicative of the malignant nature of the pleural effusion (21,24,28).

Magnetic resonance imaging (MRI) is less sensitive than CT in recognizing pleural effusion (22,29). On T1-weighted images the signal from the fluid

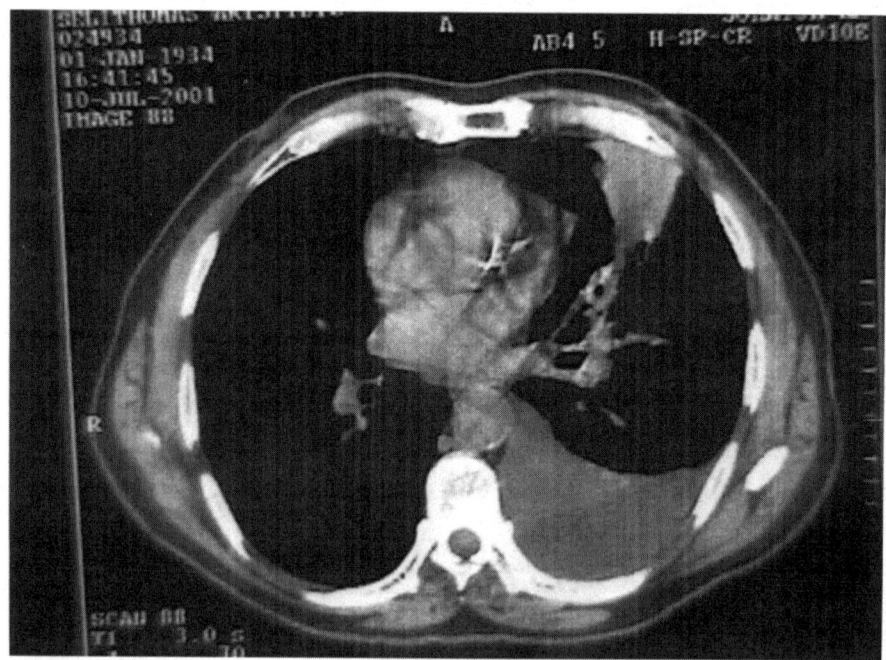

Figure 2 Chest computed tomography (mediastinal window) showing pleural effusion associated to obstructive mass and peripheral pneumonia.

is very low and may not be detected, although characteristic brightening on T2-weighted images allows detection (29,30). In addition, MRI has the same problems as CT in recognizing chest wall, mediastinal, pericardial, or diaphragmatic infiltration (23,29,30).

Ultrasound (US) is another noninvasive method to investigate the pleura. Although its major indication is loculated pleural effusions mostly due to infection, it may be helpful in patients with low performance status who are unable to perform a more sophisticated examination, such as CT of the thorax (31,32). Ultrasound sensitivity in case of pleural effusion is 92% alone, and combined with the standard chest radiograph is 98% (32,33). It also helps in the diagnosis of associated findings, such as pleural thickness, pleural or subpleural tumors, and parenchymal masses (34).

Diagnosis of lung cancer pleural effusion can only be made by finding cancer cells in the pleural fluid, as in any other malignant pleural effusion. Cytological examination of pleural fluid taken after thoracentesis is the first step in the diagnosis of pleural effusion (1,6). Cytologists face two major problems: proving the malignant origin of the pleural effusion by the existence of malignant cells and proving the organ of origin of those malignant cells. Thus, the diagnostic accuracy of cytological examination of the pleural fluid varies from series to series. It is very low for some authors, ranging from 15 to 35% (35,36), but very high for others, ranging from 80 to 90% (3,37). The blind pleural biopsy has results similar to those of pleural cytology (36).

Leukocytes in the malignant pleural fluid are relatively low, with mean values ranging from 2000 to 2500 cells/μL, with a huge range (1,9). While the total amount of leukocytes is not helpful in differential diagnosis, the type is important, as in malignant pleural effusions we find lymphocytes at a rate of >50% (9,11). Neutrophils usually represent 25% (1), while eosinophils are low (7–10%) (38,39). Other nucleated cells may be found, such as macrophages and mesothelial cells. Erythrocytes average about 4,0000–50,000 cells/μL, also with a wide range, from none to hemothorax (9,37).

When the pleural puncture shows no malignant cells and lung carcinoma is highly suspected, it is reasonable to perform fiberoptic bronchoscopy, since it may help in diagnosis (40). Indeed, pleural effusion of unknown origin after initial work-up is associated with bronchogenic carcinoma in about 30% of cases (40,41). Fiberoptic bronchoscopy is also useful in assessing the extent of the disease in the tracheobronchial tree, which is important for treatment and prognosis (40).

Thoracoscopy is a simple and safe method for the diagnosis of the cause of pleural effusion (42,43) and the assessment of the extent of lung carcinoma (7,44,45). Its sensitivity ranges from 92 to 97% (46,47) and its specificity from 99 to 100% (44,46,47) in patients with malignant pleural effusion. If thoracentesis is negative and there is suspicion of lung cancer, thoracoscopy can be performed to diagnose and to detect localized or diffused pleural infiltration, determining of non–small-cell lung carcinoma (NSCLC) T4 disease, which precludes surgical resection (7,48).

Several series have been published, showing the utility of thoracoscopy in staging NSCLC. Generally these series confirm the low rate of resectability, ranging from 0% (7) to 36% (2), and therefore the poor prognosis in patients with lung cancer and pleural effusion. Many patients, even with paramalignant pleural effusions, may be unresectable, due to the extent of the intrathoracic tumor. However, the role of thoracoscopy in lung cancer staging is limited. As thoracoscopy allows only unilateral examination, it cannot determine N3 disease and is unlikely to have an important role in distinguishing between T3 and T4 disease (48). Thus, some authors propose pleural lavage before surgical resection, even in cases without pleural effusion, since positive cytology indicates exfoliation of cancer cells in the pleural cavity and a more aggressive tumor. Positive cytological findings should be interpreted as a subclinical pleural effusion that is pathological stage T4 disease with poor prognosis (49,50).

The chemistry of pleural fluid has been the subject of many reports in patients with malignancy. There is nothing specific in pleural fluid chemistry data of patients with lung carcinoma compared to those with metastatic malignancy to the pleura (1,51). Thus, as in other malignant pleural effusions, we expect an exudative fluid, with protein concentration >3 g/dL (or pleural-to-serum protein ratio >0.5) and levels of lactate dehydrogenase (LDH) >200 IU/L (or pleural-to-serum LDH ratio >0.6) (52,53). In about 30% of the cases pH is 7.30 and glucose levels 0.6 mg/dL (or the ratio of pleural to serum glucose <0.5) (53–57). On rare occasions pleural fluid is a transudate due to associated diseases such as congestive heart failure, atelectasis from bronchial obstruction, or hypoalbuminemia (9,51). Exudate-transudate tests are not pathognomonic, but provide a probabilistic statement as to the likely nature of a pleural effusion (58).

Several tumor markers, such as carcinoembryonic antigen (CEA), CA-125, CA-19-9, CYFRA 21-1, and NSE, have been tested in patients with malignant pleural effusion (59,60,61). Although results seem to be controversial as to the usefulness of these tumor markers in the differential diagnosis of pleural effusions, even between malignant and nonmalignant, some authors propose specific tumor markers for the diagnosis of pleural effusions due to bronchogenic carcinoma (62,63). A reasonable attitude may be that tests should be performed in a selected population of patients with negative cytology and "suspect" clinical outcome (64). Recently a number of reports have been emerged, studying various novel markers, such as oncogenes (65), cytokines involved in inflammation (66), and matrix metalloproteinases (67), in differential diagnosis and prognosis of malignant pleural effusions. Until now, none of these markers proved useful even in differentiating malignant from benign pleural effusions. Generally, biochemical or biological markers in malignant pleural effusions, as well as in serum, cannot replace routine cytopathological examination in the diagnosis of disease and predict the outcome of the patient without firm diagnosis (68).

To finalize a diagnostic approach in patients with pleural effusion and suspected lung cancer, major investigations include cytopathological examination from pleural puncture or thoracoscopy in the case of failure and fiberoptic bronchoscopy. These examinations will also be useful in staging the disease and prognosis or will call for further investigations in the case of lung cancer exclusion.

IV. Therapeutic Approach

When a patient with pleural effusion due to lung carcinoma is diagnosed, one should consider certain parameters in order to decide upon treatment: the patient's performance status, the cell type of the lung carcinoma, the extent of the disease, the patient's expected survival, the patient's symptoms, needs, and quality of life before and after therapy. All of the above questions must be considered in each patient individually before treatment initiation.

An important point is the patient's performance status (69,70). Also important is the histological type of the bronchogenic carcinoma (71) and the stage of the disease (5). Surgical resection is the therapy of choice in NSCLC patients with pleural effusion and good performance status after repeated negative cytological specimen of the pleural fluid and negative thoracoscopy (7,45,72). Resectability rate of patients with NSCLC and pleural effusion is low, even after exploratory thoracotomy (2,7,45,72). This is due to the low rate of confirmed non-malignant pleural effusion and to the extent of the tumor in the chest wall, the mediastinum, and the mediastinal lymph nodes. Neoadjuvant chemotherapy in such patients has resulted in tumor response and longer survival of patients with IIIA disease (73–75), and it is now under investigation in patients with stage I-II NSCLC (76).

Postsurgical chemotherapeutic treatment is also under investigation (77,78), while postsurgical irradiation is not indicated since PORT meta-analysis showed a detrimental effect on survival of patients who received adjuvant radiotherapy (79). Results of adjuvant combination chemotherapy and radiation therapy are also controversial in patients who underwent combined treatment (80–82).

In patients with SCLC and malignant pleural effusion, the treatment of choice is systemic chemotherapy (83), since untreated patients lived only 4–6 months (84). Some authors support that survival and disease-free interval of patients with ipsilateral malignant pleural effusion and SCLC seem to be identical of those with limited disease without pleural effusion (85,86). They suggest that these patients should benefit from the same treatment as those having limited stage disease (86). However, it is generally accepted that these patients have worse survival than limited stage patients, therefore they are not included in clinical trials of limited disease.

When a malignant pleural effusion is present in a patient with NSCLC, surgical resection is not possible since the patient has stage IIIB disease (5). Systemic chemotherapy is indicated in unresectable NSCLC of good performance status, since meta-analysis has shown its benefits versus best supportive care (87,88). However, despite chemotherapy, survival of patients with IIIB disease and pleural effusion is poor, ranging from 6.9 (89) to 12 months (90). Even the new chemotherapeutic agents have not yet proven beneficial for survival in large phase III trials (91,92), despite a better response rate reported in phase II trials (93–95). Although the good response rate does not mean necessarily better survival in patients with NSCLC who underwent systemic chemotherapy, this response may be translated in gain of quality of life (80,87,88), especially in case of pleural effusion, with improvement of dyspnea (96).

Radiation therapy in pleural effusion is not indicated, since it did not prove beneficial in response rate in survival (97–99). However, in some cases the combination of irradiation with chemotherapeutic agents as radiosensitizers (100) or as multimodality treatment associating concomitant or alternating chemotherapy and irradiation may offer local control (97,101–103).

Quality of life in cancer patients is an important factor in treatment (104,105). Dyspnea is a frequent and devastating symptom among advanced cancer patients and is often difficult to control (96). Lung cancer patients with dyspnea have shorter survival than patients with other types of cancer. Palliative care assessment should be focused on dyspnea (96). We should consider pleurodesis in patients with significant and/or invalidating pleural effusion whose general condition is good and whose the expected survival is prolonged (51,106,107). Pleurodesis may be followed by systemic chemotherapy, if necessary, in order to palliate lung carcinoma. Several modalities of pleurodesis are possible, such as chemical pleurodesis through a simple thoracic drain tube or during medical thoracoscopy, VATS, thoracoscopic or surgical pleural abrasion, or pleurectomy (107,108).

Criteria for successful pleurodesis are reexpandable lung and complete removal of the pleural fluid (<100 mL drainage/24 h). Although low pleural fluid pH (<7.20) may indicate trapped lung, short expected survival, and ineffective pleurodesis (107,109,110), Aelony et al. reported that thoracoscopic talc poudrage was successful in 88% of patients with malignant pleural effusion despite low pH (111).

The choice of sclerosing agent has been the subject of many publications. More than 30 agents have been proposed as sclerosants to induce pleurodesis (1,6,107,108). Cyclins (doxycycline, minocycline, tetracycline hydrochloride) are instilled intrapleurally in a saline solution through a chest tube (112–114). Their effectiveness in malignant pleural effusion ranges from 25% (115) to 88% (116). Their advantages are the mild and rare side effects (chest pain, fever) and low cost. Tetracycline is no longer available, but minocycline and doxycycline are good alternatives (117,118).

Bleomycine has a success rate comparable to cyclins, ranging from 35% (115) to 90%, with the same side effects. However, the cost of pleurodesis with bleomycin was estimated at about 80 times the cost of talc slurry (119). New cytostatics instilled in the pleura such as taxans have also been used as sclerosing agents (120). Antimitotic drugs have been used not only for pleurodesis, but also to locally treat the underlying disease (121). However, the toxicity and current high cost of the use of cytostatics considerably limits their utilization (122–125).

Talc is most commonly used, as it is the most effective (> 90% success rate) and inexpensive agent for pleurodesis in malignant pleural effusions (1,106–108,126,127). Administration of talc in the pleura may be performed through a chest tube diluted in a saline solution (talc slurry) (117,119) or as aerosolized powder during medical (6,47,48,128–131) or surgical thoracoscopy (132,133). Both methods seem to be effective (median success rate 90%), although it seems that thoracoscopic method has advantages (111,122,126,134–137).

Side effects of talc are not different from those of other agents. Some authors do not recommend talc for pleurodesis as cases of respiratory insufficiency have been reported (138–140). However, various biases exist, explaining in a part the respiratory complications from talc such as the patient's poor performance status, respiratory comorbidities (COPD), and the extent of the pleural effusion, suggesting that the earlier pleurodesis is performed, the lower the frequency of occurrence of such manifestations (141). Another important point is the choice of the right powder in the right dose, suggesting that respiratory complications may be avoided (127). Talc is also the least expensive agent for pleurodesis currently available (122,123,127,142). *Corynebacterium parvum* injected intrapleurally without chest tube drainage has been tested as a sclerosing agent with good results and no specific side effects (143,144). Other compounds used as sclerosing agents are interferon (145) and quinacrine (146). Pleural abrasion by gauze may be an alternative when no talc is available. The method is performed during medical or surgical thoracoscopy, which requires a knowledge of the procedure (132,134,138). Pleurectomy may also be an alternative (144,147,148), but this method is aggressive in patients with advanced malignancy, considering the great number of noninvasive chemical pleurodesis possibilities.

References

1. Sahn SA. Malignancy metastatic to the pleura. Clin Chest Med 1998; 19:351–361.
2. Le Roux BT. Bronchial Carcinoma. London: E&S Livingstone.
3. Johnston WW. The malignant pleural effusion. A review of cytopathologic diagnoses of 584 specimens from 472 consecutive patients. Cancer 1985; 56:905–909.
4. Rodriguez-Panadero F, Borderas Naranjo F, Lopez Mejias J. Pleural metastatic tumours and effusions. Frequency and pathogenic mechanisms in a post-mortem series. Eur Respir J 1989; 2:366–369.
5. Mountain CF. Revisions for the international system for staging lung cancer. Chest 1997; 111:1710–1717.
6. Antony VB, Loddenkemper R, Astoul P, Boutin C, Goldstraw P, Hott J, Rodriguez-Panadero F, Sahn A. Management of malignant pleural effusions. Eur Respir J 2001; 18:402–419.
7. Rodriguez Panadero F. Lung cancer and ipsilateral pleural effusion. Ann Oncol 1995; 6(suppl 3):25–27.

8. Meyer PC. Metastatic carcinoma of the pleura. Thorax 1966; 21:437–443.
9. Chernow B, Sahn SA. Carcinomatous involvement of the pleura: an analysis of 96 patients. Am J Med 1977; 63:695–702.
10. Leff A, Hopewell PC, Costello J. Pleural effusion from malignancy. Ann Intern Med 1978; 88:532–537.
11. Domagala W, Emeson E, Kass LG. Distribution of T-lymphocytes and B-lymphocytes in peripheral blood and effusions in patients with cancer. J Natl Cancer Inst 1978; 61:295–301.
12. Kabnick EM, Sobo S, Steinbaum S, Alexander LL, Nkongho A. Spontaneous pneumothorax from bronchogenic carcinoma. J Natl Med Assoc 1982; 74:478–479.
13. Hyde L, Hyde CI. Clinical manifestations of lung cancer. Chest 1974; 65:299–306.
14. Cohen MH. Signs and symptoms of bronchogenic carcinoma. Semin Oncol 1974; 1:183–189.
15. Scagliotti GV. Symptoms and signs and staging of lung cancer. Eur Respir Mon 1995; 1:91–136.
16. Grippi MA. Clinical aspects of lung cancer. Semin Roentgenol 1990; 25:12–24.
17. White CS, Templeton PA, Belani CP. Imaging in lung cancer. Semin Oncol 1993; 20:142–152.
18. Romney BM, Austin JHM. Plain film evaluation of carcinoma of the lung. Semin Roentgenol 1990; 25:45–63.
19. Woodring JH. Pitfalls in the radiologic diagnosis of lung cancer. AJR Am J Roentgenol 1990; 154:1165–1175.
20. Steinhausling CA, Cuttat JF. Spontaneous pneumothorax a complication of lung cancer? Chest 1985; 88:709–713.
21. Woodring JH. Unusual radiographic manifestations of lung cancer. Radiol Clin North Am 1990; 28:599–618.
22. McLoud TC. CT and MRI in pleural space. Clin Chest Med 1998; 19:261–276.
23. Armstrong P, Reznek RH, Phillips RR. Diagnostic imaging of lung cancer. Eur Respir Mon 1995; 1:137–187.
24. Leung AN, Müller NL, Miller RR. CT in differential diagnosis of diffuse pleura disease. AJR Am J Roentgenol 1990; 154:487–492.
25. Glazer HS, Kaiser LR, Anderson DJ, Molina PL, Emami B, Roper CL, Sagel SS. Indeterminate mediastinal invasion in bronchogenic carcinoma: CT evaluation. Radiology 1989; 173:37–42.
26. Rato GB, Piacenza G, Frola C, Musante F, Serrano I, Giua R, Salio M, Jacovoni P, Rovida S. Chest wall involvement by lung cancer: computed tomography detection and results of operation. Ann Thorac Surg 1991; 51:182–188.
27. Pearlberg JL, Sandler MA, Beute GH. Limitations of CT in evaluation of neoplasms involving chest wall. J Comput Assist Tomogr 1987; 11:290–293.
28. Glazer HS, Duncan-Meyer J, Aronberg DJ, Moran JF, Levitt RG, Sagel SS. Pleural and chest wall invasion in bronchogenic carcinoma: CT evaluation. Radiology 1985; 157:191–194.
29. Webb WR. The role of magnetic resonance imaging in the assessment of patients with lung cancer. A comparison with computed tomography. J Thorac Imaging 1989; 4:65–75.
30. Templeton PA, Caskey CI, Zerhouni EA. Current uses of CT and MR imaging in the staging of lung cancer. Radiol Clin North Am 1990; 28:631–646.
31. O'Moore PV, Mueller PR, Simeone JF, Saini S, Butch RJ, Hahn PF, Steiner E,

Stark DD, Ferrucci JT Jr. Sonographic guidance in diagnostic and therapeutic interventions in the pleural space. AJR Am J Roentgenol 1987; 149:1–5.
32. Lipscomb DJ, Flower CD, Hadfield JW. Ultrasound of the pleural: an assessment of its clinical value. Clin Radiol 1981; 32:289–290.
33. Henschke CI, Davis SD, Romano PM, Yankelevitz DF. Pleural effusions: pathogenesis, radiologic evaluation and therapy. J Thorac Imag 1989; 4:49–60.
34. Yang PC, Luh KT, Chang DB, Wu HD, Yu CJ, Kuo SH. Value of sonography in determining the nature of pleural effusion: analysis of 320 cases. AJR Am J Roentgenol 1992; 159:29–33.
35. Storey DD, Dines DE, Coles DT. Pleural effusion: a diagnostic dilemma. JAMA 1976; 236:2183–2186.
36. Salyer WA, Eggleston JC, Erozan YS. Efficacy of pleural needle biopsy and pleural fluid cytopathology in the diagnosis of malignant neoplasm involving the pleura. Chest 1975; 67:536–538.
37. Light RW, Erozan YS, Ball WC. Cells in pleural fluid. Their value in differential diagnosis. Arch Intern Med 1973; 132:854–860.
38. Kuhn M, Fitting JW, Leuenberger P. Probability of malignancy in pleural fluid eosinophilia. Chest 1989; 96:992–994.
39. Rubins JB, Rubins HB. Etiology and prognostic significance of eosinophilic pleural effusions. A prospective study. Chest 1996; 110:1271–1274.
40. Vergnon JM, Froudarakis M. Bronchoscopy. In: Grassi C, ed. Pulmonary Diseases. London: McGraw-Hill International, 1999:39–43.
41. Poe RH, Levy PC, Israel RH, Ortiz CR, Kalley MC. Use of fiberoptic bronchoscopy in the diagnosis of bronchogenic carcinoma. A study in patients with idiopathic pleural effusions. Chest 1994; 105:1663–1667.
42. Mathur PN, Astoul P, Boutin C. Medical thoracoscopy: technical details. Clin Chest Med 1995; 16:479–486.
43. Boutin C, Astoul P. Diagnostic thoracoscopy. Clin Chest Med 1998; 19:295–309.
44. Roeslin N, Kessler R. Quelle est la place de la thoracoscopie dans le bilan d'extension pré-opératoire du cancer bronchique non à petites cellules? Rev Mal Respir 1992; 9:R247–R251.
45. Canto A, Ferrer G, Romagosa V, Moya J, Bernat R. Lung cancer and pleural effusion. Clinical significance and study of pleural metastatic locations. Chest 1985; 87:649–652.
46. Boutin C, Viallat JR, Cargnino P, Farisse P. Indications actuelles de la thoracoscopie. Compte rendu du Symposium de Marseille. Rev Fr Mal Respir 1981; 9:309–318.
47. Boutin C, Loddenkemper R, Astoul P. Diagnostic and therapeutic thoracoscopy: techniques and indications in pulmonary medicine. Tuberc Lung Dis 1993; 74:225–239.
48. Colt HG. Thoracoscopic management of malignant pleural effusions. Clin Chest Med 1995; 16:505–518.
49. Kjellberg SI, Dresler CM, Goldberg M. Pleural cytologies in lung cancer without pleural effusions. Ann Thorac Surg 1997; 64:941–944.
50. Okada M, Tsubota N, Yoshimura M, Miyamoto Y, Maniwa Y. Role of pleural lavage cytology before resection for primary lung carcinoma. Ann Surg 1999; 229:579–584.
51. Sahn SA. Pleural effusion in lung cancer. Clin Chest Med 1982; 3:443–452.

52. Light RW, Macgregor MI, Luchsinger PC, Ball WC Jr. Pleural effusions: the diagnostic separation of transudates and exudates. Ann Intern Med 1972; 77:507–513.
53. Light RW. Pleural Disease. 3rd ed. Baltimore: Williams & Wilkins, 1995:36–74.
54. Light RW, MacGregor MI, Ball WC Jr, Luchsinger PC. Diagnostic significance of pleural fluid pH and PCO_2. Chest 1973; 64:591–596.
55. Berger HW, Maher G. Decreased glucose concentration in malignant pleural effusions. Am Rev Respir Dis 1971; 103:427–429.
56. Chavalittamrong B, Angsusingha K, Tuchinda M, Habanananda S, Pidatcha P, Tuchinda C. Diagnostic significance of pH, lactic acid dehydrogenase, lactate and glucose in pleural fluid. Respiration 1979; 38:112–120.
57. Good JT Jr, Taryle DA, Sahn SA. The pathogenesis of low glucose, low pH malignant effusions. Am Rev Respir Dis 1985; 131:737–741.
58. Heffner JE. Evaluating diagnostic tests in the pleural space. Clin Chest Med 1998; 19:277–293.
59. Cascinu S, Del Ferro E, Barbanti I, Ligi M, Fedeli A, Catalano G. Tumor markers in the diagnosis of malignant serous effusions. Am J Clin Oncol 1997; 20:247–250.
60. Alatas F, Alatas O, Metintas M, Colak O, Harmanci E, Demir S. Diagnostic value of CEA, CA 15-3, CA 19-9, CYFRA 21-1, NSE and TSA assay in pleural effusions. Lung Cancer 2001; 31:9–16.
61. Miedouge M, Rouzaud P, Salama G, Pujazon MC, Vincent C, Mauduyt MA, Reyre J, Carles P, Serre G. Evaluation of seven tumour markers in pleural fluid for the diagnosis of malignant effusions. Br J Cancer 1999; 81:1059–1065.
62. Menard O, Dousset B, Jacob C, Martinet Y. Improvement of the diagnosis of the cause of pleural effusion in patients with lung cancer by simultaneous quantification of carcinoembryonic antigen (CEA) and neuron-specific enolase (NSE) pleural levels. Eur J Cancer 1993; 13:1806–1809.
63. Toumbis M, Rasidakis A, Passalidou E, Kalomenidis J, Alchanatis M, Orphanidou D, Jordanoglou J. Evaluation of CYFRA 21-1 in malignant and benign pleural effusions. Anticancer Res 1996; 16:2101–2104.
64. Falcone F, Marinelli M, Minguzzi L, Paganelli GM, Turba E, Cavalli A, Rapellino M. Tumor markers and lung cancer: guidelines in a cost-limited medical organization. Int J Biol Markers 1996; 11:61–66.
65. Stoetzer OJ, Munker R, Darsow M, Wilmanns W. P53-immunoreactive cells in benign and malignant effusions: diagnostic value using a panel of monoclonal antibodies and comparison with CEA-staining. Oncol Rep 1999; 6:455–458.
66. Alexandrakis MG, Coulocheri SA, Bouros D, Mandalaki K, Karkavitsas N, Eliopoulos GD. Evaluation of inflammatory cytokines in malignant and benign pleural effusions. Oncol Rep 2000; 7:1327–1332.
67. Hurewitz AN, Zucker S, Mancuso P, Wu CL, Dimassimo B, Lysik RM, Moutsiakis D. Human pleural effusions are rich in matrix metalloproteinases. Chest 1992; 102:1808–1814.
68. Marel M, Stastny B, Melinova L, Svandova E, Light RW. Diagnosis of pleural effusions. Experience with clinical studies, 1986 to 1990. Chest 1995; 107:1598–1603.
69. Stanley KE. Prognostic factors for survival in patients with inoperable lung cancer. JNCI 1980; 65:25–32.
70. Albain KS, Crowley JJ, LeBlanc M, Livingston RG. Survival determinants in

extensive-stage non-small cell lung cancer: the Southwestern Oncology Group experience. J Clin Oncol 1991; 9:1618–1626.
71. Mountain CF, Lukeman JM, Hammar SP, Chamberlain DW, Coulson WF, Page DL, Victor TA, Weiland LH. Lung cancer classification: the relationship of disease extent and cell type to survival in a clinical trials population. J Surg Oncol 1987; 35:147–156.
72. Decker DA, Dines DE, Payne WS, Bernatz PE, Pairolero PC. The significance of cytologically negative pleural effusion in bronchogenic carcinoma. Chest 1978; 74:640–642.
73. Rosell R, Gomez-Godina J, Camps C, Maestre J, Padille J, Canto A, Mate JL, Li S, Roig J, Olazabal A. A randomized trial comparing preoperative chemotherapy plus surgery with surgery alone in patients with non-small-cell lung cancer. N Engl J Med 1994; 330:153–158.
74. Roth JA, Fossella FV, Komaki R, Ryan MB, Putnam JB Jr, Lee S, Dhingra H, De Caro L, Chasen M, McGavran M. A randomized trial comparing perioperative chemotherapy and surgery with surgery alone in resectable stage IIIA non-small-cell lung cancer. J Natl Cancer Instit 1994; 86:673–680.
75. Rosell R, Lopez-Cabrenizo MP, Astudillo J. Preoperative chemotherapy for stage IIIA non-small-cell lung cancer. Curr Opin Oncol 1996; 9:149–155.
76. Depierre A, Milleron B, Moro-Sibilot D, Chevret S, Quoix E, Lebeau B, Braun D, Breton JL, Lemarie E, Gouva S, Paillot N, Brechot JM, Janicot H, Lebas FX, Terrioux P, Clavier J, Foucher P, Monchatre M, Coetmeur D, Level MC, Leclerc P, Blanchon F, Rodier JM, Thiberville L, Villeneuve A, Westeel V, Chastang C. Preoperative chemotherapy followed by surgery compared with primary surgery in resectable stage I (except T1N0), II, and IIIa non-small-cell lung cancer. J Clin Oncol 2002; 20:247–253.
77. The Study Group of Adjuvant Chemotherapy for Lung Cancer (Chubu Japan). A randomized trial of postoperative adjuvant chemotherapy in non-small cell lung cancer (the second cooperative study). Eur J Surg Oncol 1995; 21:69–77.
78. Keller SM. Adjuvant therapy of resected non-small-cell lung cancer. Curr Opin Oncol 2000; 12:149–155.
79. PORT Meta-analysis Trialists Group. Postoperative radiotherapy in non-small-cell lung cancer: systematic review and meta-analysis of individual patient data from nine randomised controlled trials. Lancet 1998; 352:257–263.
80. Non-Small-Cell Lung Cancer Cooperative Group. Chemotherapy in non-small cell lung cancer: a meta-analysis using updated data on individual patients from 52 randomised clinical trials. Br Med J 1995; 311:899–909.
81. Eberhardt W, Wilke H, Stamatis G, Stuschke M, Harstrick A, Menker H, Krause B, Mueller MR, Stahl M, Flasshove M, Budach V, Greschuchna D, Konietzko N, Sack H, Seeber S. Preoperative chemotherapy followed by concurrent chemoradiation therapy based on hyperfractionated accelerated radiotherapy and definitive surgery in locally advanced non-small-cell lung cancer: mature results of a phase II trial. J Clin Oncol 1998; 16:622–634.
82. Keller SM, Adak S, Wagner H, Herskovic A, Komaki R, Brooks BJ, Perry MC, Livingston RB, Johnson DH. A randomized trial of postoperative adjuvant therapy in patients with completely resected stage II or IIIA non-small-cell lung cancer. Eastern Cooperative Oncology Group. N Engl J Med 2000; 343:1217–1222.
83. Rawson N, Peto J. An overview of prognostic factors in small-cell lung cancer. Br J Cancer 1990; 61:597–604.

84. Zelen M. Keynote address on biostatistics and data retrieval. Cancer Chemoth Rep 1973; 4:31–42.
85. Shepherd FA, Ginsberg RJ, Haddad R, Feld R, Sagman U, Evans WK, DeBoer G, Maki E. Importance of clinical staging in limited small-cell lung cancer: a valuable system to separate prognostic subgroups. The University of Toronto Lung Oncology Group. J Clin Oncol 1993; 11:1592–1597.
86. Livingston RB, McCracken JD, Trauth CJ, Chen T. Isolated pleural effusion in small cell lung carcinoma: favorable prognosis. A review of the Southwest Oncology Group experience. Chest 1982; 81:208–211.
87. Souquet PJ, Chauvin F, Boissel JP, Cellerino R, Cormier Y, Ganz PA, Kaasa S, Pater JL, Quoix E, Rapp E. Polychemotherapy in advanced non small cell lung cancer: a meta-analysis. Lancet 1993; 342:19–21.
88. Souquet PJ, Chauvin F, Boissel JP, Bernard JP. Meta-analysis of randomised trials of systemic chemotherapy versus supportive treatment in non-resectable non-small cell lung cancer. Lung Cancer, 1995; (12 suppl 1):S147–154.
89. Albain KS, Hoffman PC, Little AG, Bitran JD, Golomb HM, DeMeester TR, Griem ML, Blough RR, Skosey C. Pleural involvement in stage IIIM0 non-small-cell bronchogenic carcinoma. A need to differentiate subtypes. Am J Clin Oncol 1986; 9:255–261.
90. Fujita A, Takabatake H, Tagaki S, Sekine K. Combination chemotherapy in patients with malignant pleural effusions from non-small cell lung cancer: cisplatin, ifosfamide, and irinotecan with recombinant human granulocyte colony-stimulating factor support. Chest 2001; 119:340–343.
91. Schiller JH, Harrington D, Belani CP, Langer C, Sandler A, Krook J, Zhu J, Johnson DH. Comparison of four chemotherapy regimens for advanced non-small-cell lung cancer. N Engl J Med 2002; 346:92–98.
92. Comella P, Frasci G, Panza N, Manzione L, De Cataldis G, Cioffi R, Maiorino L, Micillo E, Lorusso V, Di Rienzo G, Filippelli G, Lamberti A, Natale M, Bilancia D, Nicolella G, Di Nota A, Comella G. Randomized trial comparing cisplatin, gemcitabine, and vinorelbine with either cisplatin and gemcitabine or cisplatin and vinorelbine in advanced non-small-cell lung cancer: interim analysis of a phase III trial of the Southern Italy Cooperative Oncology Group. J Clin Oncol 2000; 18:1451–1457.
93. Jett JR, Kirschling RJ, Jung SH, Marks RS. A phase II study of paclitaxel and granulocyte colony-stimulating factor in previously untreated patients with extensive-stage small cell lung cancer: a study of the North Central Cancer Treatment Group. Semin Oncol 1995; 22(3 suppl 6):75–77.
94. Lilenbaum RC, Green MR. Novel chemotherapeutic agents in the treatment of non-small-cell lung cancer. J Clin Oncol 1993; 11:1391–1402.
95. Mattson K, Saarinen A, Jekunen A. Combination treatment with docetaxel (Taxotere) and platinum compounds for non-small cell lung cancer. Semin Oncol 1997; 24(4 suppl 14):S14-5–S14-8.
96. Ripamonti C. Management of dyspnea in advanced cancer patients. Support Care Cancer 1999; 7:233–243.
97. Werner-Wasik M, Scott C, Cox JD, Sause WT, Byhardt RW, Asbell S, Russell A, Komaki R, Lee JS. Recursive partitioning analysis of 1999 Radiation Therapy Oncology Group (RTOG) patients with locally-advanced non-small-cell lung cancer (LA-NSCLC): identification of five groups with different survival. Int J Radiat Oncol Biol Phys 2000; 48:1475–1482.

98. Wigren T, Kellokumpu-Lehtinen P, Ojala A. Radical radiotherapy of inoperable non-small cell lung cancer. Irradiation techniques and tumor characteristics in relation to local control and survival. Acta Oncol 1992; 31:555–561.
99. Scott C, Sause WT, Byhardt R, Marcial V, Pajak TF, Herskovic A, Cox JD. Recursive partitioning analysis of 1592 patients on four Radiation Therapy Oncology Group studies in inoperable non-small cell lung cancer. Lung Cancer 1997; 17(suppl 1):S59–74.
100. Koukourakis MI, Bahlitzanakis N, Froudarakis M, Giatromanolaki A, Georgoulias V, Koumiotaki S, Christodoulou M, Kyrias G, Skarlatos J, Kostantelos J, Beroukas K. Concurrent conventionally fractionated radiotherapy and weekly docetaxel in the treatment of stage IIIb non-small-cell lung carcinoma. Br J Cancer 1999; 80:1792–1796.
101. Marino P, Preatoni A, Cantoni A. Randomized trials of radiotherapy alone versus combined chemotherapy and radiotherapy in stages IIIa and IIIb nonsmall cell lung cancer. A meta-analysis. Cancer 1995; 76:593–601.
102. Baldini E, Silvano G, Tibaldi C, Campoccia S, Cionini L, Conte P. Sequential chemoradiation therapy with vinorelbine, ifosfamide, and cisplatin in stage IIIB non-small cell lung cancer: a phase II study. Semin Oncol 2000; 27(suppl 1):28–32.
103. Eberhardt W, Bildat S, Korfee S. Combined modality therapy in NSCLC. Ann Oncol 2000; 11(suppl 3):85–95.
104. Aaronson NK. Methodologic issues in assessing the quality of life of cancer patients. Semin Oncol 1991; 67:844–850.
105. Muers MF. Quality of life and symptom control. Eur Respir Mon 2001; 17:305–329.
106. Sahn SA. Pleural effusion in lung cancer. Clin Chest Med 1993; 14:189–200.
107. Rodriguez-Panadero F, Antony VB. Pleurodesis: state of the art. Eur Respir J 1997; 10:1648–1654.
108. Rodriguez-Panadero F. Current trends in pleurodesis. Curr Opin Med 1997; 3:319–325.
109. Sanchez-Armengol A, Rodriguez-Panadero F. Survival and talc pleurodesis in metastatic pleural carcinoma, revisited. Report of 125 cases. Chest 1993; 104:1482–1485.
110. Sahn SA. Malignancy metastatic to the pleura. Clin Chest Med 1998; 19:351–361.
111. Aelony Y, King RR, Boutin C. Thoracoscopic talc poudrage in malignant pleural effusions: effective pleurodesis despite low pleural pH. Chest 1998; 113:1007–1012.
112. Antony VB, Rothfuss KJ, Godbey SW, Sparks JA, Hott JW. Mechanism of tetracycline-hydrochloride-induced pleurodesis. Tetracycline-hydrochloride-stimulated mesothelial cells produce a growth-factor-like activity for fibroblasts. Am Rev Respir Dis 1992; 146:1009–1013.
113. Herrington JD, Gora-Harper ML, Salley RK. Chemical pleurodesis with doxycycline 1 g. Pharmacotherapy 1996; 16:280–285.
114. Mansson T. Treatment of malignant pleural effusion with doxycycline. Scand J Infect Dis Suppl 1988; 53:29–34.
115. Emad A, Rezaian GR. Treatment of malignant pleural effusions with a combination of bleomycin and tetracycline. A comparison of bleomycin or tetracycline alone versus a combination of bleomycin and tetracycline. Cancer 1996; 78:2498–2501.

116. Robinson LA, Fleming WH, Galbraith TA. Intrapleural doxycycline control of malignant pleural effusions. Ann Thorac Surg 1993; 55:1115–1122.
117. Grasela TH, Walawander CA, Jolson HM, Kennedy DL. Alternatives to intravenous tetracycline hydrochloride for malignant pleural effusions. Ann Pharmacother 1994; 28:968–969.
118. Light RW, Wang NS, Sassoon CS, Gruer SE, Vargas FS. Comparison of the effectiveness of tetracycline and minocycline as pleural sclerosing agents in rabbits. Chest 1994; 106:577–582.
119. Zimmer PW, Hill M, Casey K, Harvey E, Low DE. Prospective randomized trial of talc slurry vs bleomycin in pleurodesis for symptomatic malignant pleural effusions. Chest 1997; 112:430–434.
120. Perng RP, Chen YM, Wu MF, Chou KC, Lin WC, Liu JM, Whang-Peng J. Phase II trial of intrapleural paclitaxel injection for non-small-cell lung cancer patients with malignant pleural effusions. Respir Med 1998; 92:473–479.
121. Rusch VW, Figlin R, Godwin D, Piantadosi S. Intrapleural cisplatin and cytarabine in the management of malignant pleural effusions: a Lung Cancer Study Group trial. J Clin Oncol 1991; 9:313–319.
122. Diacon AH, Wyser C, Bolliger CT, Tamm M, Pless M, Perruchoud AP, Soler M. Prospective randomized comparison of thoracoscopic talc poudrage under local anesthesia versus bleomycin instillation for pleurodesis in malignant pleural effusions. Am J Respir Crit Care Med 2000; 162:1445–1449.
123. Aelony Y. Cost-effective pleurodesis. Chest 1998; 113:1731–1732.
124. Martinez-Moragon E, Aparicio J, Rogado MC, Sanchis J, Sanchis F, Gil-Suay V. Pleurodesis in malignant pleural effusions: a randomized study of tetracycline versus bleomycin. Eur Respir J 1997; 10:2380–2383.
125. Ong KC, Indumathi V, Raghuram J, Ong YY. A comparative study of pleurodesis using talc slurry and bleomycin in the management of malignant pleural effusions. Respirology 2000; 5:99–103.
126. Rodriguez-Panadero F. Malignant pleural diseases. Monaldirch Arch Chest Dis 2000; 55:17–19.
127. Bouros D, Froudarakis M, Siafakas NM. Pleurodesis: everything flows. Chest 2000; 118:577–579.
128. Mathur PN, Loddenkemper R. Medical thoracoscopy. Role in pleural and lung diseases. Clin Chest Med 1995; 16:487–496.
129. Loddenkemper R, Schonfeld N. Medical thoracoscopy. Curr Opin Pulm Med 1998; 4:235–238.
130. Loddenkemper R. Thoracoscopy—state of the art. Eur Respir J 1998; 11:213–221.
131. Aelony Y, King R, Boutin C. Thoracoscopic talc poudrage pleurodesis for chronic recurrent pleural effusions. Ann Intern Med 1991; 115:778–782.
132. Perrault LP, Gregoire J, Page A. Video-assisted thoracoscopy and thoracic surgery: the first 50 patients. Ann Chir 1993; 47:838–843.
133. Schulze M, Boehle AS, Kurdow R, Dohrmann P, Henne-Bruns D. Effective treatment of malignant pleural effusion by minimal invasive thoracic surgery: thoracoscopic talc pleurodesis and pleuroperitoneal shunts in 101 patients. Ann Thorac Surg 2001; 71:1809–1812.
134. Colt HG, Russack V, Chiu Y, Konopka RG, Chiles PG, Pedersen CA, Kapelanski D. A comparison of thoracoscopic talc insufflation, slurry, and mechanical abrasion pleurodesis. Chest 1997; 111:442–448.

135. Yim AP, Chan AT, Lee TW, Wan IY, Ho JK. Thoracoscopic talc insufflation versus talc slurry for symptomatic malignant pleural effusion. Ann Thorac Surg 1996; 62:1655–1658.
136. Cohen RG, Shely WW, Thompson SE, Hagen JA, Marboe CC, DeMeester R, Starnes VA. Talc pleurodesis: talc slurry versus thoracoscopic talc insufflation in a porcine model. Ann Thorac Surg 1996; 62:1000–1004.
137. Aelony Y. Talc pleurodesis. Talc slurry vs talc poudrage. Chest 1995; 108:289.
138. Light RW. Diseases of the pleura: the use of talc for pleurodesis. Curr Opin Pulm Med 2000; 6:255–258.
139. Brant A, Eaton T. Serious complications with talc slurry pleurodesis. Respirology 2001; 6:181–185.
140. de Campos FS, Vargas E, de Campos Werebe P, Cardoso LR, Teixeira FB, Jatene RW. Thoracoscopy talc poudrage: a 15-year experience. Chest 2001; 119:801–806.
141. Viallat F, Rey P, Astoul C. Thoracoscopic talc poudrage pleurodesis for malignant effusions. A review of 360 cases. Chest 1996; 110:1387–1393.
142. Belani CP, Pajeau TS, Bennett CL. Treating malignant pleural effusions cost consciously. Chest 1998; 113(suppl 1):78–85.
143. Walker-Renard PB, Vaughan LM, Sahn SA. Chemical pleurodesis for malignant pleural effusions. Ann Intern Med 1994; 120:56–64.
144. Vargas FS, Teixeira LR. Pleural malignancies. Curr Opin Pulm Med 1996; 2:335–340.
145. Parulekar W, Di Primio G, Matzinger F, Dennie C, Bociek G. Use of small-bore vs large-bore chest tubes for treatment of malignant pleural effusions. Chest 2001; 120:19–25.
146. Banerjee AK, Willetts I, Robertson JF, Blamey RW. Pleural effusion in breast cancer: a review of the Nottingham experience. Eur J Surg Oncol 1994; 20:33–36.
147. Keller SM. Current and future therapy for malignant pleural effusion. Chest 1993; 103(suppl 1):63–67.
148. Ruckdeschel JC. Management of malignant pleural effusion: an overview. Semin Oncol 1988; 15(suppl 3):24–28.

25

Benign Tumors of the Pleura

CAMERON D. WRIGHT and EUGENE J. MARK

Harvard Medical School
and Massachusetts General Hospital
Boston, Massachusetts, U.S.A.

Localized fibrous tumors of the pleura (LFTP) are rare, usually benign neoplasms of the pleura. This tumor has received many names, including fibrous mesothelioma, benign mesothelioma, localized mesothelioma, subpleural fibroma, solitary fibrous tumor of the pleura, and LFTP, which reflect its clinical and pathological characteristics (1). Recently the term fibrous tumor of the pleura has been preferred as it emphasizes a distinct separation from malignant mesothelioma. In contradistinction to LFTP, malignant mesothelioma is causally related to asbestos exposure, is usually diffuse in gross appearance, is of mesothelial origin and stains for cytokeratin, and is rapidly fatal. LFTP is the preferred description of this tumor rather than SFTP because several reports have documented multiple LFTP within the same patient (2,3).

I. History

The first LFTP was probably described by Wagner in 1870 (4). In 1931 Klemperer and Rabin divided primary tumors of the pleura into two types: localized and diffuse (5). The diffuse form (malignant mesothelioma) was purported to arise from the mesothelial cells, whereas the localized form (LFTP) was thought to arise from the submesothelial fibrous connective tissue. Clagett et al. reported the first large (24 patients) surgical series in 1952 from the Mayo Clinic and stressed their difference from malignant mesothelioma and the importance of resection for cure (6). Two large classic review articles summarized the clinicopathological features of fibrous tumors of the pleura a decade apart. Briselli et al., from the Massachusetts General Hospital reviewed 368 cases in 1981; 88% of the cases behaved in a benign fashion, nuclear pleomorphism and a high mitotic rate were harbingers of malignancy, and the best predictor of a good prognosis was a pedicle supporting the tumor (1). England, et al. in 1989 reviewed 223 cases from the Armed Forces Institute of Pathology in which 58% were histologically malignant, patients with malignant tumors that were cured had pedunculated or well-circumscribed tumors, and the best predictor of a good outcome was resectability (7).

II. Incidence

LFTP are rare, with only 600 cases reported up to 1989 (7). In large series of pleural tumors about 10% will be LFTP and 90% will be malignant mesotheliomas (8). The Mayo Clinic reported on 60 cases over 25 years, an incidence of 3 cases per 100,000 admissions (9). Most modern series of LFTP from thoracic surgical units report about 1 case per year emphasizing the rarity of this tumor (3,10–12).

III. Etiology

Unlike mesothelioma, asbestos is not associated with LFTP (1,7). There are no known predisposing factors for LFTP.

IV. Demographics

LFTP are most common in the sixth decade of life with more than one half of the cases over the age of 50 (1,7). A few cases have been reported in children as young as the age of five (1). LFTP are evenly distributed among men and women.

V. Clinical Features

Many patients are asymptomatic and come to medical attention because of an abnormal chest radiograph. Recent series report the incidence of symptoms from 42 to 88% (Table 1) (3,10–12). The common reported symptoms are chest pain, cough and dyspnea. Constitutional symptoms such as fever, night sweats,

Table 1 Clinical Features of Patients with LFTP

Author (Ref.)	Patients	Symptomatic	Clubbing	Hypoglycemia	Malignant
Rena (12)	21	43%	14%	14%	38%
Cardillo (3)	55	42%	ns	2%	7%
De Perrot (11)	11	70%	0	0	20%
Suter (10)	15	88%	7%	7%	60%
Briselli (1)	360	64%	35%	4%	13%
England (7)	223	48%	4%	6%	58%

ns = not stated.

and weight loss are rare. Symptoms of hypoglycemia are rare but can be dramatic and lead to an accurate clinical diagnosis if there is a known circumscribed mass in the chest. Patients with malignant and/or large tumors are more likely to be symptomatic (7). Rare patients report the sensation of a mass moving in the chest, which is highly suggestive of this tumor since many are pedunculated. Signs of a pleural effusion may be evident on chest examination and is more common in malignant than benign tumors (7). Clubbing or other manifestations of hypertrophic pulmonary osteoarthropathy are occasionally seen and were more common in older series (probably due to delayed diagnosis) than in recent reports (Table 1). Clubbing resolves with complete resection of the mass.

VI. Laboratory Features

Rarely hypoglycemia may be present (0–14%) due to the tumor secreting insulin-like growth factor II (IGF-II) (Table 1) (13). The hypoglycemia resolves after complete resection of the tumor. The pleural effusions associated with LFTP are usually clear yellow transudates, which are cytologically negative (6,12). Exudative and bloody effusions have been rarely reported (6,12). Although most effusions are small, there have been case reports of massive effusions (14).

VII. Radiographic Features

Chest radiographs usually show a well-delineated round, oval, or lobulated mass (Figs 1–3). The average size of the mass is often rather large, with two-series reporting the average size to be 8.5 or 10 cm (Table 2) (1,7). If the mass is based on the parietal pleura the angle between the mass and chest wall is characteristically obtuse. If the lesion is pedunculated, a change in patient position may lead to a change in tumor position. Evidence of a pleural effusion is present in 1–19% of patients (Table 2). Computed tomography (CT) of the chest is the next step in diagnostic evaluation and is indicated in all patients (15). CT typically

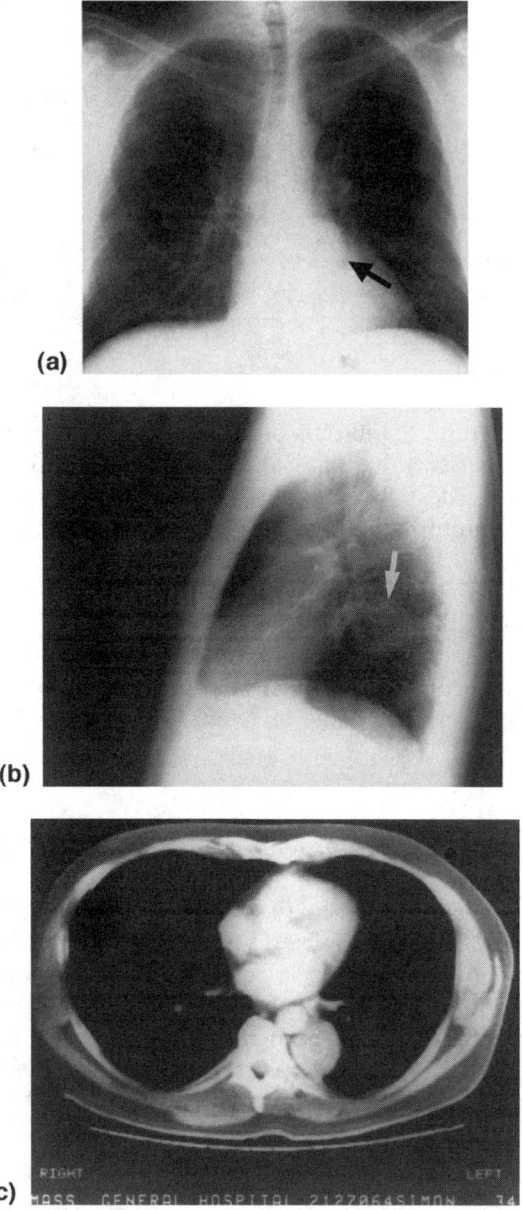

Figure 1 LFTP simulating a benign neurogenic tumor. The patient is a 51-year-old man who was asymptomatic. (a) PA chest radiograph demonstrates a 4 cm. sharply defined retrocardiac density (black arrow). (b) Lateral chest radiograph confirms posterior paravertebral gutter location and sharply defined borders (white arrow) suggest a benign etiology. (c) CT scan confirms moderately enhancing sharply defined 4 cm paravertebral mass. The preoperative diagnosis was a benign neurogenic tumor. Resection was by thoracotomy, which revealed the origin was the posterior pleura. Pathology revealed a bland LFTP, and the patient is free of recurrence 18 years after resection.

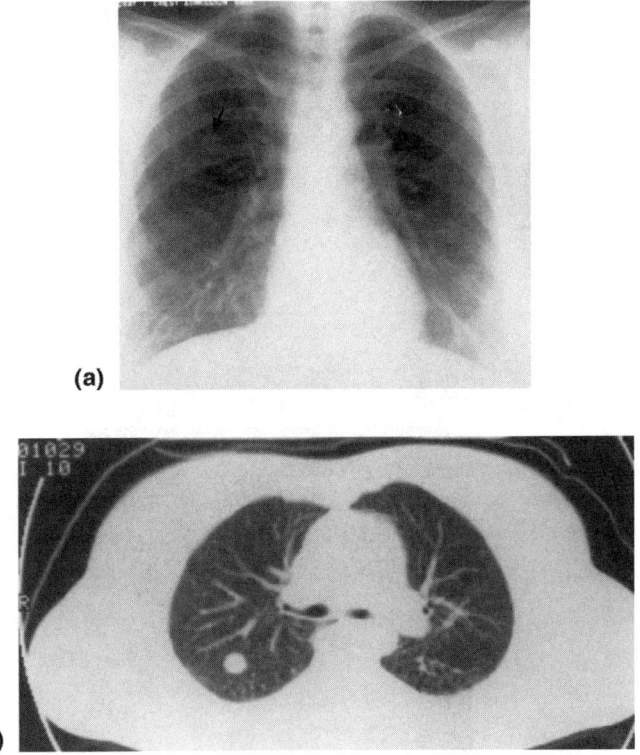

Figure 2 LFTP simulating a solitary pulmonary nodule (inverted fibroma). The patient is a healthy 41-year-old woman who was asymptomatic. The patient underwent thoracotomy and resection with a preoperative diagnosis of a solitary pulmonary nodule. (a) PA chest radiograph shows a 1.5 cm (black arrow) sharply demarcated round mass. (b) CT scan shows a 1.5 cm sharply defined mass in the posterior segment of the right upper lobe close to the major fissure. The lesion originated from the visceral pleura within the major fissure and grew into the lung (inverted fibroma). Pathology revealed a benign appearing LFTP, and follow-up has demonstrated no recurrence.

shows a sharply defined homogeneous soft tissue mass adjacent to some aspect of the pleura (Fig. 4). Calcification is occasionally noted in the mass. Heterogeneous tumors with areas of low density (which may represent areas of cystic change, hemorrhage, or necrosis) are more common in larger and malignant tumors. These tumors markedly enhance with intravenous contrast, as would be expected given their gross and microscopic findings of hypervascularity. The finding of marked enhancement with contrast can suggest the correct diagnosis of a LFTP in an unknown chest mass to the discriminating radiologist. Rarely more than one tumor is present (2,3). About two thirds of the tumors originate from the visceral pleura and one third from the parietal pleura (7). Tumors can rarely present as intraparenchymal lung tumors—the so-called inverted fibroma

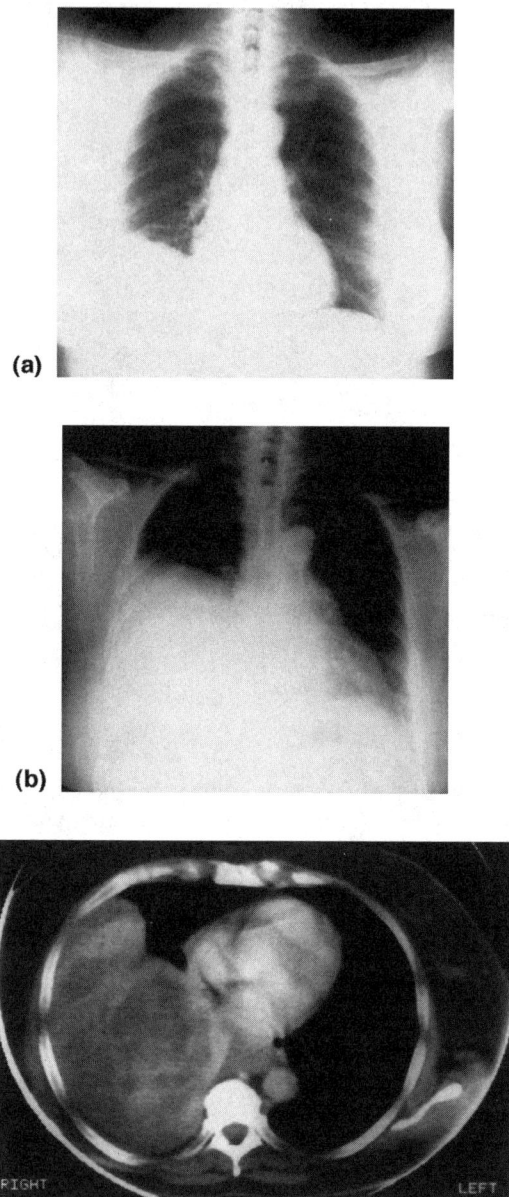

Table 2 Radiological Features of Patients with LFTP

Size (cm)	Multiple tumors (%)	Pleural effusion (%)	Sharp borders (%)	Calcification (%)	Correct FNA diagnosis (%)	Ref.
ns	0	19	76	ns	38	12
8.5 (1–28)	2	5	All	ns	36	3
10 (2.5–23)	0	0	All	27	33	11
ns	7	5	80	ns	20	10
<5 (34%), >6 (60%)	ns	17	93	ns	ns	7

ns = not stated.

(Fig. 2). Magnetic resonance (MR) imaging can be helpful in selected cases (16–18). Low signal intensity is typically seen in T1- and T2-weighted sequences, which reflects their fibrous nature (Figs. 5, 6). The tumor markedly enhances with gadolinium contrast reflecting hypervascularity of the tumor. MR is useful in assessing large tumors, tumors with extensive chest wall or diaphragm abutment, or apical tumors to better define extent of invasion and potential resectability. Angiography has been reported to be useful to define the origin of the vasculature of huge tumors and also to embolize the feeding vessels to facilitate resection (19). Massive hemorrhage has been reported during resection of large tumors, so it is prudent to consider embolization of massive tumors preoperatively.

The role of CT-guided fine needle aspiration (FNA) is controversial, and the diagnostic yield is rather low with this tumor with a reported accuracy of 10–38% in recent reports (Table 2) (3,10–12). A recent report by Okada and colleagues reported on 10 patients with LFTP, 5 of whom had attempted preoperative FNA diagnosis (20). All five biopsies were non diagnostic due to a paucity of diagnostic tumor cells recovered. At operation, intraoperative scratch

Figure 3 Huge LFTP with an unusual natural history. The patient is a 67-year-old woman who initially presented in 1991 with vague right chest discomfort. (a) PA chest radiograph revealed an apparent elevated right hemidiaphragm and an abnormal diaphragm contour. Further investigation was not undertaken. Two years later (1983) she complained of dyspnea. (b) PA chest radiograph shows a huge right chest mass occupying about one half of the hemithorax. (c) CT scan confirms a huge heterogeneous tumor with areas of central low density consistent with hemorrhage or necrosis. The borders of the mass are sharp, and there is no evidence of lung or chest wall invasion, suggesting an encapsulated tumor. Resection revealed a tumor based on the visceral pleura of the base of the right lower lobe and was a benign LFTP. Sixteen years later (1999) she represented with an apparent local recurrence on the diaphragm and she underwent reresection.

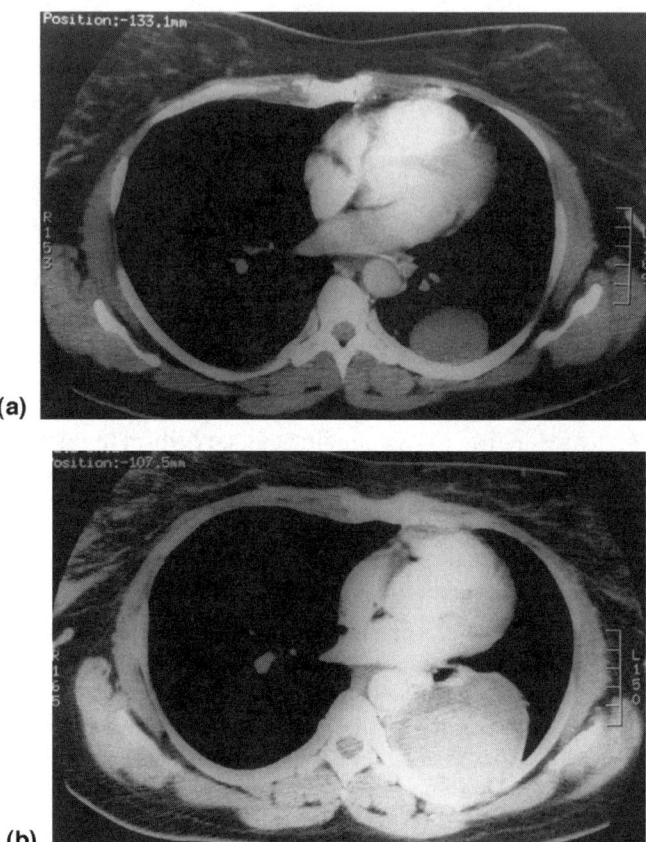

Figure 4 Recurrent invasive malignant LFTP. The patient is a 40-year-old woman who presented initially with an asymptomatic 8 cm left chest mass. Thoracotomy revealed a mediastinal pleural-based mass extending over to the lateral chest wall and adherent to the left lower lobe. Extrapleural resection of the mass with wedge resection of the lung was performed. The tumor was very cellular, had focal areas of necrosis, had minimal cytologic atypia, and had 5 mitoses per 10 high power fields. Resection margins were negative. Three years later she developed left chest pain. A CT scan was performed (a) which confined a 4 cm local recurrence in the posterior chest wall. The CT scan shows a homogeneous tumor, which does not avidly take up contrast. The patient refused surgery. Three months later the pain worsened, and a repeat CT scan (b) showed marked enlargement of the tumor to 8 cm with areas of heterogeneity. Centrally the tumor now avidly takes up contrast and there is a peripheral rim of lower density. She now consented to reresection, which involved en-bloc resection of the mass with three attached ribs and the entire left lower lobe. Pathology revealed a cellular tumor with two mitoses per 10 high power fields with about 25% of the tumor necrotic. Resections margins were negative.

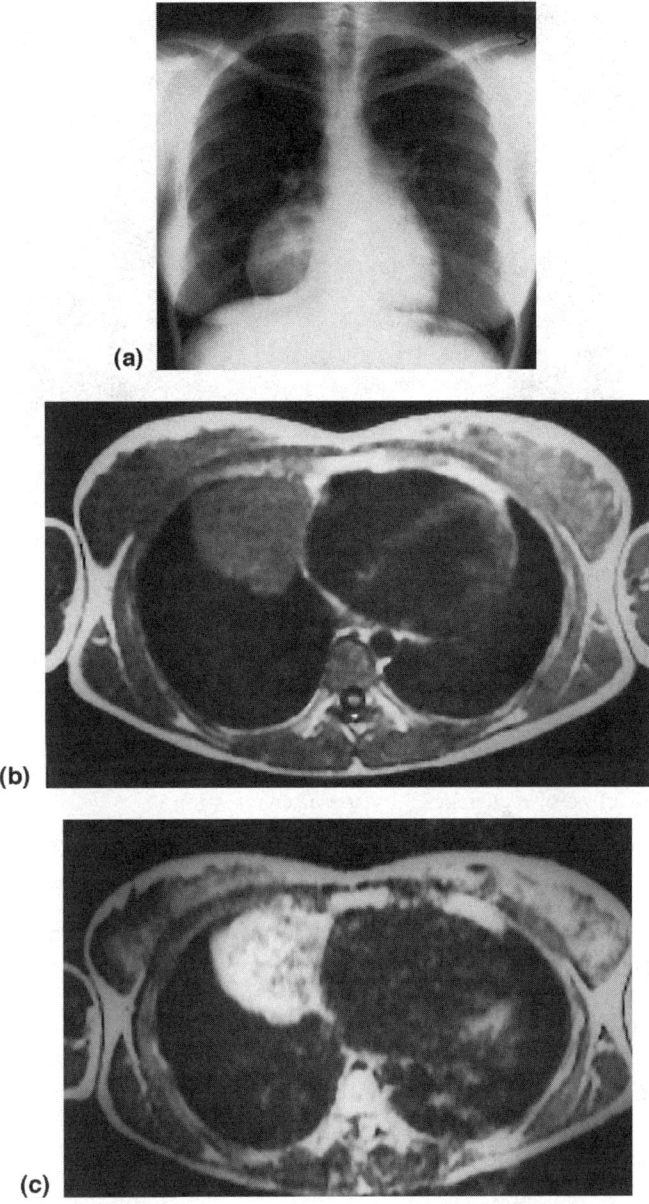

Figure 5 Magnetic resonance (MR) images of LFTP. The patient is a 31-year-old woman who presented with a cough. (a) PA chest radiograph demonstrates a right paracardiac mass with sharp lateral borders. (b) T1-weighted sequence of MR exam shows a homogeneous lesion of muscle (soft tissue) density. (c) T2-weighted sequence of MR exam demonstrates some inhomogeneity with several low-density areas. Resection showed the tumor to be based on the anterior sulcus between the chest wall and pericardium. Pathology revealed a benign LFTP.

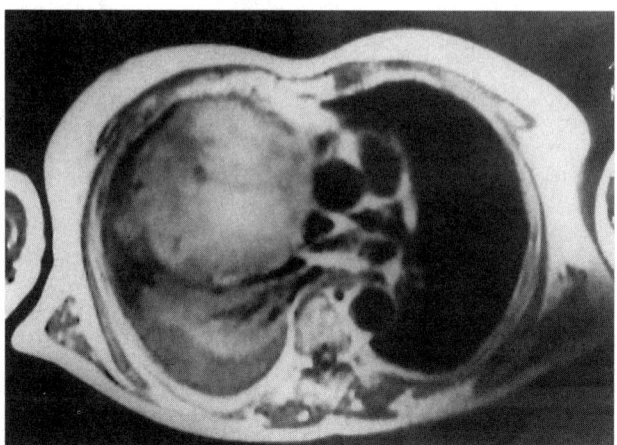

Figure 6 Huge LFTP with pleural effusion. The patient is a 56-year-old man with dyspnea and cough. A huge chest mass and a small pleural effusion were seen. The pleural effusion was tapped and was cytologically negative. Attempted resection at another hospital by a small anterior thoracotomy was met with massive bleeding and was abandoned. (a) MR exam (T1 image) shows a large anterior 10 cm tumor which is heterogeneous. Compression of the lung with a dependent pleural effusion is seen. The mediastinum and great vessels are shifted to the opposite side, and there is extensive abutment (invasion indeterminent) of the great vessels. Preoperative angiographic embolization of internal thoracic and phrenic artery branches was performed in view of the previous operative experience. Exploration through an extended posterolateral thoracotomy incision allowed easy resection of a tumor based on the mediastinal pleura. The patient remains free of recurrence 13 years after resection.

cytology was performed on all patients and a variety of cells were recovered, including spindle (bipolar, dendritic/stellate, and intermediate cells). They concluded that it was difficult to diagnose LFTP by FNA with certainty in part due to the cell morphology present resembling a heterogeneous group of spindle cell tumors and the difficulty in obtaining enough cells to review. Reports of core cutting needle biopsies suggest a higher diagnostic yield (21,22). For the routine case of an undiagnosed readily resectable chest mass, an expeditious surgical resection for diagnosis and treatment is the correct approach as the results of the needle biopsy, whether it is diagnostic or not, would not change the need for resection. Complex cases, including those that are quite large, potentially difficult to resect tumors or those where other tumors that would require a different treatment strategy (i.e., induction treatment) are high in the differential diagnosis would probably be benefited by a preoperative diagnosis. If LFTP is in the differential diagnosis of a lesion that is to be sampled preoperatively, both a FNA and a core biopsy should be requested. If the result is nondiagnostic, the clinician should remember that a LFTP is not excluded.

VIII. Pathology

A. Gross Pathology

As the name localized fibrous tumor of the pleura indicates, the typical lesion is round or oval and well circumscribed (1,7,23). The lesions may range from several millimeters to many centimeters in diameter, including examples measuring up to 36 cm and weighing up to 5000 g (Fig. 7). Larger lesions may be multilobulated. The cut surface of a resected specimen is rubbery and firm with a whorled pattern (Figs. 8, 9). Central myxoid change and hemorrhage may occasionally be seen and are more commonly encountered in large tumors. Tumors arise more commonly from the parietal than the visceral pleura. Rarely tumors arise from the thoracic surface of the diaphragm, from the mediastinum, or in the lung, where they are thought to arise from a pleural invagination in a lobular fissure. A vascular pedicle may be present, particularly on those arising from the parietal pleura.

B. Microscopic Pathology

The neoplastic cell is derived from a submesothelial fibroblast. Dark spindled nuclei may have stippled or homogeneously dense chromatin with occasional vacuolar change and inconspicuous nucleoli. Density of the nuclei varies from richly cellular to poorly cellular. The nuclei are separated by fibrillar collagen. The cells form fascicles or storiform arrays and also grow without any reproducible pattern (Figs. 10–12). Mitoses are very rare in benign tumors. Regions with numerous large blood vessels are common (Figs. 13, 14) and like, and occasional occasional admixed polygonal cells (24). Entrapment of surface

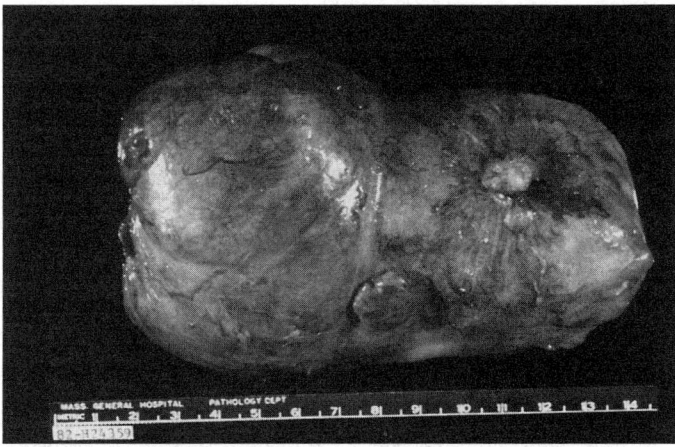

Figure 7 External surface of large localized fibrous tumor arising in the parietal pleura and presenting as a smooth bosselated mass 14 cm in greatest diameter.

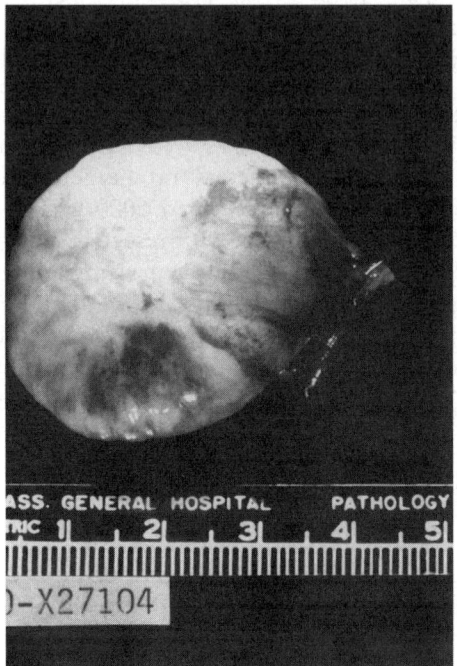

Figure 8 Cut surface of localized fibrous tumor of the pleura with a smooth homogeneous fleshy surface and focal cystic degeneration.

epithelioid mesothelial cells or entrapment of pneumocytes as the tumor grows within the lung may cause gland-like spaces, but these are not intrinsic parts of the neoplasm.

C. Electron Microscopy

The neoplastic cells have spindled nuclei with heterochromatin and occasional admixed polygonal cells (24). Nuclei may be mildly indented. Nucleoli are not prominent. Cytoplasm contains microfilaments and rough endoplasmic reticulum with cisternae. Mitochondria are generally scarce. The cells are arranged in groups and surrounded by collagen. Intercellular junctions are often discernible. The cells do not produce basement membrane.

D. Differential Diagnosis

Depending on the variety of patterns seen on routine staining, the differential diagnosis includes diffuse malignant mesothelioma of the fibrosarcomatous pattern, hemangiopericytoma, schwannoma, leiomyoma, sclerosing epithelioid fibrosarcoma, sclerosing epithelioid hemangioendothelioma, inflammatory pseudotumor, fibrous histiocytoma, sclerosing hemangioma, and carcinoid with

Benign Tumors of the Pleura

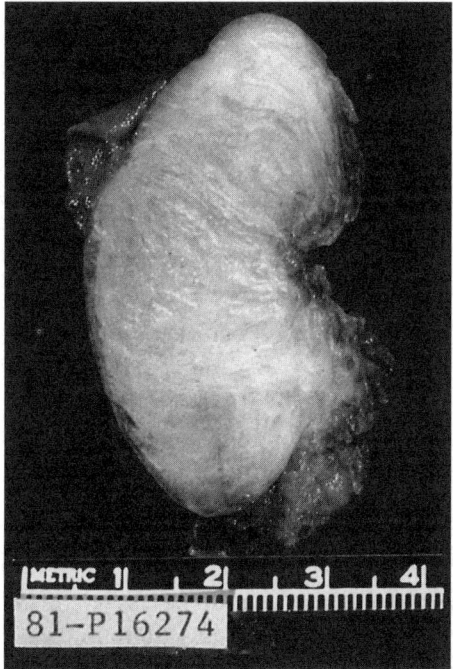

Figure 9 Cut surface of localized fibrous tumor of the pleura with dense gritty white fibrous cut surface.

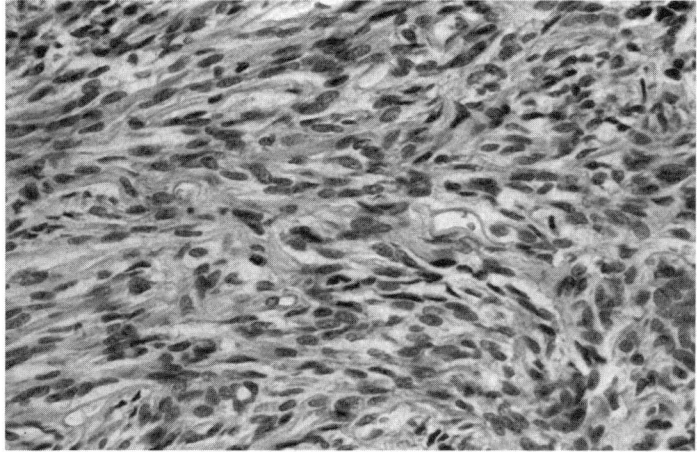

Figure 10 Localized fibrous tumor of the pleura with spindle cell proliferation, where the spindled nuclei form fascicles.

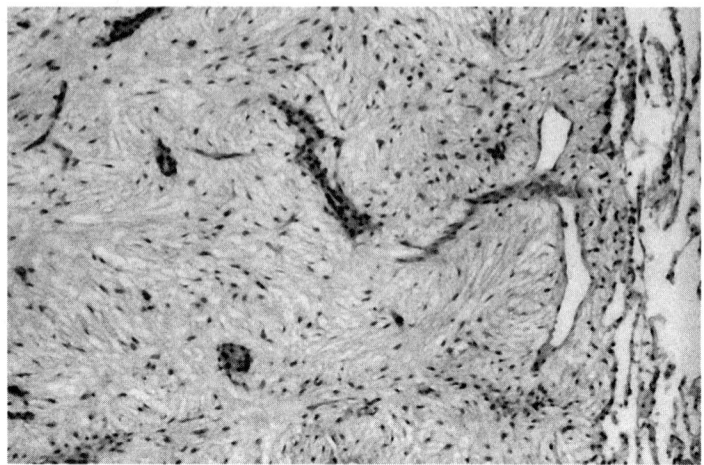

Figure 11 Localized fibrous tumor of the pleura with loose myxomatous pattern.

sclerosis. Immunochemistry is not usually necessary for diagnosis, but it may be useful in cases with one or more of these differential diagnosis. Typically the cells of the localized fibrous tumor stain for vimentin, which is a general but nonspecific marker for mesenchymal cells, and for CD34, which is a marker for fibroblasts (25,26). The cells generally do not stain for keratin or other epithelial, endothelial, or histiocytic markers.

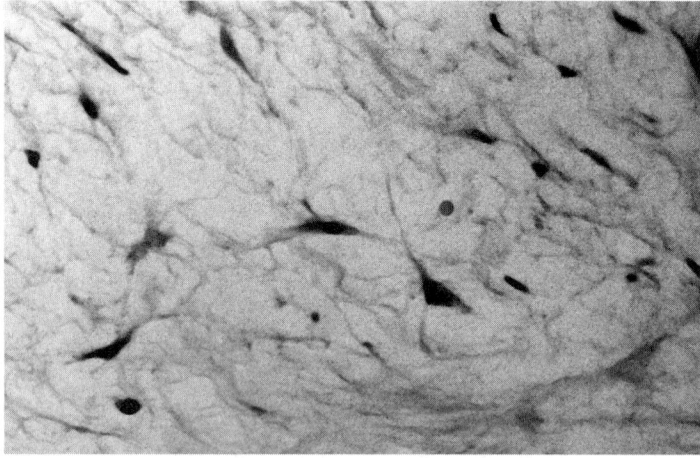

Figure 12 Individual spindled and stellate cells in myxoid region of localized fibrous tumor of the pleura.

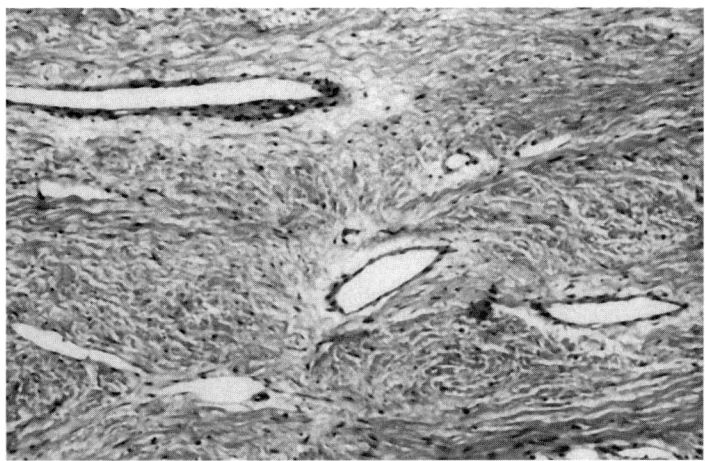

Figure 13 Ectatic thin-walled blood vessels amid proliferating spindled cells creating a pattern of angiofibroma.

IX. Malignant Fibrous Tumor of the Pleura

Approximately one third of fibrous tumors of the pleura have histological characteristics indicative of potentially malignant behavior (1,7,27). These tumors are generally grouped with fibrous tumors of the pleura and thought to be on a spectrum of variable malignancy, developing either in a benign tumor or as a progression of malignancy over time. The tumor has also been termed fibro-

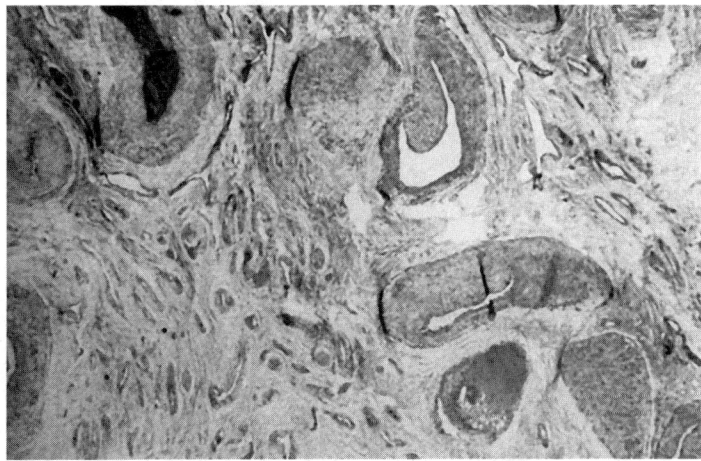

Figure 14 Large thick-walled blood vessels in the pedicle of a localized fibrous tumor attached to the parietal pleura.

sarcoma of the pleura. Resectability is the best predictor of prognosis. Approximately one half of patients whose tumors have histologic features of malignancy die with locally invasive, recurrent, or metastatic disease.

A. Gross Pathology

Necrosis and hemorrhage are visible in slightly more than half of cases malignant fibrous tumor, while uncommon in lesions with benign histology (Fig. 15). Malignant fibrous tumors of the pleura appear generally similar to localized fibrous tumor. Malignant fibrous tumors are twice as likely to be < 10 cm in size, with approximately 50% of malignant fibrous tumors reaching this size as compared to 25% of localized fibrous tumors.

B. Microscopic Pathology

The specific criteria for malignancy are (1) increased cellularity; (2) where the nuclear pleomorphism; and (3) mitoses. Increased cellularity consists of areas where the tumor appears solid with closely packed dark cells, which may be so dense as to suggest small-cell carcinoma (Fig. 16). Very highly cellular regions are seen in three fourths of malignant tumors. Nuclear pleomorphism is characterized by irregularity of the nuclei. It is seen in the great majority of cases. Mitoses are the most specific feature in the diagnosis of malignant fibrous tumor. A mitotic count of greater than four mitoses per 10 high power field has been used as a line of demarcation. By these criteria, approximately 75% of malignant fibrous tumors have this many mitoses, in contrast to 1% of solitary fibrous tumors.

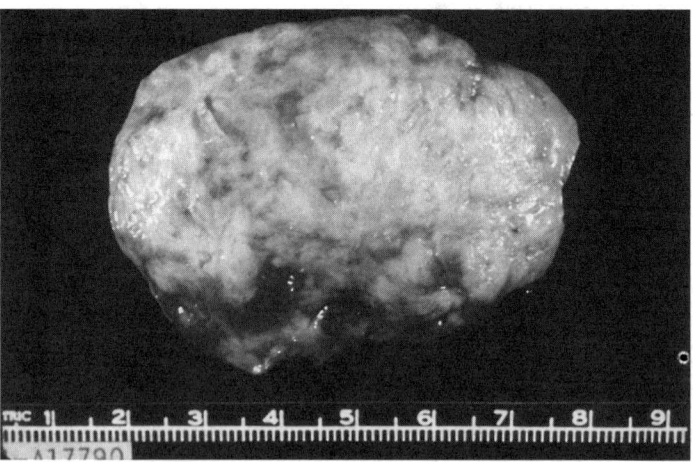

Figure 15 Malignant fibrous tumor of the pleura has cut surface with glistening myxoid gelatinous tissue and focal hemorrhagic necrosis.

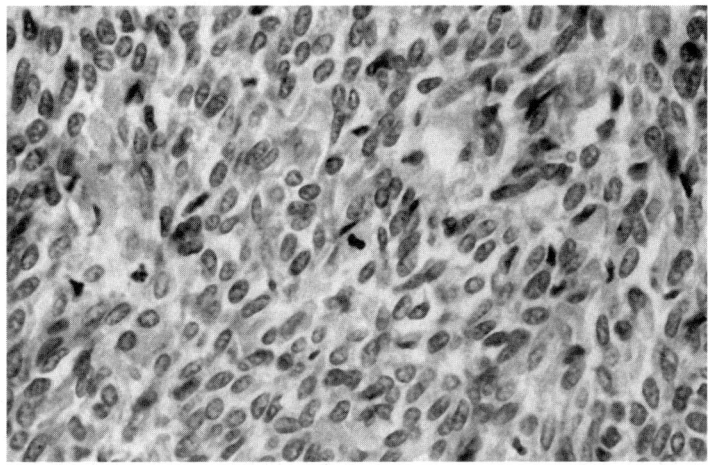

Figure 16 Malignant fibrous tumor of the pleura with closely packed, hyperchromatic, small, oval nuclei and containing several mitoses.

C. Differential Diagnosis

The differential diagnosis includes localized fibrous tumor, sarcomas in general, and the sarcomatous variant of diffuse malignant mesothelioma (28,29). The latter is sometimes referred to as desmoplastic diffuse malignant mesothelioma, which is an entirely different tumor and the most important conceptual and clinicopathological differentiation to be made.

When one is dealing with a biopsy only and not aware of whether a tumor is radiographically or clinically diffuse or localized, delineation of a spindle-cell neoplasm may be difficult. Storiform patterns can be seen in both malignant fibrous tumor and sarcomatous forms of diffuse malignant mesothelioma. Nuclear pleomorphism may not be prominent in either. Ectatic blood vessels surrounded by proliferating spindled cells creating a pattern resembling angiofibroma favor localized fibrous tumor. Any epithelioid characteristics favor a diffuse malignant mesothelioma. Immunopathology is valuable. Positive staining for keratin and calretinin favor a diffuse malignant mesothelioma, whereas positive staining for CD 34 favors malignant fibrous tumor.

D. Surgery

Large tumors are approached through a standard posterolateral thoracotomy. Small lesions can be adequately removed by video-assisted thoracic surgery (VATS) techniques if the surgeon is experienced in VATS (3). A thorough exploration should be done at the time of resection as rarely additional synchronous tumors not seen on preoperative imaging may be present (3,30). In the classic case of a pedunculated tumor of the visceral pleura, a wedge resection of normal lung should be performed to obtain an adequate margin. Local recurrences have been reported even in cases with a pedicle, so a margin of normal lung should be removed and checked with intraoperative frozen section to confirm the resection is complete (3,10–12). Pleural-based lesions are more difficult to deal with because of the difficulty in obtaining a clear margin along the chest wall. For smaller tumors that are clinically and radiologically benign, a preliminary attempt at extrapleural dissection should be performed and if the normal areolar tissue plane is present the mass should be removed in the extrapleural plane. Intraoperative frozen section evaluation should be done to asses for malignancy, evaluate the peripheral characteristics of the tumor (encapsulated or invasive), and to check the true deep margin along the extrapleural plane. If a benign encapsulated tumor is found chest wall resection is not indicated. Patients with invasive or malignant tumors should have a chest wall resection performed. Patients with large tumors that are pleural-based that do not appear invasive by CT or intraoperative findings should also have a trial of extrapleural dissection as previously mentioned. Intraoperative core cutting biopsies should be considered in doubtful cases, as the finding of atypical histologic features support more aggressive surgery. Careful evaluation of the margins is again mandatory as the completeness of the resection is the most important factor in a favorable long-term prognosis (7). Complete parietal pleurectomy is not indicated. Resection of massive tumors can be quite challenging and incisional approaches may need to be modified to fit the location of the tumor. Two incisions (i.e., median sternotomy and lateral thoracotomy) and the clamshell incision may be of use in such cases (19,21,31). Preoperative embolization has been used with success to minimize bleeding in formidable tumors (19).

E. Results of Surgery

Operative mortality is zero in most series, reflecting the straightforward nature of most resections (Table 3). Essentially all benign and most invasive tumors are resectable. Chest wall or diaphragm resections are rarely required. Benign encapsulated tumors rarely recur if adequately resected. Recurrences of benign tumors have been noted up to 18 years after the primary resection, reflecting an indolent tumor biology in these patients (10). Reresection of benign tumors for apparent cure has been reported several times and suggests the need for very long-term follow-up (3,10–12). Recurrences after resection of LFTP with benign histology have been noted sometimes to be histologically bland but sometimes are histologically malignant (3,10–12). Return of the original symptoms of either clubbing or hypoglycemia have been noted in patients with recurrent tumors. Death from recurrent tumors is extremely rare after complete resection of histologically benign tumors.

Patients with malignant or invasive tumors do not fare as well and have a more variable prognosis. Many patients with worrisome histology have encapsulated tumors, which portends an intermediate prognosis (7). In England's

Table 3 Results of Surgical Treatment of LFTP

Number	% Malignant	Operative mortality	Recurrence	Follow-up	Ref.
21	38	0	1 (10 years postop)	All alive and well, median 68 months	12
55	7	0	1 (1 year postop)	All alive and well, median 53 months	3
10	30	0	1 (6 years postop)	All alive and well, median 53 months	11
15	56	0	5 (5 mo; 10 mo, 4 y, 6 y, 18 y)	2 died with disease, rest alive and well, mean 9 y	10
223	37	ns	Benign 140; 2 recurrences Malignant 77; 39 recurrences	Survival at 15 y: benign 85%, malignant without invasion 25%, malignant with invasion 15%	7

large series, about one half of the patients in this category were apparently cured by complete resection (7). Patients with malignant histological features and invasive tumors had the worst prognosis. Table 4 contrasts clinical, radiological and pathological prognostic factors identified in collected series (1,3,7,10–12).

X. Calcifying Fibrous Pseudotumor of the Pleura

Calcifying fibrous pseudotumor is a recently described entity, which generally occurs in the extremities, scrotum, groin, neck, and axilla (32,33). A few cases

Table 4 Clinical, Radiographic, and Gross Pathological Features That Affect Prognosis

Benign	Malignant
Asymptomatic	Symptomatic
Small	Large
No pleural effusion	Pleural effusion
Pedunculated	Broad-based
Visceral pleural origin	Origin from fissure, mediastinum, or parietal pleura
Homogeneous CT appearance	Heterogeneous (necrosis and hemorrhage) CT appearance

have presented in the pleura. The lesion is benign. The histology is distinctive. Calcifying fibrous pseudotumor is characterized by dense hyalinized collagen with interspersed benign spindled cells, a sparse inflammatory infiltrate, and randomly distributed psammoma bodies as well as dystrophic calcification. The psammoma bodies and dystrophic calcification distinguish calcifying fibrous pseudotumor of the pleura from localized fibrous tumor of the pleura and from desmoid tumor of the pleura.

References

1. Briselli M, Mark EJ, Dickersin GR. Solitary fibrous tumors of the pleura: eight new cases and review of 360 cases in the literature. Cancer 1981; 47:2678–2689.
2. Tastepe I, Alper A, Ozaydin HE, Memis L, Cetin G. A case of multiple synchronous localized fibrous tumor of the pleura. Eur J Cardiothorac Surg 2000; 18:491–494.
3. Cardillo G, Facciolo F, Cavazzana AO, Capece G, Gasparri R, Martelli M. Localized (solitary) fibrous tumors of the pleura: an analysis of 55 patients. Ann Thorac Surg 2000; 70:1808–1812.
4. Wagner E. Das tuberkelähnliche Lymphadenom (der cytogene oder reticulite Tuberkel). Arch Heilk 1870; 11:497.
5. Klemperer P, Rabin CB. Pulmonary neoplasm of the pleura: a report of five cases. Arch Pathol 1931; 11:385–412.
6. Clagett OT, McDonald JR, Schmidt HW. Localized fibrous mesothelioma of the pleura. J Thorac Surg 1952; 24:213–230.
7. England DM, Hochholzer L, McCarthy M. Localized benign and malignant fibrous tumors of the pleura. A clinicopathologic review of 223 cases. Am J Surg Pathol 1989; 13:640–658.
8. Martini N, McCormack PM, Bains MS, Kraiser LR, Burt ME, Hilaris BS. Pleural mesothelioma. Ann Thorac Surg 1987; 43:113–120.
9. Okike N, Bernatz E, Woolner B. Localized mesotelioma of the pleura. J Thorac Cardiovasc Surg 1978; 75:363–372.
10. Suter M, Gebhard S, Boumghar M, Peloponisios N, Genton CY. Localized fibrous tumours of the pleura: 15 new cases and review of the literature. Eur J Cardiothorac Surg 1998; 14:453–459.
11. De Perrot M, Kurt A, Robert JH, Borisch B, Spiliopoulos A. Clinical behavior of solitary fibrous tumors of the pleura. Ann Thorac Surg 1999; 67:1456–1459.
12. Rena O, Filosso PL, Papalia E, Molinatti M, Di Marzio P, Maggi G, Oliaro A. Solitary fibrous tumour of the pleura: surgical treatment. Eur J Cardiothorac Surg 2001; 19:185–189.
13. Kishi K, Homma S, Tanimura S, Matsushita H, Nakata K. Hypoglycemia induced by secretion of high molecular weight insulin-like growth factor-II from a malignant solitary fibrous tumor of the pleura. Intern Med 2001; 40:341–344.
14. Ulrik CS, Viskum K. Fibrous pleural tumor producing 171 liters of transudate. Eur Respir J 1998; 12:1230–1232.
15. Lee KS, Im JG, Choe KO, Kim CJ, Lee BH. CT findings in benign fibrous mesothelioma of the pleura: pathologic correlation in nine patients. Am J Roentgenol 1992; 158:983–986.

16. Harris GN, Rozenshtein A, Schiff MJ. Benign fibrous mesothelioma of the pleura: MR imaging findings. Am J Roentgenol 1995; 165:1143–1144.
17. Padovani B, Mouroux J, Raffaelli C, Huys C, Chanalet S, Michiels JF, Brunner P, Bruneton JN. Benign fibrous mesothelioma of the pleura: MR study and pathologic correlation. Eur Radiol 1996; 6:425–428.
18. Ferretti GR, Chiles C, Cox JE, Choplin RH, Coulomb M. Localized benign fibrous tumors of the pleura: MR appearance. J Comput Assist Tomogr 1997; 21:115–120.
19. Khan JH, Rahman SB, Clary-Macy C, Kerlan RK, George TI, Hall TS, Jablons DM. Giant solitary fibrous tumor of the pleura. Ann Thorac Surg 1998; 65:1461–1464.
20. Okada S, Ebihara Y, Kudo M, Serizawa H, Shimizu T, Otani M, Tsuji K. Scratch cytologic findings on surgically resected solitary fibrous tumors of the pleura. Acta Cytol 2001; 45:372–380.
21. Bicer M, Yaldiz S, Gursoy S, Ulgan M. A case of giant benign localized fibrous tumor of the pleura. Eur J Cardiothorac Surg 1998; 14:211–213.
22. Weymand B, Noel H, Goncette L, Noirhomme P, Collard P. Solitary fibrous tumor of the pleura. A report of five cases diagnosed by transthoracic cutting needle biopsy. Chest 1997; 112:424–428.
23. Scharifker D, Kaneko M. Localized fibrous "mesothelioma" of pleura (submesothelial fibroma). A clinicopathologic study of 18 cases. Cancer 1979; 43:627–635.
24. Keating S, Simon GT, Alexopoulou I, Kay JM. Solitary fibrous tumor of the pleura: an ultrastructural and immunohistochemical study. Thorax 1987; 42:976–979.
25. Westra WH, Gerald WL, Rosai J. Solitary fibrous tumor. Consistent CD34 immunoreactivity and occurrence in the orbit. Am J Surg Pathol 1994; 18:992–998.
26. Van de Rijn M, Lombard CM, Rouse RV. Expression of CD34 by solitary fibrous tumors of the pleura, mediastinum, and lung. Am J Surg Pathol 1994; 18:814–820.
27. Hanau CA, Mietinen M. Solitary fibrous tumor: histochemical spectrum of benign and malignant variants presenting at different sites. Hum Pathol 1995; 26:440–449.
28. Flint A, Weiss SW. CD-34 and keratin expression distinguishes solitary fibrous tumor (fibrous mesothelioma) of pleura from desmoplastic mesothelioma. Hum Pathol 1995; 26:428–431.
29. Bai H, Aswad BI, Gaissert H, Gnepp DR. Malignant solitary fibrous tumor of the pleura with liposarcomatous differentiation. Arch Pathol Lab Med 2001; 125:406–409.
30. Tastepe I, Alper A, Ozaydin HE, Memis L, Cetin G. A case of multiple synchronous localized fibrous tumors of the pleura. Eur J Cardiothorac Surg 2000; 18:491–494.
31. Veronesi G, Spaggiari L, Mazzarol G, De Pas M, Leo F, Solli P, Pastorino U. Huge malignant localized fibrous tumor of the pleura. J Cardiovasc Surg 2000; 41:781–784.
32. Fetsch JF, Montgomery EA, Meis JM. Calcifying fibrous tumor. Am J Surg Pathol 1993; 17:502–508.
33. Pinkard NB, Wilson RW, Lawless N. Calcifying fibrous pseudotumor of the pleura: a report of three cases of a newly described entity involving the pleura. Am J Clin Pathol 1996; 105:189–194.

26

Pleurodesis

FRANCISCO RODRIGUEZ-PANADERO

Hospital Universitario Virgen del Rocío
Sevilla, Spain

Pleurodesis is defined as the symphysis between the visceral and parietal pleural surfaces that prevents accumulation of either air or fluid in the pleural space. Its main indications are malignant pleural effusions and pneumothorax, although some benign effusions may occasionally require this treatment also.

I. Pleurodesis in Malignant Pleural Effusions

Most of the patients undergoing a pleurodesis procedure have a symptomatic malignant pleural effusion (MPE). When this condition is diagnosed, palliative therapy should be considered, with special evaluation of the patient's symptoms, general health and functional status, and expected survival. The main indication for treatment in such cases is relief of dyspnea, which is dependent on both the volume of the effusion and the underlying condition of the lungs and pleura. Therapeutic thoracentesis should be performed in virtually all dyspneic patients with MPE to determine its effect on breathlessness and rate and degree of recurrence. This is especially important in patients who present with a massive pleural effusion and contralateral mediastinal shift (Fig. 1) and those patients are also the obvious candidates for a pleurodesis procedure. Also, rapid recurrence of the effusion dictates the need for immediate treatment (Fig. 2), while stability

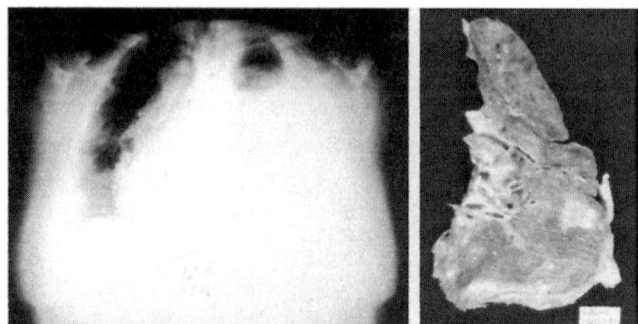

Figure 1 Contralateral mediastinal shift in a patient with lymphoma. Talc pleurodesis was successfully achieved, as shown in the autopsy specimen (on the right).

and absence of symptoms may warrant observation. If dyspnea is not relieved by thoracentesis, other causes should be investigated, such as lymphangitic carcinomatosis, atelectasis, thromboembolism, and tumor embolism.

If the effusion is small (less than one third of the hemithorax) and cytology is positive, the best choice would be to apply chemotherapy if the primary is known and it is sensitive to that treatment (breast, ovary, small-cell lung cancer,

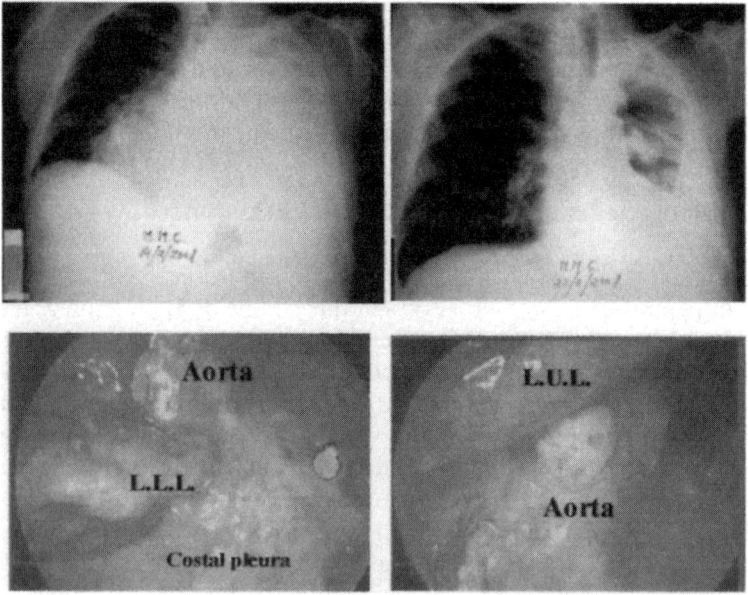

Figure 2 This patient had a rapidly recurrent effusion, and thoracoscopic talc poudrage was successfully performed. Infiltration of the costal pleura and the wall of the aorta was seen at thoracoscopy. L.L.L. = left lower lobe; L.U.L. = left upper lobe.

lymphoma, etc.) and to observe the evolution of the pleural effusion. When cytology is negative and/or the primary is unknown, thoracoscopy would be recommended, since the diagnosis yield is high, large specimens can be taken under visual control for special studies (immunohistochemistry and others), and talc poudrage for pleurodesis can be performed at the same time also.

According to our experience, pleurodesis would be required in about two thirds of patients with malignant effusion sooner or later (1). In the presence of a large and recurrent effusion the choice is clearly defined in favor of pleurodesis, preferably using talc. This should be done as early as possible in order to prevent development of a trapped lung, which could provoke a failure in lung reexpansion and pleurodesis (Fig. 3).

When the malignant effusion is relatively small (less than one third of the hemithorax), one wonders if this particular patient is ever going to need any pleurodesis procedure. The answer would be obvious if the effusion remains stable and is well tolerated, but in an undefined proportion of cases it would progress to a larger effusion, with the subsequent deterioration of the patient's condition and advance of the disease. This could lead to a trapped lung, thus making any pleurodesis attempt risky and unlikely to be successful. According to a recent prospective study from our group, serial determinations of pH and D-dimer in pleural fluid would be of help in predicting which patients are more

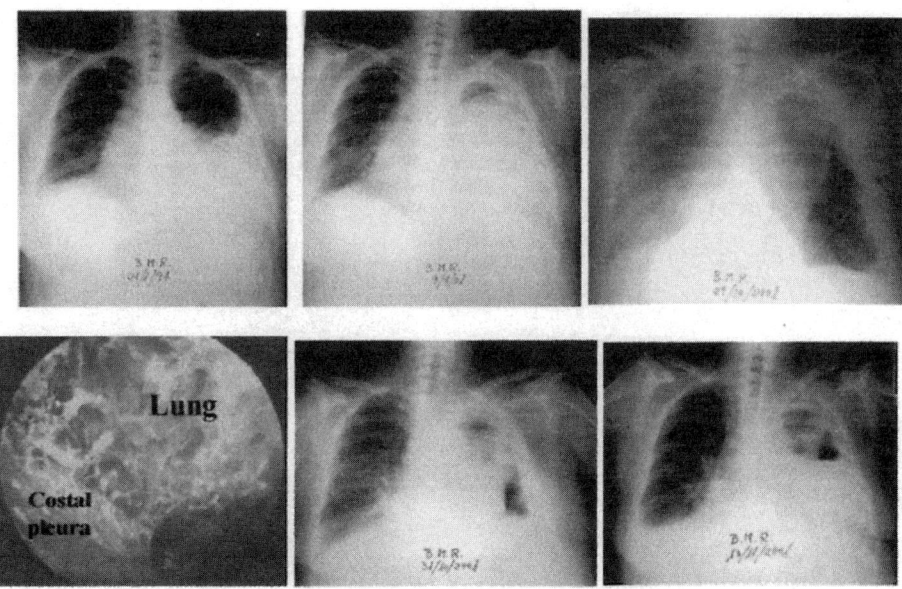

Figure 3 Left breast carcinoma was resected in 1986. A metastatic left pleural effusion was detected at the beginning of 1997, and chemotherapy was given, with partial response. Talc pleurodesis was not requested until October 2001, but a heavily trapped lung was then found at thoracoscopy, and we were unable to achieve reexpansion of the lung.

likely to need pleurodesis (2): patients requiring pleurodesis over the follow-up period showed a declining pH on serial determinations, and the pleural fluid D-dimer median levels were growing higher in the pleurodesis group than in those who never required a pleurodesis procedure.

Before attemtpting pleurodesis, complete lung reexpansion should be demonstrated. Failure of complete lung expansion occurs with mainstem bronchial occlusion by tumor or trapped lung due to extensive pleural tumor infiltration (Fig. 4). If contralateral mediastinal shift is not observed on chest radiograph with a large pleural effusion or the lung does not expand completely after pleural space drainage, an endobronchial obstruction or trapped lung should be suspected. Bronchoscopy is mandatory if the bronchial obstruction is suspected (Fig. 5), but management of trapped lung can be much more complex. It can be detected on contrast computed tomography (CT) scans, and pleural pressure measurement during thoracentesis might also be useful. In patients with mediastinum centered or with ipsilateral shift, the likelihood of a precipitous drop in pleural pressure is increased, and either pleural pressure should be monitored during thoracentesis or only a small volume of fluid should be removed. In the patient with ipsilateral mediastinal shift, it is unlikely that removal of pleural fluid will result in significant relief of dyspnea (Fig. 6), since there is either mainstem bronchial occlusion or a trapped lung. Moreover,

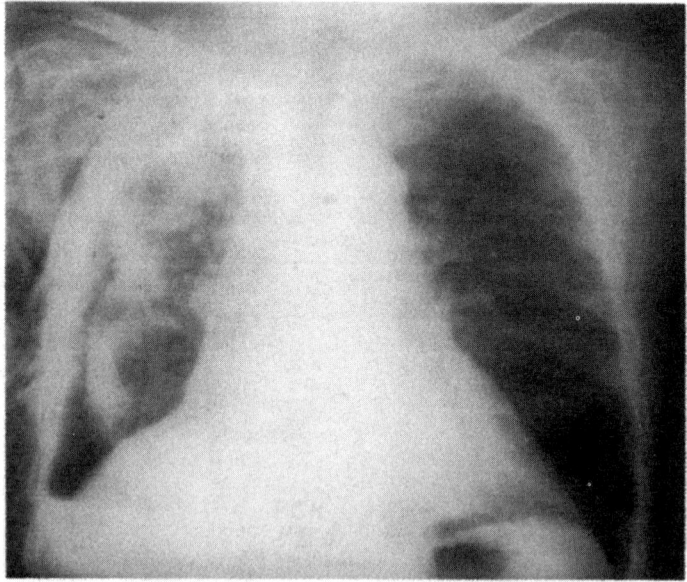

Figure 4 Metastatic pleural carcinoma of the lung. The visceral pleura is very thick and the lung could not reexpand after placement of drainage.

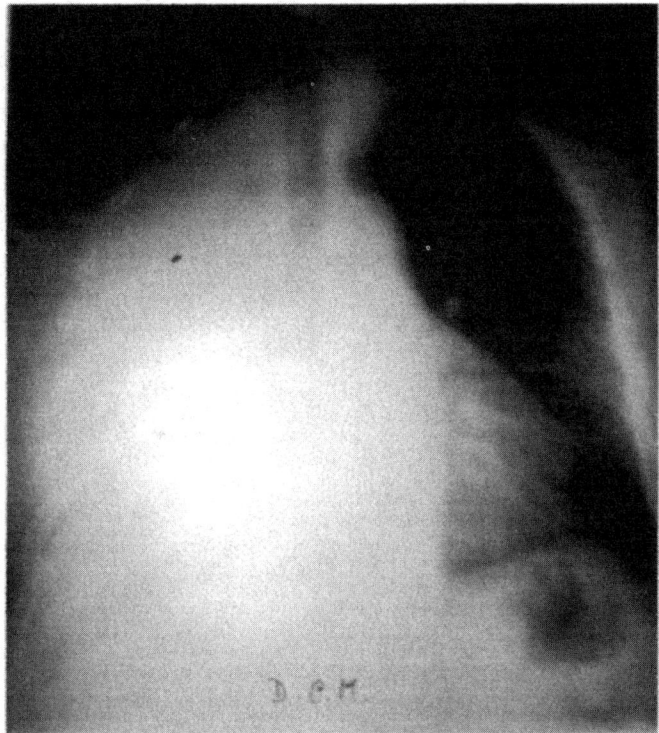

Figure 5 Pleural effusion with ipsilateral mediastinal shift and loss of volume of the right hemithorax. Bronchoscopy should be performed in these cases before attempting pleurodesis.

pleurodesis is hardly indicated in this case, and other therapeutic measures should be considered (see below).

An initial pleural fluid of -10 cmH$_2$O at thoracentesis makes trapped lung likely (3). According to Lan and coworkers (4), Pleural elastance seems to be the best predictor for trapped lung and outcome of pleurodesis, although outcome was also correlated with pH and glucose levels of the effusion (see below). Cut points of -19 cmH$_2$O with the removal of 500 mL of pleural fluid are predictive of trapped lung in the absence of endobronchial obstruction. Measurement of the pleural pressure during thoracentesis may be cumbersome, and the pressure curve profile can differ significantly between patients (5).

II. Definition of Success or Failure of Pleurodesis in MPE

Recently a Joint Task Force of the American Thoracic Society and the European Respiratory Society published a consensus statement on management of malig-

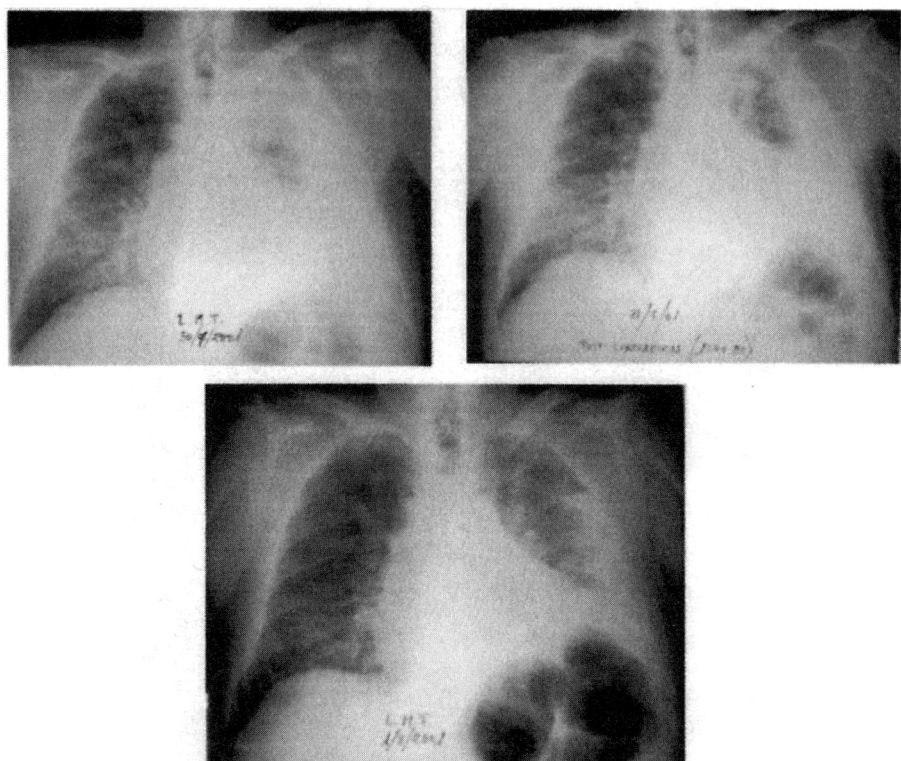

Figure 6 The left hemithorax shows a marked retraction after partial drainage of the effusion. Pleurodesis is unlikely to improve the quality of life in these patients.

nant pleural effusions. According to this statement, the following definitions are proposed (6):

Successful pleurodesis:
- Complete success. Long-term relief of symptoms related to the effusion, with absence of fluid reaccumulation on chest radiographs until death.
- Partial success. Diminution of dyspnea related to the effusion, with only partial reaccumulation of fluid (less than 50% of the initial radiographic evidence of fluid), with no further therapeutic thoracenteses required for the remainder of the patient's life.

Failed pleurodesis: Lack of success as defined above.

Comparative studies of different pleurodesis techniques should evaluate outcomes using time-to-event analyses, censoring patients who are lost to follow-up. Data should be reported with and without inclusion of patients who die within one month of pleurodesis.

A. Pleural pH and Outcome of Pleurodesis in MPE

Pleural fluid pH and glucose can be of help as a first approach to a patient in whom pleurodesis is being considered, as a low glucose/pH has been associated with short survival and poor results of pleurodesis (7,8). We found a complete successful pleurodesis in 90% of the patients with pH > 7.30, whereas it was successful only in 33% of those with pH lower than 7.20 and in none of the patients with pH < 7.15 (9). The association between pH and outcome of pleurodesis was also found by others (10,11). However, Heffner and coworkers found in a meta-analysis study that, although pH was by itself an independent predictor of survival, it has insufficient predictive accuracy for selecting patients for pleurodesis on the basis of estimated survival (12). Nevertheless, I believe that the impact of mesothelioma cases may have been underestimated in that study, since patients with mesothelioma tend to survive longer than those with metastatic pleural carcinoma (13), and they also have a tendency to show a lower pH, due to the marked pleural thickening caused by mesothelioma. Therefore, it is likely that those mesothelioma patients provoked a double-way bias on the pH-survival relationship in the Heffner studies (they survive longer and have an average lower pH than metastatic carcinomas). This bias could also explain some of the controversial reports on low pH and prolonged survival—that of Bilaceroglu and colleagues in particular (14). In the largest study reporting pleurodesis with *Corynebacterium parvum* in the literature, those authors found no correlation between pH and both survival and pleurodesis outcome in Turkey. However, a large subset of patients with mesothelioma was included in their series of 131 cases with MPE, thus making the comparison with other studies problematic.

Regarding pH and pleurodesis outcome, it must be pointed out that different procedures for pleurodesis—with repeated applications of the sclerosant in many cases—makes results hardly comparable in a "pooled" meta-analysis study. In addition, the same above-mentioned problem regarding low pH in mesotheliomas might apply here. In summary, it is my belief that pleural pH still has a role in the management of patients with malignant pleural effusion, especially those who present with low pH/glucose levels. Although I would never exclude a single patient for pleurodesis on the sole basis of his or her low pH, taking into consideration this parameter when managing patients with MPE—in conjunction with the patient's performance status, primary tumor type and response to therapeutic thoracentesis—makes things easier in clinical practice.

B. Contraindications to Pleurodesis in MPE

Like any other invasive procedure, pleurodesis, especially thoracoscopic talc poudrage, is contraindicated in cases of intractable coagulation disorders, and severe respiratory insufficiency is also a contraindication ($pCO_2 > 55$ mmHg). Moreover, pleurodesis should not be attempted in patients with a significant contralateral involvement of the lung, since they are likely to develop an acute respiratory insufficiency (Fig. 7). The presence of a bilateral pleural effusion

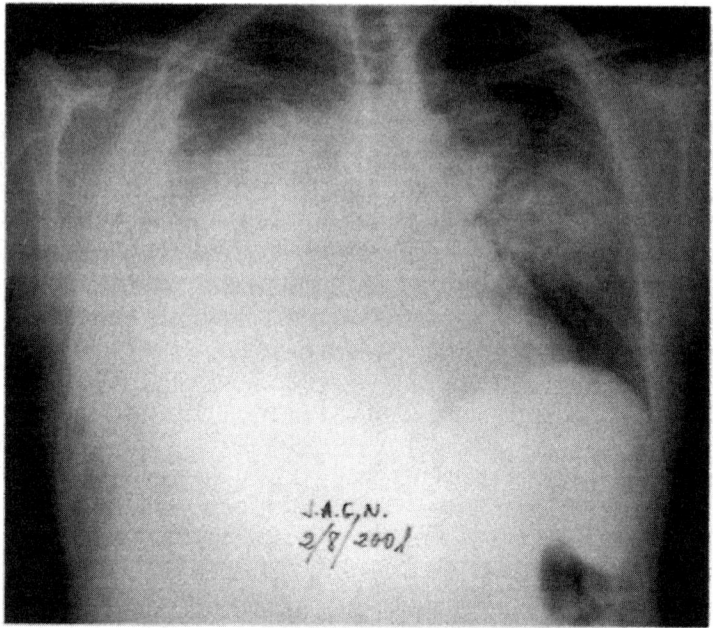

Figure 7 Extensive bilateral involvement of the lung parenchyma is a formal contraindication to talc poudrage in this patient with lymphoma.

might also be problematic, unless all the effusion is removed from the contralateral side before attempting pleurodesis on one side. Simultaneous pleurodesis should not be attempted in any case, since the likelihood of developing complications is high.

III. Pleurodesis in Pneumothorax

The main problem in managing pneumothorax—either primary or secondary—lies in the rate of recurrence, which is unacceptably high when drainage alone is used. Therefore, a pleurodesis technique is frequently required to be on the safer side and achieve a pleural symphysis. In a prospective randomized study, Almind and coworkers compared the recurrence of pneumothorax using drainage alone and drainage plus tetracycline or talc and found a rate of 36, 13, and 8%, respectively, after an average follow-up of 4.6 years (15). Alfageme and coworkers found a 9% recurrence rate with tetracycline pleurodesis as compared to 35% in patients with drainage alone (16).

Application of sclerosing agents or even thoracotomy has been done frequently to prevent recurrence in high-risk patients with pneumothorax, and it has been postulated that a previous thoracoscopic evaluation is very helpful in assigning patients to one or another procedure (17). Some controversy exists as to what would be the choice for patients with secondary spontaneous pneumothorax (i.e., with known underlying lung disease), especially those who have evidence of bullae on CT scans. There has been a growing trend to treat patients with pneumothorax using video-assisted thoracoscopic surgery (VATS), which allows for the endoscopic resection of the bullae or blebs, as well as for pleurodesis, either through mechanical abrasion of the parietal pleura or application of localized apical talc pleurodesis. In a survey conducted by the German Society for Thoracic Surgery, Hurtgen and coworkers reported the results of 1365 VATS procedures (18) and found an overall 10.2% rate of recurrence when only bleb resection was done (with no pleurodesis procedure added). Thoracoscopic pleural abrasion had also a rather high recurrence rate in their series (7.9%, but it depends on the extension of the abrasion), and coagulation of the apical zone of the parietal pleura appeared to be promising (2.7% recurrence). The VATS procedure is, however, expensive and requires general anesthesia with double-lumen tracheal intubation. According to Naunheim and coworkers (19), the rate of recurrence with VATS varies widely depending on identification and subsequent ablation of blebs. Apical talc pleurodesis should be considered as a supplement to bleb resection in select patients with high risk of recurrence of the pneumothorax.

There is some concern about the generous use of sclerosants for pleurodesis in pneumothorax, especially talc in young patients, who might require a thoracotomy for lung cancer or some other cause (i.e., lung transplantation in cystic fibrosis) in the future. Therefore, the approach to the patient with pneumothorax still remains controversial (20). In our view, VATS would be the technique of choice in young patients with recurrent pneumothorax, whereas a conventional thoracoscopic pleurodesis would be the preferred procedure in elderly patients with spontaneous pneumothorax. These patients might not tolerate VATS because the need for single-lung ventilation, and talc may be the sclerosing agent of choice in them (21,22). Pleurodesis using autologous blood "patch" appears to be effective in those difficult cases (23,24), but special care has to be taken in order to prevent development of empyema. It has been successfully used in postoperatory persistent air leak (25).

Cystic fibrosis patients have a marked tendency to develop repeated and bilateral pneumothoraces, but they can be candidates for lung transplantation as well, and they therefore need a treatment that will be efficient and yet allow for an eventual thoracotomy. Chest drainage with underwater sealing would be the choice for a few days, with subsequent VATS, bullectomy, and apical pleurodesis if the air leak persists (26,27).

IV. Pleurodesis in Benign Effusions

Although this is a rather uncommon indication for pleurodesis, there are a few occasions where patients with benign effusions, such as those with persistent effusion from cardiac, nephrotic, or cirrhotic origin that are not responsive to standard treatment, require a pleurodesis procedure. According to Sudduth and Sahn, the following three criteria should be met (28):

> The effusion must be symptomatic.
> The presence of a trapped lung should be excluded.
> Pleurodesis should be reserved for those cases where there is no other therapeutic alternative or when other measures have failed.

Vargas and coworkers reported their experience using a low dose (2 g) of talc in such conditions with a very good success rate (29). According to my own experience I would add some supplementary recommendations to those mentioned above:

> Talc pleurodesis in effusions of cardiac origin is usually successful, but a combined standard medical treatment should be applied also.
> Management of pleural effusions associated to cirrhosis of the liver is very difficult (especially when ascites is present) because some communications between the abdominal and pleural cavity frequently exist. Those peritoneal-pleural fistulas can occasionally be seen at thoracoscopy and make pleurodesis rarely successful (30).
> Patients with chylothorax are also occasionally difficult to manage, as it is absolutely necessary that chyle flux through the thoracic duct be reduced to a minimum. This can be achieved by using a special diet or, more importantly, suspending gastrointestinal feeding and giving intravenous hyperalimentation instead. Management of patients with chylothorax related to malignancy (particularly lymphoma) is especially difficult, but intravenous feeding can also be necessary in rapidly recurrent chylothorax associated with benign causes.

V. Technical Aspects of Pleurodesis

A. Choice of Sclerosing Agent

More than 30 sclerosing agents have been used to achieve pleural symphysis, including talc, tetracycline hydrochloride, or its derivatives. Bleomycin, *Corynebacterium parvum*, and silver nitrate are among the others that have been reported as effective pleurodesis agents. However, certain agents stand out for their ability to achieve pleurodesis with minimal side effects (31–33). Interested readers should consult reviews on this topic (34–37). A comprehensive review on the success obtained with the most relevant agents was provided by the ATS/ERS Consensus Statement on MPE (6). Talc had the best rate of success, and it was suggested that both poudrage and slurry applications are about equally successful, although the potential disadvantages of slurry include lack of uniform distribution and accumulation in dependent areas of the pleural cavity, with subsequent incomplete pleurodesis and multiculations (Fig. 7). Also, part of the talc instilled might come out through drainage at the time of applying suction after slurry application. In one recent randomized study comparing talc poudrage and slurry in 55 patients with malignant pleural effusion, Mañes and coworkers found a significantly higher rate of recurrences with talc slurry than with poudrage (38). Slurry is usually prepared by mixing talc in powder with different amounts of normal saline (10–250 mL). The addition of an iodide compound (thymol or povidone) has not improved the pleurodesis outcome experimentally (39). Moreover, iodide might provoke severe adverse effects when instilled into the pleural space, especially in allergic patients. Although an optimal dose of talc for poudrage has not been established, about 4 g is recommended for malignant effusions.

A dose of 2–3 g of talc should not be exceeded in pneumothorax; this dose frequently needs to be doubled in malignant effusions.

B. Drainage for Talc Pleurodesis

Several technical details should be taken into account in order to achieve good pleurodesis and avoid complications. All pleural fluid should be removed before applying talc. Removal can be easily accomplished during thoracoscopy, as air is passively entering the pleural cavity, thus creating a desirable equilibrium in pressures. Complete collapse of the lung is important, affording a good view of the pleural cavity, and the opportunity to biopsy suspicious lesions is an added bonus for thorascoscopy. Also, the wide distribution of talc can be easily checked during the procedure.

After talc insufflation, repeat inspection of the pleural cavity should be done to ensure that the powder has been evenly distributed over the pleural surface. The largely normal pleural mesothelial surface existing in pneumothorax patients leads to a significantly greater pleural responsiveness than in malignant pleural involvement.

Size of chest tube. A small-bore catheter has been sometimes proposed for pleurodesis (40–42), but I believe that a 24–32F chest tube should always be recommended whenever talc is applied in order to prevent obstruction of the drainage by clots.

Time of drainage prior to pleurodesis. Although is it frequently quoted in the literature that the amount of pleural fluid drained per day should be reduced to less than 100–150 mL before proceeding to pleurodesis, there is sufficient evidence that the only condition really needed is the ability of the lung to reexpand (43). Therefore, I would recommend applying the sclerosant as soon as possible after chest tube insertion, once the lung expandability has been demonstrated, since a prolonged drainage might provoke adhesions and multiloculations before the sclerosing procedure, thus impairing the symphysis process itself.

Rate of suction. In order to prevent reexpansion pulmonary edema, carefully graded and progressive suction should be applied and maintained until the amount of fluid aspirated per day is less than 100 mL. We usually put the drainage in water seal without suction for about 3 hours following talc poudrage, and then begin to apply gentle suction (2–5 cmH$_2$O). That suction rate can be then doubled every 3 hours until -20 to -30 cmH$_2$O are reached.

Air leak can occur during lung reexpansion (44), especially in patients who have necrotic tumor nodules in the visceral pleura. In our experience, this is more likely to occur in patients who had undergone chemotherapy previously, even if no biopsies of the lung or visceral pleura were taken during the thoracoscopy procedure.

VI. Mechanisms of Pleurodesis

The underlying, common response in the pleural space to the instillation of a pleurodesis agent is inflammation (45), and inflammation resolves with the subsequent development of fibrosis. Pleurodesis can also be achieved by abrading the pleural surface as is often done for patients with pneumothoraces following surgical removal of blebs on the surface of the lung. This implies that perturbation of normal pleural mesothelial cells allows for the initiation of an inflammatory process that eventually results in the development of symphysis between the visceral and parietal pleural surfaces. Following instillation of talc, there is a rapid neutrophil influx in the pleural space followed by an accumulation of mononuclear cells (46). In that study neutrophil accumulation reached its peak 3–24 hours following instillation of talc, and our experience is about the same (47) (Fig. 8). It appears that the chemokine interleukin-8 (IL-8) correlated with the level of neutrophils seen in the pleural space indicating that the sclerotic agent, in this instance talc, had initiated the release of neutrophil chemokines in

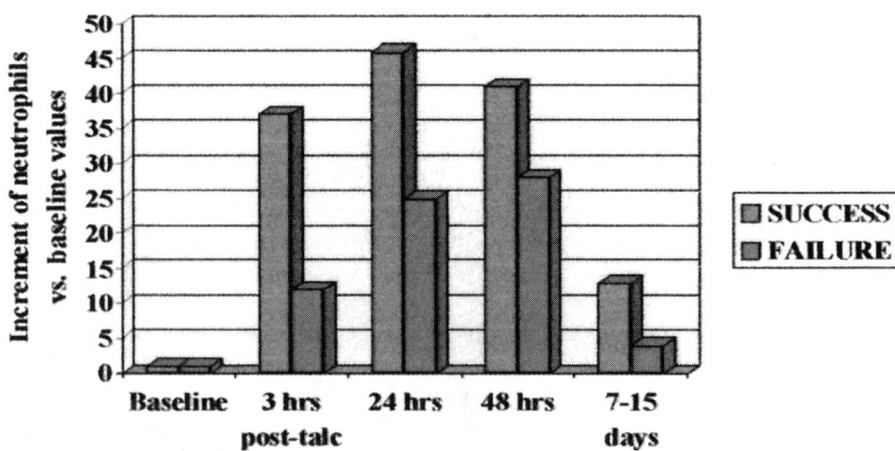

Figure 8 In patients with successful pleurodesis, neutrophils in pleural fluid increase very rapidly after intrapleural application. (Rodriguez-Panadero et al., unpublished results.)

the pleural space (48) (Fig. 9). Other chemoattractants to monocytes are also released after intrapleural instillation of the sclerosant; once neutrophils and monocytes are recruited to the pleural space, they themselves can be sources of further cytokine release, which then perpetuates the inflammatory cascade.

The inflammatory response to the sclerosant can be significantly inhibited by corticosteroids (49), and, according to our own experience, simultaneous steroid treatment is associated with an increased rate of failed pleurodesis in clinical practice (Fig. 10).

A second critical response to a sclerosing agent is the initiation of the coagulation cascade and a decrease in the pleural fibrinolytic activity. These appear to be required for the early formation of fibrin strands between the visceral and parietal pleura, which define the process of sclerosis. Fibrinolytic activity as expressed by D-dimer levels shows a decline 24 hours after talc poudrage in patients who have successful pleurodesis. In patients who have an unsuccessful pleurodesis, D-dimer activity is not decreased after talc poudrage (50). According to our investigations, this fibrinolytic activity is modulated by the expression of activators and inhibitors by the tumoral and nontumoral tissue in the pleural space (51–53). Since there are some commercial kits available to perform rapid neutrophils count and D-dimer determination, we currently use them in combination in order to monitor the ongoing biologic process after intrapleural talc instillation (Fig. 11). Thus, patients who are developing a good inflammatory response show a typical pattern with rapidly increasing neutrophils and declining D-dimer in serial samples of pleural fluid after talc poudrage. If this does not occur or the response to talc is poor, we attempt to enhance the pleurodesis process by increasing the suction rate and prolonging the drainage time in order to provoke a better pleural symphysis through mechanical irritation.

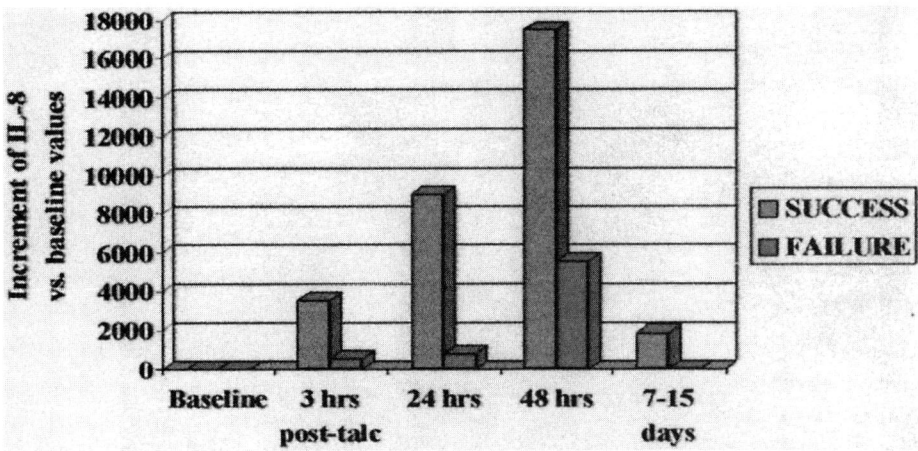

Figure 9 In a similar form to neutrophils, interleukin 8 (IL-8) increases dramatically in successful talc poudrage. (Rodriguez-Panadero et al., unpublished results.)

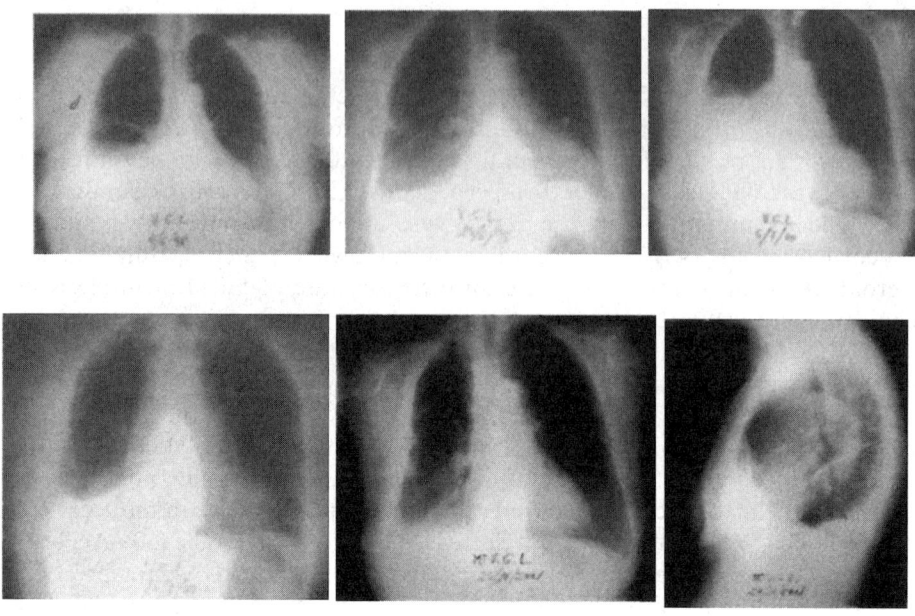

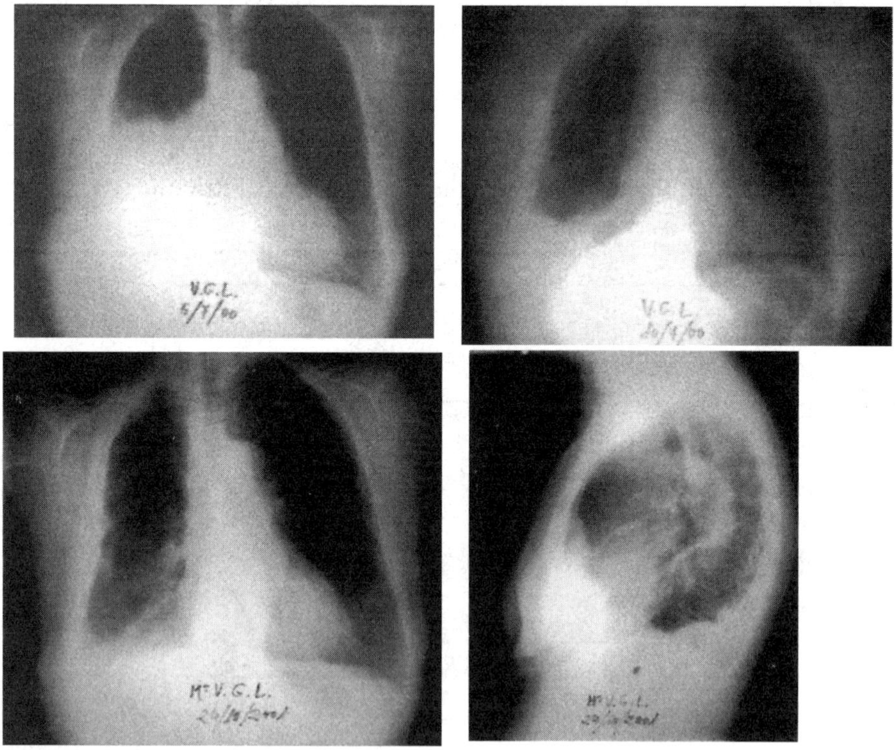

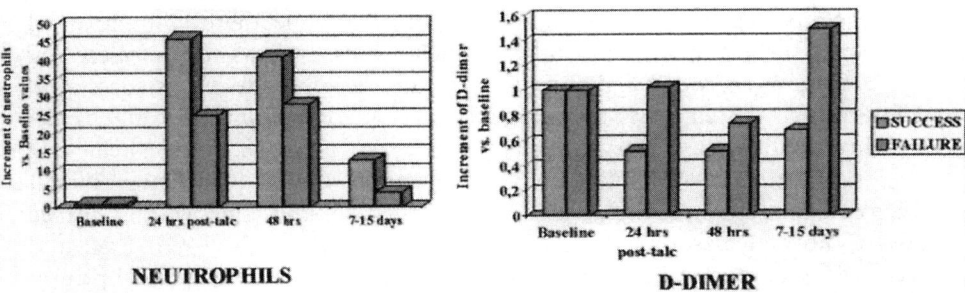

Figure 11 Monitorization of both neutrophils serial counts and D-dimer determination in pleural fluid can be very helpful in controlling the biological process that leads to pleural symphysis after talc poudrage. (Rodriguez-Panadero et al., unpublished results.)

The formation of a fine latticework of fibrin (the end product of the coagulation cascade) between the visceral and parietal pleura then allows the third step of the inflammatory cascade to be initiated. This process allows for the development of true fibrosis with the proliferation of fibroblasts, which form strong adhesive links between the visceral and parietal pleural surfaces, obliterating tissue margins. Several fibroblast growth factors have been found to be present in the pleural fluid of patients given sclerosing agents. These include platelet-derived growth factor (PDGF), basic fibroblast growth factor (bFGF), and transforming growth factor-β (TGF-β). In combined research with Antony Group at Indiana University, we evaluated pleural fluids obtained from patients who had both successful and unsuccessful pleurodesis following talc insufflation and found that patients with successful pleurodesis had a marked increase in the amount of bFGF in their pleural fluids. Patients with an unsuccessful pleurodesis had significantly lower amounts of bFGF (54). This phenomenon was also evaluated in vitro, where pleural mesothelial cells were stimulated with talc. bFGF was released in significant quantities by these mesothelial cells; however, glass beads of similar size as that of talc did not cause this exuberant response of fibroblast growth factor production (55). There appears to be a significant inverse correlation between the release of bFGF into the pleural fluids of patients who have malignant pleural effusions and the tumor size as evaluated by objective grading during thoracoscopy. Thus, patients with extensive pleural surface involvement by tumor do not have a high bFGF production by the mesothelial cells, primarily because of extensive involvement of the pleural surface by malignant implants. However, when talc was instilled into patients early

Figure 10 This patient with metastatic carcinoma of the colon was on steroids at the time of talc pleurodesis (June 15, 1998). Despite having achieved a complete lung reexpansion, pleurodesis had a late failure (a), and we had to repeat it—successfully this time—about 3 years later (b).

in the course of their malignant pleural disease while there still remained significant surface area of pleural mesothelial cells exposed to the sclerosing agent, there was a much higher level of bFGF and pleurodesis was successful. Thus, there appeared to be an inverse correlation between tumor size and bFGF level in pleural fluids. This is consistent with clinical experience where achieving sclerosis in patients with a far advanced malignant pleural involvement is difficult when compared to those early in the course of their disease. Thus, a larger surface area of normal mesothelial cells is associated with a high bFGF level and successful pleurodesis. An exuberant and vigorous response by normal pleural mesothelial cells appears to be critical for achieving pleurodesis.

In summary, initiation of pleurodesis by instillation of a sclerotic agent into the pleural space is associated with a sequence of inflammatory events leading to pleural fibrosis. These steps involve an inflammatory cascade of increased phagocytic cellular trafficking in the pleural space, the laying down of a lattice fibrin network between the visceral and parietal pleura, and finally, the exuberant growth and proliferation of pleural fibroblasts leading to loss of tissue margins between the two surfaces.

VII. Side Effects and Complications of Pleurodesis

Talc has been used widely in Europe for a long time, with only a few complications reported, but it was not so widely accepted in USA, where discontinuation of tetracycline production provoked a concerned search for other sclerosing agents (56,57). The most frequently reported side effects are pain and fever, which usually does not exceed 38°C and is related to release of acute inflammation mediators. However, more severe complications can arise after application of a sclerosant into the pleural cavity.

Pulmonary edema can occur when reexpanding the lung in pneumothorax and malignant effusions, even without application of any sclerosant. Although the edema usually appears on the ipsilateral hemithorax, Mahfood and coworkers reported three cases in which it was contralateral, with fatal outcome in two cases (58). The mechanism for this complication is not fully understood; however, a too rapid reexpansion, especially if the lung was collapsed for several weeks, may play an important role, as pointed out by several authors (59) and confirmed by our experience. We had this problem in 2 of 330 patients who underwent thoracoscopic talc poudrage, in whom a rapid increase in suction was applied (60). Nevertheless, there must be other factors involved, since no suction at all was applied in two of the patients who developed this complication in a series from Rozenman and colleagues (61). An increased protein leakage and several inflammation mediators that were chemotactic for neutrophils were found by Nakamura and coworkers in one patient who developed a reexpansion pulmonary edema following application of positive pressure through the tracheal tube during surgical treatment of pneumothorax (62). As no negative pleural pressure was used to reexpand the collapsed lung, the findings in this case support the existence of some (unclear so far) biological mechanisms involved in the development of this complication.

Acute respiratory distress or pneumonitis has been described in a few cases of talc pleurodesis (63–65). The precise pathophysiological mechanisms responsible for this severe complication are still unclear, but it appears that a high dose of talc used might have played a significant role. In their study on experimental talc slurry pleurodesis, Kennedy and coworkers found prominent perivascular infiltrates with mononuclear inflammation in the underlying lung, and they speculated that some mediators might spread through the pulmonary circulation (66). Also, they found a wide dissemination of talc particles in several distant organs, but the pathophysiological consequences of this phenomenon were not clarified in their study.

There is some concern about the systemic absorption of the sclerosing agents, and this is suspected to be the rule in almost all of the soluble agents that are instilled into the pleural space. On the other hand, talc is thought to persist for a long time in the pleural space, thus accounting, at least in part, for its better results in pleurodesis. There are, however, some disturbing reports on the finding of talc particles in distant organs after talc pleurodesis in both animals (67) and humans (68). Nevertheless, our experience with four autopsies in patients who had undergone a thoracoscopic talc poudrage is definitely different, since no talc was found beyond the pleura in any of our autopsied cases. It appears that the size of the talc particles, the technique of application (never apply strong positive pressure into the pleural space!), and perhaps some vascular openings provoked in the visceral pleura and underlying lung by the thoracoscopic biopsies might play an important role in the whole process. Recent research has demonstrated that different samples of talc show a marked variation in size or composition of particles (69,70). Another study from the same group found significant differences in experimental pleurodesis in rabbits (personal communication). In an ongoing combined study (involving samples of talc from more than 10 centers in Europe and America), we have found a significant association between some of the talc-related symptoms/complications and the size of particles. According to our findings, talc containing a significant number of particles smaller than 5 µm should be avoided for pleurodesis. Mitchem and coworkers found that talc provoked an increased angiotensin-converting enzyme activity in serum in one experimental study in rabbits (71). Although these authors did not specifically address the issue of talc particle dissemination, it is likely that this was the case, and it is therefore possible that those systemic effects were related to talc dissemination.

The possible activation of the systemic coagulation following pleurodesis is a worrying issue too. Agrenius and coworkers demonstrated an increase in pleural coagulation and inhibition of fibrinolytic activity after the instillation of quinacrine as a sclerosing agent (72,73). Since it is assumed that a fibrin mesh formation is a necessary step for the fibrotic process, these findings make sense in the context of the mechanisms that lead to pleural symphysis. We also demonstrated similar effects after talc pleurodesis in our patients (50) and were subsequently concerned about the possible systemic implications of the pleural coagulation/fibrinolysis imbalance, which is associated with the pleurodesis process itself. Prompted by this concern and by our finding of two cases of massive pulmonary embolism after talc pleurodesis, we conducted a preliminary study on simultaneous pleural/plasma determination of markers of coagulation and fibrinolysis. We found that an activation of the systemic coagulation is frequently observed after talc poudrage (74) and that this side effect can be partially controlled with prophylactic heparin (75). The relevance of this finding in clinical practice is still unclear, but it might occur that early death (less than 30 days after sclerotherapy) following some pleurodesis procedures—up to 43% in the series of Seaton and coworkers (40)—are in part related to an undetected pulmonary embolism and not only to advanced neoplastic disease, as it is commonly thought.

VIII. Alternatives to Talc Pleurodesis

A. Tetracycline Derivatives

Doxycycline

According to one experimental study done in rabbits, doxycycline is as effective as tetracycline for pleurodesis, its effect is independent of the acidity of the doxycycline solution, and moderate concentrations of the substance (10 mg/kg) can produce excellent results (76). In clinical practice, the average reported effectiveness of doxycycline is about 72%, but it often requires repeated doses, sometimes for more than 2 weeks. Pain in doxycycline application is an important issue too, and heavy analgesia is therefore recommended. Another experimental study from Mitchem and coworkers in rabbits fl found important changes in liver function enzymes and tissue toxicity.

Minocycline

Minocycline has also been proposed as a substitute for tetracycline, with an overall success rate of 86% in a few small series. However, minocycline has been reported to cause serious, albeit rare, adverse effects including serum sickness–like and hypersensitivity syndrome reactions and drug-induced lupus (77). Also, it can provoke vestibular symptoms when the doses usually required for pleurodesis are given, and a high rate of hemothorax after intrapleural application of those high doses has been reported in experimental studies (78).

B. Other Sclerosing Agents

Bleomycin

This agent does not appear to be effective in experimental animal studies (79), and it has been shown to be inferior to talc in clinical practice (80). In addition, it is expensive and also has the risk of significant systemic toxicity.

Quinacrine

Quinacrine use has been frequently reported in Scandinavia with good results. However, it can provoke serious toxicity of the central nervous system when given at high doses. Bjorkman and colleagues showed that its intrapleural administration provoked peak plasma concentrations—far above the normal therapeutic range—both in rabbits and humans and that the mean absorption half-life was approximately 7 minutes (81). The possible systemic side effects due to high absorption rate from the pleural space are likely to occur with other soluble agents, as demonstrated by Wooten and coworkers with tetracycline and lidocaine (82).

Corynebacterium Parvum Pleurodesis

This agent was widely used in a few European countries in the past but is no longer available in most institutions. Its efficacy was reported to be as high as 90% in some small series (83). However, it was effective in only 32% in another randomized study (84), and it was ineffective in creating pleural fibrosis experimentally in rabbits (85). Patient selection might have played a significant role in the wide variability of the reported results.

Sodium Hydroxide

Sodium hydroxide has been used mostly in South America, with acceptable reported effectiveness (86). As with many other sclerosants, pain is an important issue. However, according to Teixeira and coworkers (87), control of pain should not include intrapleural administration of lidocaine, since it reacts with NaOH, with subsequent partial deactivation and reduction of the sclerosing effect.

Silver Nitrate

Silver nitrate was the first reported agent injected into the pleural space to provoke pleurodesis (in pneumothorax) by Spengler in 1906 (88). Recently, an experimental study from Vargas and coworkers has shown a superiority of silver nitrate over talc slurry in producing pleurodesis in rabbits (89). However, a striking finding in their study was that the mean degree of alveolar inflammation in the silver nitrate group was significantly higher than in the talc group. If this can be extrapolated to humans, it would mean that patients submitted to silver nitrate pleurodesis would be in a greater risk of developing early pulmonary complications after its application.

TGF-β2

Recently, a few reports have appeared on the effectiveness of TGF-β2 in experimental pleurodesis studies (90,91). Although these results look promising, the cost of this treatment would likely be extremely high, and to my knowledge it has not been yet applied in humans.

IX. Other Alternatives to Pleurodesis

Repeat pleurodesis would be especially useful in patients who are in good performance status and who have a high recurrence rate of effusion. In our experience, a second talc poudrage—optionally with increased dosage of talc—can be helpful in achieving a good pleurodesis.

Pleuroperitoneal shunt can be useful in patients with good general condition and who have a trapped lung. However, they should not have a significant ascites at the time of performing the procedure (92).

Parietal pleurectomy by thoracotomy is very effective in controlling the effusion, but it is associated to a significant morbidity. Instead, thoracoscopic parietal pleural abrasion or partial pleurectomy might be attemped using VATS.

In patients with an expected short survival (poor performance status and usually very low pleural pH), placement of an indwelling pleural catheter connected to a vacuum bottle or a disposable bag can be an acceptable choice. Putnam and coworkers reported a 46% rate of spontaneous pleurodesis at a median of 26.5 days in 91 patients who were sent home with a pleural catheter. The degree of symptomatic improvement in dyspnea and the quality of life was comparable to that of a group of patients randomly assigned to doxycycline pleurodesis (93).

When the patient is in very poor general condition, repeat thoracenteses can be the only choice available. However, this option should be kept as the very last option, since discomfort, risks of infection, and protein depletion can significantly deteriorate the already poor quality of life in these patients.

Acknowledgment

Part of the research mentioned by our group was funded by grants FIS 96/0449 and FIS 98/0419.

References

1. Rodríguez-Panadero F, Anthony VB. Pleurodesis: state of the art. Eur Respir J 1997; 10:1648–1654.
2. Romero Romero B, Diaz-Cañaveral L, Laserna E, Martín Juan J, Rodríguez-Panadero F, Castillo J. The need for chemical pleurodesis in patients with malignant pleural effusion is associated to decline of pH and high levels of D-dimer in serial pleural fluid samples. Am J Respir Crit Care Med 2001; 163,5:A903.
3. Light RW, Jenkinson SG, Minh V, George RB. Observations on pleural pressure as fluid is withdrawn during thoracentesis. Am Rev Respir Dis 1980; 121:799–804.
4. Lan RS, Lo SK, Chuang ML, Yang CT, Tsao TC, Lee CH. Elastance of the pleural space: a predictor for the outcome of pleurodesis in patients with malignant pleural effusion. Ann Intern Med 1997; 126:768–774.

5. Villena V, López-Encuentra A, Pozo F, De Pablo A, Martín-Escribano P. Measurement of pleural pressure during therapeutic thoracentesis. Am J Respir Crit Care Med 2000; 162:1534–1538.
6. Antony VB, Loddenkemper R, Astoul P, Boutin C, Goldstraw P, Hott J, Rodriguez-Panadero F, Sahn SA. Management of malignant pleural effusions. Am J Respir Crit Care Med 2000; 162:1987–2001.
7. Rodriguez-Panadero F, Lopez-Mejias J. Low glucose and pH levels in malignant pleural effusions: diagnostic significance and prognostic value in respect to pleurodesis. Am Rev Respir Dis 1989; 139:663–667.
8. Sanchez-Armengol A, Rodriguez-Panadero F. Survival and talc pleurodesis in metastatic carcinoma revisited. Report on 125 cases. Chest 1993; 104:1482–1485.
9. Rodriguez-Panadero F, Sanchez Gil R, Martin Juan J, Castillo Gomez J. Prediction of results of talc pleurodesis in malignant pleural effusions. Am J Respir Crit Care Med 1994; 149,4,2:A1103.
10. Sahn SA, Good JT Jr. Pleural fluid pH in malignant effusions: diagnostic, prognostic and therapeutic implications. Ann Intern Med 1988; 108:345–349.
11. Martínez-Moragón E, Aparicio J, Sanchis J, Menéndez R, Rogado MC, Sanchis F. Malignant pleural effusion: prognostic factors for survival and response to chemical pleurodesis in a series of 120 cases. Respiration 1998; 65:108–113.
12. Heffner JE, Nietert PJ, Barbieri C. Pleural fluid pH as a predictor of survival for patients with malignant pleural effusions. Chest 2000; 117:79–86.
13. Rodríguez-Panadero F, Del Rey Pérez JJ. Survival of malignant pleural mesotheliomas as compared to metastatic carcinomas. Eur Respir Rev 1993; 3,11:208–210.
14. Bilaceroglu S, Cagirici U, Perim K, Ozacar R. *Corynebacterium parvum* pleurodesis and survival is not significantly influenced by pleural pH and glucose level. Monaldi Arch Chest Dis 1998; 53:14–22.
15. Almind M, Lange P, Viskum K. Spontaneous pneumothorax: comparison of simple drainage, talc pleurodesis, and tetracycline pleurodesis. Thorax 1989; 44:627–630.
16. Alfageme I, Moreno L, Huertas C, Vargas A, Hernandez J, Beiztegui A. Spontaneous pneumothorax. Long-term results with tetracycline pleurodesis. Chest 1994; 106:347–350.
17. Van de Brekel JA, Duurkens VAM, Vanderchueren RGJRA. Pneumothorax: results of thoracoscopy and pleurodesis with talc poudrage and thoracotomy. Chest 1993; 103:345–347.
18. Hurtgen M, Linder A, Friedel G, Toomes H. Video-assisted thoracoscopic pleurodesis. A survey conducted by the German Society for Thoracic Surgery. Thorac Cardiovasc Surg 1996; 44:199–203.
19. Naunheim KS, Mack MJ, Hazelrigg SR, Ferguson MK, Ferson FP, Boley TM, Landreneau RJ. Safety and efficacy of video-assisted thoracic surgical techniques for the treatment of spontaneous pneumothorax. J Thorac Cardiovasc Surg 1995; 109,6:1198–1204.
20. Berger R. Pleurodesis for spontaneous pneumothorax. Will the procedure of choice please stand up? Chest 1994; 106:992–994.
21. Tschopp JM, Brutsche M, Frey JG. Treatment of complicated spontaneous pneumothorax by simple talc pleurodesis under thoracoscopy and local anaesthesia. Thorax 1997; 52:329–332.
22. Noppen M, Meysman M, d'Haese J, Monsieur I, Verhaeghe W, Schlesser M, Vincken W. Comparison of video-assisted thoracoscopic talcage for recurrent

primary versus persistent secondary spontaneous pneumothorax. Eur Respir J 1997; 10:412–416.
23. Cagirici U, Sahin B, Cakan A, et al. Autologous blood patch pleurodesis in spontaneous pneumothorax with persistent air leak. Scand Cardiovasc J 1998; 32: 75–78.
24. Robinson CL. Autologous blood for pleurodesis in recurrent and chronic spontaneous pneumothorax. Can J Surg 1987; 30,6:428–429.
25. Rivas de Andres JJ, Blanco S, De la Torre M. Postsurgical pleurodesis with autologous blood in patients with persistent air leak. Ann Thorac Surg 2000; 70,1:270–272.
26. Noppen M, Dhondt E, Mahler T, Malfroot A, Dab I, Vincken W. Successful management of recurrent pneumothorax in cystic fibrosis by localized apical thoracoscopic talc poudrage. Chest 1994; 106:262–264.
27. Stringel G, Amin NS, Dozor AJ. Video-assisted thoracoscopy in the management of recurrent spontaneous pneumothorax in the pediatric population. JSLS 1999; 3:113–116.
28. Sudduth C, Sahn SA. Pleurodesis for nonmalignant pleural effusions. Recommendations. Chest 1992; 102:1855–1860.
29. Vargas FS, Milanez JRC, Filomeno LTB, Fernandez A, Jatene A, Light RW. Intrapleural talc for the prevention of recurrence in benign or undiagnosed pleural effusions. Chest 1994; 106:1771–1775.
30. Nakamura A, Kojima Y, Ohmi H, Yamada J, Yamada Y. Peritoneal-pleural communications in hepatic hydrothorax demonstrated by thoracoscopy. Chest 1996; 109:579–581.
31. Antony VB. Pathogenesis of malignant pleural effusion and talc pleurodesis. Pneumologie 1999; 53:493–498.
32. Loddenkemper R. Thoracoscopy—state of the art. Eur Respir J 1998; 11:213–221.
33. Bethune N. Pleural poudrage: a new technique for the deliberate production of pleural adhesions as a preliminary to lobectomy. J Thorac Surg 1935; 4:251–261.
34. Walker-Renard PB, Vaughan LM, Sahn SA. Chemical pleurodesis for malignant pleural effusions. Ann Intern Med 1994; 120:56–64.
35. Rodriguez-Panadero F, Antony VB. Pleurodesis: state of the art. Eur Respir J 1997; 10:1648–1654.
36. Rodriguez-Panadero F. Current trends in pleurodesis. Curr Opin Pulm Med 1997; 3:319–325.
37. Belani CP, Pajeau TS, Bennett CL. Treating malignant pleural effusions cost consciously. Chest 1998; 113,1:78S–85S.
38. Mañes N, Rodriguez-Panadero F, Bravo JL, Hernandez H, Alix A. Talc pleurodesis: prospective and randomized study. Clinical follow-up. Chest 2000; 118,4(suppl): 131S.
39. Xie C, McGovern JP, Wu W, Wang NS, Light RW. Comparisons of pleurodesis induced by talc with or without thymol iodide in rabbits. Chest 1998; 113:795–799.
40. Seaton KG, Patz EF Jr, Goodman PC. Palliative treatment of malignant pleural effusions: value of small-bore catheter thoracostomy and doxycycline sclerotherapy. Am J Roentgenol 1995; 164:589–591.
41. Clementsen P, Evald T, Grode G, Hansen M, Krag Jacobsen G, Faurschou P. Treatment of malignant pleural effusion: pleurodesis using a small percutaneous catheter. A prospective randomized study. Respir Med 1998; 92:593–596.
42. Marom EM, Patz EF Jr, Erasmus JJ, McAdams HP, Goodman PC, Herndon JE.

Malignant pleural effusions: treatment with small-bore catheter thoracostomy and talc pleurodesis. Radiology 1999; 210,1:277–281.
43. Villanueva AG, Gray AW Jr, Shahian DM, Williamson WA, Beamis JF Jr. Efficacy of short term versus long term tube thoracostomy drainage before tetracycline pleurodesis in the treatment of malignant pleural effusions. Thorax 1994; 49:23–25.
44. Chang YC, Patz EF Jr, Goodman PC. Pneumothorax after small-bore catheter placement for malignant pleural effusions. AJR Am J Roentgenol 1996; 166,5:1049–1051.
45. Sahn SA, Good JT Jr. The effect of common sclerosing agents on the rabbit pleural space. Au Rev Respir Dis 1981; 124, 1:65–67.
46. Heuvel Van Den MM, Smith JHM, Barbierato SB, Havenith CEG, Beelen RHJ, Postmus PE. Talc-induced inflammation in the pleural cavity. Eur Respir J 1998; 12:1419–1423.
47. Ayerbe R, Rodríguez Panadero F, Martín J, Segado A, Sanchez J, Antony VB. Neutrophils, IL-8 and outcome of talc pleurodesis. Eur Respir J 1994; 7(suppl 18):270s.
48. Hartman DL, Antony VB, Hott JW, Godbey SW, Yu L, Rodriguez Panadero F. Thoracoscopic talc insufflation increases pleural fluid IL-8 levels in patients with malignant pleural effusions. Am J Respir Crit Care Med 1994; 149(suppl 2,2):A974.
49. Xie C, Teixeira LR, McGovern JP, Light RW. Systemic corticosteroids decrease the effectiveness of talc pleurodesis. Am J Crit Care Med 1998; 157:1441–1444.
50. Rodriguez-Panadero F, Segado A, Martin Juan J, Ayerbe R, Torres Garcia I, Castillo J. Failure of talc pleurodesis is associated with increased pleural fibrinolysis. Am J Respir Crit Care Med 1995; 785–790.
51. Rodriguez-Panadero F, Gómez Izquierdo L, Martín Juan J, Borderas F, Vargas R, Segura DI. D-Dimer in malignant pleural effusions is associated to immunohistochemical expression for markers of fibrinolysis in non-tumoral pleural tissue. Eur Respir J 1998; 12(suppl):28:34s.
52. Rodriguez-Panadero F, Gómez Izquierdo L, Martin Juan J, Borderas F, Sánchez JF, Segura DI. The balance between expression of plasminogen activators and their inhibitor (PAI-1) in pleural tissue is associated to outcome of talc pleurodesis. Am J Respir Crit Care Med 1997; 155,4:A739.
53. Rodriguez-Panadero F, Gómez Izquierdo L, Martín Juan J, Borderas F, Díaz L, Segura DI. Expression of plasminogen activator inhibitor type-2 (PAI-2) by tumor cells or fibroblasts is inversely related to the outcome of talc pleurodesis in malignant pleural effusions. Am J Respir Crit Care Med 1999; 159,4(part 2):A384.
54. Godbey SW, Holm KA, Yu L, Hott JW, Rodriguez Panadero F, Anthony VB. Role of mesothelial cells in pleural fibrosis following successful talc poudrage: Identification of basic fibroblast growth factor (FGF-2) in pleural fluids. Am J Respir Crit Care Med 1995; 151:A353.
55. Antony VB, Kamal MA, Godbey S, Loddenkemper FW. Talc induced pleurodesis: Role of basic fibroblast growth factor (bFGF). Eur Respir J 1997; 10:403S.
56. Sahn SA. Talc should be used for pleurodesis. Am J Respir Crit Care Med 2000; 162:2023–2024.
57. Light RW. Talc should not be used for pleurodesis. Am J Respir Crit Care Med 2000; 162:2024–2026.
58. Mahfood S, Hix WR, Aaron BL, Blaes P, Watson DC. Reexpansion pulmonary edema. Ann Thorac Surg 1988; 45:340–345.

59. Critchley LA, Au HK, Yim AP. Reexpansion pulmonary edema occurring after thoracoscopic drainage of a pleural effusion. J Clin Anesth 1996; 8:591–594.
60. Rodriguez-Panadero F. Talc pleurodesis for treating malignant pleural effusions. Chest 1995; 108:1178–1179.
61. Rozenman J, Yellin A, Simansky DA, Shiner RJ. Re-expansion pulmonary oedema following spontaneous pneumothorax. Respir Med 1996; 90:235–238.
62. Nakamura H, Ishizaka A, Sawafuji M, Urano T, Fujishima S, Sakamaki F, Sayama K, Kawamura M, Kato R, Kikuchi K, Kanazawa M, Kobayashi K, Kawashiro T. Elevated levels of interleukin-8 and leukotriene B4 in pulmonary edema fluid of a patient with reexpansion pulmonary edema. Am J Respir Crit Care Med 1994; 149:1037–1040.
63. Rinaldo JE, Owens GR, Rogers RM. Adult respiratory distress syndrome following intrapleural instillation of talc. J Thorac Cardiovasc Surg 1983; 85:523–526.
64. Bouchama A, Chastre J, Gaudichet A, Soler P, Gibert C. Acute pneumonitis with bilateral pleural effusion after talc pleurodesis. Chest 1984; 86:795–797.
65. Rehse DH, Aye RW, Florence MG. Respiratory failure following talc pleurodesis. Am J Surg 1999; 177:437–440.
66. Kennedy L, Harley RA, Sahn SA, Strange C. Talc slurry pleurodesis: pleural fluid and histologic analysis. Chest 1995; 107:1707–1712.
67. Campos Werebe E, Pazetti R, Milanez de Campos JR, Pêgo Fernandez P, Capelozzi VL, Jatene FB, Vargas FS. Systemic distribution of talc after intrapleural administration in rats. Chest 1999; 115:190–193.
68. Milanez de Campos JR, Campos Werebe E, Vargas FS, et al. Respiratory failure due to inssuflated talc. Lancet 1997; 349:251–252.
69. Ferrer J, Villarino MA, Tura JM, Traveria J, Light RW. Comparison of size and composition of nine different talcs. Its relevance for pleurodesis. Am J Respir Crit Care Med 1998; 157:A66.
70. Ferrer J, Villarino MA, Tura JM, Traveria J, Light RW. Talc preparations used for pleurodesis vary markedly from one preparation to another. Chest 2001; 119:1901–1905.
71. Mitchem RE, Herndon BL, Fiorella RM, Molteni A, Battie CN, Reisz GR. Pleurodesis by autologous blood, doxycycline and talc in a rabbit model. Ann Thorac Surg 1999; 67:917–921.
72. Agrenius V, Chmielewska J, Widström O, Blombäck M. Increased coagulation activity of the pleura after tube drainage and quinacrine instillation in malignant pleural effusion. Eur Respir J 1991; 4:1135–1139.
73. Agrenius V, Chmielewska J, Widström O, Blombäck M. Pleural fibrinolytic activity is decreased in inflammation as demonstrated in quinacrine pleurodesis treatment of malignant pleural effusion. Am Rev Respir Dis 1989; 140:1381–1385.
74. Rodriguez-Panadero F, Segado A, Torres I, Martin J, Sanchez J, Castillo J. Thoracoscopy and talc poudrage induce an activation of the systemic coagulation system. Am J Respir Crit Care Med 1995; 151:A357.
75. Rodriguez-Panadero F, Segado A, Martin Juan J, Sanchez JF, Calderon E, Castillo J. Activation of systemic coagulation in talc poudrage can be (partially) controlled with prophylactic heparin. Am J Respir Crit Care Med 1996; 153:A458.
76. Hurewitz AN, Lidonicci K, Wu CL, Reim D, Zucker S. Histologic changes of doxycycline pleurodesis in rabbits: effect of concentration and pH. Chest 1994; 106:1241–1245.
77. Knowles SR, Shapiro L, Shear NH. Serious adverse reactions induced by mino-

cycline. Report of 13 patients and review of the literature. Arch Dermatol 1996; 132:934–939.
78. Light RW, Wang NS, Sassoon CSH, Gruer SE, Vargas FS. Comparison of the effectiveness of tetracycline and minocycline as pleural sclerosing agent in rabbits. Chest 1994; 106:577–582.
79. Vargas FS, Wang N-S, Lee HM, Gruer SE, Sassoon CSH, Light RW. Effectiveness of bleomycin in comparison to tetracycline as pleural sclerosing agent in rabbits. Chest 1993; 104:1582–1584.
80. Hartman DL, Gaither JM, Kesler KA, Mylet DM, Brown JW, Mathur PN. Comparison of insufflated talc under thoracoscopic guidance with standard tetracycline and bleomycin pleurodesis for control of malignant pleural effusions. J Thorac Cardiovasc Surg 1993; 105,4:743–747.
81. Bjorkman S, Elisson LO, Gabrielsson J. Pharmacokinetics of quinacrine after intrapleural instillation in rabbits and man. J Pharm Pharmacol 1989; 41:160–163.
82. Wooten SA, Barbarash RA, Strange C, Sahn SA. Systemic absorption of tetracycline and lidocaine following intrapleural instillation. Chest 1988; 94:960–963.
83. Foresti V. Intrapleural *Corynebacterium parvum* for recurrent malignant pleural effusions. Respiration 1995; 62:21–26.
84. Ostrowsky MJ, Priesstman TJ, Houston RF, Martin WM. A randomized trial of intracavitary bleomycin and *Corynebacterium parvum* in the control of malignant pleural effusions. Radiother Oncol 1989; 14:19–26.
85. Vargas FS, Wang NS, Teixeira LR, Carmo AO, Silva LMMF, Light RW. *Corynebacterium parvum* versus tetracycline as pleural sclerosing agents in rabbits. Eur Respir J 1995; 8:2174–2177.
86. Vargas FS, Carmo AO, Teixeira LR. A new look at old agents for pleurodesis: nitrogen mustard, sodium hydroxide, and silver nitrate. Curr Opin Pulm Med 2000; 6:281–286.
87. Teixeira LR, Vargas FS, Carmo AO, Cukier A, Silva LM, Light RW. Effectiveness of sodium hydroxide as a pleural sclerosing agent in rabbits: influence of concomitant intrapleural lidocaine. Lung 1996; 174:325–332.
88. Spengler L. Zur Chirurgie des Pneumothorax: Mitteilung über 10 eigene Fálle von geheilten Tuberkulosen Pneumothorax, verbunden in 6 Fällen mit gleichzeitiger Heilung der Lungentuberkulose. Beitr Z Klin Chir 1906; 49:68–89.
89. Vargas FS, Teixeira LR, Vaz MA, Carmo AO, Marchi E, Cury PM, Light RW. Silver nitrate is superior to talc slurry in producing pleurodesis in rabbits. Chest 2000; 118:808–813.
90. Light RW, Cheng DS, Lee YC, Rogers J, Davidson J, Lane KB. A single intrapleural injection of transforming growth factor-beta2 produces excellent pleurodesis in rabbits. Am J Respir Crit Care Med 2000; 162:98–104.
91. Lee YC, Lane KB, Parker RE, Ayo DS, Rogers JT, Diters RW, Thompson PJ, Light RW. Transforming growth factor beta2 (TGF-beta2) produces effective pleurodesis in sheep with no systemic complications. Thorax 2000; 55:1058–1062.
92. Petrou M, Kaplan D, Goldstraw P. The management of recurrent malignant pleural effusions: the complementary role of talc pleurodesis and pleuro-peritoneal shunting. Cancer 1995; 75:801–805.
93. Putnam JB Jr, Light RW, Rodriguez RM, Ponn R, Olak J, Pollak JS, Lee RB, Payne DK, Graeber G, Kovitz KL. A randomized comparison of indwelling pleural catheter and doxycycline pleurodesis in the management of malignant pleural effusions. Cancer 1999; 86:1992–1999.

27

Pleuroperitoneal Shunts in Malignant Effusions

GEORGE LADAS and PETER GOLDSTRAW

Royal Brompton Hospital
and Imperial College School of Medicine
London, England

I. Introduction

Pleural effusions are common during the course of malignant disease, with 16% of patients dying of malignancy found at autopsy to have a pleural effusion. Carcinomas of the lung and breast combined account for 60% of all malignant pleural effusions. These effusions can cause significant morbidity, including dyspnea in 96%, chest pain in 57%, and persistent cough in 44% of patients (1). At the same time, the prognosis for patients with malignant pleural effusions is very poor, with reported 1- and 6-month mortality rates of 54% and 85%, respectively (2,3), so that quality of life is of paramount importance. Since dyspnea in patients with advanced malignancy is often multifactorial, an initial needle aspiration will confirm diagnosis in 65% of patients, but will also help define to what extent the pleural effusion itself is responsible for the symptoms. In frail patients with very short life expectancy of 1–2 months, repeated needle aspiration can be helpful to control symptoms. In the majority of patients with recurrent symptomatic malignant effusions, lasting palliation can be achieved by one of the spectrum of techniques used to achieve chemical pleurodesis, commonly by a tube thoracostomy or video-assisted thoracoscopy under general anaesthesia for the fitter patients. The basic prerequisite for a successful chemical pleurodesis by any technique is that the lung can reexpand following drainage of the pleural effusion, so that the visceral and parietal pleura can remain apposed while adhesions are formed. However, the presence of a malignant restricting cortex on the visceral pleura prevents reexpansion of the lung and apposition to the parietal pleura. The presence of such a trapped lung (Figs. 1–3) means that any attempt at chemical pleurodesis is destined to fail. The treatment options in these circumstances are very few, and most are unattractive. Repeated aspirations require frequent hospitalization and are painful—both detrimental to quality of life of the patients. Furthermore, they carry the risk of the devastating complication of infection of the fluid and empyema formation. This is the major concern, which also limits the popularity of permanent chest drain devices like PleurX®. Thoracotomy and decortication of the lung, combined with chemical pleurodesis or pleurectomy involves major surgery with very significant morbidity and mortality, unacceptable for a palliative procedure (4). In contrast, pleuro-peritoneal shunts provide an elegant, effective, and lasting

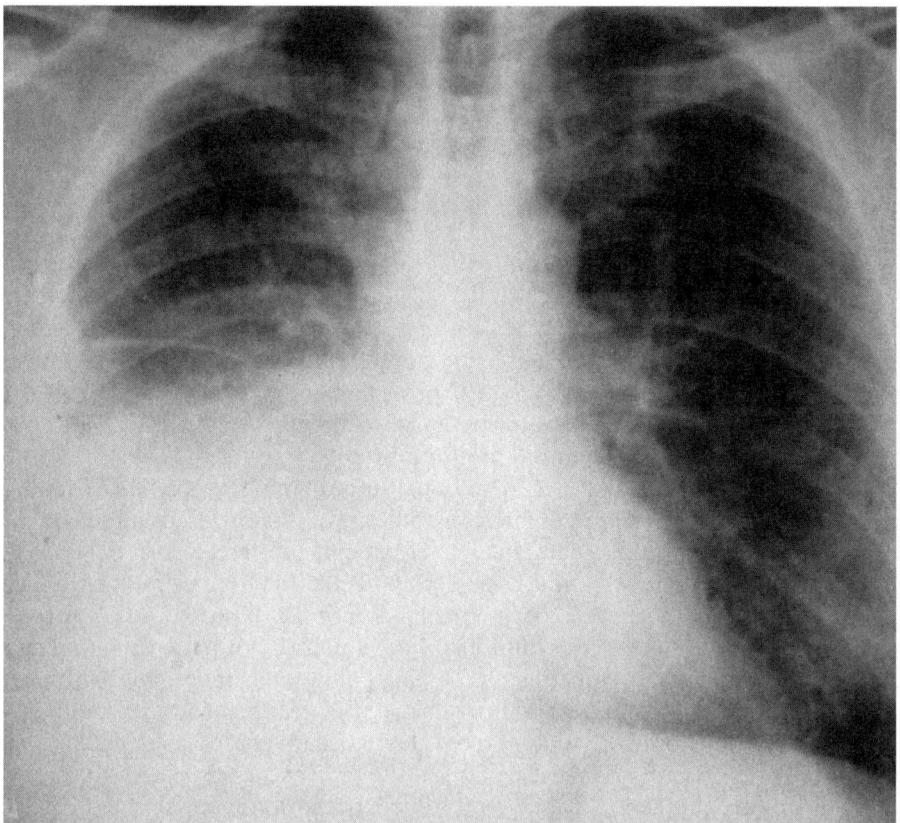

Figure 1 Chest radiograph of patient with right malignant pleural effusion.

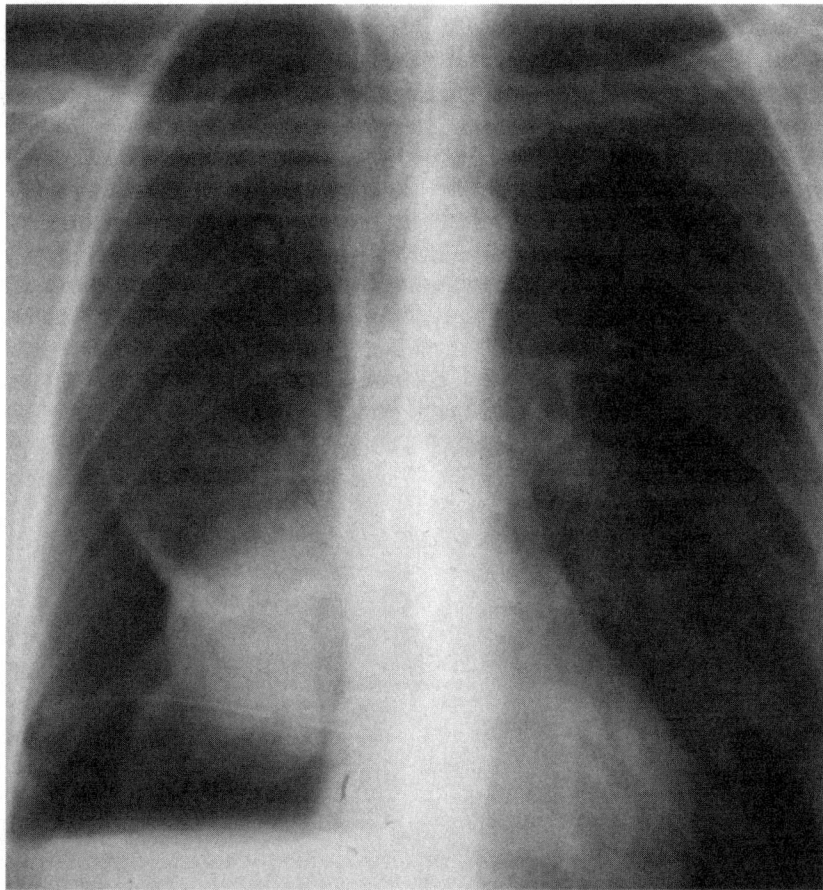

Figure 2 Chest radiograph of patient in Figure 1 following initial aspiration of the effusion. The presence of trapped lung is obvious, with a malignant cortex preventing re-expansion of the middle and lower lobes. Indication for insertion of pleuroperitoneal shunt.

solution to this difficult problem and can be used with minimal morbidity and mortality in properly selected patients (Tables 1, 2).

II. The Evolution of Pleuroperitoneal Shunts

Weese and Schouten in 1982 (5) first reported the use of a modified peritoneo-atrial Holter valve (6) as a pleuroperitoneal shunt. Since then, successful use of a purpose built device has been reported for the treatment of benign (7) but also and mainly malignant pleural effusions. The pleuroperitoneal shunt (Denver Biomedical Inc., Denver, CO) (Fig. 4) is made of inert silicone rubber. It is

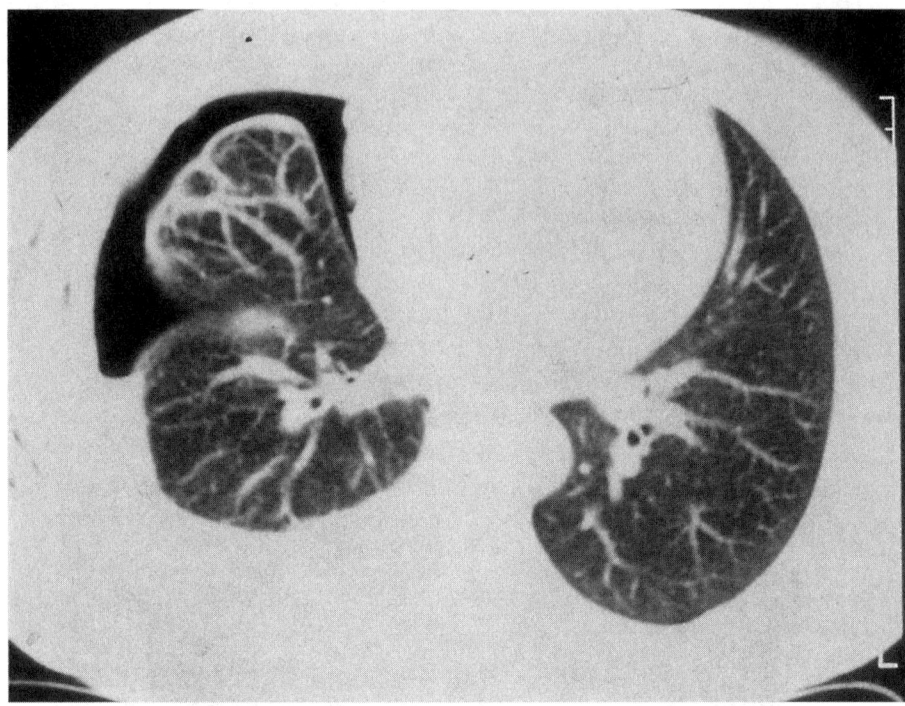

Figure 3 Computerized tomography (CT) scan appearances of patient in Figures 1 and 2. Note the thickened, restricting visceral cortex, preventing reexpansion of the lung.

composed of a central pump body, which contains two unidirectional valves. The pressure gradient required for the valves to open is 1 cm of water, and consequently spontaneous flow occurs from the pleural to the peritoneal cavity at expiration or during cough. The presence of a pleural effusion results in greater pressure gradient, which further enhances flow. The stroke volume of the pump itself is about 1 mL, and so periodic compression ensures a minimum throughput but also clears the valve leaflets from deposited fibrin. The proximal catheter of

Table 1 Indications for Use of Pleuroperitoneal Shunt

A shunt is indicated for the management of symptomatic malignant pleural effusions when:
  1. There is failure to control the effusion with other methods (particularly, recurrence of the effusion following an attempt at chemical pleurodesis)
  2. The lung fails to expand after initial drainage of the effusion (trapped lung)
  3. Reasonable expectancy of survival (>2 months)
  4. Patient or family members willing to train to operate the pump postoperatively

Table 2 Contraindications for Use of Pleuroperitoneal Shunt

Absolute
  Infected pleural effusion, empyema of the chest
  Active intraperitoneal infection, sepsis
  Congestive heart failure
Relative
  Intraperitoneal primary tumor
  Previous major abdominal surgery
  Ascites
  Pleural effusion with concomitant air leak

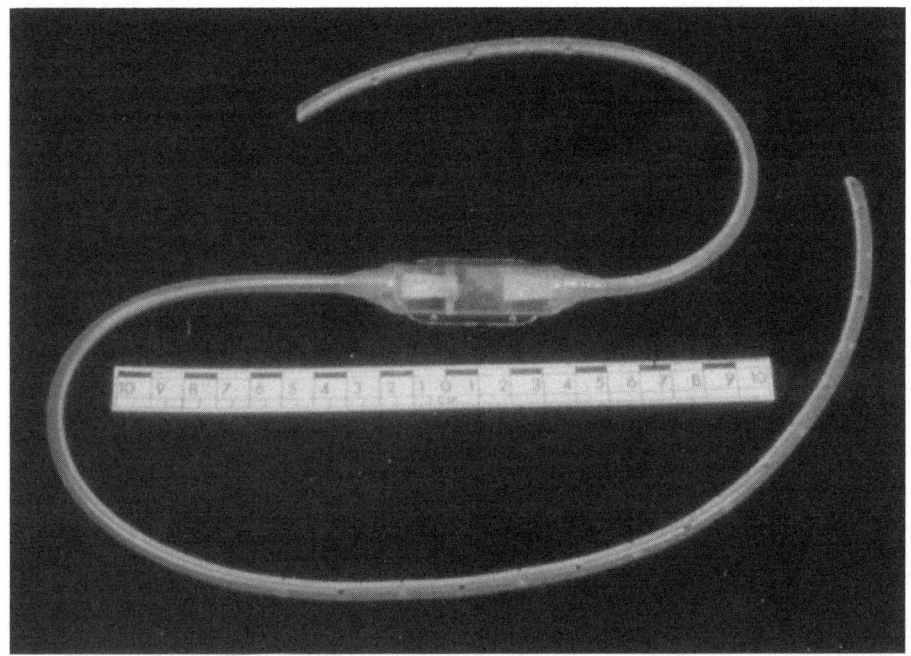

Figure 4 The pleuro-peritoneal shunt. The central compressible pump chamber with the two unidirectional valves is visible, as well as the thoracic and peritoneal limbs of the shunt.

the shunt is introduced into the pleural cavity and the distal one into the peritoneal cavity.

III. Surgical Technique

Single lung general anaesthesia is used in all our patients, with use of double lumen endotracheal tubes. The procedure is minor from the surgical point of view, but the patients are often quite frail, so good monitoring is essential. An arterial line is used as well as a neck line to allow arterial blood gases and central venous pressure measurements. We routinely insert a urinary catheter as well, since a majority of the patients will have had nephrotoxic chemotherapy at some point in the past, and close monitoring of urine output is essential in the perioperative period. We perform a rigid bronchoscopy initially to exclude the presence of airway obstruction.

This would not only account for the dyspnea to a varying extent, but might also prevent reexpansion of the lung following drainage of the effusion. If present, this is managed there and then by either endoscopic diathermy disobliteration in the case of intraluminal tumors or stent insertion in the case of external airway compression (e.g., malignant nodes), or sometimes both in obstruction of mixed aetiology. Next, the patient is positioned supine with the operated side slightly raised. A single 3 cm incision is used in most cases to insert

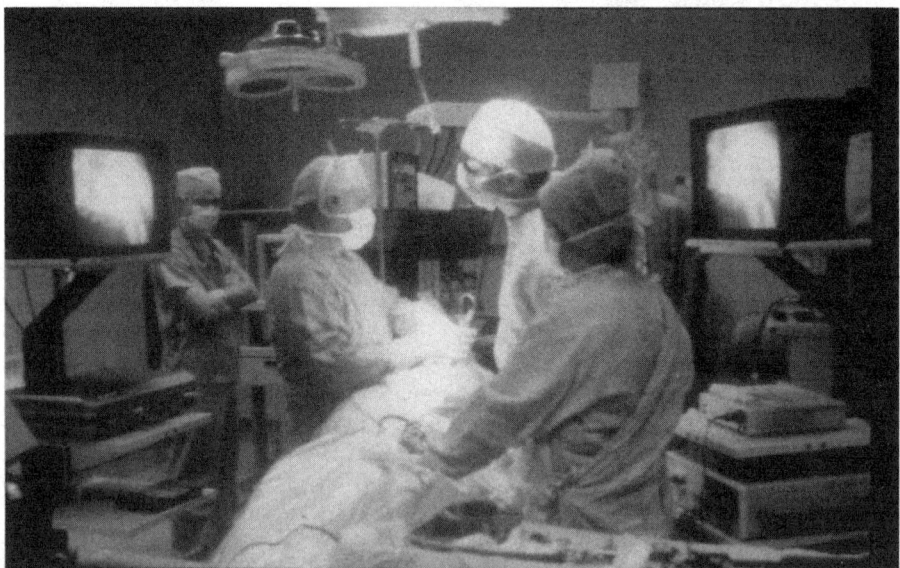

Figure 5 The operating theater arrangement during a video-assisted thoracoscopic procedure (VATS). The image captured by the rod-shaped camera is projected on the monitor screens.

an oval 22 mm port in the hemithorax and examine the pleural space with video-assisted thoracoscopy (VATS) (Fig. 5). The site of this port is chosen with the possibility of shunt insertion in mind, such that a pocket for the shunt chamber can be fashioned to lie over the costal margin. In a small minority of patients a mini-thoracotomy (5–7 cm) is used, particularly if there had been repeated pleural interventions with formation of adhesions and fibrin deposits. The pleural effusion is drained and appropriate pleural biopsies are obtained. Adhesions are divided and any fibrinous septa divided to unify the pleural cavity. The degree of lung expansion is then assessed with sustained positive pressure ventilation of up to 25 cm of water. If lung expansion is adequate, then chemical pleurodesis is performed by insufflating iodised talc. If not, then preparation is made for insertion of a shunt (Fig. 6). A second 3 cm transverse incision is made in the corresponding hypochondrium at the lateral margin of the rectus abdominis muscle, and access is gained to the peritoneal cavity via the rectus sheath. The pleuroperitoneal shunt is primed with normal saline and then tunnelled under the skin from the chest to the abdomen. The pumping chamber

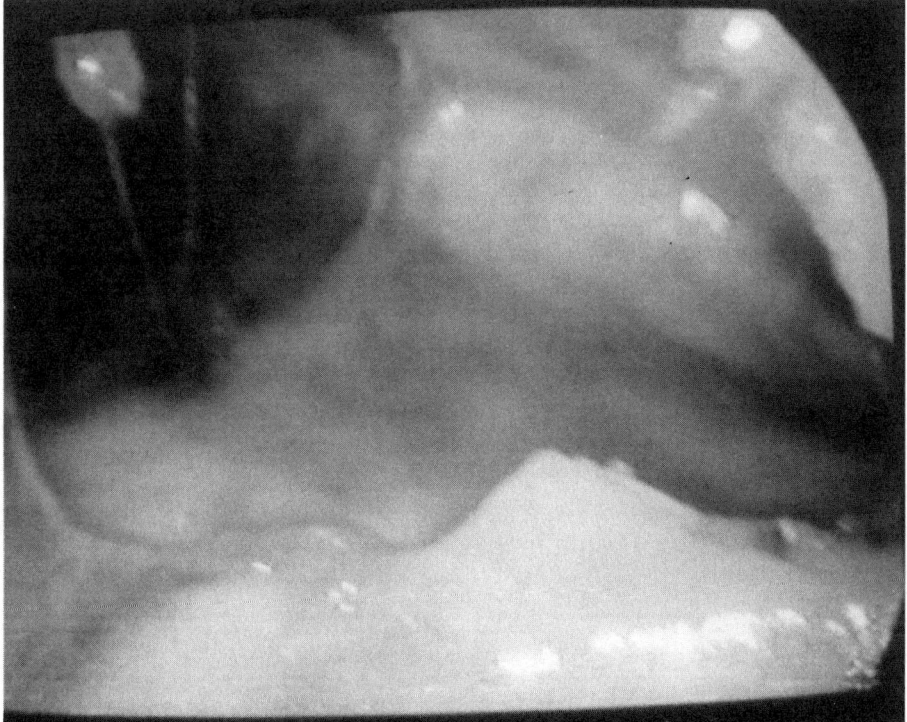

Figure 6 Appearances of the pleural cavity during VATS in a patient with trapped lung. The gross thickening of the visceral pleura is visible, with inability of the lung to reexpand.

is positioned over the costal margin in a subcutaneous pocket fashioned anteriorly to the port site and secured in place with sutures. The proximal and distal limbs of the shunt are then inserted into the respective cavities and optimal position confirmed (Fig. 7). A moderate quantity of normal saline is introduced in the pleural cavity to prime the shunt and confirm good function. The skin incisions are closed with subcuticular absorbable sutures. At the end of the

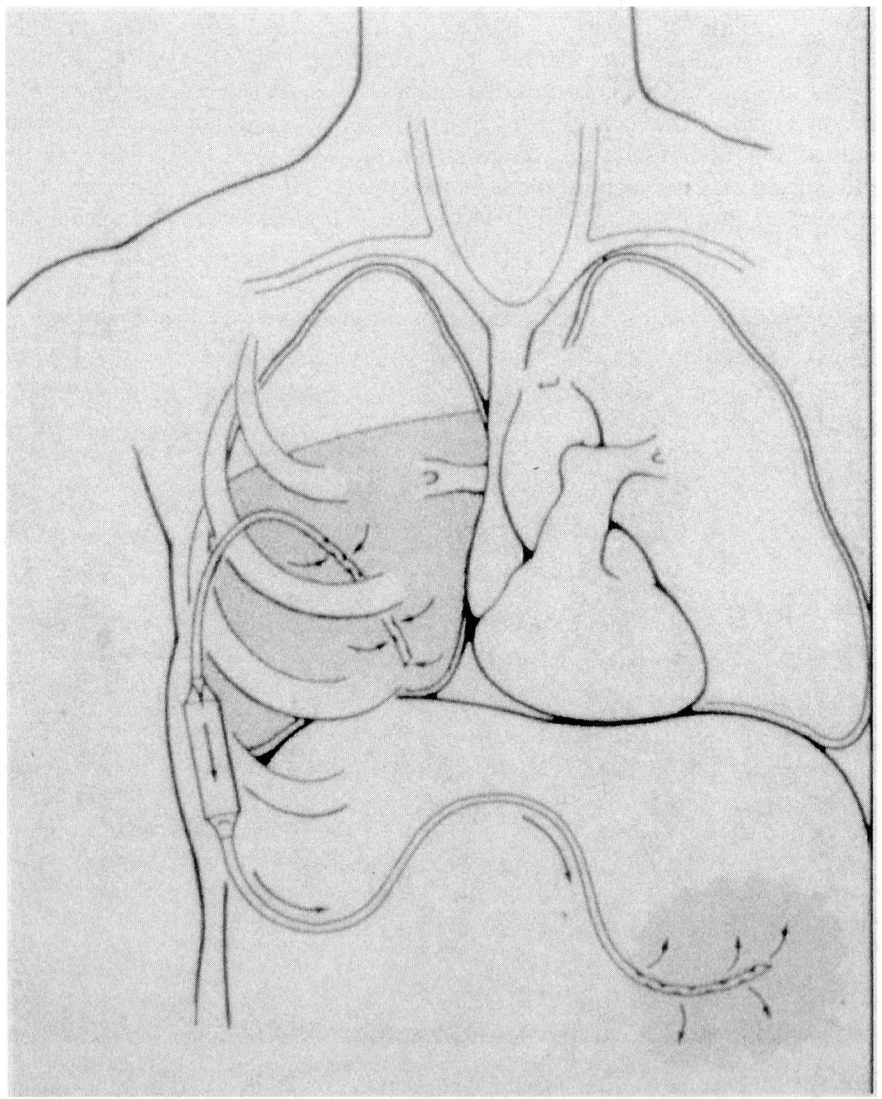

Figure 7 Schematic diagram of the function of pleuroperitoneal shunt.

procedure, the position of the pumping chamber is marked on the skin so that the nursing staff initially, and later the patient, can easily locate it.

During the initial postoperative period, the nursing staff operates the pump every 3–4 hours for 2–3 minutes at a rate of around 30 strokes per minute. With the help of appropriate audio-visual training material, the patients are able to assume responsibility for the shunt within 3–4 days postoperatively.

IV. The Royal Brompton Experience

Pleuroperitoneal shunts have been used at the Royal Brompton Hospital for more than 15 years (8,9). Between January 1983 and December 1998 there 360 patients were referred to our hospital for management of a recurrent malignant pleural effusion. Of these, 160 (44.4%) had insertion of a pleuroperitoneal shunt, while the rest had talc pleurodesis. The relatively high proportion of shunts reflects the tertiary nature of our hospital, with a large number of patients referred following failed previous interventions: 89 male and 71 female patients, with a mean age of 59.2 years (range 24–87 yr). Table 3 shows the pathology of these patients. Nearly 60% of the patients in this group had been treated prior to their referral with one or more other modalities, and oncological assessment confirmed lack of other efficient treatment options. The technique used was as described above. A larger proportion of patients were managed with minithoracotomy during the early years of our experience, while VATS has been used almost exclusively during the last 8 years.

All patients tolerated general anaesthesia well, and there were no intraoperative deaths. Local anaesthesia was never used in our practice. The hospital mortality rate was 1.87%, with 3 patients dying early due to respiratory failure. In these patients dyspnea had been multifactorial, and the nonreversible components (lymphangitis carcinomatosa, chest wall fibrosis from previous radiotherapy) outweighed the benefit from drainage of the pleural effusion.

The average hospital stay was 6.2 days (range 2–26 days). We were able to collect follow-up data for 141 patients (88%). The overall median survival was

Table 3 Pathology of Patients with Malignant Effusions Who Had Pleuroperitoneal Shunt Insertion

Tumor type	No. of patients (%)
Breast cancer	58 (36.2)
Mesothelioma	36 (22.5)
Primary lung cancer	35 (21.8)
Secondary adenocarcinoma (unknown primary)	18 (11.2)
Other	13 (8.1)
Total	160

Table 4 Survival After Shunt Insertion According to Tumor Type

Tumor type	Median survival (months)/range
Mesothelioma ($n = 36$)	10.1 (2 weeks–32 months)
Breast cancer ($n = 43$)	7.1 (2 weeks–53 months)
Others ($n = 62$)	6.8 (2 weeks–72 months)
Overall ($n = 141$)	7.7 (2 weeks–72 months)

7.7 months (range 2 weeks to 72 months). Mesothelioma patients survived longer, with a median survival of 10.1 months. Table 4 shows survival figures according to pathology.

Complications directly related to the shunt occurred in 21 patients (14.8%) and appear on Table 5 together with the action taken. This high complication rate is reasonable in such highly pretreated patients, while most complications were minor and could be treated effectively, restoring the initial good palliation. Occlusion of the shunt occurred in 12 patients (8.5%) following a mean period of 2.7 months postinsertion (range 4 days to 9 months). All patients were reoperated upon, and the shunt revised in 5 and replaced in 7, with good palliation achieved once again in all patients.

In 7 patients (4.3%) the shunt had to be removed due to infection. In only 3 of these patients was a chest drain required, as in the rest the pleural space had been spontaneously obliterated in the meantime.

One patient with metastatic breast cancer developed malignant seeding along the shunt line 7 months postinsertion, but no patient developed clinical evidence of intraperitoneal dissemination of their tumour. We would routinely refer all patients with a diagnosis of mesothelioma, though, for prophylactic irradiation of the incisions and shunt tunnel postoperatively.

Nearly 95% of our patients (153/160) experienced good palliation following insertion of the shunt, with no recurrence of symptoms and no significant reaccumulation of fluid on the chest radiograph.

Table 5 Complications of Pleuroperitoneal Shunts

Complication	No. patients	Management
Occlusion of shunt	12	Replacement 7 patients Revision 5 patients
Infection of shunt	7	Removal and chest drain in 4 patients Removal (spontaneous pleurodesis) in 3 patients
Skin erosion	1	Removal
Shunt fracture	1	Removal

V. Conclusion

Pleuroperitoneal shunts have proven in our experience to be safe and efficient in providing a lasting solution to a difficult clinical problem in a very frail patient population. The main theoretical concern of intraperitoneal tumour seeding via the shunt has failed to materialise in the clinical setting in our practice and has not been reported in the literature to our knowledge. In view of the poor overall survival of this group of patients and the lack of alternative treatment options, it certainly appears to be an acceptable risk. Our series of patients, the largest reported to date (8–10), shows very low mortality and low treatment-related morbidity combined with effective palliation in the vast majority of patients. Avoiding the need for repeated hospital admissions for thoracocentesis not only

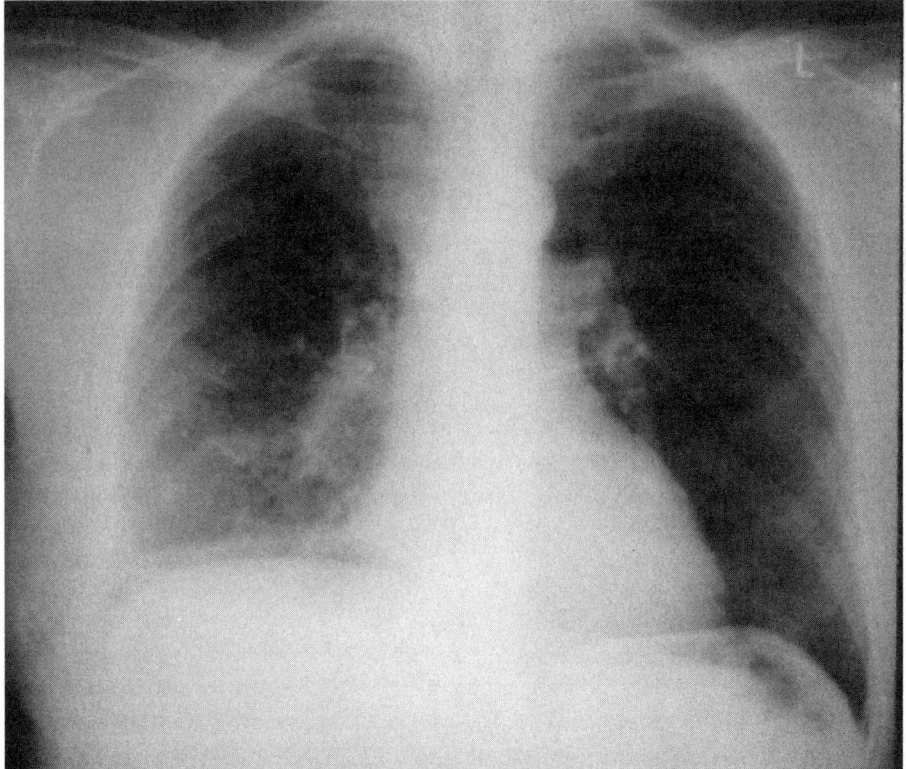

Figure 8 Early postoperative chest radiograph of a patient following insertion of a shunt on the right. The proximal limb is clearly visible within the right hemithorax, with the pump body lying in the soft tissues overlying the costal margin. The limited pneumoperitoneum resulting from air entering the peritoneal cavity intraoperatively resolves within a few days.

dramatically improves the quality of life of these patients, but also reduces the overall cost of their care (Fig. 8).

References

1. Moragon EM, Aparicio J, Sanchis J, Menendez R, Rogado MC, Sanchis F. Malignant pleural effusion: prognostic factors for survival and response to chemical pleurodesis in a series of 120 cases. Respiration 1998; 65:108–113.
2. Sahn AS. Malignancy metastatic to the pleura. Clin Chest Med 1998; 19:351–361.
3. Wong PS, Goldstraw P. Pleuroperitoneal shunts: review. Br J Hosp Med 1993; 50:16–21.
4. Martini N, Bains MS, Beattie EJ Jr. Indications for pleurectomy in malignant effusion. Cancer 1975; 35:734–738.
5. Weese JL, Schouten JT. Pleural peritoneal shunts for the treatment of malignant pleural effusions. Surg Gynaecol Obstetr 1982; 154:391–392.
6. Pollock AV. The treatment of resistant malignant ascites by insertion of a peritoneoatrial Holter valve. Br J Surg 1975; 62:104–107.
7. Milsom JW, Kron IL, Rheuban KS, Rodgers BM. Chylothorax: an assessment of current surgical management. J Thorac Cardiovasc Surg 1985; 89:221–227.
8. Tsang V, Fernando HC, Goldstraw P. Pleuroperitoneal shunt for recurrent malignant pleural effusions. Thorax 1990; 45:369–372.
9. Genc O, Petrou P, Ladas G, Goldstraw P. The long term morbidity of pleuroperitoneal shunts in the management of recurrent malignant effusions. Eur J Cardiothorac Surg 2000; 18:143–146.
10. Little AG, Kadowki MH, Ferguson MK, Staszek VM, Skinner DB. Pleuroperitoneal shunting. Alternative therapy for pleural effusions. Ann Surg 1988; 208:443–450.

28

Mesothelioma
Benign and Malignant

GUNNAR HILLERDAL

Karolinska Institute
and Karolinska Hospital
Uppsala, Sweden

I. "Benign" Mesotheliomas

Benign fibrous mesotheliomas, more correctly called solitary pleural fibrous tumors, have no connection with malignant ones or with exposure to asbestos. They seem to arise from submesothelial fibroblasts (1). These tumors arise either from the parietal or the visceral pleura, often from a small stalk. They grow slowly, do not invade any tissues but rather push them aside, and can become very big before they give symptoms or are accidentally discovered. The main symptom is dyspnea simply due to the size of the tumor. Some patients can suffer from hypoglycemic attacks, and clubbing of the fingers also occurs. Rarely, chest pain is the symptom that causes the patient to go to the doctor.

Therapy is by surgery. The tumor is easily lifted out. It is very important that the origin of the tumor is excised with a good margin; if some cells are left, the tumor will recur and then often takes a more malignant course, growing in the chest wall and causing symptoms, which requires further operation.

II. Malignant Pleural Mesothelioma

Diffuse malignant mesothelioma is a tumor that arises from mesothelial cells. It is in almost all instances an incurable disease, usually due to late effects of inhalation of asbestos fibers. It can occur in any of the body cavities covered by mesothelium; it is most frequent in the pleura or peritoneum, but may also develop in the pericardium and tunica vaginalis testis.

A. History

The existence of a malignant tumor derived from mesothelium was long doubted but was accepted during the early twentieth century. It was discovered at an early date to be more common in coastal cities than inland (2). In 1960 Wagner and coworkers proved a strong relationship between exposure to crocidolite asbestos and pleural mesothelioma, and this was soon confirmed by other reports (3,4).

B. Epidemiology

There is a large variation in the incidence of mesothelioma in different countries, but in most there has been a steady increase during the last few decades. Some of the differences are probably for diagnostic reasons; all studies have shown a considerable underdiagnosis of mesothelioma unless there is special interest in the disease. However, most of the variations can be explained by the use of asbestos in the particular society some decades earlier.

There seems to be a small spontaneous "basal" or "background" incidence of the tumor, which has been estimated to be approximately 1 per million per year (5), and the disease can even occur in children (6). However, some of these "background" cases might in fact be due to unknown occupational, domestic, or even environmental exposure, and the incidence thus may be much lower (7).

In industrialized countries the incidence is much higher. In the United States, the incidence in men was estimated to be 2.1 per million per year in 1968–81 (8), increased to 7–13 per million in 1986 (9), and has since increased further. It is estimated that there will be 21,500 deaths from malignant mesothelioma in the United States between 1985 and 2009 (10). In the United Kingdom in 1968–71 the figure was 8.4 per million per year, in 1972–76 12.6, and in 1983 17.5. The figures will rise in the United Kingdom at least until year 2010 and in the rest of the European Union (EU) until around 2020, though they might have peaked in the United States (11). The dubious record of the industrialized countries is held by Australia, where the latest figure shows a male incidence of 60.7 in 1998 (Australian Mesothelioma Registry).

Figures from the less industrialized countries, when available, are as a rule much lower. However, it is in the southeast Asian countries, Russia, and some other countries where the bulk of asbestos is used today, so one can predict great problems with mesothelioma in these countries in the future.

C. Etiology

The main cause of mesotheliomas is exposure to asbestos. The tumor can be regarded as a "signal tumor" for former asbestos exposure in a population, and it should always lead to a thorough questioning regarding exposure to asbestos. However, even with careful history taking, there remains a number of people where no exposure can be elucidated (12,13). In many of these cases environmental exposure can be suspected. Exposure to asbestos can be very difficult to ascertain, and even when it is denied, asbestos fibers can often be found in the lungs.

Asbestos is a collective name for a number of different minerals. The most important ones are chrysotile, a serpentine asbestos (i.e., with curly fibers), and the amphiboles (i.e., with straight fibers): crocidolite, amosite, tremolite, and anthophyllite. There are other types as well, more or less related, which sometimes can cause exposure to human beings.

Chrysotile accounts for 90% of the commercially used asbestos but seems to have a low potential for causing mesotheliomas (14). Most chrysotile is by nature also contaminated with amphiboles, and these "impurities" might be the tumor-causing factor. Lungs of mesothelioma patients generally contain more asbestos bodies and more amphibole fibers than control lungs but no more chrysotile, and analysis of the data strongly support the "amphibole theory," i.e., that amphiboles cause the mesotheliomas (15–19). It is difficult to find a cohort exposed to only one type of asbestos, and whether pure chrysotile can cause mesotheliomas in humans is thus controversial.

Crocidolite asbestos was the first agent proven to cause mesotheliomas (4). Its use was regulated early, but it was used in many countries up to the 1960s. There were important mines in South Africa, exporting to most of the world, and in Australia, with most of it used all over that continent. Amosite, mined in South Africa, was also exported all over the world. The problem with tremolite is different. It was (with small exceptions) never used or mined commercially, but it is a common contaminant of various ores (iron, zinc, talc, chrysotile, etc.) and has therefore been spread in our communities. In addition, it can occur in the soil or as rock outcroppings in many countries. It has been used in whitewash paint in some villages in Turkey, Greece, and New Caledonia. Such local occurrence of tremolite can cause a high rate of mesothelioma (20). Anthophyllite, finally, was mined in Finland and some other places, but never at a very large scale, and its potential to cause mesothelioma seems to be low.

Experimentally, when deposited intraperitoneally, intrapleurally, or intratracheally or when inhaled, all types of asbestos can cause mesotheliomas. The different asbestos types differ in size, chemical composition, and ability to survive in biological tissues. These factors explain why there is a big difference between them in the risk of causing mesothelioma in humans. The risk is highest for crocidolite, next highest for amosite and tremolite, and finally chrysotile, with any risk questioned by many (5,21,22). In general, in industrialized countries, amosite has been used more than crocidolite, so when investigating patients with mesothelioma amosite is often the most important fiber found, followed by tremolite (23,24). There is, nonetheless, a minority opinion that chrysotile is in fact responsible for most of the pleural mesotheliomas in society (25) or should at least be considered to carry the same risk (26).

More than 100 different minerals are known to occur in fibrous forms in the critical sizes, in addition to man-made ones. However, as far as is known, only one non-asbestos mineral fiber has been shown in epidemiological studies to be of any oncogenic significance for humans. This fiber is erionite, a fibrous zeolite, which can cause extremely high rates of mesotheliomas in environmentally exposed populations (20,27).

D. Dose-Response

Most researchers agree that there is a positive dose-response curve for mesothelioma, i.e., the heavier the exposure to asbestos, the greater the risk. It was early realized that time since first exposure was of large importance, and therefore the "cubic residence-time model" was suggested by Doll and Peto in 1985 (21). The incidence of mesothelioma was said to be proportional to 3rd or 4th power of time from first exposure. If the equation were correct, the risk would increase steeply with time, making early childhood exposure of great importance. However, there are clear indications that mineral fibers clear from the lung, albeit with different half-lives for the different types of asbestos. The half-life of crocidolite has been estimated at 7–8 years (28). This clearing of fibers would tend to actually decrease the risk of mesothelioma with older age, which is also supported by a number of studies.

The mostly accepted model today is thus a linear dose-response curve, strongly affected by the time factor. With increasing time from first exposure, the risk rises steeply but after 50 years will decline again. Even in patients with very high exposure (i.e., patients with asbestosis) only about 10% of the deaths are due to mesothelioma. Smoking does not increase the risk. On the contrary, the risk seems to be lower for smokers, perhaps due to a competitive risk of bronchial carcinoma (29).

Patients with mesotheliomas have on average increased levels of asbestos fibers in their lungs compared to controls, but there is some overlap (12,24,30). Many cases with only domestic or environmental exposure have been described, but in such cases the level of exposure is very difficult to establish. A large number of case reports with only minimal exposure exists in the literature. However, the risk with such exposure is probably low and could fit with a linear relationship. A hygiene standard for chrysotile asbestos of two fibers per cubic centimeter was often used earlier in many countries. In a group of workers exposed to this concentration from 15 to 65 years of age, it has been estimated that 2% will develop mesothelioma—a very unreliable figure, of course, based on approximations of scanty data (31).

There have been strong arguments for the existence of a threshold value (i.e., a minimal exposure required for development of mesothelioma) (32,33). Malignant mesothelioma can occur in children, and these cases could be regarded as proof of nonasbestos (i.e., spontaneous) etiology, since the latency time with necessity must be very short in these cases. Mesotheliomas also occur in animals, from baboons (34) and domestic dogs (35) to fish (36). Dogs are exposed environmentally to asbestos just like their human masters, which might explain some of the tumors, but in fish it would be difficult to blame asbestos. Thus, as in other animals, there is probably a background level of spontaneous mesotheliomas in humans. However, there is no scientific evidence for a threshold level, and with millions of people exposed at very low levels, a few mesotheliomas can be expected to occur.

E. Latency Time

The latency time from the first inhalation of asbestos to the appearance of the tumor is, on average, 30–45 years (21,37), with extremes of 8–70 years. The latency time is seldom less than 15 years, and any period less than 15 years should cast doubt on the etiology (21).

F. Other Causes

There are a number of suggested causes of mesothelioma (Table 1). Apart from mineral fibers, radiation (e.g., through the contrast Thorotrast) has been shown to be a probable cause of human mesothelioma.

Hereditary factors might be important. However, many familial cases are explained by common asbestos exposure. A recent report from the village

Table 1 Risk Factors for Mesothelioma Other Than Asbestos

Factors	Comments
Erionite	Very high incidence of mesothelioma with environmental exposure in Turkey
Radiation	Single cases after Thorotrast injection or radiotherapy
Beryllium	Two cases described
Hereditary	Familial cases explained by common environmental factors?
Immunological	Rapidly progressive cases in patients with immunological lesions (e.g., HIV infection)
Chronic inflammation	Pleural scars (TB pleurisy, therapeutic pneumothorax)
Dietary factors	Provitamin A, beta-carotene, may decrease the risk
Viruses	Mesotheliomas in animals; SV 40 in humans?

Karain, where a very high incidence of mesothelioma has been attributed to the occurrence of erionite in building stones, etc., has shown that there is a familial clustering of the tumor, suggesting a genetic basis (38). However, it is difficult to separate heredity from environment, and the exposure might differ from one house to another. Further studies are thus needed. It can be assumed, however, that, as for many other diseases, mesothelioma is the result of a combination of genetic and environmental causes.

Immunological factors could be important, as suggested by cases occurring in patients with acquired immunodeficiency syndrome (AIDS) but without any known asbestos exposure or rapidly progressive cases reported from patients with human immunodeficiency virus (HIV) infection (39).

Chronic inflammation of the pleura, as in pleural scars from tuberculous pleurisy or therapeutic pneumothorax, can in rare cases cause sarcomatous or epithelial mesotheliomas (40).

As shown with many other tumors, dietary factors seem to play a role. Consumption of vegetables, especially those containing provitamin A or β-carotene, may decrease the risk of mesothelioma.

Viruses can cause mesotheliomas in animals. Simian vacuolating virus 40 (SV40) has been very much discussed as a possible causative factor in human mesotheliomas. It was shown to be able to transform mesothelial cells in culture, and the presence of SV40-like DNA was described in malignant mesothelioma. Differing results from different laboratories added to the confusion, but with some methods up to 60% of the mesotheliomas showed such DNA (41). Some studies have suggested that SV40 might have been a contaminant of polio vaccines used in the 1950s, but others deny this, and the issue is not yet resolved (42).

In summary, as far as is known today, factors other than mineral fibers can only explain a very small number of mesotheliomas and can for practical purposes be disregarded, with the possible exception of SV40 and genetic factors, which could be important cofactors, but which need further research.

G. Histology and Pathology

Three main types of mesothelioma are recognized: the epithelial, mesenchymatous or sarcomatous, and mixed type. Large numbers of collagen fibers or areas of almost pure collagen are often present.

The epithelial type is the most common. Subgroups are also described, such as tubulopapillary, solid pleomorphic, and small cell types (43), and in the sarcomatous group fibroblastic, muscle-like, cartilaginous/osseous, angiomatoid (cystic), and fibrous (desmoplastic). Variants are seen in the peritoneum and not related to asbestos, such as the well-differentiated papillary mesothelioma and the multicystic type, which also have a fairly good prognosis. The epithelial cell type can be difficult to discriminate from metastases from an adenocarcinoma originating somewhere else in the body. One special variant of lung cancer is called the pseudomesotheliomatous type and is presumed to arise in a peripheral area of the lung and spread mainly to the pleura. Only immunohistochemical findings can show that this kind of tumor is not a mesothelioma but a peripheral lung cancer (44).

The fibrosarcomatous mesothelioma cell type is usually described as spindle-shaped. It can be difficult to differentiate from reactive mesothelial cells in unspecific inflammatory processes unless invasion is evident.

With modern immunohistological staining methods, differentiation is easier, and a diagnosis can be possible even with cytology only. The carcinoembryonic antigen (CEA) is in principle negative with mesotheliomas but positive with epithelial metastases.

Pleural mesotheliomas are mainly found in males and are commonly diagnosed at 50–70 years of age. At least in theory, the tumor can arise from both pleural layers, but early cases have more involvement of the parietal than of the visceral layer. The tumor fills out the cavity in which it originates and envelops the viscera. The large fibrous component of the tumor will shrink and cause a very typical diminishing of the affected hemithorax, which becomes contracted and immobile. In the later stages, invasion of contiguous tissues takes place and the other lung and/or the peritoneum will be invaded.

Lymphatic and bloodborne metastases are found in 50–70% at autopsy but are usually clinically silent (45,46). However, symptom-giving metastases have been described from, for instance, the brain (47). Metastasis to the lungs can give a miliary picture (48).

Speaking against major surgical procedures is the tendency for the tumor to invade scars. This can lead to sometimes painful and troublesome metastases. Some authors therefore recommend giving prophylactic radiation postoperatively. With such radiation to scars, the incidence of invasion can be considerably reduced (49). Needle channels are also sometimes invaded by tumor tissue.

A rare variant of mesothelioma is the localized malignant pleural tumor. It is also associated with asbestos exposure and can often be treated with surgery (50).

H. Diagnosis

Cytology has a low sensitivity. Pieces of pleural tissue will most often be required for the diagnosis. Ultrasound and computed tomography (CT)-guided biopsies are possible ways to get this. However, thoracoscopy is the recommended diagnostic procedure and yields a diagnosis in more than 90% of cases (51). It is important to realize that any biopsy will make it possible for the tumor to spread in the incision, and therefore diagnostic procedures should be kept to a minimum; however, a definite diagnosis should always be the aim.

Mesothelial cells can synthesize hyaluronan. A high level of hyluronan in the exudate is more common with mesotheliomas than with other causes of pleural exudate (52). The presence of hyaluronan will make the fluid more viscous, which is obvious at higher levels. High levels of hyaluronan will support the suspicion of mesothelioma, but low or unmeasurable levels will by no means exclude the diagnosis.

Sometimes even after large biopsies the diagnosis still remains doubtful. Indeed, even after a thoracotomy this can be true, and the further clinical course will give the diagnosis.

I. Clinical and Radiological Findings

The most common first symptoms are dyspnea or chest pain. More rarely, patients present with fever, cough, and fatigue. Radiologically, fluid is usually seen. In early cases this can be massive and a mediastinal shift can occur with severe dyspnea and rapid relief by thoracocentesis. More often, the tumor has already grown along the mediastinum, which will not be shifted (a highly suggestive sign of malignancy); the dyspnea will not be as great and not as relieved by thoracocentesis.

The exudate can be bloody but is almost as often serous. Sometimes a lobulated thickening, which may reach up to the apex, can be seen on the chest x-ray. More rare initial findings are a pneumothorax or a localized mass. Signs of past exposure to asbestos, i.e., pleural plaques and/or basal parenchymal fibrosis on the other side, are of additional diagnostic value and can be seen in up to 20% or more of the cases.

The patient can adapt to functioning with only one lung and remain fairly free from symptoms for months or rarely years, but sooner or later invasion by the tumor will cause severe pain, necessitating strong analgesics. Esophageal compression with dysphagia, signs of neural involvement such as Horner's syndrome or sympathetic nerve involvement of the arm, recurrent laryngeal nerve paralysis, and even invasion of the spinal canal with acute paraplegia have all been described. Sometimes, excessive sweating involving only the affected hemithorax is reported by the patient. Laboratory findings are as a rule unspecific, such as hypergammaglobulinemia, eosinophilia, and thrombocytosis.

J. Staging

Staging is very important for prognosis and for the choice of therapy. Staging is most often done by CT scanning. However, one must be aware that a clinical and radiological staging often underestimates the disease. In particular, the bulk of the tumor is usually situated in the lower part of the thorax in the costodiaphragmatic recesses. This goes far deeper than usually realized, and the CT scan must include the upper abdomen as far down as the kidneys. It is also sometimes very difficult to judge whether the tumor stays within the pleura or has already penetrated further. Magnetic resonance imaging (MRI) can show tumor spread into the interlobar fissures, tumor invasion of and penetration of diaphragm, and invasion of skeletal structures better than can CT (53) but is not yet fully evaluated. The best staging system used today is the one recommended by the International Mesothelioma Interest Group (Table 2) (54).

Positron emission tomography (PET) has recently been shown to be of value in the diagnosis and staging of mesothelioma. The tumor readily accumu-

Table 2 Staging of Malignant Pleural Mesothelioma

T 1:	Tumor confined to ipsilateral pleura, lung or pericardium
	1a: only the parietal pleura
	1b: scattered foci on visceral pleura
T 2:	Tumor involving ipsilateral pleural surfaces with involvement of diaphragmatic muscle and/or confluent visceral tumor with or without invasion of underlying lung parenchyma
T 3:	Still potentially resectable tumor: involvement of endothoracic fascia and/or mediastinal fat and/or solitary involvement of soft tissues of the chest wall and/or nontransmural involvement of pericardium
T 4:	Unresectable tumor: extension into chest wall with or without rib destruction and/or extension *per continutatem* into the peritoneum and/or the pericardium and/or other mediastinal organs and/or spine and/or the other lung
Lymph nodes:	
Nx	Cannot be assessed
N0	No lymph nodes
N1	Metastases in the ipsilateral bronchopulmonary or hilar lymph nodes
N2	Metastases in the ipsilateral mediastinal lymph nodes and/or the carinal node
N3	Metastases in the contralateral mediastinal or supraclavicular lymph nodes
Metastases:	
Mx	Cannot be assessed
M0	No distant metastases
M1	Distant metastases
Stages:	
Ia	T1aN0M0
Ib	T1bN0M0
II	T2N0M0
III	Any T3M0; T1-3N1M0; T1-3M0
IV	Any T4; any N3; any M1

Source: Ref. 54.

lates F18-fluorodeoxyglucose, and metastatic disease is also shown (55). Further experience is needed to find its correct place in diagnosis and staging.

K. Prognosis

In general, the prognosis is poor. Median survival is around 10 months (8–14 in various studies) (37,56,57).

Some prognostic factors have been described. The most important are stage, histology of the tumor, performance status, and age. The earlier the stage, the better the prognosis; mesothelioma of the epithelial cell type has a better prognosis than the mixed and purely sarcomatous type (37), and younger patients tend to survive longer than older ones.

Apart from stage, the type of tumor has an important impact on survival. Sarcomatous components considerably shorten life span, and surgery should not be performed in patients with such type of lesions. Rarely, a patient with an epithelioid mesothelioma can survive for many years without any treatment.

L. Treatment

There is no standard therapy for treatment of malignant mesothelioma. Surgery is recommended in some centers for very early stages, radiotherapy has a small role in the treatment of mesothelioma, and the tumor is generally fairly resistant to cytostatics.

Pleurodesis

In stages where recurrent exudates is a problem, pleurodesis should be performed. Talc is at the moment the most widely used agent. Another possibility is a surgical decortication, even with thoracoscopic technique (BTS statement) but it can be technically difficult. In cases where "radical" surgery is an option, pleurodesis should not be performed until this has been discussed.

Surgery

"Radical" operation is claimed to be curative in rare, early cases, but the scientific proof of this is wanting. In most instances, curative surgery is unfortunately impossible. It should only be considered in patients with epithelioid mesothelioma in good performance status and only at early stages. Surgery is sometimes combined with aggressive chemotherapy; again, there are no controlled studies verifying this, but good results, i.e., prolonged survival, have been seen in some patients.

The most extensive operation is an extrapleural pleuropneumonectomy, often including the pericardium and/or the diaphragm. Being a large operation, the operative mortality can be fairly high. Extrapleural pneumonectomy is still controversial. With more stringent selection criteria and better methods, the operative mortality should be 5–7% (58). A very strict selection of patients with less advanced disease is needed. Consequently, the fairly good survival reported in some studies is difficult to evaluate—the survival for comparable controls might also be good.

"Radical" decortication, i.e., removal of as much pleura as possible, has also been performed in some centers. The median survival was a few months longer than in the untreated group. This difference might also be explained by selection, since a nonadvanced stage is necessary for this operation.

Radiotherapy

Radiation of hemithorax at "curative" levels has not been shown to give any important response. In fact, if such doses are given, there will be extensive radiation damage to the lung as well. If there is local pain or palpable masses, these can be treated with local radiotherapy, but only about half of the cases will respond. The main use of radiotherapy seems to be prophylactic in incision wounds to prevent seeding of cells and troublesome metastases (see above).

Chemotherapy

A number of different cytostatics, alone or in combination, have been claimed to cause some responses, usually up to 20%. Unfortunately, practically all studies have been phase I or II series, including fairly few patients, and there are no randomized studies comparing with best supportive care. Furthermore, it has not been shown that survival or quality of life has been improved by chemotherapy, and thus most studies are not conclusive (59). The conclusion is thus that there is no accepted standard regime, and consequently chemotherapy should only be given in the context of controlled studies (60).

Other Treatments

Immunotherapy, for example, with interferons, are so far only experimental. Gene therapy has not yet been shown to give any benefit. Photodynamic therapy has large practical difficulties and has been tried on a small scale by different groups, but there seems to be no great hope that this will become a treatment option in the future.

References

1. Ranfaing E, Reboulet V, Arbez-Gindre F, Clement F, Ranfaing J, Carbillet JP. Solitary fibrous tumour of the pleura: an immunohistochemical study of two cases and a review of the literature. Eur Respir Rev 1993; 3(11):53–54.
2. Glatzel H. Zur Geographie des Pleuracarcinoms. Deutsch Arch Klin Med 1943; 190:418–428.
3. Wagner JC, Sleggs CA, Marchand P. Diffuse pleural mesothelioma and asbestos exposure in the north western Cape Province. Br J Industr Med 1960; 17:260–271.
4. Wagner JC. The discovery of the association between blue asbestos and asbestos and the aftermath. Br J Industr Med 1991; 48:399–403.
5. McDonald A, McDonald JC. Malignant mesothelioma in North America. Cancer 1980; 46:1650–1656.
6. Fraire AE, Cooper S, Greenberg D, Buffler P, Langston C. Mesothelioma of childhood. Cancer 1988; 62:838–847.
7. Hillerdal G. Mesothelioma: cases associated with non-occupational and low dose exposures. Occup Environ Med 1999; 56:505–513.
8. Enterline PE, Henderson VL. Geographic patterns for pleural mesothelioma deaths in the United States, 1968–81. J Natl Cancer Inst 1987; 79:31–37.
9. Spirtas R, Beebe GW, Connelly RR, Wright WE, Peters JM, Sherwin RP, Henderson BE, Stark A, Kovasznay BM, Davies JN, et al. Recent trends in mesothelioma incidence in the United States. Am J Industr Med 1986; 9:397–407.

10. Lilienfeld DE, Mandel JS, Coin P, Schuman LM. Projection of asbestos related diseases in the United States, 1985–2009. I. Cancer. Br J Industr Med 1988; 45:283–291.
11. Peto J, Hodgson JT, Matthews FE, Jones JR. Continuing increase in mesothelioma mortality in Britain. Lancet 1995; 345:535–539.
12. Dawson A, Gibbs AR, Pooley FD, Griffiths DM, Hoy J. Malignant mesothelioma in women. Thorax 1993; 48:269–274.
13. Pairon JC, Orlowski E, Iwatsubo Y, Billon-Galland MA, Dufour G, Chamming's S, Archambault C, Bignon J, Brochard P. Pleural mesothelioma and exposure to asbestos: evaluation from work histories and analysis of asbestos bodies in bronchoalveolar lavage fluid or lung tissue in 131 patients. Occup Environ Med 1994; 51:244–249.
14. Nicholson WJ, Selikoff IJ, Seidman H, Lilis R, Formby P. Long-term mortality experience of chrysotile miners and millers in Thetford mines, Quebec. Ann NY Acad Sci 1979; 330:11–21.
15. Pooley FD. An examination of the fibrous mineral content of asbestos lung tissue from the Canadian chrysotile mining industry. Environ Res 1976; 12:281–298.
16. Churg A, Wright JL, Svedal S. Fiber burden and patterns of asbestos-related disease in chrysotile miners and millers. Am Rev Respir Dis 1993; 148:25–31.93.
17. Roggli VL, McGavran MH, Subach J, Sybers HD, Greenberg SD. Pulmonary asbestos body counts and electron probe analysis of asbestos body cores in patients with mesothelioma. Cancer 1982; 50:2423–2432.
18. Lippman M. Deposition and retention of inhaled fibres: effects on incidence of lung cancer and mesothelioma. Occup Environ Med 1994; 51:793–798.
19. McDonald JC, McDonald A. The epidemiology of mesothelioma in historical context. Eur Respir J 1996; 9:1932–1942.
20. Baris YI, Sahin AA, Ozesmi M, Kerse I, Ozen E, Kolacan B, Altinors M, Goktepeli A. An outbreak of pleural mesothelioma and chronic fibrosing pleurisy in the village of Karain/Urgup in Anatolia. Thorax 1978; 33:181–192.
21. Doll R, Peto J. Effects on health of exposure to asbestos. London: Health and Safety Commission, Her Majesty's Stationery Office, London, 1985.
22. Rogers AJ, Leigh J, Berry G, Ferguson DA, Mulder HB, Ackad M. Relationship between lung asbestos fiber type and concentration and relative risk for mesothelioma. Cancer 1991; 67:1912–1920.
23. Roggli VL, Pratt PC, Brody AR. Asbestos fiber type in malignant mesothelioma: an analytical scanning electron microscope study of 94 cases. Am J Industr Med 1993; 23:605–614.
24. Dodson RF, O'Sullivan M, Corn CJ, McLarthy JW, Hammar SP. Analysis of asbestos fiber burden in lung tissue from mesothelioma patients. Ultrastruct Pathol 1997; 21:321–336.
25. Smith AH, Wright CC. Chrysotile asbestos is the main cause of pleural mesothelioma. Am J Industr Med 1996; 30:252–266.
26. Stayner LT, Dankovic DA, Lemen RA. Occupational exposure to chrysotile asbestos and cancer risk: a review of the amphibole hypothesis. Am J Publ Health 1996; 86:179–186.
27. Baris Y. The clinical and radiological aspects of 185 cases of malignant pleural mesothelioma. In: Wagner JC, ed. Biological Effects of Mineral Fibers. Vol. 2. Lyon: IARC Scientific Publications No. 30, 1980.
28. de Klerk NH, Musk AW, Williams V, Filion PR, Whitaker D, Shilkin KB. Com-

parison of measures of exposure to asbestos in former crocidolite workers from Wittenoom Gorge, W. Australia. Am J Industr Med 1996; 30:6579–6587.
29. Tagnon I, Blot WJ, Stroube RB, Day NE, Morris LE, Peace BB, Fraumeni JF Jr. Mesothelioma associated with the shipbuilding industry in coastal Virginia. Cancer Res 1980; 40:3875–3879.
30. Churg A. Fiber counting and analysis in the diagnosis of asbestos-related disease. Hum Pathol 1982; 13:381–392.
31. Peto J. The hygiene standard for chrysotile asbestos. Lancet 1978; i:484–489.
32. Browne K. Asbestos-related mesothelioma: epidemiological evidence for asbestos as a promoter. Arch Environ Haelth 1983; 38:261–266.
33. Ilgren EB, Browne K. Asbestos-related mesothelioma: evidence for a threshold in animals and humans. Regul Toxicol Pharmacol 1991; 13:116–132.
34. Fortman JUD, Manaligod JR, Bennet RT. Malignant mesothelioma in an olive baboon (*Papio anubis*). Lab Animal Sci 1993; 48:503–505.
35. Glickman LT, Domanski LM, Maguire TG, Dubielzig R, Churg A. Mesothelioma in pet dogs associated with exposure of their owners to asbestos. Environ Res 1983; 32:305–313.
36. Herman RL. Mesothelioma in rainbow trout, *Salmo gairdneri* Richardson. J Fish Dis 1985; 8:373–376.
37. Hillerdal G. Malignant mesothelioma 1982: Review of 4710 published cases. Br J Dis Chest 1983; 77:321–343.
38. Roushdy-Hammady I, Siegal J, Emri S, Testa JR, Carbone M. Genetic-susceptibility factor and malignant mesothelioma in the Cappadocian region of Turkey. Lancet 2001; 357:444–445.
39. Behling CA, Wolf PL, Haghighi P. AIDS and malignant mesothelioma—is there a connection? Chest 1993; 103:1268–1269.
40. Hillerdal G, Berg J. Malignant mesothelioma secondary to chronic inflammation and old scars. Cancer 1985; 55:1968–1972.
41. Ramael M, Nagels J, Heylen H, De Schepper S, Paulussen J, De Maeyer M, Van Haesendonck C. Detection of SV40 like viral DNA and viral antigens in malignant pleural mesothelioma. Eur Respir J 1999; 14:1381–1386.
42. Carbone M, Rizzo P, Pass HI. Simian virus 40, poliovaccines and human cancer; a review of recent developments. Oncogene 1997; 15:1877–1888.
43. Attanoos R, Gibbs AR. Pathology of malignant mesothelioma. Histopathology 1997; 30:403–418.
44. Oka K, Otani S, Yoshimura T, Hashimoto T, Tobita T, Koyamatsu S, Hakozaki H, Yatabe Y. Mucin-negative pseudomesotheliomatous adenocarcinoma of the lung. Acta Oncol 1999; 38:119–121.
45. Adams VI, Unni KK. Diffuse malignant mesothelioma of pleura: diagnostic criteria based on an autopsy study. Am J Clin Pathol 1984; 82:15–23.
46. Law MR, Hodson ME, Heard BE. Malignant mesothelioma of the pleura: relation between histological type and clinical behaviour. Thorax 1982; 37:810–815.
47. Harrison RN. Sarcomatous pleural mesothelioma and cerebral metastases: case report and a review of eight cases. Eur J Respir Dis 1984; 65:185–188.
48. Huncharek M. Miliary mesothelioma. Chest 1994; 2106:605–606.
49. Boutin C, Rey F, Viallat JR. Prevention of malignant seeding after invasive diagnostic procedures in patients with pleural mesothelioma. Chest 1995; 108:754–758.
50. Metintas M, Gibbs AR, Harmanci E, Ozdemir N, Pasaoglu O, Isiksoy S, Arslan R,

Erginel S, Adapinar B. Malignant localized fibrous tumour of the pleura occurring in a person environmentally exposed to tremolite asbestos. Respiration 1997; 64: 236–239.
51. Boutin C, Villat JR, Rey F, Astoul Ph. Clinical diagnosis of pleural mesothelioma. Eur Respir Rev 1993; 3(11):18–21.
52. Boersma A, Degand P, Biserte G. Hyaluronic acid and the diagnosis of malignant mesothelioma. Bull Physiopathol Respir 1980; 16:41–45.
53. Knuuttila A, Halme M, Kivisaari L, Kivisaari A, Salo J, Mattson K. The clinical importance of magnetic resonance imaging versus computed tomography in malignant pleural mesothelioma. Lung Cancer 1998; 22:215–225.
54. International Mesothelioma Interest Group. A proposed new International TNM staging system for malignant pleura mesothelioma. Chest 1995; 108:1122–1128.
55. Schneider DB, Clary-Macy C, Challa S, Sasse KC, Merrick SH, Hawkins R, Caputo G, Jablons D. Positron emission tomography with F18-fluorodeoxyglocose in the staging and preoperative evaluation of malignant pleural mesothelioma. J Thorac Cardiovasc Surg 2000; 120:128–133.
56. van Gelder T, Damhuis RAM, Hoogsteden HC. Prognostic factors and survival in malignant pleural mesothelioma. Eur Respir J 1994; 7:1035–1038.
57. Yates DH, Corrin B, Stidolph PN, Browne K. Malignant mesothelioma in south east England: clinicopathological experience of 272 cases. Thorax 1997; 52:507–512.
58. Faber LP. Extrapleural pneumonectomy for diffuse malignant mesothelioma: updated in 1994. Ann Thorac Surg 1994; 58:1782–1783.
59. Kraarup-Hansen A. Phase II trials of malignant mesothelioma: a commentary and update. Lung Cancer 1994; 11:305–308.
60. BTS statement on malignant mesothelioma in the United Kingdom. Thorax 2001; 56:250–265.

29

Extrapleural Pneumonectomy for Early-Stage Diffuse Malignant Pleural Mesothelioma

LAMBROS S. ZELLOS

Harvard Medical School
and Brigham & Women's Hospital
Boston, Massachusetts, U.S.A.

DAVID J. SUGARBAKER

Brigham & Women's Hospital
Boston, Massachusetts, U.S.A.

I. Introduction

Diffuse malignant pleural mesothelioma (DMPM) is a rare disease that presents several challenges to physicians. Two thousand to 3000 cases are expected annually in the United States (1), and the incidence is rising. As a result, physicians do not routinely encounter mesothelioma, and this poses difficulties in recognizing and diagnosing mesothelioma while it is still at an early stage. Hence, many patients are diagnosed too late, resulting in a quite short time period from diagnosis to demise. Surgery, chemotherapy, radiotherapy, and immunotherapy have been tried as single modalities or in various combinations as part of multimodality regimens. Treatment with a single modality has failed to prolong the 4- to 12-month median survival that matches the natural history of the disease (2). Multimodality regimens that incorporate surgery with other therapies, on the other hand, have resulted in prolonging median survival. It should be noted that even aggressive cytoreductive surgery such as extrapleural pneumonectomy should be considered in the setting of a multimodality regimen and offered to the appropriate subset of patients. Due to the lack of a universally accepted staging system and randomized controlled studies, however, debate continues as to whether extrapleural pneumonectomy is an appropriate cytoreductive procedure for DMPM.

II. Clinical Presentation

A high index of suspicion is required to diagnose DMPM. The average time from seeking medical care because of symptoms to diagnosis is 2–3 months (3). DMPM does not cause specific symptoms. Rather, symptoms are caused by the pleural effusion such as chest pain, cough, dyspnea, fever, fatigue, and night sweats (3). Most patients tend to be male (3:1 male to female ratio), over the age of 55, and with unilateral disease (95%), which is most commonly right sided (3).

III. Diagnosis

Adequate amounts of pleural fluid and tissue need to be obtained to perform all the necessary histology, immunohistochemistry, and electron microscopy techniques (Table 1) (4). Thoracentesis, closed pleural biopsy, and video-assisted thoracic surgery (VATS) are the most commonly used methods. Cytological examination and closed pleural biopsy have a rather low diagnostic yield and high false-negative rates. Repeated attempts are often needed (5–7). In addition, mesothelioma is known to seed the biopsy needle tracts with eventual chest wall

Table 1 Staining and Microscopic Profiles of Malignant Pleural Mesotheliomas, Adenocarcinomas, and Localized Fibrous Tumors of the Pleura

Marker	MPM	AC	LFTP
Diastase-PAS	−	+ (50%)	−
Hyaluronic acid	+++	+/−	−
Mucicarmine	−	+ (50%)	−
CD34	−	−	+ (80%)
CEA	+/− (10%)	+ (>75%)	−
Cytokeratins	Diffuse cytoplasmic perinuclear	Peripheral cytoplasmic or membrane-associated	−
EMA	Membrane	Diffuse, cytoplasmic	−
Leu-M1 (CD15)	−	+ (60–70%)	
Desmosomes/tonofilaments	Abundant	−	Few
Secretory granules, glycocalyceal bodies	−	+	
Villi	Long, thin, curved, branched (LDR > 15)	Short, thick, straight, sparse (LDR < 10)	Absent
Vimentin	−	−	++

AC, adenocarcinoma; CEA, carcinoembryonic antigen; EMA, epithelial membrane antigen; LDR, length-to-diameter ratio; LFTP, localized fibrous tumors of the pleura; MPM, malignant pleural mesothelioma; PAS, periodic acid/Schiff.
Source: Ref. 4.

metastasis. VATS, on the other hand, can provide drainage of loculated effusions and obtain adequate tissue resulting in a 90% or better diagnostic yield (8). Regardless of the diagnostic procedure used, incisions or thoracentesis sites should be placed along the future thoracotomy incision so that they can be resected and chest wall metastases avoided.

IV. Staging

Along with the lack of randomized studies for the treatment of mesothelioma, there is also a lack of consensus regarding the most appropriate staging system. Several staging systems have been proposed in attempts to stratify survival based on stage, but none have been universally accepted. The Butchart (Table 2) (9), International Mesothelioma Interest Group (IMIG, TNM-based system; Table 3) (10), and the revised Brigham/Dana-Farber Cancer Institute (DFCI; Table 4) (11,12) staging systems are most commonly used. The Butchart staging system was introduced in 1976 and was based on 29 patients who underwent extrapleural pneumonectomy (EPP) (9). However, it fails to stratify survival based on stage, and Boutin et al. found a subset of stage I patients who had from 7- to almost 33-month median survival based on the degree of parietal pleural involvement (13). At the current authors' institution, a retrospective review of 183 patients who underwent EPP with adjuvant chemoradiation found that positive resection margins, N2 nodal disease, and disease extending into the pericardium, diaphragm, or surrounding structures are the most important prognostic factors (11). It found, in addition, that the revised Brigham/DFCI staging system was the most accurate staging system and the only one that stratified survival based on stage when compared to the Butchart and IMIG systems (11). The median survival according to the revised Brigham/DFCI staging system was 25, 20, and 16 months for patients with stages I, II, and III

Table 2 The Butchart Staging System

Stage	Definition
I	Tumor is confined to the capsule of the parietal pleura (i.e., involves only the ipsilateral lung, pleura, pericardium, and/or diaphragm)
II	Tumor invades the chest wall or mediastinal structures (e.g., esophagus, heart, and/or contralateral pleura), or tumor involves intrathoracic lymph nodes
III	Tumor penetrates the diaphragm to involve peritoneum, or tumor involves the contralateral pleura, or tumor involves extrathoracic lymph nodes
IV	Distant bloodborne metastases

Source: Ref. 9.

Table 3 Staging System of the International Mesothelioma Interest Group (IMIG)

Tumor (T) staging:
- T1a Tumor limited to the ipsilateral parietal pleura, including the mediastinal and diaphragmatic pleura. No involvement of the visceral pleura.
- T1b Tumor involving the ipsilateral parietal pleura, including mediastinal and diaphragmatic pleura. Scattered foci of tumor also involving the visceral pleura.
- T2   Tumor involving each of the ipsilateral pleural surfaces (parietal, mediastinal, diaphragmatic, and visceral pleura) with at least one of the following features:
  Involvement of diaphragmatic muscle
  Confluent visceral pleural tumor (including the fissures) or extension of tumor from the visceral pleura into the underlying pulmonary parenchyma
- T3   Locally advanced but potentially resectable tumor. Tumor involving all of the ipsilateral pleural surfaces (parietal, mediastinal, diaphragmatic, and visceral pleura) with at least one of the following features:
  Involvement of the endothoracic fascia
  Extension into the mediastinal fat
  A solitary, completely resectable focus of tumor extending into the soft tissues of the chest wall
  Nontransmural involvement of the pericardium
- T4   Locally advanced, technically unresectable tumor. Tumor involving all of the ipsilateral pleural surfaces (parietal, mediastinal, diaphragmatic, and visceral) with at least one of the following features:
  Diffuse extension or multifocal masses of tumor in the chest wall with or without associated rib destruction
  Direct transdiaphragmatic extension of tumor to the peritoneum
  Direct extension of tumor to the contralateral pleura
  Direct extension of tumor to one or more mediastinal organs
  Direct extension of tumor into the spine
  Tumor extending through to the internal surface of the pericardium with or without a pericardial effusion; or tumor involving the myocardium

Lymph node (N) staging
- NX   Regional lymph nodes cannot be assessed
- N0   No regional lymph node metastases
- N1   Metastases in the ipsilateral bronchopulmonary or hilar lymph nodes
- N2   Metastases in the subcarinal or ipsilateral mediastinal lymph nodes, including the ipsilateral internal mammary nodes
- N3   Metastases in the contralateral mediastinal, contralateral internal mammary, ipsilateral, or contralateral supraclavicular lymph nodes

Metastases (M) staging
- MX   Presence of distant metastases cannot be assessed
- M0   No distant metastasis
- M1   Distant metastasis present

Overall staging
- Stage I
  - Ia   T1a N0 M0
  - Ib   T1b N0 M0
- Stage II   T2 N0 M0
- Stage III   Any T3 M0
  - Any   N1 M0
  - Any   N2 M0
- Stage IV   Any T4
              Any N3
              Any M1

Source: Ref. 10.

Table 4 Revised Staging System for Malignant Pleural Mesothelioma

Stage	Definition
I	Disease completely resected within the capsule of the parietal pleura without adenopathy: ipsilateral pleura, lung, pericardium, diaphragm, or chest-wall disease limited to previous biopsy sites
II	All of stage I with positive resection margins and/or intrapleural adenopathy
III	Local extension of disease into the chest wall or mediastinum; into the heart or through the diaphragm or peritoneum; or with extrapleural lymph node involvement
IV	Distant metastatic disease

Note: Patients with Butchart stage II and III disease (9) are combined into stage III. Stage I represents patients with resectable disease and negative nodes. Stage II indicates resectable disease but positive nodes.
Source: Adapted from Refs. 11, 12.

disease, respectively. Based on these results, preoperative tests, such as CT and MRI scans, echocardiograms, positron emission tomography (PET) scans, and occasionally cervical mediastinoscopy, are useful to identify those patients with N2 disease or significant extension outside of the pleural envelope. MRI gives a more precise assessment of chest wall and diaphragmatic invasion than CT scan (14). PET scan is becoming increasingly valuable in detecting occult mediastinal nodal involvement as well as distant metastasis (15). Tumor burden as measured by standard uptake value (SUV) can also be quantified and provide prognostic information. High PET scan SUV values (mean SUV 6.6 vs. 3.2) carry a negative prognostic burden for survival (16). Cervical mediastinoscopy more accurately assesses N2 disease and is useful in patients with mixed or sarcomatous histology who have borderline cardiopulmonary function and hence a higher than average mortality risk with EPP and less derived benefit due to the unfavorable histology.

Though such an extensive use of preoperative tests is not advocated by other surgeons, use of CT scan as the main staging strategy will result in a significant number of patients at surgery with either unresectable or N2 disease. Rusch and Venkatraman found that 32 out of 131 patients (24%) staged with CT scan had technically unresectable disease and 46 patients (35%) had mediastinal nodal involvement (17).

V. EPP Versus Pleurectomy/Decortication

There is still debate regarding which procedure is the cytoreductive procedure of choice, pleurectomy/decortication (P/D) or EPP. There are no randomized controlled studies comparing these two procedures, and, in addition, all the data are derived from retrospective reviews that do not compare the two procedures within each stage of disease. Significant differences exist between P/D and EPP.

During P/D the lung is left in place while the visceral and parietal pleura, the pericardium, and the diaphragm are resected. Advantages include a technically easier procedure, less postoperative physiological strain on the patient, and, hence, a lower mortality rate than seen with EPP. Mortality rates with P/D are in the range of 1.5–5% (Table 5) (18–28). Opponents of EPP point to the lower mortality of patients undergoing P/D when compared to that published in older EPP studies, such as the Butchart series from 1976 with a mortality rate of 30%, and also to the inability of EPP to prolong survival when used alone (9). However, when one discusses surgical options for patients with mesothelioma, it should be within the setting of multimodality regimens and not as a single treatment modality. It is within the setting of multimodality regimens that EPP has prolonged survival in patients with early-stage disease.

EPP is more aggressive cytoreductive surgery. It involves removal of the lung along with the parietal pleura, pericardium, and diaphragm. Because mesothelioma tends to spread into the fissures, P/D cannot always adequately remove the entire tumor because the lung is left in place. In addition, the presence of the lung limits adjuvant radiation administration. Because local recurrence remains the dominant pattern of recurrence, adjuvant therapy is particularly important (29). The prohibitively high operative mortality of 30% seen in early studies following EPP has been reduced to less than 4% in recent large modern series (Table 6) (9,11,19,29–34). This reduction has been achieved with careful

Table 5 Results of Pleurectomy

No. of patients	% Morbidity	% Mortality	% Survival		Median (mo)	Ref.
			1-year	2-year		
56	26.8	5.4	30.4	8.9	9.0	19
45	16.0	2.2	58.0	21.0	16.0	20
105	NS	NS	52.0	23.0	12.6	21
26	NS	0	NS	NS	10.9	22
63	NS	NS	NS	NS	9.8	23
64	25.0	1.5	49.0	NS	NS	24
30	NS	0	57.0	27.0	13.0	25
13	NS	NS	NS	NS	17.0	26
28	NS	11.0	82.0	32.0	20.0[a]	27
17[b]	NS	NS	NS	NS	21.0	28
16[b]	NS	NS	NS	NS	11.0	

NS, not stated.
[a] Survival calculated from onset of symptoms rather than date of operation.
[b] Patients divided into epithelium ($n = 17$) and mixed ($n = 16$) histopathological findings.
Source: Ref. 18.

Table 6 Reported Mortality with Extrapleural Pneumonectomy

No. of patients	Epithelial cell type	Operative mortality (%)	2-Year survival (%)	5-Year survival (%)	Ref.
62	—	—	37	10	31
11	31	10	3		9
9	0	27	—		32
20	9	24	6		33
20	—	15	33	—	34
40[a]	26	7.5	22.5	10	19
183[b]	103	3.8	37	14	11

[a] Extrapleural pneumonectomy followed by chemotherapy [cyclophosphamide, adriamycin(doxorubicin), and prednisone (cisplatin) (CAP)].
[b] Extrapleural pneumonectomy followed by adjuvant radiation therapy (40.5 Gy ± 14.4 Gy boost dose to areas of residual disease, localized lymph nodes and/or localized positive resection margins) and chemotherapy [doxorubicin (9 patients), CAP (80 patients), and carbo-platin/paclitaxel (94 patients)]. The 2- and 5-year survival for 176 patients who survived surgery were 38% and 15%, respectively.
Source: Ref. 30.

preoperative selection, technical experience in the conduct of the operation, and aggressive management of the potential major complications such as bronchopleural fistula, empyema, chylothorax, patch failure, and post-EPP constrictive physiology.

VI. EPP with Adjuvant Systemic Chemoradiation

At the authors' institution, EPP is the procedure of choice for patients with early-stage disease who have good functional status. Current eligibility criteria are presence of resectable disease as documented by CT and MRI scans, presence of adequate functional and cardiopulmonary status, and the absence of significant comorbidities (35,36). The preoperative scans should show the absence of mediastinal, transdiaphragmatic, or chest wall involvement. Adequate functional and cardiopulmonary status is confirmed with a Karnofsky performance score greater than 70, predicted postoperative forced expiratory volume in one second (FEV_1) greater than 0.8 L, and ejection fraction greater than 45% (11,37).

The parietal pleura, lung, pericardium, and diaphragm are resected en bloc, and the pericardial and diaphragmatic defects are reconstructed with Gore-Tex (W.L. Gore, Flagstaff, AZ) to avoid cardiac or abdominal organ herniation (38). Other postoperative issues that need to be addressed are postpneumonectomy syndrome, excessive mediastinal shift, deep vein thrombosis, pulmonary embolism, vocal cord paralysis, and post-EPP constrictive physiology. Four to 6 weeks after the surgery, adjuvant chemoradiation is administered to patients who are judged able to tolerate it.

A review of this multimodality protocol was published in 1999 (11). Between 1980 and 1997, 183 patients underwent EPP. There were 7 deaths, for an operative mortality of 3.8%. Patients surviving the operation underwent adjuvant chemoradiation ($n = 176$). Patients treated from 1980 to 1985 received doxorubicin and cyclophosphamide; cisplatin was added from 1985 to 1994. In 1994 the protocol was revised to carboplatin [area under the curve (AUC) of 6 mg/m^2] and paclitaxel (AUC 200 mg/m^2) for two cycles followed by concurrent radiotherapy and weekly paclitaxel (60 mg/m^2) and concluded with two additional cycles of chemotherapy. Radiation was started at a dose of 30 Gy to the hemithorax and 40 Gy to the mediastinum, and an additional 14 Gy was given to positive microscopic margins or positive nodes (11). The 2- and 5-year survival rates were 38% and 15%, respectively (Fig. 1) (11). Histology (epithelial vs. nonepithelial subtype), lymph node involvement (N0 vs. N1 vs. N2), resection margins, and invasion beyond the pleural envelope (invasion into diaphragm or pericardium) were found to be important prognostic factors and make up the stage criteria of the revised Brigham/DFCI staging system (11).

Median survival for patients with epithelial histology and stage I disease by the revised Brigham/DFCI staging system was 51 months. The 5-year survival of these patients was 46%. In contrast, patients with sarcomatous histology and positive N2 nodes or positive margins did not survive to 5 years (11). Hence the

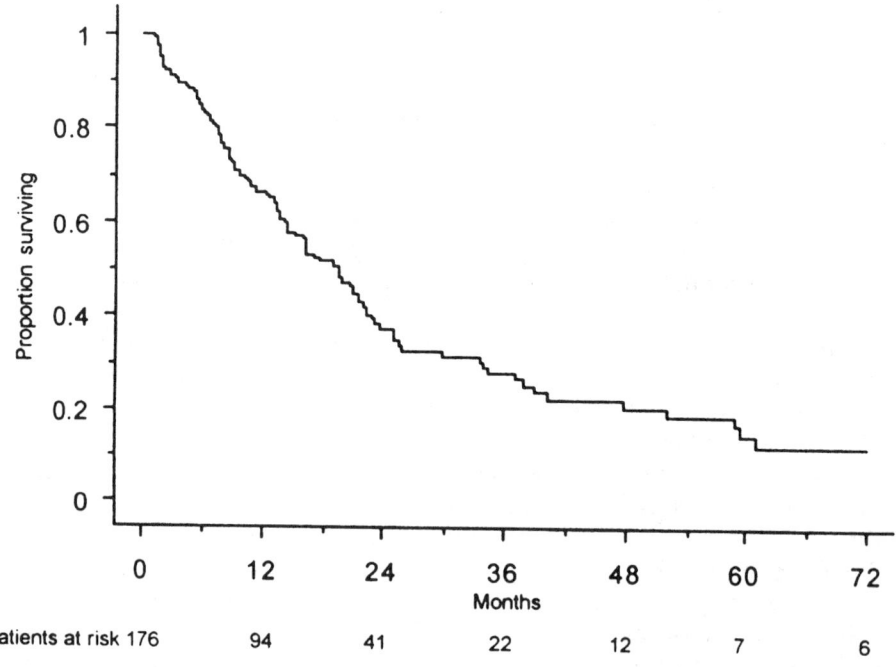

Figure 1 Kaplan-Meier survival curve for all patients surviving surgery ($n = 176$). (From Ref. 11.)

patients who benefited the most from the therapy were the ones with epithelial histology, negative nodes, and negative margins.

The Butchart and IMIG staging systems were also applied to the 176 patients. While the revised Brigham/DFCI system stratified patient survival by stage ($p = 0.0011$), the Butchart ($p = 0.09$) and the IMIG systems ($p = 0.31$) did not. Patterns of recurrence after trimodality therapy were reported on a subset of 46 patients who underwent trimodality therapy between 1987 and 1993.With a median follow-up of 18 months, 25 (54%) patients developed recurrence (ipsilateral 35%, abdominal 26%, and contralateral chest 17%) (39). While recurrence remained predominantly locoregional, distant disease was seen more often suggesting that aggressive therapy can alter the natural history.

While EPP is the procedure of choice for patients with early-stage disease, P/D is offered to patients who cannot tolerate EPP. Similar adjuvant chemotherapy is administered while radiotherapy is focused on the thoracic incision to limit chest wall metastases by intraoperative seeding. The chemotherapeutic regimen has been revised to include gemcitabine along with a platinum-based agent such as cisplatin or carboplatin.

Rusch et al. recently reported a phase II trial of EPP and P/D followed by high-dose adjuvant radiation (40). Patients were staged according to the IMIG system with CT scans. Between 1995 and 1998, 88 patients were enrolled, with 54 patients undergoing EPP and receiving 54 Gy median dose of adjuvant radiotherapy. Operative mortality was 7.9%. The median survival for patients with IMIG stages I or II disease was 33.8 months, while for patients with stage III and IV disease it was 10 months. Patterns of recurrence were also studied in this protocol, and a trend towards distant recurrence was also noted (40).

VII. EPP with Adjuvant Regional Modalities

In efforts to increase regional delivery of adjuvant therapy, several protocols have combined aggressive cytoreduction using EPP with regional administration of chemotherapy or intracavitary photodynamic therapy (PDT). A Cleveland Clinic protocol treated 19 patients, 10 of whom underwent EPP and 9 P/D. Cisplatin and mitomycin C were administered intrapleurally, immediately after P/D, and 1–2 weeks after EPP, followed by systemic adjuvant chemotherapy. Perioperative mortality was 5%. Survival was not prolonged, however, with a median survival reported of 13 months (41).

Hyperthermia increases the effectiveness of chemotherapeutic agents (42). Few studies have shown the efficacy of hyperthermic intracavitary perfusion of chemotherapeutic agents after EPP. Ratto et al. (43) reported a series of patients who underwent P/D with normothermic cisplatin perfusion ($n = 3$), P/D with hyperthermic cisplatin ($n = 3$), or EPP with hyperthermic perfusion ($n = 4$). Cisplatin perfusion was given at a dose of 100 mg/m^2. There were no deaths in this small study. Another limited study by Yellin et al. (44) tested the safety of intracavitary hyperthermic cisplatin perfusion on 8 patients who underwent EPP and another 18 patients who underwent other procedures for a variety of malignancies. There were no major complications related to the hyperthermic perfusion other than empyemas (44). A phase I dose-escalating study of intracavitary intrapleural cisplatin after EPP for mesothelioma has recently been completed at the current authors' institution to determine the maximum-tolerated dose of intrapleural cisplatin. Fifty patients underwent EPP. A range of doses of intrapleural cisplatin was given. Results are pending final follow-up.

Photodynamic therapy (PDT) is another modality that has been combined with EPP and chemotherapy. Pass et al. (45) conducted a phase III trial of EPP or P/D, adjuvant cisplatin, interferon-α-2b, and tamoxifen with and without intraoperative PDT. From 1993 to 1996, 48 of 63 patients completed the protocol. However, because most patients had advanced disease (stage III or IV), no difference in survival was noted with a median survival of 14 months (45).

VIII. Conclusions

DMPM continues to be a rare disease that poses diagnostic and treatment difficulties for physicians. A high index of suspicion is needed to diagnose DMPM in its early stages when more treatment options are available. We lack randomized studies that compare P/D to EPP for each histological subtype and within each stage. Like therapy for any other disease, the available surgical procedures need to be matched with the appropriate stages of disease. The limited retrospective and prospective trials of EPP as part of a multimodality regimen indicate that in early-stage disease significant prolongation of survival has been achieved with EPP and adjuvant therapy. Referral to a center with extensive experience in EPP is essential to avoid high operative mortality rates (4).

While distant recurrence becomes more common in DMPM, locoregional recurrence after EPP and adjuvant therapy remains a significant problem and the dominant pattern of recurrence. Intraoperative, intracavitary hyperthermic perfusion of chemotherapeutic agents has the theoretical potential to reduce the locoregional recurrence, although phase II studies are lacking. Further advances are needed in chemotherapy and immunotherapy as well studies that address the surgical procedure of choice for advanced-stage DMPM.

Acknowledgment

The authors thank Mary S. Visciano for editorial assistance.

References

1. Connelly RR, Spirtas R, Myers MH, Percy CL, Fraumeni JF Jr. Demographic patterns for mesothelioma in the United States. J Natl Cancer Inst 1987; 78:1053–1060.
2. Antman K, Shemin R, Ryan L, Klegar K, Osteen R, Herman T, Lederman G,

Corson J. Malignant mesothelioma: prognostic variables in a registry of 180 patients, the Dana-Farber Cancer Institute and Brigham and Women's Hospital experience over two decades, 1965–1985. J Clin Oncol 1988; 6:147–153.
3. Sugarbaker DJ, Garcia JP, Richards WG, Harpole DH Jr, Healy-Baldini E, DeCamp MM Jr, Mentzer SJ, Liptay MJ, Strauss GM, Swanson S. Extrapleural pneumonectomy in the multimodality therapy of malignant pleural mesothelioma. Results in 120 consecutive patients. Ann Surg 1996; 224:288–294.
4. Ho L, Sugarbaker DJ, Skarin AT. Malignant pleural mesothelioma. In: Ettinger DS, ed. Thoracic Oncology. Boston: Kluwer Academic Publishers, 2001:327–373.
5. Renshaw AA, Dean BR, Antman KH, Sugarbaker DJ, Cibas ES. The role of cytologic evaluation of pleural fluid in the diagnosis of malignant mesothelioma. Chest 1997; 111:106–109.
6. Dejmek A. Methods to improve the diagnostic accuracy of malignant mesothelioma. Respir Med 1997; 90:191–199.
7. Beauchamp HD, Kundra NK, Aranson R, Chong F, MacDonnell KFl. The role of closed pleural needle biopsy in the diagnosis of malignant mesothelioma of the pleura. Chest 1992; 102:1110–1112.
8. Boutin C, Rey F. Thoracoscopy in pleural malignant mesothelioma: a prospective study of 188 consecutive patients. Part 1: Diagnosis. Cancer 1993; 72:389–393.
9. Butchart EG, Ashcroft T, Barnsley WC, Holden MP. Pleuropneumonectomy in the management of diffuse malignant mesothelioma of the pleura: experience with 29 patients. Thorax 1976; 31:15–24.
10. Rusch VW and the International Mesothelioma Interest Group. A proposed new international TNM staging system for malignant pleural mesothelioma. From the International Mesothelioma Interest Group. Chest 1995; 108:1122–1128.
11. Sugarbaker DJ, Flores R, Jacklitsch M, Richards WG, Strauss GM, Corson JM, DeCamp MM, Swanson SJ, Bueno R, Lukanich JM, Baldini EH, Mentzer SJ. Resection margins, extrapleural nodal status, and cell type determine postoperative long-term survival in trimodality therapy of malignant pleural mesothelioma: results in 183 patients. J Thorac Cardiovasc Surg 1999; 117:54–65.
12. Sugarbaker DJ, Strauss GM, Lynch TJ, Richards W, Mentzer SJ, Lee TH, Corson JM, Antman KH. Node status has prognostic significance in the multimodality therapy of diffuse malignant mesothelioma. J Clin Oncol 1993; 11:1172–1178.
13. Boutin C, Rey F, Gouvernet J, Viallat JR, Astoul P, Ledoray V. Thoracoscopy in pleural malignant mesothelioma: a prospective study of 188 consecutive patients. Part 2: Prognosis and staging. Cancer 1993; 72:394–404.
14. Patz EF Jr, Shaffer K, Piwnica-Worms DR, Jochelson M, Sarin M, Sugarbaker DJ, Pugatch RD. Malignant pleural mesothelioma: value of CT and MR imaging in predicting resectability. AJR 1992; 159:961–966.
15. Schneider DB, Clary-Macy C, Challa S, Sasse KC, Merrick SH, Hawkins R, Caputo G, Jablons D. Positron emission tomography with f18-fluorodeoxyglucose in the staging and preoperative evaluation of malignant pleural mesothelioma. J Thorac Cardiovasc Surg 2000; 120:128–133.
16. Benard F, Sterman D, Smith RJ, Kaiser LR, Albelda SM, Alavi A. Prognostic value of FDG PET imaging in malignant pleural mesothelioma. J Nucl Med 1999; 40:1241–1245.
17. Rusch VW, Venkatraman E. The importance of surgical staging in the treatment of malignant pleural mesothelioma. J Thorac Cardiovasc Surg 1996; 111:815–825.
18. Rusch VW. Pleurectomy/decortication in the setting of multimodality treatment

for diffuse malignant pleural mesothelioma. Semin Thorac Cardiovasc Surg 1997; 9:367–372.
19. Allen KB, Faber LP, Warren WH. Malignant pleural mesothelioma. Extrapleural pneumonectomy and pleurectomy. Chest Surg Clin North Am 1994; 4:113–126.
20. Brancatisano RP, Joseph MG, McCaughan BC. Pleurectomy for mesothelioma. Med J Aust 1991; 154:455–457.
21. Mychalczak BR, Nori D, Armstrong JG, et al. Results of treatment of malignant pleural mesothelioma with surgery, brachytherapy, and external beam irradiation [abstr]. Endocurie Hypertherm Oncol 1989; 5:245.
22. Alberts AS, Falkson G, Goedhals I, Vorobiot DA, Van der Merwe CA. Malignant pleural mesothelioma: a disease unaffected by current therapeutic maneuvers. J Clin Oncol 1988; 6:527–535.
23. Ruffie R, Feld R, Minkin S, Cormier Y, Boutan-Laroze A, Ginsberg R, Ayoub J, Shepherd FA, Evans WK, Figueredo A, et al. Diffuse malignant mesothelioma of the pleura in Ontario and Quebec: a retrospective study of 332 patients. J Clin Oncol 1989; 7:1157–1168.
24. McCormack PM, Nagasaki F, Hilaris BS, Martini N. Surgical treatment of pleural mesothelioma. J Thorac Cardiovasc Surg 1982; 84:834–842.
25. Chahinian AP, Pajak TF, Hollan JF, Norton L, Ambinder RM, Mandel EM. Diffuse malignant mesothelioma. Prospective evaluation of 69 patients. Ann Int Med 1982; 96:746–755.
26. Ball DL, Cruickshank DG. The treatment of malignant mesothelioma of the pleura: review of a 5-year experience with special reference to radiotherapy. Am J Clin Oncol 1990; 13:4–9.
27. Law MR, Gregor A, Hodson ME, Bloom HJ, Turner-Warwick M. Malignant mesothelioma of the pleura: a study of 52 treated and 64 untreated patience. Thorax 1984; 39:255–259.
28. Wanebo HJ, Martini N, Melamed MR, Hilaris B, Beattie EJ Jr. Pleural mesothelioma. Cancer 1976; 38:2481–2488.
29. Rusch V, Saltz L, Venkatraman E, Ginsberg R, McCormack P, Burt M, Markman M, Kelsen D. A phase II trial of pleurectomy/decortication followed by intrapleural and systemic chemotherapy for malignant pleural mesothelioma. J Clin Oncol 1994; 12:1156–1163.
30. Swanson SJ, Grondin SC, Sugarbaker DJ. Technique of pleural pneumonectomy in diffuse mesothelioma. In: Shields TW, LoCicero J III, Ponn RB, eds. General Thoracic Surgery. 5th ed. Philadelphia: Lippincott, Williams & Wilkins, 2000:783–790.
31. Worn H. Möglichkeiten und Ergebnisse der chirurgischen Behandlung des malignen Pleuramesotheliomas. Thoraxchir Vask Chir 1974; 22:391–393.
32. DeLaria GA, Jensik R, Faber LP, Kittle CF. Surgical management of malignant mesothelioma. Ann Thorac Surg 1978; 26:375–382.
33. DaValle MJ, Faber LP, Kittle CF, Jensick RJ. Extrapleural pneumonectomy for diffuse malignant mesothelioma. Ann Thorac Surg 1986; 42:612–618.
34. Rusch VW, Piantadosi S, Holmes EC. The role of extrapleural pneumonectomy in malignant pleural mesothelioma. A Lung Cancer Study Group trial. J Thorac Cardiovasc Surg 1991; 102:1–9.
35. Sugarbaker DJ, Heher EC, Lee TH, Couper G, Mentzer S, Corson JM, Collins JJ Jr, Shemin R, Pugatch R, Weissman L, Antman KH. Extrapleural pneumonectomy, chemotherapy, and radiotherapy in the treatment of diffuse malignant pleural mesothelioma. J Thorac Cardiovasc Surg 1991; 102:10–14.

36. Sugarbaker DJ, Mentzer SJ, DeCamp M, Lynch TJ, Strauss GM. Extrapleural pneumonectomy in the setting of a multimodality approach to malignant mesothelioma. Chest 1993; 103(4 suppl):377S–381S.
37. Grondin SC, Sugarbaker DJ. Malignant mesothelioma of the pleural space. Oncology (Huntingt) 1999; 13:919–926.
38. Zellos LS, Sugarbaker DJ. Extrapleural pneumonectomy. In: Kaiser LR, Jamieson GG, eds. Rob and Smith's Operative Technique Thoracic Surgery. 5th ed. London: Arnold. Submitted.
39. Baldini EH, Recht A, Strauss GM, DeCamp MM Jr, Swanson SJ, Liptay MJ, Mentzer SJ, Sugarbaker DJ. Patterns of failure after trimodality therapy for malignant pleural mesothelioma. Ann Thorac Surg 1997; 63:334–338.
40. Rusch VW, Rosenzweig K, Venkatraman E, Leon L, Raben A, Harrison L, Bains MS, Downey RJ, Ginsberg RJ. A phase II trial of surgical resection and adjuvant high-dose hemithoracic radiation for malignant pleural mesothelioma. J Thorac Cardiovasc Surg 2001; 122:788–795.
41. Rice TW, Adelstein DJ, Kirby TJ, Saltarelli MG, Murthy SR, Van Kirk MA, Wiedemann HP, Weick JK. Aggressive multimodality therapy for malignant pleural mesothelioma. Ann Thorac Surg 1994; 58:24–29.
42. Stehlin JS Jr. Hyperthermic perfusion for melanoma of the extremities: experience with 165 patients, 1967 to 1979. Ann NY Acad Sci 1980; 335:352–355.
43. Ratto GB, Civalleri D, Esposito M, Spessa E, Alloisio A, De Cian F, Vannozzi MO. Pleural space perfusion with cisplatin in the multimodality treatment of malignant mesothelioma: a feasibility and pharmacokinetic study. J Thorac Cardiovasc Surg 1999; 117:759–765.
44. Yellin A, Simansky DA, Paley M, Refaely Y. Hyperthermic pleural perfusion with cisplatin: early clinical experience. Cancer 2001; 92(8):2197–2203.
45. Pass HI, Temeck BK, Kranda K, Thomas G, Russo A, Smith P, Friauf W, Steinberg SM. Phase III randomized trial of surgery with or without intraoperative photodynamic therapy and postoperative immunotherapy for malignant pleural mesothelioma. Ann Surg Oncol 1997; 48:628–633.

30

Benign Asbestos-Related Pleural Disease

E. BRIGITTE GOTTSCHALL and LEE S. NEWMAN

National Jewish Medical and Research Center
University of Colorado School of Medicine
Denver, Colorado, U.S.A.

I. Introduction

Asbestos has attracted attention for centuries, first because of its valuable physical properties, but sadly for the last 50–80 years, mostly because of its multiple and varied pulmonary health effects, ranging from simple pleural plaques, to extensive pleural and parenchymal fibrosis, to malignancy. The benign pleural manifestations, including circumscribed pleural plaques, benign pleural effusions, diffuse pleural thickening, and rounded atelectasis, are the focus of this chapter. Mesothelioma is discussed elsewhere in this volume.

II. History

Characteristics that made the industrial use of asbestos popular include insulation against heat, cold, and noise, incombustibility, great tensile strength, flexibility, and weavability, and resistance to corrosion by acids and alkali. Archeological studies reveal that asbestos fibers were integrated in Finnish pottery as far back as 2500 B.C. Plutarch (ca. 45–124 A.D.) wrote of asbestos wicks for oil lamps. Charlemagne (742–814 A.D.) surprised guests by cleansing asbestos napkins and tablecloths in fire. Asbestos was used in body armor in the fifteenth century. Gloves, socks, and handbags were made with asbestos in the eighteenth century. Commercial use of asbestos began in earnest with the Industrial Revolution at the end of the nineteenth century and peaked after World War II. Over 3000 commercial applications for asbestos were known in 1973 when the first ban against an asbestos product, asbestos spray-on insulation, was enacted by the U. S. Environmental Protection Agency. Further asbestos product bans and tighter asbestos exposure regulations have followed in North America, the European Union, Japan, and Australia. Regrettably, extensive asbestos usage continues in the developing world, making another epidemic of asbestos-related lung disease in the workplaces of these countries almost inevitable. The pleural and parenchymal consequences of asbestos exposure are for the most part incurable. Thus, primary prevention, especially the elimination of asbestos use, holds the key to control of the epidemic.

III. Pathogenesis

Asbestos is the name given to a group of fibrous hydrated magnesium silicates that occur naturally in the environment. Two major geological types of asbestos exist. *Serpentine* fibers are wavy and pliable and readily degrade into finer particles. Chrysotile, the only serpentine fiber, accounts for nearly 95% of commercially used asbestos worldwide. *Amphibole* fibers are needle-shaped and straight and prove to be more resistant to biological degradation. Several amphibole fibers are known, namely crocidolite, amosite, anthophyllite, tremolite, and actinolite. While crocidolite, amosite, and anthophyllite have been used commercially in small quantities, tremolite and actinolite are mostly found as contaminants of other minerals such as chrysotile, vermiculite, and talc. The mechanism by which asbestos fibers induce pleural and parenchymal disease is not completely understood; however, various pieces of the puzzle have been solved.

Fiber size has been clearly established as a deciding factor of pathogenicity. Stanton et al. in animal studies demonstrated the importance of fiber length in relation to neoplasia (1). Rats exposed to different length asbestos fibers were most likely to develop mesothelioma after the administration of fibers greater than 8 µm long and less than 0.25 µm wide. These findings were further corroborated in animal studies conducted by Pott (2).

Fibrogenicity is also linked to asbestos fiber length. King (3) exposed rabbits to different length asbestos fibers and later examined them for the development of pulmonary fibrosis. Significantly more fibrosis was produced by long (15 µm) fibers than by short (2.5 µm) ones. Other investigators subsequently confirmed these results (4,5).

The pathogenic importance of fiber size relates in part to how different length fibers are lodged in the lung tissue, processed once inhaled, and translocated to the pleura. Short fibers are often phagocytosed and moved from the lung via alveolar clearance mechanisms into the gastrointestinal tract, the hilar lymph nodes, or the pleural space (6). Macrophages are unable to fully engulf the longer fibers, triggering a complex cascade of events, including the release of oxygen radicals, cytokines, chemokines, and growth factors (7). In vitro studies have also demonstrated that long fibers interfere with the cell cytoskeleton, damage chromosomes, and interfere with the mitotic spindle during mitosis (8,9).

While fiber dimension is integral to asbestos pathogenicity, the chemical composition of a fiber plays an important role as well. Fiber composition contributes to fiber durability. When immersed into liquid environment chrysotile fibers quickly lose their magnesium content leaving behind only a silicon shell. In tissue, they readily separate into their individual fibrils. Consequently, chrysotile is removed from lung tissue much more rapidly than are amphibole fibers. This is an important phenomenon to remember when drawing conclusions regarding pathogenicity of different fiber types based on fiber counts measured in human lung tissue many years after exposure has ceased.

The surface charge of fibers varies. While crocidolite has a negative surface charge, chrysotile is positively charged, resulting in the adsorption of and interaction with different biological materials in the target organ (10).

In summary, the toxicity of asbestos appears intricately related to its morphology and physicochemical properties, but the complete cycle of the events that leads to such varied pulmonary manifestations remains patchy.

IV. Pleural Plaques

A. Epidemiology

The epidemiological evidence for a connection between asbestos exposure and the occurrence of pleural plaques is compelling. The prevalence of pleural plaques is dependent on the population studied. Most estimates of prevalence are based on radiological surveys. The highest attack rates for pleural thickening are found in villages in Turkey and Greece where outcrops contaminated with naturally occurring asbestiform fibers, namely tremolite, actinolite, or eronite, are used to prepare a whitewash or stucco applied to the inside and outside of dwellings. By the age of 70, 69% of the population of a Turkish village showed evidence of pleural thickening on chest x-ray (11). In Finland, Kiviluoto showed that the vast majority of Finns with bilateral pleural plaques lived in the vicinity of open anthophyllite asbestos pits (12). It is possible that these high rates of pleural thickening in these environmentally exposed populations can be explained by a fiber gradient, with anthophyllite and tremolite showing the strongest association with pleural plaques.

In occupational cohorts with known asbestos exposure, the prevalence of pleural thickening varies widely, ranging from 7.6 % in asbestos miners and millers (13) to 58% in insulators (14,15). The large variation in the incidence and prevalence reported in these cohorts can be explained in part by differences in mean age, length of time since first exposure (latency), and dose of exposure among the cohorts studied.

Rogan et al. estimated that 3.9% of the U.S. population aged 35–74 is afflicted with pleural thickening due to occupational asbestos exposure. They based their estimates on chest x-ray data from the National Health and Nutrition Examination Survey (NHANES) II (1976–1980) (16). This prevalence is approximately twice that estimated from NHANES I data (1971–1975) (17). Hillerdal (18) also reported an increase in pleural thickening in Uppsala county residents over the age of 40 from 0.2% in 1965 to 2.7% in 1985.

Epidemiological studies may either over- or underestimate the true incidence of pleural plaques when based on radiographs. Recently, increased body mass index (BMI >30 kg/m^2) was shown to correlate with a greater prevalence of circumscribed pleural thickening on chest radiograph in former crocidolite miners in Wittenoom, Australia (19). This was especially true for thin (<10 mm) shadows covering 25–50% of the lateral chest wall. Whether this is due to extra pleural fat or other causes is not clear at this time. However, the finding is of interest in view of the continuing increase in prevalence of obesity among the U.S. population. That chest radiographs can underestimate the presence of pleural plaques has long been known based on autopsy (20–22) and computed tomography (CT) studies (23–25).

Pleural plaques are the most common manifestation of asbestos exposure. When bilateral and partially calcified, they are virtually pathognomonic of past asbestos exposure. The plaques develop slowly over time, with an average latency period from first exposure to radiographically identifiable plaque of 20–30 years (26,27). They are not affected by smoking (28). Pleural plaques are associated with lower lung fiber counts than asbestosis (29,30). No threshold exposure has been identified for the occurrence of pleural plaques. While asbestosis has been associated with cumulative, continuous exposures, pleural disease occurs at proportionally higher rates in individuals who have had intermittent exposures (15). Nishimura et al. (31) speculated that intermittent exposures may allow more time for fiber clearance from the lung and for greater accumulation of fibers in the pleura.

Pleural plaques are not known to transform into mesothelioma. However, Hillerdall reported an increased risk for mesothelioma in those with pleural plaques on chest x-ray (32). In a necropsy-based study Bianchi et al. demonstrated that the presence of plaques >4 cm was a risk indicator for the development of mesothelioma (33). Whether radiographic evidence of pleural plaques is associated with an increased risk of developing lung cancer is controversial. The issue has been addressed in a number of studies of varying design and in reviews without a definitive conclusion. (20–22, 34–42). Plaques are not causative in the development of lung cancer, but are thought to serve as a surrogate of the magnitude of asbestos exposure. However, temporality of the exposure may play a role in addition to dose, as mentioned earlier for pleural plaques and asbestosis. Any lung cancer in an asbestos-exposed individual should be very closely examined as an asbestos-related lung cancer whether pleural plaques are present or not.

B. Pathogenesis

Inhalation of asbestos fibers results in a spectrum of thoracic manifestations unparalleled by most other toxins. For unknown reasons, the pleura is a major target. The mechanism by which asbestos fibers produce the pleural disorders discussed below is not known for certain, but increasingly sophisticated theories have been proposed. In the 1960s Kiviluoto (12) suggested that asbestos fibers poking out of the visceral pleura scratch the parietal pleura during respiration and thus induce an inflammatory reaction in the parietal pleura that eventually leads to pleural thickening. This theory has since been discarded.

Hillerdal (43) in 1980 published a report in which he suggested that some asbestos fibers that have reached the visceral pleura penetrate the pleural space and are swept up by the lymphatic flow and transported to the parietal pleura. As they pass through the parietal pleura, some fibers will actually remain there inside macrophages and initiate an inflammatory response that in time leads to pleural thickening. More recently Boutin et al. (44) published an elegant study adding to our knowledge of how pleural plaques may form. He and his coworkers obtained parietal pleura and lung biospy specimens during thoracoscopy in asbestos-exposed individuals. In the parietal pleura, they secured samples from anthracotic "black spots" and from adjacent normal pleura. Black spots are thought to be part of the lymphatic system in the pleura and correspond to Kapmeier's foci or "milky spots," which are collections of immune cells surrounding lymphatic stomata (44,45). Transmission electron microscopy (TEM) revealed high concentrations of asbestos fibers in the "black spots" and almost none in the normal pleura. In some cases, higher concentrations of fibers were found in the anthracotic areas of the pleura than in the lung tissue. One fifth of the fibers recovered from the "black spots" were >5 µm long. This study suggests that the distribution of asbestos fibers throughout the parietal pleura is heterogeneous and could explain the uneven distribution of circumscribed parietal pleural plaques.

Analysis of pleural plaques has identified mainly short, fine asbestos fibers <2 µm long. Animal studies have confirmed that fibers travel into the pleura after tracheal instillation (46,47). Pathology shows that asbestos fibers are embedded (48,49) in the pleura, and in vitro studies of disease mechanism have shown that mesothelial cells exposed to asbestos fibers promote inflammatory events leading to fibrosis (7,50–53).

C. Clinical Presentation

Macroscopically pleural plaques are discrete, raised, irregularly shaped, shiny lesions of the parietal pleura, with no associated pleural adhesions. Microscopically, on their surface is a normal appearing layer of mesothelial cells. Beneath the mesothelium is fairly acellular, dense, collagenous tissue arranged in a coarse basket weave pattern. Many submicroscopic fibers are visible in these plaques when examined by electron microscopy (54). Plaques are most often found on the posterior and lateral wall of the lower half of the thoracic cage, where they follow the course of the ribs (Fig. 1). They can also form on the domes of the diaphragm, on the mediastinal pleura (especially overlying the heart) (Fig. 2), and rarely on the pericardium itself. They spare the lung apices and costophrenic angles. As Nishimura and Broaddus (31) point out, the intriguing aspect of this distribution is that it corresponds with the distribution of the lymphatic system involved in the clearance of particles from the pleural space. This assumes that asbestos fibers can travel against the normal direction of the lymph flow, as has been reported for coal dust particles (55). Asbestos-related pleural plaques are most often bilateral and symmetrical. If unilateral, most of them seem to form in the left hemithorax based on chest x-ray (56,57). However, a recent CT study did not corroborate this left-sided predominance (58).

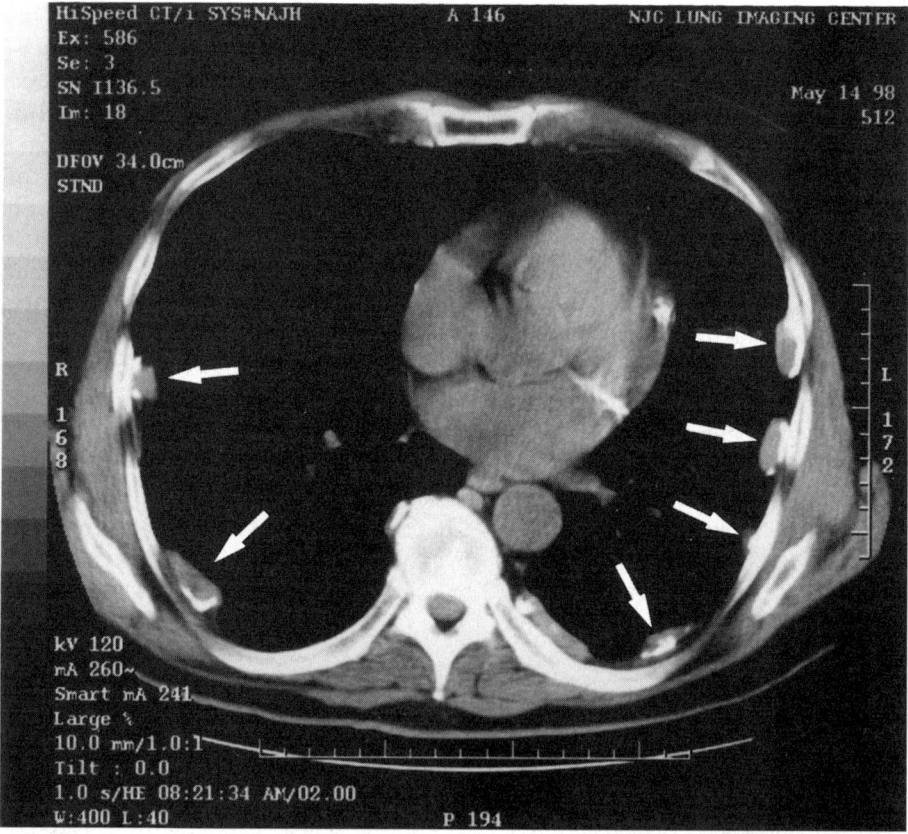

Figure 1 Chest CT with multiple large, localized, partially calcified pleural plaques (white arrows) in classic bilateral distribution along the posterior and posterolateral parietal pleura.

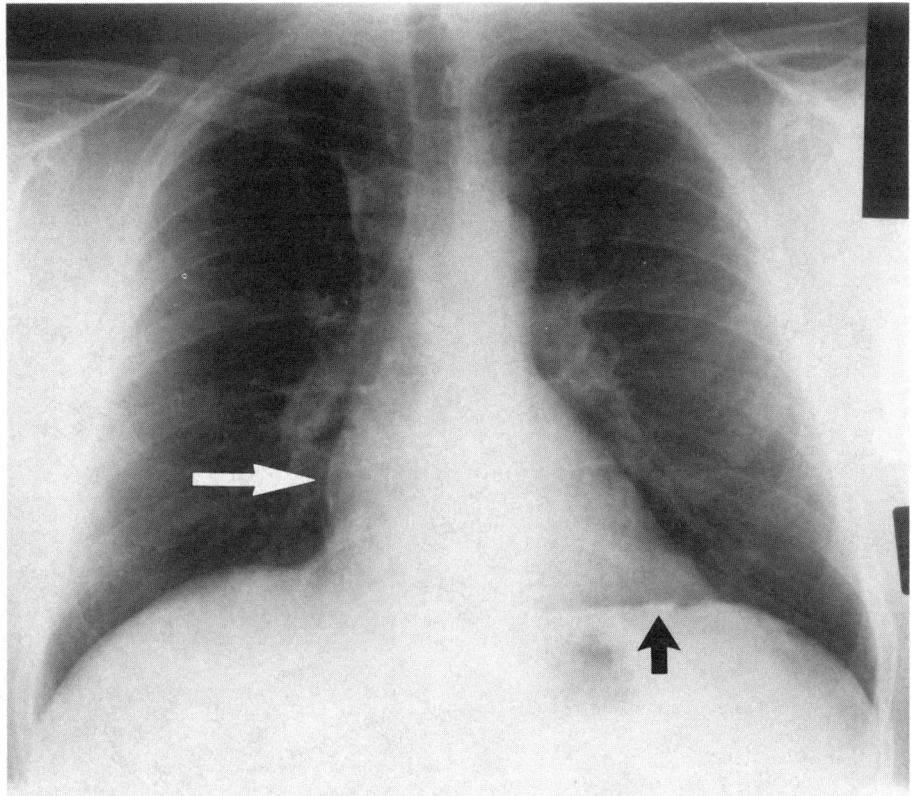

Figure 2 A former insulator with pleural plaques in multiple locations. (a) The chest radiograph shows a thin calcified plaque along the right heart border (white arrow) and overlying the dome of the left diaphragm (black arrow). (b) The chest CT also shows the delicate pleural plaque in the mediastinal pleura overlying the heart (small white arrow), but the plaque in the right paraspinous region on chest CT (large white arrow) was not visible on chest x-ray.

Chest CT scan has proven to be more sensitive than chest radiography for detecting pleural plaques and for discriminating between pleural fibrosis and extrapleural fat (23–25,59). Gevenois et al. (25) performed a conventional and high-resolution CT scan (HRCT) on 159 asbestos-exposed workers with normal chest radiographs. Of these workers, 37.1% demonstrated pleural thickening on CT scan. Conventional CT proved superior to HRCT in detecting these plaques.

Simple circumscribed asbestos-related pleural plaques usually do not produce clinical symptoms. Often they are discovered incidentally during the clinical evaluation of unrelated health problems or during participation in a screening program. Despite their subclinical presentation, pleural plaques are associated with statistically significant pulmonary function abnormalities. Most

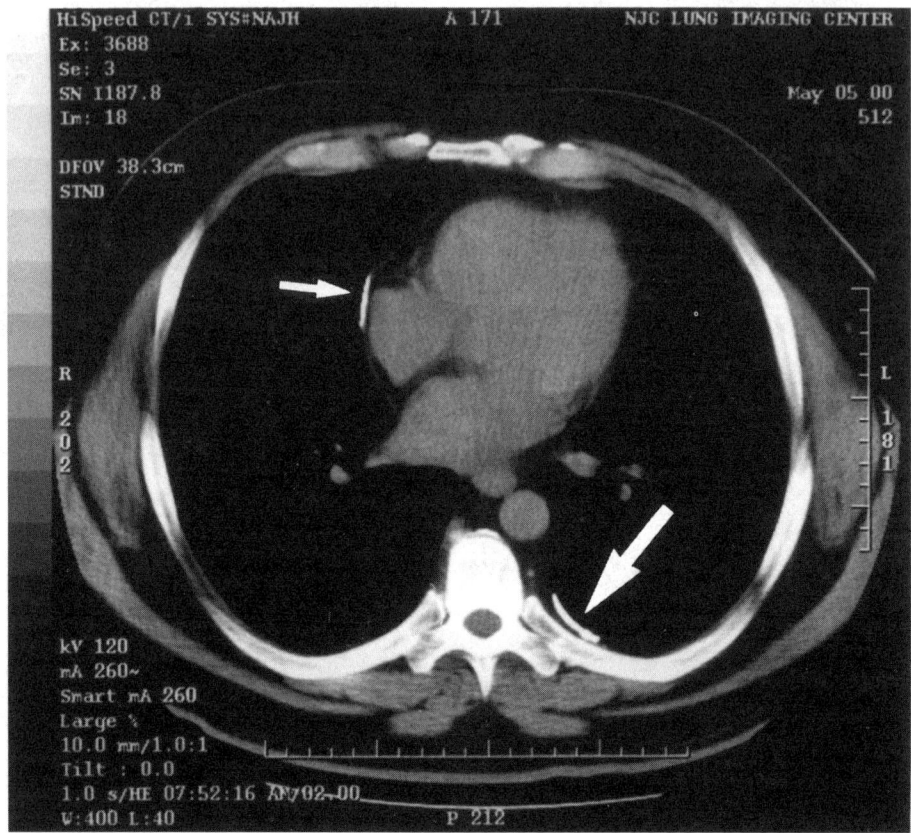

Figure 2 Continued.

consistently they lead to a reduction of the forced vital capacity (FVC) (14,60). Pleural plaques have also been associated with airflow limitation (61–65) While this can be partially attributed to the prevalence of tobacco use in asbestos-exposed cohorts, reports in nonsmokers (62) suggest an independent asbestos-related mechanism responsible for airflow limitation. The most plausible scenario is that physiological airflow limitation is a reflection of pathologically apparent, but radiographically occult peribronchiolar fibrosing alveolitis, the early tissue response to inhalation of asbestos fibers (66).

D. Treatment

No specific treatment is needed for circumscribed pleural plaques. However, since they are a marker of exposure and as such are associated with the risk of developing asbestosis and malignancy, regular follow-up of affected individuals is prudent. Recently much attention has focused on low-dose spiral CT as a lung cancer–screening tool (67–69) motivated by persistently poor 5-year survival rates (70). Asbestos-exposed workers are a well-defined high-risk group in which this screening tool has great potential. An expert panel recently met to review the advances in radiology and screening of asbestos-related disease (71). They concluded that data available do not justify broad-based lung cancer screening in asbestos-exposed cohorts. For now, the decision to screen with low-dose spiral CT must be made on a case-by-case basis.

Regular follow-up visits also offer opportunities to emphasize the importance of smoking cessation and to assist with achieving this, if necessary, and to assure updated immunization records especially for the influenza vaccine and Pneumovax.

V. Diffuse Pleural Thickening

A. Epidemiology

Diffuse pleural thickening has been recognized only recently as a distinct asbestos-related entity. For many years it was considered to be part of the spectrum of parenchymal asbestosis (48). On the other hand, it was often not clearly distinguished from circumscribed parietal pleural plaques. It is often touted as the sequel of an asbestos-related benign pleural effusion (72–75). Diffuse pleural thickening is not as specific for asbestos exposure as bilateral partially calcified pleural plaques are, since it has also been associated with other disorders, including parapneumonic exudative effusions, hemothorax, collagen vascular disease, drug exposure, especially bromocriptine (76), and Dressler's syndrome. The incidence of diffuse pleural thickening is thought to be significantly lower than that of pleural plaques. This is supported by a study conducted by Hillerdal et al. (77), who followed 891 cases with pleural thickening due to asbestos exposure and observed that 84 individuals (approximately 10%) developed diffuse pleural thickening over time. Schwartz et al. examined the chest radiographs of 1211 sheet metal workers and concluded that 260 (21.5%) had developed circumscribed pleural plaques, while again a smaller proportion, only 74 (6.1%), suffered from visceral pleural fibrosis. McLoud et al. (74) could not confirm a significantly lower incidence of diffuse pleural thickening compared to circumscribed pleural thickening when they reviewed chest radiographs of 1373 asbestos-exposed individuals. They found that 10% of the cohort had diffuse pleural thickening and only 16.5% had circumscribed pleural thickening. Some of these differences likely relate to how diffuse pleural thickening is defined by the different investigators or related to the type of asbestos fiber. De Klerk et al. studied workers exposed to crocidolite and found more diffuse pleural thickening than plaques (78).

Diffuse pleural thickening incidence increases with time since first exposure. It is associated with asbestos fiber burden levels that are intermediate between those of levels associated with pleural plaques and those of asbestosis (79–82).

B. Pathogenesis

In contrast to circumscribed pleural plaques, diffuse pleural thickening affects the visceral pleura and typically covers a much larger surface area (Fig. 3). It initially forms in the posterior and posterolateral portions of the lower visceral pleura. With time, it evolves and extends into the costophrenic angles and apices. Diffuse pleural thickening is usually bilateral, but can occur unilaterally. Adhesions between the two pleural sheaths are common. Microscopically, the visceral pleura is replaced by a layer of dense collagenous tissue with a basket-weave pattern reminiscent of that found in parietal pleural plaques. Asbestos fibers and bodies can be recovered from the pleuroparenchymal tissue, especially in the vicinity of the pleural thickening (31).

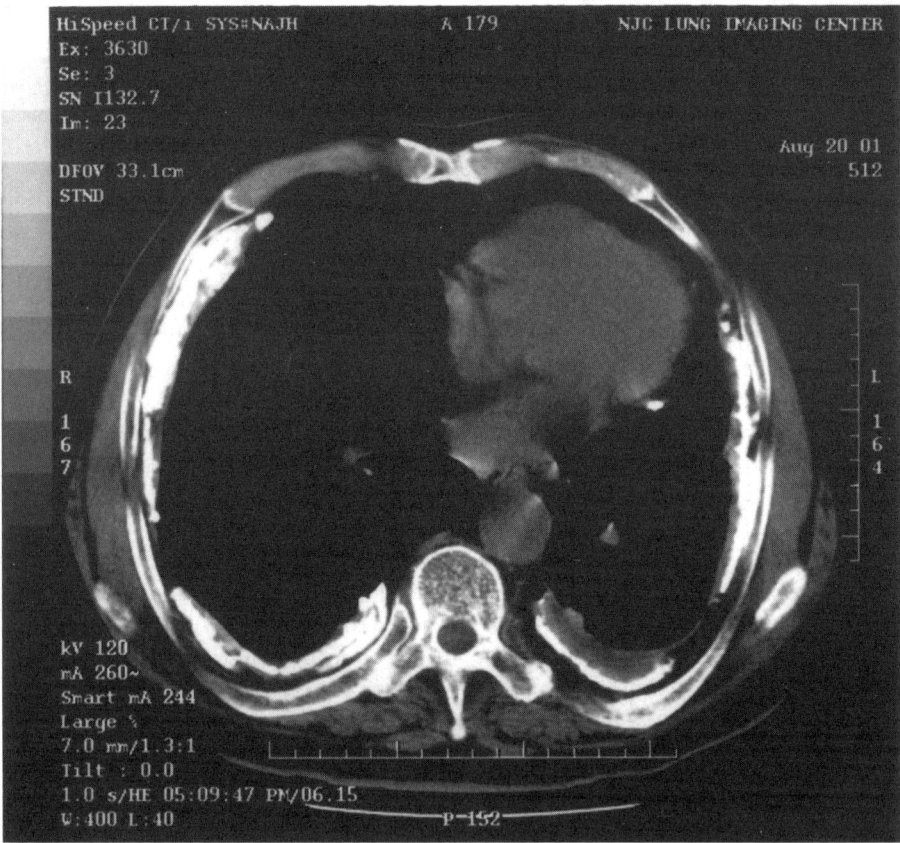

Figure 3 Chest CT depicting extensively calcified thick pleural rind extending around most of the circumference of the lung typical of diffuse pleural thickening.

The pathogenesis of diffuse pleural thickening is not precisely known. However, passage of asbestos fibers into the pleural space via lymphatics with a subsequent inflammatory response is also thought to play a role in diffuse pleural thickening. It is not known why some individuals develop circumscribed plaque while others develop diffuse pleural thickening.

C. Clinical Presentation

In contrast to simple parietal plaques, diffuse pleural thickening is often associated with respiratory symptoms. Dyspnea on exertion represents the most common complaint. In a study by Yates et al. 61 out of 64 asbestos-exposed workers with diffuse pleural thickening complained of breathlessness with exertion (83). Occasionally pleuritic chest pain occurs, most likely due to pleural adhesions in those with diffuse pleural thickening (83,84). Sometimes the pain mimics angina (85).

The physical exam in patients with diffuse pleural thickening can reveal reduced chest expansion, dullness to percussion when the pleural peel has reached significant thickness, and sometimes crackles on auscultation due to concomitant parenchymal fibrosis. Al Jarad and colleagues noted that crackles could be heard in the absence of CT evidence of asbestosis in up to 40% of subjects with diffuse pleural thickening (86).

The radiological features of asbestos-related diffuse pleural thickening have recently been reviewed (82,87). The diagnosis of diffuse pleural thickening on chest radiograph relies on the obliteration of one or both costophrenic angles (74). Based on CT scan, Lynch et al. defined diffuse pleural thickening as a "continuous sheet of pleural thickening more than 5 cm wide, more than 8 cm in craniocaudal extent, and more than 3 mm thick" (88). CT scan often detects fibrous strands, or "crow's feet," extending from the thickened pleura into the lung parenchyma. High-resolution CT scan is superior to chest radiograph in demonstrating the extent of the pleural process. It allows much better visualization of the often-involved paraspinous regions of the pleura that are otherwise obscured by mediastinal structures on chest radiographs. CT scan is also superior in distinguishing between pleural thickening and extrapleural fat.

Several studies have shown that diffuse pleural thickening impairs lung function. The most consistent findings are a decrease in FVC, total lung capacity (TLC), diffusing capacity (DLCO), and exercise tolerance (83,89). In the study by Yates et al. (83) of 64 patients with diffuse pleural thickening, FEV_1 was reduced to 62% and FVC to 77% of predicted. TLC was 71% and DLCO 74% of predicted. Similar results were reported by Kee et al. who studied 53 asbestos-exposed individuals exposed in shipyards or in the construction trades. In this study, the FVC was reduced to 68% of predicted, with a mean DLCO of 72% of predicted (90). Neither study reported DLCO corrected for lung volume, which in the absence of concomitant asbestosis would be expected to be normal.

Interestingly, Al Jarad et al. showed in 20 patients that severity of disease by CT and chest radiograph scores correlated well with the extent of their pulmonary impairment (91). Schwartz et al. also demonstrated in 60 sheet metal workers with asbestos-related pleural fibrosis that the greater the volume of pleural fibrosis derived from a three-dimensional reconstructed thoracic HRCT image, the lower the total lung capacity (92).

D. Treatment

Treatment options for those with diffuse pleural thickening and pulmonary impairment are very limited. Attempts have been made at freeing the lung with decortication, but results have been disappointing (77,93). Supportive treatment is often the best option available. Intercurrent respiratory infections should be treated aggressively. Oxygen therapy is necessary for those with hypoxemia at rest or with exertion. The importance of smoking cessation should be stressed. Immunizations are warranted.

VI. Benign Asbestos Pleural Effusion

A. Epidemiology

The epidemiology of asbestos-related benign pleural effusions mirrors that of asbestosis and the other forms of asbestos-related lung and pleural disease. Risk is associated with the same forms of inhaled asbestos that have been linked to asbestosis, asbestos-related lung cancer, mesothelioma, and other pleural disorders. Described in the 1960s (94–100), the so-called benign pleural effusion may in fact portend development of other forms of asbestos-related disease, including pleural fibrosis and possibly mesothelioma (73). In one of the largest studies of prevalence and incidence, Epler and colleagues observed 34 effusions among 1135 workers exposed in a variety of industries, including shipyards, fireproofing product manufacture, and paper mills. The prevalence was dose-related, ranging from 0.2% for peripherally exposed individuals to 7% among those with most severe exposure. It is the most common asbestos-related condition in the first 20 years after exposure, with incidence of 9.2 effusions per 1000 person-years for those exposed at the highest levels and 0.7 effusions per 1000 person-years for those with the least exposure. The effusions can occur as soon as 5 years after first exposure and have almost always occurred within the first 20 years, although studies differ in their estimates of latency, ranging from a mean of 12 to 30 years. In the Epler study, pleural effusions were five times more likely to occur in asbestos-exposed individuals compared with a nonexposed control group, including effusions related to mesothelioma and lung cancer (73). In light of the rarity of benign pleural effusions in the general population, asbestos exposure should be considered whenever an unexplained exudative effusion is detected. The studies of prevalence and incidence may, in fact, have underestimated the true frequency of asbestos effusions, since many may remain subclinical, preceding development of pleural fibrosis (77).

B. Pathogenesis

The true pathophysiology of asbestos pleural effusions is unknown. As discussed above, animal and human studies have shown that asbestos fibers can migrate to the peripheral lung parenchyma and can be demonstrated in the pleural effusions of asbestos exposed workers (101–104). These data suggest transpleural seeding of fibers in the parietal pleura (105). Alternatively, in light of the role of lymphatic drainage of asbestos fibers (106), the asbestos fibers might also gain access to the pleura by retrograde lymphatic drainage (55,107). Once in the pleural space, the fibers themselves induce an inflammatory response that results in fluid exudation and clinically obvious effusions. For example, instillation of crocidolite into the pleural space promotes neutrophil chemotaxis (98). Influx of neutrophils and macrophages in the pleural space may help promote resolution of the inflammatory response to asbestos fibers, but also may contribute to pleural fibrosis (108). This low-grade pleural fibrotic reaction is hypothesized to result in altered lymphatic clearance or increased permeability of the parietal pleural. As has been described in the lung parenchyma itself, the pleural inflammatory reaction involves a cascade of inflammatory events involving both neutrophils and macrophages and the release of neutrophil chemotactic factors, oxygen free radicals, leukotrienes, cytokines, and growth factors (7,52,109). Inflammatory changes in both the parietal and visceral pleura are observed. It is noteworthy that pleural fluid eosinophilia has also been described in approximately one fourth of patients with asbestos pleural effusions, although the role these cells may play in pathogenesis remains open to speculation. The pleural pathology seen in individuals with these effusions is typical of other acute exudative pleural responses, with biopsies demonstrating nonspecific inflammation and fibrosis in those with effusions.

C. Clinical Presentation

Benign asbestos pleural effusion is a diagnosis of exclusion. Benign asbestos effusions are defined as effusions occurring in individuals who have pleural effusion with no other known causes and who have been directly or indirectly exposed to asbestos (73). The effusion is typically exudative and may be hemorrhagic. It is important to exclude other important causes, including infection, malignancy, and pulmonary embolism. One half to two thirds are asymptomatic (73,110), detected as an incidental finding on chest radiograph or thoracic computed tomography. Notably, however, such effusions can be associated with significant pleuritic pain, with or without fever. Of those who present clinically with these effusions, approximately 17–50% report pleurisy. Other symptoms include cough and dyspnea. The effusions may be detected in the presence or absence of other findings of asbestos-related disorders such as asbestosis or diffuse pleural thickening. Pleural plaques, especially with calcification, are infrequently seen in concert with asbestos pleural effusions, probably because the effusions occur so much earlier in the course of disease. In approximately 20% of cases, severe diffuse pleural thickening will ensue. While this condition can spontaneously resolve in some cases, it should be considered a chronic condition, prone to recurrences and subsequent diffuse pleural thickening. The typical case will last for approximately one year, spontaneously clear, but then recur in approximately one third of individuals. The extent of pleural thickening often increases with each episode of effusion (75). Approximately 5% of patients with benign asbestos effusions will later develop malignant mesothelioma, necessitating careful clinical follow-up (98).

Cases are usually first suspected when a unilateral or, less commonly, bilateral pleural effusion is detected on chest radiograph. In one major series, 11% were large (>500 mL) effusions. Confirmation of this diagnosis is customarily made by thoracentesis, which reveals a typical exudative effusion profile, with elevated total protein, elevated total protein pleural:serum ratio, elevated total lactate dehydrogenase (LDH), pleural LDH:serum LDH ratio, normal glucose level, with elevated while cell count consisting principally of neutrophils, macrophages, and sometimes eosinophils (in one fourth of cases). Two thirds will contain mesothelial cells. As discussed above, the effusion is commonly hemorrhagic, even in the absence of malignancy. Nonetheless, when hemorrhagic effusions are detected, additional testing and careful clinical monitoring to rule out malignant mesothelioma or lung cancer should be considered. It is important to recognize that hemorrhagic effusions in asbestos workers do not necessarily implicate mesothelioma.

D. Treatment

There is no known treatment for asbestos pleural effusion that will alter the clinical course of this disorder. When effusions are large and associated with dyspnea, thoracentesis may help relieve shortness of breath. Anti-inflammatory medications may be prescribed for acute pleurisy symptoms. Diligent follow-up of these cases is important because of the small but significant risk of subsequent mesothelioma. Thoracoscopic pleural biopsy may be warranted in some cases to help clarify whether areas of pleural thickening are due to diffuse pleural fibrosis or malignancy. However, most cases may be followed clinically for signs of improvement, without invasive studies beyond the initial thoracentesis.

VII. Rounded Atelectasis

A. Epidemiology

Rounded atelectasis is one of the more unusual but distinctive pleural sequelae of asbestos exposure. While uncommon, it is important to recognize because it can mimic lung tumors (111) and provoke unnecessary medical and surgical interventions. The invagination of pleura with associated peripheral lobar collapse was first described in the French literature (112) in relation to infection and complications of therapeutic pneumothorax. Later, Blesovsky (113) made the link between "folded lung" and asbestos exposure when he observed this condition in a pipe fitter, a ship's engineer, and a laborer in a sugar refinery—

all of whom had exposures to asbestos and pleural plaques. While rounded atelectasis has been reported as a consequence of pulmonary infarction, Dressler's syndrome, and tuberculous effusion, asbestos is now recognized as the leading cause. Multiple published case series describe the condition and support its association with asbestos exposure, but do not provide good estimates of prevalence and incidence (111,113–122). By inference, rounded atelectasis must be a relatively late and rare event following asbestos exposure, given that Epler and colleagues reported no case in their review of 1135 asbestos workers' chest x-rays (73). Hillerdal estimated a yearly incidence of 5–15 cases per 100,000 in men older than age 40 in Sweden, although this denominator was not adjusted for history of asbestos exposure (121).

B. Pathogenesis

The pathogenesis of rounded atelectasis remains speculative. Hanke and Kretzschmar (123) suggested that the condition starts with a pleural effusion that allows infolding of a portion of the lung and the formation of a cleft around an atelectatic segment of lung. Schneider and others (116,117) have questioned this hypothesis because of the rarity with which pleural effusions are seen in cases of rounded atelectasis. However the process is initiated, the consequence is an infolding of the visceral pleura and of lung tissue subjacent to an area of pleural plaque or pleural thickening. The asbestos-induced pleural plaque itself probably contributes to the invagination of the visceral pleura. At time of thoracotomy, Blesovsky described a thick membrane covering the involved lung segment. Some cases had evidence of adhesions from the lung to the diaphragm with hyalinized plaques on the diaphragm. In another surgical series, predominantly visceral pleural thickening was observed in association with a pleuroparenchymal mass, as well as hyaline plaques on the parietal pleura (115). Histologically, the visceral and parietal pleura show fibrosis with clusters of reactive mesothelial cells and nonspecific inflammatory changes as well as laminated areas of collapsed pulmonary tissue. Some cases show evidence of interstitial pulmonary fibrosis with lymphocytic infiltration consistent with asbestosis, although in most cases the lung tissue itself appears collapsed but histologically normal (113,115).

C. Clinical Presentation

Patients with rounded atelectasis are often asymptomatic. Occasionally they may present with cough and either pleuritic or nonpleuritic chest pain. Most commonly, this condition is detected incidentally when a chest radiograph is obtained for purposes of screening for asbestos-related lung disease. The symptoms have been reported to resolve following decortication (115), although such surgical intervention is rarely warranted. Rounded atelectasis is a benign condition that can occur unilaterally or bilaterally, usually in the lower lobes.

On chest radiograph, rounded atelectasis is not necessarily round, but is a pleural-based curvilinear shadow most commonly seen along the posterior surface of the lower lobe, less frequently in the middle lobe or lingula

(111,113–117,119–121). It may have sharp or irregular borders, blurring most where the pleura intercalates with blood vessels and bronchi. Entrapment of adjacent lung may create a sweeping, "comet-tail" pattern as the segment of lung becomes compressed into the lung. These findings may be evident on chest radiograph, but usually a CT scan will be needed to provide greater confidence. Signs of lung collapse, such as diaphragmatic elevation, retraction of the fissure, or displaced hilum, are uncommon because rounded atelectasis rarely involves more than a few segments of a single lobe. Other disorders that may be confused with rounded atelectasis on chest radiograph include arteriovenous malformation, loculated effusion or empyema, mesothelioma, metastatic disease, and fibrinous pleurisy.

Rounded atelectasis is best defined by thoracic CT scan (Fig. 4) (116,119). Chronic pleural thickening will be seen adjacent to the curvilinear or oval mass. It can be shown to connect to the pleura. The degree of pleural thickening is greatest adjacent to the curvilinear mass, even in individuals who show diffuse pleural thickening or pleural plaques elsewhere in the chest.

The findings on CT scan are so characteristic that patients rarely require any form of invasive procedure to make the diagnosis. As discussed above, when the typical "comet sign" is observed, the only major consideration is to have ruled out other known causes of rounded atelectasis (116,119,124).

When followed longitudinally, the CT scan and chest radiograph will show no or very slow change over time (116,117,121). Hillerdal performed follow-up assessments in 61 of 64 patients (121), with an average observation period of 6 years. In this group, 55% had a known history of asbestos exposure. In the observation period, 24 remained stable with no other changes except slight worsening of pleural plaques. In 12 individuals, progressive diffuse pleural thickening and parenchymal changes consistent with asbestosis were observed over the next 2–15 years. Two of these individuals developed contralateral benign pleural effusions. An additional 23 patients developed bilateral progressive pleural fibrosis. The patients with rounded atelectasis who did not have asbestos exposure in Hillerdal's cohort remained stable over time, except for one case of spontaneous resolution. Notably, nine of the individuals—all of whom had asbestos exposure—died during the observation period: three from asbestosis and two due to pneumonia. Postobstructive pneumonia and pulmonary thrombosis in entrapped vessels have been reported and can result in death due to rounded atelectasis (125). On rare occasions malignancies have been masked by rounded atelectasis (126).

D. Treatment

There is no specific treatment for rounded atelectasis. In surgical series reported by Blesovsky (113) and later by Payne and colleagues (115), the surgeons were able to release the entrapped lung, resulting in reexpansion of the folded lung segment. In some individuals who had experienced chest pain, the pain resolved with this surgical intervention. In some instances the rounded atelectasis

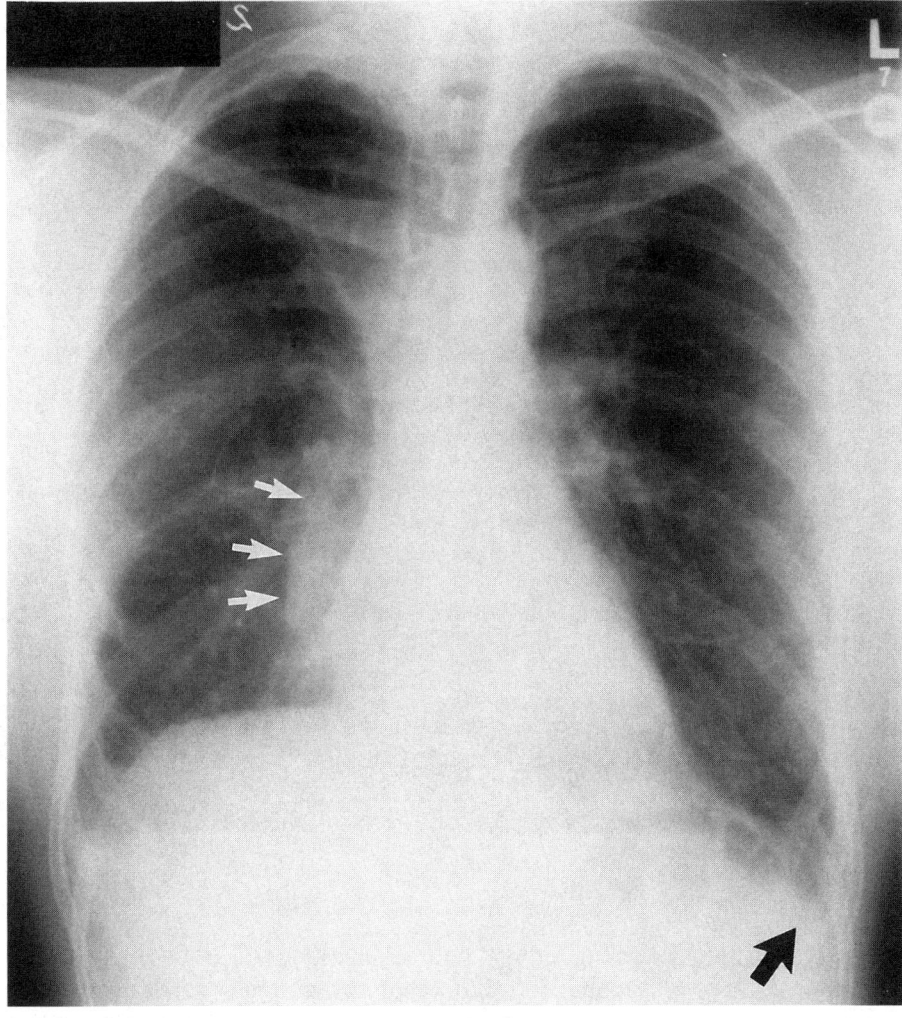

(a)

Figure 4 In a patient with past tremolite exposure, diffuse pleural thickening with rounded atelectasis has developed over time. (a) On the chest radiograph, unilateral obliteration of the left costophrenic angle (black arrow) can be seen, which is typical for diffuse pleural thickening. In addition, this radiograph depicts a right-sided mass (white arrows) located medially and at the level of the heart. (b) Computed tomography demonstrates bilateral pleural-based masses associated with pleural thickening. The right-sided mass has a "comet tail" that is pathognomonic for rounded atelectasis.

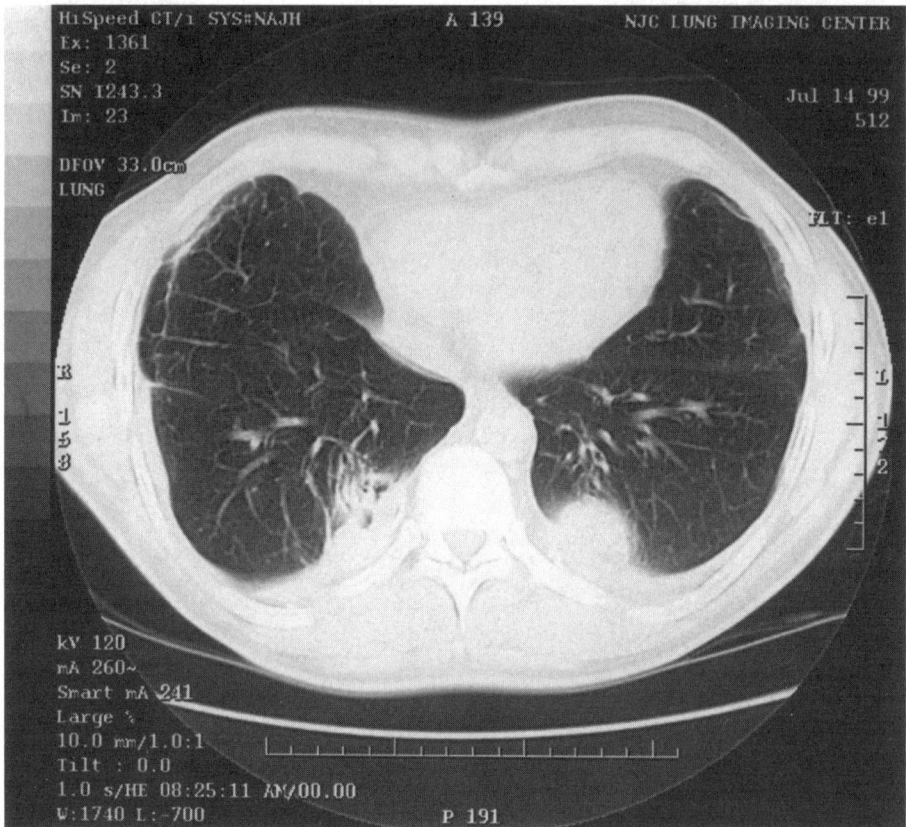

Figure 4 Continued.

reoccurred despite stripping of the lung from the pleura. Based on their experience, Payne et al. recommended thoracotomy with removal of the visceral pleura as a treatment for patients with intractable chest pain. However, when the typical CT findings are observed, unnecessary surgical intervention can be avoided in most cases. Patients should be monitored periodically for the stability of the lesion on chest radiograph or CT scan. Clinicians must remain alert for evidence of postobstructive pneumonia, intercurrent lung malignancy, mesothelioma, pulmonary thromboses, or hematoma due to rounded atelectasis, although these are all rare events.

References

1. Stanton MF, Layard M, Tegeris A, Miller E, May M, Morgan E, Smith A. Relation of particle dimension to carcinogenicity in amphibole asbestoses and other fibrous minerals. J Natl Cancer Inst 1981; 67:965–975.

2. Pott F. Some aspects on the doseometry of the carcinogenic potency of asbestos and other fibrous dusts. Staub Reinhold Luft 1978; 38:486.
3. King EJ. Effect of asbestos and asbestos and aluminium on the lungs of rabbits. Thorax 1946; 1:118.
4. Klosterkotter W. Experimentelle Untersuchungen über die Bedeutung der Faserlange für die Asbest-fibrose sowie Untersuchungen über die Beeinflussung der Fibrose durch Polyvinylpyridin-n-oxid. In: Biologische Wirkungen des Asbestos. Vol. 47. Berlin, 1968.
5. Scymczykiewicz K, Wiecek E. The effect of fibrous and amorphous asbestos on the collagen content in the lungs of guinea pigs. Proc. 13th International Conference of Occupational Hygiene, New York, 1960.
6. Hillerdal G. Nonmalignant pleural disease related to asbestos exposure. Clin Chest Med 1985; 6:141–152.
7. Robledo R, Mossman B. Cellular and molecular mechanisms of asbestos-induced fibrosis. J Cell Physiol 1999; 180:158–166.
8. Yegles M, Saint-Etienne L, Renier A, Janson X, Jaurand MC. Induction of metaphase and anaphase/telophase abnormalities by asbestos fibers in rat pleural mesothelial cells in vitro. Am J Respir Cell Mol Biol 1993; 9:186–191.
9. Jensen CG, Jensen LC, Rieder CL, Cole RW, Ault JG. Long crocidolite asbestos fibers cause polyploidy by sterically blocking cytokinesis. Carcinogenesis 1996; 17:2013–2021.
10. Desai R, Richards RJ. The absorption of biological macromolecules by mineral dusts. Environ Res 1978; 16:449–464.
11. Yazicioglu S, Ilcayto R, Balci K, Sayli BS, Yorulmaz B. Pleural calcification, pleural mesotheliomas, and bronchial cancers caused by tremolite dust. Thorax 1980; 35:564–569.
12. Kiviluoto R. Pleural calcification as a roentgenologic sign of non-occupational endemic enthophyllite-asbestosis. Acta Radiol 1960; 194:1–67.
13. Irwig LM, du Toit RS, Sluis-Cremer GK, Solomon A, Thomas RG, Hamel PP, Webster I, Hastie T. Risk of asbestosis in crocidolite and amosite mines in South Africa. Ann NY Acad Sci 1979; 330:35–52.
14. Bourbeau J, Ernst P, Chrome J, Armstrong B, Becklake MR. The relationship between respiratory impairment and asbestos-related pleural abnormality in an active work force. Am Rev Respir Dis 1990; 142:837–842.
15. Becklake MR. Asbestos and other fiber-related diseases of the lungs and pleura. Distribution and determinants in exposed populations. Chest 1991; 100: 248–254.
16. Rogan WJ, Ragan NB, Dinse GE. X-ray evidence of increased asbestos exposure in the US population from NHANES I and NHANES II, 1973-1978. National Health Examination Survey. Cancer Causes Control 2000; 11:441–449.
17. Rogan WJ, Gladen BC, Ragan NB, Anderson HA. US prevalence of occupational pleural thickening. A look at chest x-rays from the first National Health and Nutrition Examination Survey. Am J Epidemiol 1987; 126:893–900.
18. Hillerdal G. Pleural plaques in the general population. Ann NY Acad Sci 1991; 643:430–437.
19. Lee YC, Runnion CK, Pang SC, de Klerk NH, Musk AW. Increased body mass index is related to apparent circumscribed pleural thickening on plain chest radiographs. Am J Ind Med 2001; 39:112–116.
20. Fletcher DE. A mortality study of shipyard workers with pleural plaques. Br J Ind Med 1972; 29:142–145.

21. Edge JR. Incidence of bronchial carcinoma in shipyard workers with pleural plaques. Ann NY Acad Sci 1979; 330:289–294.
22. Kiviluoto R, Meurman LO, Hakama M. Pleural plaques and neoplasia in Finland. Ann NY Acad Sci 1979; 330:31–33.
23. Katz D, Kreel L. Computed tomography in pulmonary asbestosis. Clin Radiol 1979; 30:207–213.
24. Friedman AC, Fiel SB, Fisher MS, Radecki PD, Lev-Toaff AS, Caroline DF. Asbestos-related pleural disease and asbestosis: a comparison of CT and chest radiography. AJR Am J Roentgenol 1988; 150:269–275.
25. Gevenois PA, De Vuyst P, Dedeire S, Cosaert J, Vande Weyer R, Struyven J. Conventional and high-resolution CT in asymptomatic asbestos-exposed workers. Acta Radiol 1994; 35:226–229.
26. Hillerdal G. Pleural plaques in a health survey material. Frequency, development and exposure to asbestos. Scand J Respir Dis 1978; 59:257–263.
27. Becklake MR, Case BW. Fiber burden and asbestos-related lung disease: determinants of dose- response relationships. Am J Respir Crit Care Med 1994; 150:1488–1492.
28. Yano E, Tanaka K, Funaki M, Maeda K, Matsunaga C, Yamaoka K. Effect of smoking on pleural thickening in asbestos workers. Br J Ind Med 1993; 50:898–901.
29. Roggli VL, Pratt PC, Brody AR. Asbestos content of lung tissue in asbestos associated disease: a study of 110 cases. Br J Ind Med 1986; 43:18.
30. Stephens M, Gibbs AR, Pooley FD, Wagner JC. Asbestos induced diffuse pleural fibrosis: pathology and mineralogy. Thorax 1987; 42:583–588.
31. Nishimura SL, Broaddus VC. Asbestos-induced pleural disease. Clin Chest Med 1998; 19:311–329.
32. Hillerdal G. Pleural plaques and risk for bronchial carcinoma and mesothelioma. A prospective study. Chest 1994; 105:144–150.
33. Bianchi C, Giarelli L, Grandi G, Brollo A, Ramani L, Zuch C. Latency periods in asbestos-related mesothelioma of the pleura. Eur J Cancer Prev 1997; 6:162–166.
34. Hillerdal G. Pleural plaques and risk for cancer in the County of Uppsala. Eur J Respir Dis Suppl 1980; 107:111–117.
35. Thiringer G. Pleural plaques in chest x-rays of lung cancer patients and matched controls (preliminary results). Eur J Respir Dis 1980; 61:119–122.
36. Mollo F, Andrion A, Colombo A, Segnan N, Pira E. Pleural plaques and risk of cancer in Turin, northwestern Italy. An autopsy study. Cancer 1984; 54:1418–1422.
37. Wain SL, Roggli VL, Foster WL Jr. Parietal pleural plaques, asbestos bodies, and neoplasia. A clinical, pathologic, and roentgenographic correlation of 25 consecutive cases. Chest 1984; 86:707–713.
38. Harber P, Mohsenifar Z, Oren A, Lew M. Pleural plaques and asbestos-associated malignancy. J Occup Med 1987; 29:641–644.
39. Partanen T, Nurminen M, Zitting A, Koskinen H, Wiikeri M, Ahlman K. Localized pleural plaques and lung cancer. Am J Ind Med 1992; 22:185–192.
40. Weiss W. Asbestos-related pleural plaques and lung cancer. Chest 1993; 103:1854–1859.
41. Nurminen M, Tossavainen D. Is there an association between pleural plaques and lung cancer without asbestosis? Scand J Work Environ Health 1994; 20:62–64.

42. Hillerdal G, Henderson DW. Asbestos, asbestosis, pleural plaques and lung cancer. Scand J Work Environ Health 1997; 23:93–103.
43. Hillerdal G. The pathogenesis of pleural plaques and pulmonary asbestosis: possibilities and impossibilities. Eur J Respir Dis 1980; 61:129–138.
44. Boutin C, Dumortier P, Rey F, Viallat JR, De Vuyst P. Black spots concentrate oncogenic asbestos fibers in the parietal pleura. Thoracoscopic and mineralogic study. Am J Respir Crit Care Med 1996; 153:444–449.
45. Wang NS. Anatomy of the pleura. Clin Chest Med 1998; 19:229–240.
46. Viallat JR, Raybuad F, Passarel M, Boutin C. Pleural migration of chrysotile fibers after intratracheal injection in rats. Arch Environ Health 1986; 41:282–286.
47. Sahn SA, Antony VB. Pathogenesis of pleural plaques. Relationship of early cellular response and pathology. Am Rev Respir Dis 1984; 130:884–887.
48. Becklake MR. Asbestos-related diseases of the lung and other organs: their epidemiology and implications for clinical practice. Am Rev Respir Dis 1976; 114: 187–227.
49. Dodson RF, Williams MG Jr, Corn CJ, Brollo A, Bianchi C. Asbestos content of lung tissue, lymph nodes, and pleural plaques from former shipyard workers. Am Rev Respir Dis 1990; 142:843–847.
50. Kuwahara M, Verma K, Ando T, Hemenway DR, Kagan E. Asbestos exposure stimulates pleural mesothelial cells to secrete the fibroblast chemoattractant, fibronectin. Am J Respir Cell Mol Biol 1994; 10:167–176.
51. Kuwahara M, Kagan E. The mesothelial cell and its role in asbestos-induced pleural injury. Int J Exp Pathol 1995; 76:163–170.
52. Choe N, Tanaka S, Xia W, Hemenway DR, Roggli VL, Kagan E. Pleural macrophage recruitment and activation in asbestos-induced pleural injury. Environ Health Perspect 1997; 105(suppl 5):1257–1260.
53. Kinnula VL. Oxidant and antioxidant mechanisms of lung disease caused by asbestos fibres. Eur Respir J 1999; 14:706–716.
54. Herbert A. Pathogenesis of pleurisy, pleural fibrosis, and mesothelial proliferation. Thorax 1986; 41:176–189.
55. Taskinen E, Ahlamn K, Wukeri M. A current hypothesis of the lymphatic transport of inspired dust to the parietal pleura. Chest 1973; 64:193–196.
56. Withers BF, Ducatman AM, Yang WN. Roentgenographic evidence for predominant left-sided location of unilateral pleural plaques. Chest 1989; 95:1262–1264.
57. Hu H, Beckett L, Kelsey K, Christiani D. The left-sided predominance of asbestos-related pleural disease. Am Rev Respir Dis 1993; 148:981–984.
58. Gallego JC. Absence of left-sided predominance in asbestos-related pleural plaques: a CT study. Chest 1998; 113:1034–1036.
59. Gamsu G, Aberle DR, Lynch D. Computed tomography in the diagnosis of asbestos-related thoracic disease. J Thorac Imaging 1989; 4:61–67.
60. Oliver LC, Eisen EA, Greene R, Sprince NL. Asbestos-related pleural plaques and lung function. Am J Ind Med 1988; 14:649–656.
61. Hjortsberg U, Orbaek P, Aborelius M Jr, Ranstam J, Welinder H. Railroad workers with pleural plaques: I. Spirometric and nitrogen washout investigation on smoking and nonsmoking asbestos-exposed workers. Am J Ind Med 1988; 14:635–641.

62. Kilburn KH, Warshaw R. Pulmonary functional impairment associated with pleural asbestos disease. Circumscribed and diffuse thickening. Chest 1990; 98:965–972.
63. Hedenstierna G, Alexandersson R, Kolmodin-Hedman B, Szamosi A, Tollqvist J. Pleural plaques and lung function in construction workers exposed to asbestos. Eur J Respir Dis 1981; 62:111–122.
64. Kilburn KH, Warshaw RH. Abnormal pulmonary function associated with diaphragmatic pleural plaques due to exposure to asbestos. Br J Ind Med 1990; 47:611–614.
65. Kilburn KH, Warshaw RH. Abnormal lung function associated with asbestos disease of the pleura, the lung, and both: a comparative analysis. Thorax 1991; 46:33–38.
66. Brody AR. The early pathogenesis of asbestos-induced lung disease. Scan Electron Microsc, 1984; (pt 1):167–171.
67. Kaneko M, Eguchi K, Ohmatsu H, Kakinuma R, Naruke T, Suemasu K, Moriyama N. Peripheral lung cancer: screening and detection with low-dose spiral CT versus radiography. Radiology 1996; 201:798–802.
68. Henschke CI, McCauley DI, Yankelevitz DF, Naidich DP, McGuinness G, Miettinen OS, Libby DM, Pasmantier MW, Koizumi J, Altorki NK, Smith JP. Early Lung Cancer Action Project: overall design and findings from baseline screening. Lancet 1999; 354:99–105.
69. Sone S. Lung cancer screening using mobile low-dose computed tomography: results from Nagano project in Japan. Helsinki: Finnish Institute of Occupational Health, 2000.
70. Haura EB. Treatment of advanced non-small-cell lung cancer: a review of current randomized clinical trials and an examination of emerging therapies. Cancer Control 2001; 8:326–336.
71. Tossavainen A. International expert meeting on new advances in the radiology and screening of asbestos-related diseases. Scand J Work Environ Health 2000; 26:449–454.
72. Fridriksson HV, Hedenstrom H, Hillerdal G, Malmberg P. Increased lung stiffness of persons with pleural plaques. Eur J Respir Dis 1981; 62:412–424.
73. Epler GR, McLoud TC, Gaensler EA. Prevalence and incidence of benign asbestos pleural effusion in a working population. Jama 1982; 247:617–622.
74. McLoud TC, Woods BO, Carrington CB, Epler GR, Gaensler EA. Diffuse pleural thickening in an asbestos-exposed population: prevalence and causes. AJR Am J Roentgenol 1985; 144:9–18.
75. Lilis R, Lerman Y, Selikoff IJ. Symptomatic benign pleural effusions among asbestos insulation workers: residual radiographic abnormalities. Br J Ind Med 1988; 45:443–449.
76. Hillerdal G, Lee J, Blomkvist A, Rask-Andersen A, Uddenfeldt M, Koyi H, Rasmussen E. Pleural disease during treatment with bromocriptine in patients previously exposed to asbestos. Eur Respir J 1997; 10:2711–2715.
77. Hillerdal G. Non-malignant asbestos pleural disease. Thorax 1981; 36:669–675.
78. de Klerk NH, Cookson WO, Musk AW, Armstrong BK, Glancy JJ. Natural history of pleural thickening after exposure to crocidolite. Br J Indust Med 1989; 46:461–467.
79. Gibbs AR, Stephens M, Griffiths DM, Blight BJ, Pooley FD. Fibre distribution in

the lungs and pleura of subjects with asbestos related diffuse pleural fibrosis. Br J Indust Med 1991; 48:762–770.
80. Voisin C, Fisekci F, Voisin-Saltiel S, Ameille J, Brochard P, Pairon JC. Asbestos-related rounded atelectasis. Radiologic and mineralogic data in 23 cases. Chest 1995; 107:477–481.
81. Gibbs AR, Pooley FD. Analysis and interpretation of inorganic mineral particles in "lung" tissues. Thorax 1996; 51:327–334.
82. Rudd RM. New developments in asbestos-related pleural disease. Thorax 1996; 51:210–216.
83. Yates DH, Browne K, Stidolph PN, Neville E. Asbestos-related bilateral diffuse pleural thickening: natural history of radiographic and lung function abnormalities. Am J Respir Crit Care Med 1996; 153:301–306.
84. Miller A. Chronic pleuritic pain in four patients with asbestos induced pleural fibrosis. Br J Ind Med 1990; 47:147–153.
85. Mukherjee S, de Klerk N, Palmer LJ, Olsen NJ, Pang SC, William Musk A. Chest pain in asbestos-exposed individuals with benign pleural and parenchymal disease. Am J Respir Crit Care Med 2000; 162:1807–1811.
86. al Jarad N, Davies SW, Logan-Sinclair R, Rudd RM. Lung crackle characteristics in patients with asbestosis, asbestos-related pleural disease and left ventricular failure using a time-expanded waveform analysis—a comparative study. Respir Med 1994; 88:37–46.
87. Peacock C, Copley SJ, Hansell DM. Asbestos-related benign pleural disease. Clin Radiol 2000; 55:422–432.
88. Lynch DA, Gamsu G, Aberle DR. Conventional and high resolution computed tomography in the diagnosis of asbestos-related diseases. Radiographics 1989; 9:523–551.
89. Shih JF, Wilson JS, Broderick A, Watt JL, Galvin JR, Merchant JA, Schwartz DA. Asbestos-induced pleural fibrosis and impaired exercise physiology. Chest 1994; 105:1370–1376.
90. Kee ST, Gamsu G, Blanc P. Causes of pulmonary impairment in asbestos-exposed individuals with diffuse pleural thickening. Am J Respir Crit Care Med 1996; 154:789–793.
91. al Jarad N, Poulakis N, Pearson MC, Rubens MB, Rudd RM. Assessment of asbestos-induced pleural disease by computed tomography—correlation with chest radiograph and lung function. Respir Med 1991; 85:203–208.
92. Schwartz DA, Galvin JR, Yagla SJ, Speakman SB, Merchant JA, Hunninghake GW. Restrictive lung function and asbestos-induced pleural fibrosis. A quantitative approach. J Clin Invest 1993; 91:2685–2692.
93. Wright PH, Hanson A, Kreel L, Capel LH. Respiratory function changes after asbestos pleurisy. Thorax 1980; 35:31–36.
94. Eisenstadt H. Pleural asbestosis. Am Pract 1962; 13:573–578.
95. Eisenstadt H. Benign asbestos pleurisy. JAMA 1965; 192:419–421.
96. Collins TF. Pleural reaction associated with asbestos exposure. Br J Radiol 1968; 41:655–661.
97. Mattson SB, Ringqvist T. Pleural plaques and exposure to asbestos. A clinical material from a Swedish lung clinic. Scand J Respir Dis Suppl 1970; 75:1–41.
98. Gaensler EA, Kaplan AI. Asbestos pleural effusion. Ann Intern Med 1971; 74:178–191.

99. Sluis-Cremer GK, Webster I. Acute pleurisy in asbestos exposed persons. Environ Res 1972; 5:380–392.
100. Elder J. A study of 16 cases of pleurisy with effusions in ex-miners from Wittenoon Gorge. Aust NZ J Med 1972; 2:328–329.
101. Morgan A, Evans J, Holmes A. Deposition and clearance of inhaled fibrous materials in the rat: studies using radioactive tracer techniques. In: Walton W, ed. Inhaled Particles 1977; Vol. IV. Oxford: Pergamon Press, 1977:259–274.
102. Sebastien P, Fondimare A, Bignon J, NMorchaux G, Desbordes J, Bonnaud G. Topographic distribution of asbestos fibers on human lung in relation to occupational and non-occupational exposure. In: Walton W ed. Inhaled Particles 1977; Vol. IV. Oxford: Pergamon Press, 1977:433–435.
103. Sebastien P, Janson X, Gaudichet A. Asbestos retention in human respiratory tissues: comparative measurements in lung parenchyma and in parietal pleura. In: Wagner J, Davis W, eds. Biological Effects of Mineral Fibres. Vol. 1. Lyon: IARC Scientific Publications No. 30, 1980:237–246.
104. Bignon J, Jaurand M, Sebastien P, Dufour G. Interaction of pleural tissue and cells with mineral fibers. In: Chretien J, Hirsch A, eds. Diseases of the Pleural. New York: Masson, 1983:198–207.
105. Wang NS. The preformed stomas connecting the pleural cavity and the lymphatics in the parietal pleura. Am Rev Respir Dis 1975; 111:12–20.
106. Bignon J, Sebastien P, Gaudichet A. Measurement of asbestos retention in the human respiratory system related to health effects. Gaithersburg, MD: National Bureau of Standards (Special Publication), 1978:95–119.
107. Suzuki Y, Kohyama N. Translocation of inhaled asbestos fibers from the lung to other tissues. Am J Ind Med 1992; 19:701–704.
108. Schwartz DA. New developments in asbestos-induced pleural disease. Chest 1991; 99:191–198.
109. Rom WN, Travis WD, Brody AR. Cellular and molecular basis of the asbestos-related diseases. Am Revi Respir Dis 1991; 143:899–905.
110. Martensson G, Hagberg S, Pettersson K, Thiringer G. Asbestos pleural effusion: a clinical entity. Thorax 1987; 42:646–651.
111. Mintzer RA, Cugell DW. The association of asbestos-induced pleural disease and rounded atelectasis. Chest 1982; 81:457–460.
112. Roche G, Parent J, Daumet P. Atelectasies parcellaires du lobe inferieur et du lobe moyen au cours du pneumothorax therapeutique. Rev Tuberc 1956; 20:87–93.
113. Blesovsky A. The folded lung. Br J Dis Chest 1966; 60:19–22.
114. Hanke R. Rundatelektasen (Kugel- und Walzenatelektasen): ein Beitrag zur Differential Diagnose intrapulmonaler Rundherde. ROEFO 1971; 114:164–183.
115. Payne CR, Jaques P, Kerr IH. Lung folding simulating peripheral pulmonary neoplasm (Blevosky's syndrome). Thorax 1980; 35:936–940.
116. Schneider HJ, Felson B, Gonzalez LL. Rounded atelectasis. ARJ 1980; 15:174–182.
117. Mintzer RA, Gore RM, Vogelzang RL, Holz S. Rounded atelectasis and its association with asbestos-induced pleural disease. Radiology 1981; 139:567–570.
118. Stark P. Round atelectasis: another pulmonary pseudotumor. Am Rev Respir Dis 1982; 125:248–250.
119. Doyle TC, Lawler GA. CT features of rounded atelectasis of the lung. AJR 1984; 143:225–228.

120. Dernevik L, Gatzinsky P. Pathogenesis of shrinking pleuritis with atelectasis— "rounded atelectasis". Eur J Respir Dis 1987; 71:244–249.
121. Hillerdal G. Rounded atelectasis. Clinical experience with 74 patients. Chest 1989; 95:836–841.
122. Szydlowski GW, Cohn HE, Steiner RM, Edie RN. Rounded atelectasis: a pulmonary pseudotumor. Ann Thorac Surg 1992; 53:817–821.
123. Hanke R, Kretzschmar R. Round atelectasis. Semin Roentgenol 1980; 15:174–182.
124. Tylen U, Nilsson U. Computed tomography in pulmonary pseudotumors and their relation to asbestos exposure. J Comput Assist Tomogr 1982; 6:229–237.
125. Chen C, Newman LS. Rounded atelectasis complicated by obstructive pneumonia and pulmonary thrombosis. Chest 1990; 98:1283–1285.
126. Greyson-Fleg RT. Lung biopsy in rounded atelectasis. AJR 1985; 144:1316–1317.

31

Pleural Manifestations of Interstitial Lung Disease

ROBERT P. BAUGHMAN and SALLY SEYMOUR

University of Cincinnati
Cincinnati, Ohio, U.S.A.

I. Introduction

There are a wide variety of interstitial lung diseases (ILD). The broad categories include occupational interstitial diseases, infectious, collagen vascular, and unknown category. The collagen vascular diseases, especially systemic lupus erythematosus (SLE), often include pleural disease and will be discussed elsewhere in this book. Occupational lung diseases, such as asbestos-related pleural disease, will not be discussed in this chapter. We will concentrate on pleural diseases related to idiopathic diseases, such as sarcoidosis and Langerhans' cell histiocytosis (LCH).

With a few exceptions such as asbestosis and SLE, pleural disease is usually a rare manifestation of an ILD. Pleural manifestations of ILD could include pleural effusions, chylothorax, hemothorax, pleural thickening, pneumothorax, and pleural nodules or plaques. High-resolution computed tomography (HRCT) is a commonly used method to evaluate most ILD. This technique may detect subtle pleural manifestations not appreciated on plain chest roentgenogram. For example, subpleural nodules are commonly seen on HRCT of patients with sarcoidosis (1), but pleural disease is rarely seen with conventional roentgenograms for sarcoidosis. Subpleural nodules on HRCT suggest sarcoidosis rather than other ILD (1,2). We will discuss the most commonly encountered pleural manifestations, with a particular emphasis on pleural effusions.

The most common reason for pleural effusion in a patient with ILD is some other process. Table 1 lists some of the commonly encountered secondary causes of pleural disease. Congestive heart failure may be related to the underlying disease. An example is sarcoidosis, which can lead to a cardiomyopathy (3). The mean age of patients with idiopathic pulmonary fibrosis (IPF) in most series is over 60 years (4). Coexisting coronary artery disease may be encountered, and patients may thus have congestive heart failure. In addition to congestive heart failure, IPF patients appear to be at increased risk for pulmonary emboli (5). This is in part due to the cor pulmonale the patients may develop, as well as the more sedentary lifestyle they adapt as a result of their severe dyspnea. The use of immunosuppressive therapy of treatment of IPF is common (6). This is often a prolonged therapy, and the patient is at risk for acquiring an opportunistic infection either directly in the pleura or as a parapneumonic infection. Drug-induced pleural effusion may also be encountered (7). Among these is the docetaxel-associated effusion in patients being treated for lymphangitic spread of their breast cancer (8).

Some patients with ILD are at increased risk for malignancy. The increased risk of malignancy for patients with IPF was recognized by Turner-Warwick (9).

Table 1 Secondary Causes of Pleural Effusion in Interstitial Lung Diseases

Cause of effusion	Common associations	Comments
Congestive heart failure	Sarcoidosis with cardiac involvement Idiopathic pulmonary fibrosis (IPF)	Co-existing coronary artery disease may lead to CHF Echocardiogram useful to assess left ventricular performance
Parapneumonic effusion	IPF on immunosuppression	Patients receiving chemotherapy may develop complicated pneumonic process
Pulmonary embolism	IPF	Increased risk for patients with cor pulmonale
Malignancy	IPF	Need to differentiate from lymphangitic spread as cause of interstitial lung disease
Drug-induced	IPF Lymphangitic spread from cancer	Drug-induced lupus Docetaxel-associated effusion

Subsequent studies have confirmed an increased risk for malignancy in these patients (10,11). The cancers tend to be adenocarcinomas, and they have a peripheral distribution.

In patients with known IPF, the presence of a new pleural effusion should be evaluated. A secondary cause may be identified. In some cases, the secondary cause may be more treatable than the underlying IPF. Treatment of the secondary cause may lead to improvement of symptoms.

II. New Onset of ILD and Pleural Effusion

For many ILD, the mode of onset is gradual. This is particularly true for IPF (6). Detailed questioning of a patient with ILD should be performed to determine if there has been a gradual onset of symptoms over weeks to months. The abrupt onset of pulmonary symptoms and a chest roentgenogram showing both ILD and pleural disease is relatively rare except for the following two groups.

In patients with acute ILD and pleural effusion, infection is a major possibility. This includes bacterial pneumonias, such as *Legionella* and even *Streptococcus pneumoniae*. Viral pneumonia can also present this way. Opportunistic infections such as fungi and tuberculosis can cause both effusions and ILD. *Pneumocystis carinii* rarely causes pleural fluid, but it can cause pneumothoraces (12). Most infections are suggested on the basis of clinical grounds. The diagnosis of infection-associated pleural effusions are discussed elsewhere in this book.

Malignancy represents another group presenting with acute ILD with pleural effusions. With the exception of a mesothelioma, the presence of malignant cells in the pleural space implies metastases. An interstitial process in the lung can be seen with bronchioloalveolar cell carcinoma (13,14) or with a "pseudolymphoma" due to B-cell proliferation on the MALT tissue (15). Rarely will either of these processes lead to pleural disease. On the other hand, lymphangitic spread of tumor can lead to an interstitial pattern (16,17). Common malignancies causing lymphangitic spread are lung and breast. In one study of patients with lymphangitic breast cancer, pleural effusion preceded or co-existed with the lymphangitic spread in two thirds of cases (18). The HRCT scan can be highly suggestive of lymphangitic spread (17). Figure 1 shows a patient with both lymphangitic spread and pleural metastases due to breast cancer. Both bronchoscopy and thoracentesis were diagnostic in this case.

III. Chronic ILD of Unknown Cause

When a patient first presents with ILD, the clinician may not be able to determine whether the disease is chronic or not. Therefore, some of the diseases that we classify here may have been present for some time but present as acute disease. Time often clarifies whether a particular disease is chronic or not.

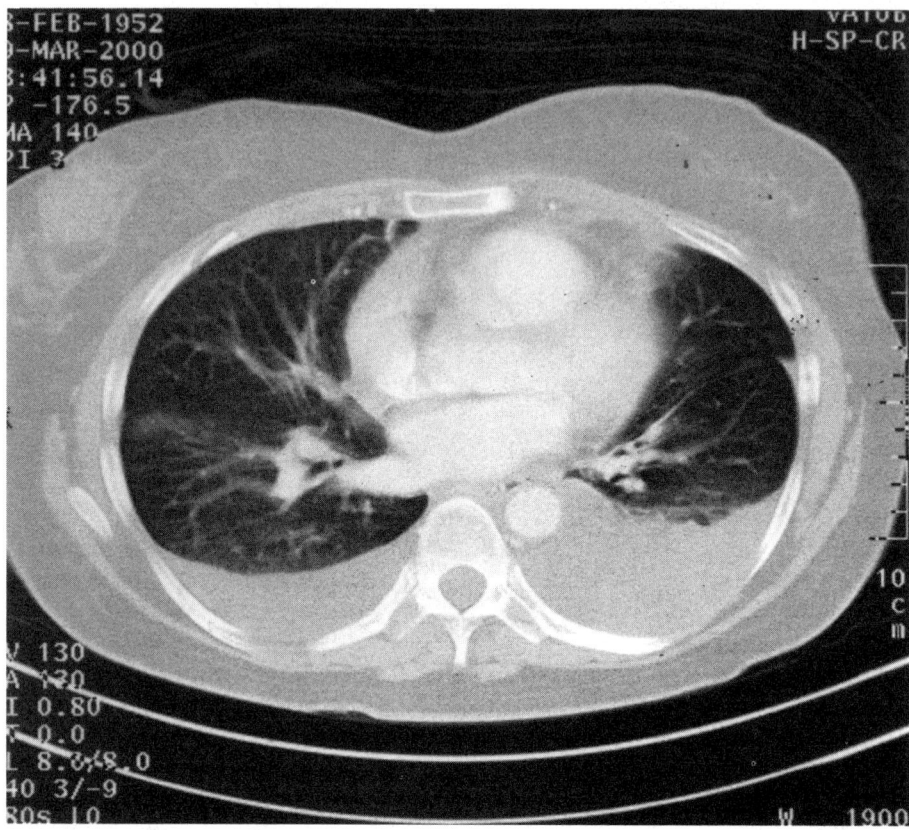

Figure 1 A 47-year-old female with a history of breast cancer who presents with increasing shortness of breath. Chest CT scan demonstrates both ILD and bilateral effusions. Samples obtained by bronchoalveolar lavage and thoracentesis were both positive for adenocarcinoma consistent with metastatic breast cancer.

A. Sarcoidosis

Sarcoidosis is a disease characterized by noncaseating granulomas in various organs of the body (19). Traditionally, pleural involvement in sarcoidosis was felt to occur in about 1–3% of cases (2,20,21). The use of HRCT has pointed out that subpleural nodules can be seen in sarcoidosis, as well as other ILD such as pneumoconiosis and lymphangitic spread (22). The subpleural nodules have been seen in at least half of the patients reported (22,23). In one series of patients with necrotizing sarcoidosis, pleural involvement was found on CT scan in six of seven cases (24).

In a pair of reviews summarizing the literature of pleural sarcoidosis, Soskel and Sharma have made several observations based on the reported cases (2,20). Figure 2 demonstrates the type of pleural involvement one can see, as

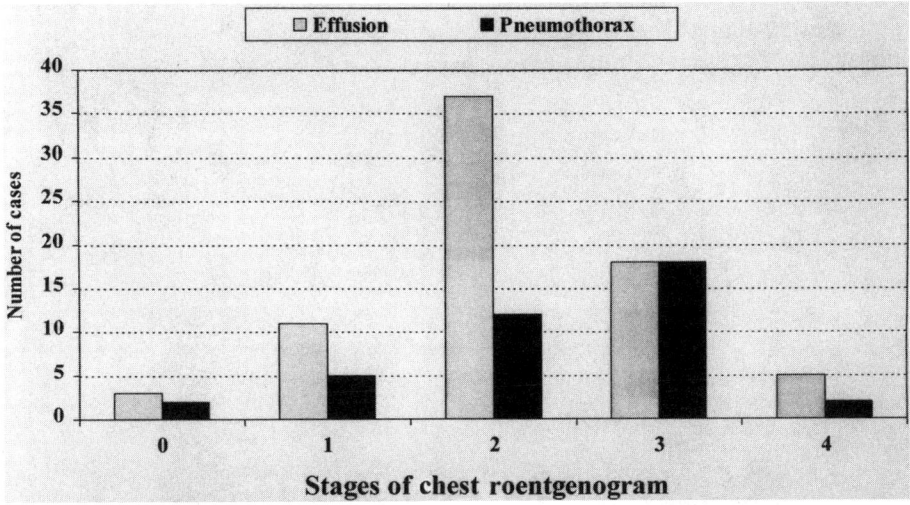

Figure 2 Number of cases of pleural effusion and pneumothorax versus Scadding chest roentgenogram stage (25) in patients with sarcoidosis. (Adapted from Refs. 2, 20.)

well as the underlying lung disease. In this figure, we use Scadding's classification of sarcoidosis lung involvement: Stage 0 is no thoracic disease, Stage 1 is hilar and mediastinal adenopathy alone, Stage 2 is adenopathy plus ILD, Stage 3 is ILD alone, and Stage 4 is fibrotic lung disease (25). Although pleural disease can be seen with any stage of the disease, patients tended to have more advanced disease when they had pleural involvement. Figure 3 is an example of a patient with pleural disease due to sarcoidosis with Stage 3—parenchymal involvement without adenopathy.

The reported average age for patients with pleural effusion was found to be 40 years (2). This is not different from the average age found in other large series of sarcoidosis patients (26). The effusions seem to be more common on the right. Despite the apparently higher prevalence of sarcoidosis in women (26), the number of cases were equal between men and women. It remains to be seen if gender has any affect on pleural involvement in large prospective studies. The pleural effusions are usually described as small to moderate in size. There have been reports of massive effusions (2,27,28). These cases often require chest tube drainage and may require systemic therapy for the sarcoidosis.

If the sarcoidosis is the direct cause of the effusion, the fluid is characteristically exudative with a predominance of lymphocytes, although increased eosinophils have been occasionally noted (2). As in other areas in which there is active sarcoidosis, such as in the bronchoalveolar lavage (BAL) and the cerebral spinal fluid, there is an increase in the CD4:CD8 lymphocyte ratio in the effusion (29,30). This lymphocyte subpopulation finding in pleural fluid may indicate pleural histological involvement similar to the lymphocytosis seen in BAL fluid in patients with alveolitis (31,32). The finding of an increased CD4:CD8 ratio is

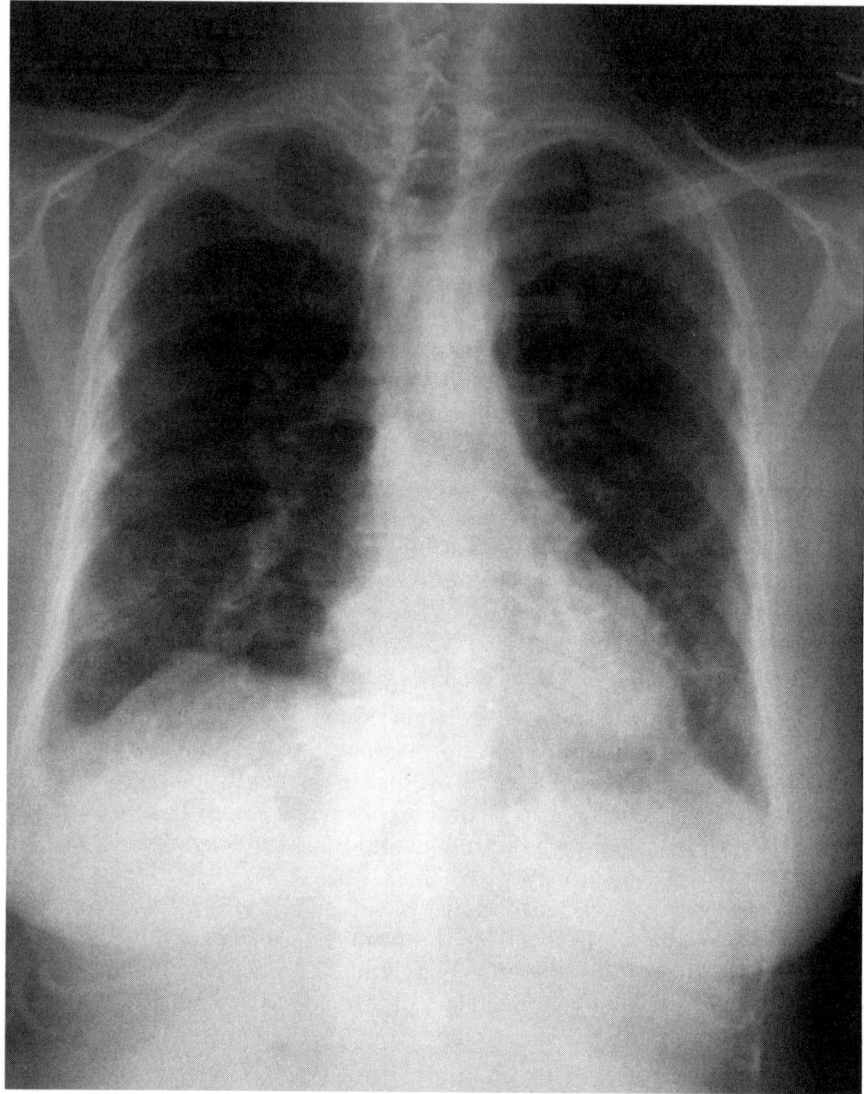

Figure 3 Fifty-one-year old woman who presented with diffuse lung and pleural disease. Open lung biopsy demonstrated granulomas in both lung and pleural space, consistent with sarcoidosis.

characteristic for sarcoidosis, but can be seen with other granulomatous diseases, such as tuberculosis (33,34). In patients with lymphocytic effusion of unknown etiology, one still has to rule out tuberculosis and fungal infections even if granulomas are identified.

In addition, the effusion may not be due to direct involvement of the pleura. Chylothorax has been reported in sarcoidosis patients (35,35). These appear to be related to mediastinal adenopathy common in sarcoidosis. In one case, a massive pleural effusion associated with sarcoidosis was secondary to brachiocephalic vein obstruction by matted sarcoidosis infiltration in mediastinal lymph nodes (36). Another cause of the pleural effusion is hemothorax, which is rare (2).

The prevalence of pneumothorax in sarcoid patients appears to be less than 5% (2,37). The proposed mechanism of pneumothorax development is unclear, but at least two conditions have been associated with pneumothorax. The first is related to the subpleural necrotizing granulomas mentioned earlier. In some cases, recurrent pneumothoraces was related to presence of necrotizing granuloma in resected pleural samples (38,39). Another mechanism is the cystic changes commonly found in patients with advanced pulmonary sarcoidosis (Fig. 4). However, patients with advanced fibrotic disease often have associated pleural reaction, as seen in Figure 4. There may be a lower risk for pneumothorax than seen in other cystic ILD. It is unclear whether systemic treatment will decrease the recurrence of spontaneous lung collapse. Most cases require systemic therapy for the treatment of their underlying lung disease. Many cases of pneumothorax from sarcoidosis respond to chest tube alone (2). Surgery is usually only necessary when the underlying diagnosis is unclear. This is different from other ILD, where surgery is often required to assure adequate sclerosis (2). This may be related to the high frequency of granulomatous inflammation present in the pleura, leading to an inflammatory reaction and sclerosis with chest tube drainage.

As illustrated by Figure 4, aspergillomas and locally invasive *Aspergillus* can occur in sarcoidosis (40,41). A pleural reaction is often associated with an aspergilloma (42). Although surgery is done in patients with recurrent pneumothoraces (43), most patients are managed medically. Itraconazole, an azole agent with high activity against *Aspergillus*, has been used with success in some cases (44,45), but not always found useful (46). The inflammatory reaction to an aspergilloma can contribute to the hemoptysis as well as bronchospasm, and some patients with symptomatic aspergillomas have been treated successfully with corticosteroids (47,48). Current treatment by our group consists of prolonged use of itraconazole and an anti-inflammatory agent such as corticosteroids or methotrexate.

B. Langerhans' Cell Histiocytosis

LCH is a spectrum of diseases characterized by Langerhans' cells infiltrating various organs of the body (49). Disease limited to the lung is pulmonary LCH,

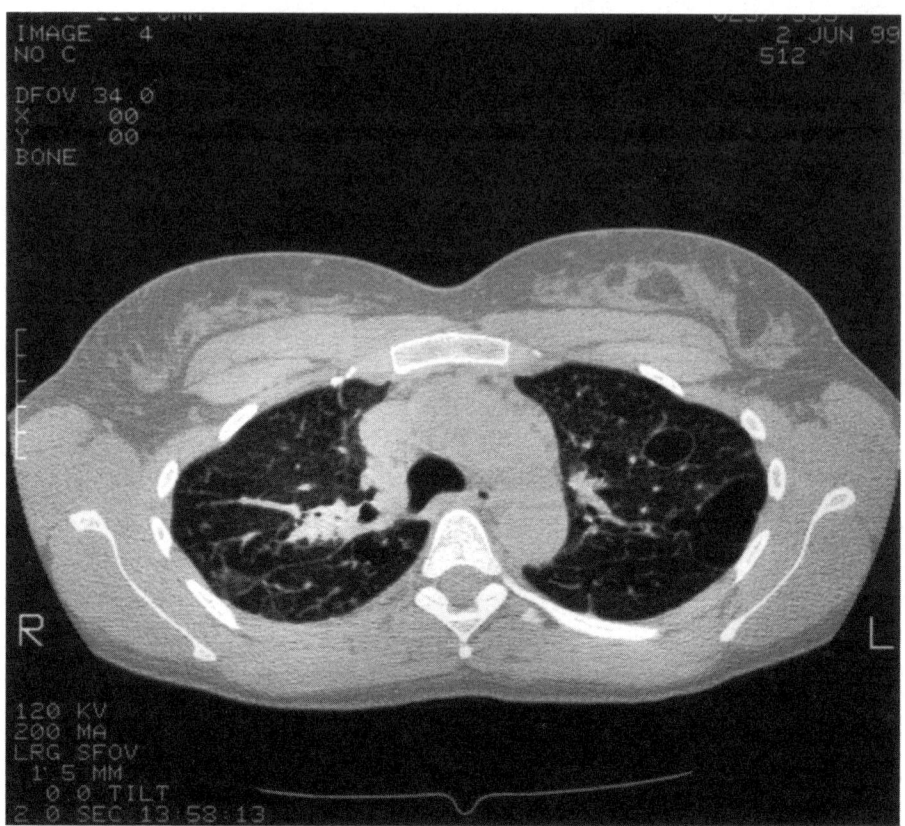

Figure 4 Patient with 10-year history of sarcoidosis presented with chest pain and hemoptysis. (a) Multiple cystic changes in upper lobe, including large subpleural lesion in left chest. (b) Mycetoma lower in chest with associated pleural reaction. Culture of bronchial washings grew *Aspergillus niger*.

previously known as eosinophilic granuloma (EG) (50–53). Pulmonary LCH is a smoking-related ILD (54,55). Pleural manifestations of the disease include pleural effusion, pneumothorax, and pleural thickening. The pleural thickening is thought to be the result of a pneumothorax. Spontaneous pneumothorax has long been recognized as an initial presentation of this disorder as well as longstanding disease, with the incidence reported between 4 and 25% (50,53,56–59). Bilateral pneumothoraces in LCH have also been reported. Because of this association, pulmonary LCH should be considered in any young adult smoker who develops a pneumothorax (53,54). The pathogenesis of spontaneous pneumothorax in LCH may be related to rupturing of subpleural blebs and cysts (53,56). In some cases, end stage honeycombing may be the cause of the pneumothorax (60).

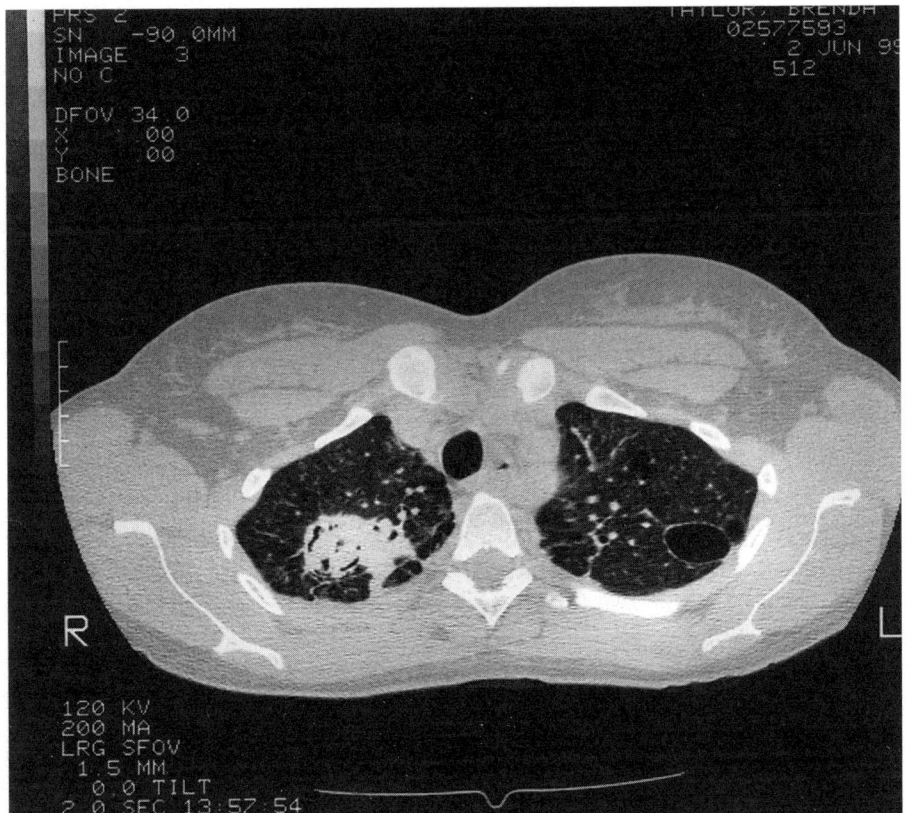

Figure 4 Continued.

There is no specific therapy for LCH. The discontinuation of smoking is associated with a high rate of remission (54,61), while those who continue to smoke may go on to to respiratory failure from the disease. Recurrence of LCH into donor lung of lung-transplanted patients has been reported in two patients who resumed smoking after transplant (62). In the patient with a significant pneumothorax from LCH, chest tube drainage alone may not be adequate. Surgical intervention with sclerosis is often required (57,59,63). Unfortunately reports of recurrent pneumothorax have been noted even following pleurodesis (57).

Pleural effusions have also been reported in LCH (64,65); however, this is a much less common manifestation, and the size of the effusion is usually small. In a patient with cystic ILD, the presence of pleural effusion is more characteristic for Erdheim-Chester disease (ECD), sarcoidosis, or lymphangioleiomyomatosis. In a patient with LCH, the presence of a moderate to large effusion should raise the concern of a secondary cause of the effusion, such as malignancy.

C. Erdheim-Chester Disease

ECD is a rare multisystem non–Langerhans' cell histiocytosis disorder of unknown etiology that occurs in adults. Manifestations include ILD, bone pain, xanthelasma, exophthalmos, and diabetes insipidus. One third of patients have pulmonary involvement (66). ECD does not have defined criteria and therefore can be difficult to distinguish from LCH, and there has been one report of both occurring in the same patient (67). One difference is the distribution of histiocytic cells in the lung. In ECD, the histiocytes accumulate in the perilymphangitic and subpleural areas. In LCH, histiocytes accumulate in peribronchial distribution (66). Immunohistochemistry identifying the Langerhans' cells (which are CD1a positive) is also useful, since there are no Langerhans' cells in the ECD lesions (67). The clinical course of the disease is variable, but pulmonary fibrosis is often reported as a cause of death (68,69).

Pleural manifestations of ECD include pleural thickening and pleural effusion. Wittenberg et al. reviewed the radiological findings of nine patients with ECD and found that four of the patients had pleural effusions and six had pericardial effusion (70). Pleural effusion appears to be a much more common finding in ECD than in LCH. Information is not available as to the characteristic of the effusion or the possible etiology.

D. Lymphangioleiomyomatosis

Lymphangioleiomyomatosis (LAM), formerly known as lymphangiomyomyotosis, is a multisystem disease primarily seen in premenopausal females (71–75). The characteristic pulmonary manifestations are diffusely distributed thin-walled cysts. Although a rare disease, recent studies have given insight into the mechanism of this disease. The abnormal cells appear to be smooth muscle cells which are under some level of estrogen control (76). There is a close association between tuberous sclerosis and LAM (77). In two prospective studies of tuberous sclerosis patients, over a third of the women had features suggesting LAM (78,79). Mutations in the tuberous sclerosis complex gene TSC2 have been found in sporadic cases of LAM (80).

Spontaneous pneumothorax is a common presentation in patients with LAM. Over half of patients with LAM develop a pneumothorax (73,81). In addition, the pneumothoraces tend to be recurrent and can be bilateral (82). Patients often require pleurodesis or pleurectomy for management of pneumothoraces (73,76,81). The mechanism of pneumothorax in LAM is again the rupture of subpleural cavities. In LAM the appearance of subpleural cystic and micronodular hyperplasia is fairly characteristic and useful for screening (79).

Chylothorax is seen in approximately 20% of patients with LAM (73,81). It may be the presenting symptom of the disease (83). The proposed mechanism is lymphatic obstruction by the LAM cells. Over half the patients with chylous effusions required pleurodesis or pleurectomy for treatment (76). There has been a report of percutaneous catheterization and subsequent embolization to successfully treat chylothorax due to LAM and other conditions (84). Chylothorax has also been reported in tuberous sclerosis (a male patient) (85).

LAM is usually a disease of women. It has been noted to worsen during pregnancy (72). Antiestrogen regimens have been used with limited success in patients with LAM (74,76,86). One difficulty is the relatively small number of cases at any one center, which has hindered the study of the new class of selective estrogen receptor modifiers (72). However, estrogen alone is not the cause of LAM. Up to 10% of female patients with LAM were diagnosed postmenopause (72). Also, LAM has been rarely reported in men (87). For end-stage disease, lung transplantation has been a successful in some patients (88).

Benign metastasizing lymphangiomyomatosis is another interstitial process that affects the lungs in premenopausal females. It can lead to interstitial changes, parenchymal nodules, and recurrent pneumothorax (Fig. 5) (86,89,90).

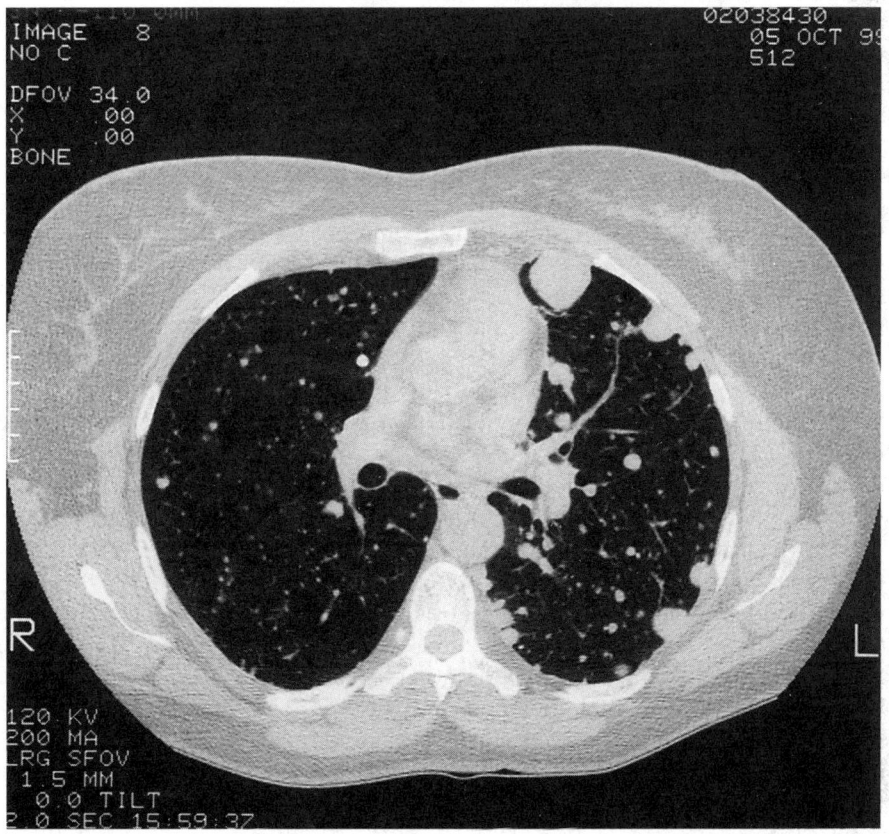

Figure 5 Thirty-year-old woman with history of recurrent pneumothoraces. Lung biopsy at time of open pleural sclerosis demonstrated benign metastasizing lymphangiomyomatosis.

There are not as many cystic changes as seen with LAM, and it is felt to represent a slow-growing variant of leiomyosarcoma (91).

E. Churg-Strauss Syndrome

Churg-Strauss syndrome (CSS) is a systemic disease that occurs in patients with a history of asthma or allergies. The syndrome is characterized by vasculitis, extravascular granulomas, eosinophilia, and fever (92,93). The most common pulmonary manifestations of CSS are fleeting infiltrates; however, patients may also develop diffuse reticulonodular opacities and interlobular septal thickening (94,95). Pleural manifestations can include pleural thickening and pleural effusion in about a quarter of patients (92,94). The pleural effusions of CSS are exudative, with a large number of eosinophils and a low glucose (96). One patient also was noted to have vasculitis of the pleura on open lung biopsy (97). The effusion may occur initially or may occur when the disease relapses, as shown in Figure 6. The disease has recently been associated with the use of antileukotriene therapy (98,99), although it clearly can occur in patients not receiving those drugs (100). Therapy is usually corticosteroids, but occasionally cytotoxic agents are used (93,101).

F. Amyloidosis

Amyloidosis is a disease characterized by the deposition of abnormal protein in the extracellular tissues (102,103). The amyloid protein characteristically exhibits apple-green birefringence under polarized microscopy and takes up Congo red stain. Typically it is categorized as primary or secondary. Secondary amyloid is often associated with neoplastic and chronic inflammatory conditions such as rheumatoid arthritis and bronchiectasis. Most often the disease affects multiple organs, but single organ involvement has been described.

Pulmonary amyloid can be isolated or can be part of systemic amyloid involvement. Autopsy studies have shown that pulmonary involvement is common in primary systemic amyloidosis but not secondary amyloidosis (104,105). In a Mayo Clinic review of 55 patients with pulmonary amyloid, ILD with or without pleural effusion was common for systemic amyloid but rare for secondary amyloid (106).

The pleural effusion of amyloidosis can be either transudate or exudate (107–109). Transudative effusions may be secondary to congestive heart failure from cardiac involvement of amyloidosis. The exudative effusions in amyloid have yet to be explained. Nodularity along the pleura has been seen at thoracoscopy in patients with amyloid (110), with direct pleural involvement documented on biopsy (107,108,110). The pleural biopsy may be positive even if the fluid is a transudate (107). Pleural involvement does not always mean systemic amyloidosis (111).

Pleural thickening without effusion has also been described as a radiological manifestation. Adams et al. described two patients who presented with dyspnea and had diffuse pleural thickening on imaging and who were thought

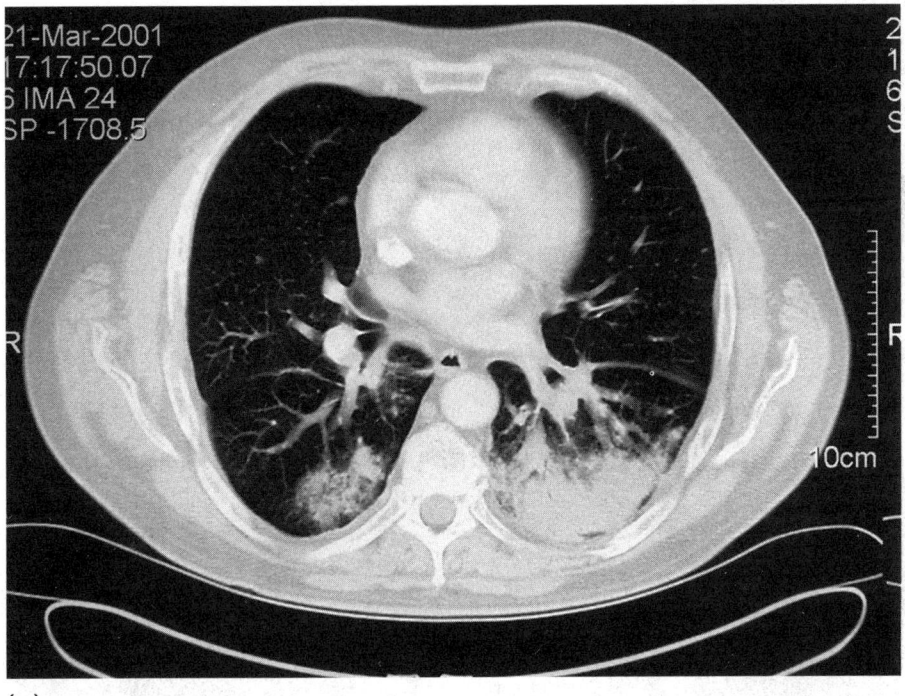

(a)

Figure 6 Fifty-year-old male asthmatic with 3-month history of cough and shortness of breath noted to have multiple pulmonary infiltrates and peripheral blood eosinophilia. (a) Multiple infiltrates prior to open lung biopsy of the right lung lesions. Patient was found to have Churg-Strauss and was treated with corticosteroids. Six months later patient was down to low dose corticosteroids when he developed worsening dyspnea. (b) New left pleural effusion and improvement of parenchymal disease. Examination of left pleural fluid demonstrated 50% eosinophils. The patient improved with increased dosage of corticosteroids.

to have mesothelioma. After surgical decortication, the diagnosis of amyloid was made by special stains of the pleura (112).

G. Idiopathic Pulmonary Fibrosis

The ILD have been reclassified based on clinical status and pathological changes (6,26). A major task for the clinician is to differentiate between nonspecific ILD and usual interstitial pneumonitis (UIP) (113,114). The term UIP refers to the pathological changes seen. Patients with consistent clinical features and a lung biopsy showing UIP are felt to have idiopathic pulmonary fibrosis (IPF) (6,26).

Pneumothorax is the most common pleural disease reported in IPF. In a study of 82 patients with pulmonary fibrosis, 3 (3.6%) of the 46 patients who

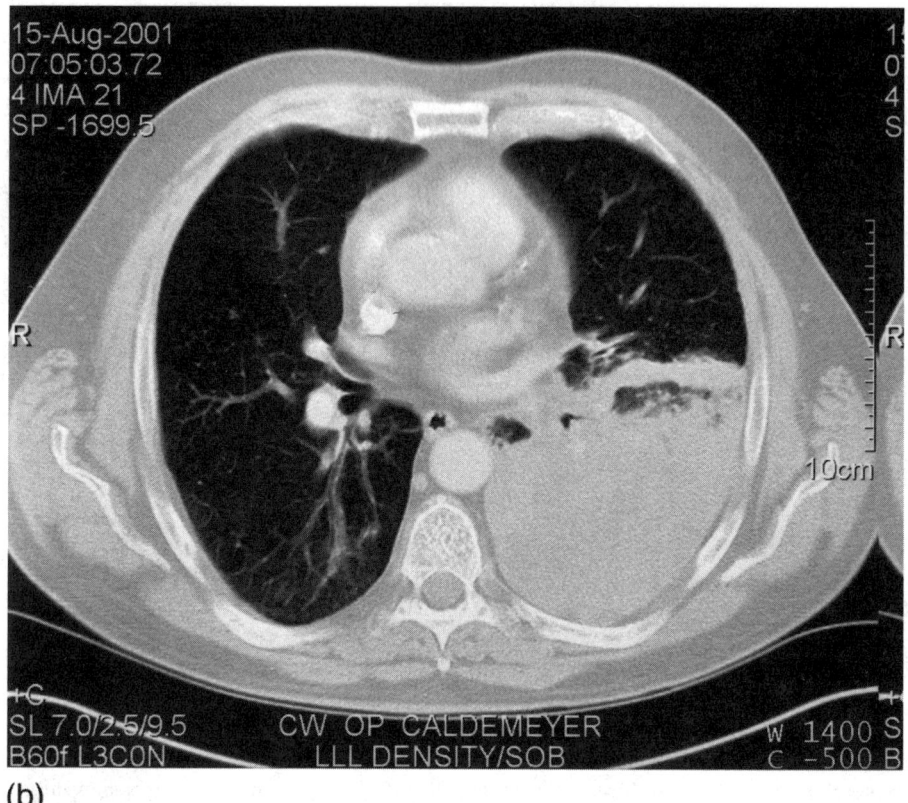

Figure 6 Continued.

meet the current criteria for IPF had a spontaneous pneumothorax (115,116). In addition, the authors found that these patients did not respond well to suction drainage and often required thoracotomy, bleb resection, and pleurectomy. In a retrospective study of the CT scans of 78 patients with UIP, 11% had extra-alveolar air, with 5 having a pneumothorax and 4 having a pneumomediastinum (117). Figure 7 shows a patient who originally presented with a spontaneous pneumothorax and was diagnosed as having UIP at the time of his open sclerosis As can be seen in the figure, the probable mechanism of the pneumothorax is rupture of the subpleural honeycombing characteristic of IPF (118). Pneumothorax can be a reason for clinical deterioration and even death in patients with IPF (5).

Pleural thickening is also commonly seen with the subpleural honeycombing characteristic of IPF (119). In a study comparing the HRCT findings of IPF to collagen vascular disease–associated pulmonary fibrosis (CVD-PF), pleural thickening was the most distinguishing feature. Of those studied, 97% of patients with IPF had pleural thickening compared to 33% of the CVD-PF

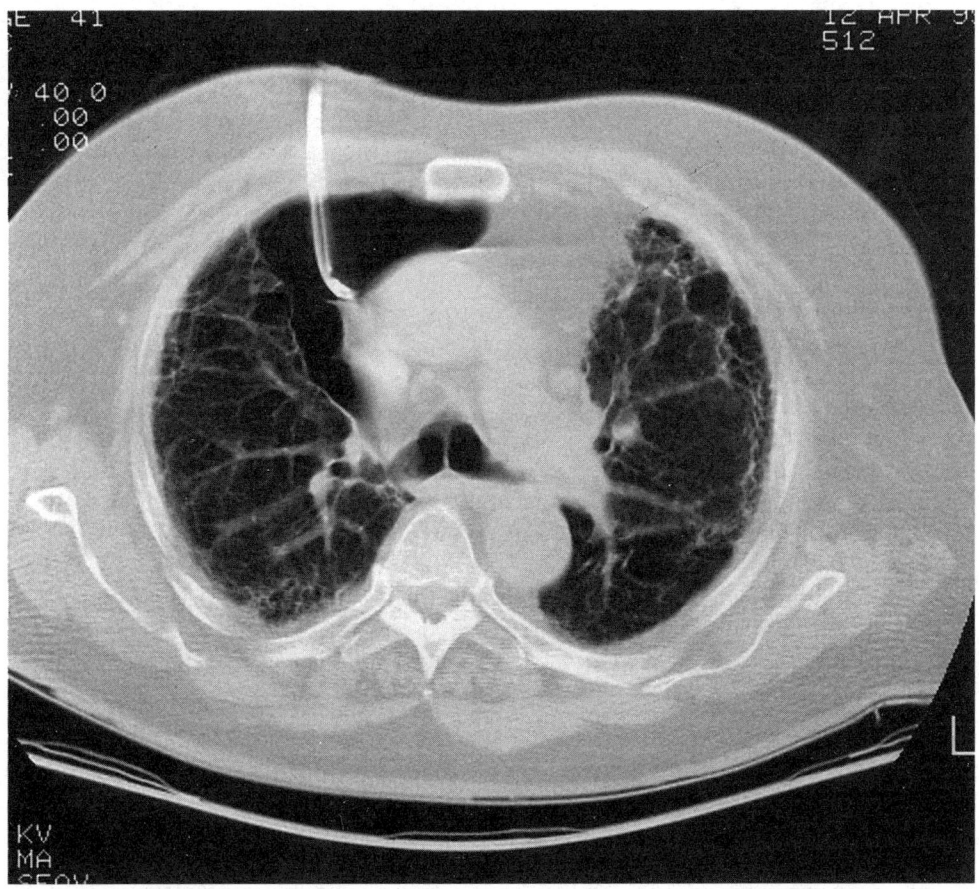

Figure 7 Seventy-year-old male who presented with dyspnea and chest pain. Chest CT scan demonstrates pneumothorax as well as subpleural honeycombing consistent with idiopathic pulmonary fibrosis. Open lung biopsy obtained at time of pleural sclerosis demonstrated usual interstitial pneumonitis.

patients. Pleural effusion was seen in only 6% of the IPF patients, but in 26% of the CVD-PF patients (120).

IV. Clinical Evaluation of Pleural Disease in ILD

In evaluating the patient with an interstitial lung process and pleural disease, one first needs to decide whether there is a possible association between the two processes. In a patient with known ILD who has developed a new pleural effusion, one has to consider secondary causes of the pleural effusion, such as congestive heart failure or infection. Workup of these pleural effusions would be similar to what one would do for a patient with a clear chest roentgenogram and a new pleural effusion.

In the patient who presents symptomatically with new effusion and ILD, one has to consider infection and congestive failure, since these are the most common and treatable conditions. In most cases, these diseases are easily determined based on the clinical evaluation of the patient. Malignancy can be a bit more obscure, but should always be considered as the cause of ILD and pleural effusion.

In the patient with a chronic interstitial lung infiltrate and pleural disease, the pattern of pleural disease may help to determine the underlying process. Table 2 summarizes the relative frequency of pleural effusion and pneumothorax for several ILD. Patients with cystic ILD such as LAM, LCH, and some with sarcoidosis can develop pneumothorax. However, the presence of a pleural effusion is more frequent in ECD, CSS, LAM, is unusual in sarcoidosis (2), and is extremely rare in LCH. The effusion in CSS usually contains a large number of eosinophils (121). The effusion associated with LAM is often chylous (83). In a patient with amyloidosis, the presence of a pleural effusion implies systemic amyloidosis (122).

The use of HRCT as part of the routine evaluation of ILD has led to recognition of pleural disease not appreciated on routine chest roentgenogram. This includes the high incidence of subpleural nodules seen in patients with

Table 2 Summary of Pleural Manifestations of Interstitial Lung Diseases

ILD	Pleural effusion	Pneumothorax	Other pleural manifestations
Sarcoidosis	+1[a]	+1	Pleural thickening, nodules, lymphocytic effusion with increased CD4:CD8 ratio
Langerhans cell histiocytosis	Rare	+2	Pleural thickening
Lymphangioleiomyomatosis	+2	+3	Chylothorax usual cause of effusion
Erdheim-Chester	+3	Rare	Pleural thickening
Churg-Strauss syndrome	+2	ND	Eosinophilic pleural effusion
Amyloidosis	+2	Rare	Effusion implies systemic amyloidosis
Idiopathic pulmonary fibrosis	Rare	+1	Pleural thickening on HRCT >90% of cases

[a] Relative score of patients reported to have pleural manifestation: $+3 = >40\%$; $+2 = 10-30\%$; $+1 = 1-10\%$; rare $= <1\%$. ND, not described.

sarcoidosis (1) and the pleural thickening seen with IPF (120). As more attention is placed on pleural disease, we are sure more of these correlations will be made.

References

1. Remy-Jardin M, Beuscart R, Sault MC, Marquette CH, Remy J. Subpleural micronodules in diffuse infiltrative lung diseases: evaluation with thin-section CT scans. Radiology 1990; 177:133–139.
2. Soskel NT, Sharma OP. Pleural involvement in sarcoidosis. Curr Opin Pulm Med 2000; 6:455–468.
3. Lynch JP, Sharma OP, Baughman RP. Extrapulmonary sarcoidosis. Semin Respir Infect 1998; 13:229–254.
4. Schwartz DA, Van Fossen DS, Davis CS, Helmers RA, Dayton CS, Burmeister LF, Hunninghake GW. Determinants of progression in idiopathic pulmonary fibrosis. Am J Respir Crit Care Med 1994; 149:444–449.
5. Panos RJ, Morrenson R, Niccoli SA, King TE. Clinical deterioration in patients with idiopathic pulmonary fibrosis. Causes and assessment. Am J Med 1990; 88: 396–404.
6. American Thoracic Society, European Respiratory Society. Idiopathic pulmonary fibrosis: diagnosis and treatment. International consensus statement. Am J Respir Crit Care Med 2000; 161:646–664.
7. Antony VB. Drug-induced pleural disease. Clin Chest Med 1998; 19:331–340.
8. Shapiro JD, Millward MJ, Rischin D, Davison JD, Michael M, Francis PA, Ganju V, Toner GC. Activity and toxicity of docetaxel (Taxotere) in women with previously treated metastatic breast cancer. Aust NZ J Med 1997; 27:40–44.
9. Turner-Warwick M, Lebowitz M, Burrows B, Johnson A. Cryptogenic fibrosing alveolitis and lung cancer. Thorax 1980; 35:496–499.
10. Lee HJ, Im JG, Ahn JM, Yeon KM. Lung cancer in patients with idiopathic pulmonary fibrosis: CT findings. J Comput Assist Tomogr 1996; 20:979–982.
11. Mizushima Y, Kobayashi M. Clinical characteristics of synchronous multiple lung cancer associated with idiopathic pulmonary fibrosis. A review of Japanese cases [see comments]. Chest 1995; 108:1272–1277.
12. Sepkowitz KA, Telzak EE, Gold JW, Bernard EM, Blum S, Carrow M, Dickmeyer M, Armstrong D. Pneumothorax in AIDS. Ann Intern Med 1991; 114:455–459.
13. Adler B, Padley S, Miller RR, Muller NL. High-resolution CT of bronchioloalveolar carcinoma. AJR Am J Roentgenol 1992; 159:275–277.
14. Greco RJ, Steiner RM, Goldman S, Cotler H, Patchefsky A, Cohn HE. Bronchoalveolar cell carcinoma of the lung. Ann Thorac Surg 1986; 41:652–656.
15. McCulloch GL, Sinnatamby R, Stewart S, Goddard M, Flower CD. High-resolution computed tomographic appearance of MALToma of the lung. Eur Radiol 1998; 8:1669–1673.
16. Honda O, Johkoh T, Ichikado K, Yoshida S, Mihara N, Higashi M, Tomiyama N, Maeda M, Hamada S, Naito H, Takeuchi N, Yamamoto S, Nakamura H. Comparison of high resolution CT findings of sarcoidosis, lymphoma, and lymphangitic carcinoma: is there any difference of involved interstitium? J Comput Assist Tomogr 1999; 23:374–379.
17. Johkoh T, Ikezoe J, Tomiyama N, Nagareda T, Kohno N, Takeuchi N, Yamagami

H, Kido S, Takashima S, Arisawa J, et al. CT findings in lymphangitic carcinomatosis of the lung: correlation with histologic findings and pulmonary function tests. AJR Am J Roentgenol 1992; 158:1217–1222.
18. Lower EE, Baughman RP. Pulmonary lymphangitic metastasis from breast cancer. Lymphocytic alveolitis is associated with favorable prognosis. Chest 1992; 102:1113–1117.
19. Hunninghake GW, Costabel U, Ando M, Baughman R, Cordier JF, du Bois R, Eklund A, Kitaichi M, Lynch J, Rizzato G, Rose C, Selroos O, Semenzato G, Sharma OP. ATS/ERS/WASOG statement on sarcoidosis. American Thoracic Society/European Respiratory Society/World Association of Sarcoidosis and other Granulomatous Disorders. Sarcoid Vasc Diffuse Lung Dis 1999; 16:149–173.
20. Soskel NT, Sharma OP. Pleural involvement in sarcoidosis. Semin Respir Med 1992; 13:492–514.
21. Blackmon GM, Raghu G. Pulmonary sarcoidosis: a mimic of respiratory infection. Semin Respir Infect 1995; 10:176–186.
22. Remy JM, Beuscart R, Sault MC, Marquette CH, Remy J. Subpleural micronodules in diffuse infiltrative lung diseases: evaluation with thin-section CT scans. Radiology 1990; 177:133–139.
23. Nishimura K, Itoh H, Kitaichi M, Nagai S, Izumi T. Pulmonary sarcoidosis: correlation of CT and histopathologic findings [published erratum appears in Radiology 1994; 190:907]. Radiology 1993; 189:105–109.
24. Chittock DR, Joseph MG, Paterson NA, McFadden RG. Necrotizing sarcoid granulomatosis with pleural involvement. Clinical and radiographic features. Chest 1994; 106:672–676.
25. Scadding JG. Prognosis of intrathoracic sarcoidosis in England. Br Med J 1961; 4:1165–1172.
26. ACCESS Research Group. Design of a case controlled etiologic study of sarcoidosis (ACCESS). J Clin Epidemiol 1999; 52:1173–1186.
27. Carter AB, Hunninghake GW. Massive pleural effusion in diffuse granulomatous disease. Chest 1997; 112:284–288.
28. Claiborne RA, Kerby GR. Pleural sarcoidosis with massive effusion and lung entrapment. Kans Med 1990; 91:103–105.
29. Groman GS, Castele RJ, Altose MD, Scillian J, Kleinhenz ME, Ehlers R. Lymphocyte subpopulations in sarcoid pleural effusion. Ann Intern Med 1984; 100:75–77.
30. Flammangd'Ortho MP, Cadranel J, Milleron BJ, Akoun GM. Pleural, alveolar and blood T-lymphocyte subsets in pleuropulmonary sarcoidosis. Chest 1990; 98:782–783.
31. Semenzato G, Zambello R, Trentin L, Agostini C. Cellular immunity in sarcoidosis and hypersensitivity pneumonitis. Recent advances. Chest 1993; 103:S139–S143.
32. Hunninghake GW, Crystal RG. Pulmonary sarcoidosis: a disorder mediated by excess helper T-lymphocyte activity at sites of disease activity. N Engl J Med 1981; 305:429–432.
33. Hoheisel GB, Tabak L, Teschler H, Erkan F, Kroegel C, Costabel U. Bronchoalveolar lavage cytology and immunocytology in pulmonary tuberculosis. Am J Respir Crit Care Med 1994; 149(2 Pt 1):460–463.
34. Baughman RP. Sarcoidosis. Usual and unusual manifestations. Chest 1988; 94:165–170.

35. Parker JM, Torrington KG, Phillips YY. Sarcoidosis complicated by chylothorax. South Med J 1994; 87:860–862.
36. Javaheri S, Hales CA. Sarcoidosis: a cause of innominate vein obstruction and massive pleural effusion. Lung 1980; 157:81–85.
37. Soskel NT, Sharma OP. Pleural involvement in sarcoidosis. Semin Respir Med 1992; 13:492–514.
38. Froudarakis ME, Bouros D, Voloudaki A, Papiris S, Kottakis Y, Constantopoulos SH, Siafakas NM. Pneumothorax as a first manifestation of sarcoidosis. Chest 1997; 112:278–280.
39. Lake KB, Sharma OP, VanDyke JJ. Pneumothorax in sarcoidosis. Rev Interam Radiol 1978; 3:33–36.
40. Waldhorn RE, Tsou E, Kerwin DM. Invasive pulmonary aspergillosis associated with aspergilloma in sarcoidosis. South Med J 1983; 76:251–253.
41. Israel HL, Ostrow A. Sarcoidosis and aspergilloma. Am J Med 1969; 47:243–250.
42. Nakahira M, Saito H, Miyagi T. Left vocal cord paralysis as a primary manifestation of invasive pulmonary aspergillosis in a nonimmunocompromised host. Arch Otolaryngol Head Neck Surg 1999; 125:691–693.
43. Wex P, Utta E, Drozdz W. Surgical treatment of pulmonary and pleuro-pulmonary *Aspergillus* disease. Thorac Cardiovasc Surg 1993; 41:64–70.
44. Kawana A, Yamauchi Y, Kudo K. Anti-fungal chemotherapy for symptomatic pulmonary aspergilloma. Jpn J Infect Dis 2000; 53:29–30.
45. Campbell JH, Winter JH, Richardson MD, Shankland GS, Banham SW. Treatment of pulmonary aspergilloma with itraconazole. Thorax 1991; 46:839–841.
46. Kawamura S, Maesaki S, Tomono K, Tashiro T, Kohno S. Clinical evaluation of 61 patients with pulmonary aspergilloma. Intern Med 2000; 39:209–212.
47. Rosenberg IL, Greenberger PA. Allergic bronchopulmonary aspergillosis and aspergilloma. Long-term follow-up without enlargement of a large multiloculated cavity. Chest 1984; 85:123–125.
48. Ein ME, Wallace RJ, Williams TJ. Allergic bronchopulmonary aspergillosis-like syndrome consequent to aspergilloma. Am Rev Respir Dis 1979; 119:811–820.
49. Lieberman PH, Jones CR, Steinman RM, Erlandson RA, Smith J, Gee T, Huvos A, Garin-Chesa P, Filippa DA, Urmacher C, Gangi MD, Sperber M. Langerhans cell (eosinophilic) granulomatosis. A clinicopathologic study encompassing 50 years. Am J Surg Path 1996; 20:519–552.
50. Hoffman L, Cohn JE. Respiratory abnormalities in eosinophilic granuloma of the lung. N Engl J Med 1962; 267:577–589.
51. Tazi A, Soler P, Hance AJ. Adult pulmonary Langerhans' cell histiocytosis. Thorax 2000; 55:405–416.
52. Friedman PJ, Liebow AA, Sokoloff J. Eosinophilic granuloma of lung. Clinical aspects of primary histiocytosis in the adult. Medicine 1981; 60:385–396.
53. Colby TV, Lombard C. Histiocytosis X in the lung. Hum Pathol 1983; 14:847–856.
54. Murin S, Bilello KS, Matthay R. Other smoking-affected pulmonary diseases. Clin Chest Med 2000; 21:121–137.
55. Hance AJ, Basset F, Saumon G, Danel C, Valeyre D, Battesti JP, Chretien J, Georges R. Smoking and interstitial lung disease. The effect of cigarette smoking on the incidence of pulmonary histiocytosis X and sarcoidosis. Ann NY Acad Sci 1986; 465:643–656.
56. Travis WD, Borok Z, Roum JH, Zhang J, Feuerstein I, Ferrans VJ, Crystal RG.

Pulmonary Langerhans cell granulomatosis (histiocytosis X). A clinicopathologic study of 48 cases. Am J Surg Pathol 1993; 17:971–986.
57. Roland A. Recurrent spontaneous pneumothorax. N Engl J Med 1964; 270:73–77.
58. Minghini A, Trogdon SD. Recurrent spontaneous pneumothorax in pulmonary histiocytosis X. Am Surg 1998; 64:1040–1042.
59. Roland AS. Recurrent spontaneous pneumothorax. N Engl J Med 1964; 270:73–77.
60. Gore RM, Port RB, Fry WJ. Spontaneous pneumothorax in a patient with honeycomb lung. Chest 1981; 80:215–216.
61. Von Essen S, West W, Sitorius M, Rennard SI. Complete resolution of roentgenographic changes in a patient with pulmonary histiocytosis X. Chest 1990; 98:765–767.
62. Etienne B, Bertocchi M, Gamondes JP, Thevenet F, Boudard C, Wiesendanger T, Loire R, Brune J, Mornex JF. Relapsing pulmonary Langerhans cell histiocytosis after lung transplantation. Am J Respir Crit Care Med 1998; 157:288–291.
63. Gelfand ET, Sheiner NM. Pneumothorax in pulmonary eosinophilic granuloma. Can Med Assoc J 1974; 110:937.
64. Pappas CA, Rheinlander HF, Stadecker MJ. Pleural effusion as a complication of solitary eosinophilic granuloma of the rib. Hum Pathol 1980; 11:675–677.
65. Nagaoka S, Maruyama R, Koike M, Fujihara S, Shirakawa R, Furuya H, Tanaka N. Cytology of Langerhans cell histiocytosis in effusions: a case report. Acta Cytol 1996; 40:563–566.
66. Shamburek RD, Brewer HJ, Gochuico BR. Erdheim-Chester disease: a rare multisystem histiocytic disorder associated with interstitial lung disease. Am J Med Sci 2001; 321:66–75.
67. Kambouchner M, Colby TV, Domenge C, Battesti JP, Soler P, Tazi A. Erdheim-Chester disease with prominent pulmonary involvement associated with eosinophilic granuloma of mandibular bone. Histopathology 1997; 30:353–358.
68. Egan AJ, Boardman LA, Tazelaar HD, Swensen SJ, Jett JR, Yousem SA, Myers JL. Erdheim-Chester disease: clinical, radiologic, and histopathologic findings in five patients with interstitial lung disease. Am J Surg Pathol 1999; 23:17–26.
69. Veyssier-Belot C, Cacoub P, Caparros-Lefebvre D, Wechsler J, Brun B, Remy M, Wallaert B, Petit H, Grimaldi A, Wechsler B, Godeau P. Erdheim-Chester disease. Clinical and radiologic characteristics of 59 cases. Medicine 1996; 75:157–169.
70. Wittenberg KH, Swensen SJ, Myers JL. Pulmonary involvement with Erdheim-Chester disease: radiographic and CT findings. AJR Am J Roentgenol 2000; 174:1327–1331.
71. Ferrans VJ, Yu ZX, Nelson WK, Valencia JC, Tatsuguchi A, Avila NA, Riemenschn W, Matsui K, Travis WD, Moss J. Lymphangioleiomyomatosis (LAM): a review of clinical and morphological features. J Nippon Med Sch 2000; 67:311–329.
72. Urban T, Lazor R, Lacronique J, Murris M, Labrune S, Valeyre D, Cordier JF. Pulmonary lymphangioleiomyomatosis. A study of 69 patients. Groupe d'Etudes et de Recherche sur les Maladies "Orphelines" Pulmonaires (GERM"O"P). Medicine (Baltimore) 1999; 78:321–337.
73. Chu SC, Horiba K, Usuki J, Avila NA, Chen CC, Travis WD, Ferrans VJ, Moss J. Comprehensive evaluation of 35 patients with lymphangioleiomyomatosis. Chest 1999; 115:1041–1052.
74. Kitaichi M, Nishimura K, Itoh H, Izumi T. Pulmonary lymphangioleiomyoma-

tosis: a report of 46 patients including a clinicopathologic study of prognostic factors. Am J Respir Crit Care Med 1995; 151(2 pt 1):527–533.
75. Taylor JR, Ryu J, Colby TV, Raffin TA. Lymphangioleiomyomatosis. Clinical course in 32 patients. N Engl J Med 1990; 323:1254–1260.
76. Johnson S. Rare diseases. Lymphangioleiomyomatosis: clinical features, management and basic mechanisms. Thorax 1999; 54:254–264.
77. Costello LC, Hartman TE, Ryu JH. High frequency of pulmonary lymphangioleiomyomatosis in women with tuberous sclerosis complex. Mayo Clin Proc 2000; 75:591–594.
78. Moss J, Avila NA, Barnes PM, Litzenberger RA, Bechtle J, Brooks PG, Hedin CJ, Hunsberger S, Kristof AS. Prevalence and clinical characteristics of lymphangioleiomyomatosis (LAM) in patients with tuberous sclerosis complex. Am J Resp Crit Care Med 2001; 164:669–671.
79. Franz DN, Brody A, Meyer C, Leonard J, Chuck G, Dabora S, Sethuraman G, Colby TV, Kwiatkowski DJ, McCormack FX. Mutational and radiographic analysis of pulmonary disease consistent with lymphangioleiomyomatosis and micronodular pneumocyte hyperplasia in women with tuberous sclerosis. Am J Respir Crit Care Med 2001; 164:661–668.
80. Carsillo T, Astrinidis A, Henske EP. Mutations in the tuberous sclerosis complex gene TSC2 are a cause of sporadic pulmonary lymphangioleiomyomatosis. Proc Natl Acad Sci USA 2000; 97:6085–6090.
81. Johnson SR, Tattersfield AE. Clinical experience of lymphangioleiomyomatosis in the UK. Thorax 2000; 55:1052–1057.
82. Berkman N, Bloom A, Cohen P, Deviri E, Bar-Ziv Y, Shimon D, Kramer MR. Bilateral spontaneous pneumothorax as the presenting feature in lymphangioleiomyomatosis. Respir Med 1995; 89:381–383.
83. Chuang ML, Tsai YH, Pang LC. Early chylopneumothorax in a patient with pulmonary lymphangioleiomyomatosis. J Formos Med Assoc 1993; 92:278–282.
84. Cope C, Salem R, Kaiser LR. Management of chylothorax by percutaneous catheterization and embolization of the thoracic duct: prospective trial. J Vasc Interv Radiol 1999; 10:1248–1254.
85. Foresti V, Casati O, Zubani R, Villa A. Chylous pleural effusion in tuberous sclerosis. Respiration 1990; 57:398–401.
86. Banner AS, Carrington CB, Emory WB, Kittle F, Leonard G, Ringus J, Taylor P, Addington WW. Efficacy of oophorectomy in lymphangioleiomyomatosis and benign metastasizing leiomyoma. N Engl J Med 1981; 305:204–209.
87. Aubry MC, Myers JL, Ryu JH, Henske EP, Logginidou H, Jalal SM, Tazelaar HD. Pulmonary lymphangioleiomyomatosis in a man. Am J Respir Crit Care Med 2000; 162(2 pt 1):749–752.
88. Boehler A, Speich R, Russi EW, Weder W. Lung transplantation for lymphangioleiomyomatosis. N Engl J Med 1996; 335:1275–1280.
89. Shin MS, Fulmer JD, Ho KJ. Unusual computed tomographic manifestations of benign metastasizing leiomyomas as cavitary nodular lesions or interstitial lung disease. Clin Imag 1996; 20:45–49.
90. Uchida T, Tokumaru T, Kojima H, Nakagawaji K, Imaizumi M, Abe T. A case of multiple leiomyomatous lesions of the lung: an analysis of flow cytometry and hormone receptors. Surg Today 1992; 22:265–268.
91. Kayser K, Zink S, Schneider T, Dienemann H, Andre S, Kaltner H, Schuring MP, Zick Y, Gabius HJ. Benign metastasizing leiomyoma of the uterus: documenta-

tion of clinical, immunohistochemical and lectin-histochemical data of ten cases. Virchows Archiv 2000; 437:284–292.
92. Lanham JG, Elkon KB, Pusey CD, Hughes GR. Systemic vasculitis with asthma and eosinophilia: a clinical approach to the Churg-Strauss syndrome. Medicine 1984; 63:65–81.
93. Guillevin L, Cohen P, Gayraud M, Lhote F, Jarrousse B, Casassus P. Churg-Strauss syndrome. Clinical study and long-term follow-up of 96 patients. Medicine (Baltimore) 1999; 78:26–37.
94. Choi YH, Im JG, Han BK, Kim JH, Lee KY, Myoung NH. Thoracic manifestation of Churg-Strauss syndrome: radiologic and clinical findings. Chest 2000; 117:117–124.
95. Worthy SA, Muller NL, Hansell DM, Flower CD. Churg-Strauss syndrome: the spectrum of pulmonary CT findings in 17 patients. AJR Am J Roentgenol 1998; 170:297–300.
96. Erzurum SC, Underwood GA, Hamilos DL, Waldron JA. Pleural effusion in Churg-Strauss syndrome. Chest 1989; 95:1357–1359.
97. Choi YH, Im JG, Han BK, Kim JH, Lee KY, Myoung NH. Thoracic manifestation of Churg-Strauss syndrome: radiologic and clinical findings. Chest 2000; 117:117–124.
98. Wechsler ME, Finn D, Gunawardena D, Westlake R, Barker A, Haranath SP, Pauwels RA, Kips JC, Drazen JM. Churg-Strauss syndrome in patients receiving montelukast as treatment for asthma. Chest 2000; 117:708–713.
99. Wechsler ME, Garpestad E, Flier SR, Kocher O, Weiland DA, Polito AJ, Klinek MM, Bigby TD, Wong GA, Helmers RA, Drazen JM. Pulmonary infiltrates, eosinophilia, and cardiomyopathy following corticosteroid withdrawal in patients with asthma receiving zafirlukast. JAMA 1998; 279:455–457.
100. Bili A, Condemi JJ, Bottone SM, Ryan CK. Seven cases of complete and incomplete forms of Churg-Strauss syndrome not related to leukotriene receptor antagonists. J Allergy Clin Immunol 1999; 104:1060–1065.
101. Genereau T, Lortholary O, Leclerq P, Grenet D, Tubery M, Sicard D, Caubarrere I, Guillevin L. Treatment of systemic vasculitis with cyclophosphamide and steroids: daily oral low-dose cyclophosphamide administration after failure of a pulse intravenous high-dose regimen in four patients. Br J Rheumatol 1994; 33: 959–962.
102. Westermark P. The pathogenesis of amyloidosis: understanding general principles. Am J Pathol 1998; 152:1125–1127.
103. Cohen AS, Wegelius O. Classification of amyloid: 1979–1980. Arthr Rheum 1980; 23:644–645.
104. Celli BR, Rubinow A, Cohen AS, Brody JS. Patterns of pulmonary involvement in systemic amyloidosis. Chest 1978; 74:543–547.
105. Smith RR, Hutchins GM, Moore GW, Humphrey RL. Type and distribution of pulmonary parenchymal and vascular amyloid. Correlation with cardiac amyloid. Am J Med 1979; 66:96–104.
106. Utz JP, Swensen SJ, Gertz MA. Pulmonary amyloidosis. The Mayo Clinic experience from 1980 to 1993. Ann Intern Med 1996; 124:407–413.
107. Kavuru MS, Adamo JP, Ahmad M, Mehta AC, Gephardt GN. Amyloidosis and pleural disease. Chest 1990; 98:20–23.
108. Knapp MJ, Roggli VL, Kim J, Moore JO, Shelburne JD. Pleural amyloidosis. Arch Pathol Lab Med 1988; 112:57–60.

109. Graham DR, Ahmad D. Clinical aspects of pulmonary amyloidosis. Chest 1987; 92:576–577.
110. Bontemps F, Tillie-Leblond I, Coppin MC, Frehart P, Wallaert B, Ramon P, Tonnel AB. Pleural amyloidosis: thoracoscopic aspects. Eur Respir J 1995; 8:1025–1027.
111. Smith FB, Brown RB, Maguire G, Oliver J. Localized pleural microdeposition of type A amyloid in a patient with rheumatoid pleuritis. Histologic distinction from pleural involvement in systemic amyloidosis. Am J Clin Pathol 1993; 99:261–264.
112. Adams AL, Castro CY, Singh SP, Moran CA. Pleural amyloidosis mimicking mesothelioma: a clinicopathologic study of two cases. Ann Diagn Pathol 2001; 5: 229–232.
113. Katzenstein AL, Myers JL. Idiopathic pulmonary fibrosis: clinical relevance of pathologic classification. Am J Respir Crit Care Med 1998; 157(4 pt 1):1301–1315.
114. Katzenstein AL, Fiorelli RF. Nonspecific interstitial pneumonia/fibrosis. Histologic features and clinical significance. Am J Surg Pathol 1994; 18:136–147.
115. Picado C, Gomez dA, Xaubet A, Montserrat J, Letang E, Sanchez-Lloret J. Spontaneous pneumothorax in cryptogenic fibrosing alveolitis. Respiration 1985; 48:77–80.
116. Picado C, Gomez DA, Xaubet A, Montserrat J, Letang E, Sanchez-Lloret J. Spontaneous pneumothorax in cryptogenic fibrosing alveolitis. Respiration 1985; 48:77–80.
117. Franquet T, Gimenez A, Torrubia S, Sabate JM, Rodriguez-Arias JM. Spontaneous pneumothorax and pneumomediastinum in IPF. Eur Radiol 2000; 10:108–113.
118. Hunninghake GW, Zimmerman MB, Schwartz DA, King TE Jr, Lynch J, Hegele R, Waldron J, Colby T, Muller N, Lynch D, Galvin J, Gross B, Hogg J, Toews G, Helmers R, Cooper JA Jr, Baughman R, Strange C, Millard M. Utility of a lung biopsy for the diagnosis of idiopathic pulmonary fibrosis. Am J Respir Crit Care Med 2001; 164:193–196.
119. Nishimura K, Kitaichi M, Izumi T, Nagai S, Kanaoka M, Itoh H. Usual interstitial pneumonia: histologic correlation with high-resolution CT. Radiology 1992; 182:337–342.
120. Lim MK, Im JG, Ahn JM, Kim JH, Lee SK, Yeon KM, Han MC. Idiopathic pulmonary fibrosis vs. pulmonary involvement of collagen vascular disease: HRCT findings. J Korean Med Sci 1997; 12:492–498.
121. Erzurum SC, Underwood GA, Hamilos DL, Waldron JA. Pleural effusion in Churg-Strauss syndrome. Chest 1989; 95:1357–1359.
122. Utz JP, Swensen SJ, Gertz MA. Pulmonary amyloidosis. The Mayo Clinic experience from 1980 to 1993. Ann Intern Med 1996; 124:407–413.

32

Immunological Diseases of the Pleura

DEMETRIOS A. VASSILAKIS

Rethymnon General Hospital
Rethymnon, Crete, Greece

ATHOL U. WELLS

Royal Brompton Hospital
London, England

DEMOSTHENES BOUROS

Demokritos University of Thrace
 Medical School
and University Hospital of Alexandroupolis
Alexandroupolis, Greece

I. Introduction

Pleural disease in connective tissue disease occurs most frequently in rheumatoid arthritis (RA) and systemic lupus erythematosus (SLE), but there is considerable variation in the reported prevalence, natural history and treated course of pleural involvement in both diseases. The definition of pleural disease in other connective tissue disorders is necessarily imprecise. Many of the systemic diseases covered in this chapter are, themselves, rare, and pleural involvement is infrequent; thus, the spectrum of pleural disease is not captured in the medical literature to two standard deviations of disease behavior. It is foolhardy to attempt to generalize from single case reports or very small series.

There are other problems that apply equally to RA, SLE, and other connective tissue diseases. The prevalence and severity of an individual pulmonary feature is likely to be critically dependent upon the nature of the population studied. Potentially important selection biases include evaluation of patients at the onset of disease (following which clinical features may evolve significantly) and presentation to a subspecialty respiratory unit (leading to the selection of patients with particularly vexing pulmonary complications). Furthermore, as clinical experience of unusual diseases accumulates, patients with milder disease are increasingly recognized, especially if ancillary diagnostic tests are developed.

A good example of this phenomenon is the widespread determination of serum antineutrophil cytoplasmic antibody levels, leading to a lower diagnostic threshold for Wegener's granulomatosis in patients with mild or even subclinical disease and a corresponding change in the reported clinical spectrum of disease. In pleural disease, this problem is exacerbated by increasingly sophisticated imaging techniques, allowing the detection of previously unsuspected small effusions of doubtful clinical significance. Plainly the apparent prevalence of pleural disease will depend utterly upon whether patients are investigated for symptomatic pleural disease, screened radiographically, or undergo computed tomography (CT) by protocol.

Concurrent pathological processes also complicate the definition of pleural disease in connective tissue disorders. Pleural abnormalities may result from renal or cardiac disease, pulmonary emboli, and, especially, pneumonia or empyema, both of which tend to be more prevalent in connective tissue disease. Thus, in many cases, apparent pleural involvement does not, in fact, represent active autoimmune pleuritis, and it becomes increasingly difficult to interpret the significance of occasional case reports of pleural involvement in diseases other than SLE or RA. A further problem is the existence of overlap autoimmune syndromes. For example, pleural disease in patients with apparently isolated systemic sclerosis (SSc) or polymyositis/dermatomyositis (PM/DM) may, in fact, represent incipient overlap with RA or SLE, and the clinical heterogeneity of Churg-Strauss syndrome and Wegener's granulomatosus is notorious.

Finally, treatment is largely anecdotal, with no controlled data, even in cohorts of patients with RA or SLE. This reflects the fact that pleural involvement is often clinically trivial and does not require treatment, a fact not always captured in statements of prevalence.

In this chapter, pleural disease in RA and SLE is covered in greater detail, and the reported experience of pleural disease is summarized briefly in other connective tissue diseases.

II. Rheumatoid Arthritis

Pleural disease (pleuritis, with or without pleural effusion) is the most common intrathoracic manifestation of RA. It usually affects middle-aged men and is characterized by a low pleural fluid glucose level.

A. Incidence

Pleural involvement in RA, first reported in the mid nineteenth century (1), is found at autopsy in approximately 50% of patients (2). However, only 20% of RA patients experience pleuritic pain at some stage, and many pleural effusions are found incidentally on chest radiography, with overt clinical evidence of pleural disease in less than 5% (3–5). In a study of 516 patients with RA, only 17 (3.3%) had pleural effusions, with the prevalence higher in males (7.9%) than females (1.6%) (3). By contrast, in a controlled study of 309 RA patients, chest radiographic evidence of preexisting pleural disease was seen in 24% of males and 16% of females (compared to 16% and 8% of controlled subjects) (6). Pleuritic pain is also more prevalent in male patients (3,6).

B. Histological Features

The most consistent finding is replacement of the normal mesothelial cell covering by a pseudo-stratified layer of epithelioid cells, with focal multinucleated giant cells (which differ from foreign body giant cells), regular small papillae containing branching capillaries and occasional cholesterol clefts, but no necrosis or granulomata (7–9). Typical rheumatoid nodules are an occasional finding (9). These findings are pathognomonic for rheumatoid pleuritis, but histological appearances are nonspecific in many cases and needle biopsy specimens generally show nonspecific evidence of chronic pleuritis (10).

C. Clinical Manifestations

Most patients are asymptomatic, but breathlessness may result from pulmonary compression in large effusions. Fever, cough, and pleuritic pain are occasional complaints (11), and respiratory failure has been precipitated by a large effusion in a patient with preexisting chronic obstructive pulmonary disease (12). Ninety-two of 113 patients (81%) with rheumatoid pleural effusions, reported before 1968, were male, and the average age of onset was 51 years (range 35–69 years) (3). Rheumatoid effusions are associated with subcutaneous nodules in over 50% (3,10,11) and usually develop after the onset of joint manifestations; in only 6% do effusions precede arthritis and in 11%, pleural and systemic disease present concurrently. Pleural effusions are a late manifestation (i.e., developing 10 or more years after the onset of systemic disease) in 20% (3). The presence of pleural disease has not been linked to more severe systemic disease, although associated with a higher prevalence of cardiac and ocular lesions (3).

D. Radiographic Imaging

On chest radiography, effusions are bilateral in 25% (3), with no predilection for either side (10). Effusions are usually small or moderate, but are occasionally massive (12,13), and may be transient, chronic, or recurrent (14). Up to 30% of patients have simultaneous parenchymal lesions (interstitial lung disease or necrobiotic nodules) (3,14), and concurrent pneumothoraces occur in approximately 5% (15).

E. Diagnosis

The diagnosis of a rheumatoid pleural effusion is made by the exclusion of other causes, although male gender, age in excess of 50, longstanding arthritis, and the presence of subcutaneous nodules all increase the diagnostic likelihood. Effusions are exudative and characterized by high titers of rheumatoid factor, low glucose levels, low pH, and high lactate dehydrogenase levels.

F. Differential Diagnosis

In patients with coexisting arthritis and pleural effusions, the major differential diagnosis is systemic lupus erythematosus. Lupoid effusions are distinguished from rheumatoid effusions by absent or low (1:40) titers of rheumatoid factor, glucose concentrations in excess of 80 mg/dL, lactic dehydrogenase levels of 500 IU/L or less, and pH > 7.35.

Rheumatoid pleural effusions are seldom a prolonged source of diagnostic uncertainty. In a study of 40 consecutive patients with exudative pleural effusions, undiagnosed after exhaustive evaluation and followed, on average, for 5 years, no underlying cause was identified in 32 cases (80%), but rheumatoid arthritis was eventually diagnosed in only one case (16).

G. Fluid Analysis

The fluid is exudative and nonodorous and may be cloudy, greenish-yellow, or opalescent (7). Glucose levels exceed 3 g/100 mL in 20–30%, but normal glucose concentrations reduce the likelihood of rheumatoid pleural disease (10). Other biochemical findings include pH < 7.2, lactate dehydrogenase (LDH) levels more than twice the upper limit of the normal serum value, low complement and immune complexes levels, and rheumatoid factor titers (>1:320) that exceed serum titers (11). Whole complement activity and C3, C4 levels are lower in RA pleural fluid than in nonrheumatoid effusions (17). The complement cascade is activated through both classic and alternative pathways in rheumatic pleurisy; in one study, determinations of SC5b-9 and C4d/C4 content in pleural fluid most accurately distinguished between rheumatic, tuberculous, and malignant effusions (18).

As in empyema and tuberculous effusions, the activity of adenosine deaminase in rheumatoid effusions is higher in pleural fluid than in serum, indicating local synthesis of ADA by cells within the pleural cavity in RA (19).

H. Fluid Cytology

Cytological examination may disclose a characteristic triad of giant multinucleated macrophages, elongated macrophages, and a background of granular debris (8,14). One or more of these features was present in 24 patients with RA pleuritis (granular necrotic material, $n = 23$; multinucleated giant macrophages, $n = 17$; elongated macrophages, $n = 15$), but in none of 10,000 non-rheumatoid effusions (20). "RA cells" ("ragocytes" with characteristic inclusion bodies, representing phagocytic vacuoles or phagosomes, larger than lysosomes seen in granular leukocytes) are sometimes present (21), but may also be seen in tuberculous effusions and empyema (14), and have no diagnostic value (20,22).

I. Glucose

Pleural fluid glucose concentrations of 25 mg/100 mL or less, despite normal serum glucose concentrations, are virtually diagnostic of RA, in the absence of bacteria and acid-fast bacilli (23). In a study of 76 rheumatoid effusions, pleural glucose levels were less than 20 mg/dL in 63%, and less than 50 mg/dL in 83% (10). The mechanism for low pleural glucose levels in RA is unknown. The administration of glucose increases serum but not pleural glucose concentrations (5,23). However, pleural glucose is not utilized rapidly; the addition of glucose to pleural fluid in vitro is not associated with significant cellular glucose utilization (5). It has been suggested that the rheumatoid inflammatory process may influence the activity of enzymes contributing to cellular membrane carbohydrate transport (23) or produces substances interfering with glucose entry into pleural fluid (5).

J. Cholesterol

High concentrations of total lipids and cholesterol have been observed in some rheumatoid effusions (5,9,10), and cholesterol crystal formation, an occasional finding, may give rise to an "opalescent sheen" (10). Chronicity or high cellularity are probably necessary for the development of a high pleural fluid lipid or cholesterol content (unless the effusion is a true chylothorax) (5,10).

K. Infection

Empyema may complicate rheumatoid pleural disease, but the reported prevalence is highly variable. Five of 10 patients with RA pleural effusions observed during a 5-year period developed empyema and these patients made up 16% of all adult cases with empyema at that institution (24). By contrast, only one of 19 patients with pleural effusions in RA had empyema (3). In a study of 67 patients with nontuberculous empyema, three were associated with RA (25). It appears that empyema in RA may be associated with nodular pleuropulmonary disease and the formation of pyopneumothoraces, but may also occur in the absence of other pleuropulmonary complications of RA. Middle-aged males seem to be particularly susceptible (25). Possible causative factors include corticosteroid therapy, a rheumatoid susceptibility to infection, preexisting chronic bronchopulmonary infection, preexisting rheumatoid effusions, altered biochemical characteristics of pleural fluid and the formation of broncho-pleural fistulas though necrotic rheumatoid nodules (24).

L. Pneumothorax

This rare complication of RA, thought to occur in approximately 5% of patients with rheumatoid lung (26) and found on chest radiography in 6% of patients with rheumatoid effusions (25), may be bilateral (15) or recurrent (27). The pleural fluid cholesterol content is often increased (9). Pneumothoraces are thought to result from perforation of cavitating rheumatoid nodules into the pleural space, creating continuous leakage. Prolonged chest tube drainage or surgical intervention may be required (28). A triad of rheumatoid lung disease, pneumothorax, and peripheral eosinophilia has been described (29,30).

M. Biopsy

Needle biopsy of the pleura has proved disappointing: in most cases nonspecific granulomatous or fibrotic changes are reported (3,31). On rare occasions pleural rheumatoid nodules are demonstrated, which are diagnostic (31,32).

Thoracoscopy sometimes offers an invaluable supplement to other laboratory data in the evaluation of suspected rheumatoid effusions (7,32,33). The thoracoscopic granular appearance of the parietal pleura and the histopathological changes in tissue gained from thoracoscopic biopsies are often diagnostic (7).

N. Treatment

There is little reported information on the efficacy of therapy in rheumatoid pleural disease. Most effusions are asymptomatic and do not require specific treatment. Initial treatment of pleuritic with nonsteroidal anti-inflammatory agents may suffice. Some patients respond to corticosteroids (3,9,14,34), but others do not (2,35,36), and effusions may recur despite maintenance steroid therapy. Repeated aspirations have been used to control effusions. Occasionally, persistent symptomatic effusions or pleural thickening necessitate decortication (37–39).

Intrapleural installation of corticosteroids has been attempted. In two patients with large persistent, asymptomatic pleural effusions, intrapleural injection was ineffective (35), but a further patient has responded to an injection of 10 mg of depo-methylprednisolone (40).

Decortication should be considered in patients with symptomatic pleural thickening. The significance of pleural thickening can be estimated by serial pleural pressure measurements during therapeutic thoracocentesis; a rapid drop in pleural pressure is noted denotes trapping of the lung by thickened pleura (41). However, decortication may be technically difficult in rheumatoid pleural disease (39).

O. Long-Term Outcome

Rheumatoid effusions resolve within 4 weeks in 50% and within 4 months in two thirds of patients (3), but persist for years in approximately 20% (2).

III. Systemic Lupus Erythematosus

A. Incidence

Pleural effusions are common in SLE and are included in the American Rheumatism Association diagnostic criteria for SLE (42). Approximately 30–50% of patients develop a pleural effusion during the course of their illness (2,43–46). Pleural abnormalities are found at autopsy in 40–93% (47–50), but represent secondary cardiopulmonary complications of SLE, such as heart failure, infection, and pulmonary emboli, rather than lupus pleuritis, in some cases (49). Pleural effusions are variably reported to be more prevalent in females (43) and males (51), with no clear evidence overall of a major association with gender. Pleuritic pain was reported in 60 of 138 patients in one series, with 14 experiencing repeated episodes (52), and a chest radiographic study disclosed a prevalence of pleural effusion of approximately 35% (53). However, the exact prevalence is difficult to determine, because many patients with transient pleural disease are asymptomatic and may not come to medical attention. Moreover, the clinical features of SLE, including the frequency of pleural disease, vary significantly between ethnic groups (54–59).

B. Histology

Little has been written about the histological features of pleural disease in SLE, perhaps because findings at autopsy represent the end result of multiple episodes, with fibrotic ablation of preceding lesions (53). In an autopsy study of 54 patients, acute fibrinous pleuritis was present in 40%. In 33% of cases, there was evidence of previous inflammation, as shown by pleural fibrosis. Hematoxylin bodies, considered diagnostic by some, were infrequent (60).

C. Clinical Manifestations

Pleuritic pain is the most frequent pleural symptom in SLE, occurring in most patients with lupus pleuritis, although dyspnea and cough are also common (45). Pleuritic pain is often distressing and may be prolonged (52), occasionally necessitating pleurectomy after failure of conservative treatment (61). Frequent findings on examination include fever, pleural rub, and tachycardia (45). Lupus pleuritis is the first manifestation of SLE in only 5–10%, but is an early feature in 25–30%, usually preceded by arthralgia, and is sometimes associated with pneumonitis and pericarditis (53). Other patients present with painless pleural effusions (62). The prevalence of pleural disease at presentation increases in the elderly (sixth decade or later) (63), but pleural involvement is also frequent in children (64–66), and fatal lupus pleuritis has occurred during pregnancy (67). Pleuritis is also a frequent feature of drug-induced lupus syndromes (not covered in this chapter). Finally, pleural effusions may represent complications of SLE (rather than representing primary disease activity), including lupus nephritis, uremia, pneumonia, pulmonary emboli, congestive heart failure, empyema, and other disorders.

D. Radiographic Imaging

On chest radiography, pleural effusions are generally small, but are occasionally massive (68–74). Effusions are bilateral in about 50% of patients, with no major predilection for the right or left side (2), and serial chest radiographs often disclose a change in side (52). Although pleural involvement was invariably associated with pneumonitis in one study (52), pleural abnormalities are more prevalent than radiographic evidence of interstitial lung disease in other reports (46,53). Other chest radiographic findings include nonspecific alveolar infiltrates, atelectasis, and cardiomegaly, representing cardiomyopathy or pericardial effusions (45,75).

E. Diagnosis

SLE pleuritis should be considered in any patient with an exudative pleural effusion of unknown etiology (53). The diagnosis is often obvious in patients with overt SLE, but in patients with pleuritis in association with nonspecific arthritis, the major differential diagnosis is rheumatoid pleural disease. Laboratory data distinguishing between rheumatoid and lupus pleuritis (45) are covered in the section on rheumatoid arthritis. Measurement of lactic acid has been proposed a rapid tool to distinguish between bacterial pleural inflammation and other causes of exudative effusions (76), but the measurement of adenosine deaminase isoenzymes does not enhance the overall diagnostic value of adenosine deaminase activity in pleural effusions (77).

F. Pleural Fluid Analysis

The pleural fluid is usually exudative, yellow, or seroanguineous (45,53), with rare reports of hemothorax (74,78), and tends to be neutrophilic in patients with pleurisy, but lymphocytic in chronic effusions (44,45). A pleural fluid eosinophilia is generally considered to rule out underlying SLE (79) but has been reported in a single SLE patient (80). Generally, the pH is higher than 7.20, glucose concentrations are slightly decreased (45,81), although usually higher than 60 mg/dL, and LDH levels are lower than 500 IU (44). However, occasional exceptions exist to all three observations (44,45). The clinical features of pleural disease are not linked to pleural pH and glucose levels (45).

As in rheumatoid arthritis, reductions in pleural fluid complement levels have been observed (3,42–44,82,83), possibly reflecting complement conversion by immune complexes (17,44,45,82,83). Immune complex deposition may engender pleural effusions by increasing capillary permeability (84). Low titer rheumatoid factor positivity is an occasional finding in a lupoid effusion (44). Elevated CA125 levels have been reported in the pleural fluid of a number of connective tissue diseases, including SLE (85,86); elevated serum CA125 levels are an indicator or pleural disease in connective tissue disease.

In patients with nondiagnostic serum antinuclear antibody, rheumatoid factor, anti-DNA antibody, and hemolytic complement levels, the measurement of corresponding pleural levels is diagnostically valueless (87). Similarly, serum antinuclear and associated antibody positivity is not diagnostically useful, although there is a weak association in SLE between anti-RNP positivity and pleuritis (88,89).

G. Pleural Fluid Antinuclear Antibodies

Pleural fluid antinuclear antibodies (ANA) titers >1:60 and pleural fluid to serum ANA ratios >1 are suggestive but not diagnostic of SLE pleuritis; high pleural fluid titers (up to 1:640) are seen occasionally in patients with nonlupoid exudative effusions (90). Most patients with SLE also have higher ANA titers for ssDNA, dsDNA, smooth muscle, and ribonucleoprotein (90,91), although demonstrable pleural fluid ANA are occasionally absent (92). Pleural fluid ANA titer levels may be useful in distinguishing between lupus pleuritis and other causes of pleural disease in SLE patients, in which ANA titers tend to be low or absent (93).

H. Fluid Lupus Cells

Lupus erythematosus (LE) cells are found occasionally in serous effusions in SLE (45,94–100) and may appear at the onset or later in the disease course (101). LE cells also occur in drug-induced lupus pleuritis (94,95). Some have regarded the presence of LE cells in serous effusions as virtually diagnostic of SLE (94–97), although LE cells are occasionally present in malignant pleural effusions (102), rheumatoid joint effusions (103), and have also been reported in pleural fluid, without clinical evidence of SLE (101). However, LE cells are not found in the pleural fluid of all patients with lupoid pleuritis (93) and are usually associated with the presence of serum LE cells; thus, the added value of pleural fluid LE cell positivity is questionable (93). Moreover, the detection of LE cells is not straightforward technically, and may be subject to significant observer variation (96). Thus, the diagnostic identification of LE cells has largely fallen out of favor.

I. Biopsy

In pleural biopsy specimens from three patients with drug-induced lupus pleural effusions (104) and autopsy pleural specimens from patients with SLE (105), a specific immunofluorescent pattern has been observed, characterized by diffuse and speckled staining of cell nuclei with antiimmunoglobulin G, anti-IgM, or anti-C3 (104).

J. Pneumothorax

Pneumothoraces and pneumohemathoraces have been described in adults with SLE (78,106).

K. Treatment

Pleuritic pain in SLE may respond to nonsteroidal anti-inflammatory agents and almost always responds strikingly to corticosteroid therapy, although high doses may be needed for severe pleuritis or large effusions (107). In refractory cases, immunosuppressive agents such as azathioprine and hydroxychloroquine are sometimes but not always efficacious (70,108,109), and monthly cyclosporin courses have been used, with a good outcome (109). Recurrent pleural effusions usually respond to tetracycline (110,111) or talc (70) pleurodesis.

L. Prognosis

Asymptomatic lupoid effusions require no treatment, usually resolve spontaneously (53), and have no known prognostic significance. However, pleuritic pain appears to be an adverse prognostic marker (53,112,113), with a mean survival of less than 4 years in affected cases in one study (53).

IV. Systemic Sclerosis

Pleural effusions have been reported in both diffuse (85,114,115) and limited (116) scleroderma, but are rare. In a formal evaluation of the prevalence of serositis in SSc, none of 37 patients (including 19 with limited SSc) had a pleural effusion, and on review of medical records, pleural effusions were identified in only 4 of 58 other SSc patients (7%) (117). By contrast, pericardial effusions were present in 17% (117). The very low prevalence of pleural effusions in SSc makes the association uncertain, as a proportion of patients with SSc eventually develop SLE overlap. Thus, an evolving overlap syndrome might give rise to pleural involvement in some patients, including the recently reported case of an 88-year-old woman with SSc and a pleural effusion, eventually diagnosed as an SSc/SLE overlap (118).

In two cases, pleural effusions in SSc have been associated with elevated serum and pleural fluid CA125 levels (85,114), which were seen to decrease with resolution of the effusion in one case (85). CA125 levels are usually normal in collagen vascular disease, in the absence of pleural involvement (85), and, thus, it has been suggested that CA125 levels might reflect the activity of serositis (114).

V. Polymyositis/Dermatomyositis

Polymyositis/dermatomyositis are grouped disorders, categorized under the idiopathic inflammatory myopathies and characterized by symmetrical proximal muscle weakness, elevated serum levels of skeletal muscle enzymes, electrophysiological changes consistent with myopathy, and evidence of non-suppurative inflammation in skeletal muscle tissue (119,120). Dermatomyositis consists of all the manifestations of polymyositis with additional cutaneous features.

Although pleuritic pain is occasionally reported (121–123), overt clinical or radiographic evidence of pleural disease is exceedingly rare. None of 65 patients with polymyositis ($n = 24$) or dermatomyositis ($n = 41$) had pleural effusions clinically or at autopsy, although histological evidence of fibrinous pleuritis was seen occasionally (121). Two patients with massive pleural effusions have been described, both presenting with marked pyrexia and a good response to corticosteroid therapy (124). Although cardiomyopathy and hypothyroidism might have contributed to pleural fluid accumulation in one case, no confounding features were present in the second patient, a 34-year-old man with dermatomyositis and coexisting interstitial lung disease.

VI. Sjögren's Syndrome

Sjögren's syndrome (SS) is a chronic inflammatory disease characterized by dryness of the mouth (xerostomia), eyes (keratoconjunctivitis sicca), and other mucous membranes (2). SS may be primary or secondary (when associated with rheumatoid arthritis, systemic lupus erythrematosus, dermatomyositis/polymyositis, or systemic sclerosis). Respiratory involvement in primary SS is often clinically mild, although severe symptoms occasionally arise from desiccation of the tracheobronchial tree or lymphocytic infiltration of the lung parenchyma (125). Pleurisy, with or without a pleural effusion, is exceedingly rare in primary SS, but sometimes occurs in secondary SS with accompanying rheumatoid arthritis or systemic lupus erythematosus, in keeping with the high prevalence of pleural involvement in those disorders (126).

Overall, pleural effusions have been reported in none of 62 patients with SS (127) in none of 36 patients with primary SS (128), in only 5 of 349 patients with SS, including 2 with primary SS (129), and in none of 40 patients with primary SS or 26 with secondary SS (130). Pleuritic pain was confined to patients with secondary SS and a control cohort with rheumatoid arthritis (130).

In a handful of reported pleural effusions associated with primary SS, disease is more often bilateral (126,131,132), but may be unilateral (133), and the fluid is lymphocytic and exudative, with normal glucose levels and pH, and low adenosine deaminase levels (132–134). Studies of serum and pleural fluid in one patient disclosed rheumatoid factor and anti-SS-A antibody, immune complexes, and activation of complement, all localized to pleural fluid (126). Analysis of pleural fluid T-cell receptor β-chain variable (V β) regions revealed overexpression of V β gene products, including V β 2 and V β 13, previously shown to be overrepresented in salivary glands of SS patients (126). In two instances pleural effusions associated with primary SS have regressed with corticosteroid therapy (131,132), or improved spontaneously until complete resolution (134).

VII. Ankylosing Spondylitis

Ankylosing spondylitis (AS) is an inflammatory disease involving entheses and joints, especially those in and around the spine, and resulting in chest wall pain, diminished chest wall movement, and a dorsal stoop. Pleural involvement is most frequently associated with apical fibro-bullous lung disease, found in a small proportion of AS patients. The initial, mainly fibrotic changes become fibro-bullous as the condition progresses, with evolution to prominent cavitation being an occasional feature. Cavities developing within apical fibrotic tissue in AS have a particular predilection for mycobacterial or fungal colonization, especially *Aspergillus fumigatus*, isolated in up to 60% of AS patients with apical cavitation (135). Infection of a cavity may lead to underlying pleural thickening or even empyema.

Other forms of pleural disease in AS are exceedingly rare (136), consisting of a handful of cases with pleural effusions (137–139). In population studies, pleural disease has been identified in 2 of 53 patients (one tuberculous, one nontuberculous effusion) (140), 2 of 255 patients (idiopathic bilateral pleural calcification) (141), and one of 200 patients (unexplained pleural thickening) (142). These findings are difficult to interpret, as they might have represented the pleural sequelae of tuberculous or nontuberculous infection, rather than a direct complication of AS. A chest radiographic study of 2080 patients with AS disclosed nonapical pleural disease in 10 patients, which did not differ significantly in prevalence from control subjects and included 3 transient pleural exudates with normal pleural fluid glucose concentrations and one patient with empyema (143).

VIII. Mixed Connective Tissue Disease

The term mixed connective tissue disease (MCTD), or Sharp's syndrome (144), applies to patients exhibiting a mixture of clinical features of SLE, SSc, and PM/DM, in association with high titers of a circulating antinuclear antibody, with specificity for a nuclear ribonucleoprotein antigen (snRNP) (145). Pleuropulmonary manifestations, reported to occur in 20–80%, include interstitial pneumonitis and fibrosis (20–65%), and pulmonary hypertension (10–45%) (146). Pleural effusions develop during the course of the illness in 50% (146) and pleuritic chest pain is reported in approximately 40% (147). However, despite a high overall prevalence of inflammatory pleural disease, often associated with pericarditis, pleural involvement is seldom an initial manifestation of disease (unlike SLE) (148). In the few reported cases of MCTD, in which pleural involvement is the cardinal presenting feature, pleural effusions are sometimes but not always associated with pericarditis (144,148) and may be bilateral (149) or unilateral (150). In general, pleural effusions are small and resolve spontaneously (146).

IX. Eosinophilia-Myalgia Syndrome

Eosinophilia-myalgia syndrome (EMS), a recently defined disorder reaching epidemic proportions in 1989 (151,152), is almost always associated with ingestion of manufactured tryptophan, although occasional idiopathic cases occur (153). Diagnostic criteria are debilitating myalgia and an absolute blood eosinophil count >1.0 (10 × 9) cells/L. The syndrome usually affects Caucasian women older than 35, and clinical data suggest a multisystem disorder, with frequent arthralgia, rash, peripheral edema, elevated aldolase level, and deranged liver function tests. Neuropathy or neuritis occur in 25% (151) and occasionally end in paralysis or death. Cough or dyspnea are present in 60%, although less than 10% have pleural effusions on chest radiography (151).

Although the exact pathogenesis of the syndrome remains uncertain (154), cessation of tryptophan ingestion, with or without the addition of corticosteroids, may lead to a rapid complete response, although recovery is often incomplete or prolonged (152) and several deaths have occurred (151,155). Following withdrawal of commercially available preparations of tryptophan, the incidence of EMS has fallen dramatically (151).

Pleural effusions have been reported on chest radiography in 12% of 178 cases (151) and in six of 18 patients (156). Effusions are usually bilateral and the fluid is sterile and exudative (153,156). Pleural involvement is not necessarily clinically significant and has no documented therapeutic or prognostic implication.

X. Angio-Immunoblastic Lymphadenopathy

Angio-immunoblastic lymphadenopathy (AIL), a disease of unknown etiology and pathogenesis, has variable features of hyperimmunity and immune deficiency. It often resembles Hodgkin's disease (157,158), presenting with fever, true drenching sweats, weight loss, and, often, a rash, generalized lymphadenopathy and hepatosplenomegaly. Polyclonal hypergammaglobulinaemia is usual and hemolytic anemia is frequent (2,157). AIL is uncommon, with 200 cases being reported (158) in the 6 years following the initial definition of the disease in 1973 (157). The diagnosis is made by histological examination of an enlarged lymph node. The course of the disease is usually progressive, with a median survival of 15 months in 18 fatal cases out of 32 studied in one series (157). Treatments have included prednisone and cyclophosphamide (158), but survival beyond 2 years is exceedingly rare, and failure to achieve complete remission is associated with a mortality at one year of 90%. More intensive chemotherapy is usually unsuccessful and very hazardous, as the risk of severe infection is high.

Histologically, AIL is characterized by a morphological triad: proliferation of arborizing small vessels, prominent immunoblastic proliferation, and amorphous acidophilic interstitial material, with benign appearances (2,157). Progression of disease is thought to represent a nonneoplastic hyperimmune proliferation of B lymphocytes, possibly related to a lack of suppressor T lymphocytes (158,159). Transformations to immunoblastic lymphoma (158) and immunoblastic sarcoma (157) have been reported.

Pleural effusions occur in AIL in at least 10% of cases, with a higher prevalence in some reports. In a Japanese series, pleural effusions were found in 50%, including all five index cases and 8 of 21 patients previously reported in the Japanese literature (160). In a study of 10 patients, 5 where found to have a pleural effusion eventually associated with ascites and pedal edema (158). Surprisingly, the characteristics of the pleural fluid (including fundamental features such as protein content) are not well described.

XI. Churg-Strauss Syndrome

Churg-Strauss syndrome (CSS) is characterized by asthma, hypereosinophilia, and necrotizing systemic vasculitis with extravascular eosinophil granulomas. Diagnosis requires satisfaction of at least four American College of Rheumatology criteria: asthma, hypereosinophilia $>1,500/mm^3$ or $>10\%$, paranasal sinusitis, pulmonary infiltration, histological evidence of vasculitis, and mononeuritis multiplex; asthma is the most prevalent clinical manifestation at presentation (161). Although not included in formal diagnostic criteria, weight loss, fever, myalgia, skin involvement, arthralgia, and gastrointestinal involvement are also common (161). The most common thin-section CT findings include bilateral ground-glass attenuation, airspace consolidation (predominantly subpleural and surrounded by ground-glass attenuation), centri-lobular nodules (mostly within ground-glass attenuation) bronchial wall thickening; and increased vessel caliber (162).

CSS is often difficult to diagnose, due to striking variations in clinical behavior between patients, and a high frequency of clinical and histological features that overlap with other granulomatous, vasculitic, and eosinophilic disorders (163). "Typical" histological features (necrotizing vasculitis, eosinophilic tissue infiltration, extravascular granulomas) are not consistently captured at biopsy. The significance of an association between leukotriene receptor antagonist administration and CSS remains uncertain (164–168).

Corticosteroid therapy, with or without an immunosuppressive agent (usually cyclophosphamide during initial treatment) results in remission in 90%, although 25% of patients relapse (161); plasma exchange is sometimes warranted in refractory disease. The long-term prognosis is good, although low-dose oral steroid therapy is usually required for asthma for many years, even when clinical evidence of vasculitis regresses rapidly (161).

Although pleural involvement is generally regarded as rare, as shown in a long-term follow-up study of 96 patients (161); a review of the English literature before 1984 disclosed a prevalence of pleural effusions of 30% in 61 patients with documented chest radiograph (163). In a more recent study of 9 patients with CSS, pleural effusions were detected in two (as well as two pericardial effusions) (162). In one case with diagnostic features at lung biopsy, thoracocentesis yielded an acidotic exudative effusion with low glucose, low C3, eosinophilia, and a markedly increased rheumatoid factor (169), and in a second case, histological features diagnostic of CSS were present on pleural biopsy (170). Thus, pleural involvement is an occasional feature of CSS.

XII. Wegener's Granulomatosis

Wegener's granulomatosis (WG) is a disease of unknown etiology, characterized histologically by necrotizing granulomatous angiitis. The nose, lungs, and kidneys are classical sites of involvement on which a clinical diagnosis was based historically, but the disease can affect almost all other organ systems (171). Based on a series of 77 patients, pulmonary symptoms (cough, mild dyspnea, hemoptysis, chest pain) occur in over 95% (172). However, reported cohorts vary greatly, due to selection bias and a major increase in the detection of sub-clinical disease with characterization of serological features. Most patients with WG have serum antineutrophil cytoplasmic antibodies, with granular immunofluorescence staining in the cytoplasm (c-ANCA) (173); the measurement of c-ANCA titers is now widespread in suspected autoimmune disease, and less severe WG is increasingly diagnosed

Characteristic imaging features include nodules and pulmonary infiltrates (172), but chest radiographic appearances often understate the extent of pulmonary involvement and CT is sometimes invaluable (174), especially when it discloses previously undetected cavitation within opacities (172). The course of WG has been dramatically improved by daily treatment with cyclophosphamide and glucocorticoids. Nonetheless, relapses are common (175).

Based upon studies of small groups of patients, minor pleural involvement is not infrequent. In studies of small groups of patients, effusions were present on chest radiography in 6 of 11, 4 of 11, 4 of 77, and 4 of 18 cases (172,176–178). Pleural thickening is occasionally evident on chest radiography (178) or CT (179), and pneumothorax has been reported (180). Pleural aspiration has shown an exudative neutrophilic content, with protein levels 38–57 g/L in 4 with an effusion out of 77 cases (172).

Pleural effusions in WG are seldom clinically important and generally resolve spontaneously, or regress with the introduction of corticosteroid and/or immunosuppressive treatment.

XIII. Miscellaneous Diseases

Pleural effusions occasionally accompany other connective tissue diseases, including polyarteritis nodosa (181), temporal arteritis (182), giant cell arteritis (183,184), Kawasaki disease (185), Adamantiadis-Bechet syndrome (186), human adjuvant disease (187), and adult-onset Still's disease (188–190). The major difficulty in characterizing pleural involvement in these disorders is the paucity of cases of diseases which are, themselves, rare. Thus, steroid-responsive exudative effusions have been reported in temporal arteritis in a handful of cases, but little more is known about this complication (182,191,192). In giant cell arteritis, pulmonary involvement is similarly rare and consists of interstitial infiltration, pulmonary nodules, pulmonary artery vasculitis, granuloma formation, and, in a few cases (183,184), pleural effusions.

Pleuro-pulmonary complications are more prevalent in Kawasaki disease. In a series of 129 patients, chest radiographic abnormalities were identified in 15%, invariably within 10 days of the onset, and included reticulonodular patterns, peribronchial cuffing, atelectasis, and air trapping; pleural effusions were found in only 3% of the population (185). The pathological basis of radiographic abnormalities remains uncertain in the absence of histological evaluation, but heart failure was not implicated, and it appears likely that the abnormalities represented lower respiratory tract inflammation and/or pulmonary arteritis, both features of Kawasaki disease (185).

Human adjuvant disease is a connective tissue disease occurring after cosmetic surgery with silicone injections or implants. There is a single report of a chylous effusion developing in association with a lupus-like syndrome, after mammary augmentation with silicone gel-filled prostheses (187).

Adult-onset Still's disease (AOSD) is a rare splenic disorder of unknown cause, which may involve other organs, including the liver, kidney, bone marrow, and, less frequently, the lungs. Pulmonary involvement usually consists of pleural effusion or transient pulmonary infiltrates; life-threatening progression to the acute respiratory distress syndrome has been reported. High-dose corticosteroid therapy tends to be used as first line treatment of pulmonary complications, although responses have also been achieved with cyclophosphamide, azathioprine, and intravenous immunoglobulin (190).

References

1. Fuller HM. On Rheumatism, Rheumatic Gout and Sciatica: Their Pathology, Symptoms and Treatment. New York: S. S. and W. Wood, 1854.
2. Hunninghake GW, Fauci AS. Pulmonary involvement in the collagen vascular diseases. Am Rev Respir Dis 1979; 119:471–503.
3. Walker WC, Wright V. Pulmonary lesions and rheumatoid arthritis. Medicine (Baltimore) 1968; 47:501–520.
4. Hyland RH, Gordon DA, Broder I, Davies GM, Russell ML, Hutcheon MA, Reid GD, Cox DW, Corey PN, Mintz S. A systematic controlled study of pulmonary abnormalities in rheumatoid arthritis. J Rheumatol 1983; 10:395–405.
5. Dodson WH, Hollingsworth JW. Pleural effusion in rheumatoid arthritis. Impaired transport of glucose. N Engl J Med 1966; 275:1337–1342.
6. Jurik AG, Davidsen D, Graudal H. Prevalence of pulmonary involvement in rheumatoid arthritis and its relationship to some characteristics of the patients. A radiological and clinical study. Scand J Rheumatol 1982; 11:217–224.
7. Faurschou P, Francis D, Faarup P. Thoracoscopic, histological, and clinical findings in nine case of rheumatoid pleural effusion. Thorax 1985; 40:371–375.
8. Aru A, Engel U, Francis D. Characteristic and specific histological findings in rheumatoid pleurisy. Acta Pathol Microbiol Immunol Scand A 1986; 94:57–62.
9. Ferguson GC. Cholesterol pleural effusion in rheumatoid lung disease. Thorax 1966; 21:577–582.
10. Lillington GA, Carr DT, Mayne GJ. Rheumatoid pleurisy with pleural effusion. Arch Intern Med 1971; 128:764–768.

11. Halla JT, Schronhenloher RE, Volanakis JE. Immune complexes and other laoratory features of pleural effusions. Ann Intern Med 1980; 92:748–752.
12. Pritikin JD, Jensen WA, Yenokida GG, Kirsch CM, Fainstat M. Respiratory failure due to a massive rheumatoid pleural effusion. J Rheumatol 1990; 17:673–675.
13. Brennan SR, Daly JJ. Large pleural effusions in rheumatoid arthritis. Br J Dis Chest 1979; 73:133–140.
14. Joseph J, Sahn SA. Connective tissue diseases and the pleura. Chest 1993; 104:262–270.
15. Ayzenberg O, Reiff DB, Levin L. Bilateral pneumothoraces and pleural effusions complicating rheumatoid lung disease. Thorax 1983; 38:159–160.
16. Ferrer JS, Munoz XG, Orriols RM, Light RW, Morell FB. Evolution of idiopathic pleural effusion: a prospective, long-term follow-up study. Chest 1996; 109:1508–1513.
17. Hunder GG, McDuffie FC, Hepper NG. Pleural fluid complement in systemic lupus erythematosus and rheumatoid arthritis. Ann Intern Med 1972; 76:357–363.
18. Salomaa ER, Viander M, Saaresranta T, Terho EO. Complement components and their activation products in pleural fluid. Chest 1998; 114:723–730.
19. Pettersson T, Ojala K, Weber TH. Adenosine deaminase in the diagnosis of pleural effusions. Acta Med Scand 1984; 215:299–304.
20. Naylor B. The pathognomonic cytologic picture of rheumatoid pleuritis. Acta Cytol 1990; 34:465–473.
21. Sahn SA. Immunologic diseases of the pleura. Clin Chest Med 1985; 6:103–112.
22. Faurschou P. Decreased glucose in RA-cell-positive pleural effusion: correlation of pleural glucose, lactic dehydrogenase and protein concentration to the presence of RA-cells. Eur J Respir Dis 1984; 65:272–277.
23. Carr DT, McGuckin WF. Pleural fluid glucose. Am Rev Respir Dis 1968; 97:302–305.
24. Jones FL, Blodget RC. Empyema in rheumatoid pleuropulmonary disease. Ann Intern Med 1971; 74:665–671.
25. Dieppe PA. Empyema in rheumatoid arthritis. Ann Rheum Dis 1975; 34:181–185.
26. Martel W, Abell MR, Mikkelsen WM, Whitehouse WM. Pulmonary and pleural lesions in rheumatoid disease. Radiology 1968; 90:641–653.
27. Adelman HM, Dupont EL, Flannery MT, Wallach PM. Case report: recurrent pneumothorax in a patient with rheumatoid arthritis. Am J Med Sci 1994; 308:171–172.
28. Sharma SS, Reynolds PM. Broncho-pleural fistula complicating rheumatoid lung disease. Postgrad Med J 1982; 58:187–189.
29. Portner MM, Gracie WAJ. Rheumatoid lung disease with cavitary nodules, pneumothorax and eosinophilia. N Engl J Med 1966; 275:697–700.
30. Crisp AJ, Armstrong RD, Grahame R, Dussek JE. Rheumatoid lung disease, pneumothorax, and eosinophilia. Ann Rheum Dis 1982; 41:137–140.
31. Anonymous. Pleural effusion in rheumatoid arthritis (editorials). Lancet 1972; I:480–481.
32. Faurschou P. Rheumatoid pleuritis and thoracoscopy. Scand J Respir Dis 1974; 55:277–283.

33. Faurschou P. Thoracoscopy in rheumatoid pleural effusion. Pneumologie 1989; 43:69–71.
34. Ward R. Pleural effusion and rheumatoid disease. Lancet 1961; 2:1336.
35. Russell ML, Gladman DD, Mintz S. Rheumatoid pleural effusion: lack of response to intrapleural corticosteroid. J Rheumatol 1986; 13:412–415.
36. Emerson RA. Pleural effusion complicating rheumatoid arthritis. Br Med J 1956; 1:428.
37. Walker WC, Wright W. Rheumatoid pleuritis. Ann Rheum Dis 1967; 26:467.
38. Brunk JR, Drash EC, Swineford O. Rheumatoid pleuritis successfully treated with decortication. Am J Med 1966; 251:545.
39. Yarbrough JW, Sealy WC, Miller JA. Thoracic surgical problems associated with rheumatoid arthritis. J Thorac Cardiovasc Surg 1975; 69:347–354.
40. Chapman PT, O' Donnell JL, Moller PW. Rheumatoid pleural effusion: response to intrapleural corticosteroid. Rheumatology 1992; 19:478–480.
41. Light RW, Jenkinson SG, Minh VD, George RB. Observations on pleural pressures as fluid is withdrawn during thoracentesis. Am Rev Respir Dis 1980; 121:799–804.
42. Cohen AS, Reynolds WE, Franklin EC. Preliminary criteria for the classification of systemic lupus erythematosus. Bull Rheum Dis 1971; 21:643–648.
43. Pines A, Kaplinsky N, Olchovsky D, Rozenman J, Frankl O. Pleuro-pulmonary manifestations of systemic lupus erythematosus: clinical features of its subgroups. Prognostic and therapeutic implications. Chest 1985; 88:129–135.
44. Halla JT, Schrohenloher RE, Volanakis JE. Immune complexes and other laboratory features of pleural effusions: a comparison of rheumatoid arthritis, systemic lupus erythematosus, and other diseases. Ann Intern Med 1980; 92:748–752.
45. Good JT Jr, King TE, Antony VB, Sahn SA. Lupus pleuritis. Clinical features and pleural fluid characteristics with special reference to pleural fluid antinuclear antibodies. Chest 1983; 84:714–718.
46. Alarcon-Segovia D, Alarcon DG. Pleuro-pulmonary manifestations of systemic lupus erythematosus. Dis Chest 1961; 39:7–17.
47. Ropes MW. Systemic Lupus Erythematosus. Cambridge: Harvard University Press, 1976.
48. Miller LR, Greenberg SD, McLarty JW. Lupus lung. Chest 1985; 88:265–269.
49. Haupt HM, Moore GW, Hutchins GM. The lung in systemic lupus erythematosus. Analysis of the pathologic changes in 120 patients. Am J Med 1981; 71:791–798.
50. Gross M, Esterly JR, Earle RH. Pulmonary alterations in systemic lupus erythematosus. Am Rev Respir Dis 1972; 105:572–577.
51. Miller MH, Urowitz MB, Gladman DD, Killinger DW. Systemic lupus erythematosus in males. Medicine (Baltimore) 1983; 62:327–334.
52. Harvey AM, Shulman LE, Tumulty PA, et al. Systemic lupus erythematosus: a review of the literature and clinical analysis of 138 cases. Medicine 1954; 33:291–437.
53. Winslow WA, Ploss LN, Loitman B. Pleuritis in systemic lupus erythematosus: its importance as an early manifestation in diagnosis. Ann Intern Med 1958; 49:70–88.
54. Segasothy M, Phillips PA. Systemic lupus erythematosus in Aborigines and Caucasians in central Australia: a comparative study. Lupus 2001; 10:439–444.

55. Camilleri F, Mallia C. Male SLE patients in Malta. Adv Exp Med Biol 1999; 455:173–179.
56. Molina JF, Molina J, Garcia C, Gharavi AE, Wilson WA, Espinoza LR. Ethnic differences in the clinical expression of systemic lupus erythematosus: a comparative study between African-Americans and Latin Americans. Lupus 1997; 6:63–67.
57. Chang CC, Shih TY, Chu SJ, Kuo SY, Chen CM, Hsu CM, Chang ML, Chang DM. Lupus in Chinese male: a retrospective study of 61 patients. Chung Hua I Hsueh Tsa Chih (Taipei) 1995; 55:143–150.
58. Costallat LT, Coimbra AM. Systemic lupus erythematosus in 18 Brazilian males: clinical and laboratory analysis. Clin Rheumatol 1993; 12:522–525.
59. Al Rawi Z, Al Shaarbaf H, Al Raheem E, Khalifa SJ. Clinical features of early cases of systemic lupus erythematosus in Iraqui patients. Br J Rheumatol 1983; 22:165–171.
60. Gueft B, Laufer A. Futher cytochemical studies in systemic lupus erythematosus. Arch Path 1954; 57:201.
61. Bell R, Lawrence DS. Chronic pleurisy in systemic lupus erythematosus treated with pleurectomy. Br J Dis Chest 1979; 73:314–316.
62. Wang DY, Chang DB, Kuo SH, Yang S, Shiah DC, Chou HT, Luh KT. Systemic lupus erythematosus presenting as pleural effusion: report of a case. J Formos Med Assoc 1995; 94:746–749.
63. Baker SB, Rovira JR, Campion EW, Mills JA. Late onset systemic lupus erythematosus. Am J Med 1979; 66:727–732.
64. Chantarojanasiri T, Sittirath A, Preutthipan A, Tapaneya-Olarn W, Suwanjutha S. Pulmonary involvement in childhood systemic lupus erythematosus. J Med Assoc Thai 1999; 82(suppl 1):S144–S148.
65. Gedalia A, Molina JF, Molina J, Uribe O, Malagon C, Espinoza LR. Childhood-onset systemic lupus erythematosus: a comparative study of African Americans and Latin Americans. J Natl Med Assoc 1999; 91:497–501.
66. Nadorra RL, Landing BH. Pulmonary lesions in childhood onset systemic lupus erythematosus: analysis of 26 cases, and summary of literature. Pediatr Pathol 1987; 7:1–18.
67. Katz VL, Kuller JA, McCoy MC, Hansen WF. Fatal lupus pleuritis presenting in pregnancy. A case report. J Reprod Med 1996; 41:537–540.
68. Bouros D, Panagou P, Papandreou L, Kottakis I, Tegos C. Massive bilateral pleural effusion as the only first presentation of systemic lupus erythematosus. Respiration 1992; 59:173–175.
69. Elborn JS, Conn P, Roberts SD. Refractory massive pleural effusion in systemic lupus erythematosus treated by pleurectomy. Ann Rheum Dis 1987; 46:77–80.
70. Kaine JL. Refractory massive pleural effusion in systemic lupus erythematosus treated with talc poudrage. Ann Rheum Dis 1985; 44:61–64.
71. Bulgrin JG, Dubois EL, Jacobson G. Chest roentgenographic changes in systemic lupus erythematosus. Radiology 1960; 74:42.
72. Taylor TL, Ostrum H. The roentgen evaluation of systemic lupus erythematosus. Am J Roentgenol 1959; 82:95.
73. Mathlouthi A, Ben M'rad S, Merai S, Kovitz KL, Slabbynck H, Djenayah F. Massive pleural effusion in systemic lupus erythematosus: thoracoscopic and immunohistological findings. Monaldi Arch Chest Dis 1998; 53:34–36.

74. Mulkey D, Hudson L. Massive spontaneous unilateral hemothorax in systemic lupus erythematosus. Am J Med 1974; 56:570.
75. Gould DM, Dayes ML. Roentgenologic findings in systemic lupus erythematosus. J Chronic Dis 1955; 2:136–145.
76. Brook I. Measurement of lactic acid in pleural fluid. Respiration 1980; 40:344–348.
77. Carstens ME, Burgess LJ, Maritz FJ, Taljaard JJ. Isoenzymes of adenosine deaminase in pleural effusions: a diagnostic tool? Int J Tuberc Lung Dis 1998; 2:831–835.
78. Passero FC, Myers AR. Hemopneumothorax in systemic lupus erythematosus. J Rheumatol 1980; 7:183–186.
79. Lakhotia M, Mehta SR, Mathur D, Baid CS, Varma AR. Diagnostic significance of pleural fluid eosinophilia during initial thoracocentesis. Indian J Chest Dis Allied Sci 1989; 31:259–264.
80. Wysenbeek AJ, Pick AI, Sella A, Beigel Y, Yeshurun D. Eosinophilic pleural effusion with high anti-DNA activity as a manifestation of systemic lupus erythematosus. Postgrad Med J 1980; 56:57–58.
81. Carr DT, Lillington GA, Mayne JG. Pleural-fluid glucose in systemic lupus erythematosus. Mayo Clin Proc 1970; 45:409–412.
82. Hunder GG, McDuffie FC, Huston KA, Elveback LR, Hepper NG. Pleural fluid complement, complement conversion, and immune complexes in immunologic and nonimmunologic diseases. J Lab Clin Med 1977; 90:971–980.
83. Glovsky MM, Louie JS, Pitts WH Jr, Alenty A. Reduction of pleural fluid complement activity in patients with systemic lupus erythematosus and rheumatoid arthritis. Clin Immunol Immunopathol 1976; 6:31–41.
84. Andrews BS, Arora NS, Shadforth MF, Goldberg SK, Davis JS. The role of immune complexes in the pathogenesis of pleural effusions. Am Rev Respir Dis 1981; 124:115–120.
85. Kimura K, Ezoe K, Yokozeki H, Katayama I, Nishioka K. Elevated serum CA125 in progressive systemic sclerosis with pleural effusion. J Dermatol 1995; 22:28–31.
86. Yucel AE, Calguneri M, Ruacan S. False positive pleural biopsy and high CA125 levels in serum and pleural effusion in systemic lupus erythematosus. Clin Rheumatol 1996; 15:295–297.
87. Small P, Frank H, Kreisman H, Wolkove N. An immunological evaluation of pleural effusions in systemic lupus erythematosus. Ann Allergy 1982; 49:101–103.
88. Swaak AJ, Huysen V, Nossent JC, Smeenk RJ. Antinuclear antibody profiles in relation to specific disease manifestations of systemic lupus erythematosus. Clin Rheumatol 1990; 9:82–94.
89. Camilleri F, Mallia C. RNP positivity in Maltese SLE patients. Adv Exp Med Biol 1999; 455:161–166.
90. Khare V, Baethge B, Lang S, Wolf RE, Campbell GD Jr. Antinuclear antibodies in pleural fluid. Chest 1994; 106:866–871.
91. Riska H, Fyhrquist F, Selander RK, Hellstrom PE. Systemic lupus erythematosus and DNA antibodies in pleural effusions. Scand J Rheumatol 1978; 7:159–160.
92. Ferreiro JE, Reiter WM, Saldana MJ. Systemic lupus erythematosus presenting as chronic serositis with no demonstrable antinuclear antibodies. Am J Med 1984; 76:1100–1105.
93. Wang DY, Yang PC, Yu WL, Shiah DC, Kuo HW, Hsu NY. Comparison of

different diagnostic methods for lupus pleuritis and pericarditis: a prospective three-year study. J Formos Med Assoc 2000; 99:375–380.
94. Carel RS, Shapiro MS, Cordoba O, Taragan R, Gutman A. LE cells in pleural fluid. Arthritis Rheum 1979; 22:936–937.
95. Keshgegian AA. Lupus erythematosus cells in pleural fluid. Am J Clin Pathol 1978; 69:570–571.
96. Naylor B. Cytological aspects of pleural, peritoneal and pericardial fluids from patients with systemic lupus erythematosus. Cytopathology 1992; 3:1–8.
97. Yoshiyuki OR, Shioya S, Handa K, Shimizu K. Lupus erythematosus cells in pleural fluid cytologic diagnosis in two patients. Acta Cytol 1977; 21:215–217.
98. Reda MG, Baigelman W. Pleural effusion in systemic lupus erythematosus. Acta Cytol 1980; 24:553–557.
99. Makashir R, Jayaram G. Lupus erythematosus cells in pleural fluid. Diagn Cytopathol 1988; 4:273–274.
100. Sethi S, Pooley RJ, Yu GH. Lupus erythematosus (LE) cells in pleural fluid: initial diagnosis of systemic lupus erythematosus by cytologic examination. Cytopathology 1996; 7:292–294.
101. Chao TY, Huang SH, Chu CC. Lupus erythematosus cells in pleural effusions: diagnostic of systemic lupus erythematosus? Acta Cytol 1997; 41:1231–1233.
102. Greis M, Atay Z. Zytomorphologische Begleitreaction bei malignen Pleuraerguessen. Pneumonologie 1990; 44(suppl):262–264.
103. Hunder GG, Pierre RV. In vivo LE cell phenomenon. Arthritis Rheum 1970; 13:570–571.
104. Chandrasekhar AJ, Robinson J, Barr L. Antibody deposition in the pleura: a finding in drug–induced lupus. J Allergy Clin Immunol 1978; 61:399–402.
105. Pertschuk LP, Moccia LF, Rosen Y, Lyons H, Marino CM, Rashford AA, Wollschlager CM. Acute pulmonary complications in systemic lupus erythematosus. Immunofluorescence and light microscopic study. Am J Clin Pathol 1977; 68:553–557.
106. Jay MS, Jerath R, Van Derzalm T, Freeman D. Pneumothorax in an adolescent with fulminant systemic lupus erythematosus. J Adolesc Health Care 1984; 5:142–144.
107. Brasington RD, Furst DE. Pulmonary disease in systemic lupus erythematosus. Clin Exp Rheumatol 1985; 3:269–276.
108. Ben Chetrit E, Putterman C, Naparstek Y. Lupus refractory pleural effusion: transient response to intravenous immunoglobulins. J Rheumatol 1991; 18:1635–1637.
109. Sherer Y, Langevitz P, Levy Y, Fabrizzi F, Shoenfeld Y. Treatment of chronic bilateral pleural effusions with intravenous immunoglobulin and cyclosporin. Lupus 1999; 8:324–327.
110. McKnight KM, Adair NE, Agudelo CA. Successful use of tetracycline pleurodesis to treat massive pleural effusion secondary to systemic lupus erythematosus. Arthritis Rheum 1991; 34:1483–1484.
111. Gilleece MH, Evans CC, Bucknall RC. Steroid resistant pleural effusion in systemic lupus erythematosus treated with tetracycline pleurodesis. Ann Rheum Dis 1988; 47:1031–1032.
112. Cook RJ, Gladman DD, Pericak D, Urowitz MB. Prediction of short term mortality in systemic lupus erythematosus with time dependent measures of disease activity. J Rheumatol 2000; 27:1892–1895.

113. Cervera R, Khamashta MA, Font J, Sebastiani GD, Gil A, Lavilla P, Aydintug AO, Jedryka-Goral A, de Ramon E, Fernandez-Nebro A, Galeazzi M, Haga HJ, Mathieu A, Houssiau F, Ruiz-Irastorza G, Ingelmo M, Hughes GR. Morbidity and mortality in systemic lupus erythematosus during a 5-year period. A multicenter prospective study of 1,000 patients. European Working Party on Systemic Lupus Erythematosus. Medicine (Baltimore) 1999; 78:167–175.
114. Funauchi M, Ikoma S, Yu H, Sugiyama M, Ohno M, Kinoshita K, Hamada K, Kanamaru A. A case of progressive systemic sclerosis complicated by massive pleural effusion with elevated CA125. Lupus 2000; 9:382–385.
115. Hiramatsu K, Takeda N, Okumura S, Takuno H, Yasuda K. [Progressive systemic sclerosis associated with massive pleural and pericardial effusion in a 90-year-old woman]. Nippon Ronen Igakkai Zasshi 1996; 33:535–539.
116. Lee YH, Ji JD, Shim JJ, Kang KH, Song GG. Exudative pleural effusion and pleural leukocytoclastic vasculitis in limited scleroderma. J Rheumatol 1998; 25: 1006–1008.
117. Thompson AE, Pope JE. A study of the frequency of pericardial and pleural effusions in scleroderma. Br J Rheumatol 1998; 37:1320–1323.
118. Takeda N, Teramoto S, Ihn H, Arao T, Matsuse T, Toba K, Tamaki K, Ouchi Y. [A case of very late onset overlap syndrome of systemic sclerosis and systemic lupus erythematosus]. Nippon Ronen Igakkai Zasshi 2000; 37:74–79.
119. Pearson CM, Bohan A. The spectrum of polymyositis and dermatomyositis. Med Clin North Am 1977; 61:439–457.
120. Kagen LJ. Polymyositis/dermatomyositis. In: McCarthy DJ, Koopman WJ, eds. Arthritis and Related Conditions. Philadelphia: Lee and Febiger, 1993:1225.
121. Lakhanpal S, Lie JT, Conn DL, Martin WJ. Pulmonary disease in polymyositis/ dermatomyositis: a clinicopathological analysis of 65 autopsy cases. Ann Rheum Dis 1987; 46:23–29.
122. Ozawa Y, Kurosaka D, Hashimoto N. [An autopsy case of dermatomyositis with rapidly progressive interstitial pneumonia]. Nihon Rinsho Meneki Gakkai Kaishi 1995; 18:552–558.
123. Schwarz MI, Matthay RA, Sahn SA, Stanford RE, Marmorstein BL, Scheinhorn DJ. Interstitial lung disease in polymyositis and dermatomyositis: analysis of six cases and review of the literature. Medicine (Baltimore) 1976; 55:89–104.
124. Miyata M, Fukaya E, Takagi T, Watanabe K, Saito H, Ito M, Yoshioka R, Kazuta Y, Yusa Y, Irisawa A, Sato Y, Nishimaki T, Kumakawa H, Kasukawa R. Two patients with polymyositis or dermatomyositis complicated with massive pleural effusion. Intern Med 1998; 37:1058–1063.
125. Constantopoulos SH, Tsianos EV, Moutsopoulos HM. Pulmonary and gastrointestinal manifestations of Sjögren's syndrome. Rheum Dis Clin North Am 1992; 18:617–635.
126. Kawamata K, Haraoka H, Hirohata S, Hashimoto T, Jenkins RN, Lipsky PE. Pleurisy in primary Sjögren's syndrome: T cell receptor beta-chain variable region gene bias and local autoantibody production in the pleural effusion. Clin Exp Rheumatol 1997; 15:193–196.
127. Bloch KJ, Buchanan WW, Wohl MJ, Bunim JJ. Sjögren's syndrome. A clinical, pathological, and serological study of sixty-two cases. Medicine (Baltimore) 1992; 71:386–401.
128. Constantopoulos SH, Papadimitriou CS, Moutsopoulos HM. Respiratory mani-

festations in primary Sjögren's syndrome. A clinical, functional, and histologic study. Chest 1985; 88:226–229.
129. Strimlan CV, Rosenow EC III, Divertie MB, Harrison EG Jr. Pulmonary manifestations of Sjögren's syndrome. Chest 1976; 70:354–361.
130. Papathanasiou MP, Constantopoulos SH, Tsampoulas C, Drosos AA, Moutsopoulos HM. Reappraisal of respiratory abnormalities in primary and secondary Sjögren's syndrome. A controlled study. Chest 1986; 90:370–374.
131. Kashiwabara K, Kishi K, Narushima K, Nakamura H, Yagyu H, Kiguchi T, Syohda S, Kusama H, Matsuoka K. [Primary Sjögren's syndrome accompanied by pleural effusion]. Nihon Kyobu Shikkan Gakkai Zasshi 1995; 33:1325–1329.
132. Tanaka A, Tohda Y, Fukuoka M, Nakajima S. [A case of Sjögren's syndrome with pleural effusion]. Nihon Kokyuki Gakkai Zasshi 2000; 38:628–631.
133. Ogihara T, Nakatani A, Ito H, Irokawa M, Ban S, Takahashi A, Nishinarita M, Oka Y. Sjögren's syndrome with pleural effusion. Intern Med 1995; 34:811–814.
134. Alvarez-Sala R, Sanchez-Toril F, Garcia-Martinez J, Zaera A, Masa JF. Primary Sjögren syndrome and pleural effusion. Chest 1989; 96:1440–1441.
135. Davies D. Ankylosing spondylitis and lung fibrosis. Q J Med 1972; 41:395–417.
136. Haslock I. Ankylosing spondylitis. Baillieres Clin Rheumatol 1993; 7:99–115.
137. Tanaka H, Itoh E, Shibusa T, Chiba H, Hirasawa M, Abe S. Pleural effusion in ankylosing spondylitis: successful treatment with intra-pleural steroid administration. Respir Med 1995; 89:509–511.
138. Dudley-Hart F, Bogdanovich A, Nichol WD. The thorax in ankylosing spondilitis. Ann Rheum Dis 1950; 9:116–131.
139. Kinnear WJ, Shneerson JM. Acute pleural effusions in inactive ankylosing spondylitis. Thorax 1985; 40:150–151.
140. Zorab PA. The lungs in ankylosing spondylitis. Q J Med 1962; 31:267–280.
141. Crompton GK, Cameron SJ, Langlands AO. Pulmonary fibrosis, pulmonary tuberculosis and ankylosing spondylitis. Br J Dis Chest 1974; 68:51–56.
142. Spencer DG, Park WM, Dick HM, Papazoglou SN, Buchanan WW. Radiological manifestations in 200 patients with ankylosing spondylitis: correlation with clinical features and HLA B27. J Reumatol 1979; 6:305–315.
143. Rosenow E, Strimlan CV, Muhm JR, Ferguson RH. Pleuropulmonary manifestations of ankylosing spondylitis. Mayo Clin Proc 1977; 52:641–649.
144. Richard P, Sabouret P, Vayre F, Desrame J, Ollivier JP. [Pleuropericarditis complicated of tamponade disclosing mixed connective tissue disease. Remission with non-steroidal anti-inflammatory agents. Apropos of a case]. Ann Cardiol Angeiol (Paris) 1996; 45:513–515.
145. Prakash UB. Lungs in mixed connective tissue disease. J Thorac Imaging 1992; 7:55–61.
146. Prakash UB. Respiratory complications in mixed connective tissue disease. Clin Chest Med 1998; 19:733–746, ix.
147. Sullivan WD, Hurst DJ, Harmon CE, Esther JH, Agia GA, Maltby JD, Lillard SB, Held CN, Wolfe JF, Sunderrajan EV. A prospective evaluation emphasizing pulmonary involvement in patients with mixed connective tissue disease. Medicine (Baltimore) 1984; 63:92–107.
148. Beier JM, Nielsen HL, Nielsen D. Pleuritis-pericarditis—an unusual initial manifestation of mixed connective tissue disease. Eur Heart J 1992; 13:859–861.
149. Hoogsteden HC, van Dongen JJ, van der Kwast TH, Hooijkaas H, Hilvering C.

Bilateral exudative pleuritis, an unusual pulmonary onset of mixed connective tissue disease. Respiration 1985; 48:164–167.
150. Ilan Y, Ben Yehuda A, Okon E, Breuer R. Mixed connective tissue disease presenting as a left sided pleural effusion. Ann Rheum Dis 1992; 51:1157–1158.
151. Swygert LA, Maes EF, Sewell LE, Miller L, Falk H, Kilbourne EM. Eosinophilia-myalgia syndrome. Results of national surveillance. JAMA 1990; 264:1698–1703.
152. Martin RW, Duffy J, Engel AG, Lie JT, Bowles CA, Moyer TP, Gleich GJ. The clinical spectrum of the eosinophilia-myalgia syndrome associated with L-tryptophan ingestion. Clinical features in 20 patients and aspects of pathophysiology. Ann Intern Med 1990; 113:124–134.
153. Killen JW, Swift GL, White RJ. Eosinophilic fasciitis with pulmonary and pleural involvement. Postgrad Med J 2000; 76:36–37.
154. Strumpf IJ, Drucker RD, Anders KH, Cohen S, Fajolu O. Acute eosinophilic pulmonary disease associated with the ingestion of L-tryptophan-containing products. Chest 1991; 99:8–13.
155. Andre M, Canon JL, Levecque P, Dermine P, Mortier C, Leveau F. Eosinophilia-myalgia syndrome associated with L-tryptophan. A case report with pulmonary manifestations and review of the literature. Acta Clin Belg 1991; 46:178–182.
156. Williamson MR, Eidson M, Rosenberg RD, Williamson SL. Eosinophilia-myalgia syndrome: findings on chest radiographs in 18 patients. Radiology 1991; 180:849–852.
157. Lukes RJ, Tindle BH. Immunoblastic lymphadenopathy. A hyperimmune entity resembling Hodgkin's disease. N Engl J Med 1975; 292:1–8.
158. Cullen MH, Stansfeld AG, Oliver RT, Lister TA, Malpas JS. Angio-immunoblastic lymphadenopathy: report of ten cases and review of the literature. Q J Med 1979; 48:151–177.
159. Shaw RA, Schonfeld SA, Whitcomb ME. A perplexing case of hilar adenopathy. Clinical conference in pulmonary disease from the Ohio State University College of Medicine. Chest 1981; 80:736–740.
160. Sugiyama H, Kotajima F, Kamimura M, Yoshizawa A, Hojo M, Horiuchi T, Kudo K, Kabe J. [Pulmonary involvement in immunoblastic lymphadenopathy: case reports and review of literature published in Japan]. Nihon Kyobu Shikkan Gakkai Zasshi 1995; 33:1276–1282.
161. Guillevin L, Cohen P, Gayraud M, Lhote F, Jarrousse B, Casassus P. Churg-Strauss syndrome. Clinical study and long-term follow-up of 96 patients. Medicine (Baltimore) 1999; 78:26–37.
162. Choi YH, Im JG, Han BK, Kim JH, Lee KY, Myoung NH. Thoracic manifestation of Churg-Strauss syndrome: radiologic and clinical findings. Chest 2000; 117:117–124.
163. Lanham JG, Elkon KB, Pusey CD, Hughes GR. Systemic vasculitis with asthma and eosinophilia: a clinical approach to the Churg-Strauss syndrome. Medicine (Baltimore) 1984; 63:65–81.
164. Ben Noun L. Drug-induced respiratory disorders: incidence, prevention and management. Drug Saf 2000; 23:143–164.
165. Wechsler ME, Garpestad E, Flier SR, Kocher O, Weiland DA, Polito AJ, Klinek MM, Bigby TD, Wong GA, Helmers RA, Drazen JM. Pulmonary infiltrates, eosinophilia, and cardiomyopathy following corticosteroid withdrawal in patients with asthma receiving zafirlukast. JAMA 1998; 279:455–457.
166. Wechsler ME, Pauwels R, Drazen JM. Leukotriene modifiers and Churg-Strauss

syndrome: adverse effect or response to corticosteroid withdrawal? Drug Saf 1999; 21:241–251.
167. Wechsler ME, Drazen JM. Zafirlukast and Churg-Strauss syndrome. Chest 1999; 116:266–267.
168. Wechsler ME, Finn D, Gunawardena D, Westlake R, Barker A, Haranath SP, Pauwels RA, Kips JC, Drazen JM. Churg-Strauss syndrome in patients receiving montelukast as treatment for asthma. Chest 2000; 117:708–713.
169. Erzurum SC, Underwood GA, Hamilos DL, Waldron JA. Pleural effusion in Churg-Strauss syndrome. Chest 1989; 95:1357–1359.
170. Hirasaki S, Kamei T, Iwasaki Y, Miyatake H, Hiratsuka I, Horiike A, Ogita Y, Matsuhashi Y, Yamamoto S. Churg-Strauss syndrome with pleural involvement. Intern Med 2000; 39:976–978.
171. Bambery P, Sakhuja V, Behera D, Deodhar SD. Pleural effusions in Wegener's granulomatosis: report of five patients and a brief review of the literature. Scand J Rheumatol 1991; 20:445–447.
172. Cordier JF, Valeyre D, Guillevin L, Loire R, Brechot JM. Pulmonary Wegener's granulomatosis. A clinical and imaging study of 77 cases. Chest 1990; 97:906–912.
173. Homer RJ. Antineutrophil cytoplasmic antibodies as markers for systemic autoimmune disease. Clin Chest Med 1998; 19:627–639, viii.
174. Papiris SA, Manoussakis MN, Drosos AA, Kontogiannis D, Constantopoulos SH, Moutsopoulos HM. Imaging of thoracic Wegener's granulomatosis: the computed tomographic appearance. Am J Med 1992; 93:529–536.
175. Hoffman GS, Kerr GS, Leavitt RY, Hallahan CW, Lebovics RS, Travis WD, Rottem M, Fauci AS. Wegener granulomatosis: an analysis of 158 patients. Ann Intern Med 1992; 116:488–498.
176. Gonzalez L, Van Ordstr HS. Wegener's granulomatosis. Review of 11 cases. Radiology 1973; 107:295–300.
177. Bambery P, Katariya S, Sakhuja V, Kaur U, Behera D, Malik SK, Deodhar SD. Wegener's granulomatosis in north India. Radiologic manifestations in eleven patients. Acta Radiol 1988; 29:11–13.
178. Fauci AS, Wolff SM. Wegener's granulomatosis: studies in eighteen patients and a review of the literature. Medicine (Baltimore) 1973; 73:315–324.
179. Weir IH, Muller NL, Chiles C, Godwin JD, Lee SH, Kullnig P. Wegener's granulomatosis: findings from computed tomography of the chest in 10 patients. Can Assoc Radiol J 1992; 43:31–34.
180. Jaspan T, Davison AM, Walker WC. Spontaneous pneumothorax in Wegener's granulomatosis. Thorax 1982; 37:774–775.
181. Bosch X, Ramirez J. [Bilateral lung images and respiratory insufficiency in an 86-year-old man with polyarteritis nodosa]. Med Clin (Barc) 1999; 113:189–197.
182. Turiaf J, Valere PE, Gubler MC. [Recurrent pleurisy during temporal arteritis]. Poumon Coeur 1967; 23:633–652.
183. Ramos A, Laguna P, Cuervas V. Pleural effusion in giant cell arteritis. Ann Intern Med 1992; 116:957.
184. Gur H, Ehrenfeld M, Izsak E. Pleural effusion as a presenting manifestation of giant cell arteritis. Clin Rheumatol 1996; 15:200–203.
185. Umezawa T, Saji T, Matsuo N, Odagiri K. Chest x-ray findings in the acute phase of Kawasaki disease. Pediatr Radiol 1989; 20:48–51.
186. Tunaci A, Berkmen YM, Gokmen E. Thoracic involvement in Behcet's disease:

pathologic, clinical, and imaging features. AJR Am J Roentgenol 1995; 164:51–56.
187. Walsh FW, Solomon DA, Espinoza LR, Adams GD, Whitelocke HE. Human adjuvant disease. A new cause of chylous effusions. Arch Intern Med 1989; 149: 1194–1196.
188. Pasteur M, Laroche C, Keogan M. Pleuropericardial effusion in a 50 year old woman. Pleuropericardial effusion caused by adult inset Still's disease. Postgrad Med J 2001; 77:346, 355–346, 357.
189. Nishio J, Koike R, Iizuka H, Nanki T, Mizushima N, Kohsaka H, Kubota T, Miyasaka N. [A refractory case of adult-onset Still's disease]. Nihon Rinsho Meneki Gakkai Kaishi 1997; 20:191–198.
190. Cheema GS, Quismorio FP Jr. Pulmonary involvement in adult-onset Still's disease. Curr Opin Pulm Med 1999; 5:305–309.
191. Romero S, Vela P, Padilla I, Rosas J, Martin C, Aranda I. Pleural effusion as manifestation of temporal arteritis. Thorax 1992; 47:398–399.
192. Garcia-Alfranca F, Solans R, Simeon C, Gomez-Lozano A, Perez-Bocanegra C, Bosch JA. Pleural effusion as a form of presentation of temporal arteritis. Br J Rheumatol 1998; 37:802–803.

33

Pleural Effusions in Blood Diseases

DESPINA S. KYRIAKOU

University of Thessalia Medical School
and University Hospital of Larissa
Larissa, Thessalia, Greece

MICHAEL G. ALEXANDRAKIS

University of Crete Medical School
and University Hospital of Heraklion
Heraklion, Crete, Greece

DEMOSTHENES BOUROS

Demokritos University of Thrace Medical School
and University Hospital of Alexandroupolis
Alexandroupolis, Greece

I. Non-Hodgkin's Lymphomas and Hodgkin's Disease

Pleural effusions occur in up to 20% of patients with non-Hodgkin's lymphomas (NHL) (1). On the other hand, up to 10% of malignant (positive cytology) pleural effusions are due to NHL (2). However, the majority of information in the literature is based on minor observational studies or case reports (1–13). In the majority of patients the pleural effusion is present at diagnosis, and it has not been proved to affect complete remission or survival (1,10,14). Pleural effusion usually occurs as a part of widespread disease (mainly associated with mediastinal involvement) (4,6,9,10,14). It may be unilateral or bilateral, and as a rule it causes symptoms such as dyspnea, cough, and chest pain. The majority of cases belong to the intermediate grade of malignancy group, a small proportion belongs to the low-grade group, and an even smaller proportion belongs to the high-grade group. The latter has the most unfavorable prognosis (5–14).

In the majority of cases the pleural effusion is due to infiltration of the pleura, is exudate (15–18), and appears serous or serosanguineous on aspiration. The rate of chylous pleural effusions is reported to be about 12% (1). Infections (especially tuberculosis), central lymphatic obstruction, pleural damage due to previous irradiation or chemotherapy, and infiltration by other neoplasms should also be considered in the differential diagnosis (19–23). In rare cases, especially in advanced stages of low-grade lymphomas with multiple organ infiltration, the pleural effusion is a transudate due to venous compression, cardiac or renal failure and hypoalbuminemia (23). Transudative or exudative reactive pleural effusions have also been reported to accompany lung involvement in lymphomas (5,9,13,24–28). In Hodgkin's disease pleural effusion is rarely attributed to infiltration, and is most commonly due to other causes (19,20,29).

When an effusion is the result of infiltration, the lymphocytes in the pleural fluid are usually identical to the cells in involved lymph nodes and in circulating blood, if present (2,3,16,18,20,30–32). Thoracocentesis results in a positive cytological diagnosis in 60–90% of patients with NHL and pleural involvement. The diagnostic yield may be further increased by thoracoscopy (15–17,33–35). In the cases of reactive pleural effusions, lymphocytes are small, mature, polyclonal, and predominantly of the T-cell subset (16,28,36,37). Difficulties in distinguishing morphologically neoplastic from reactive lymphocytes arise in low-grade lymphomas where the involved cell in both cases is a small mature lymphocyte, and whenever a mixed population of neoplastic and reactive lymphocytes exists (16). Cytological, immunological, and molecular methods are available for differentiation between reactive and neoplastic involvement in pleural effusions (15,16,33,38–42).

Primary effusion lymphoma (PEL) is a rare but interesting entity initially observed in HIV-positive patients. It accounts for 1–2% of NHL in these patients (26,43–51). It is a peculiar type of B-cell lymphoma associated with human herpesvirus–8 (HHV-8) (also termed Kaposi sarcoma-HHV) infection that preferentially grows in liquid phase in serous body cavities (51–57). In no case has evidence of extensive disease or dissemination existed. About half of the cases of PEL are also associated with Epstein-Barr virus (EBV) infection (48,52–54,58). Genetic analysis of immunoglobulin heavy-chain (IgH) gene sequences in PEL cases revealed clonal IgH gene rearrangements, inserted HHV-8 sequences, and in many cases inserted EBV DNA sequences (54). No alterations of known oncogenes have been reported in PEL, except for BCL-6, which is found mutated in a large percentage of cases. In addition, complex hyperdiploid karyotypes with multiple structural abnormalities are seen in PEL cell lines. In almost all cases, the cells of PEL express CD138/syndecan-1 antigen, suggesting a possible role of this molecule in the serosal preference of these cells (59). Of note, this lymphoma sometimes originates from HIV-positive/EBV-negative cells in HIV-positive/HBV-positive patients, as proved by genetic studies (52,54,60). In addition, there is evidence that the development of PELs may not be restricted to a specific stage in B-cell differentiation but may occur at different stages of B-cell ontogeny (35,38). PEL has also been reported in non-HIV patients presenting HHV-8 positivity. In these cases, the lymphoma is usually non-T, non-B of high grade of malignancy (46,48,50), while in most other cases it belongs to the intermediate grade. Immunophenotype markers of malignant clones in PEL can be diverse in different cases, but expression of activation markers (CD30, CD38, HLA-DR) is almost universal (7,38,40,61). Cases with T-cell markers are very rare

(45). PEL has also been reported in childhood (30,44). The distinct features of PEL has led some specialists to recommend that it should be considered for inclusion as a new entity in the Revised European-American Lymphoma (REAL) classification.

HHV-8 has been associated with Kaposi's sarcoma, multicentric Castelman's disease, and, as mentioned above, primary effusion lymphoma. Kaposi's sarcoma and multicentric Castelman's disease patients may develop body cavity effusions that either fulfill the criteria of HHV-8–positive PEL or may represent an HHV-8–associated nonneoplastic process (46). In the latter cases, effusions are rich in monocytes/macrophages rich and in some cases harbor B-cell monoclonal proliferation. These observations support the hypothesis of multistage PEL development and that a prelymphomatous effusion may precede overt body cavity lymphoma. Because HHV-8 contains DNA sequences of several protein homologs, the HHV-8 (+) cell lines produce various cytokines, cytokine receptors, chemokines, cell cycle and antiapoptotic modulators, which are upregulated upon stimulation. Indeed, some cell lines produce high levels of IL-6, IL-6–soluble receptor, and IL-10. However, PEL cells do not respond proliferatively to these cytokines, although their proliferation is inhibited by blocking the IL-6 receptor's signaling pathway. The aforementioned cytokines seems to play a role in effusion development (54).

Pyothorax associated lymphoma (PAL) occurs in a clinical setting of longstanding pyothorax or chronic inflammation of the pleura (62). Like the primary effusion lymphoma, it has an association with Epstein-Barr virus (EBV), is confined to the pleural cavity, but has different morphological and phenotypic features. HHV-8 is not an obligate pathogen in PAL, as it is not detected in all cases (62).

II. Acute Leukemias

Pleural effusions during the course of acute leukemias are rare events, although they are a common finding at autopsy (63). They are mostly due to pleural infiltration by extramedullary leukemia development (64,65). Pleural disease, as an initial finding in acute leukemia, has also been reported in very rare cases (66–69). In contrast, unusual extramedullary sites of relapse, such as pleural involvement, are being recognized with increasing frequency as long-term survival improves. Most cases reported in the literature concern acute lymphocytic leukemia (ALL) and very few cases of acute nonlymphocytic leukemia (AML) (Fig. 1). The same applies to extramedullary granulocytic sarcoma of the thorax with pleural involvement, which is an extremely rare entity (69–75).

Adult T-cell leukemia-lymphoma is a distinct lymphoid malignancy presenting with four types: smoldering, chronic, lymphoma, and acute. In the active stage of acute and lymphoma types, pleural (and/or ascitic) effusion may be present (76). In rare cases this disease may be localized to the pleura and/or peritoneum without involvement of other sites. Diagnosis is established by detection

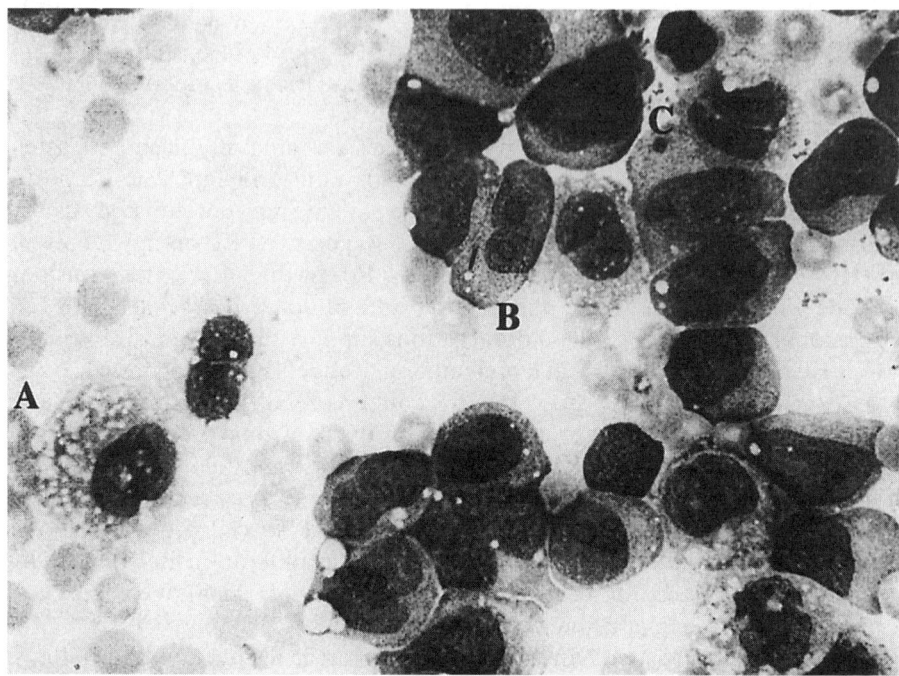

Figure 1 A case of acute nonlymphocytic leukemia. This 60-year-old man presented with chest pain and pleural effusion and no other finding. The effusion contained numerous myeloblasts with Auer bodies and Auer rods. Peroxidase staining was positive. Bone marrow aspiration revealed 60% infiltration with myeloblasts, while the peripheral blood did not contain immature granulocytes. The effusion disappeared after chemotherapy and reappeared at relapse. A, pleural macrophages; B, blast cell with Auer rods; C, blast cell with Auer body.

of specific surface markers for T lymphocytes and the determination of HTLV-1 viral DNA in mononuclear cells on the effusion (74,75).

Unusual cases of hairy cell leukemia and plasma cell leukemia may present with pleural effusions with typical leukemic cells in the fluid (68,73). In all the above situations, the possibility of other causes for the pleural effusion should be excluded. Infections (bacterial or viral), solid tumors (most commonly adenocarcinoma), and complications of therapy should also be kept in mind when dealing with pleural effusions in leukemic patients. In addition, reactive pleural effusions may also be seen in lung diseases of various etiologies in these patients (64,76). Immunocytochemistry, flow cytometry, electron microscopy, and PCR applied to cytology specimens can contribute to the differential diagnosis, and the findings sometimes need to be confirmed by pleuroscopy and surgical biopsy (64,76). Cytological examination of pleural effusions has a higher yield in leukemia-lymphoma compared to solid tumors (16). This is explained by the tendency of leukemic blasts to infiltrate tissues and pass through serosal membranes easily due to the lack of adhesion molecules, while cells of most solid tumors usually cluster due to the presence of specialized adhesion mechanisms.

The development of pleural effusion in acute leukemia is rare, and its prognostic significance is obscure. Some investigators have found that the presence of a pleural effusion at diagnosis in acute leukemia does not affect the rate of remission and survival. However, others report a worse prognosis, especially in plasmacytic and hairy cell leukemias (68,73).

A pleural effusion in patients with acute leukemias usually disappears quickly after induction chemotherapy if the patient achieves complete remission and may reappear at relapse. If the patients do not achieve remission, they may present with respiratory failure due to fluid accumulation, necessitating local treatment of the pleural disease. This treatment involves intrapleural chemotherapy, pleurodesis, or frequent drainage (30,77,78).

III. Bone Marrow Transplantation

Serous effusions are rare complications of bone marrow transplantation (BMT) and result mainly from infections or tumor relapse (79). In the remaining patients with pleural effusion after bone marrow transplantation, acute or chronic graft-versus-host disease (GVHD) is the most common cause (80–82). In these cases CD8+/HLA-DR+ lymphocytes with CD57 expression predominate in the fluid (80). Other causes include the conditioning regimens with high-dose cytotoxic drugs or total body irradiation, posttransplant veno-occlusive disease, and capillary-leakage syndrome (83–87).

A distinguishable entity called posttransplantation lymphoproliferative disorder has been associated with the reactivation of EBV or cytomegalovirus (CMV) infection. This condition is accompanied by pleural effusion and sometimes by CD4+ lymphocyte expansion. It is a serious and sometimes fatal complication in these patients, who usually are resistant to immunosuppressive therapy (81).

Capillary leakage syndrome occurs frequently after bone marrow transplantation in addition to GVHD and infections. The underlying pathophysiology is poorly understood, but the clinical manifestations of excessive weight gain, ascites, and edema associated with kidney and liver abnormalities suggest tissue injury in multiple organs. About 50% of allogeneic or autologous transplant recipients develop noncardiogenic pulmonary edema with or without pleural effusions; half of them are accompanied by hepatic dysfunction or renal dysfunction or central nervous system abnormalities. These observations suggest that circulating leukocytes may play a role in the development of the syndrome (84,85).

Hepatic veno-occlussive disease (VOD) following bone marrow transplantation is associated with high-dose combination cytoreductive therapy during conditioning. Experimental models have suggested that drug-induced injury to hepatic sinusoidal endothelial cells is involved in the pathogenesis. About 50%

of patients with VOD develop pleural fluid. VOD nearly always resolves after treatment (86).

IV. Myelodysplastic Syndromes

Pleural effusions in myelodysplastic syndromes (MDS) are rare and, as in most hemopoietic diseases, is a consequence of infections. Rarely, pleural infiltration with the malignant clone is observed especially during transformation to acute leukemia. Immune disorders are observed in MDS patients with increased frequency but are rarely accompanied by pleural effusion. These cases display systemic vasculitis or eosinophilic infiltration of the lung as the underlying cause (88,89).

V. Chronic Leukemias

In chronic leukemias the incidence of effusions, although rare, is higher than in acute leukemias (90–105). In chronic lymphocytic leukemia (CLL) the most common cause of pleural effusion is pleural infiltration. These infiltrations may predispose to the transformation to more aggressive lymphoid neoplasms such as Richter's syndrome and prolymphocytic transformation (93). In CLL the fluid may be hemorrhagic or not and contains numerous lymphocytes identical to those in the blood and bone marrow.

Lymphocytic pleural effusions, cytologically indistinguishable from those in CLL, are well recognized in tuberculous and other nonneoplastic conditions (22,97). Small lymphocytic infiltrations of the pleura are difficult to evaluate histopathologically. Usually, involvement of the pleura in B-CLL may lead to increased proportion of B cells in the pleural effusion with light-chain class restriction and monoclonal IgG heavy-chain rearrangements (98). In most reactive pleural effusions, T cells predominate and a small proportion of polyclonal B cells may be found. A high proportion of T cells, with monoclonal TCR rearrangements, may be found in T-cell neoplasms. Although some investigators suggest that the study of clonality and immunocytochemistry could provide a definite diagnosis, there are case reports where neoplastic infiltration by B-CLL leads to a reactive pleural effusion with predominant polyclonal T cells (96,98).

It is difficult to elucidate the precise pathophysiology of effusion development in each case. Increased lymphatic permeability associated with an active inflammatory type response, pleural lymphatic obstruction, or more central mediastinal nodal involvement resulting in lymphatic obstruction or obstruction of the thoracic duct with chylothoraces and changes induced by other therapies may be possible mechanisms of effusion development. In cases with reactive effusions, cytotoxic T cells predominate, suggesting a possible antitumor effect of these cells (91,92,95,96).

In chronic myelocytic leukemia (CML) and chronic myelomonocytic leukemia (CMML), the most common cause of pleural effusions is extramedullary hemopoiesis, although pleura is the most uncommon site of extramedullary hemopoiesis in these patients (100–105). Hemopoiesis resembles that of the bone marrow. All the three hemopoietic lineages are present, and the degree of maturation is similar to that of the bone marrow. In Philadelphia-positive cases the Philadelphia chromosome is detected in the pleural granulocytic cells by conventional cytogenetics and FISH method (102–104). In some cases the extramedullary hemopoiesis consists of normal hemopoietic tissue only. In some other cases, pleural effusion is due to CML development in the pleura. In the latter case, the predominant cells are mature and immature granulocytes, monocytes, and variable numbers of blasts. The leukemic population is accompanied by variable numbers of reactive lymphocytes, macrophages, and activated mesothelial cells. The differential diagnosis usually presents difficulties, especially when the proportion of blasts is low. The fluid is usually hemorrhagic. Leukocyte alkaline phosphatase, known to be low in CML granulocytes in peripheral blood, has been reported to be normal in leukemic granulocytes of pleural effusions in the same patients. Pleural infiltration in CML and CMML sometimes appears shortly before transformation to acute leukemia, and in these cases the pleural effusion contains a greater proportion of myeloblasts (100,102).

In some cases the development of pleural effusions is difficult to explain. Patients with CML and CMML may develop pleural fluid during uncontrolled leukocytosis. These effusions may develop without clinical evidence of extramedullary hemopoiesis or leukemic infiltration and are very responsive to conventional chemotherapy (101). Possible obstruction of pleural capillaries or infiltration of interstitial tissue by leukemic cells, increased capillary permeability due to cytokine production, and other nonspecific mechanisms may be responsible for the development of pleural effusions in these patients (101).

In other myeloproliferative disorders (myelofibrosis, polycythemia), the most common cause of pleuritis, other than infection, is extramedullary hemopoiesis and infiltration at the stage of leukemic transformation (100).

Rare conditions, belonging to chronic hematopoietic neoplasms, may be associated with serosal effusions including pleural effusions. Such conditions include systemic mastocytosis, chronic eosinophilic leukemia, and chronic granulocytic leukemia. The effusions in these patients are due to infiltration of the pleura with malignant cells or are reactive with predominantly macrophages, mesothelial cells, and T lymphocytes (70,106,107).

VI. Pleural Effusions Related to the Treatment of Hematological Malignancies

All-*trans*-retinoic acid (ATRA) is a differentiation agent that can induce complete remission in acute promyelocytic leukemia (APL). Unfortunately, about 50% of patients treated with ATRA may develop a life-threatening complication of uncertain pathogenesis (108). The main clinical signs are respiratory distress, fever, pulmonary infiltrates, weight gain, pleural effusion, renal failure, pericardial effusion, cardiac failure, edema, thromboembolic events, and hypotension. Some patients require mechanical ventilation or dialysis. The lung disease has been ascribed to infiltration of the parenchyma with leukemic or maturing myeloid cells to pulmonary capillaritis and pleuritis. The incidence of death in ATRA syndrome is 1.2% of the total APL patients treated with ATRA, but its occurrence has been associated with shorter remission duration and overall survival. The development of pleural effusion in most cases is of undetermined etiology. Pleural infiltration or pleural inflammation is sometimes the case (108–113).

Other chemotherapeutic regimens have been reported to induce pleural effusion in leukemia patients. High-dose regimens of cytosino-arabinoside, cyclophosphamide, and busulfan and other megatherapies have been reported to be associated with pleural effusions of undetermined pathophysiology. Irradiation of the mediastinum or the total body irradiation that is applied for conditioning in bone marrow transplantation is associated with pleural damage that may lead to pleural effusion (83,114). In addition, pleural effusions have rarely been reported after administration of GM-CSF and high-dose antiglobulin therapy (115,116).

VII. Multiple Myeloma

Pleural effusions in multiple myeloma may be due to nephrotic syndrome, pulmonary embolism, congestive heart failure, second neoplasms, and infiltration by the myeloma cells. In a large series of 958 multiple myeloma patients (117), 58 developed pleural effusions of various etiologies. In only 6 of them was the effusion attributed to infiltration by the myeloma. In other reports the incidence of myelomatous pleural effusions is estimated to be <1% (118). Almost the whole remaining literature consists of case reports of various types of multiple myelomas or plasmatocytomas infiltrating the pleura. IgA multiple myeloma is responsible for 80% of the cases of multiple myeloma pleural effusions in the literature (119–124).

In most cases the effusion contains numerous plasma cells secreting monoclonal immunoglobulin (M-component). M-component is identified in the cell free effusion and is identical to that identified in the serum of the patients. Plasma cells in the effusion are also identical, in morphology and kinetics, to those of the bone marrow of the patients. In rare cases of nonsecreting myeloma, M-component is not found in the effusion. In these cases the differential diagnosis from lymphomas and undifferentiated carcinomas is normally easy based on cell morphology and immunocytochemistry. In light-chain myeloma, immunoelectrophoresis of the pleural fluid reveals light chains. Immunocytochemistry and molecular biology may also be helpful (118–124).

A well-recognized complication of multiple myeloma is amyloidosis. Amyloidosis may also present as a complication of other chronic diseases or as the primary type. In exceptional cases, where amyloidosis involves the pleura, an effusion may develop with transudative or exudative features without any characteristic cell type. Diagnosis is made by pleuroscopy and pleural biopsy (125,126).

Waldenström's macroglobulinemia is a rare disorder with lymphoplasmacytic monoclonal proliferation and a high amount of monoclonal IgM immunoglobulin. In rare cases of pleural involvement, lymphoid and plasmatocytoid cells are found in the effusion and monoclonal IgM immunoglobulin in the cell free fluid (127).

VIII. Thalassemias

Thalassemia major is characterized by severe anemia that needs to be treated with regular transfusions (124). In homozygous β-thalassemia, anemia develops at about the sixth month after birth because until then fetal hemoglobin (Hb F) effectively replaces hemoglobin A (Hb A). In homozygous α-thalassemia (with four genes affected), severe anemia is obvious at 16 weeks gestational age leading to hydrops fetalis and intrauterine death in most cases. In less severe cases, with nonzero homozygous α-thalassemia, the child may develop hydrops with bilateral pleural and ascitic effusions and grow further even until birth. Today with prenatal diagnosis of thalassemia in areas with high prevalence of the disease, cases with hydrops fetalis due to thalassemia are very rarely seen. In hemoglobinopathy H, a variety of α-thalassemia with three α genes affected, the symptoms of anemia are obvious at birth (128). In β-thalassemia major, chronic anemia and iron overload lead to cardiovascular damage and insufficiency. In addition, viral infections (HCV, HBV) together with iron overload may lead to liver insufficiency. Heart and liver insufficiency with hypoalbuminemia are the most common causes of transudative effusions in these patients. Other possible cause of effusions in these patients are venous compression by extramedullary hemopoiesis in the mediastinum, extramedullary hemopoietic tumors in the lung with parapneumonic transudates, and direct infiltration of the pleura by hemopoietic masses producing exudates with erythropoietic precursors in the fluid (129–136). Some microorganisms grow preferentially in iron-rich environments producing infections in these patients at a higher frequency. Effusions may develop during the course of these infections (130,137).

Sickle cell disease is a common disorder in special communities. Sickle cell crisis, a predominant feature of this disease, may be accompanied by pleural effusion because of pulmonary infarction and/or subsequent infections (137–139).

IX. Anemias and Coagulation Disorders

In severe anemias (like megaloblastic anemia or aplastic anemia), cardiac failure is a cause of pleural effusion. Infections are also a common cause of effusions in many anemias such as Fanconi's anemia, hereditary spherocytosis, other red cell membrane disorders, aplastic anemia, autoimmune anemias treated with corticosteroids, etc. In these cases treatment of the underlying cause leads to improvement of the effusion. Pleural effusions in coagulation disorders are almost always due to hemothorax (140-143).

References

1. Elis A, Blickstein D, Mulchanov I, Manor Y, Radnay J, Shapiro H, Lishner M. Pleural effusion in patients with non-Hodgkin's lymphoma: a case control study. Cancer 1998; 83:1607-1611.
2. Johnston WW. The malignant pleural effusion. A review of cytopatologic diagnosis of 584 specimens from 472 consecutive patients. Cancer 1985; 56:905-909.
3. Yasuda H, Nakao M, Kanemasa H, Ueha T, Mori T, Fujino H, Oishi T, Ohta M, Inada Y, Tanigawa H, Horiike S, Yokota S, Misawa S, Kashima K. T-cell lymphoma presenting with pericardial and pleural effusion as the initial and primary lesion: cytogenetic and molecular evidence. Intern Med 1996; 35:150-154.
4. Raina V, Boyd G, Soukop M. Longstanding pleural effusion in an elderly man due to non-Hodgkin's lymphoma (multilobulated nuclear cell type). Aust NZ J Med 1990; 20:826-827.
5. Mizuki M, Ueda S, Tagawa S, Shibayama H, Nishimori Y, Shibano M, Asada H, Tanaka m, Nagata S, Koudera U, Suzuki K, Machii T, Ohsawa M, Aozasa K, Kitani Y. Natural killer-cell derived large granular lymphocyte lymphoma of lung developed in a patient with hypersensitivity to mosquito bites and reactivated Epstein-Barr virus infection. Am J Hematol 1998; 59:309-315.
6. Suster S, Moran CA. Pleomorphic large cell lymphoma of the mediastinum. Am J Surg Pathol 1996; 20:224-232.
7. Dunphy CH, Collins B, Ramos R, Grosso LE. Secondary pleural involvement by an AIDS related anaplastic large cell (CD30+) lymphoma simulating metastatic adenocarcinoma. Diagn Cytopathol 1998; 18:113-117.
8. Patriarcha F, Ermacora A, Skert C. Pleural involvement in a case of monocytoid B-cell lymphoma. Haematologica 1999; 84:949-950.
9. Kodama K, Yokose T, Takahashi K, Minami H, Nagai K, Matsuno Y, Nishiwaki Y, Ochiai A. Low-grade B-cell lymphoma of mucosa-associated lymphoid tissue in the lung: a report of a case with pleural dissemination. Lung Cancer 1999; 24:175-178.
10. Siegert W, Nerl C, Agthe A, Engelhard M, Brittinger G, Tiemann M, Lennert K, Huhn D. Angioimmunoblastic lymphadenopathy (AILD)-type-T cell lymphoma: prognostic impact of clinical observations and laboratory findings at presentation. The Kiel Lymphoma Study Group. Ann Oncol 1995; 6:659-664.
11. Shepherd SF, A'Hern RP, Pinkerton CR. Childhood T-cell lymphoblastic lymphoma. Does early resolution of mediastinal mass predict for final outcome? The United Kingdom Children's Cancer Study Group (UKCCSG). Br J Cancer 1995; 72:752-756.
12. Naschitz JE, Lazarow N, Yeshurun D. Unilateral chest wall edema with associated pleural effusion: unusual sign of primary retroperitoneal lymphoma. Lymphology 1984; 17:34-36.

13. Berkman N, Breuer R, Kramer MR, Polliack A. Pulmonary involvement in lymphoma. Leuk Lymphoma 1996; 20:237–299.
14. Snalund JT, Crist WM, Abromowitch M, Fairclogh D, Berard CW, Rafferty M, Pui CH. Pleural effusion is associated with a poor outcome in stage III small non-cleaved cell lymphoma. Leukemia 1991; 5:71–74.
15. Moriki T, Wada M, Takahashi T, Ueda S, Miyazaki E. Pleural effusion cytology in a case of cytophagic histiocytic panniculitis (subcutaneous panniculitic T-cell lymphoma). A case report. Acta Cytol 2000; 44:1040–1044.
16. Bangerter M, Hildebrand A, Griesshammer M. Combined cytomorphologic and immunophenotypic analysis in the diagnostic workup of lymphomatous effusions. Acta Cytol 2001; 45:307–312.
17. Gulzman J, Bross KJ, Costabel U. Malignant lymphoma in pleural effusions: an immunohistochemical cell surface analysis. Diagn Cytopathol 1991; 7:113–118.
18. Chagnaud BE, Bonsack TA, Kozakewich HP, Shamberger RC. Pleural effusions in lymphoblastic lymphoma: a diagnostic alternative. J Pediatr Surg 1998; 33:1355–1357.
19. Rondriguez-Garcia JL, Frail G, Moreno MA, Sanchez-Corral JA, Penalver R. Recurrent massive pleural effusion as a late complication of radiotherapy in Hodgkin's disease. Chest 1991; 100:1165–1166.
20. Bishop PC, Elwood PC. Images in clinical medicine. Chylous effusion in Hodgkin's disease. N Engl J Med 1998; 339:1515.
21. Van Renterghem DM, Pauwels RA. Chylothorax and pleural effusions as a late complications of thoracic irradiation. Chest 1995; 108:884–886.
22. Valdes L, Alvarez D, Valle JM, Pose A, San Jose E. The etiology of pleural effusions in an area with high incidence of tuberculosis. Chest 1996; 109:158–162.
23. Sakemi T, Uchida M, Ikeda Y, Shouno Y. Acute renal failure and nephrotic syndrome in a patient with T-cell lymphoma. Nephron 1996; 72:326–327.
24. Collins J, Muller NL, Leung AN, McGuinness G, Mergo PJ, Flint JD, Warner TF, Poirier C, Theodore J, Zander D, Yee HT. Epstein-Barr-virus associated lymphoproliferative disease of the lung: CT and histological findings. Radiology 1998; 208:749–759.
25. Ooi GC, Chim CS, Lie AK, Tsang KW. Computed tomography features of primary pulmonary non-Hodgkin's lymphoma. Clin Radiol 1999; 54:438–443.
26. Ray P, Antoine M, Mary-Krause M, Lebrette MG, Wislez M, Duvivier C, Meyoha MC, Girard PM, Mayaud C, Cadranel J. AIDS-related primary pulmonary lymphoma. Am J Respir Crit Care Med 1998; 158:1221–1229.
27. Bazot M, Cadranel J, Benayoun S, Tassart M, Bigot JM, Carette MF. Primary pulmonary AIDS-related lymphoma: radiographic and CT findings. Chest 1999; 11:1282–1286.
28. Aquino SL, Chen MY, Kuo WT, Chiles C. The CT appearance of pleural and extrapleural disease in lymphoma. Clin Radiol 1999; 54:647–650.
29. Moritani T, Aihara T, Oguma E, Shimanuki Y, Oishi T, Hanada R. Spectrum of Epstein-Barr virus infection in Japanese children. A pictorial essay. Clin Imaging 2001; 25:1–8.
30. Das DK, Chowdhury V, Kishore B, Chachra K, Bhatt NC, Kakar AK. CD-30 (Ki-1)-positive anaplastic large cell lymphoma in a pleural effusion. Case report with diagnosis by cytomorphologic and immunocytochemical studies. Acta Cytol 1999; 43:498–502.
31. Bangerter M, Hildebrand A, Griesshammer M. Immunophenotypic analysis of

simultaneous specimens from different sites of the same patient with malignant lymphoma. Cytopathology 2001; 12:168–176.
32. Ohori NP, Whisnant RE, Nalesnik MA, Swerdlow SH. Primary pleural effusion post-transplant lymphoproliferative disorder: distinction from secondary involvement and effusion lymphoma. Diagn Cytopathol 2001; 25:50–53.
33. Pietsch JB, Whitlock JA, Ford C, Kinney MC. Management of pleural effusions in children with malignant lymphoma. J Pediatr Surg 1999; 34:635–638.
34. Sahn SA. Malignancy metastatic to the pleura. Clin Chest Med 1998; 19:351–361.
35. Alifano M, Guggino G, Gentile M, Elia S, Vernaglia A. Management of concurrent pleural effusion in patients with lymphoma: thoracoscopy a useful tool in diagnosis and treatment. 1031 Monaldi Arch Chest Dis 1997; 52:330–334.
36. Laurini JA, Garcia A, Elsner B, Belloti M, Rescia C. Relation between natural killer cells and neoplastic cells in serious fluids. Diagn Cytopathol; 22: 347–350.
37. Green LK, Griffin J. Increased natural killer cells in fluids. A new, sensitive means of detecting carcinoma. Acta Cytol 1996; 40:1240–1245.
38. Matolsky A, Nador RG, Cesarman E, Knowles DM. Immunoglobulin VH gene mutational analysis suggests that primary effusion lymphomas derive from different stages of B cell maturation. Am J Pathol 1998; 153:1609–1614.
39. Gaidano G, Carbone A, Dalla-Favera R. Pathogenesis of AIDS-related lymphomas: molecular and histogenetic heterogeneity. Am J Pathol 1998; 152:623–630.
40. Falzetti D, Crescenzi B, Matteuci C, Falini B, Martelli MF, Van Den Berghe H, Mecucci C. Genomic instability and recurrent breakpoints are main cytogenetic findings in Hodgkin's disease. Haematologica 1999; 84:298–305.
41. Drexler HG, Uphoff CC, Gaidano G, Carbone A. Lymphoma cell lines: in vitro models for the study of HHV-8(+) primary effusion lymphomas (body cavity-based lymphomas). Leukemia 1998; 12:1507–1517.
42. Peterson IM, Raible M. Malignant pleural effusion in Hodgkin's lymphoma. Report of a case with immunoperoxidase studies. Acta Cytol 1991; 35:300–305.
43. Afessa B. Pleural effusions and pneumothoraces in AIDS. Curr Opin Pulm Med 2001; 7:202–209.
44. Karadeniz C, Guven MA, Ruacan S, Demirbilek S, Sagbil S, Akhan O. Primary pleural lymphoma: an unusual presentation of childhood non-Hodgkin lymphoma. Pediatr Hematol Oncol 2000; 17:695–699.
45. Iwahashi M, Iida S, Sako S, Inoue S, Kikuchi H, Otsuka E, Nasu M. Primary effusion lymphoma with B-cell phenotype. Am J Hematol 2000; 64:317–318.
46. Casado Farinas I, Alonso Martin MJ, Gomez Aguado F, Picazo Talavera A, Corcuera Pindado MT, Blanco Quintana F. Primary effusion lymphoma associated with type-8 human herpes virus infection. Ann Med Interna 2000; 17:366–368.
47. Ferrozi F, Tognini G, Mulonzia NW, Bova D, Pavone P. Primary effusion lymphomas in AIDS: CT findings in two cases. Eur Radiol 2001; 11:623–625.
48. Ascoli V, Siriani MC, Mezzaroma I, Mastroianni CM, Vullo V, Andreoni M, Narciso P, Scalzo CC, Nardi F, Pistilli A, Lo Coco F. Human herpesvirus-8 in lymphomatous and nonlymphomatous body cavity effusions developing in Kaposi's sarcoma and multicentric Castelman's disease. Ann Diagn Pathol 1999; 3:357–363.
49. Ibrahimbacha A, Farah M, Saluza J. An HIV-infected patient with pleural effusion. Chest 1999; 116:1113–1115.
50. Nador RG, Cesarman E, Chadburn A, Dawson DB, Ansari MQ, Sald J, Knowles DM. Primary effusion lymphoma: a distinct clinicopathologic entity associated with Kaposi's sarcoma-associated herpes virus. Blood 1996; 88:645–656.

51. Light RW, Hamm H. Pleural disease and acquired immune deficiency syndrome. Eur Respir J 1997; 10:2638–2643.
52. Ascoli V, Mastroianni CM, Galati V, Sirianni MC, Fruscalzo A, Pistilli A, Lo Coco F. Primary effusion lymphoma containing human herpesvirus 8 DNA in two AIDS patients with Kaposi's sarcoma. Haematologica 1998; 83:8–12.
53. Beck JM. Pleural disease in patients with acquired immune deficiency syndrome. Clin Chest Med 1998; 19:341–349.
54. Lacost V, Judde JG, Bestett G, Cadranel J, Antoine M, Valensi F, Delabesse E, Macintyre E, Gessain A. Virological and molecular characterization of a new B lymphoid cell line, established from an AIDS patient with primary effusion lymphoma, harboring both KSHV/HHV8 and EBV viruses. Luk Lymph 2000; 38:401–409.
55. Perez MT, Cabanello-Inchausti B, Viamonte M Jr, Nixon D. Pleural body cavity-based lymphoma. Ann Diagn Pathol 1998; 2:127–134.
56. Vince A, Begovac J, Kessler H, Rabenau HF, Poljiak M, Siftar Z, Zidovec S, Jeren T. AIDS-related body cavity-based lymphoma. A case report. Acta Cytol 2001; 45:420–424.
57. Lankester KJ, Lishman S, Ayliffe U, Kocjan G, Spittle MF, Miller RF. Primary effusion lymphoma and Kaposi's sarcoma in an HIV-infected man. Int J STD AIDS 1998; 9:616–618.
58. Arvanitakis L, Mesri EA, Nador RG, Said JW, Asch AS, Knowles DM, Cesarman E. Establishment and characterization of a primary effusion (body cavity - based) lymphoma cell line (BC-3) harboring Kaposi's sarcoma-associated herpes virus (KSHV/HHV-8) in the absence of Epstein-Barr virus. Blood 1996; 88:2648–2654.
59. Kuwabara H, Nagai m, Shibanushi T, Ohmori M, Kawakami K, Asakura H. CD138-positive and Kaposi's sarcoma-associated herpesvirus (KSHV)-negative B-cell lymphoma with serosal spreading of the body cavity and lymphadenopathy: an autopsy case. Human Pathol 2000; 31:1171–1175.
60. Carbone A, Cilia AM, Gloghini A, Canzonieri V, Pastore C, Todesco M, Cozzi M, Perin T, Volpe R, Pinto A, Gaidano G. Establishment of HHV-8-positive and HHV-8-negative lymphoma cell lines from primary lymphomatous effusions. Int J Cancer 1997; 73:562–569.
61. Hocqueloux L, Agbalika F, Oksenhendler E, Molina JM. Long-term remission of an AIDS-related primary effusion lymphoma with antiviral therapy. AIDS 2001; 26:15: 280–282.
62. O'Donovan M, Silva I, Uhlam V, Bermingham N, Luttich K, Martin C, Sheils O, Killalea A, Kenny C, Pileri S, O'Leary JJ. Expression profile of human herpesvirus 8 (HHV-8) in pyothorax associated lymphoma and in effusion lymphoma. Mol Pathol 2001; 54:80–85.
63. Zhang SF, Guo BY, Wang HL. Clinicopathologic changes in leukemic lung lesions. Zhonghua Nei Ke Za Zhi 1994; 33:99–102.
64. Mitchel CD, Gordon I, Chessells JM. Clinical, haematological, and radiological features in T-cell lymphoblastic malignancy in childhood. Clin Radiol 1986; 37:257–261.
65. Rege K, Powles C, Norton J, Malendra P, Mitchel P, Agrawal S, Metha J, Treleaven J. An unusual presentation of acute myeloid leukemia with pericardial and pleural effusions due to granulocytic sarcoma. Leuk Lymph 1993; 11:305–307.
66. Saha PK, Agrawal BV, Mishra SK, Vaish SK, Agrawal SK. Pleuropericardial

effusion: a presenting manifestation of acute myeloblastic leukemia. Indian Heart J 1977; 29:165–169.
67. Mital OP, Sacham AS, Singh RP, Katiyar SK, Nath N. Acute myelogenous leukemia presenting as massive pleural effusion. Indian J Chest Dis 1975; 17:179–181.
68. Fukushima Y, Miyakumi T, Yoshida K, Miura AB, Watanuki T. Pleural effusion in a case of plasma cell leukemia after undergoing simple total hysterectomy for uterine cervical carcinoma. Review of multiple myeloma and plasma cell leukemia effusion in Japan. Rinsko Ketsueki 1987; 28:1424–1429.
69. Mufti GJ, Oscier DG, Hamblin TJ, Nightingale A, Darlow S. Serous effusions in monocytic leukemias. Br J Hematol 1984; 58:547–552.
70. Yam LT. Granulocytic sarcoma with pleural involvement. Identification of neoplastic cells with cytometry. Acta Cytol 1985; 29:63–66.
71. Dix DB, Anderson RA, McFadden DE, Wadsworth LD. Pleural relapse during hemopoietic remission in childhood acute lymphoblastic leukemia. J Pediatr Hematol Oncol 1997; 19:470–472.
72. Igarashi T, Shimizu S, Morishita K, Ohtsu T, Itoh K, Minami H, Fujii H, Sasaki Y, Mukai K. Acute myelogenous leukemia with monosomy 7, inv(3)(q21q26) involving activated EVI 1 gene occurring after a complete remission of lymphoblastic lymphoma: a case report. Jpn J Clin Oncol 1998; 28:688–695.
73. Bouronchle BA. Unusual presentations and complications of hairy cell leukemia. Leukemia 1987; 1:288–293.
74. Takasugi JE, Godwin JD, Marglin SI, Petersdorf SH. Intrathoracic granulocytic sarcomas. J Thor Imaging 1996; 11:223–230.
75. Scmetzer HM, Williams W, Gerhartz HH. Detection of acute myeloid leukemia cells in complete remission and in extramedullary sites by clonal analysis. Acta Haematol 1996; 96:83–87.
76. Shimoyama M. Diagnostic criteria and classification of clinical subtypes of adult T-cell leukemia-lymphoma. A report from the Lymphoma Study Group (1984-87). Br J Haematol 1991; 79:428–437.
77. Aasebo U, Norum J, Sager G, Slordal L. Intrapleurally instilled mitoxanthrone in metastatic pleural effusions: a phase II study. J Chemother 1997; 9:106–111.
78. Bronner GM, Baas P, Beijnen JH. Pleurodesis in malignant pleural effusion. Ned Tijdschr Geneeskd 1997; 141:1810–1814.
79. Ueda T, Manabe A, Kikuchi A, Yoshino H, Ebihara Y, Ishii T, Yagasaki H, Mitsui T, Hisakawa H, Masunaga A, Tsuji K, Nakahata T. Massive pericardial and pleural effusion with anasarca following allogeneic bone marrow transplantation. Int J Hematol 2000; 71:394–397.
80. Lechapt-zalcman E, Rieux C, Cordonnier C, Desvaux D. Post-transplantation lymphoproliferative disorder mimicking nonspecific lymphocytic pleural effusion in a bone marrow transplant recipient. A case report. Acta Cytol 1999; 43:239–242.
81. Hashino S, Mori A, Kobayashi S, Tanaka J, Musashi M, Asaka M, Immanura M. Proliferation of CD4+ Lymphocytes in a patient with chronic graft-versus-host disease after allogeneic bone marrow transplantation. Int J Hematol 2000; 71:389–393.
82. Seber A, Khan SP, Kersey JH. Unexplained effusions: association with allogeneic bone marrow transplantation and acute or chronic graft-versus-host disease. Bone Marrow Transplant 1996; 17:207–211.
83. Schaap N, Raymakers R, Schattenberg A, Ottevanger JP, de Witte T. Massive

pleural effusion attributed to high-dose cyclophosphamide during conditioning for BMT. Bone Marrow Transplant 1996; 18:247–248.
84. Cahill RA, Spitzer TR, Mazumder A. Marrow engraftment and clinical manifestations of capillary leak syndrome. Bone Marrow Transplant 1996; 18:177–184.
85. Oeda E, Shinohara K, Kamei S, Nomiyama J, Inoue H. Capillary leak syndrome likely the result of granulocyte colony stimulating factor after high-dose chemotherapy. Intern Med 1994; 33:115–119.
86. Ozkaynak MF, Weinberg K, Kohn D, Sender L, Parkman R, Lenarsky C. Hepatic veno-occlusive disease post-bone marrow transplantation in children conditioned with busulphan and cyclophosphamide: incidence risk factors, and clinical outcome. Bone Marrow Transplant 1991; 7:467–474.
87. Veys PA, McAvinchery R, Rothman MT, Mair GH, Newland AC. Pericardial effusion following conditioning for bone marrow transplantation in acute leukemia. Bone Marrow Transpl 1987; 2:213–216.
88. Hicsonmez G, Tuncer AM, Sayli T, Guler E, Cetin M, Ozbek N, Mufti GJ. High-dose methylprednisolone, low-dose cytosine arabinoside, and mitoxanthrone in children with myelodysplastic syndromes. Hematol Pathol 1995; 9:185–193.
89. Matsushima T, Murakami H, Kim K, Uchiumi H, Murata N, Tamura J, Sawamura M, Karasawa M, Naruse T, Tsuchiya J. Steroid-responsive pulmonary disorders associated with myelodysplastic syndromes with der(1q; 7p) chromosomal abnormality. Am J Hematol 1995; 50:110–115.
90. Bourantas KL, Tsiara S, Panteli A, Milionis C, Christou L. Pleural effusion in chronic myelomonocytic leukemia. Acta Hematolol 1998; 99:34–37.
91. Sivakumaran M, Qureshi H, Chapman CS. Chylous effusions in CLL. Leuk Lymphoma 1995; 18:365–366.
92. Andrieu V, Encaoua R, Carbon C, Couvelard A, Grange MJ. Leukemic pleural effusion in B-cell prolymphocytic leukemia. Hematol Cell Ther 1998; 40:275–278.
93. Shimoni A, Shvidel L, Shtalrid M, Klepfish A, Berrebi A. Prolymphocytic transformation of B-chronic lymphocytic leukemia presenting as malignant ascites and pleural effusion. Am J Hematol 1998; 59:316–318.
94. Jacobson RJ, Jacobson HJ, Derman DP. Leukemic involvement of the pleura. A case report. S Afr Med J 1977; 52:938–940.
95. Horn KD, Penchansky L. Chylous pleural effusions simulating leukemic infiltrate associated with thoracoabdominal disease and surgery in infants. Am J Clin Pathol 1999; 111:99–104.
96. Ben-Gherit E, Assaf Y, Shnar E. Predominant T-cells in pleural effusion of a patient with B-cell CLL. Acta Hematol 1985; 73:101–103.
97. Cooper C, Watts EJ, Smith AG. Salmonella septicemia and pleural effusion as presenting features of hairy cell leukemia. Br J Clin Pract 1987; 41:670–671.
98. Miyahara M, Shimamoto Y, Sano M, Nakano K, Matsuzaki. Immunoglobulin gene rearrangement in T-cell-rich reactive pleural effusion of a patient with B-cell chronic lymphocytic leukemia. Acta Haematol 1996; 96:41–44.
99. Bouronch BA. Unusual presentations and complications of hairy cell leukemia. Leukemia 1987; 1:288–293.
100. Chubachi A, Wakui H, Miura I, Saitoh M, Nishinary T, Nishimura S, Miura AB. Extramedullary megakaryoblastic tumors following an indolent phase of myelofibrosis. Leuk Lymphoma 1995; 17:351–354.
101. Hicsonmez G, Cetin M, Tunc B, Tuncer AM, Gumruk F, Yenicesu I. Dramatic

resolution of pleural effusion in children with chronic myelomonocytic leukemia following short-course high-dose methylprednisolone. Leuk Lymphoma 1998; 29: 617–623.
102. Bourantas KL, Repousis P, Tsiara S, Christou L, Konstantinidou P, Bai M. Chronic myelogenous leukemia terminating in acute megakaryoblasting leukemia. Case report. J Exp Clin Cancer Res 1998; 17:234–235.
103. Lancon JP, Charve P, Favre JP, Caillaux D. Pleural myeloid metaplasia revealing chronic myelogenous leukemia. Crit Care Med 1986; 14:834–835.
104. Mohapatra MK, Das SP, Mohanty NC, Dash PC, Bastia BK. Hemopericardium with cardiac tamponade and pleural effusion in chronic myeloid leukemia. Indian Heart J 2000; 52:209–211.
105. De Renzo A, Micera V, Vaglio S, Luciano L, Selleri C, Rotoli B. Induction of alkaline phosphatase activity in chronic myeloid leukemia cells: in vitro studies and speculative hypothesis. Am J Hematol 1990; 35:278–280.
106. Petit A, Pulik M, Gaulier A, Lionnet F, Mahe A, Sigal M. Systemic mastocytosis associated with chronic myelomonocytic leukemia: clinical features and response to interferon alpha therapy. J Am Acad Dermatol 1995; 32:850–853.
107. Farrell SA, Warda LJ, LaFlair P, Szymonowicz W. Adams-Oliver syndrome: a case with juvenile chronic myelogenous leukemia and chylothorax. Am J Med Genet 1993; 47:1175–1179.
108. Davis BA, Cervi P, Amin Z, Moshi G, Shaw P, Porter J. Retinoic acid syndrome: pulmonary computed tomography (CT) findings. Leuk Lymph 1996; 23:113–117.
109. Schaap N, Raymakers R, Schattenberg A, Ottevanger JP, de Witte E. Massive pleural effusion attributed to high dose cyclophosphamide during conditioning for BMT. Bone Marrow Transplant 1996; 18:247–248.
110. Camacho LH, Soignet SL, Chanel S, Heller G, Scheinberg DA, Ellison, Warrell RP. Leukocytosis and the retinoic acid syndrome in patients with acute promyelocytic leukemia treated with arsenic trioxide. J Clin Oncol 2000; 18:2620–2625.
111. Tallman MS, Andersen JW, Schiffer CA, Appelbaum FR, Feusner JH, Ogden A, Shepher L, Rowe JM, Francois C, Larson RS, Wiernik PH. Clinical description of 44 patients with acute promyelocytic leukemia who developed retinoic acid syndrome. Blood 2000; 95:90–95.
112. Nicolls MR, Terada LS, Tuder RM, Prindiville SA, Schwarz MS. Diffuse alveolar hemorrhage with underlying pulmonary capillaritis in the retinoic acid syndrome. Am J Respir Crit Care Med 1998; 158:1302–1305.
113. De Botton S, Dombret H, Sanz M, Miguel JS, Caillot D, Zittoun R, Gardenbas M, Stamatoulas A, Conde E, Guerci A, Gardin C, Geiser K, Mackhoul DC, Rema O, de la Serna J, Lefrere F, Chomienne C, Chastang C, Degos L, Fenaux P. Incidence, clinical features, and outcome of all trans-retinoic acid syndrome in 413 cases of newly diagnosed acute promyelocytic leukemia. The European APL Group. Blood 1998; 92:2712–2718.
114. Woods T, Vidarson B, Mosher D, Stein JH. Transient effusive constrictive pericarditis due to chemotherapy. Clin Cardiol 1999; 22:316–318.
115. Sebach J, Speich R, Fehr J, Tuchschmid P, Russi E. GM-CSF induced acute eosinophilic pneumonia. Br J Haematol 1995; 90:963–965.
116. Bolanos-Meade J, Keung YK, Cobos E. Recurrent lymphocytic pleural effusion after intravenous immunoglobulin. Am J Hematol 1999; 60:248–249.

117. Kintzer JS, Rosenow EC, Kyle RA. Thoracic and pulmonary abnormalities in a multiple myeloma. A review of 958 cases. Arch Intern Med 1978; 138:727–730.
118. Elloumi M, Frikha M, Masmoudi H, Maeddi S, Ben Ayed M, Bouaziz M, Makni F, Souissi T. Plasmocytic pleural effusion disclosing multiple myeloma. Rev Mol Respir 2000; 17:495–497.
119. Rodriguez JN, Pereira A, Martinez JC, Conde J, Pujol E. Pleural effusion in multiple myeloma. Chest 1994; 105:622–624.
120. Pacheco A, Perpina A, Eschribano L, Sanz I, Bellas C. Pleural effusion as the first sign of extramedullary plasmatocytoma. Chest 1992; 102:296–297.
121. Palmer HE, Wilson CS, Bardales RH. Cytology and flow cytometry of malignant effusions of multiple myeloma. Diagn Cytopathol 2000; 22:147–151.
122. Manley R, Monteath J, Patton WN. Co-incidental presentation of IgA lambda multiple myeloma and pleural involvement with IgM kappa non-Hodgkin's lymphoma. Clin Lab Haematol 1999; 21:61–63.
123. Nagai K, Ando K, Yoshida H, Kusaka S, Hinuma Y, Hakamata Y, Ishi K, Kume N, Ochi H, Wakatsuki Y, Yokode M, Murakami M, Kita T. Response of the extramedullary lung plasmatocytoma with pleural effusion to chemotherapy. Ann Hematol 1997; 74:279–281.
124. Meoli A, Willsie S, Fiorella R. Myelomatous pleural effusion. South Med J 1997; 90:65–68.
125. Maeno T, Sando Y, Tsukagoshi M, Suga T, Endo M, Seki R, Ooyama Y, Yamagishi T, Kaneko Y, Kanda T, Iwasaki T, Kurabayashi m, Nagai R. Pleural amyloidosis in a patient with intractable pleural effusion and multiple myeloma. Respirology 2000; 5:79–80.
126. Knapp MJ, Roggli VL, Kim J, Moore JO, Shelburn JD. Pleural amyloidosis. Arch Pathol Lab 1988; 112:57–60.
127. Stevenet P, Stevenet A, Helias A, D'Arlhac M, Maurisset O. Pleural manifestations of secondary monoclonal dysproteinemia (apropos of 4 cases). Poumon Coeur 1977; 33:143–148.
128. Weatherall DJ, Higgs DR, Bunch C, Old JM, Hunt DM, Pressley L, Clegg JB, Bethlenfalvay NC, Sjolin S, Koler RD, Magenis E, Francis JL, Bebbington D. Hemoglobin H disease and mental retardation: a new syndrome or a remarkable coincidence? N Engl J Med 1981; 305:607–612.
129. Srair HA, Owa JA, Aman HA, Madan MA. Acute chest syndrome in children with sickle cell disease. Indian J Pediatr 1995; 62(2):201–205. Bilateral pleural effusions in a beta-thalassemia intermediate patient with posterior mediastinal extramedullary hemopoietic masses. Hemoglobin 1999; 23:249–253.
130. Urbaniak-Kujda D, Cielinska S, Kapelko-Slowik K, Mazur G, Bronowicz A. Disseminated nocardiosis as a complication of Evans' syndrome. Ann Hematol 78:385–387.
131. Peng MJ, Kuo HT, Chang MC. A case of intrathoracic extramedullary hematopoiesis with massive pleural effusion: successful pleurodesis with intrapleural minocycline. J Formos Med Assoc 1994; 93:445–447.
132. Longaker MT, Laberge JM, Dansereau J, Langer JC, Crombleholme TM, Callen PW, Golbus MS, Harrison MR. Primary fetal hydrothorax: natural history and management. J Pediatr Surg 1989; 24:573–576.
133. Smoleniec J, James D. Predictive value of pleural effusions in fetal hydrops. Fetal Diagn Ther 1995; 10:95–100.

134. Ries M, Beinder E, Gruner C, Zenker M. Rapid development of hydrops fetalis in the donor twin following death of the recipient twin in twin-twin transfusion syndrome. J Perinat Med 1999; 27:68–73.
135. Tongsong T, Wanapirak C, Srisomboon J, Piyamongkol W, Sirichotiyakul S. Antenatal sonographic features of 100 alpha-thalassemia hydrops fetalis fetusis. J Clin Ultrasound 1996; 24:73–77.
136. Smoleniec J, James D. Predictive value of pleural effusions in fetal hydrops. Fetal Diagn Ther 1995; 10:95–100.
137. Becton DL, Friedman HS, Kurtzberg J, Chaffee S, Falletta JM, Kinney TR. Severe mycoplasma pneumonia in three sisters with sickle cell disease. Pediatr Hematol Oncol 1986; 3:259–265.
138. Oestreich AE. Pleural effusions in sickle cell disease. J Natl Med Assoc 1977; 69:579–580.
139. Dekker A, Graham T, Bupp PA. The occurrence of sickle cells in pleural fluid: report of a patient with sickle cell disease. Acta Cytol 1975; 19:251–254.
140. Butterfield JH, Schwenk NM, Colville DS, Kuipers BJ. Severe generalized reactions to ibuprofen: report of a case. J Rheumatol 1986; 13:649–650.
141. Clark JH, Fitzgerald JG. Hemorrhagic complications of Henoch-Schonlein syndrome. J Pediatr Gastroenterol Nutr 1985; 4:311–315.
142. Oppermann HC, Wille L. Hemothorax in the newborn. Pediatr Radiol 1980; 9:129–134.
143. Levo Y, Pick Al, Avidor I, Ben-Bassat M. Clinicopathological study of a patient with procainamide-induced systemic lupus erythematosus. Ann Rheum Dis 1976; 35:181–185.

34

Pleural Effusions in HIV

KRISTINA CROTHERS and LAURENCE HUANG

University of California, San Francisco
San Francisco, California, U.S.A.

I. Introduction

The approach to the evaluation of a pleural effusion in a human immunodeficiency virus (HIV)–infected patient begins with a differential diagnosis that includes all of the causes of both exudative and transudative pleural effusions found in non–HIV-infected individuals. As in all patients, helpful details in investigating the etiology of a pleural effusion can be obtained from historical and physical exam findings. In particular, duration of illness, symptoms, and other medical problems can provide significant clues as to the underlying process. For example, a pleural effusion in the setting of the acute onset of fever, cough, and purulent sputum would point towards a bacterial parapneumonic process, whereas increasing dyspnea and cough in a patient with cutaneous Kaposi's sarcoma (KS) could suggest pleuropulmonary KS. As in non–HIV-infected individuals, evaluation of concomitant radiographic abnormalities and sampling of pleural fluid are crucial diagnostic steps.

In addition to HIV immune status, the underlying HIV risk factors of the patient and the prevalence of different diseases in the community influence the likelihood of a specific cause of pleural effusion. Certain diagnoses will be more common in specific populations, such as parapneumonic effusion in injection drug users and KS in men who have sex with men (MSM). In areas endemic for *Mycobacterium tuberculosis*, for instance, many more cases of pleural effusion will be caused by tuberculous pleurisy. Therefore, consideration of community, HIV disease state, and risk factors for HIV infection, as well as clinical presentation and concomitant chest radiographic abnormalities, are all integral factors in evaluating the etiology of a pleural effusion in an HIV-infected patient.

This chapter will provide an overview of the epidemiology of pleural effusions in hospitalized HIV-infected patients, general diagnostic procedures, and patient outcomes. Individual causes of exudative pleural effusions, namely infectious and malignant causes, will then be discussed in more detail, followed by a brief review of transudative effusions in HIV-infected patients. Features characteristic of pleural effusions in HIV-infected patients that may be distinct from features seen in HIV-negative patients will be emphasized.

II. Epidemiology of Pleural Effusion in Hospitalized HIV-Infected Patients

In five recent retrospective studies, the prevalence of pleural effusion in hospitalized HIV patients ranged widely, from 1.7 to 27% of all HIV admissions (1–5). The most frequent etiologies are infectious, with the majority of cases parapneumonic in origin. In addition to parapneumonic effusions, tuberculous effusions and malignant effusions due to KS are the three most common causes of pleural effusion in HIV-infected patients (Table 1) (1–9). Other less frequently reported causes of effusion in these descriptive studies of hospitalized HIV patients are processes that can be seen in HIV-negative patients as well, including exudative effusions related to pancreatitis or other intraabdominal processes, pulmonary embolism, or trauma, and transudative effusions related to congestive heart failure, renal failure, or liver disease.

The patient population studied and specific HIV risk factors affect the proportion of various etiologies of pleural effusion. In a study by Afessa, the population of injection drug users was more likely to present with pleural effusion (1). While 21% of patient admissions with the risk factor of injection drug use had pleural effusions, only 7% of admissions with heterosexual contact ($p = 0.0001$) and 10% of admissions with homosexual contact ($p = 0.0097$) had pleural effusion (1). In the population of HIV-infected patients who inject drugs, the most common cause of a pleural effusion is likely to be infectious, given the increased risk for bacterial pneumonia in this population, especially if CD4+ T-cell counts are below 200 cells/μL (10,11). In a large retrospective study from Spain, records of 86 hospitalized HIV-infected patients with a pleural effusion were reviewed (8). Ninety-four percent of the patients were injection drug users, and 54% had AIDS. Overall, 88% of effusions were attributed to infectious causes, and 69% were parapneumonic. In another study from England, 58 consecutive hospitalized HIV-infected admissions with pleural effusion were prospectively evaluated (4). In this study, only 3.4% of patients were injection

Table 1 Causes of Pleural Effusion in Hospitalized HIV-Infected Patients

	Ref. 1	Ref. 4	Ref. 7	Ref. 8	Ref. 2	Ref. 3	Ref. 5	Ref. 6	Ref. 9
No. of patients	160	58	30	86	28	30	59	75	91
Incidence per HIV ADMITS	14.6%	5.6%	NS	NS	7.2%	1.7%	26.6%	NS	NS
Infectious	42%	55%	70%	88%	71%	60%	66%	35%	95%
Parapneumonic	31%	28%	47%	69%	32%	33%	30%	11%	4%
Empyema	1%	—	—	—	—	7%	3%	—	—
M. tuberculosis	6%	14%	3%	17%	21%	20%	9%	12%	90%
P. carinii	3%	10%	—	2%	7%	—	15%	1%	—
Noninfectious	38%	45%	30%	6%	29%	27%	31%	47%	6%
Malignancy	6%	40%	30%	1%	25%	10%	2%	47%	4%
KS	1%	33%	10%	—	7%	7%	2%	43%	3%
Lymphoma	1%	7%	17%	1%	14%	—	—	3%	1%
Lung cancer	3%	—	3%	—	3%	3%	—	1%	—
CHF	3%	2%	—	1%	3%	—	5%	—	—
Renal insufficiency	9%	—	—	1%	—	10%	2%	—	—
Liver failure	3%	—	—	2%	—	—	—	—	—
Hypoalbuminemia	8%	—	—	—	—	—	19%	—	—
Other[a]	9%	3%	—	—	—	7%	5%	—	1%
Unknown etiology	21%	—	—	6%	—	10%	3%	19%	—

NS = Not stated.
[a] Other causes include pulmonary embolism, pancreatitis, pericarditis, thoracic surgery, chest trauma, atelectasis, ARDS, and subcapsular splenic hematoma.

drug users and 69% were MSM. As result, only 55% of all effusions were attributed to infectious causes, and 28% were parapneumonic. Given the low percentage of injection drug users and the high percentage of patients who were MSM, it is not surprising that more effusions proved to be due to KS than to pneumonia, illustrating the importance of patient population and specific HIV risk factors in influencing disease presentation.

The etiology of a pleural effusion will also vary with geography and disease prevalence in the community. In areas with a high rate of tuberculosis, a greater proportion of HIV patients will present with pleural effusion due to tuberculosis. In an investigation of 127 cases of undiagnosed pleural effusion in patients in Rwanda, 86% of effusions were due to *M. tuberculosis*; 83% of these patients who underwent testing were HIV seropositive, indicating a strong association between HIV and tuberculous pleurisy in Africa (9). Other etiologies, such as parapneumonic effusion and KS, were much less frequent in this population. In contrast, in reports from the United States, at most, 20% of effusions in HIV-infected patients were due to *M. tuberculosis* (Table 1) (3).

In addition, the degree of immunosuppression will impact the etiology of a pleural effusion, as the incidence of opportunistic infections and other processes such as AIDS-related lymphoma will rise with a decreasing CD4+ T-cell count. The majority of patients included in these studies had AIDS. Whether patients with a lower CD4+ T-cell count are more likely to have a pleural effusion as a complication of underlying disease is unclear. In an earlier study, Joseph et al. found that HIV-infected patients with pleural effusion had significantly lower CD4+ T-cell counts than patients without effusion (72 ± 12 cells/μL vs. 274 ± 26 cells/μL; $p < 0.001$) (5). However, a later study by Afessa found that HIV-infected patients with pleural effusion had marginally higher CD4+ T-cell counts (152 ± 186 cells/μL vs. 147 ± 218 cells/μL; $p = 0.0382$) (1).

Finally, the percentages reported in these studies may not be representative of the entire HIV-infected population, because all of these studies have included only hospitalized patients. Therefore, the incidence of effusions secondary to infectious processes may be overestimated in these series, as these patients are likely to be hospitalized more frequently. Effusions related to malignancy, heart failure, or other less acute processes might be underestimated in these series. These effusions may go unnoticed until the size or other systemic complications cause symptoms, or they may be managed on an outpatient basis.

III. Outcome of HIV-Infected Patients with Pleural Effusion

HIV-infected patients may have a worse outcome if a pleural effusion is present. In the prospective, observational study by Afessa HIV-infected admissions with pleural effusion had significantly higher APACHE (acute physiology and chronic health evaluation) II predicted mortality rates than HIV-negative admissions (29% vs. 23%; $p = 0.0001$) (1). The length of hospitalization was on median one day longer (7.6 ± 8.2 days vs. 6.4 ± 6.4 days; $p = 0.0064$), and the in-hospital mortality rate was significantly higher in admissions with pleural effusion than without (10.0% vs. 5.4%; $p = 0.0407$). However, the presence of pleural effusion was not found to be an independent risk factor for increased mortality [odds ratio (OR) 1.5, 95% confidence interval (CI) 0.8–2.8] (1), suggesting that this may instead be a marker for the severity of underlying disease.

Pleural effusions related to parapneumonic effusion or tuberculosis do not appear to result in significantly more morbidity or mortality in HIV-infected patients than in HIV-negative patients (8,12). Specifically, there have been no differences in the proportion of cases with residual fibrosis, in the time to resolution of the effusion, or in overall mortality.

IV. Diagnostic Evaluation of the HIV-Infected Patient with Pleural Effusion

Evaluation of the HIV-infected patient with a pleural effusion includes routine history, physical exam, and radiographic studies as in the HIV-negative individual. In particular, important clues can be obtained from the presence of bilateral versus unilateral effusions and from concomitant pulmonary abnormalities detected on chest imaging. The presence of bilateral versus unilateral effusions can be suggestive of different diagnoses: bilateral effusions are more commonly seen in KS, lymphoma, and congestive heart failure than in parapneumonic effusion (4). Unilateral effusions are more likely to be of parapneumonic (4) or tuberculous origin (13,14). The size of a pleural effusion has not generally been helpful in ascertaining its etiology (1,4,5,7,8).

In addition, underlying pulmonary parenchymal abnormalities and mediastinal lymphadenopathy can provide diagnostic clues. Bilateral pleural effusions with ill-defined peribronchovascular nodules and septal thickening suggest KS (15). A unilateral effusion with focal air space consolidation suggests parapneumonic effusion, while a unilateral effusion with miliary nodules and/or mediastinal lymphadenopathy suggests tuberculosis (4).

Pleural fluid should be sampled promptly and analyzed for cell differential, protein, lactate dehydrogenase (LDH) and glucose and sent for detailed microbiological analysis. In addition to routine smears and cultures for bacteria, mycobacteria, and fungi, a Wright-Giemsa stain can detect fungal elements. Cytological analysis for malignancy should always be performed. Closed pleural biopsy can be particularly useful in the evaluation of tuberculosis as well as lymphoma in HIV-infected patients (13,16). Thoracoscopic evaluation with biopsy can be performed in the evaluation of an undiagnosed effusion and can be particularly useful if confirmation of KS is required, as thoracentesis and closed pleural biopsy will not yield a diagnosis of KS (17). Further procedures to consider in working up the undiagnosed pleural effusion include flow cytometry and measurement of pleural fluid adenosine deaminase and cryptococcal antigen; these can be suggestive of the diagnoses of malignancy, tuberculosis, and cryptococcus, respectively (18,19).

V. Infectious Causes of Pleural Effusion in HIV-Infected Patients

A. Parapneumonic Effusions

Among the infectious causes of exudative effusions, parapneumonic effusions account for the majority of pleural effusions in HIV-infected hospitalized patients, ranging from 27 to 69% in recent large studies (1,4,8). The high frequency of parapneumonic effusions is not surprising, given the increased susceptibility to bacterial pneumonia (10,11,20) and the high rate of bacteremia in HIV-infected populations with community-acquired pneumonia (CAP), particularly if CD4+ T-cell counts are below 200 cells/µL (21,22). HIV-infected patients appear to be at increased risk of developing a parapneumonic effusion in association with CAP: in a study of 137 patients with CAP, the rate of developing a parapneumonic effusion was higher in the HIV-infected patients than in the

HIV-negative patients (21% vs. 13%; $p < 0.05$) (23). Blood cultures and pleural fluid cultures were more likely to be positive in this HIV-infected population (23).

Of microbiological causes, *Staphylococcus aureus* is the most frequently reported cause of parapneumonic effusion in a number of retrospective studies (Table 2) (4,7,8). Seen particularly in HIV-infected injection drug users due to increased risk of *S. aureus* infections, *S. aureus* pneumonia is frequently complicated by pleural effusions in HIV-infected patients. In one study, nearly one third of cases were associated with pleural effusion (24). Pleural effusion due to *S. aureus* infection can be related to community-acquired pneumonia as well as to septic embolism from infectious endocarditis and may cause uncomplicated parapneumonic effusion as well as empyema (8,23–25).

Another very common cause of pneumonia in HIV patients (20,22,26–28), *Streptococcus pneumoniae*, is likewise one of the most common causes of parapneumonic pleural effusion in HIV patients (Table 2) (7,8). Although the rate of pneumococcal bacteremia may be up to 100 times greater in HIV-infected patients compared to age-matched HIV-negative patients (28), increased rates of empyema in HIV-infected patients have not been reported (23,28). However,

Table 2 Infectious Causes of Pleural Effusion in HIV-Infected Hospitalized Patients

	Ref. 4	Ref. 7	Ref. 8	Ref. 5
Infectious effusions	32/58 (55%)	21/30 (70%)	76/86 (88%)	39/59 (66%)
Presumed bacterial	12 (38%)	6 (29%)	16 (21%)	6 (15%)
S. aureus	2 (6%)	4 (19%)	26 (34%)	1 (3%)
S. pneumoniae		4 (19%)	5 (7%)	8 (21%)
S. epidermidis			4 (5%)	
H. influenzae	1 (3%)			
K. pneumoniae			1 (1%)	
L. pneumophila				1 (3%)
M. pneumoniae				1 (3%)
P. aeruginosa	1 (3%)		6 (8%)	
E. coli				2 (5%)
Enterobacter spp.				1 (3%)
C. jejuni			1 (1%)	
Gram-negative bacilli		3 (14%)		
Nocardia spp.		1 (5%)		2 (5%)
M. tuberculosis	8 (25%)	1 (5%)	15 (17%)	5 (13%)
M. avium		2 (10%)		1 (3%)
P. carinii	6 (19%)		2 (3%)	9 (23%)
Aspergillus spp.	1 (3%)[a]			
Cryptococcus neoformans	1 (3%)			2 (5%)
Leishmania	1 (3%)[a]			

[a] One patient had both *Aspergillus* and *Leishmania*.

individual cases of more unusual and aggressive manifestations of pneumococcal infection in the pleural space have been reported in HIV patients, including recurrent exudative pleural effusions and pyopneumothorax (29).

Numerous other bacteria have been documented to cause pleural effusion in HIV-infected individuals, including *Staphylococcus epidermidis* and gram-negative organisms such as *Pseudomonas aeruginosa* and *Escherichia coli* (5,7,8). *P. aeruginosa* has been reported particularly in injection drug users and in those with more advanced immunosuppression from HIV (8,30). Although a common cause of pneumonia in HIV patients (26,27), *Haemophilus influenzae* has been infrequently reported as a cause of pleural effusion (4). More unusual organisms can also infect the pleural space, such as *Campylobacter jejuni*, *Salmonella* species, *Nocardia* species, and, rarely, *Rhodococcus equi* (31–34). Pulmonary nocardiosis in HIV-infected patients has been associated with pleural effusion in 10–33% of cases, most commonly as a unilateral effusion associated with underlying parenchymal abnormalities such as consolidation, mass-like or cavitary lesions (32,35). *Nocardia* empyema requiring tube thoracostomy for drainage has also been described (32).

HIV-infected patients may be more likely to develop complicated parapneumonic pleural effusions than HIV-negative patients. In the study by Gil Suay et al. comparing HIV-infected to HIV-negative patients with CAP and parapneumonic effusion, the HIV-infected patients were more likely to have a complicated clinical course and to develop complicated parapneumonic effusions (23). The HIV-infected patients were younger and were also found to have a significantly longer duration of symptoms prior to admission and a higher fever on admission. Although no differences were observed in pleural fluid pH, protein, LDH, or absolute number of cells, patients with HIV had significantly lower levels of pleural fluid glucose and were more likely to require chest tube drainage. Furthermore, the duration of fever and of intravenous antibiotic treatment and the number of antibiotics were all higher in the HIV-infected group. These findings may be related to the increased frequency of *S. aureus* parapneumonic effusions observed in this study, which included a high proportion of injection drug users, and the increased complications typically observed with this organism (23). No increase in the number of cases of empyema was reported, however, nor was a difference in mortality demonstrated. In another study, no significant difference was detected in the outcome of HIV-infected and HIV-negative patients with either complicated or uncomplicated parapneumonic effusions (8).

Management of parapneumonic effusion in an HIV-infected patient should be the same as in immunocompetent individuals (17). If the patient is an injection drug user, choice of empiric antibiotics should include consideration of antistaphylococcal coverage, given the high percentage of parapneumonic effusions in these patients. Antipseudomonal coverage may also be considered, particularly in more severely immunosuppressed patients. Sampling of pleural fluid is integral in deciding therapy. Given the increased potential for complicated parapneumonic effusions, tube thoracostomy and surgical interventions for drainage are appropriate procedures to consider (36). In cases of empyema not resolving with chest tube drainage, early thoracoscopy for pleural debridement has been advocated (37).

B. Mycobacterial Pleural Effusions

Mycobacterium Tuberculosis

Mycobacterium tuberculosis is a frequent cause of pleural effusion in HIV. Prevalence varies according to the background rate of tuberculosis in the population reported. *M. tuberculosis* accounts for between 3 to 21% of pleural effusions in HIV-infected hospitalized patients in the United States and Europe (Table 1) (1–8). In contrast, in an area endemic for tuberculosis, up to 90% of effusions in HIV-infected patients in Kigali, Rwanda, were caused by tuberculosis (9).

Tuberculous pleural effusion tends to occur more commonly in patients with HIV infection, despite substantial overlap in the frequency of disease reported in HIV-infected and HIV-negative populations. Of patients with TB, 8–43% of cases in HIV-infected patients have been reported to present with pleural effusion (14,38–42), compared to approximately 4–20% of cases in HIV-negative patients in studies from the United States, Europe, and Africa (14,38–41,43). In a review comparing 963 HIV-infected adults to 1000 HIV-negative adults in sub-Saharan Africa, significantly more HIV-infected patients presented with pleural effusion on chest x-ray (16% vs. 6.8%; $p = 0.001$) (40). These results are consistent with the findings in other studies of tuberculosis in South Africa (39, 41) and Rwanda (38).

Clinical presentation is similar, although compared to HIV-negative patients, HIV-infected patients with TB pleural effusion were noted to be younger in one study from New York City; this may potentially reflect more cases of primary infection as opposed to reactivation tuberculosis (13). HIV-infected patients with TB pleurisy have also been reported to present with more prolonged symptoms such as dyspnea, fever, nights sweats, and fatigue (44). On radiograph, pleural effusions associated with tuberculosis are usually unilateral and are frequently associated with underlying pulmonary parenchymal abnormalities (13,38–41). However, pleural effusion may also be the only finding (13). As in HIV-negative patients, 5–10% of HIV-infected patients may present with bilateral pleural effusions (13,14,44).

The CD4+ T-cell count influences the presentation of tuberculosis in HIV-infected patients. Although features such as mediastinal adenopathy are more common in patients with CD4+ T-cell counts below 200 cells/μL, manifestations such as cavitary lesions and pleural effusions tend to be more common in patients with higher CD4+ T-cell counts (42,45,46). Although in one well-designed study by Jones et al., a higher percentage of patients with CD4+ T-cell counts above 200 cells/μL had pleural effusions, this has not been a consistent finding in other studies (Table 3) (38,42,45). As tuberculous pleuritis is postulated to represent a delayed-type hypersensitivity reaction, with immune response mediated by CD4+ T cells in the pleural fluid, an increased number

Table 3 Relationship Between Degree of Immunosuppression and Presence of Tuberculous Pleural Effusion in HIV-Infected Patients

CD4+ T cells ≤200 (AIDS)	CD4+ T cells >200 (non-AIDS)	p-value	Ref.
15/35 (42%)	6/13 (46%)	0.83	38
6/58 (10%)	8/30 (27%)	0.05	45
7/98 (7%)	3/30 (10%)	0.70	42

of effusions could be explained in patients with higher CD4+ T-cell counts (13,45).

As in the non–HIV-infected patient, a unilateral exudative effusion with lymphocyte predominance and an elevated protein should prompt consideration of tuberculosis. No significant differences between pleural fluid cell differential, protein concentration, or glucose levels have been found between HIV-seropositive and -seronegative individuals with pleural tuberculosis (44). Although usually scarce in tuberculous pleural effusions, an elevated mesothelial cell count can be an unreliable predictor in HIV-infected patients, as increased mesothelial cells have been reported in a small number of cases in HIV-infected patients with pleural tuberculosis (47).

If routine cultures are nondiagnostic, a pleural biopsy should be strongly considered. Pleural fluid smears, culture and pleural biopsy specimens may have a higher yield in HIV-infected patients related to an increased burden of microorganisms in the pleural space (13), although this has not been consistently demonstrated. In one study pleural biopsy specimens were significantly more likely to be AFB smear positive in HIV-infected patients compared to HIV-negative patients with pleural tuberculosis (69% vs. 21%; $p < 0.01$) (13), although in other reports no significant differences in the microbiological yield of pleural specimens could be demonstrated (Table 4) (34,44). The percentage of positive results varies greatly between the studies, as it does for HIV-negative patients, related to factors such as amount of fluid sampled, culture techniques, and number of biopsy specimens (48).

Used less commonly in the United States, additional pleural fluid assays to aid in the diagnosis of tuberculosis in immunocompetent patients include measurements of adenosine deaminase (ADA), interferon-gamma (IFN-γ), and lysozyme and polymerase chain reaction (PCR) to detect *M. tuberculosis*. The role of these studies in HIV-infected patients is not clearly defined. ADA is an enzyme that is found in highest concentrations in stimulated T-lymphocytes, with elevated levels observed in tuberculous pleural effusions as well as in empyema. It has been shown to have a sensitivity ranging from 90 to 100%, and a specificity of 85–100% in immunocompetent patients (43,49,50). In prior studies on HIV patients, the ADA had a lower sensitivity due to increased false-negative results (51). However, in a recent analysis that included the largest

Table 4 Positive Microbiological Results on Pleural Specimens in Tuberculosis According to HIV Status

	Pleural fluid		Pleural biopsy		
Ref.	Smear	Culture	Histology	Smear	Culture
9					
($N = 90$)[a]	1%	46%	52%	NS	50%
13					
HIV$^+$ ($N = 43$)	15%	91%	88%	69%[b]	47%[c]
HIV$^-$ ($N = 27$)	8%	78%	71%	21%	86%
34					
HIV$^+$ ($N = 22$)	NS	13.6%	68.2%	NS	18.2%
HIV$^-$ ($N = 30$)	NS	6.7%	53.3%	NS	10%
14					
HIV$^+$ ($N = 22$)	6%	64%	78%	44%	40%
HIV^{-d}		53%			

NS = not stated.
[a] Results for HIV$^+$ and HIV$^-$ patients combined; HIV positivity rate 83% in the total of 110 patients with pleural TB.
[b] $p < 0.01$ compared to HIV$^-$.
[c] $p < 0.05$ compared to HIV$^-$.
[d] Rate of pleural fluid AFB culture was taken from control cases seen in HIV$^-$ patients within the same state during the study period.

number of HIV-infected patients with pleural tuberculosis reported thus far (37 patients), the ADA values did not differ significantly from HIV-negative patients, suggesting that it may be equally sensitive in HIV patients (52).

IFN-γ has also been investigated as a diagnostic marker for tuberculous pleural effusion. A lymphokine produced by T lymphocytes in response to antigen stimulation, IFN-γ levels increase in tuberculous pleuritis. High sensitivity and specificity of up to 99% and 98%, respectively, have been reported (53). The sensitivity did not differ significantly when compared between 9 HIV-infected and 41 HIV-negative patients. Although the level of IFN-γ tended to be lower in the HIV-infected patients, it remained well above the cut-off point of 3.7 U/mL (53). Interestingly, PCR has been reported to have a much lower sensitivity of 42% but a high specificity of 99%, with no significant difference in sensitivity reported in the small number of HIV-infected and HIV-negative patients in which it was studied (54).

HIV-infected patients with pleural tuberculosis can be treated with a standard 6-month antituberculous regimen, substituting rifabutin for rifampin if patients are on protease inhibitors or nonnucleoside reverse-transcriptase inhibitors. Provided appropriate clinical response, prolonged treatment for pleural disease is not required (55).

Nontuberculous Mycobacteria

Large pleural effusions due to nontuberculous mycobacteria are uncommon features in HIV-infected as well as HIV-negative patients. Although *Mycobacterium avium* complex is the most frequent cause of nontuberculous disease (56) and is often disseminated in AIDS patients, pleural involvement is a rare feature (57). Other pulmonary pathogens in HIV patients, namely *M. kansasii* and *M. xenopi*, are associated with pleural effusions in 8–18% of cases (58–60), with no significant differences reported between the proportion of cases with pleural involvement in AIDS versus non-AIDS patients (61). Pulmonary disease caused by atypical mycobacteria usually occurs in HIV-infected patients with advanced immunosuppression, often with CD4+ T-cell counts averaging 50 cells/μL (56, 60,61). Unlike *M. tuberculosis*, the atypical mycobacteria are unlikely to cause large effusions or isolated pleurisy. This may be related to the profound immunosuppression of patients with these pathogens, as other features that are usually associated with higher CD4+ T-cell counts in patients with *M. tuberculosis* infection, such as cavitation, are also seen less frequently (60,62,63).

C. Fungal Pleural Effusions

Numerous cases of fungal pleural effusion in HIV-infected patients have been reported. Now classified as a fungus, *Pneumocystis carinii* is a frequent cause of opportunistic pneumonia in HIV-infected patients, but is rarely associated with pleural effusion. However, a relatively large proportion of cases of pleural effusion have been attributed to *P. carinii* on retrospective review (Table 1) (1,2,4–6). In the study by Joseph et al., a particularly high incidence (15%) of pleural effusions was attributed to *P. carinii* (5). This is likely to be an overestimation, as no cytological stains were done on pleural fluid specimens to confirm the presence of cysts or trophozoites of *P. carinii*. Rather, the presence of pleural effusion in a patient with *P. carinii* pneumonia may be due to a second infection or underlying illness or may be related to factors associated with the pneumonic process that affect the intrapleural pressure, lymphatic clearance, and permeability of the microcirculation (5).

Rare individual cases that document *P. carinii* by cytological exam in the pleural space have been reported (64–66). Of note, all of these cases have been associated with aerosolized pentamidine use, frequently in combination with a pneumothorax, raising the possibility that pleural pneumocystis may be an anatomical extension of subpleural infection that erodes into the pleural space (64).

Another fungus not infrequently reported to cause pleural effusions in HIV-infected patients is *Cryptococcus neoformans* (18,67–71). Pleural effusions in cryptococcal disease are more common in HIV-infected than non–HIV-infected individuals (72). Reported in association with 5–20% of cases of cryptococcal pneumonia (67, 68), pleural effusion due to *Cryptococcus* has also preceded disseminated disease and has been seen in the absence of concomitant pulmonary parenchymal disease (18,69–71,73). Methods for diagnosis include fungal smear and culture, as well as closed pleural biopsy and assay for cryptococcal antigen in the pleural fluid (18,70).

In rare cases, disseminated histoplasmosis has been associated with pleural effusion in HIV-infected patients, with microbiological confirmation on thoracentesis as well as a pleural biopsy specimen (74,75). Pleural effusion is an uncommon finding in coccidiomycosis (76,77) and invasive pulmonary aspergillosis (2,4,78).

D. Other Infectious Causes of Pleural Effusion

Parasitic causes of pleural effusion in HIV-infected patients include invasive amebiasis (79), as well as *Leishmania* (4,6,80). Consideration of these more unusual infections would depend upon the patient's presentation, exposures, and travel history. For example, the cases of amebiasis were reported from an endemic area in Taiwan and were seen in association with liver abscesses. Although a rare disease, pulmonary toxoplasmosis can be associated with pleural effusion in 7% of cases (81).

VI. Malignant Pleural Effusions in HIV-Infected Patients

Malignant pleural effusions in HIV-infected patients can result from tumors that are seen in HIV-negative patients as well as those that are particular to an HIV-infected population. The two most prevalent malignancies in HIV patients, KS and non-Hodgkin's lymphoma (NHL), are the most common causes of malignant effusion in HIV-infected patients (82). Bronchogenic carcinoma accounts for approximately 3% of effusions in HIV-infected hospitalized patients (1–3,6,7). Metastatic cancer and rare diseases, as in a case report of a malignant mesothelioma in the absence of asbestos exposure, can also be encountered in the AIDS patient (83). Certain malignant effusions, such as primary effusion lymphoma and KS, are seen nearly exclusively in those with HIV infection. The characteristics of three causes of malignant pleural effusion particular to AIDS patients are discussed in more detail below.

A. Kaposi's Sarcoma

An angioproliferative tumor, KS is seen nearly exclusively in MSM (84), affecting 15–20% of this population (85). Pulmonary involvement is evident in 6–49% of patients with known mucocutaneous KS, with a higher prevalence of 47–75% noted in autopsy series (85). Although uncommon, pulmonary disease can also be seen in up to 15% of patients in the absence of mucocutaneous lesions (84). Pleural involvement in KS is a frequent complication, with effusions present in approximately 50% of cases (4,84–86). Correspondingly, KS is the most common malignant effusion in HIV patients, accounting for up to 43% of effusions in HIV-infected patients who present with pleural effusion; the reported frequency varies depending on the patient population under study (Table 1) (1–4,6,7).

The most common clinical symptoms of pulmonary KS are dyspnea, nonproductive cough, and fever (84,87). Patients with pulmonary KS have advanced HIV, with CD4+ T-cell counts below 150 cells/μL in most series (85). Pleural fluid is commonly a serosanguineous or bloody exudate with a mononuclear cell predominance (87), although serosanguineous transudates can be found (85,86). Pleural effusion due to KS can present as a chylothorax, presumably related to lymphatic obstruction of the thoracic duct (86–88).

In 65–76% of cases, the pleural effusions related to KS are bilateral (4,15,86). Most effusions are small to moderate in size and, if bilateral, tend to be symmetrical (15). Pleural effusions are reported nearly exclusively in patients with parenchymal lung involvement related to KS (84,89). In the series by O'Brien and Cohn, 3 of 13 cases of pleuropulmonary KS were reported as having pleural involvement alone on the basis of chest x-ray findings (87), although a CT scan may have detected parenchymal involvement in these patients.

Diagnosis of pleural effusions related to KS can be problematic, as pleural fluid cytology is either negative or reveals only reactive or atypical cells (87,90). Pleural biopsies likewise are usually negative, as KS is confined to the visceral pleura (85,87). Other diagnostic procedures include thoracoscopic evaluation with visualization or biopsy of lesions on the visceral pleura (17). Identification of the KS-associated virus human herpesvirus-8 by PCR from involved tissue offers a promising approach for diagnosis (85), although its performance in pleural fluid has not been studied (17). In current practice, the attribution of a pleural effusion to KS is largely based on the combination of clinical presentation, physical exam, and radiographic findings. Although infectious causes should always be considered, the findings of pleural effusion in association with typical parenchymal abnormalities, namely ill-defined peribronchovascular nodules, perihilar infiltrates, and septal thickening, are suggestive of KS (15,86,91).

Treatment options include chemotherapy, radiation therapy, and highly active antiretroviral therapy (HAART). Tumors have been reported to shrink as patients experience an immunological and virological response to HAART (85). Historically, in the pre-HAART era, prognosis has been poor, with median survival ranging between 4 and 12 months in patients with pulmonary KS. Survival appears to be significantly improved, however, in current reports of patients treated with HAART (85). Recurrent pleural effusions can be problematic and may require repeated drainage; although sclerotherapy is usually ineffective, pleurodesis and pleuroperitoneal shunts are alternative options (82).

B. Non-Hodgkin's Lymphoma

The second most common malignancy in HIV-infected patients (92), non-Hodgkin's lymphoma (NHL), occurs in 2–5% of HIV-infected patients (90).

Most of these tumors are of B-cell origin and can be classified into one of three histological subtypes: large-cell immunoblastic, small noncleaved cell or Burkitt's, and diffuse large cell (93). Frequently a disseminated disease with extranodal spread at the time of diagnosis, pulmonary involvement occurs in 5–31% of patients with AIDS-related NHL based on clinical grounds (16,94,95), although a significantly higher proportion have pulmonary involvement documented on autopsy (16).

Pleural effusions are common in AIDS-related NHL. In a retrospective review of 38 cases of pulmonary involvement in NHL in AIDS patients, pleural effusions were detected on chest x-ray in 44%, and in 68% of patients by CT scan (16). In patients with HIV who present with pleural effusion, NHL accounts for approximately 1–17% of cases (Table 1) (1,2,4,6–8). NHL is distinct from AIDS-related primary pulmonary lymphoma, also typically a B-cell tumor, which excludes patients with pleural effusion and includes only those patients with pulmonary parenchymal involvement in the absence of thoracic lymphadenopathy or extrathoracic spread (96,97).

As in many pulmonary illnesses, common presenting features are nonspecific and include dyspnea and cough (16). Most patients have advanced HIV infection, with median CD4+ T-cell counts below 100 cells/μL (16). Pleural fluid is exudative, often with very high levels of LDH (16). Thoracentesis and pleural biopsy are useful diagnostic steps. The yield of pleural cytology is significantly higher in HIV-associated pulmonary lymphoma as opposed to HIV-negative cases (7). In one report, as few as 11% of cases in HIV-negative individuals had positive results on fluid cytology, with only a 16% yield on closed pleural biopsy (98). In contrast, up to 45–75% of cases in HIV-infected individuals had positive results on pleural fluid cytology (16,94), with a 100% yield on closed pleural biopsy specimens reported (16). Flow cytometry of pleural fluid can also be used for diagnosis (19).

Pleural effusions tend to be bilateral in 41–55% of cases, with more bilateral effusions detected on CT scan as opposed to chest x-ray (16,94). Associated parenchymal radiographic findings consist primarily of nodules, lobar consolidation, masses, and hilar or mediastinal lymphadenopathy (16,95). Rare prior cases of primary pleural involvement in the absence of detectable systemic lymphadenopathy or parenchymal involvement have been reported as a manifestation of AIDS-associated NHL (94,99). These cases may actually represent primary effusion lymphoma, a subset of AIDS-associated pulmonary lymphomas, which is discussed further below.

AIDS-related NHL are generally aggressive tumors with a poor prognosis; median survival has historically been approximately 4–10 months prior to HAART (90,100). Although previous studies have indicated that intensive chemotherapy was associated with increased deaths due to infection (90), current studies suggest that combining HAART with more intensive chemotherapy can improve disease-free survival in these patients (100). Pulmonary involvement is treated as a part of systemic disease.

C. Primary Effusion Lymphoma

A subset of NHL, primary effusion lymphomas (PEL) or body-cavity-based lymphomas are tumors that grow exclusively in the pleural, pericardial, or peritoneal cavities as lymphomatous effusions (101). Although immunophenotypically indeterminate, they are of B-cell genotype with clonal rearrangements of the immunoglobulin gene (101). These tumors are found nearly exclusively in HIV-infected patients (102) who are MSM with advanced disease (103,104). The KS-associated human herpesvirus 8 is found in all cases of PEL, with Epstein-Barr virus demonstrated in nearly all of the tumors as well (101–104). A rare disease, PEL represents about 3% of all AIDS-related NHL (105).

Pleural effusions due to PEL can be unilateral or bilateral; by definition, no pulmonary parenchymal or nodal disease is evident (102,104). Pleural disease can include diffuse thickening of the parietal pleura, but no plaque-like or nodular thickening is demonstrable on CT scan (102). Pleural fluid cytology is positive, consistent with the liquid phase growth pattern of these tumors (102). Prognosis is poor, with median survival on the order of 2–3 months (101,104).

VII. Causes of Transudative Effusions in HIV-Infected Patients

Most transudative effusions in HIV-infected patients result from the same etiologies as are seen in HIV-negative individuals, namely congestive heart failure (CHF), renal insufficiency, and liver disease (Table 1). Treatment consists of management of the underlying medical conditions, as in HIV-negative patients. Whether HIV-infected patients are more likely to develop effusions related to these disease processes has not been studied.

A significant number of transudative effusions in hospitalized HIV-infected patients have been attributed to hypoalbuminemia. In one study, nearly 20% of effusions were attributed to hypoalbuminemia, which was defined as a serum albumin concentration ≤1.8 g/dL with no other identifiable cause for the effusion (5). Whether hypoalbuminemia alone is sufficient to cause a clinically

Table 5 Association of Hypoalbuminemia with Pleural Effusion in HIV-Infected Patients

Patients with pleural effusion		Patients without pleural effusion			
No. patients	Serum albumin (g/dL)	No. patients	Serum albumin (g/dL)	p-value	Ref.
48	2.5 ± 0.1	96	3.4 ± 0.1	<0.001	5
160	2.4 ± 0.8	937	2.9 ± 1.8	<0.0001	1

Source: Adapted from V. C. Broaddus, personal communication.

significant pleural effusion, however, is unclear; rather, hypoalbuminemia is likely to act in concert with another pathological cause in contributing to the formation of an effusion (106) (Broaddus VC, personal communication). In agreement with this, two studies have reported a significantly increased prevalence of pleural effusion in HIV-infected patients with lower serum albumin values (Table 5) (1,5).

VIII. Conclusion

The causes of pleural effusion in HIV-infected patients are diverse. Etiologies to consider include all the causes of transudative and exudative effusions that can be seen in HIV-seronegative patients. Certain infectious agents such as parapneumonic effusions and tuberculosis are encountered very commonly in the HIV-infected patient as well as in the HIV-negative patient. Other etiologies such as KS or PEL will be encountered nearly exclusively in the HIV-infected patient. Key features to consider in addition to routine history and physical examination include degree of immunosuppression, HIV risk factors and behaviors, regional variability in disease prevalence, and concomitant radiographic abnormalities. Diagnostic evaluation and management choices are generally the same as in HIV-negative individuals.

References

1. Afessa B. Pleural effusion and pneumothorax in hospitalized patients with HIV infection: the Pulmonary Complications, ICU support, and Prognostic Factors of Hospitalized Patients with HIV (PIP) Study. Chest 2000; 117:1031–1037.
2. Armbruster C, Schalleschak J, Vetter N, Pokieser L. Pleural effusions in human immunodeficiency virus-infected patients. Correlation with concomitant pulmonary diseases. Acta Cytol 1995; 39:698–700.
3. Lababidi HMS, Gupta K, Newman T, Fuleihan FJD. A retrospective analysis of pleural effusion in human immunodeficiency virus infected patients [abstr]. Chest 1994; 106:86S.
4. Miller RF, Howling SJ, Reid AJ, Shaw PJ. Pleural effusions in patients with AIDS. Sex Transm Infect 2000; 76:122–125.
5. Joseph J, Strange C, Sahn SA. Pleural effusions in hospitalized patients with AIDS. Ann Intern Med 1993; 118:856–859.
6. Cadranel JL, Chouaid C, Denis M, Lebeau B, Akoun GM, Mayaud CM. Causes of pleural effusion in 75 HIV-infected patients. Chest 1993; 104:655.
7. Soubani AO, Michelson MK, Karnik A. Pleural fluid findings in patients with the acquired immunodeficiency syndrome: correlation with concomitant pulmonary disease. South Med J 1999; 92:400–403.
8. Trejo O, Giron JA, Perez-Guzman E, Segura E, Fernandez-Gutierrez C, Garcia-Tapia A, Clavo AJ, Bascunana A. Pleural effusion in patients infected with the human immunodeficiency virus. Eur J Clin Microbiol Infect Dis 1997; 16:807–815.

9. Batungwanayo J, Taelman H, Allen S, Bogaerts J, Kagame A, Van de Perre P. Pleural effusion, tuberculosis and HIV-1 infection in Kigali, Rwanda. AIDS 1993; 7:73–79.
10. Hirschtick RE, Glassroth J, Jordan MC, Wilcosky TC, Wallace JM, Kvale PA, Markowitz N, Rosen MJ, Mangura BT, Hopewell PC. Bacterial pneumonia in persons infected with the human immunodeficiency virus. Pulmonary Complications of HIV Infection Study Group. N Engl J Med 1995; 333:845–851.
11. Wallace JM, Hansen NI, Lavange L, Glassroth J, Browdy BL, Rosen MJ, Kvale PA, Mangura BT, Reichman LB, Hopewell PC. Respiratory disease trends in the Pulmonary Complications of HIV Infection Study cohort. Pulmonary Complications of HIV Infection Study Group. Am J Respir Crit Care Med 1997; 155:72–80.
12. Cohen M, Sahn SA. Resolution of pleural effusions. Chest 2001; 119:1547–1562.
13. Relkin F, Aranda CP, Garay SM, Smith R, Berkowitz KA, Rom WN. Pleural tuberculosis and HIV infection. Chest 1994; 105:1338–1341.
14. Frye MD, Pozsik CJ, Sahn SA. Tuberculous pleurisy is more common in AIDS than in non-AIDS patients with tuberculosis. Chest 1997; 112:393–397.
15. Gruden JF, Huang L, Webb WR, Gamsu G, Hopewell PC, Sides DM. AIDS-related Kaposi sarcoma of the lung: radiographic findings and staging system with bronchoscopic correlation. Radiology 1995; 195:545–552.
16. Eisner MD, Kaplan LD, Herndier B, Stulbarg MS. The pulmonary manifestations of AIDS-related non-Hodgkin's lymphoma. Chest 1996; 110:729–736.
17. Beck JM. Pleural disease in patients with acquired immune deficiency syndrome. Clin Chest Med 1998; 19:341–349.
18. de Lalla F, Vaglia A, Franzetti M, Manfrin V, Pellizzer GP, Fabris P. Cryptococcal pleural effusion as first indicator of AIDS: a case report. Infection 1993; 21:192.
19. Lee AM, Katner HP. AIDS-related lymphoma diagnosed by flow cytometry of a pleural effusion. South Med J 1991; 84:1278–1279.
20. Selwyn PA, Feingold AR, Hartel D, Schoenbaum EE, Alderman MH, Klein RS, Friedland GH. Increased risk of bacterial pneumonia in HIV-infected intravenous drug users without AIDS. AIDS 1988; 2:267–272.
21. Clavo-Sanchez AJ, Giron-Gonzalez JA, Lopez-Prieto D, Torres-Tortosa M, Sanchez-Porto A. Influence of CD4+ status on the invasiveness of pneumococcal pneumonia in HIV patients. Eur J Clin Microbiol Infect Dis 1996; 15:959–960.
22. Falco V, Fernandez de Sevilla T, Alegre J, Barbe J, Ferrer A, Ocana I, Ribera E, Martinez-Vazquez JM. Bacterial pneumonia in HIV-infected patients: a prospective study of 68 episodes. Eur Respir J 1994; 7:235–239.
23. Gil Suay V, Cordero PJ, Martinez E, Soler JJ, Perpina M, Greses JV, Sanchis J. Parapneumonic effusions secondary to community-acquired bacterial pneumonia in human immunodeficiency virus-infected patients. Eur Respir J 1995; 8:1934–1939.
24. Tumbarello M, Tacconelli E, Lucia MB, Cauda R, Ortona L. Predictors of *Staphylococcus aureus* pneumonia associated with human immunodeficiency virus infection. Respir Med 1996; 90:531–537.
25. Hernandez Borge J, Alfageme Michavila I, Munoz Mendez J, Campos Rodriguez F, Pena Grinan N, Villagomez Cerrato R. Thoracic empyema in HIV-infected patients: microbiology, management, and outcome. Chest 1998; 113:732–738.
26. Mundy LM, Auwaerter PG, Oldach D, Warner ML, Burton A, Vance E, Gaydos CA, Joseph JM, Gopalan R, Moore RD, et al. Community-acquired pneumonia: impact of immune status. Am J Respir Crit Care Med 1995; 152:1309–1315.

27. Burack JH, Hahn JA, Saint-Maurice D, Jacobson MA. Microbiology of community-acquired bacterial pneumonia in persons with and at risk for human immunodeficiency virus type 1 infection. Implications for rational empiric antibiotic therapy. Arch Intern Med 1994; 154:2589–2596.
28. Janoff EN, Breiman RF, Daley CL, Hopewell PC. Pneumococcal disease during HIV infection. Epidemiologic, clinical, and immunologic perspectives. Ann Intern Med 1992; 117:314–324.
29. Rodriguez M, Barradas C, Musher DM, Hamill RJ, Dowell M, Bagwell JT, Sanders CV. Unusual manifestations of pneumococcal infection in human immunodeficiency virus-infected individuals: the past revisited. Clin Infect Dis 1992; 14: 192–199.
30. Kielhofner M, Atmar RL, Hamill RJ, Musher DM. Life-threatening *Pseudomonas aeruginosa* infections in patients with human immunodeficiency virus infection. Clin Infect Dis 1992; 14:403–411.
31. Wolday D, Seyoum B. Pleural empyema due to *Salmonella paratyphi* in a patient with AIDS. Trop Med Int Health 1997; 2:1140–1142.
32. Uttamchandani RB, Daikos GL, Reyes RR, Fischl MA, Dickinson GM, Yamaguchi E, Kramer MR. Nocardiosis in 30 patients with advanced human immunodeficiency virus infection: clinical features and outcome. Clin Infect Dis 1994; 18: 348–353.
33. Calore EE, Vazquez CR, Perez NM, Cavaliere MJ, Curti R Jr, Campos Salles PS, Araujo MF. Empyema with malakoplakic-like lesions by *Rhodococcus equi* as a presentation of HIV infection. Pathologica 1995; 87:525–527.
34. Owino EA, McLigeyo SO, Gathua SN, Nyong'o A. Prevalence of human immunodeficiency virus infection: its impact on the diagnostic yields in exudative pleural effusions at the Kenyatta National Hospital, Nairobi. East Afr Med J 1996; 73: 575–578.
35. Kramer MR, Uttamchandani RB. The radiographic appearance of pulmonary nocardiosis associated with AIDS. Chest 1990; 98:382–385.
36. Feins RH. The role of thoracoscopy in the AIDS/immunocompromised patient. Ann Thorac Surg 1993; 56:649–650.
37. Flum DR, Steinberg SD, Bernik TR, Bonfils-Roberts E, Kramer MD, Adams PX, Wallack MK. Thoracoscopy in acquired immunodeficiency syndrome. J Thorac Cardiovasc Surg 1997; 114:361–366.
38. Batungwanayo J, Taelman H, Dhote R, Bogaerts J, Allen S, Van de Perre P. Pulmonary tuberculosis in Kigali, Rwanda. Impact of human immunodeficiency virus infection on clinical and radiographic presentation. Am Rev Respir Dis 1992; 146:53–56.
39. Saks AM, Posner R. Tuberculosis in HIV positive patients in South Africa: a comparative radiological study with HIV negative patients. Clin Radiol 1992; 46: 387–390.
40. Tshibwabwa-Tumba E, Mwinga A, Pobee JO, Zumla A. Radiological features of pulmonary tuberculosis in 963 HIV-infected adults at three central African hospitals. Clin Radiol 1997; 52:837–841.
41. Lawn SD, Evans AJ, Sedgwick PM, Acheampong JW. Pulmonary tuberculosis: radiological features in West Africans coinfected with HIV. Br J Radiol 1999; 72: 339–344.
42. Perlman DC, el-Sadr WM, Nelson ET, Matts JP, Telzak EE, Salomon N, Chirgwin K, Hafner R. Variation of chest radiographic patterns in pulmonary tuberculosis

by degree of human immunodeficiency virus-related immunosuppression. The Terry Beirn Community Programs for Clinical Research on AIDS (CPCRA). The AIDS Clinical Trials Group (ACTG). Clin Infect Dis 1997; 25:242–246.
43. Valdes L, San Jose E, Alvarez D, Sarandeses A, Pose A, Chomon B, Alvarez-Dobano JM, Salgueiro M, Rodriguez Suarez JR. Diagnosis of tuberculous pleurisy using the biologic parameters adenosine deaminase, lysozyme, and interferon gamma. Chest 1993; 103:458–465.
44. Richter C, Perenboom R, Mtoni I, Kitinya J, Chande H, Swai AB, Kazema RR, Chuwa LM. Clinical features of HIV-seropositive and HIV-seronegative patients with tuberculous pleural effusion in Dar es Salaam, Tanzania. Chest 1994; 106: 1471–1475.
45. Jones BE, Young SM, Antoniskis D, Davidson PT, Kramer F, Barnes PF. Relationship of the manifestations of tuberculosis to CD4 cell counts in patients with human immunodeficiency virus infection. Am Rev Respir Dis 1993; 148:1292–1297.
46. Post FA, Wood R, Pillay GP. Pulmonary tuberculosis in HIV infection: radiographic appearance is related to CD4+ T-lymphocyte count. Tuber Lung Dis 1995; 76:518–521.
47. Jones D, Lieb T, Narita M, Hollender ES, Pitchenik AE, Ashkin D. Mesothelial cells in tuberculous pleural effusions of HIV-infected patients. Chest 2000; 117: 289–291.
48. Morehead RS. Tuberculosis of the pleura. South Med J 1998; 91:630–636.
49. Roth BJ. Searching for tuberculosis in the pleural space. Chest 1999; 116:3–5.
50. Villena V, Navarro-Gonzalvez JA, Garcia-Benayas C, Manzanos JA, Echave J, Lopez-Encuentra A, Arenas Barbero J. Rapid automated determination of adenosine deaminase and lysozyme for differentiating tuberculous and nontuberculous pleural effusions. Clin Chem 1996; 42:218–221.
51. Hsu WH, Chiang CD, Huang PL. Diagnostic value of pleural adenosine deaminase in tuberculous effusions of immunocompromised hosts. J Formos Med Assoc 1993; 92:668–670.
52. Riantawan P, Chaowalit P, Wongsangiem M, Rojanaraweewong P. Diagnostic value of pleural fluid adenosine deaminase in tuberculous pleuritis with reference to HIV coinfection and a Bayesian analysis. Chest 1999; 116:97–103.
53. Villena V, Lopez-Encuentra A, Echave-Sustaeta J, Martin-Escribano P, Ortuno-de-Solo B, Estenoz-Alfaro J. Interferon-gamma in 388 immunocompromised and immunocompetent patients for diagnosing pleural tuberculosis. Eur Respir J 1996; 9:2635–2639.
54. Villena V, Rebollo MJ, Aguado JM, Galan A, Lopez Encuentra A, Palenque E. Polymerase chain reaction for the diagnosis of pleural tuberculosis in immunocompromised and immunocompetent patients. Clin Infect Dis 1998; 26:212–214.
55. Small PM, Fujiwara PI. Management of tuberculosis in the United States. N Engl J Med 2001; 345:189–200.
56. Chin DP, Hopewell PC. Mycobacterial complications of HIV infection. Clin Chest Med 1996; 17:697–711.
57. Rigsby MO, Curtis AM. Pulmonary disease from nontuberculous mycobacteria in patients with human immunodeficiency virus. Chest 1994; 106:913–919.
58. Bankier AA, Stauffer F, Fleischmann D, Kreuzer S, Strasser G, Mossbacher U, Mallek R. Radiographic findings in patients with acquired immunodeficiency

syndrome, pulmonary infection, and microbiologic evidence of *Mycobacterium xenopi*. J Thorac Imaging 1998; 13:282–288.
59. Fishman JE, Schwartz DS, Sais GJ. Mycobacterium kansasii pulmonary infection in patients with AIDS: spectrum of chest radiographic findings. Radiology 1997; 204:171–175.
60. Campo RE, Campo CE. Mycobacterium kansasii disease in patients infected with human immunodeficiency virus. Clin Infect Dis 1997; 24:1233–1238.
61. El-Solh AA, Nopper J, Abdul-Khoudoud MR, Sherif SM, Aquilina AT, Grant BJ. Clinical and radiographic manifestations of uncommon pulmonary nontuberculous mycobacterial disease in AIDS patients. Chest 1998; 114:138–145.
62. Juffermans NP, Verbon A, Danner SA, Kuijper EJ, Speelman P. *Mycobacterium xenopi* in HIV-infected patients: an emerging pathogen. AIDS 1998; 12:1661–1666.
63. Laissy JP, Cadi M, Cinqualbre A, Boudiaf ZE, Lariven S, Casalino E, Wolff M, Schouman-Claeys E. *Mycobacterium tuberculosis* versus nontuberculous mycobacterial infection of the lung in AIDS patients: CT and HRCT patterns. J Comput Assist Tomogr 1997; 21:312–317.
64. Horowitz ML, Schiff M, Samuels J, Russo R, Schnader J. *Pneumocystis carinii* pleural effusion. Pathogenesis and pleural fluid analysis. Am Rev Respir Dis 1993; 148:232–234.
65. Jayes RL, Kamerow HN, Hasselquist SM, Delaney MD, Parenti DM. Disseminated pneumocystosis presenting as a pleural effusion. Chest 1993; 103:306–308.
66. Schaumberg TH, Schnapp LM, Taylor KG, Golden JA. Diagnosis of *Pneumocystis carinii* infection in HIV-seropositive patients by identification of *P. carinii* in pleural fluid. Chest 1993; 103:1890–1891.
67. Batungwanayo J, Taelman H, Bogaerts J, Allen S, Lucas S, Kagame A, Clerinx J, Montane J, Saraux A, Muhlberger F, et al. Pulmonary cryptococcosis associated with HIV-1 infection in Rwanda: a retrospective study of 37 cases. AIDS 1994; 8: 1271–1276.
68. Friedman EP, Miller RF, Severn A, Williams IG, Shaw PJ. Cryptococcal pneumonia in patients with the acquired immunodeficiency syndrome. Clin Radiol 1995; 50:756–760.
69. Grum EE, Schwab R, Margolis ML. Cryptococcal pleural effusion preceding cryptococcal meningitis in AIDS. Am J Med Sci 1991; 301:329–330.
70. Katz AS, Niesenbaum L, Mass B. Pleural effusion as the initial manifestation of disseminated cryptococcosis in acquired immune deficiency syndrome. Diagnosis by pleural biopsy. Chest 1989; 96:440–441.
71. Newman TG, Soni A, Acaron S, Huang CT. Pleural cryptococcosis in the acquired immune deficiency syndrome. Chest 1987; 91:459–461.
72. Fungal infection in HIV-infected persons. American Thoracic Society. Am J Respir Crit Care Med 1995; 152:816–822.
73. Miller WT Jr, Edelman JM, Miller WT. Cryptococcal pulmonary infection in patients with AIDS: radiographic appearance. Radiology 1990; 175:725–728.
74. Ankobiah WA, Vaidya K, Powell S, Carrasco M, Allam A, Chechani V, Kamholz SL. Disseminated histoplasmosis in AIDS Clinicopathologic features in seven patients from a non-endemic area. NY State J Med 1990; 90:234–238.
75. Marshall BC, Cox JK Jr, Carroll KC, Morrison RE. Histoplasmosis as a cause of pleural effusion in the acquired immunodeficiency syndrome. Am J Med Sci 1990; 300:98–101.
76. Fish DG, Ampel NM, Galgiani JN, Dols CL, Kelly PC, Johnson CH, Pappagianis

D, Edwards JE, Wasserman RB, Clark RJ, et al. Coccidioidomycosis during human immunodeficiency virus infection. A review of 77 patients. Medicine (Baltimore) 1990; 69:384–391.
77. Singh VR, Smith DK, Lawerence J, Kelly PC, Thomas AR, Spitz B, Sarosi GA. Coccidioidomycosis in patients infected with human immunodeficiency virus: review of 91 cases at a single institution. Clin Infect Dis 1996; 23:563–568.
78. Staples CA, Kang EY, Wright JL, Phillips P, Muller NL. Invasive pulmonary aspergillosis in AIDS: radiographic, CT, and pathologic findings. Radiology 1995; 196:409–414.
79. Hung CC, Chen PJ, Hsieh SM, Wong JM, Fang CT, Chang SC, Chen MY. Invasive amoebiasis: an emerging parasitic disease in patients infected with HIV in an area endemic for amoebic infection. AIDS 1999; 13:2421–2428.
80. Chenoweth CE, Singal S, Pearson RD, Betts RF, Markovitz DM. Acquired immunodeficiency syndrome-related visceral leishmaniasis presenting in a pleural effusion. Chest 1993; 103:648–649.
81. Rabaud C, May T, Lucet JC, Leport C, Ambroise-Thomas P, Canton P. Pulmonary toxoplasmosis in patients infected with human immunodeficiency virus: a French National Survey. Clin Infect Dis 1996; 23:1249–1254.
82. Afessa B. Pleural effusions and pneumothoraces in AIDS. Curr Opin Pulm Med 2001; 7:202–209.
83. Behling CA, Wolf PL, Haghighi P. AIDS and malignant mesothelioma—is there a connection? Chest 1993; 103:1268–1269.
84. Huang L, Schnapp LM, Gruden JF, Hopewell PC, Stansell JD. Presentation of AIDS-related pulmonary Kaposi's sarcoma diagnosed by bronchoscopy. Am J Respir Crit Care Med 1996; 153:1385–1390.
85. Aboulafia DM. The epidemiologic, pathologic, and clinical features of AIDS-associated pulmonary Kaposi's sarcoma. Chest 2000; 117:1128–1145.
86. Khalil AM, Carette MF, Cadranel JL, Mayaud CM, Bigot JM. Intrathoracic Kaposi's sarcoma. CT findings. Chest 1995; 108:1622–1626.
87. O'Brien RF, Cohn DL. Serosanguineous pleural effusions in AIDS-associated Kaposi's sarcoma. Chest 1989; 96:460–466.
88. Judson MA, Postic B. Chylothorax in a patient with AIDS and Kaposi's sarcoma. South Med J 1990; 83:322–324.
89. Sivit CJ, Schwartz AM, Rockoff SD. Kaposi's sarcoma of the lung in AIDS: radiologic-pathologic analysis. AJR Am J Roentgenol 1987; 148:25–28.
90. White DA. Pulmonary complications of HIV-associated malignancies. Clin Chest Med 1996; 17:755–761.
91. Padley SP, King LJ. Computed tomography of the thorax in HIV disease. Eur Radiol 1999; 9:1556–1569.
92. Powles T, Matthews G, Bower M. AIDS related systemic non-Hodgkin's lymphoma. Sex Transm Infect 2000; 76:335–341.
93. Sandler AS, Kaplan L. AIDS lymphoma. Curr Opin Oncol 1996; 8:377–385.
94. Sider L, Weiss AJ, Smith MD, VonRoenn JH, Glassroth J. Varied appearance of AIDS-related lymphoma in the chest. Radiology 1989; 171:629–632.
95. Blunt DM, Padley SP. Radiographic manifestations of AIDS related lymphoma in the thorax. Clin Radiol 1995; 50:607–612.
96. Bazot M, Cadranel J, Khalil A, Benayoun S, Milleron B, Bigot JM, Carette MF. Computed tomographic diagnosis of bronchogenic carcinoma in HIV-infected patients. Lung Cancer 2000; 28:203–209.

97. Ray P, Antoine M, Mary-Krause M, Lebrette MG, Wislez M, Duvivier C, Meyohas MC, Girard PM, Mayaud C, Cadranel J. AIDS-related primary pulmonary lymphoma. Am J Respir Crit Care Med 1998; 158:1221–1229.
98. Celikoglu F, Teirstein AS, Krellenstein DJ, Strauchen JA. Pleural effusion in non-Hodgkin's lymphoma. Chest 1992; 101:1357–1360.
99. Alonso-Villaverde C, Hernandez Flix S, Tomas Mas R, Masana Marin L. Pleural involvement as a manifestation of AIDS-associated lymphoma. AJR Am J Roentgenol 1994; 163:993–994.
100. Tirelli U, Spina M, Gaidano G, Vaccher E, Franceschi S, Carbone A. Epidemiological, biological and clinical features of HIV-related lymphomas in the era of highly active antiretroviral therapy. Aids 2000; 14:1675–1688.
101. Cesarman E, Chang Y, Moore PS, Said JW, Knowles DM. Kaposi's sarcoma-associated herpesvirus-like DNA sequences in AIDS-related body-cavity-based lymphomas. N Engl J Med 1995; 332:1186–1191.
102. Morassut S, Vaccher E, Balestreri L, Gloghini A, Gaidano G, Volpe R, Tirelli U, Carbone A. HIV-associated human herpesvirus 8-positive primary lymphomatous effusions: radiologic findings in six patients. Radiology 1997; 205:459–463.
103. Nador RG, Cesarman E, Chadburn A, Dawson DB, Ansari MQ, Sald J, Knowles DM. Primary effusion lymphoma: a distinct clinicopathologic entity associated with the Kaposi's sarcoma-associated herpes virus. Blood 1996; 88:645–656.
104. Ansari MQ, Dawson DB, Nador R, Rutherford C, Schneider NR, Latimer MJ, Picker L, Knowles DM, McKenna RW. Primary body cavity-based AIDS-related lymphomas. Am J Clin Pathol 1996; 105:221–229.
105. Ibrahimbacha A, Farah M, Saluja J. An HIV-infected patient with pleural effusion. Chest 1999; 116:1113–1115.
106. Eid AA, Keddissi JI, Kinasewitz GT. Hypoalbuminemia as a cause of pleural effusions. Chest 1999; 115:1066–1069.

35

Pneumothorax

CHARLIE STRANGE

Medical University of South Carolina
Charleston, South Carolina, U.S.A.

MICHAEL A. JANTZ

University of Florida Health Sciences Center
Gainesville, Florida, U.S.A.

I. Introduction

Pneumothorax is defined as air in the pleural space. Traumatic pneumothoraces can occur following both blunt and penetrating injuries to the chest, although the most common traumatic pneumothorax occurs following iatrogenic needle puncture of the lung. Spontaneous pneumothoraces are divided into primary and secondary subtypes. Primary spontaneous pneumothorax occurs in the absence of underlying lung disease, while secondary spontaneous pneumothorax occurs with increased frequency compared to the general population in nearly every lung disease.

Spontaneous pneumothorax incidence has been estimated at 13.7/100,000 per year for men and 3.2/100,000 per year for women from data extracted from Olmsted County, Minnesota, where 141 cases were seen from 1950 to 1974 (1). The incidence in females is likely higher today, since chronic obstructive pulmonary disease (COPD) and smoking incidence has risen. Approximately equal numbers of patients will have primary and secondary spontaneous pneumothorax.

This chapter is designed to cover the breadth of literature on pneumothorax while keeping the focus on the clinical presentation of disease, appropriate diagnostic testing, and stratified treatment approaches. Recent consensus studies have provided an approach to disease that will need confirmation of algorithms and objective trials to establish appropriate therapy.

II. Traumatic Pneumothorax

Traumatic pneumothorax from blunt or penetrating injury to the thorax occurs commonly. In one recent series of major trauma cases, pneumothorax was present in approximately 20% of cases and was associated with more clinical instability than cases without pneumothorax (2). Any pneumothorax, regardless of size, should receive a chest tube since the extent of organ injuries are usually incompletely known at the time of presentation. Observation makes little sense if there is a remote chance of tension pneumothorax since the threshold for thoracotomy is low for hemodynamic instability. Although a few chest tubes may be placed for small pneumothoraces that may not have progressed, the single case with hemodynamic instability from pneumothorax that could have been prevented while cardiac contusions, aortic dissections, and pericardial tamponade remain in the differential diagnosis suggests that an aggressive treatment algorithm is warranted.

III. Iatrogenic Pneumothorax

Iatrogenic pneumothoraces most commonly follow needle punctures of the lung. When needle aspiration cytology of the lung is performed for lung cancer diagnosis, the frequency of pneumothorax is related to the degree of airway obstruction, the depth of needle puncture, needle size, and the number of fissures crossed. Other common causes of iatrogenic pneumothorax include complications of central venous catheter placement (3), tracheostomy (4), thoracentesis, bronchoscopy, gastric tube placement (5), and pericardiocentesis. Rare cases associated with acupuncture (6) and from self-inflicted needle puncture in Münchausen's syndrome (7) have been reported.

The natural history of iatrogenic pneumothoraces is different than in other forms of pneumothorax since the needle puncture site usually heals within 24 hours. Pneumothorax is radiographically evident within an hour of needle puncture in the majority of cases (8), and onset more than 4 hours after intervention is rare. Therefore, observation is used more frequently than in other pneumothoraces, and short-term interventions such as small-caliber chest tubes with Heimlich valves have become popular.

IV. Primary Spontaneous Pneumothorax

Approximately half of all pneumothoraces occur in the absence of clinically apparent underlying lung disease. The demographics of this population include disproportionate representation of individuals age 15–30 years, of tall stature, and with thin body habitus (9). This body habitus produces a larger gradient in pleural pressure and greater distending pressure in apical alveoli, which may be important in pneumothorax development.

Some evidence from case reports of siblings with disease suggests that genetic factors may predispose some individuals to develop pneumothorax (10). In most series, more than 90% smoke cigarettes (11). Pneumothorax incidence is related to the number of cigarettes smoked, with relative risk >50 for smokers who consume more than one pack per day (12). Lung function tests after resolution of pneumothorax are usually normal.

In some aspects, the primary designation is a misnomer, since high-resolution chest computed tomography (CT) has suggested the presence of subpleural areas of air space enlargement in the majority of these patients (13). These "emphysema-like changes" are commonly bilateral and rarely present in nonsmoking, age-matched controls. Lung density measurements in areas not involved were normal in one study (14). This finding has generated considerable controversy, but no data exist proving that the site of pneumothorax generation is from these lesions. Furthermore, contralateral pneumothorax is no more common in patients who have contralateral emphysema-like changes than in those without contralateral CT abnormalities (15). Because the frequency of bullae is high, a tendency to stratify patients on the basis of their lung anatomy has become more common. The stratification scheme of Vanderschueren is presented in Table 1.

This controversy extends itself into treatment decisions, since staple bullectomy has been recommended for patients with bullae seen on radiograph or CT. It should be noted that no randomized controlled trials of bullectomy versus nonbullectomy pleurodesis have been performed for either primary or secondary spontaneous pneumothorax.

The physiological factor that induces pneumothorax development is an increased transpleural pressure. Epidemiological trials have demonstrated that atmospheric pressure changes are associated with increased pneumothorax incidence (16,17). Pneumothoraces associated with compressed air diving or skydiving have been described. Patients whose occupation requires contact with swings in barometric pressure should consider pleurodesis.

Table 1 Pneumothorax Classification

Stage 1: Anatomically normal lungs
Stage 2: Pleural adhesions
Stage 3: Blebs < 2 cm
Stage 4: Blebs > 2 cm

Source: Ref. 62.

V. Secondary Spontaneous Pneumothorax

A variety of lung diseases can be complicated by pneumothorax. Although the most common disease in case series is usually chronic obstructive lung disease, the heterogeneity of other diseases makes specific diagnosis a particularly important aspect of pneumothorax management.

Many diseases have established diagnoses at the time of pneumothorax presentation. Cystic fibrosis patients have a 1% yearly risk of pneumothorax that presents following exacerbations. Asthmatic patients have been noted to have significant risks for pneumothorax if mechanically ventilated (18). Increased pneumothorax frequency in idiopathic pulmonary fibrosis (IPF) generally occurs in established disease with extensive subpleural honeycomb change.

Pneumothorax occurs most commonly in the obstructive lung diseases. Because of expiratory airflow obstruction, the path of least resistance for subpleural air may remain across the visceral pleural surface, perpetuating the air leak. The other factor favoring pneumothorax development in these diseases is that elastin destruction is common in both the airway and visceral pleura.

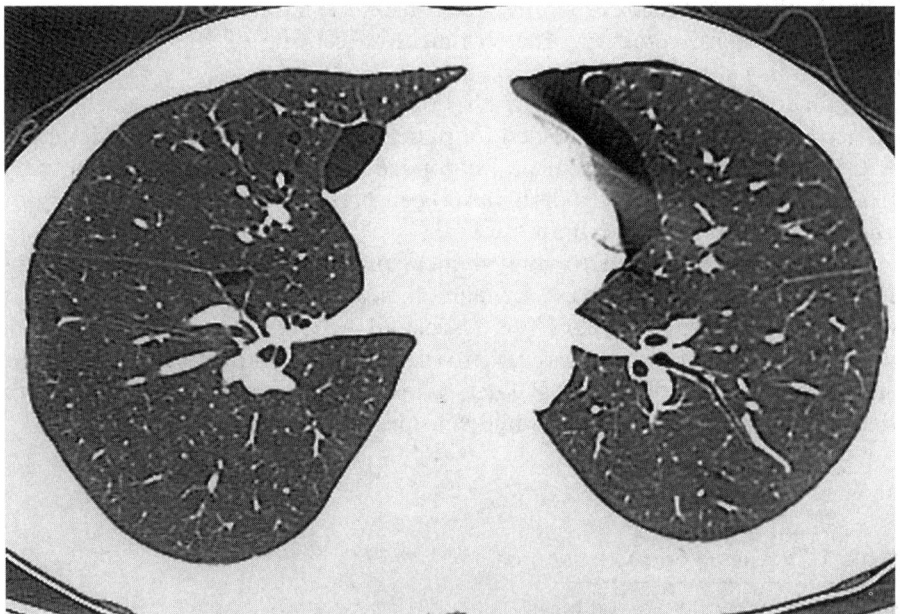

Figure 1 Chest CT scan of 35-year-old male occasional smoker with Birt-Hogg-Dube syndrome who presented with pneumothorax. His father had had five previous pneumothoraces and renal cell carcinoma. Unilateral thoracotomy was performed for definitive recurrence prevention. Note the multiple cysts within the lung and left pneumothorax.

Although no comprehensive studies of human pleural histology following pneumothorax have been performed, some small case series have suggested that visceral pleural connective tissue is reduced.

Some rare diseases are associated with an increased pneumothorax risk. Birt-Hogg-Dube syndrome is an autosomal dominant disease characterized by large lung cysts and increased risk for renal cell carcinoma (19). Pneumothorax is often the herald symptom in an affected patient (Fig. 1). Pneumothorax has been seen with Marfan syndrome and Ehlers-Danlos syndrome (20).

A particularly morbid form of pneumothorax is seen in the acquired immunodeficiency syndrome (AIDS). When pneumothorax occurs it is usually the consequence of subpleural cysts caused by *Pneumocystis carinii*, often being prophylaxed with inhaled pentamidine. Pneumothorax is often protracted, and home chest tubes have been used with frequency in this disorder (21,22).

When pneumothorax occurs with an undiagnosed interstitial lung disease seen on radiograph, the possibilities of Langerhans cell granulomatosis and lymphangioleiomyomatosis should be considered. Both of these diseases carry pneumothorax prevalences of greater than 30%. CT can help in differential diagnosis. Other interstitial lung diseases that have some component of obstruction also carry increased incidence of pneumothorax. These diseases include sarcoidosis, berylliosis, bronchiolitis obliterans with organizing pneumonia, and Sjögren's bronchiolitis (23), among others.

VI. Bronchopleural Fistula

A pneumothorax in which the pleural airleak continues is designated a bronchopleural fistula (BPF). Although any pneumothorax with an occasional bubble through a water seal chamber technically qualifies for the formal definition, most clinicians reserve BPF to designate a patient on mechanical ventilation with significant air leak through the chest tube sufficient to impair alveolar ventilation.

Bronchopleural fistulae are most commonly seen postoperatively following thoracic operations and as complications of acute respiratory distress syndrome (ARDS) (24). Although few randomized trials of therapy have been performed, these patients are often sufficiently ill that elective thoracoscopy for pleural closure is precluded. Nonoperative interventions include optimizing mechanical ventilation to keep airflow across the fistula as low as possible to assist pleural healing. Figure 2 demonstrates the effect of altering mechanical ventilation parameters to lessen bronchopleural airflow. Keeping positive end expiratory pressure as low as possible is usually the best strategy.

Recognizing that significant CO_2 is eliminated by some BPFs (25), aggressive closure of these airleaks is not always indicated. When insufficient alveolar ventilation results despite optimal ventilatory management, options of timed chest tube pressurization can limit the amount of ventilated air traversing the pleura (26,27). Double lumen endotracheal tubes may also be used (28). Of

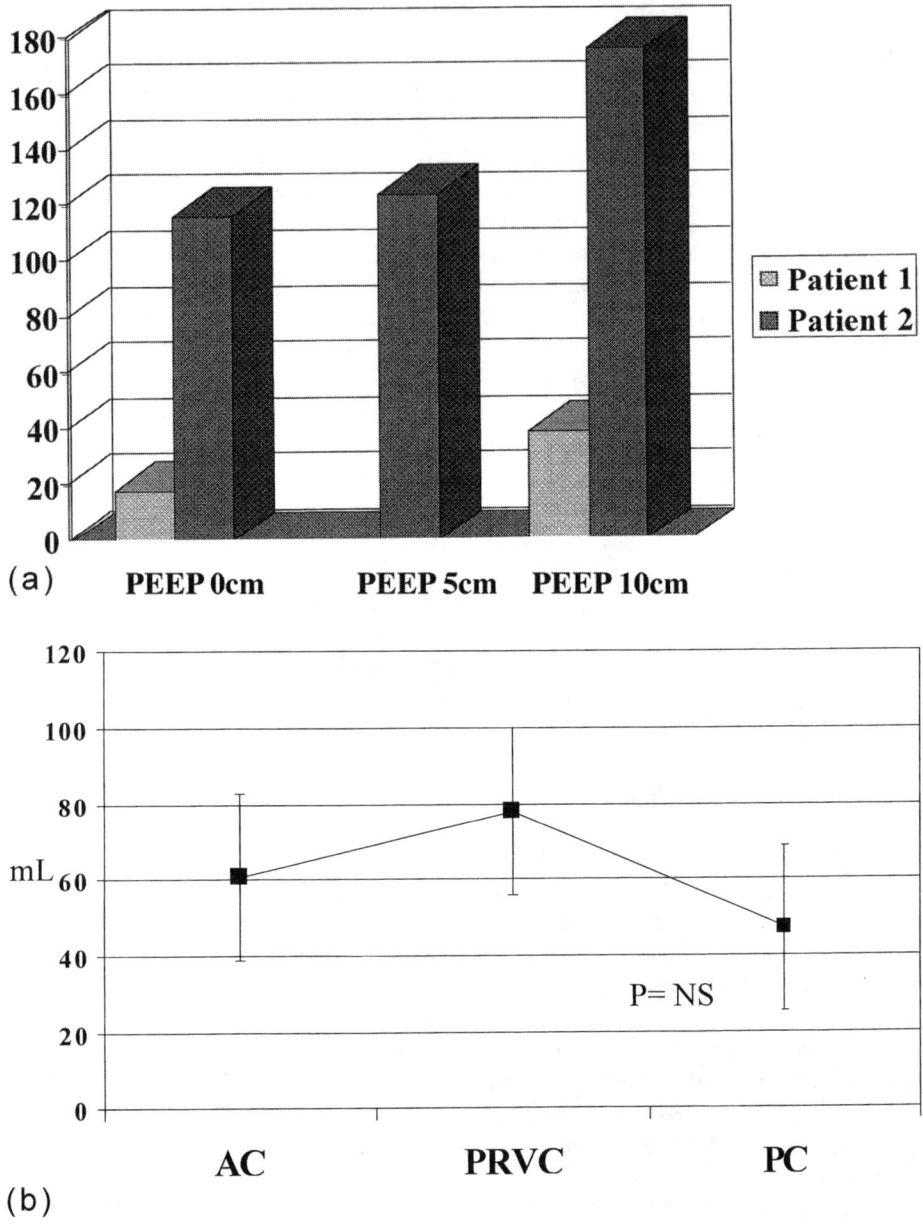

Figure 2 Two patients with bronchopleural fistulae of varying size received mechanical ventilation while measuring the air leak through the chest tube by a chest tube pneumotachometer. Changes in peak airway pressure, tidal volume, minute ventilation, and I:E ratio failed to consistently produce decreases in airleak. (a) Increasing PEEP was shown to increase the size of airleak (mL/breath). (b) Pressure-controlled (PC) ventilation was associated with trends in lowered airleak (mL/breath) compared to pressure-regulated volume controlled (PRVC), and assist-controlled (AC) modes. (c) CO_2 tensions in chest tube gases fell as BPF flow (mL/min) increased.

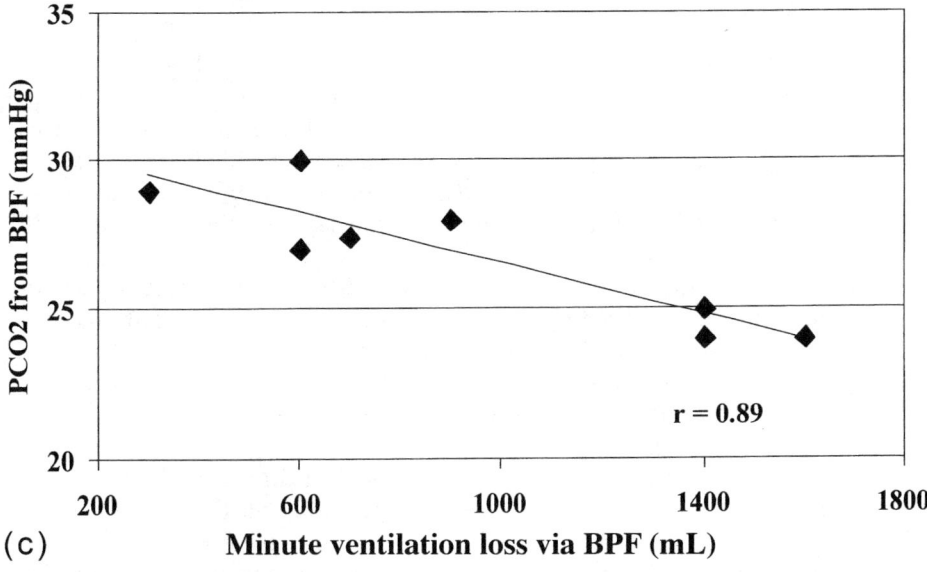

Figure 2 Continued.

interest is that patients with ARDS have no difference in mortality when stratified for the presence or absence of pneumothorax (29).

A. Clinical Presentation

Pleuritic chest pain is the most common symptom at pneumothorax presentation but is present in only 90% of patients (30). The onset of pain can be abrupt or indolent. Radiation to the ipsilateral shoulder is common. Occasionally patients can feel unusual fluttering sensations within the chest that correspond to Hampton's crunch, an unusual sound heard on physical exam suspected to arise from air escaping from within trapped spaces in the major or minor fissures.

Dyspnea is nearly universal in secondary spontaneous pneumothorax (31) and in COPD is often out of proportion to the size of the pneumothorax (32). Because alveolar ventilation drops as lung volumes are reduced, hypercapnea is common (31). Hypoxemia results from both ventilation-perfusion mismatch and shunt that can be as large as 20% (33).

Presentation to medical care can be at times distant from symptom onset. In some series more than 50% of patients waited more than 24 hours before emergency room arrival (34). Presentation after lung transplant can be catastrophic since both pleural spaces may communicate (35).

B. Diagnosis

Although CT is the most specific diagnostic modality, the chest radiograph usually demonstrates pleural air. The optimal technique to obtain chest radiography has been the subject of extensive study. Upright radiographs are superior to supine films. Although expiratory films should theoretically increase visceral pleural density and enhance pneumothorax detection, clinical trials have shown no difference between detection rates from radiographs obtained in full inspiration.

Some series have noted that physicians tend to underestimate the size of pneumothorax from chest radiography (36). Current treatment algorithms have therefore attempted to simplify recommendations using the distance from the lung apex to the thoracic apex as a surrogate measure for percentage lung collapse (37). These recommendations have recently been validated with computed tomography (38).

Plain radiographs in supine patients in the ICU carry significant risks of missed pneumothorax (39–41). In the supine position two thirds of pneumothoraces are found in the subpulmonic space or along the mediastinal pleura (39). Although lateral decubitus views can help clarify some cases, CT remains superior if available. The consequences of a missed pneumothorax in the ICU are significant since 50% may advance to tension (39).

Thoracic ultrasound is also a useful test to detect pneumothorax. The test is not sensitive when subcutaneous air is present but is otherwise both sensitive and specific in the hands of a trained operator (42–43). Lightweight portable ultrasound machines now in common medical use can be used to detect pneumothorax in aerospace medicine and terrestrial trauma patients.

VII. Tension Pneumothorax

Tension pneumothorax is a condition most often seen in hospitalized patients. Although radiographic signs of a positive intrapleural pressure are often seen in pneumothorax, the definition is usually reserved for those patients with physiological manifestations of tension. Radiographic signs include the deep sulcus sign, mediastinal shift, rib splaying, and diaphragmatic depression. Physiological signs of tension include dyspnea, increased pulsus paradoxus, tachycardia (44), hypoxemia, and hypotension (45).

Tension pneumothorax occurs more commonly under positive pressure ventilation. The diagnosis in these patients is often made at bedside before radiographic conformation by the absence of breath sounds and asymmetrical ventilation on chest observation. If the lung is consolidated and therefore unable to collapse, tension physiology can occur with a small or localized pneumothorax (46). A rush of air should accompany the placement of an intravenous catheter through the intercostal space. More formal chest thoracostomy tube placement can be performed electively.

Since tension pneumothorax is frequently catastrophic, any pneumothorax seen in mechanically ventilated patients should receive chest tube drainage. It is reassuring to know that properly treated pneumothoraces do not seem to increase mortality in ARDS (29).

VIII. Therapy

Therapy for pneumothorax remains complicated. Any discussion of therapeutic options must include a discussion of recurrence prevention. In the largest prospective clinical trial of pneumothorax therapy, the VA Cooperative Trial randomized 520 patients to pleural tetracycline or placebo (47). The 5-year recurrence risk for the placebo patients was 32% for primary spontaneous pneumothorax and 41% for secondary spontaneous disease. The majority of pneumothoraces occurred within the first year after the herald event. Although intrapleural tetracycline decreased the pneumothorax recurrence rate to 25%, commercial unavailability and alternatives such as intrapleural talc make this study of historical importance for the natural history of pneumothorax.

IX. Observation

Observation is the recommended treatment modality for stable patients in the recent American College of Chest Physicians Delphi Consensus Statement of Management of Spontaneous Pneumothorax (37). Some criteria must be met before a pneumothorax can be safely observed (Table 2). The pneumothorax should be small enough so that progression in size can be detected (48). Although judging the size of a pneumothorax from an upright chest radiograph is not very accurate, pneumothoraces that are smaller than 3 cm from the lung apex to the apex of the thoracic cavity can usually be watched safely. The patient should be

Table 2 Criteria Necessary for Pneumothorax Observation

Clinical stability
  Stable vital signs
  Ability to speak in full sentences
  Normal oxygenation
Lack of progression
  Unchanging pneumothorax size over 4 hours
Access to emergency care
  Proximity to emergency care
  Sufficient resources to return for worsening

Source: Ref. 37.

symptomatically stable without dyspnea. In secondary spontaneous pneumothoraces, this criterion is rarely met because of the underlying cardiopulmonary reserve. Lastly, sufficient resources should be immediately available for lung reexpansion should the patient decompensate. This might occur at home if the patient has been watched without pneumothorax progression for at least 4 hours and the patient has ready access to emergency services for worsening.

Observation allows for intrapleural air to be resorbed through the pleural vasculature. If the patient is on supplemental oxygen at the time of pneumothorax, the pleural air may contain sufficient oxygen for rapid resorption. More commonly, pleural air rich in nitrogen is resorbed at 1.25% of the pleural volume per day, suggesting a usual course of a few weeks for pneumothorax resolution (49). Oxygen speeds pleural nitrogen resorption by increasing the transvascular gradient for nitrogen resorption by at least a factor of 4 (50,51).

Few clinical series have systematically used observation. In one series of 40 patients in which observation was used for with pneumothorax, 9 of 40 required subsequent chest tube placement. A 32% recurrence rate was recorded with 2 deaths (52).

X. Aspiration

Small catheter aspiration is a procedure that is often used when lung collapse is large, the onset of symptoms is distant from presentation, and patients are stable. The technique of aspiration involves placement of a small catheter into the pleural space to withdraw air. Serial aliquots of air can be withdrawn by 50 mL syringe until gentle pressure is felt or 3–4 L of air has been aspirated. The catheter is withdrawn or a Heimlich valve is attached until a chest radiograph confirms reexpansion. If no subsequent air leak is seen through the Heimlich valve when placed to water seal, a stopcock can close the catheter. Subsequent radiographs in 4 hours show completely expanded lungs in approximately 65% of cases.

The advantage of leaving the small-bore catheter in place during the aspiration procedure is to avoid a second intervention should the lung leak be persistent. Conversion to a water-sealed chest tube is as simple as connecting the catheter to a pleural drainage device.

XI. Chest Thoracostomy Tubes

Chest tube placement should be performed for any patient with clinical instability or when a large pneumothorax complicates secondary spontaneous pneumothorax. Chest tube size is usually adequate with thoracostomy tubes >20 French, although the largest bronchopleural fistulae during ARDS have been measured at 16 L/min, a flow that requires tubes of at least 32 French to handle. Chest tubes should be placed on water seal and not suction since airleak cessation occurs more quickly when suction is avoided (53). The exception occurs when the lung is not expanded on water seal alone or when a large air leak (bubbles ≥4/7 on the water seal chamber of most closed system chest drainage devices) is ongoing (53).

Intercostal tube removal remains somewhat controversial, with some physicians believing that tube clamping improves the ability to accurately detect ongoing pleural airleak. What is clear from several studies is that recurrence rates are substantial if chest tubes are pulled immediately after air bubbles stop traversing the water seal chamber. By waiting an additional 12–48 hours, chest tube removal is usually successful (54,55).

XII. Chest Thoracotomy Tube Pleurodesis

Since pneumothorax recurrence is common, procedures that decrease the risk have been used. It should be noted that a chest tube alone does not alter the recurrence rate of pneumothorax (56). Options for pleurodesis include thoracoscopy, thoracotomy, and application of chemical sclerosing agents through a chest tube (57). The VA Cooperative Study was the first trial to demonstrate the efficacy of intrapleural tetracycline in a prospective, randomized controlled trial. Although pleural tetracycline decreased pneumothorax recurrence, the recurrence rate still remained unacceptably high. Since the removal of tetracycline from the market, doxycycline has been used with similar results.

Talc pleurodesis through a chest tube has been performed by mixing 5 g of talc in sterile saline as a slurry. When administered through the chest tube and allowed to dwell in the thorax for 2 hours, significant amounts of talc are deposited on the pleural surface. Although larger trials of talc slurry pleurodesis have been performed in malignant pleural effusions, the efficacy in preventing pneumothorax recurrence from small case series appears to approach 90% (58). Thoracoscopy that has followed talc slurry pleurodesis failures has noted an asymmetrical talc deposition with most of the substance localized to lung fissures.

XIII. Thoracoscopy and Pleuroscopy

Thoracoscopy for pneumothorax allows inspection of the pleural surface, electrocautery of persistent areas of airleak, application of talc poudrage that dusts the surface of the lung and parietal pleura under visualization, abrasion of one or more pleural surfaces, and resection of bullae. The difficulty in evaluating the efficacy of thoracoscopy for pneumothorax is that different combinations of interventions have been used in different series and no randomized trials have been completed.

The most controversial intervention is the issue of whether bullectomy is indicated for patients in whom bullae are noted on CT scan or at time of thoracoscopy that exceed 2 cm in greatest diameter. Although pleurodesis success has been noted to be less when large bullae are seen, longer duration of airleak usually complicates a bullectomy procedure. Furthermore, the success rate of talc poudrage alone appears to be equally effective when compared to bullectomy/abrasion procedures. Other comparisons between talc poudrage and abrasion have suggested that talc is the more successful intervention (59).

Some controversy has developed over the safety of talc administration. Sterile asbestos-free talc is available in multiple formulations in the United States and abroad. Particle size generally remains proprietary information. Although there is good evidence that some talc particles are removed from the pleural space and traverse pleural lymphatics to the mediastinal lymph nodes and to the systemic circulation, no evidence of organ injury has been suggested. The possible exception is a perivascular lymphocytic infiltrate that has been seen in the lung of animal models of intrapleural talc (60). The rare cases of respiratory failure that have been seen after talc administration (discussed in more detail in other chapters) appear more common when large doses of talc are administered. Although no increased incidence of cancer has been seen 30 years after pleural talc administration, some practitioners use these data to suggest that young individuals should avoid talc pleurodesis. The last concern is that the pneumothorax risk factor of cigarette smoking is also a risk factor for lung cancer or lung transplant that may need subsequent chest surgery. Although surgery is not precluded by previous talc, the operations are more difficult and have more associated morbidity.

XIV. Thoracotomy

Some practitioners still suggest that thoracotomy remains the procedure of choice for recurrent pneumothoraces, since recurrence rates remain less than 2% in most case series. Series using thoracoscopy have slightly higher rates of recurrence. The major morbidity of thoracotomy includes a postthoracotomy pain syndrome that usually resolves over time. For patients with bilateral disease, the option of a median sternotomy has been used.

XV. Timing of Interventions

Considerable controversy surrounds the timing of pneumothorax intervention for pleurodesis. In primary spontaneous pneumothorax in which the risk of death is low because the cardiopulmonary reserve is high, pneumothorax has often been viewed as a nuisance disease. Because the recurrence rate is approximately 30%, any intervention to effect pleurodesis will result in unnecessary treatment of 70% of patients. The counterargument is that pneumothorax death is a tragedy in young individuals and is likely underreported. Primary economic analyses suggest that money can be saved by intervening with talc poudrage by thoracoscopy in first presentations of disease (61).

In the ACCP consensus document, pleurodesis was recommended after the first secondary spontaneous pneumothorax and after the second primary spontaneous pneumothorax.

XVI. Future Research

Since little can be done—other than smoking cessation initiatives—as primary prevention, most research will need to focus on the best treatment modalities. Unfortunately, trials performed in the past have been retrospective case series or small nonrandomized prospective trials. The next generation of pneumothorax research will require prospective, randomized clinical trials. The likelihood of such trials being performed is not high since pneumothorax remains a sporadic disease in which therapy must be initiated rather quickly in most cases. No obvious economic incentives are likely to emerge to foster clinical trials in this area.

High on the list of priorities for research is whether bullectomy is needed when thoracoscopy is performed for continuing bronchopleural fistula or for recurrence prevention. The needed trial would require computed tomography to stratify patients and randomize comparable groups to bullectomy with talc poudrage and talc poudrage alone. At issue is whether interventional pulmonologists should be performing therapy in all patients in the absence of bullectomy capabilities.

References

1. Melton LJ III, Hepper NG, Offord KP. Incidence of spontaneous pneumothorax in Olmsted County, Minnesota: 1950 to 1974. Am Rev Respir Dis 1979; 120:1379–1382.
2. Di Bartolomeo S, Sanson G, Nardi G, Scian F, Michelutto V, Lattuada L. A population-based study on pneumothorax in severely traumatized patients. J Trauma 2001; 51:677–682.
3. Eerola R, Kaukinen L, Kaukinen S. Analysis of 13 800 subclavian vein catheterizations. Acta Anaesthesiol Scand 1985; 29:193–197.
4. Arola MK. Tracheostomy and its complications. A retrospective study of 794 tracheostomized patients. Ann Chir Gynaecol 1981; 70:96–106.
5. Wendell GD, Lenchner GS, Promisloff RA. Pneumothorax complicating small-bore feeding tube placement [see comments]. Arch Intern Med 1991; 151:599–602.
6. Ernst E, White AR. Prospective studies of the safety of acupuncture: a systematic review. Am J Med 2001; 110:481–485.
7. Urschel JD, Miller JD, Bennett WF. Self-inflicted pneumothoraces. Ann Thorac Surg 2001; 72:280–281.
8. Dennie CJ, Matzinger FR, Marriner JR, Maziak DE. Transthoracic needle biopsy of the lung: results of early discharge in 506 outpatients. Radiology 2001; 219:247–251.
9. Melton LJ III, Hepper NG, Offord KP. Influence of height on the risk of spontaneous pneumothorax. Mayo Clin Proc 1981; 56:678–682.
10. Koivisto PA, Mustonen A. Primary spontaneous pneumothorax in two siblings suggests autosomal recessive inheritance. Chest 2001; 119:1610–1612.
11. Light R. Pleural Diseases. 2d ed. Philadelphia: Lea & Febiger, 1990:331.
12. Bense L, Eklund G, Wiman LG. Smoking and the increased risk of contracting spontaneous pneumothorax. Chest 1987; 92:1009–1012.

13. Bense L, Lewander R, Edlund G, Hedenstierna GC, Wiman LG. Nonsmoing, non-alpha1-antitrypsin deficiency-induced emphysema in nonsmokers with healed spontaneous pneumothorax, identified by computed tomography of the lungs. Chest 1993; 103:433–438.
14. van Belle AF, Lamers RJ, ten Velde GP, Wouters EF. Diagnostic yield of computed tomography and densitometric measurements of the lung in thoracoscopically-defined idiopathic spontaneous pneumothorax. Respir Med 2001; 95:292–296.
15. Schramel FM, Zanen P. Blebs and/or bullae are of no importance and have no predictive value for recurrences in patients with primary spontaneous pneumothorax. Chest 2001; 119:1976–1977.
16. Bense L. Spontaneous pneumothorax related to falls in atmospheric pressure. Eur J Respir Dis 1984; 65:544–546.
17. Scott GC, Berger R, McKean HE. The role of atmospheric pressure variation in the development of spontaneous pneumothoraces. Am Rev Respir Dis 1989; 139:659–662.
18. Afessa B, Morales I, Cury JD. Clinical course and outcome of patients admitted to an ICU for status asthmaticus. Chest 2001; 120:1616–1621.
19. Schmidt LS, Warren MB, Nickerson ML, Weirich G, Matrosova V, Toro JR, Turner ML, Duray P, Merino M, Hewitt S, Pavlovich CP, Glenn G, Greenberg CR, Linehan WM, Zbar B. Birt-Hogg-Dube syndrome, a genodermatosis associated with spontaneous pneumothorax and kidney neoplasia, maps to chromosome 17p11.2. Am J Hum Genet 2001; 69:876–882.
20. Nishiyama Y, Nejima J, Watanabe A, Kotani E, Sakai N, Hatamochi A, Shinkai H, Kiuchi K, Tamura K, Shimada T, Takano T, Katayama Y. Ehlers-Danlos syndrome type IV with a unique point mutation in COL3A1 and familial phenotype of myocardial infarction without organic coronary stenosis. J Intern Med 2001; 249:103–108.
21. Afessa B. Pleural effusions and pneumothoraces in AIDS. Curr Opin Pulm Med 2001; 7:202–209.
22. Vricella LA, Trachiotis GD. Heimlich valve in the management of pneumothorax in patients with advanced AIDS. Chest 2001; 120:15–18.
23. Wu S, Sagawa M, Suzuki S, Kumagai-Braesch M, Honda Y, Sato M, Kondo T. Pulmonary fibrosis with intractable pneumothorax: new pulmonary manifestation of relapsing polychondritis. Tohoku J Exp Med 2001; 194:191–195.
24. Gammon RB, Shin MS, Groves RH Jr, Hardin JM, Hsu C, Buchalter SE. Clinical risk factors for pulmonary barotrauma: a multivariate analysis. Am J Respir Crit Care Med 1995; 152:1235–1240.
25. Bishop MJ, Benson MS, Pierson DJ. Carbon dioxide excretion via bronchopleural fistulas in adult respiratory distress syndrome. Chest 1987; 91:400–402.
26. Blanche PB, Koens JC, Layon AJ. A new device that allows synchronous intermittent inspiratory chest tube occlusion with any mechanical ventilator. Chest 1990; 97:1426–1430.
27. Carvalho P, Thompson WH, Riggs R, Carvalho C, Charan NB. Management of bronchopleural fistula with a variable-resistance valve and a single ventilator. Chest 1997; 111:1452–1454.
28. Strange C. Double-lumen endotracheal tubes. Clin Chest Med 1991; 12:497–506.
29. Weg JG, Anzucto A, Balk RA, Wiedemann HP, Pattishall EN, Schork MA, Wagner LA. The relation of pneumothorax and other air leaks to mortality in the acute respiratory distress syndrome [see comments]. N Engl J Med 1998; 338:341–346.

30. Seremetis MG. The management of spontaneous pneumothorax. Chest 1970; 57:65–68.
31. Dines DE, Clagett OT, Payne WS. Spontaneous pneumothorax in emphysema. Mayo Clin Proc 1970; 45:481–487.
32. Shields TW, Oilschlager GA. Spontaneous pneumothorax in patients 40 years of age and older. Ann Thorac Surg 1966; 2:377–383.
33. Norris RM, Jones JG, Bishop JM. Respiratory gas exchange in patients with spontaneous pneumothorax. Thorax 1968; 23:427–433.
34. O'Hara VS. Spontaneous pneumothorax. Mil Med 1978; 143:32–35.
35. Slebos DJ, Elting-Wartan AN, Bakker M, van der Bij W, van Putten JW. Managing a bilateral pneumothorax in lung transplantation using single chest-tube drainage. J Heart Lung Transplant 2001; 20:796–797.
36. Engdahl O, Toft T, Boe J. Chest radiograph—a poor method for determining the size of a pneumothorax [see comments]. Chest 1993; 103:26–29.
37. Baumann MH, Strange C, Heffner JE, Light R, Kirby TJ, Klein J, Luketich JD, Panacek EA, Sahn SA. Management of spontaneous pneumothorax: an American College of Chest Physicians Delphi consensus statement. Chest 2001; 119:590–602.
38. Noppen M, Alexander P, Driesen P, Slabbynck H, Verstraete A. Quantification of the size of primary spontaneous pneumothorax: accuracy of the Light index. Respiration 2001; 68:396–399.
39. Tocino IM, Miller MH, Fairfax WR. Distribution of pneumothorax in the supine and semirecumbent critically ill adult. AJR Am J Roentgenol 1985; 144:901–905.
40. Kollef MH. The effect of an increased index of suspicion on the diagnosis of pneumothorax in the critically ill. Mil Med 1992; 157:591–593.
41. Kollef MH. Risk factors for the misdiagnosis of pneumothorax in the intensive care unit. Crit Care Med 1991; 19:906–910.
42. Dulchavsky SA, Schwarz KL, Kirkpatrick AW, Billica RD, Williams DR, Diebel LN, Campbell MR, Sargysan AE, Hamilton DR. Prospective evaluation of thoracic ultrasound in the detection of pneumothorax. J Trauma 2001; 50:201–205.
43. Lichtenstein DA, Menu Y. A bedside ultrasound sign ruling out pneumothorax in the critically ill. Lung sliding. Chest 1995; 108:1345–1348.
44. Gustman P, Yerger L, Wanner A. Immediate cardiovascular effects of tension pneumothorax. Am Rev Respir Dis 1983; 127:171–174.
45. Rutherford RB, Hurt HH, Brickman RD. The pathophysiology of progressive tension pneumothorax. J Trauma 1968; 8:212–227.
46. Gobien RP, Reines HD, Schabel SI. Localized tension pneumothorax: unrecognized form of barotrauma in adult respiratory distress syndrome. Radiology 1982; 142:15–19.
47. Light RW, O'Hara VS, Moritz TE, McElhinney AJ, Butz R, Haakenson CM, Read RC, Sassoon CS, Eastridge CE, Berger R. Intrapleural tetracycline for the prevention of recurrent spontaneous pneumothorax. Results of a Department of Veterans Affairs cooperative study. JAMA 1990; 264:2224–2230.
48. Wolfman NT, Myers WS, Glauser SJ, Meredith JW, Chen MY. Validity of CT classification on management of occult pneumothorax: a prospective study [In Process Citation]. AJR Am J Roentgenol 1998; 171:1317–1320.
49. Kircher L, Swartzel R. Spontaneous pneumothorax and its treatment. JAMA 1954; 155:24–29.
50. Northfield TC. Oxygen therapy for spontaneous pneumothorax. Br Med J 1971; 4:86–88.

51. England GJ, Hill RC, Timberlake GA, Harrah JD, Hill JF, Shahan YA, Billie M. Resolution of experimental pneumothorax in rabbits by graded oxygen therapy. J Trauma 1998; 45:333–334.
52. O'Rourke JP, Yee ES. Civilian spontaneous pneumothorax. Treatment options and long-term results. Chest 1989; 96:1302–1306.
53. Cerfolio RJ, Bass C, Katholi CR. Prospective randomized trial compares suction versus water seal for air leaks. Ann Thorac Surg 2001; 71:1613–1617.
54. Sharma TN, Agnihotri SP, Jain NK, Madan A, Deopura G. Intercostal tube thoracostomy in pneumothorax—factors influencing re-expansion of lung. Indian J Chest Dis Allied Sci 1988; 30:32–35.
55. So SY, Yu DY. Catheter drainage of spontaneous pneumothorax: suction or no suction, early or late removal? Thorax 1982; 37:46–48.
56. Andrivet P, Djedaini K, Teboul JL, Brochard L, Dreyfuss D. Spontaneous pneumothorax. Comparison of thoracic drainage vs immediate or delayed needle aspiration. Chest 1995; 108:335–339.
57. Almind M, Lange P, Viskum K. Spontaneous pneumothorax: comparison of simple drainage, talc pleurodesis, and tetracycline pleurodesis. Thorax 1989; 44:627–630.
58. Kennedy L, Sahn SA. Talc pleurodesis for the treatment of pneumothorax and pleural effusion. Chest 1994; 106:1215–1222.
59. Cardillo G, Facciolo F, Regal M, Carbone L, Corzani F, Ricci A, Martelli M. Recurrences following videothoracoscopic treatment of primary spontaneous pneumothorax: the role of redo-videothoracoscopy. Eur J Cardiothorac Surg 2001; 19:396–399.
60. Kennedy L, Harley RA, Sahn SA, Strange C. Talc slurry pleurodesis. Pleural fluid and histologic analysis. Chest 1995; 107:1707–1712.
61. Torresini G, Vaccarili M, Divisi D, Crisci R. Is video-assisted thoracic surgery justified at first spontaneous pneumothorax? Eur J Cardiothorac Surg 2001; 20:42–45.
62. Vanderschueren RG. Pleural talcage in patients with spontaneous pneumothorax. Poumon Coeur 1981; 37:273–276.

36

Tuberculous Pleuritis

PETER D. O. DAVIES

The Cardiothoracic Centre
Liverpool NHS Trust
Liverpool, England

I. Introduction

At the age of 65, Nelson Mandela, while imprisoned on Robbin Island off the coast of Cape Town, South Africa, developed tuberculous pleuritis. He gives a very graphic account of his diagnosis and treatment in his book: "Without any preliminaries he tapped me roughly on my chest and then said gruffly, 'There is water in your lung.' He asked a nurse to bring him a syringe and without further ado he poked it into my chest and drew out some brownish liquid" (1). Tuberculous pleuritis can strike the old as well as the young, but once treated it does not usually affect the health or longevity of the individual.

II. Definition

Tuberculous pleurisy is the development of pleurisy and/or a pleural effusion as a result of infection with a bacterium of the *Mycobacterium tuberculosis* complex. It is a fairly benign form of tuberculosis, being usually self-limiting and only occasionally causing complications. It should always be treated, as nearly half of patients will subsequently go on to develop postpleuritic tuberculosis.

It may be difficult to confirm the diagnosis, but a strongly positive tuberculin test in the presence of symptoms and signs is highly suggestive. The isolation of *M. tuberculosis* from the fluid or pleural biopsy confirms the diagnosis.

Treatment is with the standard 6-month regimen, and the prognosis is good.

III. Epidemiology

The precise incidence of tuberculous pleuritis is difficult to determine, as it is not routinely separated from other forms of respiratory tuberculosis when being notified. Two notification surveys of tuberculosis in England and Wales investigated the chest radiographic pattern of disease (2,3), providing an estimate of the frequency of tuberculosis effusion. There was a remarkable consistency across the two surveys. In the 1978/9 survey, 80 of 1267 (6%) patients for whom a chest radiograph was available and who had a diagnosis of respiratory tuberculosis had a pleural effusion only, and a further 6 (<1%) had an effusion and enlarged hilar nodes. The figures for the 1983 survey were 129 of 2001 patients (6%). The proportions were slightly higher in those of Indian subcontinent ethnic origin (patients originating form India, Pakistan and Bangladesh)—51 of 670 (8%)—compared with white patients—66 of 1201 (5%).

A separate analysis of children in the same surveys was undertaken (4). This showed that in 1978/9, 3 of 119 children had enlarged nodes and an effusion and 2 an effusion only. The figures for 1983 were 9 (3%) and 12 (4%) of 301. The percentages for the Indian subcontinent and White groups were similar—4% and 3% and 2% and 5%, respectively.

Based on the numbers of tuberculosis cases in the 6-month surveys, these figures would give an overall proportion of 5% of all notified cases having tuberculous pleurisy, or a rate of 0.5 per 100,000. Because the radiographic results from the two sequential surveys were so similar, further notification surveys did not include a radiographic assessment. This means that a more up-to-date incidence of tuberculous pleurisy in the United Kingdom is not possible until results of the enhanced notification system, which started in 2000, are published.

These data compare with an incidence of 4.9% in a 20-year retrospective review of 1738 cases reported from the United States and 2.2% incidence from New York (5,6). Coexistent HIV infection may be expected to increase the overall incidence of tuberculosis and the pattern of presentation. However, one study did not show any difference in the proportion of patients with tuberculous pleuritis (7).

In a large study of 5480 patients with pulmonary and pleural tuberculosis from Turkey, 343 (6.7%) had a pleural effusion. This was right sided in 193, left sided in 141, and bilateral in 9. A pneumothorax was present in 78 (1.5%). The incidence of HIV positivity in these patients was not known but at the time of the study was generally low in Turkey (probably less than 3%) (8).

An extensive study of tuberculous pleurisy from Romania showed a decrease from 30.7/100,000 to 4.2/100,000 between 1958 and 1985, followed by a "stagnation" at 4.3/100,000 for 1986–1989. In 1990, the incidence of tuberculous pleurisy increased to 6.8/100,000. The proportion of pleural involvement in respiratory disease was maintained at 13–15% for 1960–1980, with a subsequent diminution to 7.9% in 1989. By age groups, the incidence of tuberculous pleurisy was at its highest level (19.1/100,000) at the age of 20–24 years in 1990 (9).

IV. Tuberculous Pleurisy and HIV

In a prospective study, 94 patients presenting at two large Harare hospitals with clinically suspected pleural TB were enrolled over a 10-month period. Pleural TB was diagnosed in 90 individuals (median age 33 years; range 18–65; 64 males); the seroprevalence of HIV was 85%. HIV-positive patients were older than HIV-negative individuals and had a significantly lower median CD4+ count. A CD4+ count of $< 200 \times 10^6/L$ was associated with a length of illness >30 days, a positive pleural fluid smear and a positive pleural biopsy Ziehl-Neelsen stain. However, a relationship between CD4+ count and either pleural granuloma formation or radiological evidence of disseminated disease was not observed. The authors concluded that in sub-Saharan Africa, TB pleural effusions have become associated with older age, a chronic onset, an increased mycobacterial load, and a low CD4+ count (10).

All cases of pleural tuberculosis in AIDS patients in South Carolina from 1988 through 1994 were reviewed. Twenty-two (11%) of the 202 AIDS patients with tuberculosis had pleural involvement compared to 6% in non-AIDS patients ($p = 0.01$). Associated features of AIDS tuberculous pleurisy included substantial weight loss (7.65 ± 1.35 kg) and lower lobe infiltrates (12/22; 55%). No difference in pleural fluid characteristics was found when comparing AIDS patients with a serum CD4 count >200/µL to patients with CD4 count <200/µL. Two (9%) of the 22 patients died of tuberculosis. Chest radiograph follow-up of 20 patients showed complete resolution in 7, improvement in 10, and no improvement in 3. The authors concluded that in South Carolina, pleural involvement is more common in AIDS patients than in non-AIDS patients with tuberculosis. Tuberculous pleurisy has several atypical features in AIDS patients such as substantial weight loss and lower lobe infiltrates. The outcome of treatment is good for most patients (11).

V. Pathophysiology

Probably the most comprehensive overview of TB pleuritis is given by Patiala's monograph reviewing 2816 men with TB pleuritis from the Finnish army (12).

Patiala was able to follow all but a few of these patients for a period of between 7 and 9 years. The great majority was between 18 and 20 years as they were mostly young recruits to the army. The main weakness of the paper is that tuberculous pleuritis was defined only as the presence of and exudative pleural effusion in the presence of a positive tuberculin test.

During the follow-up period, 43.1% of the series developed postpleuritic tuberculosis, the great majority of whom (70%) developed pulmonary or (10%) bone and joint tuberculosis. He found that the time interval between tuberculous pleurisy and the development of postpleuritic tuberculosis was short, 75% of patients proceeding to disease within 2 years. Progress to postpleuritic tuberculosis was more likely the older the patient at age of onset of pleurisy. Development of postpleuritic tuberculosis was also more common in urban than in rural settings, as was the presence of a family history of tuberculosis.

The prognosis of uncomplicated pleuritis was good. Within one year after the onset of the disease, three quarters of the group were considered fit for work, and at the end of the follow-up period only a few showed slight disabilities due to pleural thickening.

Of the group with subsequent development of postpleuritic tuberculosis, only a quarter was fully fit for work 9 years after the onset of pleurisy. The death rate for this group was 37.3%, while that for the entire pleuritis series was 15.6%.

The incidence of the development of tuberculous pleuritis was age related, being most common at age 18 and declining exponentially thereafter.

Patiala describes three forms of tuberculous pleuritis:

1. Pleuritis associated with the acute primary stage. This may be more common in adults incurring primary infection than children.
2. Pleuritis occurring after apparent healing of the primary focus in the lung. This may be due to direct spread from enlarged hilar lymph nodes.
3. Pleuritis occurring simultaneously with lung changes. This is presumed to be caused by direct spread from the lung or lymphatic infection following the development of postprimary lung disease. If pleuritis is the first sign of disease, this may be difficult to distinguish from acute primary pleuritis. It is this form that may be associated with a pneumothorax.

Tuberculous pleurisy is a result of the discharge of mycobacterial antigens from a subpleural node into the subpleural space of a hypersensitive host. The clinical syndrome arises from the delayed-type hypersensitivity reaction in which plasma proteins are exuded into the pleural space and CD4+ cells accumulate, multiply, and release inflammatory mediators, particularly IFN-γ. These may provide a means of diagnosis (see below) (13–16).

The occasional anergic response to PPD in a patient suffering from tuberculous pleural effusion has been explained by the sequestration of the antigen-specific T cells into the pleural space, and so being unable to mount a peripheral hypersensivity response, IL-2 is also released from macrophages within the pleural fluid (13,17,18). High vitamin D concentrations (cholecalciferol) have also been reported, representing enhanced macrophage activation (19).

VI. Case Study 1: A Breathless Man

A. Presenting Complaint

A 47-year-old barman presented with a 3-month history of breathlessness.

B. Medical History

The patient, who worked part time in a social club bar, complained that for 3 months he had had progressive breathlessness. He had a persistent smoker's cough, which had not changed, and had lost no weight. There was no significant past history. He drank in excess of 50 units of alcohol a week.

C. Examination and Tests

He was obese (105 kg) and there was clinical evidence of a right-sided pleural effusion. He had a low-grade fluctuating pyrexia. The presence of an effusion was confirmed on chest x-ray (Fig. 1). A liter of straw-colored fluid was aspirated from the chest, which was an exudate. This was negative on direct smear for AAFB, but a pleural biopsy done at the same time showed a few granulomata. A Mantoux test was strongly positive (25 mm induration to 10 TU).

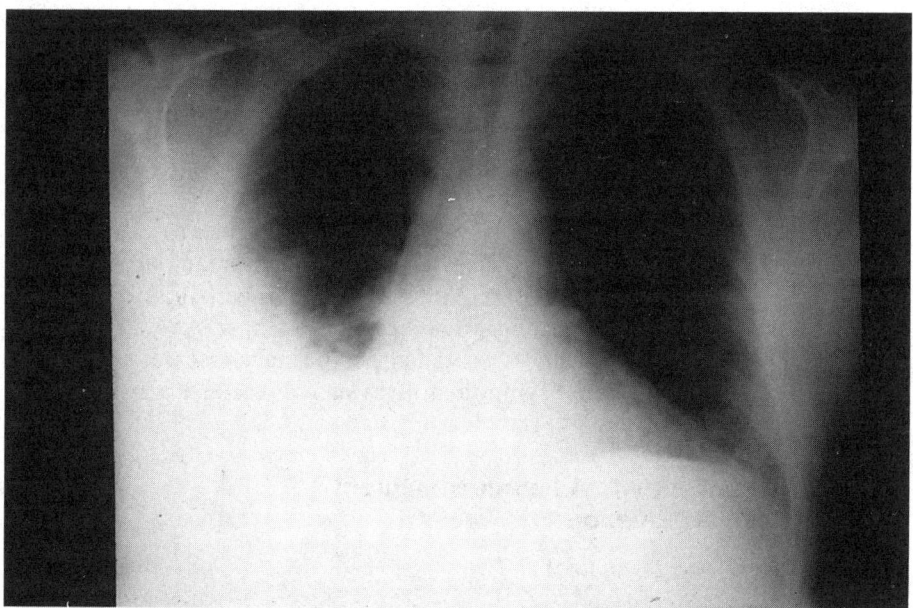

Figure 1 Chest x-ray of a 47-year-old British white barman showing a right-sided pleural effusion. See text for details.

D. Outcome

He was started on triple antituberculous chemotherapy comprising isoniazid, rifampicin, and pyrazinamide. Initially there was no apparent response. The pyrexia continued, and he showed no symptomatic improvement. After a week of continuing pyrexia he was started on oral prednisolone (60 mg). Within 24 hours the temperature had returned to normal and he felt considerably better. He was discharged from hospital and continued on steroids in addition to full antituberculous chemotherapy for 4 months. The effusion had resolved by the end of the third month of treatment. Antituberculous drugs were continued for 6 months.

E. Comment

Depending on the epidemiological context, pleural effusions are usually associated with primary tuberculosis, as was the case in this man. Bacilli in the fluid are sparse so that smear is usually negative and negative culture is not uncommon. Rarely they may become heavily contaminated with bacilli and a tuberculous empyema may result. This is usually the result of reactive, not primary disease. Histology and culture of the pleura are usually needed to make the diagnosis. If pleural fluid can be removed, then a pleural biopsy can and should be carried out. Standard chemotherapy for 6 months is sufficient, and steroids are said to speed the resorption of fluid, though recent evidence suggests that they make no difference to the final outcome.

This patient had continuing pyrexia despite several days of treatment. The fact that steroids immediately suppressed this suggests a hypersensitivity phenomenon, though whether this was due to the initial pathology or the antituberculous chemotherapy is not clear. Steroids have an important role in suppressing the hypersensitivity reaction of tuberculosis itself or of the drugs used in treatment and should be considered if pyrexia persists beyond a week of treatment in the presence of a firm diagnosis of tuberculosis.

The absence of weight loss or of any symptoms other than those caused by the effusion itself suggests a primary disease in this patient. In fact, he was one of several patients to be identified as part of an outbreak of tuberculosis around the bar in which he worked. Pleural effusion in the elderly is more likely to be due to reactivation of a primary infection, so-called postprimary disease, and in this situation weight loss and other sympomatology such as malaise is usual.

VII. Case Study 2: A Febrile Immigrant with an Effusion

A. Presenting Complaint

An 18-year-old Pakistani woman presented with fever, dry cough, and breathlessness, which had persisted for 2 weeks.

B. History of Presenting Complaint

The patient had been in the United Kingdom for 12 months. She had experienced fever and "flu-like" symptoms for 2 weeks, with weight loss of 7 kg. She had also had a dry nonproductive cough and had developed breathlessness on moderate effort. There was no past history of note.

C. Examination

The patient was toxic, with a temperature of 39.0°C and signs of a large right pleural effusion.

D. Tests

The chest x-ray showed a left-sided pleural effusion (Fig. 2) Hemoglobin was 10.0 g/dL normochromic, and ESR was 123 mm/h. Serum proteins showed an albumen level of 29 g/L and a globulin level of 37 g/L. The tuberculin test was strongly positive. Pleural aspiration, biopsy, and drainage were performed. The fluid showed an exudate (protein 51 g/L), which was heavily lymphocytic on cytology. Pleural biopsy showed multiple necrotic granulomata with palisaded epithelioid histiocytes and lymphocytes. Pleural fluid was later culture positive at 6 weeks for *M. tuberculosis* fully sensitive to first-line drugs.

E. Progress

A total of 4 L of fluid was drained, and treatment recommended on the basis of the lymphocytic exudates. Treatment was started with rifampicin, isoniazid, and pyrazinamide orally. The patient remained toxic and was vomiting despite normal transaminases. Treatment with IV rifampicin and isoniazid, together with streptomycin and hydrocortisone, was given for 4 days. This stopped the vomiting and reduced the fever. Treatment was then switched back to oral rifampicin, isoniazid, and pyrazinamide with prednisolone (30 mg/day). Treatment with steroids was gradually withdrawn over 2 months. Pyrazinamide was stopped when full sensitivity was confirmed, and treatment was continued with rifampicin/isoniazid as combination tablets for a total of 6 months. At the end of treatment the chest x-ray showed only minimal basal pleural reaction, and the ESR was 4 mm/h.

F. Comment

The immediate working diagnosis here was tuberculosis. Any person in an ethnic minority group with a pleural effusion, particularly if a recent immigrant, should be regarded as having tuberculosis until proved otherwise. Treatment was commenced on the basis of a lymphocytic exudate and a positive tuberculin test. Pleural fluid is positive on culture in up to 50% of cases but is rarely microscopy positive, and it usually takes 4–6 weeks to yield a positive culture. Similarly,

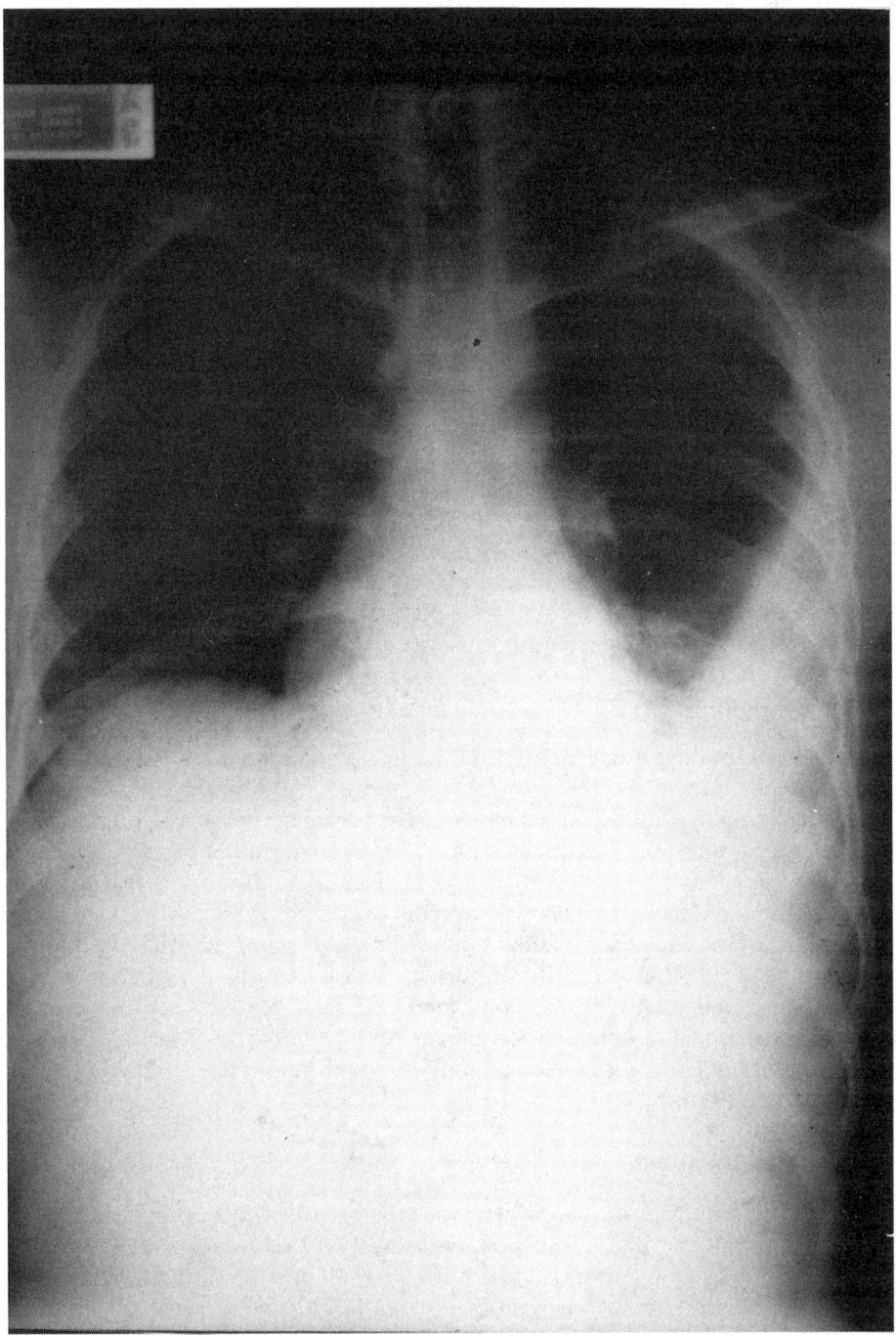

Figure 2 Chest x-ray of an 18-year-old immigrant Pakistani woman showing a left-sided pleural effusion. See text for details.

pleural biopsy is not positive in all cases due to the patchy distribution of granulomata. The biopsy is more likely to be positive if multiple samples are taken, the operator is experienced, or the biopsy is under direct vision (e.g., a thoracoscopy). Standard short-course chemotherapy is appropriate for pleural disease. Corticosteriods may be needed in addition for systemic effects, and there are some data to support more rapid clearance of fluid with corticosteroids. Large pleural effusions need to be drained, while smaller amounts can be aspirated or left to resolve on medication. Continued fluid production or the need for repeated fluid aspirations is an indication for corticosteroids. In low-income countries treatment based on clinical findings and a positive tuberculin test may be appropriate. In HIV-coinfected patients there is an increase in pleural disease, but the tuberculin test is more likely to be negative (20,21).

VIII. Case Study 3: A Breathless Woman

A. Presenting Complaint

A 69-year-old white woman was seen with malaise and a pleural effusion.

B. History of Presenting Complaint

The patient had had flu-like symptoms 4 months earlier and had then been admitted to hospital 8 weeks earlier with right pleuritic plan and fever. She had been treated for pneumonia and showed clinical improvement, but 50 mL of bloodstained fluid had been aspirated at that time. She had been a nonsmoker for over 20 years, but she had had some exposure to industrial asbestos 45 years earlier. Persistent pleural shadowing was seen on the chest x-ray, and the patient was referred to the chest clinic.

C. Past Medical History

Appendectomy and cholecystectomy were the only features of the history.

D. Examination

The patient's weight was 65 kg, with signs of a small right pleural effusion.

E. Tests

Chest x-ray showed right basal shadowing, which was mainly pleural. Hemoglobin was 12.1 g/dL and ESR was 37 mm/h. The pleural fluid that was removed several weeks earlier had shown no malignant cells and had a protein content of 46 g/L. Liver function and biochemical profile was normal.

F. Progress

A computed tomography scan (CT) of the thorax was arranged, but within a few days the pleural fluid aspirated earlier was reported to be culture positive for

AFB, later confirmed as *M. tuberculosis*, which was sensitive to all drugs. The CT was canceled, and treatment with Rifater was started. The patient now recalled that a cousin had died of tuberculosis 22 years earlier. Her treatment was uneventful until week 8, when vomiting and jaundice developed. Treatment was stopped with an ALT concentration of 3690 IU/L. There had been considerable improvement in the chest x-ray. Liver function had returned to normal after 3 weeks, so rifampicin/isoniazid was restarted, but the ALT concentration decreased to 165 IU/L and bilirubin rose to 32 mmol/L within 10 days. The drugs were again stopped. Liver function returned to normal within 5 days, ethambutol (15 mg/kg) was started and isoniazid was reintroduced, initially at 50 mg/day for 3 days and then at 300. Ethambutol was continued for a further 7 months. The chest x-ray showed only minimal blunting of the right costophrenic angle on completion of treatment.

G. Comment

Tuberculosis was not suspected in the older white woman, and secondary malignancy or mesothelioma was considered more likely. However, pleural fluid had been sent for culture despite the small probability of infection. Pleural tuberculosis usually gives straw-colored lymphocyte-rich exudates, but the effusion can be heavily bloodstained. Pleural biopsy might have given the diagnosis, but may only yield granulomata in 50% of cases, multiple biopsies being more likely to give a positive result. Tuberculous pleural effusion is usually an immediate postprimary phenomenon, but can occur as a reactivation phenomenon in older age (22).

IX. Case Study 4: A Case of Empyema

A. Presenting Complaint

A 38-year-old Pakistani man was seen with a 5-day history of fever.

B. History of Presenting Complaint

The patient had returned 1 week earlier from a 7-week visit to Pakistan, and the fever had developed 2 days after his return. He had lost 4 kg in weight over a 6-month period.

C. Past Medical History

The patient was a nonsmoker but admitted to drinking 90 units of alcohol a week until 3 months before presentation.

D. Examination

The patient was febrile at between 38.5 and 39.0°C, and showed signs of a right pleural effusion.

E. Tests

Hemoglobin was 11.7 g/dL normochromic and the white cell count was 6.1×10^6/mL. Bilirubin was normal but ALT at 56 IU/L (normal range < 45 IU/L) and alkaline phosphatase at 161 IU/L (normal range < 145 IU/L) were slightly elevated. Chest x-ray showed a right pleural effusion with some widening of the upper mediastinum. Aspiration of the plural effusion showed 400 mL of purulent fluid, which was sent for culture.

F. Progress

Because of the purulent fluid the patient was treated as an empyema case, with intravenous cefotaxime, gentamycin, and metronidazole. A right basal chest drain was inserted and a further 800 mL of purulent fluid were drained. His fever did not respond to 7 days of the above antibiotics. The pleural fluid showed predominantly lymphocytes on cytology, was negative on standard and anaerobic cultures, and was an exudate (protein 55 mg/L). The pleural fluid was negative on direct microscopy for AFB. A trial of antituberculosis treatment with Rifater 5 tablets (for weight 63 kg) was given, and the fever responded within 7 days. The drain was removed and the patient began to regain weight. His dose of Rifater was increased to 6 tablets when he reached 65 kg in weight. After 5 weeks positive cultures were received for *M. tuberculosis*, later shown to be fully sensitive. Liver function monitoring because of the patient's history of abnormal liver function tests and previous excessive alcohol consumption showed improvement to normal over 4 weeks. The pyrazinamide was stopped when full sensitivity was confirmed. He was treated with a further 4 months of rifampicin/isoniazid and weighed 76 kg on completion of treatment. There was some residual pleural scarring, and the patient's spirometry showed a mild restrictive defect (FEV_1 2.35/2.75 L, compared to predicted value of 3.40/4.21 L).

G. Comment

In view of the short history and purulent pleural fluid, a nontuberculous empyema was first suspected. The lack of response to broad-spectrum antibiotics and particularly the finding of a lymphocytosis in the purulent fluid, rather than a polymorph leukocytosis, suggested tuberculosis. Pleural fluid was negative on microscopy, but was later culture positive. Tuberculous empyemas may be microscopy positive, whereas this is very rarely the case for "standard" tuberculous pleural effusions. A tuberculous empyema should be managed in the same was as any other empyema, with appropriate antibiotics, drainage of pus, and consideration of decortication. It is possible in this case that the lung function at the end of treatment might have been better if a decortication had been performed, but the patient was reluctant to consider surgery (23).

X. Case Study 5: Untreated Tuberculous Pleuritis Leads to Something Worse

A. Presenting Complaint

A 29-year-old woman was seen in the TB contact clinic having been in close and frequent contact with an aunt who had developed pulmonary tuberculosis. The contact had a grade IV Heaf test but no follow-up was carried out. She presented to the same chest clinic 6 months later with a large right-sided pleural effusion.

B. Progress

The patient was seen on three occasions in the next 2 months and sputum taken for AFB. The effusion gradually resolved and the sputum was negative for AFB on smear and culture. The patient was discharged from the clinic. Five months later the patient presented with a month of increasingly severe headaches. When seen she had signs of meningitis. Within 48 hours she had a rapid deterioration, became unrousable and required ventilation. A CSF sample was negative on direct smear but grew *M. tuberculosis*. Though the patient survived she remains severely handicapped.

C. Comment

The fact that the patient had tuberculous pleuritis was not recognized in the chest clinic. This was despite a previously strongly positive tuberculin test and a history of contact with a potentially infectious patient. The attempted exclusion of tuberculosis by sending sputum for smear and culture is often inappropriate in tuberculous pleuritis, which may be a complication of primary tuberculosis and will therefore have relatively few bacilli. The appropriate investigation would have been aspiration of the fluid and pleural biopsy for histology and culture. Even in the absence of a clear diagnosis by these means a pleural effusion following TB contact and a positive tuberculin test in a relatively young person should have been treated as a case of tuberculous pleurisy with appropriate antibiotics. Had this been done the subsequent development of tuberculous meningitis and the severe disability that resulted would have been avoided. The fact that this was not done was negligent on the part of the consulting doctor.

This patient exhibited the classic sequence of primary disease manifesting initially as tuberculous pleuritis. This resolved spontaneously with no treatment, but as a result a much more serious form of tuberculosis, tuberculous meningitis, developed approximately 6 months later.

XI. Diagnosis

Isolating the organism from a sample taken from the patient is the only way to prove a diagnosis of a tuberculous pleural effusion. The problem is that bacteria may be scarce in this condition. The pleural fluid is very rarely smear positive for organisms, and cultures may be negative. It is often necessary to rely on nonspecific diagnostic criteria, particularly while cultures are awaited.

A. Characteristics of the Pleural Fluid

When the fluid is tapped, it usually has a clear yellow, "straw"-colored appearance but may be brown as a result of light blood staining or dark red due to heavy blood staining (1).

Most tuberculous pleural effusions are exudates with a pleural fluid-to-serum protein ratio of >0.5. Glucose concentration is usually low. Lymphocytes usually comprise more than half of the cellular material. None of these factors is particularly useful in differentiating a tuberculous pleural effusion from other causes, specifically malignant, parapneumonic, or rheumatoid (24,25).

Biopsying the pleura will be more productive in producing a diagnosis than simply aspirating the pleural fluid. Wherever fluid can be aspirated, a pleural biopsy is technically possible and should be attempted. Histological examination of the pleura revealed granulomas in 60% of tuberculous effusions in one series. The diagnostic yield rises to 90% if pleural biopsies are cultured (26,27).

Using these diagnostic criteria, only 10% (7 of 70) patients required a presumptive diagnosis of a tuberculous pleural effusion based the criteria of, a positive skin test, a lymphocytic effusion, and successful treatment with antituberculosis chemotherapy (5).

Some authors distinguish between tuberculous pleuritis as a result of primary disease, where no lung infiltrates are present on chest x-ray, and reactivated disease, where infiltrates are present. In one series a positive sputum was obtained from only 4/35 (11.4%) of cases with no infiltrates but 31/35 (88.6%) of cases with infiltrates. A positive culture result, however, was obtained from pleural fluid in 18/30 (60%) and from pleural biopsy in 6/9 (67%) of noninfiltrate cases. Positive results from pleural fluid and biopsy specimens from those patients with infiltrates was similar (5).

In another series from Spain with 129 patients, positive smear from sputum samples was obtained from 7% of the 98 patients with no infiltrates but 28% of the 31 with infiltrates. A positive microbiological culture was obtained from 64% and 63% of patients from the two groups, respectively (28). Results of diagnostic tests from a series of 88 patients from Malaysia showed a positive histological diagnosis (granuloma present) in 80% of patients with no lung infiltrate designated primary disease and 70% of those with infiltrates designated reactive disease (29).

Despite 90% efficacy of diagnosis based on traditional histological and microbiological techniques, an enormous literature around biochemical diagnostic tests for tuberculous pleurisy has evolved. The presence of high concentrations of adenosine deaminase (ADA) in the pleural fluid has received the most attention. A review in 1995 concluded that DNA tests would be of more value (30).

B. Adenosine Deaminase Activity

ADA activity has been proposed as a diagnostic test for tuberculous pleurisy since 1978 (31). ADA is an enzyme involved in purine catabolism found in most cells, but particularly in lymphocytes, where its concentration is inversely related to the degree of differentiation. High levels of ADA have been found in patients with lung cancer and tuberculosis. Levels of ADA activity show a significant correlation with the number of CD4+ cells in the pleural effusion (32,33).

False-positive tests can be found in patients with rheumatoid disease, chronic lymphatic leukaemia, and undifferentiated carcinoma (34,35). The reviewer goes on to ask whether the measurement of ADA activity would be useful in deciding which of the 10–20% of patients who have negative histological or bacteriological results should have empirical therapy. Also, this method of diagnosing tuberculous pleurisy differs from others, such as IFN-γ, serum antibody to the 38 kDA antigen, and detection of bacterial DNA. The last method has achieved sensitivities of 60–80%, depending on which sequencing within the bacterial DNA is used for detection (36,37).

Studies trying to differentiate the isoenzymes of ADA as a diagnostic test for tuberculous pleurisy have not been shown to be useful (38).

C. DNA Methods

A more recent study on the sensitivity of PCR for DNA amplification to diagnose tuberculous pleuritis showed that, based on microbiological and histological diagnosis, the sensitivity could be improved to 89% and specificity to 100%. However, there were no cases in this series, which were undiagnosed by traditional methods, so it was not possible to determine whether PCR could be of use in the diagnosis of microbiological and histologically negative tuberculous pleuritis (39).

In a recent study from Thailand, 98 patients with symptomatic exudative lymphocytic pleural effusion were enrolled in a study to evaluate the diagnostic sensitivity of polymerase chain reaction (PCR) assay. Pleural fluid was sent for gram staining, AFB staining, aerobic culture, culture of *Mycobacterium tuberculosis* on LJ media, and cytology. Additional fluid was used for a PCR assay of the 16 S-23 S rRNA gene spacer sequences and for a nested PCR of the 16 S rRNA gene as a blind control. Overall etiologies comprised malignancy 53.1%, tuberculosis 36.7%, lymphoma 2.0%, and chronic nonspecific inflammation 8.2%. The sensitivity and specificity of AFB-staining were 6% and 79%, respectively; while cultures on LJ media were 17% and 100%, respectively. The sensitivity of the PCR assay was 50% and the specificity was 61%. When PCR was nested, the sensitivity was 72% and specificity was 53%. Two thirds (26/36) of tuberculous pleural effusion cases underwent pleural biopsy, and 62% were diagnosed by histopathology. There were no complications from thoracocentesis or pleural biopsy in any of the patients. The authors concluded that PCR assay was more sensitive than AFB staining and mycobacteria culture for diagnosis tuberculous pleural effusion, but its specificity was quite low (40).

A South American study evaluated ADA activity, IFN-γ levels, and PCR in 140 cases of pleural effusion, 42 with confirmed pleural TB, 19 with probable pleural TB, 70 with a nontuberculous aetiology, and 9 having an undetermined aetiology. ADA activity, IFN-γ levels, and PCR were 88%, 85.7%, and 73.8% sensitive, respectively, and 85.7%, 97.1%, and 90% specific, respectively, for pleural TB that had been confirmed by either culture or pleural biopsy specimens. The combination of PCR, IFN-γ measurement, and ADA activity determination allowed the selective increase of sensitivity and specificity for probable and confirmed cases compared to individual methods. Positive and negative predictive values for these individual or combined methods were maintained over a wide range of prevalence of pleural TB in the patient population presenting with pleural effusions. These clinical variables, together with the use of ADA activity determination, PCR, and measurement of IFN-γ levels, provide the basis for the rapid and efficient diagnosis of pleural TB in different clinical settings (41).

In practice about 90% of cases of tuberculous pleural effusion can be diagnosed using the conventional techniques of pleural fluid and biopsy smear, culture, and histology. In the younger patient with a positive tuberculin test a trial of therapy if the diagnosis remains unclear is probably warranted. In the older patient where malignancy is likely, further diagnostic procedures including thoracoscopy and even thoracotomy to obtain adequate tissue samples should be carried out.

D. Radiographic Diagnosis

The radiography of a tuberculous pleural effusion is essentially nonspecific. Unusually, a nodular picture seen on CT scanning has been reported. Contrast enhanced CT examination of a 22-year-old male with pleuritic chest pain showed pleural-based nodular thickening and masses without any parenchymal involvement or mediastinal lymphadenopathy. Pathological examination following right parietal pleural decortication showed multiple granulomas with caseating necrosis typical of tuberculosis (42).

E. Differential Diagnosis of Pleurisy

The differential diagnosis of pleurisy will depend on the epidemiological circumstances.

Cardiac causes
  Congestive cardiac failure (often bilateral and transudate)
Malignancy (malignant cells may be present in the fluid)
  Bronchogenic carcinoma
  Mesothelioma
  Lymphoma

Autoimmune disease (may be a transudate, reduced glucose concentration)
    Rheumatoid arthritis
    Systemic lupus erythematosis
    Polyserositis
Infections (parapneumonic)
    Bacterial
    Tuberculosis
    Any other bacteria
    Viral
    Bornholm disease
Circulatory
    Pulmonary embolus
Renal disease (transudate)
    Nephrotic syndrome
    Peritoneal dialysis
Trauma

XII. Management of Tuberculous Pleural Effusion

All patients believed to be suffering from tuberculous pleurisy should be treated with antituberculosis chemotherapy. The standard short-course chemotherapy of 2 months of isoniazid, rifampicin, and pyrazinamide followed by 4 months of isoniazid and rifampicin has shown to be adequate (43,21). Although using only 2 drugs for 6 months has also been shown to have no relapse, this approach can no longer be recommended because of the increased danger of drug resistance in recent years (44). In fact it is now recommended that a fourth drug be added, usually ethambutol for the initial two months or until sensitivity results are available (45,46). Doses for children should be adjusted by weight (47). It is generally assumed that the addition of steroids speeds the time of resolution of the effusion but makes no difference to the overall outcome (48,49).

A recent Cochrane review concluded that there was insufficient evidence to know whether steroids are effective in tuberculosis. Only three small trials totaling 236 patients met the criteria for inclusion in the analysis (50).

In a study from Malawi, 296 patients with smear-negative and 138 with pleural TB were enrolled: 366 (84%) of patients were HIV-positive; 220 (51%) completed treatment, and 144 (33%) died by 12 months. Significantly higher case fatality rates were found in older patients, HIV-positive patients, and patients with pulmonary parenchymal lung disease. The treatment regimens compared three times weekly isoniazid, rifampicin, and pyrazinamide for 2 months followed by isoniazid and ethambutol or Thiacetazone for 2 months followed by isoniazid alone for four months, against the "standard" regimen of streptomycin, Thiacetazone (or ethambutol), and isoniazid for one month followed by isoniazid and ethambutol or Thiacetazone for 11 months. They found no difference in outcomes between the regimens. In resource-poor settings the ability of a regimen that excludes rifampicin to cure the patient is an advantage in cost saving. However, in areas where HIV infection is high, ethambutol should be used instead of Thiacetazone to avoid serious adverse effects (51).

Paradoxical worsening of disease, in spite of effective chemotherapy for tuberculosis, has been reported to occur in cases of intracranial tuberculoma, lymph node, and pulmonary tuberculosis. However, only rare case reports describe such paradoxical response in tuberculosis pleurisy. Sixty-one patients with a proven tuberculous pleural effusion were retrospectively screened in Riyadh, Saudi Arabia. Paradoxical increase in the size of the effusion was detected in 10 of 61 patients. In 6 patients the effusion became massive with worsening of dyspnea requiring the use of corticosteroids in 5 patients and therapeutic aspiration in all 6. However, complete resolution occurred in all 10 patients within 1–3 months. Three out of the 10 patients developed residual pleural thickening (52).

XIII. Management of Complications of Pleural Tuberculosis

Tuberculous empyema represents a chronic, active infection of the pleural space with a large number of tubercle bacilli. It is rare compared with tuberculous pleural effusions. The inflammatory process may be present for years with few symptoms. Patients often come to clinical attention at the time of a routine chest radiograph or after the development of bronchopleural fistula. The diagnosis of tuberculous empyema is suspected on computed tomography imaging by finding a thick, calcific pleural rind and rib thickening surrounding loculated pleural fluid. The pleural fluid is grossly purulent and smear positive for acid-fast bacilli. Treatment consists of pleural space drainage and antituberculous chemotherapy. Problematic treatment issues include the inability to reexpand the trapped lung and difficulty in achieving therapeutic drug levels in pleural fluid, which can lead to drug resistance. Surgery, which is often challenging, should be undertaken by experienced thoracic surgeons (53).

From a study in Saudi Arabia, 26 patients (23 male and three female) with an average age of 33.8 years (range 18–61 years) presented with tuberculous empyema. The empyema was right-sided in 13, left-sided in 12, and bilateral in one patient. Patients presented with respiratory symptoms for a mean duration of 4.43 months (range 1–48 months). In patients with exudative empyema ($n = 4$) the fluid was aspirated, but one patient required intercostal tube (ICT) drainage for 6 days. There were four patients with fibrinopurulent empyema treated with thoracoscopic drainage with a mean postoperative stay of 8 days (range 4–12 days). In the organizing stage ($n = 18$), initial drainage with large ICT was performed. The pleura was less than 2 cm in thickness in eight patients, for which repeated installation of streptokinase was performed (three to seven times). Satisfactory results were achieved in six patients (75%), and the remaining two required decortication. Of the 10 patients with thick cortex, one required a window and nine had decortication, two of which had additional lobectomy and two had pneumonectomy. All patients fully recovered with no mortality and with a mean duration of drainage of 18 days (range 3–61 days). The stage and the state of the underlying lung should guide surgical treatment for tuberculous empyema (54).

Twelve patients suffering from posttuberculous chronic empyema were reviewed. There was an average latency period of 44.83 years between the acute tuberculous illness and the clinical manifestation of the empyema. Nine of the patients had been treated with collapse therapy, induced by artificial intrapleural pneumothorax, 1 with thoracoplasty, and 2 only with late and inadequate antimycobacterial chemotherapy. Eleven patients (91.6%) also had a cutaneous fistula (7 cases) and/or a bronchopleural fistula (4 cases). Late tuberculous sequelae are significant not only from a numerical standpoint, but also for the seriousness of the caused pathological conditions, often posing problems for differential diagnosis. Tuberculosis should never be neglected or considered last in the differential diagnosis of empyema and pyopneumothorax (55).

References

1. Mandela N. Long Walk to Freedom. 1994 Abacus 646.
2. Medical Research Unit Tuberculosis and Chest Diseases Unit. National Survey of Tuberculosis Notifications in England and Wales 1978–9. Br Med J 1980; 281:895–898.
3. Medical Research Unit Tuberculosis and Chest Diseases Unit. National survey of tuberculosis notifications in England and Wales in 1983: characteristics of disease. Tubercle 1987; 68:19–32.
4. Medical Research Unit Tuberculosis and Chest Diseases Unit. Tuberculosis in children: a national survey of notifications in England and Wales in 1983. Arch Dis Child 1988; 63:19–32.
5. Seibert AF, Haynes J Jr, Middleton R, Bass JB Jr. Tuberculous pleural effusion— twenty year experience. Chest 1991; 99:883–886.
6. Tuberculosis in New York City 1992. New York: Bureau of Tuberculosis Control, New York City Department of Health, 1993.
7. Ankobiah WA, Finch P, Powell S, Heurich A, Shivaram I, Kamholz SL. Pleural tuberculosis in patients with and without AIDS. J Assoc Acad Minority Physicians 1990; 1:20–23.
8. Akotgu S, Yorgancioglu A, Cirak K, Dereli SM. Clinical spectrum of pulmonary and pleural tuberculosis: a report of 5,480 cases. Eur Respir J 1996; 9:2031–2035.
9. Didilescu C, Marica M, Jalba M. The epidemiological aspects of tuberculous pleurisy in Romania. Pneumoftiziologia 1992; 41:83–87.
10. Heyderman RS, Makunike R, Muza T, Odwee M, Kadzirange G, Manyemba J, Muchedzi C, Ndemera B, Gomo ZA, Gwanzura LK, Mason PR. Pleural tuberculosis in Harare, Zimbabwe: the relationship between human immunodeficiency virus, CD4 lymphocyte count, granuloma formation and disseminated disease. Trop Med Intern Health 1998; 3:14–20.

11. Frye MD, Pozsik CJ, Sahn SA. Tuberculous pleurisy is more common in AIDS than in non-AIDS patients with tuberculosis. Chest 1997; 112:393–397.
12. Patiala J. Initial Tuberculous Pleuritis in the Finnish Armed Forces in 1939–45 with Special Reference to Eventual Postpleuritic Tuberculosis. Copenhagen: Enjar Munksgaard, 1955.
13. Ellner JJ, Barnes PF, Wallis RS, Modlin RL. The immunology of tuberculous pleurisy. Semin Respir Inf 1988; 3:335–342.
14. Ribera E, Ocaana I, Martinez-Vazquez JM, Rossell M, Espanol T, Ruibal A. High levels of interferon gamma in tuberculous pleural effusions. Chest 1988; 93:308–311.
15. Shimakata K, Kishimoto H, Takagi E, Tsunekawa H. Determination of the T-cell subset producing gamma-interferon in tuberculous pleural effusion. Microbiol Immunol 1986; 30:353–361.
16. Rossi GA, Balbi B, Manca F. Tuberculous pleural effusions. Am Rev Respir Dis 1987; 138:575–579.
17. Ota T, Okubo Y, Sekiguchi M. Analysis of immunological mechanisms of natural killer cell activity in tuberculous pleural effusions. Am Rev Respir Dis 1990; 142:29–33.
18. Ito M, Kojiro N, Shirasaka T, Moriwaki Y, Tachhibana I, Kokubu T. Elevated levels of soluble interleukin-2 receptors in tuberculous pleural effusions. Chest 1990; 97:1141–1143.
19. Barnes PF, Modlin RL, Bikle DD, Adams JS. Transpleural gradient of 1,25-dihydroxyvitamin D in tuberculous pleuritis. J Clin Invest 1989; 83:1527–1532.
20. Lee CH, Wang WJ, Lan RS, Tsai YH, Chiang YC. Corticosteroids in the treatment of tuberculous pleurisy. A double blind, placebo controlled, randomized study. Chest 1988; 94:1256–1259.
21. Ormerod LP, McCarthy OR, Rudd RM, Horsfield N. Short course chemotherapy for tuberculous pleural effusions and culture negative tuberculosis. Tuberc Lung Dis 1995; 76:25–27.
22. Mungall IP, Cowen PN, Cooke NT, Roach TC, Cooke NJ. Multiple pleural biopsy with the Abrams needle. Thorax 1980; 35:600–602.
23. Davies PDO, Ormerod LP. Case Presentations in Clinical Tuberculosis. London: Arnold, 1999.
24. Light RW, Erozan YS, Ball WC. Cells in pleural fluid: their value in differential diagnosis. Arch Intern Med 1973; 132:854–860.
25. Yam LT. Diagnostic significance of lymphocytes in pleural effusions. Ann Int Med 1967; 66:972–982.
26. Levine H, Metzger W, Lacera D, Kay L. Diagnosis of tuberculous pleurisy by culture of pleural biopsy specimen. Arch Intern Med 1970; 126:269–271.
27. Scharer L, McClement JH. Isolation of tubercle bacilli from needle biopsy specimens of parietal pleura. Am Rev Respir Dis 1968; 97:466–468.
28. Arriero JM, Romero S, Hernandez L, Candela A, Martin C, Gil J, Fernandez C. Tuberculous pleurisy with and without radiographic evidence of disease. Is there a difference? Int J Tuberc Lung Dis 1998; 2:513–517.
29. Liam CK, Lim KH, Wong MM. Tuberculous pleurisy as a manifestation of primary and reactivation disease in a region with a high prevalence of tuberculosis. Int J Tuberc Lung Dis 1999; 3:816–822.
30. Bothamley GH. Tuberculous pleurisy and adenosine deaminase. Thorax 1995; 50:593–594.

31. Piras MA, Gakis C, Budroni M, Andreoni G. Adenosine deaminase activity in pleural effusions: an aid to differential diagnosis. Br Med J 1978; 2:1751–1752.
32. Baganha MF, Pego A, Lima MA, Gaspar EV, Cordeiro AR. Serum and pleural adenosine deaminase. Correlation with lymphocytic populations. Chest 1990; 97:605–610.
33. Nishihara H, Akedo H, Okada H, Hattori S. Multienzyme patterns of serum adenosine deaminase by agar gel electrophoresis: an evaluation of the diagnostic value in lung cancer. Clin Chim Acta 1970; 30:251–258.
34. Ocana I, Ribera E, Martinez-Vazquez JM, Ruiz I, Bejarano E, Pigrau C, Pahissa A. Adenosine deaminase activity in rheumatoid pleural effusion. Ann Rheum Dis 1988; 47:394–397.
35. Valdes L, San Jose E, Alvarez D, Sarandeses A, Pose A, Chomon B, Alvarez-Dobano JM, Salgueiro M, Rodriguez Suarez JR. Diagnosis of tuberculous pleurisy using the biologic parameters adenosine deaminase, lysozyme, and interferon gamma. Chest 1993; 103:458–465.
36. de Wit D, Maartens G, Steyn L. A comparative study of the polymerase chain reaction and conventional procedures for the diagnosis of tuberculous pleural effusion. Tuberc Lung Dis 1992; 73:262–267.
37. de Lassence A, Lecossier D, Pierre C, Cadranel J, Stern M, Hance AJ. Detection of mycobacterial DNA in pleural fluid from patients with tuberculous pleurisy by means of the polymerase chain reaction: comparison of two protocols. Thorax 1992; 47:265–269.
38. Carstens ME, Burgess LJ, Martiz FJ, Taljaard JJF. Isoenzymes of adenosine deaminase in pleural fluid: a diagnostic tool? Int J Tuberc Lung Dis 1998; 2:831–835.
39. Takagi N, Hasegawa Y, Ichiyama S, Shibagaki T, Shimokata K. Polymerase chain reaction of pleural biopsy specimens for rapid diagnosis of tuberculous pleuritis. Int J Tuberc Lung Dis 1998; 2:338–341.
40. Reechaipichitkul W, Lulitanond V, Sungkeeree S, Patjanasoontorn B. Rapid diagnosis of tuberculous pleural effusion using polymerase chain reaction. Southeast Asian J Trop Med Public Health 2000; 31:509–514.
41. Villegas MV, Labrada LA, Saravia NG. Evaluation of polymerase chain reaction, adenosine deaminase, and interferon-gamma in pleural fluid for the differential diagnosis of pleural tuberculosis. Chest 2000; 118:1355–1364.
42. Ariyurek OM, Cil BE. Atypical presentation of pleural tuberculosis: CT findings. Br J Radiol 2000; 73:209–210.
43. Ormerod LP, Horsfield N. Short-course antituberculosis chemotherapy for pulmonary and pleural disease: 5 years experience in clinical practice. Br J Dis Chest 1987; 81:268–271.
44. Dutt AK, Moers D, Stead WW. Tuberculous pleural effusion: six-month therapy with isoniazid and rifampicin. Am Rev Respir Dis 1992; 145:1429–1432.
45. Joint Tuberculosis Committee of the British Thoracic Society. Chemotherapy and management of tuberculosis in the United Kingdom: recommendations 1998. Thorax 1998; 53:536–548.
46. Migliori GB, Raviglione MC, Schaberg T, Davies PDO, Zellweger JP, Grzemska M, Mihaescu T, Clancy L, Casali L. Tuberculosis management in Europe. Recommendations of a working group of the European Respiratory Society (ERS), the World Health Organisation (WHO) and the International Union Against Tuberculosis and Lung Disease, European Region (IUATLD). Eur Respir J 1999; 14:978–992.

47. Donald PR, Byers N. Tuberculosis in childhood. In: Clinical Tuberculosis. 2d ed. Chapman and Hall London, 1998.
48. Wyser C, Walzl G, Smedema JP, Swart F, van Schalkwyk EM, van de Wal BW. Corticosteroids in the treatment of tuberculous pleurisy. A double-blind, placebo-controlled, randomized study. Chest 1996; 110:333–338.
49. Galarza I, Canete C, Granados A, Estopa R, Manresa F. Randomised trial of corticosteroids in the treatment of tuberculous pleurisy. Thorax 1995; 50:1305–1307.
50. Matchaba PT, Volmink J. Steroids for Treating Tuberculous Pleurisy. Cochrane database of systemic reviews DC0018876, 2000.
51. Harries AD, Nyangulu DS, Banda H, Kang'ombe C, Van der Paal L, Glynn JR, Subramanyam VR, Wirima JJ, Salaniponi FM, Maher D, Nunn P. Efficacy of an unsupervised ambulatory treatment regimen for smear-negative pulmonary tuberculosis and tuberculous pleural effusion in Malawi. Int J Tuberc Lung Dis 1999; 3:402–408.
52. Al-Majed SA. Study of paradoxical response to chemotherapy in tuberculous pleural effusion. Respir Med 1996; 90:211–214.
53. Sahn SA, Iseman MD. Tuberculous empyema. Semin Respir Inf 1999; 14:82–87.
54. Al-Kattan KM. Management of tuberculous empyema. Eur J Cardiothor Surgery 2000; 17:251–254.
55. Mancini P, Mazzei L, Zarzana A, Biagioli D, Sposato B, Croce GF. Post-tuberculosis chronic empyema of the "forty years after." Eur Rev Med Pharmacol Sciences 1998; 2:25–29.

37

Pleural Effusions in Children

JOHN N. TSANAKAS and ELPIS HATZIAGOROU

Aristotelian University of Thessaloniki
and Hippokration General Hospital
Thessaloniki, Greece

I. Introduction

Pleural effusions (PE) in children are caused by the same factors as in adults, but they appear with a different incidence, related to age. In the neonate, PE are usually present either as part of a generalized disease, like hydrops fetalis or congenital heart disease, or as an isolated finding, like chylothorax, intrauterine or perinatal infection, transient tachypnea of the newborn, persistent hypertension of the newborn, etc. (1). In older children the most common cause is bacterial pneumonia, followed by heart failure, rheumatic disorders, and malignancies (2). Tuberculus effusions are also increasing in frequency (3). In this chapter we will focus on the most common causes of pleurisy in the pediatric population, the diagnostic approach, and management.

Pleural space is the space formed between the parietal and visceral pleura. It is a continuous compartment, covering the lung as an envelope filled with a relatively acellular fluid (4,5). This pleural fluid is mainly formed by filtration of fluid from subpleural capillaries at a quantity, which is estimated between 0.1 and 0.2 mL/kg under normal conditions. It acts as a lubricant between the two pleural layers, moves actively from the visceral to the parietal pleura, and is drained there by small openings, called stomata (6–9). Stomata communicate

Table 1 Classification of Pleural Effusions in Children

Transudate	Exudate
Congestive heart failure	Infection
Nephrotic syndrome	Malignancy
Chylothorax	Hemothorax
Collagen vascular disease	Pancreatitis
Pulmonary emboli	Perforation of esophagus
Hypothyroidism	Pulmonary infarction
Liver cirrhosis	
Iatrogenic	

with the pulmonary lymphatics, which drain into the mediastinum, into the thoracic duct, and finally into the venous circulation. Therefore, the pleural fluid quantity is influenced by changes in its production (e.g., increased vascular permeability in pneumonia) or removal (e.g., increased lymphatic pressure in heart failure, mediastinal tumors).

According to its content, the pleural fluid can be classified as transudate, exudate, and empyema. Transudates are noninflamed fluids, which result from an imbalance between hydrostatic and oncotic pressures. They contain little protein and few mononuclear cells, and their concentrations of glucose, pH, and LDH are similar to those in serum [10]. Exudates are the result of inflammation of pleura or obstruction of lymphatic flow. Empyemas, (Greek εν + πύον = pus within a space), are heavily infected exudates. The distinction between the three categories of pleural fluid is based on certain markers. A practical classification of PE in children is based on the assessment of the pleural fluid (Table 1).

II. Clinical Presentation

The clinical presentation is related to the cause and the size of the effusion. If, for example, the underlying disease is pneumonia, then cough, fever, and malaise, or even lethargy and cyanosis may precede the development of dyspnea (11). Noninfectious diseases like malignancies may not cause any symptoms if the amount of pleural fluid is small. On the other hand, large infusions may cause cough, respiratory distress of various degree, and orthopnea. Pain on inspiration may be the first sign of an effusion, originating from the sensitive innervation of the parietal pleura (12). The pain may be referred to the ipsilateral shoulder or the abdomen (13). In some cases abdominal symptoms may mimic acute appendicitis and gastroenteritis (14).

Specific signs include asymmetrical movement of the affected side, dullness to percussion, decreased tactile and voice fremitous, diminished breath sounds, and voice egophony above the effusions. Large effusions may cause scoliosis, contralateral cardiac and tracheal displacement, and/or hepatomegaly, signs that are more prominent in young infants and babies (10). However, the younger the child is, the more difficult to elicit and relay on the physical findings. This is due to the poor cooperation of the sick infant and the small size of the rib cage, which transmits the auscultatory findings to the unaffected side.

III. Investigation

The clinical suspicion of a PE will be confirmed by various image techniques and examination of the pleural fluid. A chest radiograph in the upright position may show blunting of the costophrenic angle if the amount of fluid is more than 100–200 mL, depending on the size of the child. A chest film in the supine position may not show any abnormality if the amount of fluid is small or may appear as a "diffuse haziness" in the affected side (15). Lateral decubitus films, taken with the child lying on the affected side, are more sensitive as they can detect the presence of smaller amounts of fluid, but are applicable only in cooperative patients. A sign of fluid loculation is the inability of the liquid to shift from the upright to decubitus position. The amount of fluid adequate for thoracentesis is considered if the fluid layer is at least 10 mm thick in the decubitus film. Large collections may also cause a shift of the mediastinum to the opposite site (Fig. 1a).

Ultrasonography is a very helpful method for the detection of the amount of fluid and its composition in the pleural space (16). It can also distinguish pleural thickening or lung abscess from clear fluid (17). Ultrasound can distinguish the serous anechoic fluid, with no evidence of fibrinous organization from the thick purulent fluid formatting septations (Figs. 1,2). Repeated sonographs are also helpful in monitoring the progress of the disease (16).

Computed tomography (CT) is helpful for the assessment of atelectasis or probable lung compression. However, being an expensive and time-consuming method, needing a lot of cooperation, it is not routinely used in children with PE [18]. Its application is justified only in selected cases with complicated PE, where there is a need to discriminate abscess formation from empyema, or when an underlying lung disorder is suspected (19).

Pleural tap (thoracentesis) and pleural fluid analysis are necessary investigations for the majority of children with PE, with an exception of minor effusions of obvious cause, like uncomplicated viral infections, congestive heart failure, nephrotic syndrome, and ascites (20). Some investigators advocate pleural tap in every child with PE, while others reserve it only to those with a suspicion of an infection (21,22). In our institution we perform thoracentesis in all children presenting with PE, excluding those with very little fluid and those who need drainage tubes.

Thoracentesis is a relatively safe procedure in children, with no absolute contraindications and rare complications, the most common of which is pain at

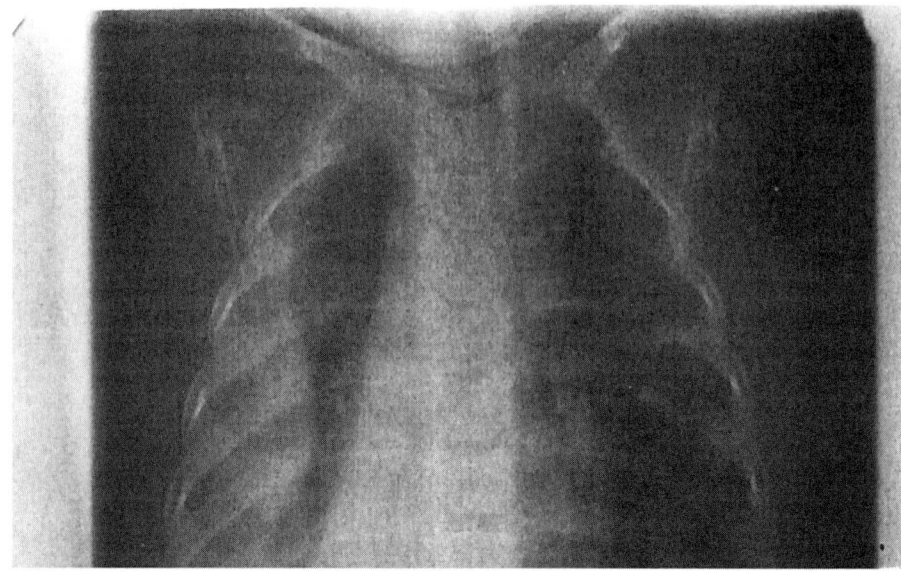

(a)

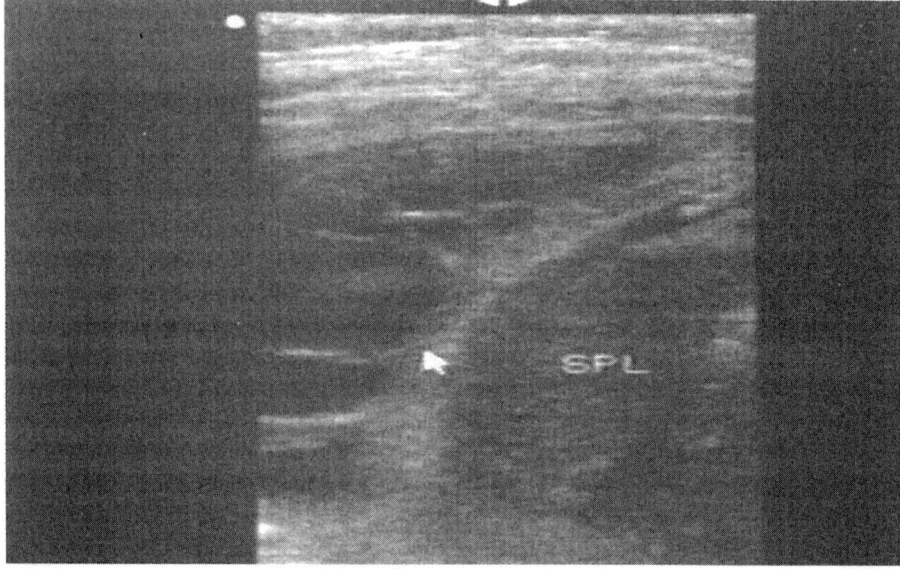

(b)

Figure 1 (a) A 2-year-old girl with right side empyema pushing the trachea to the left. (b) Ultrasonography shows difference in echogenicity of the pleural fluid, indicating the presence of septated membranes and loculated areas in the pleural space. Tube drainage plus fibrinolysis were necessary.

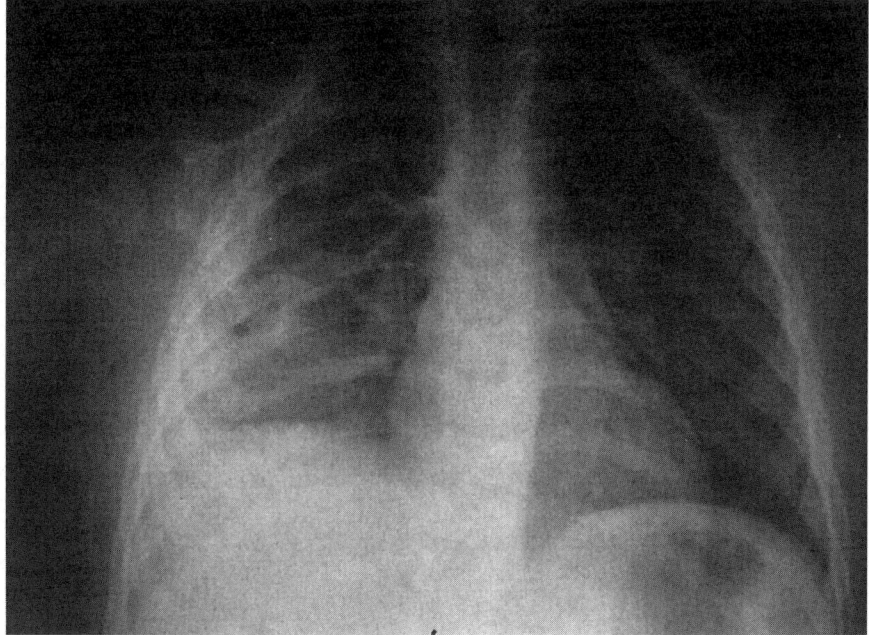

(a)

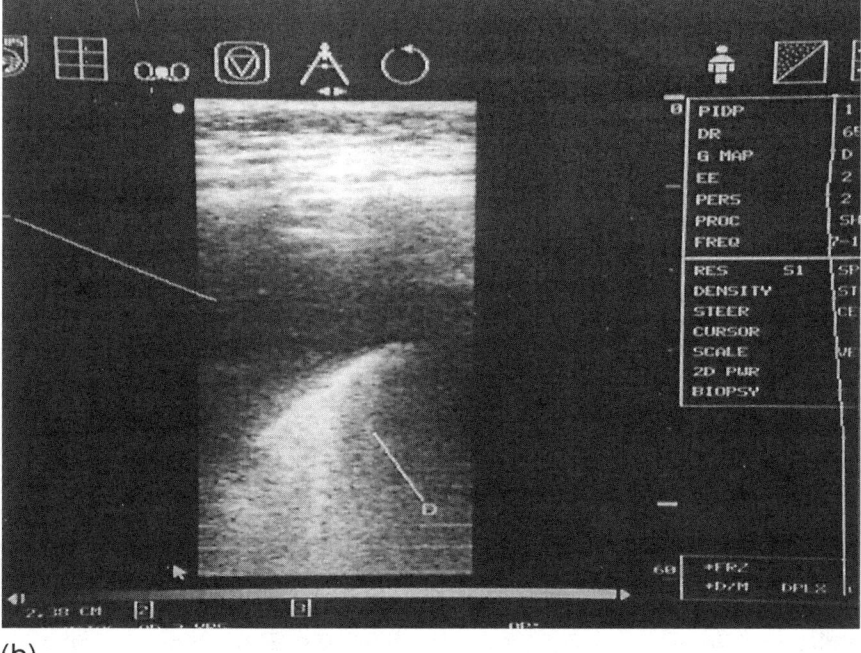

(b)

Figure 2 (a) A 6-year old boy with right-side pleurisy. (b) Ultrasonography shows homogeneous echogenicity of the pleural fluid, a sign of uncomplicated effusion. No need for tube drainage or fibrinolysis.

the insertion site. Other complications include iatrogenic pneumothorax, infection, intercostal nerve damage, and puncture of the liver or spleen (23). Ultrasounds help to determine the exact location for thoracentesis, which is usually 1–2 cm below the onset of dullness to percussion (21,24).

The procedure (Table 2) must be followed up carefully under strictly aseptic conditions to avoid contamination of the pleural space. Examination of the pleural fluid is of outmost importance for the majority of PE in children. The gross appearance of the fluid will help to distinguish the milky fluid of chylothorax from the purulent fluid of empyema or from the pale yellow liquid of a transudate or an exudate. Bloody fluid may be due to trauma or malignancy. Further chemical and cellular analysis are necessary to confirm the diagnosis (Table 3).

The diagnostic value of these tests for the differentiation between transudates and exudates is not as strong as in adults, and the results should always be interpreted in relation to the clinical findings (25,26). Pleural fluid pH in discriminating transudates from exudates and empyemas in children has been proposed by some authors (21) with the additional advantage of rapid diagnosis (27).

IV. Diagnostic and Therapeutic Approach

A rational approach to the child with PE is presented in Figure 3.

A. Parapneumonic Effusions (Exudates of Infectious Origin)

These are by far the most common cause of PE in the pediatric population. They are usually complications of pneumonias and may be caused by viruses like influenza, parainfluenza, adenovirus, and rhinovirus or by bacteria like *Staphylococcus aureus*, *Streptococcus pneumoniae*, and *Haemophilus influenzae*. Other less common organisms include *Streptococcus pyogenes*, Enterobacteriaceae, anaerobes, *Legionella,* and *Histoplasma*. The incidence of infectious PE in hospitalized children varies between 50% and 78%, with a recent increase in empyemas [28–30]. *S. aureus* used to be the predominant causative organism of empyema, but recently has been replaced by *S. pneumoniae*, followed by *H. influenzae* [31]. In a number of cases the bacterial pathogen cannot be isolated.

The clinical presentation of parapneumonic effusions varies, with empyema being the worst end. Cough, chest pain, progressive dyspnea, and high fever not responding to antibiotics is highly suggestive of empyema. Examination of the pleural fluid will help to establish the diagnosis. With no proper treatment, the pleural fluid passes within hours from the *exudative stage* (clear, serous, sterile fluid) to the fibrinopurulent stage (thick pus with fibrin clots, formatting fibrin membranes, with collections of fluid between), and finally within 1–3

Table 2 Procedure for Thoracentesis

Parental information:	Inform the parents and the child (if possible) of the procedure and the need for it.
Sedation:	Use chloral hydrate or midazolam to relieve agitation.
Position of patient:	Older children may be comfortably seated, leaning forward over a pillow. Young infants and babies must be supine leaning on the affected side, supported by an assistant.
Analgesia:	Is achieved with topical application of xylocaine.
Technique:	The exact site for thoracentesis will be decided with the aid of ultrasonography, which must be performed immediately before the procedure. The needle is usually inserted at the 7th interspace in the mid-axillary or the posterior axillary line, aiming toward the center of the rib below the interspace. Upon entering the skin, move the needle and the skin up so that the needle passes over the top of the rib and into the pleural space. Aspirate a small amount of fluid and gently remove the needle.

Source: Modified from Ref. 13.

weeks to the *organizational stage* (invasion of fibroblasts and formation of a thick nonelastic pleura) (32).

The management of a parapneumonic effusion involves eradication of the causative organism using the proper antibiotics and drainage of the pleural cavity at the earliest possible stage.

The choice of proper antibiotics largely depends on the results of the pleural fluid or blood culture, which are not always positive (14,33). As a first-line combination the use of a third-generation cephalosporin plus antistaphylococcal β-lactamase–resistant penicillin is recommended in all cases with empyema (31). In cases of resistant streptococci or anaerobic pathogens, clindamycin should be used, while vancomycin should be reserved for the very severe life-

Table 3 Laboratory Studies for Pleural Fluid Specimens

Chemistry:	Glucose, protein, pH, LDH, amylase, cholesterol, triglycerides
Cytology:	Total and differential cell count; cytological examination for malignancy
Microbiology:	Gram stain, bacterial culture

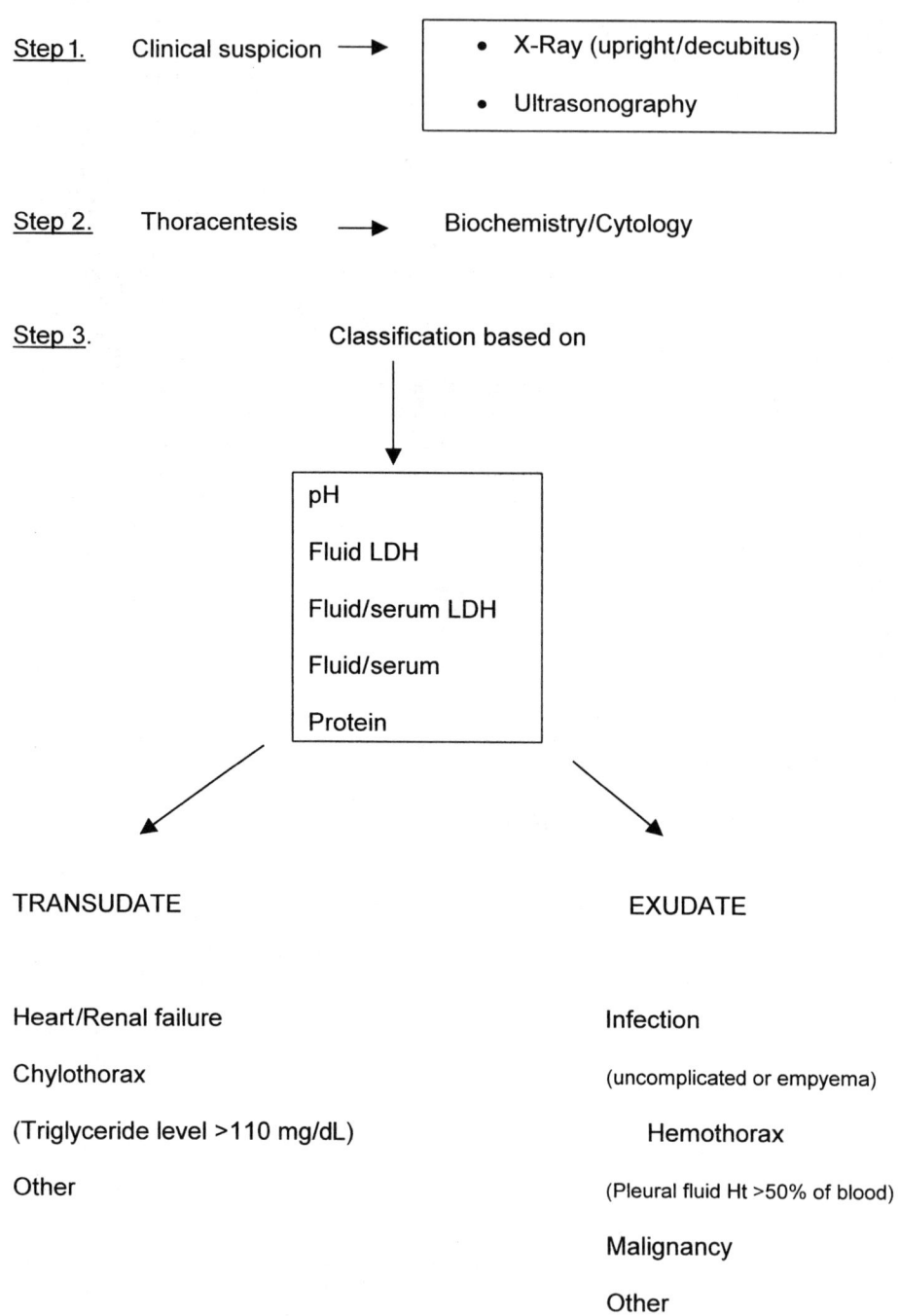

Figure 3 Steps for the diagnosis of common PE in children.

threatening cases of methicillin-resistant *S. aureus*. Once the causative organism is identified, the proper antibiotic should replace the empirical regime.

Drainage of the pleural cavity has changed during the last decade from a more conservative policy to an earlier operative treatment (14,33,34). The treatment of choice is related to the phase of the plural fluid. During the exudative or early fibropurulent stage a tube drainage plus fibrinolytics may be effective, whereas at the organizational stage, interventional thoracoscopy or thoracotomy is necessary.The accuracy of ultrasonography in the detection of the location and the quantity and the quality of the pleural fluid has led to a more rational treatment and reduced hospitalization (16). Computed tomography may be helpful, but may not be adequate to differentiate between the fibrinopurulent and organizing phases of empyema (35).

In case of chest drainage, the tube should be kept in place until the fluid drainage is less than 15 mL per 24 hours. It is important that the child be encouraged not to stay immobilized in bed while having the tube, as this may lead to impaired pulmonary toilet and retardation of clearing the pleural space. Gentle physiotherapy and even taking a few steps in the ward corridor after provisional clapping of the drainage system will help.

The efficacy of fibrinolysis as an adjunct treatment in complicated pleural effusions has been well documented in adult studies (36,37), with negligible adverse reactions in the recommended doses (38). Some authors, however, believe that when compared with video-assisted thoracoscopic surgery, fibrinolysis is inferior (39). Experience with children is limited. Small studies have shown considerable improvement in children with empyema who received urokinase therapy (40–42). In none of these studies were major adverse reactions, such as bleeding, changing of the clotting parameters, or anaphylaxis, reported. Transient fever or chest pain during the administration of the drug were the only minor reactions, reported in some patients. We are expecting the results of large double-blind ongoing studies in children to confirm these encouraging reports.

Some centers recommend the use of tube placement at an early stage (43), while others advocate early surgical intervention (either thoracotomy or video-assisted thoracoscopic surgery) as a first-line intervention in children with empyema (44–46) Others recommend the use of surgical treatment 10 days after the beginning of medical treatment, providing there is no improvement (47) (Fig. 4). We believe that while surgical treatment is the method of choice for selected cases, like complicated empyemas, following necrotizing pneumonitis (48) for the great majority of parapneumonic effusions, tube drainage and fibrinolytics should be the first-line treatment. An algorithm for a rational approach to treatment of parapneumonic effusions is shown in Figure 5.

In our institution we routinely use ultrasonography for the diagnosis and follow-up of all parapneumonic effusions. Diagnostic thoracentesis is performed in the great majority of children with PE, followed by tube drainage plus fibrinolytics in every case with purulent loculated fluid.

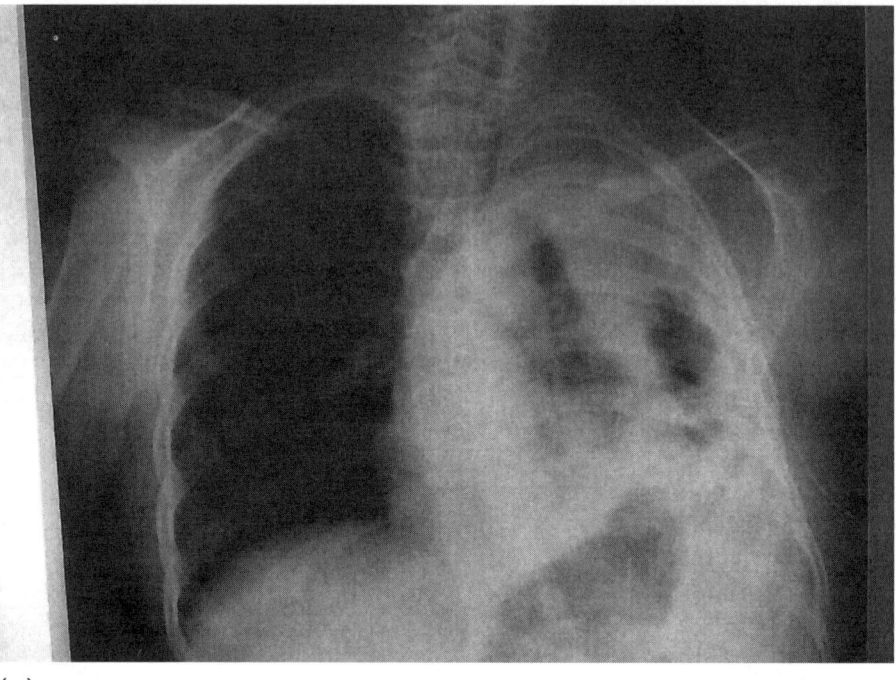

(a)

Figure 4 (a) An 8-year-old girl with left-sided staphylococcal empyema. Note the displacement of the trachea to the right. Tube drainage and fibrinolytics were tried for 10 days with no definite improvement. Lung decortication was decided upon. (b) The same patient immediately after the lung decortication. (c) The patient 3 months later. (d) Ventilation scan before the surgical intervention. (e) Ventilation scan 3 months following the lung decortication.

We use urokinase 100,000 units diluted in 100 mL of normal saline for children older than 12 years or 30,000–50,000 units diluted in 30–50 ml normal saline for children younger than 3 years. Children aged 3–12 years receive an intermediate dose depending on their size. Children with coagulation disorders or with hemorrhagic pleural fluid are excluded. Urokinase is injected in the pleural cavity through the drainage tube, which remains clamped for the following 4 hours. Then the pleural fluid is drained with gentle suction via a negative pressure pump (we apply continuous negative pressure -18 mmHg for children older than 12 years and -10 mmHg for the younger ones). The above is repeated for 4 days, with serial daily sonograms for evaluation. If the condition is not improving after 4 days, we proceed to open thoracotomy and lung decortication. Of 54 chidren with parapneumonic effusions treated in our clinic in the last 2 years, in 12 cases urokinase was added to treatment, while in one case open thoracotomy was necessary. In contrast to adults, most parapneumonic effu-

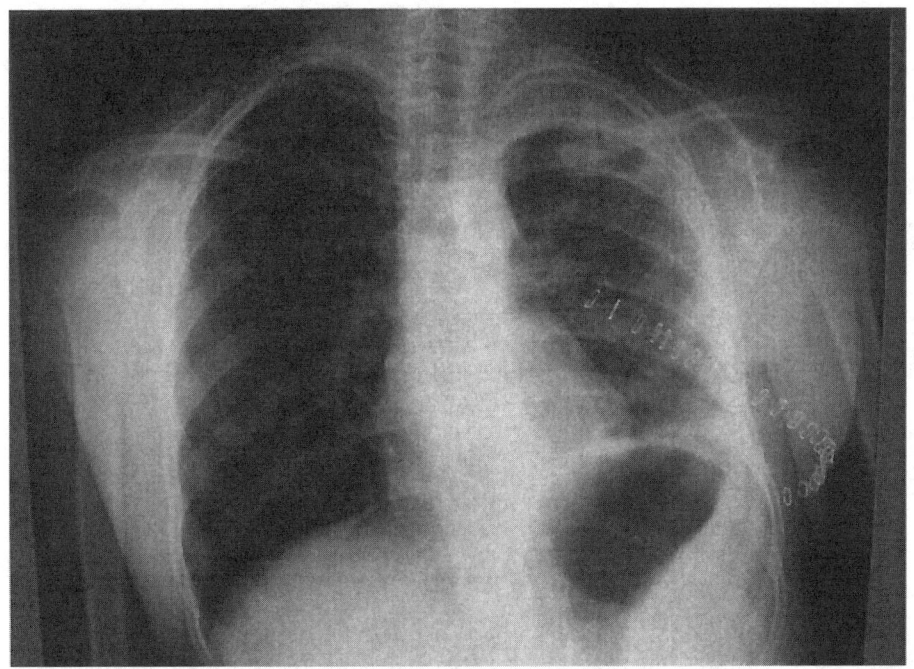

(b)

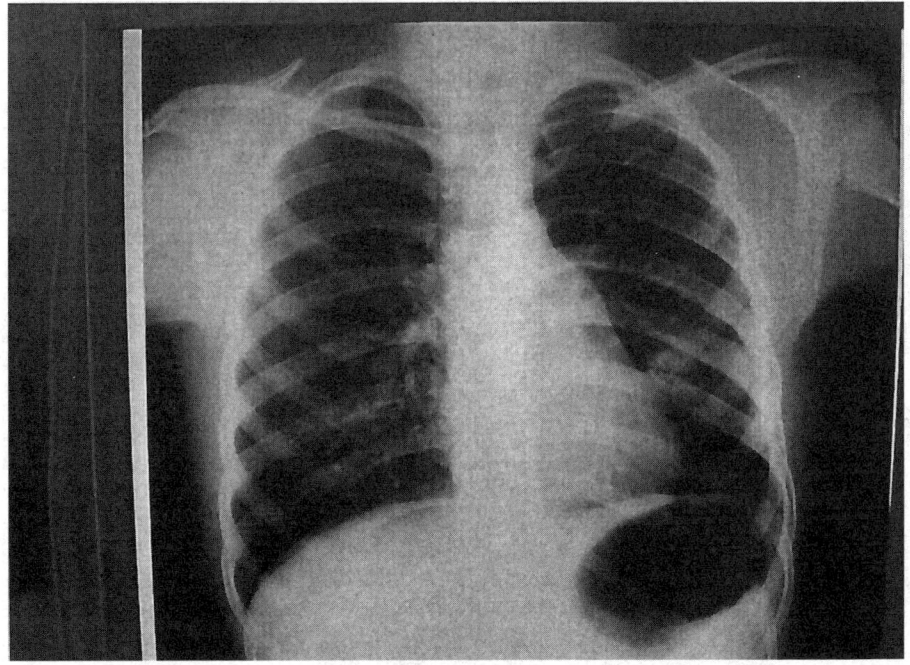

(c)

Figure 4 Continued.

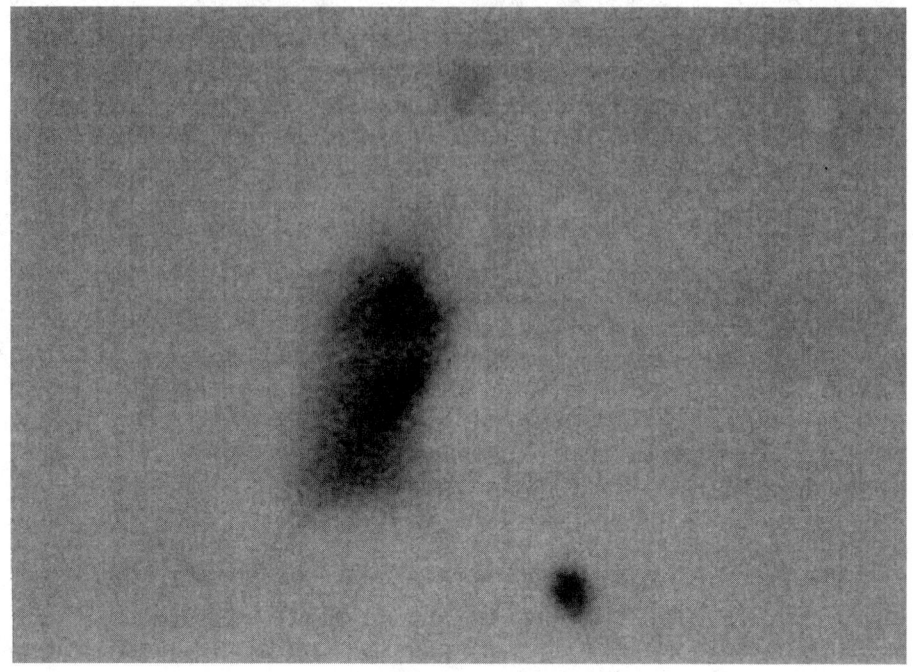

(d)

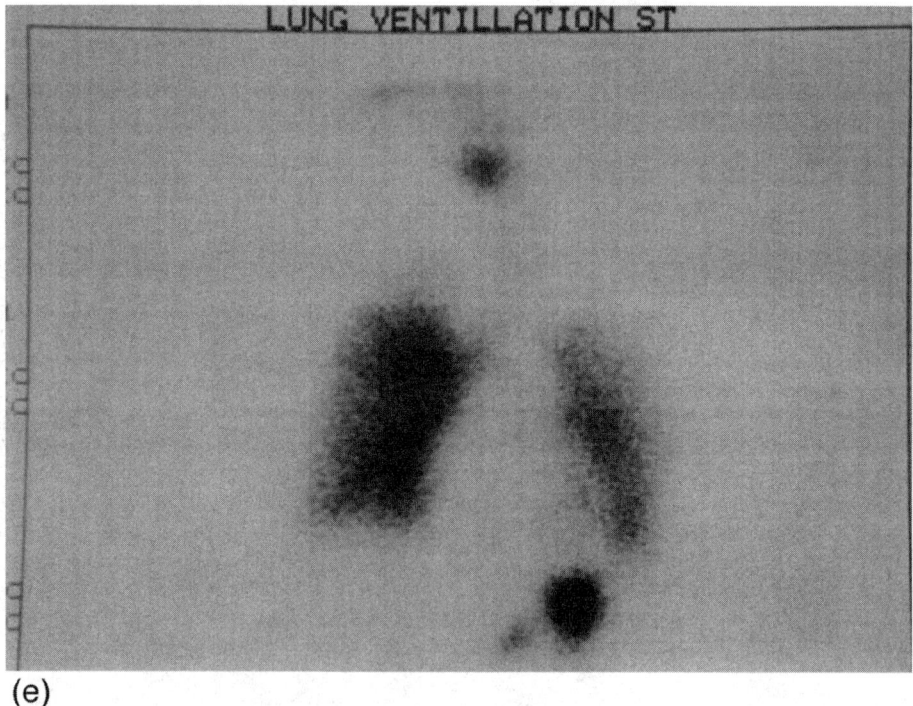

(e)

Figure 4 Continued.

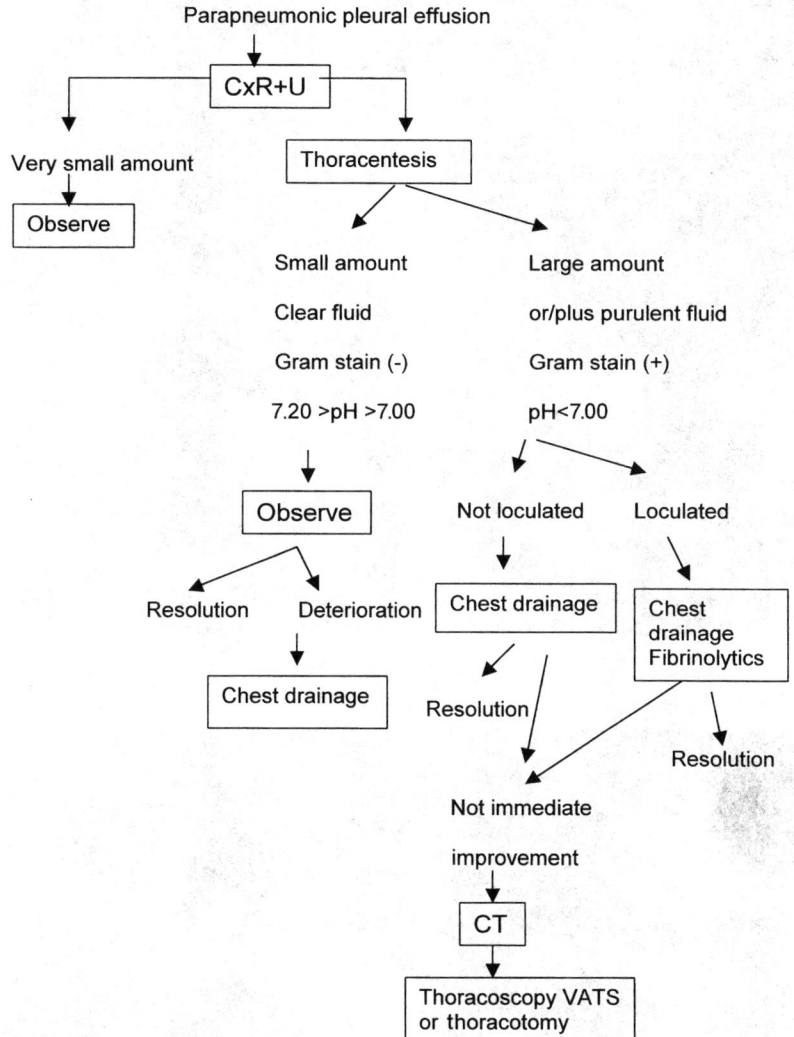

Figure 5 Algorithm for the management of parapneumonic effusions in children. CXR: Chest x-ray; US: ultrasonography; CT: computed tomography; VATS: video-assisted thoracoscopic surgery. (Modified from Refs. 32,35.)

sions in children resolve, with no serious complications. A residual pleural thickening with mild abnormalities on lung function, either obstructive or restrictive, have been reported, mainly in younger children (49,50). Mortality rates for complicated empyemas are between 6% and 9%, mainly in young infants less than 2 years of age. With rational antibiotic therapy and prompt intervention, most children are absolutely well after a period of 3–18 months (Fig. 6).

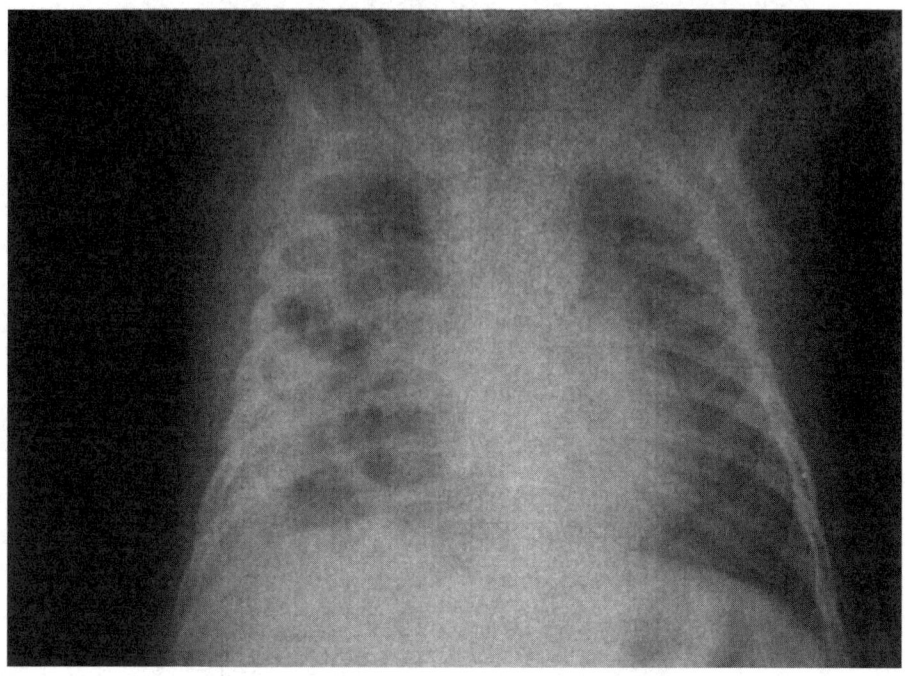
(a)

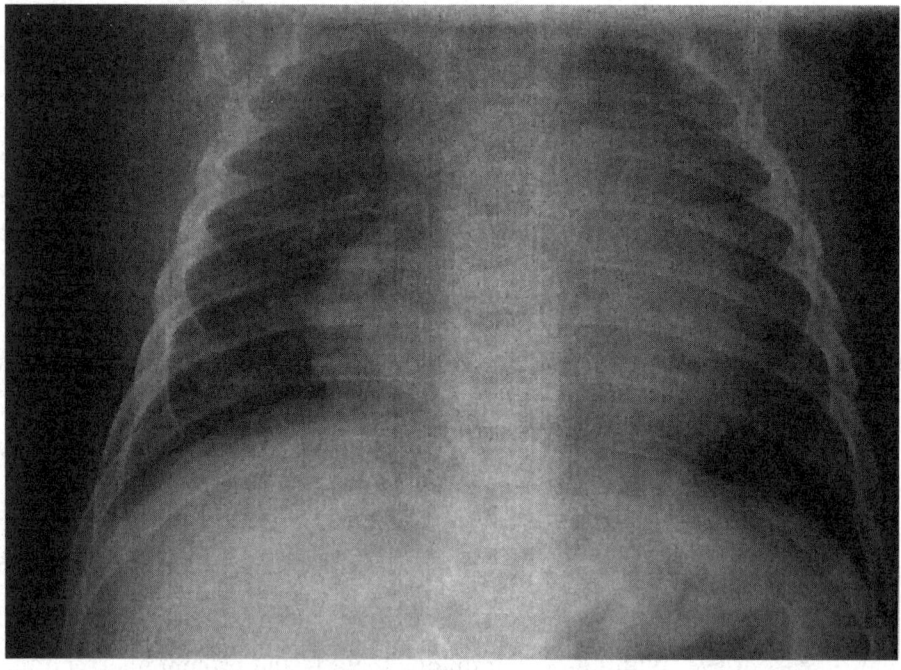
(b)

B. Tuberculous Effusions

Tuberculosis (TB) remains a worldwide disease, increasing recently especially in Africa, Asia, and urban areas of Europe and North America (51). It is estimated that 450,000 children under the age of 15 years die annually from TB [52]. Tuberculous pleurisy is not uncommon in children, particularly adolescents. It is usually the consequence of subpleural granulomata or hematogenous spread of tubercle bacilli.

The combination of pleural and hilar adenopathy found in the majority of cases is highly suggestive of tuberculosis, but in some patients pleurisy is the only presenting manifestation of the disease. TB effusions are usually unilateral, presenting suddenly with fever, chest pain on inspiration, and shortness of breath of various severity, depending on the amount of the accumulated pleural fluid. Tuberculin tests have a high sensitivity and should be used to confirm the diagnosis in all suspicious cases [53]. Examination of the fluid shows a lymphocytic predominance, low glucose, and pH between 7.0 and 7.3. Tubercle bacilli are found in almost half of the fluid cultures. Presence of TB granulomata is found in 50–80% of pleural biopsies (54). However, a biopsy should be performed only in case of diagnostic difficulty. Other specific diagnostic tests like adenosine deaminase activity test (ADA) or interferon gamma levels have very high sensitivity and specificity, which reaches the level of 95%. They are recommended for routine use in countries with a high incidence of TB (55,56). Most children with TB pleurisy respond excellent to antituberculous treatment. However, adding a course of steroids for 2–4 weeks causes a dramatic improvement in symptoms in patients with large effusions and shift of the mediastinum (Fig. 7).

C. Malignant Effusions

Malignancies are the third most common cause of pleural effusions in children, with lymphomas predominating (Fig. 8). They are usually unilateral, resulting from obstruction of the lymphatics in the lung or from direct invasion of pleura by malignant cells. Respiratory distress with increasing dyspnea is the main presenting symptom. The pleural fluid may be hemorrhagic, with lymphocytic predominance, or containing malignant cells. Glucose and pH are within normal limits (57). Immunochemical stain studies are necessary in some cases for making the diagnosis (58). Malignant effusions generally respond well to chemotherapy and irradiation. Thoracocentesis, though helpful for temporary relief of symptoms, should be carried out with caution, as aggressive removal of the pleural fluid may be followed by reexpansion pulmonary edema (59).

Figure 6 (a) A 2-month-old boy with multiple bullae formation and pleural effusion due to *Staphylococcus aureus*. Tube drainage and prolonged antistaphylococcus treatment (4 weeks) were given. (b) Complete recovery 3 months later.

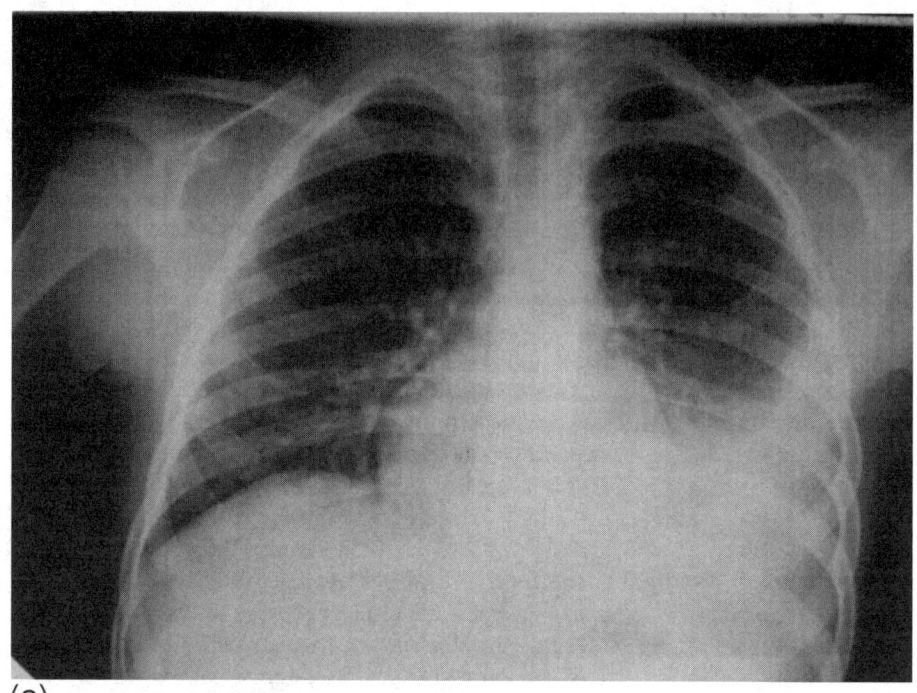

(a)

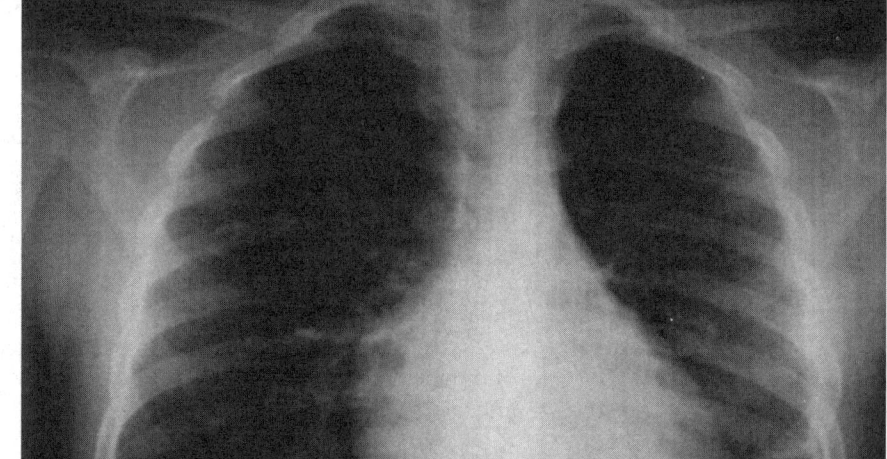

(b)

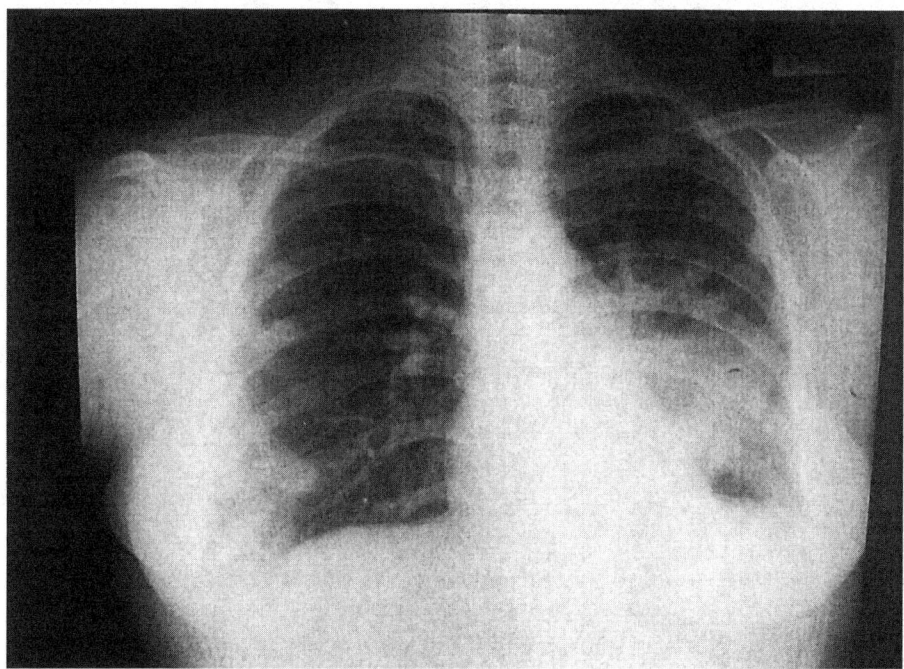

Figure 8 A 4-year-old girl with b-cell lymphoma and bilateral pleural effusion.

D. Chylothorax

By this term we mean the accumulation of lymph fluid within the pleural cavity. Accumulation of chylous may appear during the fetal period (congenital) or later in childhood (60).

Congenital chylothorax is the most common cause of pleural effusion in the neonate, with an incidence of 1:10000 deliveries. Among the most common cause is a congenital abnormality of lymph vessels (lymphangiomatosis or lymphangiectasia) or congenital heart disease. Less common causes are lobar sequestration or mediastinal malignancies (61). Neonates with chylothorax present immediately at birth with difficulty to establish adequate respiration. Resuscitation is cumbersome and sometimes intense effort causes pneumothorax to the neonatal lung. On examination, the trachea and mediastinum are shifted to the contralateral side, with dullness to percussion of the ipsilateral thorax.

Ultrasonography helps to identify the presence of chylothorax even antenatally. However, the diagnosis is established by finding large numbers of

---

Figure 7 (a) A 9-year-old girl with tuberculous pleural effusion with no hilar adenopathy. Note that the findings are not specific. (b) The same patient after 3 months of antituberculous treatment. No tube drainage was necessary.

lymphocytes (>90%) in the pleural fluid together with high triglyceride levels (>110 mg/dL).

Thoracostomy and tube drainage is the immediate treatment for all neonates with chylothorax to facilitate the expansion of the compressed lung. If the accumulation of chyle persists for long, management of fluids, nutrition, and electrolytes becomes necessary (62).

Chylothorax beyond the neonatal period is usually a postoperative complication, related to cardiothoracic interventions or central venous catheterizations (63,64). Rarely it may be the result of obstruction of the thoracic duct by a tumor. The presentation and diagnosis is the same as in congenital chylothorax. Management is a combination of pleural drainage and special diet with medium-chain triglyceride oil, fat-free oral foods, and/or total parenteric nutrition. If the situation is not improving in 2–4 weeks, then pleurodesis is attempted.

V. Summary

Pleural effusions in children have similar etiology as in adults, but they appear with a different incidence according to the age of presentation. The most common PE in the pediatric population are those of infectious origin, usually presenting as complications of pneumonias. Fibrinolysis for complicated PE seems to be effective in children, but we are waiting for the results of large studies to confirm this impression. Moreover, though conservative treatment with tube drainage and fibrinolysis remains the first-choice approach for complicated parapneumonic effusions, surgical intervention like video-assisted thoracoscopy or open thoracotomy and lung decortication should not be delayed if there is no immediate improvement.

Acknowledgments

We thank Dr. Maria Badouraki, Senior Register in Pediatric Radiology, Hippokration Hospital, for her critical review and helpful comments on x-Ray and ultrasound films, used in the manuscript.

References

1. Greenough A. Pleural effusion. In: Greenough A, Roberton NRC, Milner AD, eds. Neonatal Respiratory Disorders. London: Arnold Publishers, 1996:426–435.
2. Orenstein D. Diseases of the pleura. In: Behram R, Kliegman R, Jenson H, eds. Nelson Textbook of Pediatrics. 16th ed. Philadelphia: W.B. Saunders Co, 2000: 1329–1331.
3. Dinwiddie R. Diagnosis and Management of Paediatric Respiratory Disease. 2nd ed. New York: Churchill Livingstone, 1997:121.

4. Albertine KH, Wiener KJ, Bastacky J, Staub NC. No evidence for mesothelial cell contact across the costal pleural space of sheep. J Appl Physiol 1991; 10:123–134.
5. Kobzik L. The lung. In: Cortan R, Kumar V, Collins T, eds. Pathologic Basis of Disease. Philadelphia: WB Saunders Co, 1999:749–751.
6. Wang NS. The performed stomas connecting the pleural cavity and the lymphatics in the parietal pleura. Am Rev Respir Dis 1975; 11:12–20.
7. Miserocchi G, Venturoli D, Negrini D, Gilardi MC, Bellina R. Intrapleural fluid movements described by a porous flow model. J Appl Physiol 1992; 73:2511–2516.
8. Rusch V, Ginsberg R. Chest wall, pleura lung and mediastinum. In: Schwartz S, ed. Principles of Surgery. 7th ed. New York: McGraw-Hill, 1999:669–670.
9. Sahn SA. State of the art: the pleura. Am Rev Respir Dis 1988; 138:184–234.
10. Panitch HB, Papastamelos C, Schidlow V. Abnormalities of the pleural space. In: Taussig LM, Landau LI, eds. Pediatric Respiratory Medicine. St Louis: Mosby, 1999:1178–1196.
11. Maziah W, Choo KE, Ray JG. Empyema thoracis in hospitalized children in Kelantan, Malaysia. J Trop Pediatr 1995; 41:185–188.
12. Givan DC, Eigen H. Common pleural effusions in children. Clin Chest Med 1998; 19:363–371.
13. Zeitlin PL. Pleural effusions and empyema. In: Loughlin GM, Eigen H, eds. Respiratory Disease in Children. Philadelphia: Williams &Wilkins, 1994:453–463.
14. Shankar KR, Kenny SE, Okoye BO, Carty HML, Loyd DA, Losty PD. Evolving experience in the management of empyema thoracis. Acta Pediatr 2000; 89:417–420.
15. Woodring JH. Recognition of pleural effusions on supine radiographs. How much fluid is required? Am J Roentgenol 1984; 142:59–64.
16. Ramnath RR, Heller RM, Ben-Ami T, Miller M, Campell P, Neblett W, Holcomb G, Hernanz-Schulman M. Implications of early sonographic evaluation of parapneumonic effusions in children with pneumonia. Pediatrics 1998; 101:68–71.
17. Libscomb DJ, Flower CDR, Hadfield JW. Ultrasound of the pleura: an assessment of its clinical value. Clin Radiol 1981; 32:289–290.
18. Donnelly LF, Klosterman LA. CT appearance of parapneumonic effusions in children: findings are not specific for empyema. AJR Am J Roentgenol 1997; 169:179–182.
19. Moon WK, Kim WS, Kim IO, Im JG, Kim JH, Yeon KM, Han MC. Complicated pleural tuberculosis in children: CT evaluation. Pediatr Radiol 1999; 29:153–157.
20. Butani L, Polinsky MS, Kaiser BA, Baluarte HJ. Pleural effusion complicating acute peritoneal dialysis in haemolytic uremic syndrome. Pediatr Nephrol 1998; 12:772–774.
21. Montgomery M. Air and liquid in pleural space. In: Chernick V, Boat T, Kending E, eds. Disorders of the Respiratory Tract in Children. 6th ed. Philadelphia: W.B. Saunders Co., 1998:389–411.
22. Papastamelos C. Pleural effusions. In: Schidlow DV, Smith DS, eds. A Practical Guide to Pediatric Respiratory Disease. Philadelphia: Hanley and Belfus, Inc., 1994:436–445.
23. Haddad G, Palazzo R. Diagnostic approach to respiratory disease. In: Behram R, Kliegman R, Jenson H, eds. Nelson Textbook of Pediatrics. 16th ed. Philadelphia: W.B. Saunders Co., 2000:1257.

24. Ghaye B, Dondelinger RF. Imaging guided thoracic interventions. Eur Respir J 2001; 17:507–528.
25. Alkrinawi S, Chernick V. Pleural fluid in hospitalized pediatric patients. Clin Pediatr 1996; 35:5–9.
26. Heffner JE. Evaluating diagnostic tests in the pleura. Diseases of the Pleura, Clinics in Chest Medicine. Vol. 19. Philadelphia: Saunders, 1998:277–293.
27. Azoulay E, Farthoukh M, Galliot R, Bauud F, Simonneau G, Gall JR, Schellmer B, Chevret S. Rapid diagnosis of infectious pleural effusions by use of reagent strips. Clin Infect Dis 2000; 31:914–919.
28. Hardie W, Bokulic R, Garcia VF, Reising SF, Christie C. Pneumococcal pleural empyemas in children. Clin Infect Dis 1996; 22:1057–1063.
29. Rees JHM, Spencer DA, Parikh D, Weller P. Increase in incidence of childhood empyema in West Midlands, U.K. Lancet 1997; 349:342.
30. Alkrinawi S, Chernick V. Pleural infection in children. Semin Respir Infect 1996; 11:148–154.
31. Campbell JD, Nataro JP. Pleural empyema. Pediatr Infect Dis J 1999; 18:725–726.
32. Ham H, Light RW. Parapneumonic effusion and empyema. Eur Respir J 1997; 10:1150–1156.
33. Meier AH, Smith B, Raghavan A, Moss L. Rational treatment of empyema in children. Arch Surg 2000; 135:907–912.
34. Doski J, Lou D, Hicks B, Megison SM, Sanchez P, Contitor M, Guzzetta P. Management of parapneumonic collections in infants and children. J Pediatr Surg 2000; 35:265–270.
35. Cassina PC, Hauser M, Hillejan L, Greschuchna D, Stamatis G. Video-assisted thoracoscopy in the treatment of pleural empyema: stage-based management and outcome. J Thorac Cardiovasc Surg 1999; 117:234–238.
36. Davies RJ, Traill ZC, Gleeson FV. Randomised controlled trial of intrapleural streptokinase in community acquired pleural infection. Thorax 1997; 52:416–421.
37. Bouros D, Schiza S, Tzanakis N, Drositis J, Siafakas N. Intrapleural urokinase versus normal saline in the treatment of complicated parapneumonic effusions and empyema. Am J Respir Crit Care Med 1999; 159:37–42.
38. Davies CW, Lok S, Davies RJO. The systematic fibrinolytic activity of intrapleural streptokinase. Am J Respir Crit Care Med 1998; 157:328–330.
39. Wait M, Sharma S, Hohn J, Nogare AD. A Randomized trial of empyema therapy. Chest 1997; 111:1548–1551.
40. Krishnan S, Amin N, Dozor A, Stringel G. Urokinase in the management of complicated parapneumonic effusions in children. Chest 1997; 112:1579–1583.
41. Benedictis FM, Glori G, Niccoll A, Troiani S, Rizzo F, Lemml A. Treatment of complicated leural effusion with intracavity urokinase in children. Pediatr Pulmonol 2000; 29:438–442.
42. Hull J, Thomson A. Empyema thoracis: a role for open thoracotomy and decortication. Arch Dis Child 1999; 80:581.
43. Sasse S, Nguyen T, Mulligan M, Wang N, Mahutte K, Light R. The effects of early chest tube placement on empyema resolution. Chest 1997; 111:1679–1683.
44. Patton RM, Abrams RS, Gauderer MWL. Is thoracoscopically aided pleural debridement advantageous in children? Am Surgeon 1999; 65:69–72.
45. Kercher K, Attori R, Hoover D, Morton D. Thoracoscopic decortication as first-line therapy for pediatric parapneumonic empyema. Chest 2000; 118:24–27.

46. Rescola FJ, West KW, Gingalewski CA, Engum SA, Scherer LR, Grosfeld JL. Efficacy of primary and secondary video-assisted thoracic surgery in children. J Pediatr Surg 2000; 35:134–138.
47. Balquet M, Larroquet M, Gruner M. Current surgical treatment for pleural empyema in children. Pediatr Pulmon 1999; 18(suppl):109.
48. Wong KS, Chiu CH, Yeow KM, Huang YC, Liu HP, Lin TY. Necrotising pneumonitis in children. Eur J Pediatr 2000; 159:684–688.
49. Redding GJ, Walund LD, Jones JW, Stamey DC, Gibson RL. Lung function in children following empyema. Am J Dis Child 1990; 144:1337–1342.
50. Hoff SJ, Neblett WW, Heller RM, Pietch JB, Holcomb GW, Sheller JR, Harmon T. Postpneumonic empyema in childhood: selecting appropriate therapy. J Pediatr Surg 1989; 24:659–664.
51. Enarson DA, Ait-Khaled N. Tuberculosis. Annesi-Maesano I, Gulsvic A, Viegi G, eds. Respiratory Epidemiology in Europe (Monograph) 2000; 5:67–91.
52. Gremin BJ. Tuberculosis—the resurgence of our most lethal infectious disease—a review. Pediatr Radiol 1995; 25:620–626.
53. Merino JM, Carpintero I, Alvarez T, Rodrigo J, Sanchez J, Coello J. Tuberculous pleural effusion in children. Chest 1999; 115:26–30.
54. Seibert AF, Haynes J Jr, Middleton R. Tuberculous pleural effusion: twenty-year experience. Chest 1991; 99:883–886.
55. Burgess LJ, Maritz FJ, Le Roux I, Taljaard JJ. Use of adenosine deaminase as a diagnostic tool for tuberculous pleurisy. Thorax 1995; 50:593–594.
56. Wongtim S, Silachamroon U, Ruxrungtham K, Udompanich V, Limthongkul S, Charoenlap P, Nuchprayoon C. Interferon gamma for diagnosing tuberculous pleural effusions. Thorax 1999; 54:921–924.
57. Strings AI, Van Hegan RI. Cytologic diagnosis of lymphomas of serous effusion. J Clin Pathol 1981; 34:1311–1325.
58. Cohen I, Loberant N, King E, Herskovits M, Sweed Y, Jerushalmi J. Rhabdomyosarcoma in a child with massive pleural effusion: cytological diagnosis from pleural fluid. Diagn Cytopathol 1999; 21:125–128.
59. Pietsch JB, Whitlock JA, Ford C, Kinney MC. Management of pleural effusions in children with malignant lymphoma. J Pediatr Surg 1999; 34:635–638.
60. Chernick V, Reed MH. Pneumothorax and chylothorax in the neonatal period. J Pediatr 1970; 76:624–632.
61. Hilliard RI, Mckendry JB, Phillips MJ. Congenital abnormalities of the lymphatic system: a new clinical classification. Pediatrics 1990; 86:988–994.
62. Dubin PJ, King IN, Gallagher PG. Congenital chylothorax. Curr Opin Pediatr 2000; 12:505–509.
63. Buttiker V, Fanconi S, Burger R. Chylothorax in children. Guidelines for diagnosis and management. Chest 1999; 116:682–687.
64. Madhavi P, Jameson R, Robinson MJ. Unilateral pleural effusion complicating central venous catheterisation. Arc Dis Chid Fetal Neonatal Ed 2000; 82:F248–F249.

38

Pleural Effusions in Cardiac Disease

JOHN F. MURRAY

University of California, San Francisco
San Francisco, California, U.S.A.

I. Introduction

The most common cause of pleural effusion in the industrialized countries of the world is heart disease. Classically, the fluid accumulates in both pleural spaces and the effusion is a transudate, but, as will be discussed in this chapter, there are important exceptions to these generalities that depend on the kind of heart disease that is present as well as on its treatment. Most patients with cardiogenic pleural effusions have congestive failure from some variety of left-sided heart disease; less commonly, pericardial disease and various types of cardiac injury may be associated with pleural effusion. Patients with heart disease may also develop pleural effusions of noncardiac origin, especially those caused by pulmonary emboli and bacterial pneumonia. The diagnosis of cardiac-related pleural effusions is typically straightforward, and treatment is focused on the underlying heart disease; there are, however, certain pitfalls that may worsen the patient's clinical manifestations, confuse the attending physician, and delay the institution of appropriate therapy.

II. Prevalence

Cardiac disease has been recognized as one of the three most important causes of pleural effusion in virtually all large series of cases reported during the last 50 years; whether cardiac disease leads the ranking or follows malignancy and/or tuberculosis depends on the location and type of institution in which the survey was carried out. In one community-based epidemiological study of the incidence and etiology of pleural effusion in central Bohemia, congestive heart failure was the most common diagnosis and caused nearly half of all the effusions identified (1). According to Light (2), congestive heart failure also heads the list of estimates of the annual incidence of pleural effusion of various types in the United States, accounting for 500,000 of the 1,337,000 total anticipated cases. In some referral institutions, however, malignancies predominate (3), and it must be remembered that tuberculosis remains the most common cause of pleural effusion in countries with a high prevalence of that disease (4).

The frequency of hydrothorax in patients with cardiac disease, as might be expected, depends on two factors: the presence and severity of associated heart failure, and the sensitivity of the method used to detect whether or not effusion is present. These two factors account for the considerable variation in prevalence that appears in published reports. For example, using the radiological techniques available in 1941, Bedford and Lovibond (5) found pleural effusions in 39% of 356 patients with overt congestive failure; in 1963, Logue and coworkers (6) conducted a careful radiological study, which included tomography in an unspecified number and reported a prevalence of pleural effusion of 58% in 114 patients with a diagnosis of pulmonary edema; finally, using modern techniques of computed tomography, Kataoka (7) identified pleural effusion(s) in 87% of 60 patients with congestive heart failure. Among 71 patients awaiting cardiac transplantation who were selected by their physicians to have computed tomography, the prevalence of pleural effusion was 44% (8). In patients with heart failure of sufficient magnitude to warrant hospitalization in an intensive care unit, the prevalence of pleural effusions detected by sonography varied from 51% (9) to 67% (10).

The great majority of cardiogenic pleural effusions occur in patients with congestive heart failure from disorders that affect the left ventricle, chiefly ischemic heart disease, mitral or aortic valve disorders, and cardiomyopathy. As described in the next section, these particular afflictions create the physiological abnormalities that ultimately lead to pleural effusion(s).

III. Pathogenesis

The mechanisms that underlie the formation of the characteristic transudative pleural effusions that are found in patients with congestive heart failure are now reasonably well understood and have been completely revised during the last 20 years. The small amount of fluid that is normally present in the pleural spaces of healthy humans originates from branches of the systemic circulation that perfuse the parietal pleural lining of the outer surface of both pleural cavities; once formed from the capillaries and other tiny blood vessels (collectively known as "microvessels"), the low-protein ultrafiltrate traverses the parietal surface membrane into the pleural spaces; ordinarily, none of the fluid emanates from the lungs and enters the pleural space through the visceral pleura. Pleural fluid is removed by bulk flow—with an unchanged protein concentration—through lymphatic channels that drain the pleural space through stomata, microscopic openings that are present only on the parietal pleura (11).

The fluid that collects in the pleural spaces of patients with congestive heart failure arises from within the lungs, and its formation is governed by forces that affect the microvessels of the pulmonary circulation. Pleural effusion occurs late in the evolution of the underlying heart disease, after the onset of congestive failure. Once left ventricular filling pressure is increased, pulmonary capillary hydrostatic pressure rises correspondingly and fluid filtration increases in the lungs. In a study by Wiener-Kronish and Matthay (9), mean pulmonary arterial wedge pressure was 24 ± 1 mmHg in the 19 patients with cardiogenic pleural effusions compared with 17 ± 2 mmHg in the 18 patients without effusions.

Several inherent safety factors serve to protect the lungs by preventing the development of pulmonary edema, thereby preserving gas exchange. But when these mechanisms are overwhelmed, fluid begins to accumulate, first in the large peribronchovascular interstitial space and last in the alveoli (12). No one knows exactly when along the continuum of worsening edema the fluid begins to spill over into the pleural spaces. Judging from experiments in which the lungs were made progressively edematous, it took time for the lungs to start to leak (13); presumably, this means that the peribronchovascular interstitium has to be at least partially filled with fluid before it seeps from the subpleural interstitial space into the pleural space owing to the prevailing pressure gradient across the visceral pleura (14).

Cardiogenic pleural effusions, therefore, represent pulmonary edema that has leaked across the visceral pleura, an obvious way to rid the lungs of fluid that would otherwise accumulate within them; in other words, the development of pleural effusions retards the onset of alveolar flooding and helps to preserve gas exchange. The amount of edema that flows into the pleural space is substantial. In one experimental preparation, 25% of the total amount of pulmonary edema that formed oozed through the visceral pleura and was recovered (13).

The debate about the relative importance and contributions of pressures in the right-sided and left-sided chambers of the heart to the formation of pleural effusion(s) has now been settled—firmly—in favor of pressures in the left ventricle–left atrium–pulmonary veins, all of which affect pulmonary capillary pressure. This conclusion was derived from a pair of important clinical studies in patients with heart disease in whom pressures in the left and right sides of the heart were measured and the presence or absence of pleural effusion was documented by ultrasonography (15,16). This reinforces my earlier statement that patients with congestive heart failure and pleural effusion(s) are apt to have left ventricular dysfunction.

The concentration of protein in pleural fluid sampled from patients with heart failure is low, but not as low as is presumed to exist in the small amount of fluid of systemic origin that is normally present in the pleural spaces of healthy persons. (No satisfactory measurements have been made in healthy humans, but there is no reason to believe that the value would differ greatly from that found in sheep.) Moreover, the ratio of the concentration of protein in the hydrothorax to that in the plasma is also low and satisfies one of Light's criteria of a transudate (17). Measurements in experimental animals showed that the protein concentrations in pulmonary edema fluid within the lungs, fluid in the pleural space, and fluid in the lymphatics that drain the lungs were identical (13); these results corroborate the belief that pleural effusions in patients with congestive heart failure are formed by movement of pulmonary edema from the lungs into the pleural spaces.

Although the routes of formation of pleural fluid in healthy subjects and in patients with congestive heart failure differ, the routes of spontaneous clearance appear to be the same—by bulk flow via lymphatic channels that drain the parietal pleura. (The effect of treatment with diuretics on clearance and protein concentration is considered later.) In theory, then, an increase in pressure in the systemic veins into which lymphatic channels drain might serve to decrease lymph flow; this, in turn, would augment the rate of pleural effusion accumulation by retarding the rate of its clearance. Studies in experimental animals, however, are not clear-cut. Mellins and coworkers (18) were able to produce large pleural effusions by raising systemic venous pressure and lowering plasma oncotic pressure; in contrast, in the experiments of Broaddus et al. (13), an artificial hydrothorax was absorbed even when superior vena caval pressure was elevated. From a clinical point of view, it seems likely that an increase in systemic venous pressure, a common occurrence in congestive heart failure, which by itself is insufficient to cause effusions, will slow the removal of fluid leaking from the lungs into the pleural space, thereby contributing to the formation of cardiogenic pleural effusions as well as to the duration of their presence.

IV. Congestive Heart Failure

A. Characteristics

For the reasons just discussed, the majority of patients with cardiogenic pleural effusion(s) have congestive heart failure from left ventricular dysfunction, which may be predominantly systolic, diastolic, or mixed. The most common causes of these circulatory abnormalities in industrialized countries are ischemic heart disease from coronary artery involvement or hypertension, cardiomyopathy of any etiology, and acquired mitral or aortic valve disease.

There is an oft-repeated clinical maxim dating from the nineteenth century that says that pleural effusions in congestive heart failure are right-sided or bilateral (for review and references, see Ref. 5). This led to the belief and exaggerated recommendation that a unilateral left hydrothorax in a patient with congestive failure was presumed to be unrelated to heart disease and required special workup. Table 1 shows the results of six studies that used chest radiography or computed tomography to detect and localize pleural effusions in patients with congestive heart failure. Nearly half of the effusions were bilateral, and right-sided effusions predominated over left-sided by a ratio of 1.7 to 1. But solitary left hydrothorax was not uncommon and accounted for 20% of the total.

There is no satisfactory explanation for a large localized effusion in either pleural space in the face of left-sided heart disease with pulmonary vascular congestion. Regardless of its origin, an increase in pulmonary capillary pressure should increase fluid filtration equally in both lungs. Obliterative pleuritis and regional differences in intrapulmonary vascular pressures or lymph flows may occasionally influence laterality, but are inadequate causes overall. It has been speculated that cardiogenic effusions may be unilateral in mild congestive heart failure and become bilateral as failure worsens (5). But a more likely explanation relates to the accuracy of the method used to define whether or not an effusion is present. Table 1 shows that when computed tomography is employed, a much higher number of identifiable effusions proves to be bilateral than when less sensitive standard radiographic techniques are used.

We would expect, therefore, that postmortem examination of patients who died with or of congestive heart failure should demonstrate a preponderance of bilateral hydrothorax; as expected, 290 such patients autopsied at the Mayo Clinic showed that the great majority, 88%, had bilateral pleural effusions larger than 250 mL (22). Of additional interest was the observation that the average quantity of fluid found in the right hemithorax (1084 mL) exceeded that in the left hemithorax (913 mL) by about 16%. In 1935, Dock (23) described the anatomical and hydrostatic forces controlling blood flow from the

Table 1 Radiographic Studies of Laterality of Pleural Effusions in Congestive Heart Failure

Authors (Ref.)	Method	No. patients	Location of effusion(s)		
			Right	Left	Bilateral
Bedford and Lovibond (5)	Standard	136	68	42	26
McPeak and Levine (19)	Standard	52	20	4	28
Peterman and Brothers (20)	Standard	54	18	17	19
Weiss and Spodick (21)	Standard	70	13	6	51
Kataoka (7)	CT	52	5	2	45
Lewin et al. (8)	CT	31	7	8	16
Total		395	131	79	185
Percent		100	33	20	47

CT = computed tomography.

pulmonary venous bed to the left ventricle that he believed strongly favored the predominance of right over left hydrothorax. Broaddus (24), however, has proposed that the difference may well be explained by the simple facts that the volume, visceral pleural surface area, and leakage rates from the right lung are greater than those from the left lung.

B. Diagnosis

In most instances the diagnosis of cardiogenic hydrothorax is obvious because the effusion(s) are but one manifestation of the familiar constellation of clinical and radiographic findings that typify the presence of congestive failure in a patient with known left-sided heart disease. Other associated features are cardiac enlargement, gallop rhythm, systolic or diastolic murmurs, basilar crackles, venous engorgement, hepatic tenderness, and edema of the lower extremities. It is important to remember that pleural effusions, a sign of left ventricular dysfunction, may develop in the absence of peripheral edema and other signs of right-sided heart disease; this clinical event usually occurs in new-onset left ventricular failure, which most commonly accompanies myocardial infarction. Conversely, pure right-sided heart failure (e.g., from cor pulmonale or pulmonary hypertension) should not be accepted as a sole cause of cardiogenic pleural effusion(s).

Physical examination is not a sensitive way of detecting pleural effusion unless it is large. Most effusions are discovered by standard posteroanterior and lateral radiographic examination, which may be taken as part of a routine checkup or for evaluation of worsening symptoms. Even with high-quality films, pleural fluid collections are likely to be missed unless they are larger than 300 mL; lateral decubitus projections should detect 100 mL or more of fluid (25). The results of a recent study that used thoracic computed tomography as the gold standard for identifying pleural effusions in patients with congestive heart failure indicated that routine radiography missed about 60% of the effusions found by the more sensitive method (26). Portable anteroposterior radiographs, which are often taken with patients in the supine position in intensive care units, are considerably worse; such films cannot be relied on to detect even moderate-sized pleural effusions.

Ultrasonography is clearly superior to standard radiography, particularly for the identification of small pleural effusions, and can be used at the bedside of seriously ill patients, including those in intensive care units (27). Ultrasonography, because of its relatively low cost, ready availability, and accuracy, would appear to be the method of choice for detecting pleural effusions, if clinically indicated, in patients whose standard films are negative or who cannot be taken to the radiology department. Most of the time, however, it is not necessary to determine if small effusions are present or not because the information does not affect how the patient is treated.

The great majority of cardiogenic hydrothoraces do not need to be verified by thoracentesis, provided they occur in an appropriate clinical setting. In patients with known or obvious cardiac disease, the presence of unilateral or bilateral pleural effusions can be regarded as one of the associated findings of overt congestive heart failure, which should be evident. The indications for thoracentesis are listed in Table 2; none is particularly common. Apart from the occasional need to relieve breathlessness from a massive fluid collection, the chief reasons for tapping the chest relate to the importance of finding a noncardiogenic cause for an effusion that requires specific treatment. This is especially true for pulmonary embolism and infection.

Classically, cardiogenic pleural effusions are transudates, but owing to the efficacy of diuretic treatment of congestive heart failure, that old dictum needs to be qualified. I have already noted that the pulmonary edema fluid that seeps across the visceral pleura and collects in the pleural space has a low protein concentration; typically, it also has a low lactate dehydrogenase (LDH) concentration, thus satisfying Light's criteria for a transudate (17). In untreated cardiogenic effusions that resolve spontaneously by bulk flow, the concentrations of protein, LDH, and other constituents in the hydrothorax remain constant. In contrast, in patients treated with diuretics, water is removed at a faster rate than protein; this phenomenon causes the pleural-plasma concentration ratio of protein in the remaining fluid to increase, sometimes to levels that mimic those of an exudate (for recent review and references, see Refs. 28, 29).

In theory, LDH concentration in pleural fluid should rise proportionate to the rise in protein concentration during diuresis, but in reality, LDH may rise higher than expected owing to the added influence of cell lysis and trauma from multiple thoracenteses. This effect may be accompanied by a reduction in serum LDH from the diuresis-induced relief of hepatic congestion that follows improvement of the underlying heart failure; the increase in pleural fluid and the decrease in serum LDH concentrations may occasionally cause the pleural-serum ratio to rise to levels consistent with an exudate. To circumvent this problem, several authors have proposed that when evaluating a hydrothorax in a patient with congestive heart failure, especially after diuresis has begun, if the protein and LDH concentration ratios are slightly in the exudative range, one should examine the pleural-serum albumin difference; if the difference is greater than 1.2 g/dL, the effusion is most likely a transudate of cardiac origin (29–31).

Table 2 Indications for Thoracentesis in Patients with Pleural Effusion(s) and Congestive Heart Failure

When effusion(s) is/are large and patient is severely breathless
When congestive failure improves with treatment but effusion either does not respond or worsens
When patient is febrile and/or has pleuritic pain, especially if the effusion is unilateral
When effusion occurs in pure right-sided heart failure (e.g., from cor pulmonale or pulmonary hypertension)

C. Treatment

Therapy of cardiogenic hydrothorax should be directed at the underlying heart disease. Essential elements of treatment include arrhythmia control, preload and afterload reduction, diuresis, sodium restriction, and inotropic agents. Pleural effusions generally respond to these measures, although there may be a lag between improvement in cardiac function and clearing of the chest radiograph. The key feature is that the effusions diminish rather than increase in volume.

Congestive heart failure is apt to wax and wane in severity, and with these changes pleural effusions often worsen and remit. When respiratory function is compromised by a large hydrothorax, thoracentesis is warranted to improve breathlessness and gas exchange. The role of sclerotherapy in patients with persistent or recurrent symptomatic hydrothorax—despite maximum medical therapy—is controversial. According to one recent review of the subject, 12 patients have been treated by pleurodesis, with a successful outcome in 10 of them (32). Concern has been expressed about the possibility of worsening the magnitude of pleural effusion in the opposite hemithorax (33), but that should not happen. Because the development of pleural effusions in congestive heart failure serves to minimize the accumulation of fluid within the lungs, obliterating one pleural space would be expected to worsen pulmonary edema in the affected lung and have no effect on the opposite side.

V. Pericarditis

Sporadic case reports and small series of cases leave no doubt that hydrothorax occurs in patients with either acute or chronic (constrictive) pericarditis. Owing to the infrequency of the two conditions, however, it is impossible to make firm statements about the prevalence of associated pleural effusions, their location, and the composition of the fluid.

A. Acute Pericarditis

Weiss and Spodick (34) reviewed the charts and radiographs of 133 consecutively discharged patients with any form of pericardial disease; of these, 35 (26%) had pleural effusion(s). Among the 21 patients with evidence of acute pericarditis (etiology not specified), 15 had only left-sided pleural effusions; 3 had bilateral effusions, left larger than right; and 3 had bilateral effusions of equal size. No patient had either an isolated right-sided effusion or bilateral effusions that were predominately right-sided. Unfortunately, no thoracenteses were performed.

Our experience at San Francisco General Hospital agrees with that of Weiss and Spodick about the frequency of left-only or left-sided predominance of bilateral pleural effusions, usually small, in patients with acute idiopathic, presumably viral, pericarditis. Thoracenteses in a few patients revealed exudative, usually lymphocytic fluid that was similar, when both spaces were sampled, to the fluid obtained from within the pericardium. We have assumed the mechanism of pleural fluid formation to be direct extension of the inflammatory process from within the pericardium to the contiguous pleural membrane(s).

The presence of a small left-sided or bilateral pleural effusion in a patient with acute pericarditis usually poses no diagnostic difficulty. The clinical manifestations are dominated by fever, precordial pain, and dyspnea related to the pericarditis, which can be diagnosed by hearing a friction rub or by characteristic electrocardiographic changes. Pericardiocentesis is indicated if echocardiography reveals a significant amount of pericardial fluid. Thoracentesis is seldom warranted unless the pleural collection is huge or does not subside as the pericardial disease resolves.

Treatment is directed at the pericardial disease if a specific cause can be identified, which is seldom the case. Symptomatic treatment with anti-inflammatory agents such as indomethacin is generally effective; corticosteroids are used in refractory cases.

B. Chronic (Constrictive) Pericarditis

Pleural effusion is said to be common in patients with chronic constrictive pericarditis, but data are scant. The largest series to date was reported by Plumb and coworkers (35); of 35 surgically proven cases, 21 (60%) had pleural effusion(s), which were bilateral in 12 patients and right-sided in 9; unilateral left-sided effusion was never observed. Tomaselli and colleagues (36) also found a 60% prevalence of hydrothorax in 30 patients with constrictive pericarditis of several different causes. The size was not specified, but in 12 patients the effusions were bilateral and symmetrical; in the remaining 6 patients, 3 had right-sided involvement and 3 left-sided. Thus, the left-sided predominance noted in acute pericarditis clearly does not obtain in chronic (constrictive) pericarditis.

There are few reports of thoracentesis findings. Of the four patients studied by Tomaselli and colleagues (36), three had exudates and one a transudate, presumably related to contiguous inflammation and congestive failure, respectively, although the precise mechanisms were not specified.

Diagnostic attention is directed toward examination of the heart by echocardiography and computed tomography. Cardiac catheterization is indicated to detect the presence and severity of hemodynamic impairment. In occasional patients, the effusions may be so large and clinically dominant as to obscure the underlying cardiac diagnosis (36,37).

VI. Postcardiac Injury Syndrome

In 1956, Dressler (38) reported 10 cases of a postmyocardial infarction syndrome, which was characterized by fever, pericarditis, pleurisy, and pneumonitis, a constellation of findings that had been previously recognized after mitral valve commissurotomy (39). As the indications for and use of open-heart surgery proliferated during the 1960s and thereafter, the onset of fever, pericarditis, and pleural effusion within a few weeks, occasionally months, of the operation was called the postpericardiotomy syndrome, a serious complication that has led to bypass graft closure and fatal cardiac tamponade (40). Similar sequelae have been reported following blunt chest trauma (41), percutaneous left ventricular puncture (42), implantation of a pacemaker (43), and even radiofrequency ablation for cardiac arrhythmias when complicated by self-limited cardiac perforation (44). Owing to the similarities in clinical manifestations and, presumably, in etiology, these disorders are now known collectively as the postcardiac injury syndrome (45), the prevalence of which varies with the type of injury to the heart. Following open-heart surgery the syndrome occurs in 10–50% of patients (40). The incidence is lower following myocardial infarction, varying from about 1% in a series of 500 cases (46) to as high as 15% among a highly selected group of 40 patients who had detectable postmyocardial infarction pericarditis shortly after having their infarcts (47).

Patients with the postcardiac injury syndrome usually complain of precordial pain and nearly always have fever and evidence of pericarditis (audible friction rub and/or typical echocardiographic or electrocardiographic abnormalities); pleural effusion is common but not invariable; pneumonitis is less frequent. In Dressler's original series, 6 of 10 patients (60%) with the syndrome following myocardial infarction had pleural effusions (38); of 38 postoperative surgical patients analyzed by Kaminsky and coworkers (48), 68% had pleural effusions. The hydrothorax is left-sided in the majority of patients and bilateral in the remainder; isolated right-sided involvement is rare. The exudative fluid is bloody in 30% of cases. Either monocytes or polymorphonuclear cells may predominate. The etiology of the postcardiac injury syndrome remains mysterious, but appears to be immunological in origin; antimyocardial antibodies, which were found in the serum of a high percentage of postsurgical patients who developed the syndrome (49), have also been identified in the pleural fluid of one afflicted patient (50); such antibodies, though, are nonspecific, so their diagnostic significance is uncertain.

The onset of fever with symptoms of pericarditis in association with pleural effusion and sometimes pneumonitis a week or two after some sort of cardiac trauma, most frequently open-heart surgery, is now so common and easy to recognize that the diagnosis should present no problem. Neither pericardiocentesis nor thoracentesis is usually indicated. Symptomatic treatment with antiinflammatory agents is generally all that is required and works well, although recurrences may occur.

VII. Coronary Artery Revascularization

Pulmonary complications, such as pleural effusion, hemothorax, atelectasis, pulmonary edema, diaphragmatic dysfunction, and pneumonia, are frequent after coronary artery revascularization surgery (51). Of these, pleural effusions are among the most common, with a reported prevalence of 42% (52). One study found no difference in the prevalence of postoperative hydrothoraces when saphenous vein grafts were used compared with when internal mammary (thoracic) artery grafts were used (52); a later study, however, reported nearly twice as many pleural effusions with internal mammary (84%) as with saphenous vein (47%) grafts (53). Surprisingly, there was no difference in the prevalence of hydrothorax after coronary artery surgery with unilateral compared with bilateral internal mammary artery grafting (54). Most revascularization-related effusions, however, are small, confined to the left hemithorax, asymptomatic, and resolve spontaneously (52,55).

A recent survey by Light and coworkers (55) of 3707 patients, most of whom also had at least one internal mammary artery bypass, identified 29 patients (0.9%) who developed pleural effusions that occupied 25% or more of the hemithorax. Seven of these effusions accompanied congestive heart failure, two were associated with constrictive pericarditis, and one was caused by pulmonary embolism. Attention was focused on the remaining 19 patients whose hydrothoraces had "no discernible cause"; these effusions, which were invariably exudates, were unilateral on the left or bilateral with left-sided predominance in 17 of the 19 patients.

Differences were found in the clinical course and outcome between the 8 patients whose unexplained effusions were bloody and the 11 patients whose effusions were nonbloody (55). Bloody effusions were thought to be related to bleeding into the pleural space during or soon after the operation because they occurred early, reached a maximum 13 days after the operation, and tended to subside, with few exceptions, without intervention. In contrast, nonbloody effusions developed late, reaching a maximum 49 days after surgery, and required more intensive therapy, including treatment with anti-inflammatory agents, multiple thoracenteses, tube thoracostomy, pleural sclerosis, and pleurectomy. Nonbloody effusions were also differentiated from bloody ones by having a lower concentration of LDH and an abundance of small lymphocytes.

The origin of nonbloody effusions remains obscure. Postcardiac injury syndrome is an obvious explanation for some of the cases, but usually there is no evidence of pericarditis, which is generally considered a sine qua non for a diagnosis of postcardiac injury. Also, there is a discrepancy of timing: effusions following cardiac injury typically occur within the first few weeks of trauma, whereas those following revascularization are apt to develop several weeks after the operation. For both conceptual and therapeutic reasons, a specific diagnostic test is needed to differentiate (or to link) postcardiac injury syndrome and revascularization sequelae.

VIII. Other Causes

Most pleural effusions in patients with heart disease are related to one of the cardiac abnormalities just described. But patients with heart disease also have an increased susceptibility to certain other—noncardiogenic—causes of pleural effusion.

A. Pulmonary Embolism

Patients hospitalized for congestive heart failure or acute myocardial infarction are at increased risk of developing pulmonary embolism (56), which, as discussed in Chapter 43, is often associated with pleural effusion. Data are conflicting whether congestive failure in nonhospitalized patients is (57) or is not (58) a risk factor for venous thromboembolism. Patients with cardiac disease who undergo surgical procedures on their hearts or elsewhere in the body are considered at high risk for pulmonary embolism. The presence of a transvenous pacemaker is another recently described risk factor for the development of venous thrombosis and pulmonary embolism in patients with heart disease (58).

B. Pneumonia

Community-acquired pneumonia occurs with increased frequency in patients with heart disease and failure. In a review of 300 consecutive patients hospitalized for congestive heart failure, Flint (59) documented that over half of them had some form of respiratory infection, chiefly acute bronchitis and pneumonia; in most cases, the infection was the precipitating cause of admission. In another study, heart disease was the most frequent underlying condition associated with hospitalization for community-acquired pneumonia, exceeding even the contribution of alcoholism, chronic lung disease, and diabetes mellitus as risk factors (60). The mechanism by which cardiac disease predisposes to pneumonia is unknown, but presumably an impairment of antibacterial defenses, particularly alveolar macrophage function, plays an important role (61). Confusion may occur because pneumonia is often complicated by a parapneumonic effusion or empyema (see Chapter 21), which may be mistaken for a cardiogenic hydrothorax.

C. Antiarrhythmia Agents

Two drugs used to treat arrhythmias in patients with heart disease are known to induce pleural effusions. Amiodarone causes multiorgan toxicity, of which fibrosing interstitial pneumonitis is the most serious and sometimes fatal; although uncommon, pleural effusions coexisting with parenchymal involvement have also been reported (62,63). Similarly, procainamide can cause pleural effusions as part of a drug-induced lupus reaction (64,65).

IX. Summary

Hydrothorax from congestive heart failure, the most common cause of pleural effusion in the industrialized countries of the world, is usually easily diagnosed by the presence of the many clinical and radiographic features of underlying cardiac dysfunction. Cardiogenic effusions are caused by leakage of pulmonary edema fluid from the lungs into the pleural spaces. Acute and chronic pericarditis, injury to the myocardium and pericardium, and revascularization surgical procedures are also frequently complicated by the development of pleural effusions. The mechanisms of fluid formation in these disorders remain obscure, but contiguous spread of cardiac inflammation to the neighboring pleural surfaces and/or an immunologically mediated reaction are believed to be responsible.

References

1. Marel M, Zrustova M, Stasmy B, Light RW. The incidence of pleural effusion in a well-defined region. Epidemiologic study in central Bohemia. Chest 1993; 104:1486–1489.
2. Light RW. Pleural Diseases. 4th ed. Baltimore: Lippincott, Williams & Wilkins, 2001:89.
3. Storey DD, Dines DE, Loles DT. Pleural effusion: a diagnostic dilemma. JAMA 1976; 236:2183–2186.
4. Valdes L, Alvarez D, Valle JM, Pose A, San Jose E. The etiology of pleural effusions in an area with high incidence of tuberculosis. Chest 1996; 109:158–162.
5. Bedford DE, Lovibond JL. Hydrothorax in heart failure. Br Heart J 1941; 3:93–111.
6. Logue RB, Rogers JV, Gay BB. Subtle roentgenographic signs of left heart failure. Am Heart J 1963; 65:464–473.
7. Kataoka H. Pericardial and pleural effusions in decompensated chronic heart failure. Am Heart J 2000; 139:918–923.
8. Lewin S, Goldberg L, Dec GW. The spectrum of pulmonary abnormalities on computed chest tomographic imaging in patients with advanced heart failure. Am J Cardiol 2000; 86:98–100.
9. Wiener-Kronish JP, Matthay MQ. Pleural effusions associated with hydrostatic and increased permeability pulmonary edema. Chest 1988; 93:852–858.
10. Mattison LE, Coppage L, Alderman DF, Herlong JO, Sahn SA. Pleural effusions in the medical ICU. Prevalence, causes, and clinical implications. Chest 1997; 111:1018–1023.
11. Staub NC, Wiener-Kronish JP, Albertine KH. Transport through the pleura. Physiology of normal liquid and solute exchange in the pleural space. In: Chrétien J, Bignon J, Hirsh A, eds. The Pleura in Health and Disease. New York: Marcel Dekker, Inc., 1985:169–193.
12. Staub NC. Pathophysiology of pulmonary edema. In: Staub NC, Taylor AE, eds. Edema. New York: Raven Press, 1984:719–746.
13. Broaddus VC, Wiener-Kronish JP, Staub NC. Clearance of lung edema into the pleural space of volume-loaded, anesthetized sheep. J Appl Physiol 1990; 68:2623–2630.
14. Bhattacharya J, Gropper MA, Staub NC. Interstitial fluid pressure gradient measured by micropuncture in excised dog lung. J Appl Physiol 1984; 56:271–277.
15. Wiener-Kronish JP, Matthay MA, Callen PW, Filly RA, Gamsu G, Staub NC. Relationship of pleural effusions to pulmonary hemodynamics in patients with heart failure. Am Rev Respir Dis 1985; 132:1253–1256.
16. Wiener-Kronish JP, Goldstein R, Matthay RA, Bionidi JW, Broaddus VC, Chatterjee K, Matthay MA. Lack of association of pleural effusion with chronic pulmonary arterial and right atrial hypertension. Chest 1987; 92:967–970.

17. Light RW, MacGregor MI, Luchsinger PC, Ball WC Jr. Pleural effusions: the diagnostic separation of transudates and exudates. Ann Intern Med 1972; 77:507–513.
18. Mellins RB, Levine DR, Fishman AP. Effect of systemic and pulmonary venous hypertension on pleural and pericardial fluid accumulation. J Appl Physiol 1970; 29:564–569.
19. McPeak EM, Levine SA. The preponderance of right hydrothorax in congestive heart failure. Ann Intern Med 1946; 25:916–927.
20. Peterman TA, Brothers SK. Pleural effusion in congestive heart failure and in pericardial disease. N Engl J Med 1983; 309:313.
21. Weiss JM, Spodick DH. Laterality of pleural effusions in chronic congestive heart failure. Am J Cardiol 1984; 53:951.
22. Race GA, Scheifley CH, Edwards JE. Hydrothorax in congestive heart failure. Am J Med 1957; 22:83–89.
23. Dock W. The anatomical and hydrostatic basis of orthopnea and of right hydrothorax in cardiac failure. Am Heart J 1935; 10:1047–1055.
24. Broaddus VC. Transudative pleural effusions. In: Loddenkemper R, Antony VB, eds. Pleural Disease. Eur Respir Mon 2002; 22:157–176.
25. Paré JA, Fraser RG. Synopsis of Diseases of the Chest. Philadelphia: WB Saunders, 1983:104.
26. Kataoka H, Takada S. The role of thoracic ultrasonography for evaluation of patients with decompensated chronic heart failure. J Am Coll Cardiol 2000; 35:1638–1646.
27. Goodman LR. Cardiopulmonary disorders in the critically ill. In: Goodman LR, Putman CE, eds. Intensive Care Radiology: Imaging of the Critically Ill. Philadelphia: WB Saunders, 1983:77–78.
28. Romero-Candeira SY, Fernandez C, Martin C, Sanchez-Paya J, Hernandez L. Influence of diuretics on the concentration of proteins and other components of pleural transudates in patients with heart failure. Am J Med 2001; 110:681–686.
29. Broaddus VC. Diuresis and transudative effusions—changing the rules of the game. Am J Med 2001; 110:732–735.
30. Roth BJ, O'meara TF, Cragun WH. The serum-effusion albumin gradient in the evaluation of pleural effusions. Chest 1990; 98:546–549.
31. Burgess LJ, Maritz FJ, Taljaard JJF. Comparative analysis of the biochemical parameters used to distinguish between pleural transudates and exudates. Chest 1995; 1604–1609.
32. Glazer M, Berkman N, Lafair JS, Kramer MR. Successful talc slurry pleurodesis in patients with nonmalignant pleural effusion. Report of 16 cases and review of the literature. Chest 2000; 117:1404–1409.
33. Sudduth CD, Sahn SA. Pleurodesis for nonmalignant pleural effusions. Recommendations. Chest 1992; 102:1855–1860.
34. Weiss JM, Spodick DH. Association of left pleural effusion with pericardial disease. N Engl J Med 1983; 308:696–697.
35. Plumb GE, Bruwer AJ, Clagett OT. Chronic constrictive pericarditis: roentgenologic findings in 35 surgically proven cases. Mayo Clin Proc 1957; 32:555–566.
36. Tomaselli G, Gamsu G, Stulbarg JS. Constrictive pericarditis presenting as pleural effusion of unknown origin. Arch Intern Med 1989; 149:201–203.
37. Sadikot RT, Fredi JL, Light RW. A 43-year old man with a large recurrent right-sided pleural effusion. Chest 2000; 117:1191–1194.

38. Dressler W. A post-myocardial-infarction syndrome. Preliminary report of a complication resembling idiopathic, recurrent, benign pericarditis. JAMA 1956; 160: 1379–1383.
39. Janton DH, Glover RP, O'Neil THE, Gregory JE, Frois GF. Results of the surgical treatment of mitral stenosis. Circulation 1952; 6:321–333.
40. Miller RH, Horneffer PJ, Gardner TJ, Rykiel MF, Pearson TA. The epidemiology of the postpericardiotomy syndrome: a common complication of surgery. Am Heart J 1988; 116:1323–1329.
41. Tabatznik B, Isaacs JP. Postpericardiotomy syndrome following traumatic hemopericardium. Am J Cardiol 1961; 7:83–96.
42. Peters RH, Whalen RE, Orgain ES, McIntosh HD. Postpericardiotomy syndrome as a complication of percutaneous left ventricular puncture. Am J Cardiol 1966; 17:86–90.
43. Terada Y, Mitsui T, Kaminishi Y, Yoshimura Y. Postpericardiotomy syndrome after pacemaker implantation. Ann Thorac Surg 1995; 59:1272–1273.
44. Turitto G, Abordo MG Jr, Mandawat MK, Togay VS, El-Sherif N. Radiofrequency ablation for cardiac arrhythmias causing postcardiac injury. Am J Cardiol 1998; 81:369–370.
45. Khan AH. The postcardiac injury syndromes. Clin Cardiol 1992; 15:67–72.
46. Broch OJ, Ofstad J. The post-myocardial-infarction. Acta Med Scand 1960; 166: 281–290.
47. Toole JC, Silverman ME. Pericarditis of acute myocardial infarction. Chest 1975; 67:647–653.
48. Kaminsky ME, Rodan BA, Chen JTT, Sealy WC, Putman CE. Postpericardiotomy syndrome. AJR 1982; 138:503–508.
49. Engle MA, McCabe JC, Ebert PA, Zabriskie J. The post-pericardiotomy syndrome and antiheart antibodies. Circulation 1974; 49:401–406.
50. Kim S, Sahn SA. Postcardiac injury syndrome. An immunologic pleural fluid analysis. Chest 1996; 109:570–572.
51. Schuller D, Morrow LE. Pulmonary complications after coronary revascularization. Curr Opin Cardiol 2000; 15:309–315.
52. Peng MJ, Vargas FS, Cukler A, Terra-Filho M, Teixeira LR, Light RW. Postoperative pleural changes after coronary revascularization. Comparison between saphenous vein and internal mammary artery. Chest 1992; 101:327–330.
53. Hurlbert D, Myers ML, Lefcoe M, Goldbach M. Pleuropulmonary morbidity: internal thoracic artery versus saphenous vein graft. Ann Thorac Surg 1990; 50:959–964.
54. Daganou M, Dimopoulou I, Michalopoulos N, Papadoupoulos K, Karakatsani A, Geroulanos S, Tzelpis GE. Respiratory complications after coronary artery bypass surgery with unilateral or bilateral internal mammary artery grafting. Chest 1998; 113:1285–1289.
55. Light RW, Rogers JT, Cheng D-C, Rodriquez M. Cardiovascular Associates. Large pleural effusions occurring after coronary artery bypass grafting. Ann Intern Med 1999; 130:891–896.
56. Hull RD, Pineo GF. Prophylaxis of deep venous thrombosis and pulmonary empolism. Current recommendations. Med Clin North Am 1998; 82:477–493.
57. Cogo A, Bernardi E, Prandoni P, Girolani B, Noventa F, Simioni P, Girolani A. Acquired risk factors for deep-vein thrombosis in symptomatic outpatients. Arch Intern Med 1994; 154:164–168.

58. Heit JA, Silverstein MD, Mohr DN, Petterson TM, O'Fallon M, Melton LJ. Risk factors for deep vein thrombosis and pulmonary embolism. Arch Intern Med 2000; 160:809–815.
59. Flint FJ. The factor of infection in heart failure. Br Med J 1954; 2:1018–1022.
60. Sullivan RJ Jr, Dowdle WR, Marine WM, Hierholzer JC. Adult pneumonia in a general hospital. Etiology and host risk factors. Arch Intern Med 1972; 129:935–942.
61. LaForce FM, Mullane JF, Boehme RF, Kelly WJ, Huber GL. The effect of pulmonary edema on antibacterial defenses of the lung. J Lab Clin Med 1973; 82:634–648.
62. Gonzalez-Rothi RJ, Hannan SE, Hood CI, Franzini DA. Amiodarone pulmonary toxicity presenting as bilateral exudative pleural effusions. Chest 1987; 92:179–182.
63. Akoun GM, Milleron BJ, Badaro DM, Mayaud CM, Liote HA. Pleural T-lymphocyte subsets in amiodarone-associated pleuropneumonitis. Chest 1989; 95:596–597.
64. Kaplan AI, Zakher F, Sabin S. Drug-induced lupus erythematosus with in vivo lupus erythematosus cells in pleural fluid. Chest 1978; 73:875–876.
65. Smith PR, Nacht RI. Drug-induced lupus pleuritis mimicking pleural space infection. Chest 1992; 101:268–269.

39

Pleural Effusions in Pregnancy and Gynecological Diseases

NIKOLAOS E. TZANAKIS and KATERINA ANTONIOU

University of Crete Medical School
and University Hospital of Heraklion
Heraklion, Crete, Greece

I. Introduction

Pulmonary effusion (PE) has been reported to accompany several gynecological conditions, mostly as a clinical feature of a systemic abnormality or seldom as an isolated extragynecological sign of a heterogeneous group of disorders (Table 1). The PEs related to pregnancy are rare in overall incidence, although they remain as a particularly devastating problem affecting not only the health of a young and presumably previously healthy and productive member of society, but also very often the life of the fetus or newborn infant. Pregnant women may potentially be at risk for misdiagnosis of pleural disease. The main reason for this is the obscure clinical features masked by the main event of pregnancy. The classical approach to differential diagnosis of PE can be missed if women avoid essential diagnostic techniques (e.g., chest x-ray) out of concern for the health of the fetus. However, the serious consequences of certain pleural diseases for maternal and fetal well-being require effective management of these unusual complications.

In this chapter, we discuss PE associated with special gynecological diseases or with the intrapartum and postpartum periods either resulting from a primary pleural disease or representing an important clinical manifestation of a pregnancy-related systemic or pulmonary abnormality (Table 1). Secondary PE

Table 1 PE in Gynecology and Obstetrics

I. Related to gynecological conditions
   a. Ovarian hyperstimulation syndrome (OHSS)
   b. Meigs' syndrome
   c. Endometriosis
II. Related to obstetrics and pregnancy
   a. Benign postpartum effusion
   b. Antiphospholipase antibody–related PE
   c. Choriocarcinoma
   d. Chylothorax
      i. Associated with lymphangiomyomatosis
      ii. Traumatic
   e. Other
      i. Hemothorax related to neurofibromatosis
      ii. Ruptured diaphragm
      iii. Hominis empyema
      iv. Urinothorax
   f. Specific
      i. Tuberculosis pleural effusion
      ii. Parapneumonic pleural effusion

due to specific disorders, e.g., tuberculous PE, will be discussed within the framework of the particularity of coexistence with pregnancy.

II. Pleural Effusion in Gynecology

A. Ovarian Hyperstimulation Syndrome

Pharmacological ovarian stimulation, a well-established therapeutic procedure in the field of infertility, has been widely used in the last decade (1). This treatment modality consists of ovulation induction with human chorionic gonadotropin (hCG) alone or in combination with clomiphene. It has become the gold standard method since the introduction of in vitro fertilization. One of the more common complications of this treatment is the development of the ovarian hyperstimulation syndrome (OHSS), characterized by ovarian enlargement, ascites, pleural effusion, hypovolemia, hemoconcentration, oliguria, and rarely thromboembolism. The incidence of OHSS is rising, and this increase is associated with the treatment of women with polycystic ovaries or with the induction of pregnancy (2). The syndrome can fall into four clinical stages of increasing severity: (1) mild, with abdominal distension and discomfort; (2) moderate, with ascites on ultrasound examination; (3) severe, with ascites clinically apparent with or without another effusion (pleural, rarely pericardial), and a hemoconcentration (hematocrit >45% and WBC count >15 000 cells/mL); and (4) critical, with, in addition to the above signs, hypovolemic shock, an acute renal and respiratory cells/mL failure, a marked hemoconcentration (hematocrit

>55% and WBC count >25 000), and thrombotic disorders (3). It can be extremely severe, with a morbidity reaching 5% of in vitro fertilizations (1).

The pathogenesis of OHSS has yet to be elucidated. This syndrome represents an overexpression of the normal ovulatory process described in normal pregnancy. The mechanisms underlying the clinical manifestations of OHSS involve an increased permeability of the ovarian capillaries and other mesothelial vessels triggered by the release of vasoactive substances of the ovaries under HCG stimulation (4). Recent evidence argues for the critical role of several mediators, including the angiotensin cascade components and various cytokines such as interleukins (IL)-1, -6, -8, tumor necrosis factor-α, vascular endothelial growth factor (VEGF), and endothelin 1 (5,6). A direct correlation between plasma rennin levels and the clinical severity of OHSS has been reported by Bergh and Navot (7).

The origin of pleural effusion is believed to be secondary to fluid shift from abdominal ascites. In patients with bilateral effusions, the probable mechanism that has been suggested is capillary leak into the pleural space itself. In the particular cases of isolated pleural effusions, the pathogenesis is more complex, with the unilaterally increased permeability remaining unexplained. The pleural effusions with OHSS are usually right sided. In the series of 33 patients with pleural effusion reported by Abramov et al. (8), 17 effusions (52%) were right sided, 9 (27%) were bilateral, and 7 (21%) were left sided. Two recently reported studies included a total of seven cases of isolated pleural effusions with OHSS, six of which were unilaterally right sided (9,10). Some authors suggest that this preferential location might be explained by a capillary leak and exudation into the pleural space due to the decreased right lymphatic drainage as compared to the left side (9). In addition, ascitic-related pleural effusions are also predominant in the right side because of the transfer through diaphragmatic defect or hiatus (6,11). The pleural fluid in patients with OHSS is an exudate. In the case-series of Abramov et al. (12), the mean pleural fluid protein was 4.1 g/dL, whereas the mean plasma protein was 4.4 g/dL.

The unpredictable individual responses to ovulation inducers make the prevention of OHSS very difficult. The following risk factors have been identified: age <35 years, presence of a polycystic ovarian disease prior to stimulation, a number of follicles >10, estradiol plasma concentration >2000 pg/mL, and an ongoing active pregnancy (10). Several recent studies reported the possible prognostic importance of serial cytokines as markers of this syndrome. Chen and colleagues have reported that the levels of VEGF and IL-6 in ascites dropped significantly during the course of OHSS and levels of VEGF were significantly correlated with levels of IL-1β, IL-8, and TNF-α, as well as progesterone concentrations, hematocrit, and white blood cell counts (WBC) (13). A similar study suggests that follicular fluid IL-6 concentrations at the time of oocyte retrieval and serum IL-8 concentrations on the day of embryo transfer may serve as early predictors of this syndrome (14).

Patients with OHSS initially develop abdominal discomfort and distension, followed by nausea, vomiting, and diarrhea. As the syndrome worsens, the patients develop evidence of ascites and then hydrothorax or breathing difficulties. In the most severe stages, the patient develops increased blood viscosity owing to hemoconcentration, coagulation abnormalities, and diminished renal function (12,15). Respiratory symptoms develop 7–14 days after the hCG injection (15,16). The ovarian hyperstimulation syndrome as a complication of hormonal treatment is usually mild in degree. In cases of increased risk, the patients' monitoring should be very cautious, with repeated ultrasonographic examinations and plasma hormonal determinations. The severity of OHSS varies with the delay between the onset of symptoms and the stimulation: within 3–7 days of hCG administration, it is often moderate to severe, while a later onset (12–17 days) often signals a more severe clinical form (10). The treatment is mainly supportive (bed rest and avoidance of further hormonal treatment), and the symptoms usually resolve spontaneously. Hemoconcentration should be treated with intravenous fluids to avoid acute renal failure. Large pleural effusions with respiratory discomfort should be treated by intercostal drainage. In conclusion, chest physicians should be more aware of this syndrome in order to ensure a better and minimally invasive management of these potentially pregnant women. The OHSS has to be considered in the differential diagnosis of pleural effusion in young women undergoing ovulation induction for in vitro fertilization, because of its increasing prevalence (12).

B. Endometriosis

Although endometriosis is generally confined to the pelvis, it may occur at remote sites with unusual manifestations. Thoracic endometriosis is a relatively rare condition, with a varying clinical presentation and is usually diagnosed from a history of recurrent chest pain with or without hemoptysis termed as catamenial hemoptysis. This monthly presentation coincides with the menstrual cycle, with the pain occurring at the time of menstruation. The most common presentation of the disease is right-sided pneumothorax (17). Hemothorax, recurrent hemoptysis, chest pain, and asymptomatic pulmonary nodules occur less commonly (18–20).

Ectopic endometrium in distant sites from the pelvis is well described. It causes symptoms relative to the site where the bleeding occurs. Rare examples include pulmonary endometriosis and endometriosis associated with ascites. Muneyyirci-Delale et al. (21) presented 4 cases, reviewed the literature of 23 additional cases, and found that 8 of the 27 patients (30%) also presented with pleural effusion. Bhojawala et al. (22) published 12 cases of both bloodstained ascites and pleural effusion with endometriosis since the first report by Meigs (23). The ascitic and/or pleural fluid are described as a bloodstained or chocolate-colored fluid (22). The etiology of thoracic endometriosis remains speculative, with two possible theories having been suggested. The first of these is a vascular theory whereby endometrial cells are transported via the venous system to the right side of the heart and thereafter via the pulmonary artery to peripheral sites of the lungs. Ascites may result from rupture of endometriosis or chocolate cysts leading to peritoneal irritation (24), or it may occur in a similar way to that in Meigs' syndrome (25,26). However, evidence in human and nonhuman primates suggests a genetic basis for endometriosis (26). The pleural effusion generally occurs on the right [although Yu and Grimes reported bilateral pleural effusions (27)] and is thought to be due to ascitic fluid gaining entrance to the pleural cavity through the diaphragm.

The treatment of massive ascites, pleural effusion, and endometriosis is difficult. The medical treatment of this syndrome is temporary and merely confirms the fact that the hypo-estrogenic state is the desired curative course. The use of the hypothalamus-derived gonadorelin releasing hormone (GnRH) agonists in the treatment of endometriosis would seem to be extremely helpful in establishing a course of therapy. A case report by Shek et al. recommended a GnRH analog agonist (nafarelin acetate) administered through nasal route and thoracentesis as the initial treatment for endometriosis related ascites and/or pleural effusion (28). Of the 31 patients reviewed by Muneyyirci-Delale et al., only 3 were managed without laparotomy (21). Total abdominal hysterectomy and bilateral salpingo-oophorectomy are the most commonly performed procedures (21). At operation, endometriosis usually involved surrounding structures such as the fallopian tubes, ovaries, appendix, sigmoid colon, and omentum (21).

C. Meigs' Syndrome

In 1937, Meigs and Cass (29) reported the clinical picture of ovarian fibroma associated with ascites and pleural effusion in seven patients. Thereafter, the syndrome was referred to as Meigs' syndrome (23). Meigs proposed that the true Meigs' syndrome be limited to benign and solid ovarian tumors (fibroma, thecoma, and granulose cell tumor) (23). In contrast, pseudo-Meigs' syndrome is a condition characterized by nonmalignant ascites and/or pleural effusion due to pelvic tumors other than solid benign ovarian tumors (e.g., other benign cysts of the ovary, leiomyomas of the uterus, teratomas) (30,31). Meigs still prefers to reserve his name for only those cases in which the primary neoplasm is a benign solid ovarian tumor (23). Light classifies any patient with a pelvic neoplasm associated with ascites and pleural effusion, in whom surgical removal of the tumor results in permanent disappearance of the ascites and pleural effusion, as having Meigs' syndrome (32).

Fibromas are associated with ascites in approximately 10–15% of all cases. Ascites probably occurs by means of a transudative mechanism through the tumor surface that exceeds the peritoneum's capacity to reabsorb the fluid (33). Other possible mechanisms include obstruction of peritoneal lymphatics by tumor or increased permeability of the neovasculature with protein leakage. The plausible theory is that the pressure on the lymphatic vessels in the tumor itself causes the escape of fluid through the surface lymphatics, which are situated just beneath the single-layered cuboid epithelium covering the tumor. CA125 has been demonstrated to be elevated in benign conditions, such as pelvic inflammatory disease, endometriosis, uterine leiomyoma, and early pregnancy (33).

There are 11 reports (14 patients) of Meigs' syndrome with elevated CA125 levels. All these cases prove that elevated CA125 levels are common in patients with this syndrome (33). Results of immunoperoxidase stains suggest that serum elevation of CA125 antigen is caused by mesothelial expression of the antigen rather than by the fibroma (33). A recent report found differences in changes in VEGF levels in pleural effusion and ascites after removal of ovarian tumor complicated by Meigs' syndrome. Postoperative VEGF levels decreased in the patient's pleural fluid but not in the peritoneal fluid. Although the mechanism of this phenomenon is clear thus far, the possibility of differences in kinetics of fluid in the peritoneal and pleural cavity has been shown. This finding may provide a clue that the mechanism of the development of the pleural effusion and ascites in Meigs' syndrome may differ (34). The findings of a recent report suggest the involvement of vasoactive growth factors such as fibroblast growth factor (FGF) and VEGF and of the inflammatory cytokine IL-6 in the pathogenesis of Meigs' syndrome (5). All three factors possess potent vascular permeability–enhancing properties, and all have been associated with capillary leakage and with the formation of ascites and pleural effusion in other gynecological abnormalities, such as the ovarian hyperstimulation syndrome (8).

Patients with Meigs' syndrome usually have a chronic illness characterized by weight loss, pleural effusion, ascites, and a pelvic mass (23). The pleural effusion is right sided in about 70% of the patients, left sided in 10%, and bilateral in 20% (35). The only symptom referable to the pleural effusion is shortness of breath. The ascites may not be evident on physical examination. The pleural fluid is usually an exudate. Most pleural fluids secondary to Meigs' syndrome have a protein level above 3.0 g/dL (11). The pleural fluid has usually low WBC (fewer than $1.000/mm^3$) and is occasionally bloody (36). The diagnosis of Meigs' syndrome should be considered in all women who have pelvic masses, ascites, and pleural effusions. Laparotomy is required for the correct diagnosis of ovarian tumors since peritoneal cytology, tumor markers, and other indicators of malignant pathology may be misleading. The diagnosis is confirmed when the ascites and the pleural effusion resolve postoperatively and do not reoccur. Postoperatively, the pleural fluid disappears rapidly and is usually completely gone within 2 weeks (37).

III. Pregnancy-Related Pleural Effusion

A. Benign Postpartum PE

Asymptomatic PE presented in the immediate postpartum period is a benign condition that is not clinically significant but should be included in the differential diagnosis of diseases occurring in the postpartum period. Benign PE may develop in the immediate postpartum period within a week after delivery. Hessen reported the first prospective clinical study of the presentation of PE in 23% of a group of 92 women 7–12 days after a normal delivery (38). Another 14% of the population under study had radiographic findings compatible with a probable

PE. In the study of Hessen, a control group of 300 healthy individuals, including 163 nonpregnant women and 137 men, underwent a similar radiographic evaluation. Radiographic findings of a small effusion were identified in 12 subjects (4%) and a probable small effusion in 18 (6%). In the above study, no information is reported on the cardiorespiratory status of the studied patients. Subsequently, several investigators examined, either prospectively or retrospectively, women with uncomplicated labor and delivery. Hughson et al. (39) studied retrospectively 112 women who had delivered vaginally and had posteroanterior and lateral chest x-ray within 24 hours of delivery. Two independent radiologists reviewed the radiographs using a scoring system that reflected the degree of costophrenic angle blunting. None of the patients had evidence of cardiorespiratory disease. The authors reported moderate-sized PE in 4% of the patients and small in 46%, which were bilateral in 75% (39). Based on this observation, the same group conducted a prospective study wherein 30 similar patients were evaluated using the same methodology. PE was reported in 20 (67%) and in 11 (36%) was bilateral. In both studies, retrospective and prospective of Hughson and colleagues (39) reported that the presence of the PE was not correlated with any of the clinical features they analyzed including age, weight gain during pregnancy, hematocrit, serum protein, existence of preeclampsia, duration and difficulty of labor, use of intravenous fluids, or administration of oxytocin. The presence of postpartum PE was also not correlated with a major obstetric complication or with an adverse fetal outcome.

In another study Stark and Pollack (40) reviewed chest radiographs of 45 women within 48 hours of labor and delivery. Forty-four of the 45 patients had radiographic evidence of small PE. However, the case series design (women were evaluated for fever or respiratory symptoms) and the high proportion of delivery by cesarean section are particular biases not allowing acceptance of the high incidence of the postpartum PE reported in this study (40).

The plain chest radiographs without decubitus views have a low sensitivity and specificity for the detection of PE (41). In contrast, thoracic ultrasonographic scans provide a sensitive and specific method for the detection of PEs in very low volumes—3–5 mL (41–43). Thus, Udeshi and colleagues examined women postpartum for the presence of PE using thoracic ultrasonography (44). Of the 50 patients studied, all examined within 48 hours of labor and delivery, 29 had delivered by the vaginal route and the other 21 underwent a cesarean section. Only one of the 50 patients evaluated had ultrasonic evidence of PE. Since this patient had experienced severe preeclampsia complicated by pulmonary edema, the authors concluded that PEs rarely occur after an uncomplicated vaginal or cesarean delivery (44). In contrast to the above report, Gourgoulianis et al. (45) in a case-control study examined 31 postpartum women delivered vaginally and normally and 22 healthy nonpregnant women as control group with thoracic ultrasonography. They reported ultrasonic evidence of PE in 7 out of the 31 patients (23%) and in none of the 22 healthy controls (45). The authors concluded that the physiological conditions of pregnancy, labor, and normal delivery could promote transudation of fluid into the pleural space because of the increased hydrostatic pressure in the systemic circulation and the decreased colloid osmotic pressure. Moreover, the repeated Valsava maneuvers of parturition may further promote pleural effusion through an increase of intrathoracic pressure and an impairment of the lymphatic drainage of the pleural space.

In a subsequent study, Wallis et al. (46) designed a case series study aiming to determine the incidence of the postpartum PE in patients with moderate to severe preeclampsia. Nine of the 34 individuals (26.5%) had ultrasonic findings of PE. There was no difference in the severity of the preeclampsia, radiographic appearance of pulmonary edema, or the amount of intravenous fluids between those with and without PE. However, the investigators reported a 10-fold higher incidence of perinatal fetal mortality in women who experienced a postpartum PE (46).

Since thoracic ultrasonography is more sensitive than chest radiography (41,42), it is likely that the true incidence of postpartum PE related to normal labor and delivery is closer to the case series and case control studies (44–46) that have used ultrasound evaluation. Postpartum small size, asymptomatic PE is not clinically significant but should be included in the differential diagnosis of the pleural diseases occurring in the postpartum period. However, moderate to large effusions, particularly if accompanied by signs and symptoms of a complicated disease, should be evaluated and managed as pleural effusions similar to other clinical settings.

B. Antiphospholipid Antibody–Related PE

In addition to the "normal" phenomenon of the benign postpartum pleural effusion, which usually occurs immediately after labor and delivery, there have been two studies (47,48) reporting a systemic disease with pulmonary effusion and pulmonary infiltrates a few weeks after delivery. In the first study, Kochenour et al. (47) presented a series of three women with antiphospholipid antibodies and a postpartum syndrome of pleuropulmonary disease, fever, and cardiac manifestations. Each patient had either lupus anticoagulant or anticardiolipin antibodies or both. However, none of the patients had antinuclear antibodies or fulfills the criteria for the diagnosis of systemic lupus erythematosus (47). Two of the three patients experienced thromboembolic episodes. Based on the association between antiphospholipid antibodies and fetal loss, fetal growth retardation, and preeclampsia, investigators suggested that patients with antiphospholipid antibodies are at risk for a serious autoimmune postpartum syndrome. The second report is a case report of a patient at 29 weeks' gestation who had elevated blood pressure, proteinuria, and early intrauterine growth retardation (48). Studies were positive for the presence of both lupus anticoagulant and anticardiolipin antibodies. After delivery, chest pain and a pleural effusion developed as further manifestations of the patient's autoimmune disease. In addition to the known association between antiphospholipid syndrome and instances of fetal death (49,50), the above studies (47,48) demonstrate another important relationship between these immunological markers and serious pleuropulmonary and cardiac disorders in the postpartum period. The authors propose that antiphospholipid antibody syndrome be considered if patients experience serious pleuropulmonary or/and cardiac disease in the first month after delivery (47). On the other hand, pregnant women with positive antiphospholipid antibodies may benefit from immunosuppressive therapy and prophylactic anticoagulation to prevent life-threatening thromboembolic disease (47,48).

C. Choriocarcinoma

Choriocarcinoma is a form of gestational trophoblastic disease (GTD), a heterogeneous group of interrelated lesions that may occur after any gestational experience (e.g., abortion, ectopic, or term pregnancy). The pathogenesis is unique because the maternal tumor arises from fetal, not maternal, tissue. It is commonly metastatic to several organs such as lung, brain, liver, pelvis, vagina, spleen, intestine, and kidney (51). Pulmonary metastatic gestational trophoblastic disease poses problems in diagnosis and management and has a poorer prognosis than the nonmetastatic variant. The overall survival rate at 2 years after diagnosis in the series of Kumar et al. (51) was 65%. Pleural effusion may occur mostly as a consequence of a metastatic disease to the pleura or to the neighboring subpleural lung parenchyma. Rarely, the vascular dissemination of the trophoblastic tissue undergoes pulmonary infarction secondary to tumor emboli presenting as pleural effusion.

In many patients of the case series study of Kumar et al. (51), the pulmonary lesions were asymptomatic. However, patients may present with the following signs and symptoms (51,52):

Dyspnea secondary to tumor emboli and pulmonary infarction
Cough and hemoptysis due to bronchial or parenchymal lesions
Persistent gradually worsening dyspnea secondary to lung parenchyma metastases
Pleuritic pain as a result of pleural metastatic disease

Most patients with choriocarcinoma and pulmonary lesion have an antecedent molar pregnancy, although an associated choriocarcinomatous lesion in the uterus is absent in the majority of them (51). Fewer than 5% of patients have other gestational experience such as abortion, ectopic, immediate-term or term pregnancy. However, a higher mortality has been observed when the antecedent pregnancy ended at term (51,52). Choriocarcinomatous pleural effusion may be due to the metastatic pleural disease or to the pulmonary tumor embolism and is usually hemorrhagic. The pleural involvement frequently causes large hemothorax (pleural fluid/blood hematocrit >50%) (53,54) leading to severe dyspnea and respiratory failure.

Since the clinical presentation of the metastatic choriocarcinoma in pleura and lungs is the same as in pulmonary embolism, these two entities should be carefully sorted out, taking into account that metastatic choriocarcinoma treated wrongly with anticoagulants may lead to fatal spontaneous hemorrhage from the brain. Several management options are available for patients who are symptomatic and require some form of therapy, such as chest tube drainage, outpatient thoracentesis for recurrent effusions to prevent respiratory stress and the development of fibrothorax and trapped lung.

D. Chylothorax

Associated with Lymphangiomyomatosis

Pulmonary lymphangiomyomatosis (LAM) is a rare idiopathic lung disease that afflicts women of childbearing age (55–57). It is characterized pathologically by the proliferation of atypical pulmonary interstitial smooth muscle in the pulmonary blood vessels, airways, and lymphatic channels and by cysts formation (57). Pulmonary LAM presents almost exclusively in premenopausal women (57,58). More than 70% of the patients are between 20 and 40 years of age at the onset of the disease. Only 6% are more than 50 years of age at presentation, many of them associated with hormone replacement therapy (58). The disease causes dyspnea, pneumothorax, chylous pleural effusion, hemoptysis, and eventually respiratory failure. At presentation most patients have airflow obstruction, relatively normal lung volumes, and a low diffusing capacity of the lung (I_{LCO}) (57,58).

Extrapulmonary manifestations include abdominal and pelvic masses occurring along axial lymphatics (now termed lymphangioleiomyoma), chylous ascites, and in more than 80% renal angiomyolipomas (59). The pathogenesis of LAM is unknown, but data are accumulating that suggest a role for abnormalities in proteins involved in the synthesis of catecholamines (55,60). It is likely that estrogen plays a central role in disease progression, since the disease does not present prior to menarche and only rarely after menopause (57). Estrogen and progesterone receptors have been demonstrated in biopsy tissue (61,62). Furthermore, the disease is known to accelerate during pregnancy (63–68), and there is some evidence that women with LAM are less likely to become pregnant (58). Of the 50 cases of the study of Johnson and Tattersfield (58), 28 had been pregnant and 27 had had children. Seven out of the 50 developed their first symptom of LAM when pregnant or postpartum ($n = 4$). Of the seven patients, one pregnancy was uncomplicated and one was terminated. The other five patients had complications during pregnancy while two developed a chylous pleural effusion and three experienced one or more pneumothoraces. The overall incidence of complications was 11 times higher during pregnancy than at other times (58). In the same study the two patients with chylous pleural effusion (one bilateral and one unilateral) were treated initially by aspiration and intercostal drainage. One woman with unilateral effusion needed further procedures including thoracotomy, thoracic duct ligation, and pleurectomy (58). On the basis of observations that women with LAM present an increased incidence of complications during pregnancy, patients should be aware of this before conception.

Traumatic

Chylothorax nonassociated with LAM has been rarely reported in pregnancy (69,70). It can be classified as traumatic etiology because the condition seems to be a consequence after a prolonged difficult vaginal delivery with the obstructed expiratory effort of the Valsalva maneuver transmitting high intrathoracic pressures to thoracic structures. This mechanism causes main lymphatic duct rupture and chylothorax. Difficult childbirth has been reported as an unusual etiology for the formation of chylothorax. Doctors should take into account this diagnosis when lymphoma, lymphangiomyomatosis, malignancies, and miscellaneous other causes of chylothorax are not evident. The management of this condition is the same as with any other traumatic chylothorax (71).

E. Other

Neurofibromatosis-Related Hemothorax

Massive spontaneous intrathoracic hemorrhage related to neurofibromatosis has been reported in two cases during the first week after delivery (72). Neurofibromatosis is an idiopathic disease characterized by abnormal proliferation of fibrous tissue in the skin and viscera. Effects of pregnancy on the clinical course of neurofibromatosis are known to include worsening of cutaneous lesions, increased incidence of hypertension, and renal artery rupture. Vessel wall rupture in areas of vascular neurofibromatous infiltration is the possible mechanism of hemorrhagic pleural effusion.

Ruptured Diaphragm

Prolonged and tiring vaginal delivery generates high intrathoracic and intraabdominal pressures with rapid acceleration and deceleration during the effort to utilize the Valsalva maneuvers. This delivery mechanism may cause rupture of the diaphragm, a rare but serious complication of pregnancy commonly associated with hemorrhagic pleural effusion (73–77). Onset of the rupture usually presents with acute abdominal pain with varying degree of dyspnea nausea and emesis because of the herniated bowel (73,74). In the case of a strangulated herniated bowel, serious manifestations may occur such as cyanosis and shock (73). Chest roentgenography and computed tomography revealed bowel in the left hemithorax, compatible with a left-sided diaphragmatic rupture. Delayed rupture of diaphragm not related with labor but associated with intrauterine pregnancy has seldom been reported (78,79). In one case report, this delayed ruptured diaphragm presented as pleural empyema (80). Surgical therapy is the cornerstone of management, particularly when a diaphragmatic defect is symptomatic. The route of delivery may be individualized for patients with diaphragmatic repairs in whom there has been sufficient time for healing (77).

Mycoplasma Hominis *Empyema*

Mycoplasma hominis frequently colonizes the genital tract, but is rarely isolated from the respiratory tract (81). The significance of *M. hominis* in respiratory infections must be interpreted with caution. *M. hominis* has been isolated from respiratory secretions in 1–3% of healthy persons, 8% of patients with chronic respiratory complaints, and 14% of persons engaging in orogenital sex (82). Thus, *M. hominis* is probably rarely capable of causing lower respiratory tract infection. Dissemination of *M. hominis* has been documented in women with a febrile illness after delivery (81). Occasional reports exist in which *M. hominis* has been isolated from pure culture from empyema fluid (83,84). Intrathoracic infection with *M. hominis* has been reported to cause complicated pleural empyema in two case reports. The first involved a postpartum 16-year-old patient (85) with complicated pleural empyema, and the second was the case of a 32-year-old woman in her 29th week of pregnancy with persistent pleural effusion (86).

Urinothorax

Relaxation of ureteral smooth muscle induced by hormones producing ureteral atony and pressure on the ureters by the gravid uterus may result in mild to moderate dilatation of the collecting systems of the kidney (87). This functional hydronephrosis, which tends to be more prominent on the right, is not usually associated with renal dysfunction (87). However, moderate or severe hydronephrosis is a well-recognized complication in the previously pregnant women (87,88). The degree of obstruction is rarely sufficient to cause acute renal failure due to ureteral obstruction by the gravid uterus (89). In some cases the normalization of renal function in the lateral recumbent position relieves pressure on the ureters by the uterus, and its recurrence when supine confirms the diagnosis. Occasionally, pyelonephritis coexists with pregnancy because of a moderate to severe ureteral obstruction (90). Acute oliguric renal failure associated with bacterial pyelonephritis is a rarely recognized clinical entity in pregnancy (91).

Pleural effusion related either to functional hydronephrosis and/or pyelonephritis has been reported during pregnancy (87,89,92,93). In some reports patients presented with large pleural effusion and renal failure (89,92). In most cases, the pleural fluid is transudate. In some case reports, the transudative pleural effusion may represent urinothoraces (94). The diagnosis of urinothorax is confirmed by demonstrating a pleural fluid–to–serum creatinine ratio of greater than one (95).

F. Pleural Effusion of Specific Etiology

When a pleural effusion of specific etiology such as tuberculous or parapneumonic is diagnosed in coexistence with pregnancy, a number of challenging clinical problems should promptly managed. The complete review of these conditions is discussed elsewhere in this book. We will focus here on available important clinical evidence of management of tuberculosis and infectious pleural effusions relevant for the maternal and infant well-being.

Tuberculous Pleural Effusion

The prevalence of tuberculosis (TB), especially extrapulmonary tuberculosis, is increasing worldwide (96). Despite the fact that extrapulmonary tuberculosis does not affect the course of pregnancy, labor, or the perinatal outcome, a higher rate of antenatal maternal hospitalization along with low Apgar scores and low birth weight in infants has been reported (96). The clinical manifestations of tuberculous pleural effusion in the pregnant woman are no different from those in nonpregnant individuals, and the same is true concerning the treatment modalities. Thus, the treatment rationale in established TB pleural effusion is recommended in pregnancy, although it is not verified in this group of women (97). None of the first-line drugs has been shown to be teratogenic (98). Streptomycin should be avoided, as it may be ototoxic (98). In the United States, caution is recommended regarding the use of pyrazinamide. The American Thoracic Society guidelines state that pyrazinamide should be avoided in pregnancy but can be given after first trimester (97). In summary, isoniazid in combination with ethambutol and rifampicin is recommended for a pregnant woman with tuberculosis (99). If a fourth drug is warranted, then pyrazinamide could be added after the third trimester. Routine therapeutic abortion is not medically indicated for a pregnant woman who is taking first-line antituberculosis drugs (97). Pregnant women with suspected TB pleural effusion should be targeted for tuberculin skin testing (100). There are some cases when the pregnant women have positive tuberculin test but the pleural effusion finally is diagnosed as of a different cause than tuberculosis. In this case, the patient is diagnosed as having latent tuberculosis infection (LTBI) (100). Although the recommended treatment scheme for active tuberculosis pleural effusion is likely valid in pregnancy, the treatment of LTBI is rather controversial (100). Some experts agree that treatment can wait until after delivery since pregnancy does not increase the risk of disease progression (100). On the other hand, some reports have emphasized isoniazid hepatotoxicity observed in pregnancy (100). However, many experts suggested that pregnant women with LTBI at risk of conditions that promote progression to the disease or hematogenous spread of organisms to the placenta [recent TB infection, immunodeficiency (e.g., HIV infection)] should be treated during pregnancy (100). Pregnant women receiving isoniazid must undergo careful clinical and laboratory monitoring for hepatitis.

Parapneumonic Pleural Effusion

An important predisposing factor to the development of severe pneumonic infections and parapneumonic pleural effusion or empyema during pregnancy is the altering of the maternal immune system. This altering affects primarily cell-mediated immunity, explaining why certain microorganisms are related to respiratory infections during pregnancy. Whereas the clinical features of bacterial pneumonia during pregnancy are not dramatically different from those seen in the nonpregnant patient, complications are more frequently reported, reflecting a possible delay of recognition of pneumonia. Madinger et al. reported a case series study of 25 patients in whom diagnoses of bacterial pneumonia were initially overlooked in five cases. This delay was possibly related to the increased incidence of serious complications, including empyema, in nearly half of all the patients in this series (101).

A detailed discussion of the clinical manifestations and the diagnosis of parapneumonic pleural effusion or empyema are beyond the scope of this review. Generally, the presentation and diagnosis of parapneumonic effusion or empyema does not differ between nonpregnant and pregnant patients, although the physiological changes of pregnancy make it difficult for the pregnant woman to tolerate a large parapneumonic effusion. The management of parapneumonic effusion or empyema in pregnant women is similar to the free-of-pregnancy situation, taking into account the basic recommendations regarding using antibiotic therapy in pregnancy (102,103). Chest tube for evacuation of large or complicated parapneumonic effusions is not contraindicated. Intrapleural instillation of fibrinolytic agents has been shown in a number of studies to be an effective and safe mode of treatment in complicated parapneumonic effusions and empyema, minimizing the need for surgical intervention (104). However, fibrinolysis in the management of complicated multiloculated empyemas is generally not recommended in pregnancy because of limited experience (104–106).

References

1. Golan A, Ron-el R, Herman A, Soffer Y, Weinraub Z, Caspi E. Ovarian hyperstimulation syndrome: an update review. Obstet Gynecol Surv 1989; 44:430–440.
2. Schenker JG, Ezra Y. Complications of assisted reproductive techniques. Fertil Steril 1994; 61:411–422.
3. Navot D, Bergh PA, Laufer N. Ovarian hyperstimulation syndrome in novel reproductive technologies: prevention and treatment. Fertil Steril 1992; 58:249–261.
4. Varma TR, Patel RH. Ovarian hyperstimulation syndrome. A case history and review. Acta Obstet Gynecol Scand 1988; 67:579–584.
5. Abramov Y, Anteby SO, Fasouliotis SJ, Barak V. Markedly elevated levels of vascular endothelial growth factor, fibroblast growth factor, and interleukin 6 in Meigs syndrome. Am J Obstet Gynecol 2001; 184:354–355.
6. Loret de Mola JR. Pathophysiology of unilateral pleural effusions in the ovarian hyperstimulation syndrome. Hum Reprod 1999; 14:272–273.
7. Bergh PA, Navot D. Ovarian hyperstimulation syndrome: a review of pathophysiology. J Assist Reprod Genet 1992; 9:429–438.
8. Abramov Y, Barak V, Nisman B, Schenker JG. Vascular endothelial growth factor plasma levels correlate to the clinical picture in severe ovarian hyperstimulation syndrome. Fertil Steril 1997; 67:261–265.
9. Man A, Schwarz Y, Greif J. Pleural effusion as a presenting symptom of ovarian hyperstimulation syndrome. Eur Respir J 1997; 10:2425–2426.

10. Roden S, Juvin K, Homasson JP, Israel-Biet D. An uncommon etiology of isolated pleural effusion. The ovarian hyperstimulation syndrome. Chest 2000; 118:256–258.
11. Light RW. Pleural diseases. Dis Mon 1992; 38:261–331.
12. Abramov Y, Elchalal U, Schenker JG. Febrile morbidity in severe and critical ovarian hyperstimulation syndrome: a multicentre study. Hum Reprod 1998; 13: 3128–3131.
13. Chen CD, Wu MY, Chen HF, Chen SU, Ho HN, Yang YS. Prognostic importance of serial cytokine changes in ascites and pleural effusion in women with severe ovarian hyperstimulation syndrome. Fertil Steril 1999; 72:286–292.
14. Chen CD, Chen HF, Lu HF, Chen SU, Ho HN, Yang YS. Value of serum and follicular fluid cytokine profile in the prediction of moderate to severe ovarian hyperstimulation syndrome. Hum Reprod 2000; 15:1037–1042.
15. Levin MF, Kaplan BR, Hutton LC. Thoracic manifestations of ovarian hyperstimulation syndrome. Can Assoc Radiol J 1995; 46:23–26.
16. Gregory WT, Patton PE. Isolated pleural effusion in severe ovarian hyperstimulation: a case report. Am J Obstet Gynecol 1999; 180:1468–1471.
17. Carter EJ, Ettensohn DB. Catamenial pneumothorax. Chest 1990; 98:713–716.
18. Wilkins SB, Bell-Thomson J, Tyras DH. Hemothorax associated with endometriosis. J Thorac Cardiovasc Surg 1985; 89:636–638.
19. Elliot DL, Barker AF, Dixon LM. Catamenial hemoptysis. New methods of diagnosis and therapy. Chest 1985; 87:687–688.
20. Horsfield K. Catamenial pleural pain. Eur Respir J 1989; 2:1013–1014.
21. Muneyyirci-Delale O, Neil G, Serur E, Gordon D, Maiman M, Sedlis A. Endometriosis with massive ascites. Gynecol Oncol 1998; 69:42–46.
22. Bhojawala J, Heller DS, Cracchiolo B, Sama J. Endometriosis presenting as bloody pleural effusion and ascites-report of a case and review of the literature. Arch Gynecol Obstet 2000; 264:39–41.
23. Meigs JV. Fibroma of the ovary with ascites and hydrothorax. Meigs' syndrome. Am J Obstet Gynecol 1954; 67:962–987.
24. Joseph J, Sahn SA. Thoracic endometriosis syndrome: new observations from an analysis of 110 cases. Am J Med 1996; 100:164–170.
25. Chervenak FA, Greenlee RM, Lewenstein L, Tovell HM. Massive ascites associated wth endometriosis. Obstet Gynecol 1981; 57:379–381.
26. Kennedy S. Is there a genetic basis to endometriosis? Semin Reprod Endocrinol 1997; 15:309–318.
27. Yu J, Grimes DA. Ascites and pleural effusions associated with endometriosis. Obstet Gynecol 1991; 78:533–534.
28. Shek Y, De Lia JE, Pattillo RA. Endometriosis with a pleural effusion and ascites. Report of a case treated with nafarelin acetate. J Reprod Med 1995; 40: 540–542.
29. Meigs JV, Cass JW. Fibroma of the ovary with ascites and hydrothorax. Am J Obstet Gynecol 1937; 33:249–267.
30. Chen FC, Fink RL, Jolly H. Meigs' syndrome in association with a locally invasive adenocarcinoma of the fallopian tube. Aust NZ J Surg 1995; 65:761–762.
31. Ryan RJ. PseudoMeigs syndrome. Associated with metastatic cancer of ovary. NY State J Med 1972; 72:727–730.
32. Light RW. Diagnostic principles in pleural disease. Eur Respir J 1997; 10:476–481.
33. Abad A, Cazorla E, Ruiz F, Aznar I, Asins E, Llixiona J. Meigs' syndrome with

elevated CA125: case report and review of the literature. Eur J Obstet Gynecol Reprod Biol 1999; 82:97–99.
34. Ishiko O, Yoshida H, Sumi T, Hirai K, Ogita S. Vascular endothelial growth factor levels in pleural and peritoneal fluid in Meigs' syndrome. Eur J Obstet Gynecol Reprod Biol 2001; 98:129–130.
35. Majzlin G, Stevens FL. Meigs' syndrome: case report and review of literature. J Int Coll Surg 1964; 42:625–630.
36. Neustadt JE, Levy RC. Hemorrhagic pleural effusion in Meig's syndrome. JAMA 1968; 204:81–82.
37. Jimerson SD. Pseudo-Meigs's syndrome. An unusual case with analysis of the effusions. Obstet Gynecol 1973; 42:535–537.
38. Hessen I. Roentgen examination of pleural fluid. Acta Radiol 1951; 86:62–64.
39. Hughson WG, Friedman PJ, Feigin DS, Resnik R, Moser KM. Postpartum pleural effusion: a common radiologic finding. Ann Intern Med 1982; 97:856–858.
40. Stark P, Pollack MS. Pleural effusions in the postpartum period. Radiologe 1986; 26:471–473.
41. Eibenberger KL, Dock WI, Ammann ME, Dorffner R, Hormann MF, Grabenwoger F. Quantification of pleural effusions: sonography versus radiography. Radiology 1994; 191:681–684.
42. Lipscomb DJ, Flower CD, Hadfield JW. Ultrasound of the pleura: an assessment of its clinical value. Clin Radiol 1981; 32:289–290.
43. Matalon TA, Neiman HL, Mintzer RA. Noncardiac chest sonography. The state of the art. Chest 1983; 83:675–678.
44. Udeshi UL, McHugo JM, Crawford JS. Postpartum pleural effusion. Br J Obstet Gynaecol 1988; 95:894–897.
45. Gourgoulianis KI, Karantanas AH, Molyvdas PA. Peripartum pleural effusion. Chest 1997; 111:1467–1468.
46. Wallis MG, McHugo JM, Carruthers DA, Selwyn Crawford J. The prevalence of pleural effusions in pre-eclampsia: an ultrasound study. Br J Obstet Gynaecol 1989; 96:431–433.
47. Kochenour NK, Branch DW, Rote NS, Scott JR. A new postpartum syndrome associated with antiphospholipid antibodies. Obstet Gynecol 1987; 69:460–468.
48. Ayres MA, Sulak PJ. Pregnancy complicated by antiphospholipid antibodies. South Med J 1991; 84:266–269.
49. Backos M, Rai R, Baxter N, Chilcott IT, Cohen H, Regan L. Pregnancy complications in women with recurrent miscarriage associated with antiphospholipid antibodies treated with low dose aspirin and heparin. Br J Obstet Gynaecol 1999; 106:102–107.
50. Caruso A, De Carolis S, Di Simone N. Antiphospholipid antibodies in obstetrics: new complexities and sites of action. Hum Reprod Update 1999; 5:267–276.
51. Kumar J, Ilancheran A, Ratnam SS. Pulmonary metastases in gestational trophoblastic disease: a review of 97 cases. Br J Obstet Gynaecol 1988; 95:70–74.
52. Libshitz HI, Baber CE, Hammond CB. The pulmonary metastases of choriocarcinoma. Obstet Gynecol 1977; 49:412–416.
53. Johnson TR Jr, Comstock CH, Anderson DG. Benign gestational trophoblastic disease metastatic to pleura: unusual cause of hemothorax. Obstet Gynecol 1979; 53:509–511.
54. Sudduth CD, Strange C, Campbell BA, Sahn SA. Metastatic choriocarcinoma of the lung presenting as hemothorax. Chest 1991; 99:527–528.

55. Kalassian KG, Doyle R, Kao P, Ruoss S, Raffin TA. Lymphangioleiomyomatosis: new insights. Am J Respir Crit Care Med 1997; 155:1183–1186.
56. Sullivan EJ. Lymphangioleiomyomatosis: a review. Chest 1998; 114:1689–1703.
57. NHLBI W Summary. Report of workshop on lymphangioleiomyomatosis. National Heart, Lung, and Blood Institute. Am J Respir Crit Care Med 1999; 159: 679–683.
58. Johnson SR, Tattersfield AE. Clinical experience of lymphangioleiomyomatosis in the UK. Thorax 2000; 55:1052–1057.
59. Urban T, Lazor R, Lacronique J. Pulmonary lymphangioleiomyomatosis. A study of 69 patients. Groupe d'Etudes et de Recherche sur les Maladies "Orphelines" Pulmonaires (GERM"O"P). Medicine (Baltimore) 1999; 78:321–337.
60. Beck GJ, Sullivan EJ, Stoller JK, Peavy HH. Lymphangioleiomyomatosis: new insights. Am J Respir Crit Care Med 1997; 156:670.
61. Berger U, Khaghani A, Pomerance A, Yacoub MH, Coombes RC. Pulmonary lymphangioleiomyomatosis and steroid receptors. An immunocytochemical study. Am J Clin Pathol 1990; 93:609–614.
62. Ohori NP, Yousem SA, Sonmez-Alpan E, Colby TV. Estrogen and progesterone receptors in lymphangioleiomyomatosis, epithelioid hemangioendothelioma, and sclerosing hemangioma of the lung. Am J Clin Pathol 1991; 96:529–535.
63. Brunelli A, Catalini G, Fianchini A. Pregnancy exacerbating unsuspected mediastinal lymphangioleiomyomatosis and chylothorax. Int J Gynaecol Obstet 1996; 52:289–290.
64. Hughes E, Hodder RV. Pulmonary lymphangiomyomatosis complicating pregnancy. A case report. J Reprod Med 1987; 32:553–557.
65. Lieberman J, Agliozzo CM. Intrapleural nitrogen mustard for treating chylous effusion of pulmonary lymphangioleiomyomatosis. Cancer 1974; 33:1505–1511.
66. Monteforte WJ Jr, Kohnen PW. Angiomyolipomas in a case of lymphangiomyomatosis syndrome: relationships to tuberous sclerosis. Cancer 1974; 34:317–321.
67. Silverstein EF, Ellis K, Wolff M, Jaretzki A III. Pulmonary lymphangiomyomatosis. Am J Roentgenol Radium Ther Nucl Med 1974; 120:832–850.
68. Yockey CC, Riepe RE, Ryan K. Pulmonary lymphangioleiomyomatosis complicated by pregnancy. Kans Med 1986; 87:277–278, 293.
69. Cammarata SK, Brush RE, Hyzy RC Jr. Chylothorax after childbirth. Chest 1991; 99:1539–1540.
70. Tornling G, Axelsson G, Peterffy A. Chylothorax as a complication after delivery. Acta Obstet Gynecol Scand 1987; 66:381–382.
71. Valentine VG, Raffin TA. The management of chylothorax. Chest 1992; 102:586–591.
72. Brady DB, Bolan JC. Neurofibromatosis and spontaneous hemothorax in pregnancy: two case reports. Obstet Gynecol 1984; 63:35S–38S.
73. Bernhardt LC, Lawton BR. Pregnancy complicated by traumatic rupture of the diaphragm. Am J Surg 1966; 112:918–922.
74. Diddle AW, Tidrick RT. Diaphragmatic hernia associated with pregnancy. Am J Obstet Gynecol 1941; 41:317–318.
75. Wolfe CA, Peterson MW. An unusual cause of massive pleural effusion in pregnancy. Thorax 1988; 43:484–485.
76. Rajapaksa DS. Traumatic diaphragmatic hernia in pregnancy. Ceylon Med J 1986; 31:153–155.

77. Flick RP, Bofill JA, King JC. Pregnancy complicated by traumatic diaphragmatic rupture. A case report. J Reprod Med 1999; 44:127–130.
78. Dudley AG, Teaford H, Gatewood TS Jr. Delayed traumatic rupture of the diaphragm in pregnancy. Obstet Gynecol 1979; 53:25S–27S.
79. Henzler M, Martin ML, Young J. Delayed diagnosis of traumatic diaphragmatic hernia during pregnancy. Ann Emerg Med 1988; 17:350–353.
80. Goldstein AI, Gazzaniga AB, Ackerman ES, Rajcher WJ, Kent DR, Campbell R. Strangulated diaphragmatic hernia in pregnancy presenting as an empyema. J Reprod Med 1972; 9:135–139.
81. Platt R, Lin JS, Warren JW, Rosner B, Edelin KC, McCormack WM. Infection with Mycoplasma hominis in postpartum fever. Lancet 1980; 2:1217–1221.
82. Mufson MA. Mycoplasma hominis: a review of its role as a respiratory tract pathogen of humans. Sex Transm Dis 1983; 10:335–340.
83. Vogel U, Luneberg E, Kuse ER, Neulinger AL, Frosch M. Extragenital Mycoplasma hominis infection in two liver transplant recipients. Clin Infect Dis 1997; 24:512–513.
84. Madoff S, Hooper DC. Nongenitourinary infections caused by Mycoplasma hominis in adults. Rev Infect Dis 1988; 10:602–613.
85. Word BM, Baldridge A. Mycoplasma hominis pneumonia and pleural effusion in a postpartum adolescent. Pediatr Infect Dis J 1990; 9:295–296.
86. Fabbri J, Tamm M, Frei R, Zimmerli W. Mycoplasma hominis empyema following pleuropneumonia in late pregnancy. Schweiz Med Wochenschr 1993; 123: 2244–2246.
87. Fried AM. Hydronephrosis of pregnancy: ultrasonographic study and classification of asymptomatic women. Am J Obstet Gynecol 1979; 135:1066–1070.
88. Brandes JC, Fritsche C. Obstructive acute renal failure by a gravid uterus: a case report and review. Am J Kidney Dis 1991; 18:398–401.
89. Weiss Z, Shalev E, Zuckerman H, Shental J, Barzilay E. Obstructive renal failure and pleural effusion caused by the gravid uterus. Acta Obstet Gynecol Scand 1986; 65:187–189.
90. Heffner JE, Sahn SA. Pleural disease in pregnancy. Clin Chest Med 1992; 13:667–678.
91. Thompson C, Verani R, Evanoff G, Weinman E. Suppurative bacterial pyelonephritis as a cause of acute renal failure. Am J Kidney Dis 1986; 8:271–273.
92. Corriere JN Jr, Miller WT, Murphy JJ. Hydronephrosis as a cause of pleural effusion. Radiology 1968; 90:79–84.
93. Carey MP, Ihle BU, Woodward CS, Desmedt E. Ureteric obstruction by the gravid uterus. Aust N Z J Obstet Gynaecol 1989; 29:308–313.
94. Kamble RT, Bhat SP, Joshi JM. Urinothorax: a case report. Indian J Chest Dis Allied Sci 2000; 42:189–190.
95. Sahn SA. The diagnostic value of pleural fluid analysis. Semin Respir Crit Care Med 1995; 1:269–276.
96. Jana N, Vasishta K, Saha SC, Ghosh K. Obstetrical Outcomes among Women with Extrapulmonary Tuberculosis. N Engl J Med 1999; 341:645–649.
97. Diagnostic Standards and Classification of Tuberculosis in Adults and Children. Am J Respir Crit Care Med 2000; 161:1376–1395.
98. BTS-Guidelines. Chemotherapy and management of tuberculosis in the United Kingdom: recommendations 1998. Joint Tuberculosis Committee of the British Thoracic Society Thorax 1998; 53:536–548.

99. Snider DE Jr, Layde PM, Johnson MW, Lyle MA. Treatment of tuberculosis during pregnancy. Am Rev Respir Dis 1980; 122:65–79.
100. Targeted tuberculin testing and treatment of latent tuberculosis infection. Am J Respir Crit Care Med 2000; 161:S221–S247.
101. Madinger NE, Greenspoon JS, Ellrodt AG. Pneumonia during pregnancy: has modern technology improved maternal and fetal outcome? Am J Obstet Gynecol 1989; 161:657–662.
102. Montella KR. Pulmonary pharmacology in pregnancy. Clin Chest Med 1992; 13:587–595.
103. Rubin P. Fortnightly review: drug treatment during pregnancy. BMJ 1998; 317:1503–1506.
104. Bouros D, Schiza S, Siafakas N. Fibrinolytics in the treatment of parapneumonic effusions. Monaldi Arch Chest Dis 1999; 54:258–263.
105. Bouros D, Schiza S, Siafakas N. Utility of fibrinolytic agents for draining intrapleural infections. Semin Respir Infect 1999; 14:39–47.
106. Bouros D, Schiza S, Tzanakis N, Chalkiadakis G, Drositis J, Siafakas N. Intrapleural urokinase versus normal saline in the treatment of complicated parapneumonic effusions and empyema. A randomized, double-blind study. Am J Respir Crit Care Med 1999; 159:37–42.

40

Pleural Disease in the Intensive Care Unit

SPYRIDON A. PAPIRIS and CHARIS ROUSSOS

National and Capodistrian University of Athens
Athens, Greece

I. Pleural Effusions in the Intensive Care Unit

A. Introduction

Pleural effusions can occur as complications of many different diseases (pulmonary or extrapulmonary) and almost always constitute a matter of concern for the physician (1). Concern primarily derives from what pleural effusions represent (infection, malignancy, embolism, hemothorax, or other) as well as from the difficulties of their diagnostic approach and rarely from the physiological consequences of fluid collection on lung mechanics and gas exchange. Patients in the intensive care unit (ICU) are rarely admitted for primary pleural disease causing respiratory insufficiency (hemothorax, hydropneumothorax, massive effusions) (2). However, in the medical ICU setting, pleural effusions are common but frequently benign and, when analyzed, only occasionally require or alter treatment, but this may be not the case in the surgical or trauma ICU (2). Furthermore, pleural effusions in the ICU frequently go unrecognized on supine radiographs (especially if small to moderate and bilateral) and occasionally when remain undiagnosed may add to morbidity and mortality.

The diagnostic approach to the critically ill patient with pleural effusion is difficult for obvious reasons. Radiographic examination, in order to detect pleural effusion in the ICU, should include bilateral lateral decubitus films (only available for special circumstances) and frequently other diagnostic techniques such as ultrasonography and/or computed tomography. Furthermore, thoracentesis in the critically ill patient is far more hazardous than in the cooperative patient and may be associated with significant morbidity. Decisions regarding the diagnostic approach to the critically ill patient with pleural effusion are dictated by the balance between the possibility of missing the diagnosis of a disease that is present and requires treatment and the possibility of treating a disease that does not significantly contributes to morbidity (3).

B. Pathogenesis and Etiology of Pleural Effusions in the ICU

Fluid movement between the pleural capillaries and the pleural space is considered to obey Starling's law of transcapillary exchange according to the equation

$$Q_f = L_p \cdot A[(P_{cap} - P_{pl}) - \sigma_d(\pi_{cap} - \pi_{pl})]$$

where Q_f is the liquid movement, L_p is the filtration coefficient per unit or the hydraulic water conductivity of the membrane, A is the surface area of the membrane, P and π are the hydrostatic and oncotic pressures, respectively, of the capillary (cap) and pleural (pl) space, and σ_d is the solute reflection coefficient for protein, a measure of the membrane's ability to restrict the passage of large molecules (1). In humans under homeostatic conditions, it is currently believed that pleural fluid enters the pleural space from the capillaries of the parietal pleura mainly in the less dependent parts of the cavity (4). Pleural fluid turnover is estimated to be ~0.15 mL/kg/h. Pleural fluid reabsorbs from the lymphatic vessels in the parietal pleura in the most dependent regions of the cavity, on the diaphragmatic surface, and in the mediastinal regions (4). The absorbing capacity of the parietal pleural is of the order of 30 mL/h of fluid, equivalent to ≅700 mL/day (4).

Abnormal quantities of pleural fluid can originate in both sites of the diaphragm or from external sources (e.g., parenteral feeding) (Table 1). Intrathoracic sources are, the pleural capillaries, the interstitial space of the lung, the thoracic lymphatics, the intrathoracic blood vessels, and the thoracic portion of the subarachnoid space. Extrathoracic sources are the peritoneal cavity and its content and the retroperitoneal space. Pleural effusions form when the rate of pleural fluid formation exceeds the rate of pleural fluid absorption (Table 1). Pleural effusions are classically divided into transudates and exudates. A transudative pleural effusion develops when the systemic factors that influence the formation or absorption of pleural fluid are altered so that pleural fluid accumulates. In contrast, an exudative pleural effusion develops when the pleural surfaces or the capillaries are altered such that fluid accumulates (1).

Exudative pleural effusions meet at least one of the following (Light's) criteria, whereas transudative pleural effusions meet none:

1. Pleural fluid protein divided by serum protein greater than 0.5
2. Pleural fluid lactate dehydrogenase (LDH) divided by serum LDH greater than 0.6

Table 1 Pathogenesis of Pleural Effusions

Increased pleural fluid formation	Decreased pleural fluid absorption
Increased interstitial fluid in the lung (high or low protein pulmonary edema): left heart failure, pneumonia, ARDS, embolism, lung transplantation Increased intravascular pressure in pleura: right or left heart failure, pericardial effusion, superior vena cava syndrome Increased permeability of the pleural capillaries: pleural inflammation Increased pleural oncotic pressure: high-protein pulmonary edema, hemothorax, pleural inflammation Decreased pleural pressure: lung atelectasis, trapped lung Abnormal fluid in peritoneal cavity or retroperitoneal space: ascites, peritoneal dialysis, urinoma Thoracic duct disruption Blood vessel disruption in the thorax External sources (e.g., central line in the pleural space) Subarachnoid pleural fistula	Obstruction of the lymphatics draining the parietal pleural Elevation of systemic vascular pressures: superior vena cava syndrome, right or left heart failure

3. Pleural fluid LDH greater than two thirds of the upper limit of normal for the serum LDH

Occasionally, Light's criteria may label some patients with transudative pleural effusions as having exudative effusions. In those patients the serum to pleural fluid albumin gradient has been measured. If this gradient is greater than 1.2 g/dL, then the patient has a transudative pleural effusion (5). Pleural effusions in the ICU are frequently occurring with both transudates and exudates but may not invariably require thoracentesis (Table 2).

C. Imaging of Pleural Effusions in the ICU

Critically ill patients are difficult to assess for complicating pleural effusions because of their altered sensorium, multiple monitoring devices, supine or semi-recumbent position, and immobility. In the supine position, the most dependent pleural spaces are the apex and the posterior basilar space, where fluid is difficult to detect. Furthermore, technical factors in the supine radiograph, including poor beam alignment, rotation, underpenetration, artifacts from scattered radiation, respiratory motion artifacts, small lung volumes, spreading of the fluid over a larger area than in the erect position, and the commonly occurring lower

Table 2 Etiology of Pleural Effusions in the ICU

Transudative pleural effusions	Exudative pleural effusions
Congestive heart failure[a]	Infection (pneumonia, mediastinitis, abdominal sepsis)
Hepatic hydrothorax[a]	Systemic sepsis (endocarditis, line sepsis)
Peritoneal dialysis[a]	Malignancy[a]
Nephrotic syndrome[a]	Embolism[a]
Superior vena cava syndrome	Gastrointestinal disease (pancreatitis, esophageal perforation, postabdominal surgery, diaphragmatic hernia)
Urinothorax	Autoimmune disorders (systemic lupus erythematosus, vasculitis)
Glomerulonephritis	Hemothorax
Myxedema[b]	Chylothorax
Subarachnoid pleural fistula	Heart disease (coronary bypass surgery, Dressler's syndrome, pericarditis)
Hypoalbuminemia[a]	Uremia
Meigs' syndrome[b]	Trapped lung[a]
Embolism[b]	ARDS
Sarcoidosis	Electrical burns
Central line in the pleural space[c]	Therapeutic radiation exposure
	Iatrogenic

[a] May not require tap.
[b] Can be an exudate or a transudate.
[c] Composition similar to the infusate.

lobe infiltrates and/or atelectasis, add to the difficulty in diagnosing pleural effusion (6). The radiographic appearance of pleural effusion in the posterior basilar pleural space without additional lung infiltrates or atelectasis is characterized early on by blunting of the costophrenic angle and subsequently by a homogeneous increase in density in the lower hemithorax without obliteration of the normal bronchovascular markings and in some patients with loss of hemidiaphragmatic silhouette (Figs. 1 and 2). Fluid in the apex of the hemithorax in the supine position is readily recognized as a pleural cap and when increases spread in the lateral as well the medial apical pleura. The medial spreading of the fluid is of some importance in patients with trauma, since obliterating the mediastinal contour may simulate mediastinal widening, and needs further assessment. Subpulmonic effusions are frequently occurring in the critically ill patient and again may be undetectable in the supine films. Subpulmonic effusions may extend into the paramediastinal gutter and when large enough can displace the gastric air bubble and splenic flexure of the colon inferiorly. Intrafissural spreading of a pleural effusion is not uncommon and renders the fissures more apparent. However, the radiographic appearance of intrafissural spreading depends on many different factors, among them the size of the effusion, the

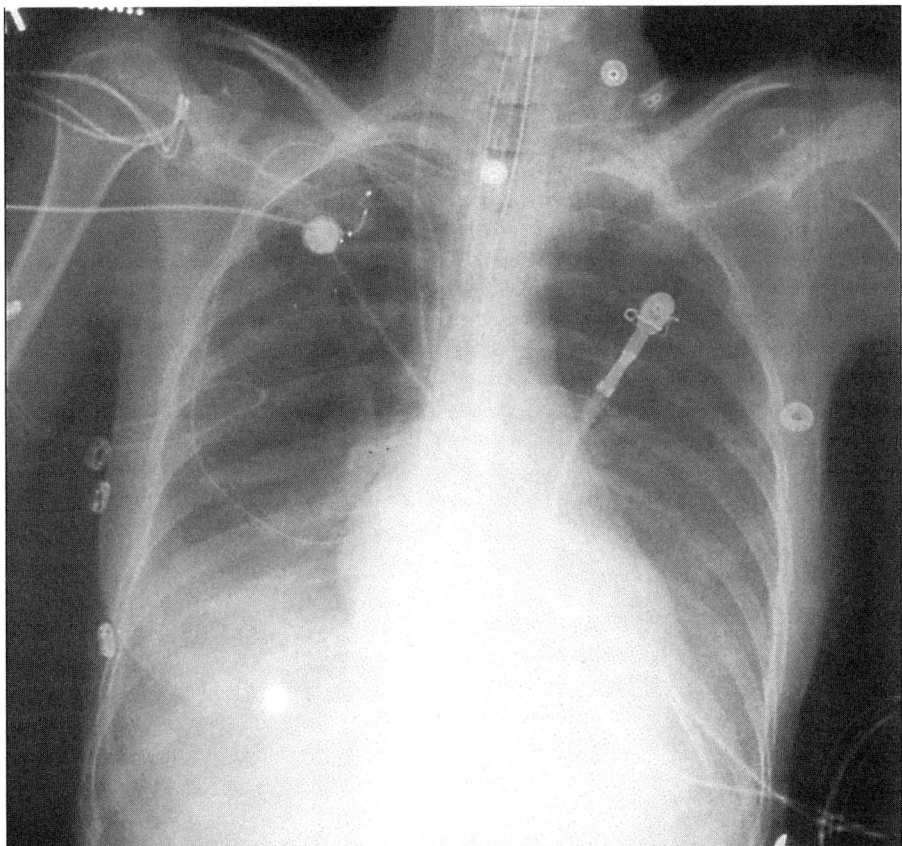

Figure 1 Chest radiograph of a critically ill patient in the semirecumbent position reveals typical features of bilateral pleural effusion. There is opacification of the lower zones of both hemithoraces, more evident on the right. Note that the pulmonary vascular markings are not obliterated. Endotracheal tube, central venous lines, and esophageal tube are in good position. (Courtesy of Dr. K. Malagari.)

location of the fluid, and the shape, orientation, and completeness of the fissure. Radiographic manifestations of intrafissural spreading of the fluid that can be observed are the "pseudotumor" sign, the "middle lobe step" sign, the appearance of sharp perihilar lucency when the fluid enters the plane of an incomplete major fissure, and the "pseudocavity" sign when a small quantity of fluid in a fissure coexists with parenchymal volume loss. Bilateral lateral decubitus films and erect radiographs may help to confirm or rule out the presence of effusion, but in some patients these cannot be obtained.

Computed tomography of the chest can play an important adjunctive role in bedside chest radiography in critically ill patients (7,8). Computed tomography shows findings undetected with bedside chest radiography in the majority

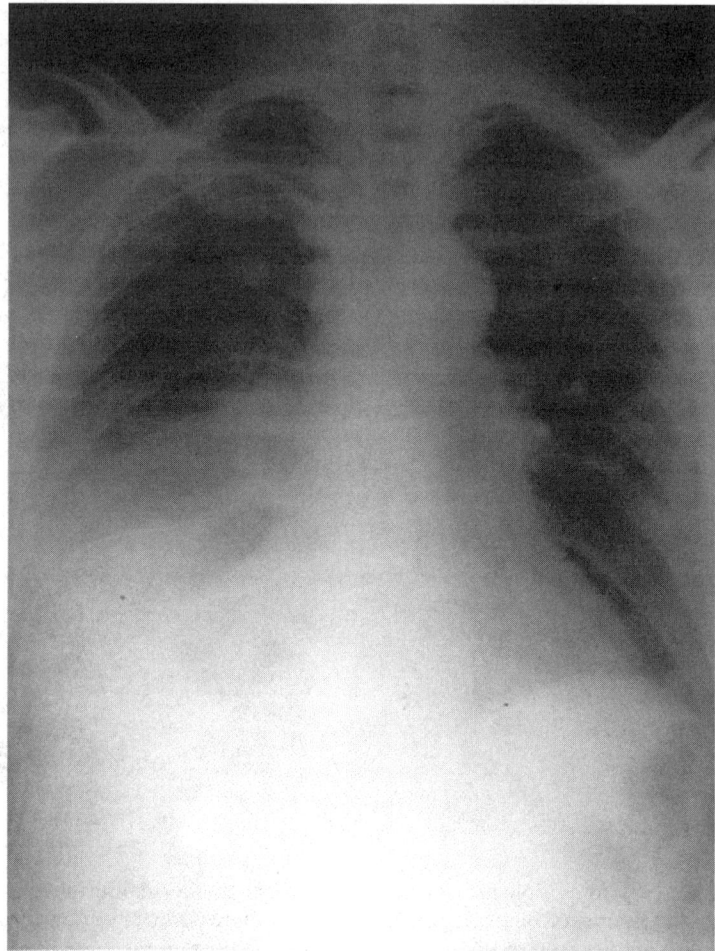

Figure 2 Chest radiograph in the semirecumbent position reveals pleural effusion on the right hemithorax in a critically ill patient with a bullet wound and a bleeding liver lesion. The effusion causes loss of contour of the right hemidiaphragm and homogeneous opacification of the lower hemithorax. (Courtesy of Dr. K. Malagari.)

of patients, although part of these findings may prove to be clinically unimportant (7,8). Computed tomography can readily detect pleural effusions, estimate their extension, loculations, and their relationship to other intrathoracic structures (Figs. 3, 4). Computed tomography studies frequently detect pleural effusions not visible in the supine chest radiograph. Although computed tomography cannot discriminate exudative from transudative fluid collection, the presence of blood can be recognized by the increased density values. However, hemothorax may present low-density values in patients with low hematocrit

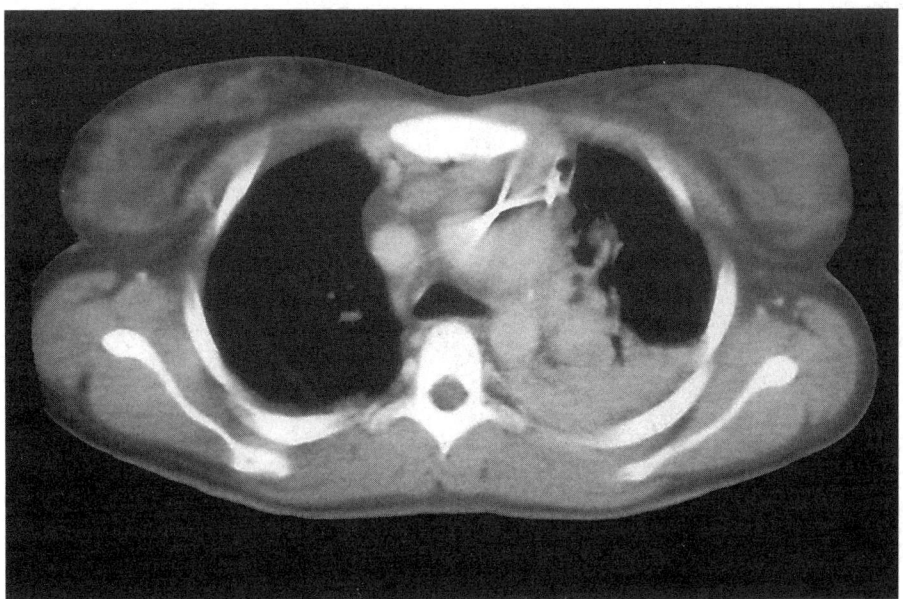

Figure 3 Computed tomography reveals pleural effusion in a patient with chest trauma and aortic rupture. The effusion is of increased density due to the presence of hemoglobin (hemothorax). (Courtesy of Dr. K. Malagari.)

(Fig. 5). Intravenous contrast administration is advisable for the early detection of pleural thickening and loculations. Ultrasonography may enhance the physical examination of the critically ill patient and provide for an early detection of select complications (9). Ultrasonography is very useful in the study of pleural effusions and, in particular, in the detection of internal loculations, the distinction between pleural effusion and pleural thickening, and is a valuable tool to perform safely thoracentesis at bedside (10). Magnetic resonance imaging of the chest can identify pleural effusions but at the present time is less satisfactory than ultrasound or computed tomography for the evaluation of pleural effusions (1). Nevertheless, magnetic resonance imaging may offer additional information in the patient with trauma, pleural effusion (hemothorax), and vessel injury (Fig. 6).

D. Diagnosis of Pleural Effusions in the ICU

Once a pleural effusion has been recognized by physical examination and the assistance of the above-described imaging modalities, the decision must be taken whether or not to perform a thoracentesis. The need for thoracentesis in the ICU is based on history, physical examination, laboratory data, and hospital course (3). Pleural effusions usually require expedient thoracentesis when the fluid is suspected infected, or suspected blood, and when large enough to cause

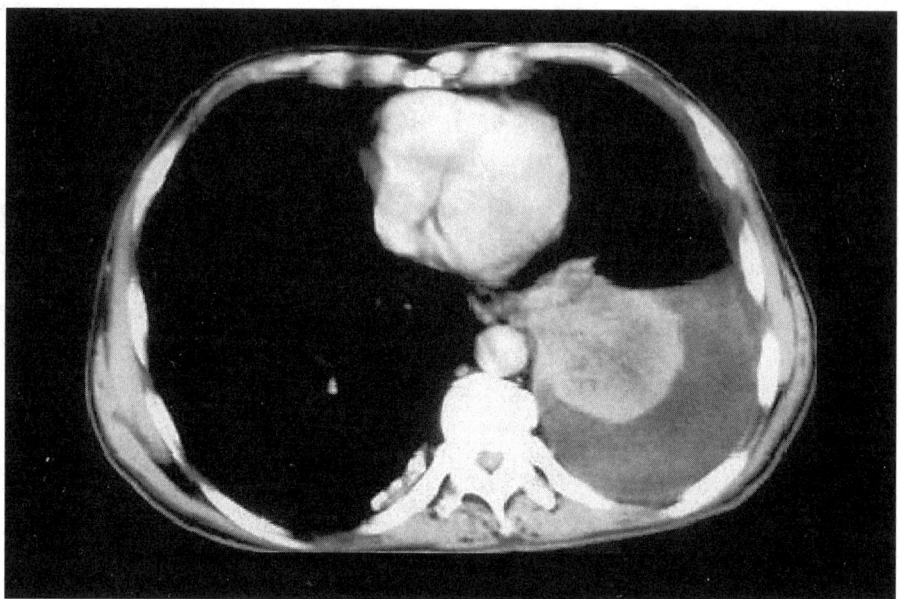

Figure 4 Computed tomography reveals a pleural effusion and pneumonia. The effusion is of low density compared to the enhancing consolidated lower lobe. No enhancement of the pleura is noted, indicating that there is no pleural thickening or compartmentalization. Pleural calcifications are evident on the opposite side. (Courtesy of Dr. K. Malagari.)

ventilatory compromise (3). Diagnostic or therapeutic thoracentesis in the critically ill patient in supine position can be performed through a posterolateral approach with the head of the bed elevated as close to 90-degree angle as possible. In this position thoracentesis is approached along the posterior axillary line (11). The level of thoracentesis should be one or two interspaces below the percussed fluid level but not lower than the eighth intercostal space. However, ultrasound- or computed tomography–guided thoracentesis could be a safer option. Chest radiograph is always necessary after completion of the procedure. The most common complication of thoracentesis is pneumothorax. Other complications include infection of the pleural space, hemothorax, splenic or hepatic laceration, soft tissue infection, and seeding of the needle tract with tumor cells in case of malignancy of the pleural space. The main indications of therapeutic thoracentesis in the critically ill patient are (1) to remove empyema, (2) to remove blood, (3) to improve ventilatory compromise in case of massive effusions, (4) to evaluate the status of the underlying lung in case of massive effusions, and (5) to perform pleurodesis in case of recurrent and symptomatic malignant or even nonmalignant effusions.

The gross appearance of thoracentesis fluid frequently offers diagnostic information. The color, turbidity, viscosity, and odor should be described (1).

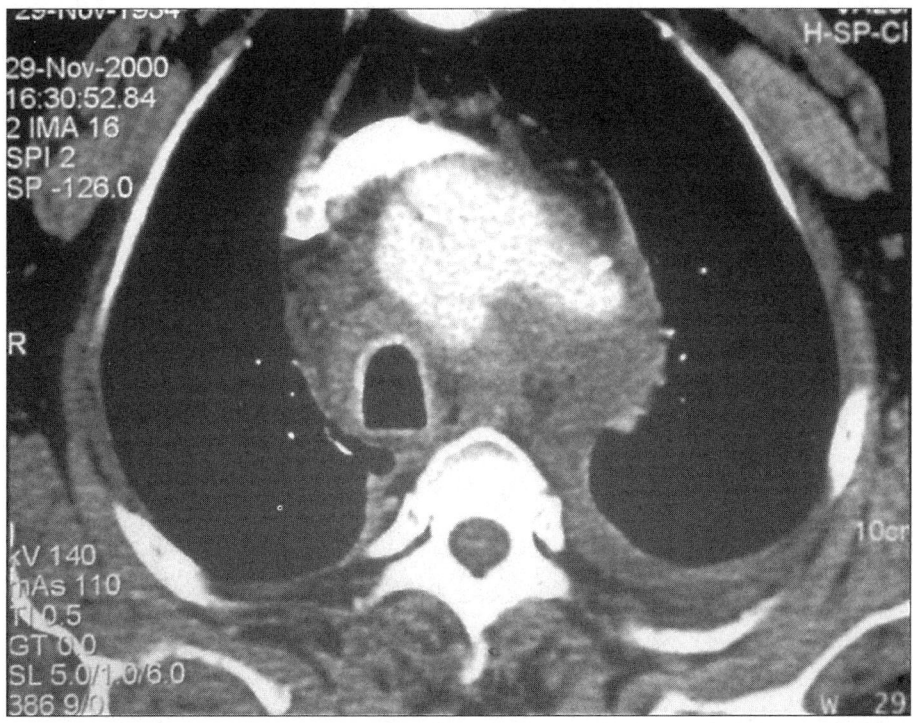

Figure 5 Contrast enhanced spiral computed tomography of the chest at the level of the aortic arch. There is gross irregularity of the aortic wall demonstrating a contained aortic rupture associated with hemomediastinum and displacement of the trachea and esophagus to the right. Note that the associated left pleural effusion is of low density despite the presence of blood due to the low hematocrit of the patient. (Courtesy of Dr. K. Malagari.)

Many effusions are clear, straw-colored, nonviscid, and odorless. A reddish color indicates blood, and a brownish color indicates chronicity of blood presence. When the effusion appears bloody, a hematocrit will define if the effusion is hemothorax. Fluid should be sent for blood cell count, Gram's stain, Ziehl-Nielsen and fungal smears, culture (aerobic, anaerobic, fungal, and mycobacterium), cytology, pH, and to determine the levels of protein, glucose, lactate dehydrogenase (LDH), adenosine deaminase (ADA), and amylase. Under special clinical circumstances, additional tests may prove useful, such as rheumatoid factor (RF) in the unusual case of a patient with rheumatoid arthritis, antinuclear antibodies (ANA), lupus erythematosus cells (LE cell test) and complement levels in the diagnostic possibility of systemic lupus erythematosus, lipid studies in the differential diagnosis between chylothorax and pseudochylothorax, creatinine levels in case of urinothorax, and flow cytometry

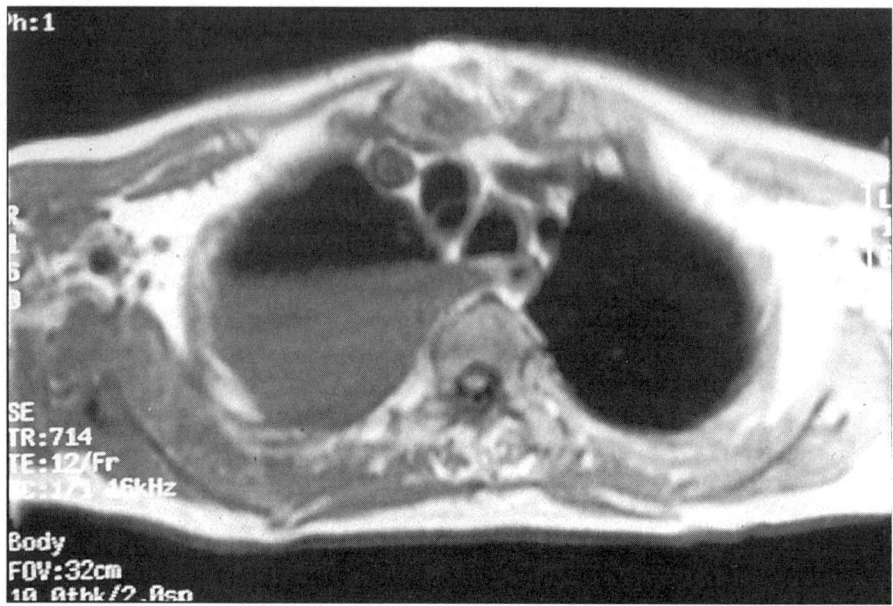

Figure 6 Magnetic resonance imaging appearance of a pleural effusion: In this T1-weighted sequence pleural fluid is of low intensity compared to the high signal of the subcutaneous fat. MRI was performed for the evaluation of aortic dissection extending to the anonymous artery. (Courtesy of Dr. K. Malagari.)

to define T-lymphocytic subpopulations in the diagnostic possibility of lymphoma.

Infection of the Pleural Space

Infection in the pleural space (empyema thoracis = pus in the pleural space) may be parapneumonic or nonparapneumonic, and infected pleural fluid may be free or loculated (1,12). Loculated effusions may be uniloculated or multiloculated and, if untreated, may drain spontaneously through the chest wall (empyema necessitatis) or into the lung (bronchopleural fistula). Parapneumonic effusions are those associated with pneumonia, lung abscess, and bronchiectasis (1). Furthermore, a multitude of hyper- and subdiaphragmatic medical and surgical conditions may be associated with empyema (Table 3). Although a multitude of conditions frequently encountered in the ICU can cause empyemas, their occurrence in this setting are not common since many patients are early treated with antibiotics for pneumonia or extrathoracic sepsis (13). Empyema when diagnosed should be treated promptly with broad-spectrum coverage with antibiotics (most empyemas are caused by mixtures of aerobic and anaerobic organisms) and tube thoracostomy (1,13,14). Additional treatment modalities such as intrapleural injection of a fibrinolytic agent, lysis of adhesions by video-

Table 3 Etiology of Empyema Thoracis in the ICU

Parapneumonic empyemas	Nonparapneumonic empyemas
Pneumonia	Mediastinitis
Lung abscess	Esophageal perforation
Bronchiectasis	Postthoracentesis
	Postthoracostomy
	Postthoracotomy
	Chest trauma
	Sepsis
	Abdominal sepsis
	Abdominal trauma

assisted thoracoscopy, and decortication for an uncontrolled infection may become necessary in selected patients (1).

Hemothorax

Hemothorax (blood in the pleural space) exists when the hematocrit level of the pleural effusion is greater or equal of the 50% of the serum value (1). Hemothorax may be traumatic (penetrating and nonpenetrating chest trauma), iatrogenic, nontraumatic, and rarely idiopathic. In the ICU setting hemothorax may result from different procedures such as the perforation of central vein by a percutaneously inserted catheter, venous bleeding after thoracentesis, pleural biopsy and chest tube placement, percutaneous lung aspiration and biopsy, sclerotherapy for esophageal varices, insertion of a Swan-Ganz catheter, transbronchial biopsy, and others. Once recognized, in the critically ill patient the existence of a hemothorax should be treated promptly with the insertion of a chest tube. Chest tubes are necessary among other reasons, to: (1) allow the complete evacuation of the pleural space, (2) help to stop bleeding because the apposition of the pleural surfaces will produce a tamponade, (3) allow the reexpansion of the lung and help to improve gas exchange, (4) allow to quantitate and monitor bleeding, (5) decrease the likelihood of infection in the pleural space, and (6) decrease the incidence of subsequent fibrothorax (1). Complications of hemothorax are (1) the retention of clotted blood, (2) empyema, (3) pleural effusion, and (4) fibrothorax. Thoracotomy in order to control bleeding may become necessary in different conditions, both traumatic and nontraumatic.

Chylothorax

Chylothorax is formed when the thoracic duct is damaged or blocked and chyle (lymph) enters the pleural space (1). Chylothorax occurs infrequently in the ICU, and, when it occurs, it is almost always traumatic. This trauma is usually a cardiovascular, pulmonary, or esophageal procedure. Penetrating and nonpenetrating trauma and a multitude of different conditions have also been described as causing of chylothorax. Rarely, chylothorax may be idiopathic. Diagnosis is made by analysis of the pleural fluid, which contains high levels of triglycerides, and is confirmed by the presence of chylomicrons. Besides treatment of the underlying disease, the management of chylothorax includes conservative and surgical measures (1,15). Conservative measures include repeated thoracenteses, continuous drainage, dietary modifications (low-fat diet, medium-chain triglyceride diet, or total parenteral nutrition), and pleurodesis (15). Surgical measures include pleuroperitoneal shunt, fibrin glue to close the leak in the duct, ligation of the thoracic duct by thorascopy or thoracostomy, and pleurectomy (15).

Exudative Pleural Effusions Secondary to Abdominal and Pelvic Diseases

Several medical and surgical conditions of the abdomen and pelvis can be associated with exudative (benign or malignant) pleural effusions (Table 4) (1). A

Table 4 Exudative Pleural Effusions Secondary to Abdominal and Pelvic Diseases

Pancreatic disease
    Acute pancreatitis
    Pancreatic abscess
    Pancreatic abscess and chronic
      pancreatic pleural effusion
    Pancreatic ascites
Subphrenic abscess
Intrahepatic abscess
Intrasplenic abscess
Esophageal perforation
Abdominal surgical procedures
Diaphragmatic hernia
Endoscopic variceal sclerotherapy
Bilious pleural effusions
Pleural effusions after liver transplantation
Abdominal trauma
Primary and secondary peritoneal
    malignancies
Obstetric and gynecological disorders
    Ovarian hyperstimulation syndrome
    Postpartum pleural effusion
    Meigs' syndrome
    Endometriosis

multitude of mechanisms are implicated in the pathogenesis of the pleural fluid formation, including transdiaphragmatic transfer (through pores in the diaphragm) of the ascitic fluid, diaphragmatic inflammation and pleural irritation, transfer of abnormal abdominal fluid through the aortic and/or esophageal hiatus into the mediastinum and subsequent decompression of the mediastinal collection into the pleural space, direct sinus tract formation (fistula) between the affected abdominal organs (pancreas, biliary tract) and the pleural space, and others. In the ICU setting, abdominal and pelvic diseases causing pleural effusions may significantly contribute to the deterioration of patient's clinical condition, and prompt diagnosis is necessary. Diagnostic approach and treatment are usually dictated by the specific clinical contest.

E. Conclusions

In the medical ICU setting, pleural effusions are common (both transudative and exudative) but frequently benign and, when analyzed, only occasionally require or alter treatment, but this may be not the case in the surgical or trauma ICU. The diagnostic approach to critically ill patients with pleural effusion is difficult because of their altered sensorium, multiple monitoring devices, supine or semirecumbent position, and immobility. In addition, pleural effusions frequently go unrecognized on supine radiograms and may, when undiagnosed, add to morbidity and mortality. In order to detect pleural effusions in some patients, radiographic examination should include bilateral lateral decubitus films and frequently ultrasonography and/or computed tomography. Thoracentesis in the critically ill patient is more hazardous than in the cooperative patient and may be associated with significant morbidity. The decision for diagnostic thoracentesis should be based on history, physical examination, laboratory data, and hospital course. Expedient thoracentesis is usually required when the fluid is suspected infected, or suspected blood, and when large enough to cause ventilatory compromise. Prompt diagnosis and adequate treatment of pleural effusions in the ICU may help to ensure a successful outcome for the patient.

II. Pneumothorax and Related Conditions Secondary to Pulmonary Barotrauma in the ICU

A. Introduction

Barotrauma (air leak) is the presence of extra-alveolar air in locations where it is not normally seen in patients who are mechanically ventilated (16). Barotrauma includes a multitude of conditions such as tension lung cysts, hyperinflated lobe, subpleural air cysts, pulmonary interstitial emphysema, pneumothorax, pneumopericardium, subcutaneous emphysema, pneumomediastinum, pneumoretroperitoneum, pneumoperitoneum, and air embolism (16). However, in this era in the ICU setting, the term barotrauma also includes the most recently emerged, early installed ventilation-induced lung injury, characterized by microscopic

Table 5 Baro-volutrauma, Ventilation-Induced Lung Injury

Microscopic lesions of epithelial disruption and a resulting permeability edema
Tension lung cysts
Hyperinflated lobe
Subpleural air cysts
Pulmonary interstitial emphysema
Pneumothorax
Pneumopericardium
Subcutaneous emphysema
Pneumomediastinum
Pneumoretroperitoneum
Pneumoperitoneum
Air embolism

---

lesions of epithelial disruption and a resulting permeability edema (Table 5) (17). It has been suggested that any ventilatory modality or maneuver that induces any form of overinflation generates barotrauma, and the word volutrauma would be more appropriate (18,19). Furthermore, recent studies have identified that the main determinant of volutrauma seems to be the end-inspiratory volume (the overall lung distension), rather than the tidal volume or functional residual capacity (20). In ICU patients mechanical ventilation is not the only cause of barotrauma. Pneumothorax and related conditions may follow blunt or open thoracic trauma as well as several diagnostic or therapeutic maneuvers such as intubation, central venous catheterization, cardiopulmonary resuscitation, and others.

Pneumothorax and some related conditions in the ICU may go undetected on supine radiograms, and when they remain undiagnosed they have the potential to add to morbidity and mortality. Indeed, patients with unrecognized pneumothoraces who are receiving mechanical ventilation are those most likely to develop a tension pneumothorax (1). The incidence of pneumothorax and related conditions in the ICU patient is difficult to estimate but is not infrequent. It appears to be relatively high in patients with ARDS (21) where it frequently occurs during the resolution phase, when lung volume and compliance are improving. Thus, adjusting of the ventilatory modes to the lowest levels compatible with adequate oxygenation and ventilation may help to reduce the incidence of pulmonary volu-barotrauma.

B. Pathogenesis and Pathophysiology

In the ICU setting pneumothorax and related conditions may result from penetrating and nonpenetrating lung injuries that involve the parietal or the visceral pleura and the alveoli or from internal forces associated with mechanical ventilation. All forms of ventilator-induced barotraumas develop after rupture of overdistended alveoli. When the alveoli rupture, air is introduced into the bronchovascular sheath, which results in interstitial emphysema and may dissect towards the periphery to produce pneumothorax or the mediastinum to produce pneumomediastinum (22). After the development of pneumomediastinum, air may decompress along the cervical fascial planes into the subcutaneous tissue of the neck, face, and thorax, to produce subcutaneous emphysema or escape retroperitoneally to produce pneumoretroperitoneum and eventually burst into the peritoneal cavity to cause pneumoperitoneum. If large quantities of air are accumulating into the mediastinal space and decompression is not possible to relieve the tension, the mediastinal parietal pleura may rupture, resulting in pneumothorax. In this situation pneumopericardium is also possible. Alternatively, air may enter directly into the pleural space from rupture of alveoli or blebs and pneumatoceles without the previous formation of pneumomediastinum.

In the mechanically ventilated patient, when pneumothorax develops it will likely become a tension pneumothorax. The mechanism by which a tension pneumothorax develops in the intubated patient with positive end-expiratory pressure is obvious since the alveolar pressure is positive throughout the respiratory cycle (1). Tension pneumothorax can produce life-threatening pulmonary and cardiovascular deterioration. When tension pneumothorax develops, the increased tension causes the ipsilateral lung to be compressed and displaced to the opposite side. Mediastinum shift causes not only deterioration of ventilation and gas exchange in both lungs, but also compression of the major vessels of blood return at both the thoracic inlet of the neck and the diaphragmatic entrance leading to severe compromise of the venous return and consequently marked decrease in cardiac output. This combination of hypoxemia and decrease in cardiac output can be rapidly lethal, and immediate treatment is required.

C. Diagnosis

The diagnosis of pneumothorax in critically ill patients may prove problematic since symptoms are unlikely to be specific and patients are unable to speak. A high index of suspicion and knowledge of the dynamic of injuries that predispose to barotrauma is imperative. Agitation, deterioration of hypoxemia, hypotension, or cardiovascular collapse should suggest the possibility of a pneumothorax, especially a tension pneumothorax. Physical signs may be subtle (decreased breath sounds ipsilaterally) or obvious (crepitations in the neck, face, chest, axillae, or abdomen suggesting subcutaneous emphysema). A mediastinal "crunch" is reported in some patients with emphysema. The presence of subcutaneous emphysema and/or pneumomediastinum is rarely associated with cardiorespiratory compromise but may herald an imminent (tension) pneumothorax.

D. Imaging of Pneumothorax and Related Conditions in the ICU

The bedside chest radiography in the supine or in the semirecumbent position may be not fully sensitive for the diagnosis of pneumothorax (23). The earliest radiographic finding associated with volu-barotrauma is pulmonary interstitial emphysema. In this condition, radiographic findings include linear streaks of air radiating toward the hila, perivascular halos, intraseptal air collections, small parenchymal air cysts, pneumatoceles, and more or less large subpleural air collections (blebs) (6). The streaks of air radiating toward the hila and the perivascular halos represent air in the peribronchovascular loose connective tissue. Intraseptal air collections can also be described as the negative image of the Kerley's A and B lines. Air cysts are mainly recognized in perihilar and subpleural distribution. The subpleural air collections (blebs) represent the finding most likely to progress to pneumothorax. Additionally, the chest radiograph may provide diagnostic results for subcutaneous emphysema, pneumomediastinum, pneumopericardium, and tension pneumothorax. Pneumomediastinum is evident on the radiograph when air outlines the edges of anatomical structures not normally visible (Figs. 7–9). However, since similar findings may be observed in pneumopericardium and anteromedial pneumothorax, the most specific signs of pneumomediastinum are the presence of air dissecting the great vessels of the

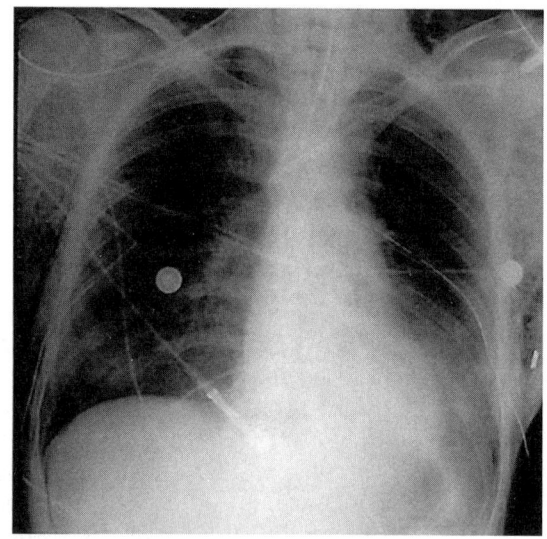

(a)

Figure 7 Chest radiograph of a 44-year-old male patient posttrauma. (a) Bilateral pneumothoraces were present effectively evacuated by chest tubes. The lungs appear completely reexpanded. Pneumomediastinum is present and is indicated by the linear lucencies in the neck. (b) The closest view demonstrates at better advantage the linear, low-density lucencies in the soft tissues of the neck. (Courtesy of Dr. K. Malagari.)

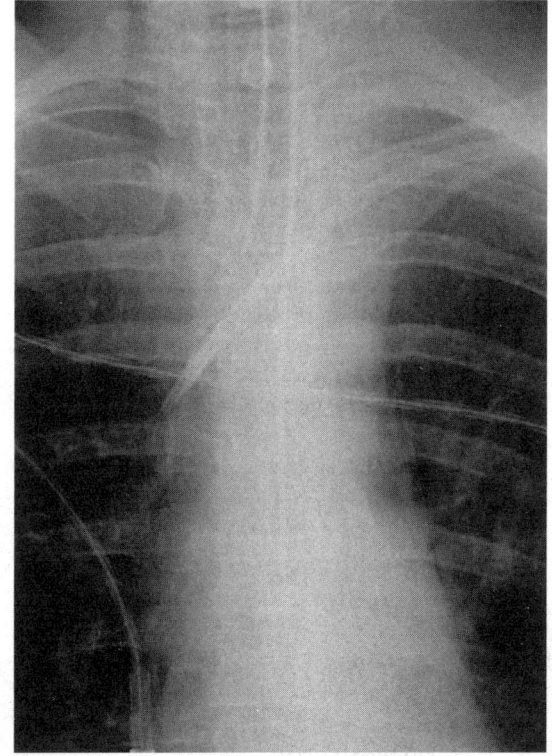

Figure 7 Continued.

chest and neck (6). Furthermore, air can outline the central portion of the diaphragm under the cardiac silhouette. Pneumomediastinum in the ICU patient is not only related to barotraumas since it may also originate from rupture of the esophagus or other intra-abdominal hollow viscera, and in some patients with retropharyngeal abscess or facial trauma, air may dissect from the soft tissues of the face and neck into the mediastinum. Subcutaneous emphysema is easy to detect and is usually the first radiographic sign of barotrauma. In some patients air may extend from the subcutaneous tissues of the face and neck to the chest (including the muscular bundles of the major chest wall muscles) (Fig. 8), retroperitoneum, and abdomen. From the mediastinum air may dissect to the retroperitoneum through the diaphragmatic hiatus, forming pneumoretroperitoneum. Its diagnosis is made when the psoas muscle, the pararenal fascia, or the diaphragmatic crura is outlined by air (6).

Pneumothorax may be secondary to pneumomediastinum or may result from the direct entry of air into the pleural space from the rupture of alveoli or blebs and pneumatoceles. The radiographic appearance of the pneumothorax is influenced by the patient's position as well as by the underlying pleuropulmonary condition. Both the clinician and the radiologist can miss small pneumothoraces. More than half of missed pneumothoraces progress to tension pneumothorax (23). In the critically ill supine patient, location of the pneumothorax includes, in addition to the classical apicolateral location (relatively uncommon), the anteromedial and subpulmonic (that represent the majority) and also the posteromedial pleural recesses (Figs. 9, 10). In the supine patient the two more classical signs of pneumothorax are (1) "the deep sulcus sign," which is intrapleural air ascending into the anterior costophrenic sulcus producing a

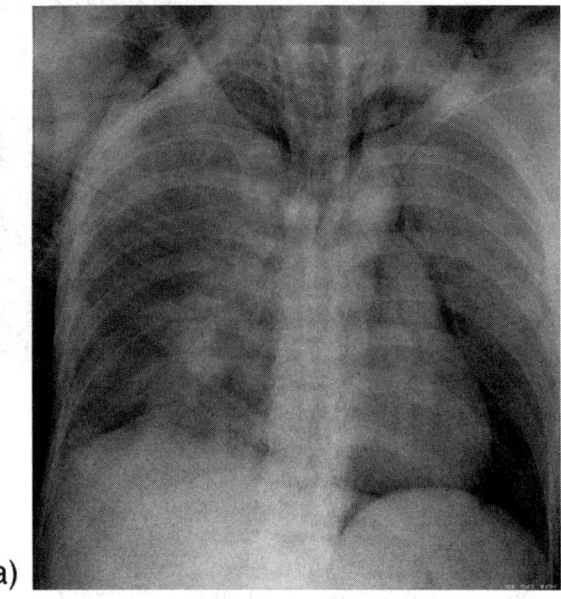

(a)

Figure 8 Chest radiograph (a) of a 22-year-old male patient posttrauma, which reveals linear lucencies along the mediastinal structures indicating pneumomediastinum. The thin line seen on the left of the left cardiovascular border represents the visceral pleura (pneumothorax): extensive lucencies in the supraclavicular fossae and along the muscle fibers of the major pectoralis muscles represent extensive subcutaneous emphysema. Contrast enhanced computerized tomography of the chest of the same patient. At the level of the upper mediastinum (b) air lucencies are seen surrounding the mediastinal vascular structures and the left wall of the trachea. There is extensive subcutaneous emphysema extending within almost all muscles of the chest wall, particularly in the nondependent sites. CT slice at a lower level (c) reveals bilateral pneumothorax, more extensive on the right. Parenchymal consolidations are seen in the dependent lung portions. Again, pneumomediastinum is indicated by the lucencies surrounding the mediastinal structures. Slice at the level above the diaphragm (d). Decreased compliance of the consolidated lung on the right prevents complete reexpansion despite the presence of the chest tube. (Courtesy of Dr. K. Malagari.)

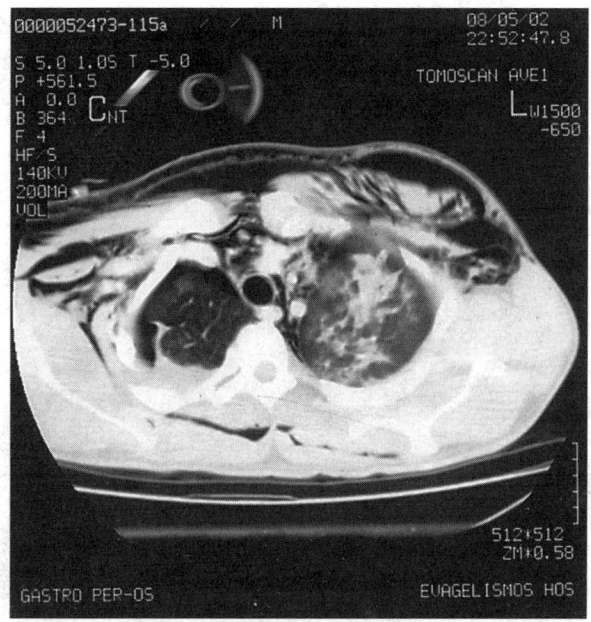

(b)

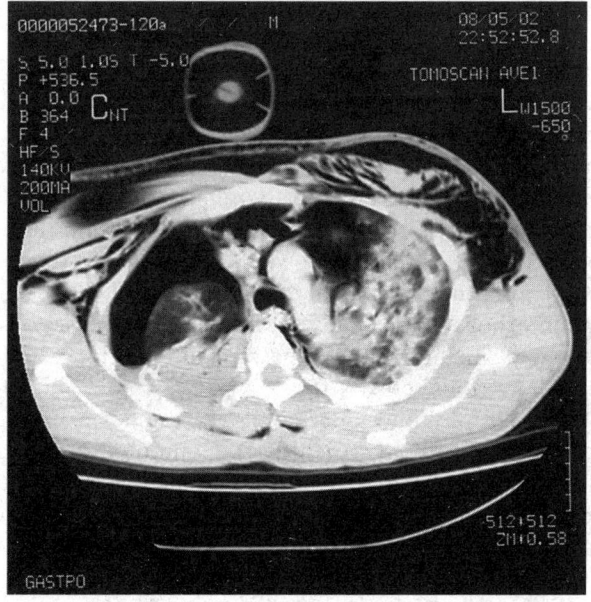

(c)

Figure 8 Continued.

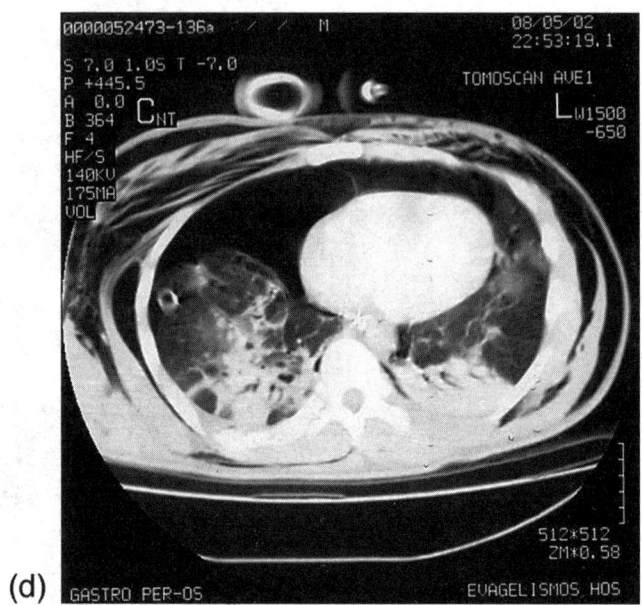

Figure 8 Continued.

"deep" lateral costophrenic angle (subpulmonary location), and (2) the presence of a dark, lucent band between the medial lung and the mediastinum (anteromedial pneumothorax).

Tension pneumothorax is primarily a clinical diagnosis since there may not be a radiographic equivalent. The most common radiographic signs of tension pneumothorax are contralateral shift of the mediastinum, ipsilateral diaphragmatic depression, and ipsilateral chest wall expansion. However, these signs may not be fully evident in the critically ill patient with ARDS. The most specific sign of tension pneumothorax is probably the flattening of the heart border and other vascular structures, including the superior and inferior vena cava, reflecting impairment of the venous return (6).

Digital radiography may offer some advantages over standard portable radiographs in the critically ill patient (24). Computed tomography is the gold standard for the diagnosis of pneumothorax in the ICU but is not easy to perform, necessitates transfer of the critically ill patient, and exposes the patient to significantly higher irradiation. The utility of ultrasound to rule out pneumothorax is currently under investigation (25,26).

E. Prophylaxis and Treatment

All patients treated with mechanical ventilation are at risk to develop pulmonary barotrauma. Methods to reduce its frequency include measures to decrease alveolar inflation and pressures, end-inspiratory volume, positive end-expiratory pressure (PEEP), and intrinsic PEEP. Controlled hypoventilation as well as effective patient sedation and good coordination with the ventilator may be helpful.

Specific treatment modalities for pulmonary baro-volutrauma vary with the type. Pulmonary interstitial emphysema, pneumomediastinum, and subcutaneous emphysema are considered benign and do not need treatment. In special situations decompression with subcutaneous catheters may be helpful for severe subcutaneous emphysema. The issue of placement of chest tubes for "prophylaxis" in patients with this type of barotrauma but without pneumothorax remains unresolved. In individual patients with extremely high PEEP requirements, bilateral chest tube placement may be warranted. Tension pneumopericardium should be treated with pericardiocentesis.

In patients with suspected pneumothorax, confirmation and temporary relieve may be achieved by catheter aspiration via the placement of an intravenous cannula (16 gauge, 6.4 cm long) in the second anterior intercostal space. When a pneumothorax is present, especially if a tension one, the treatment is the placement of a large-bore chest tube (32–36 French) for immediate decompression, at the second intercostal space in the midclavicular line or the fourth to fifth intercostal space anterior to the midaxillary line. In some patients radiography and/or computerized tomography may be required to guide effective drainage of

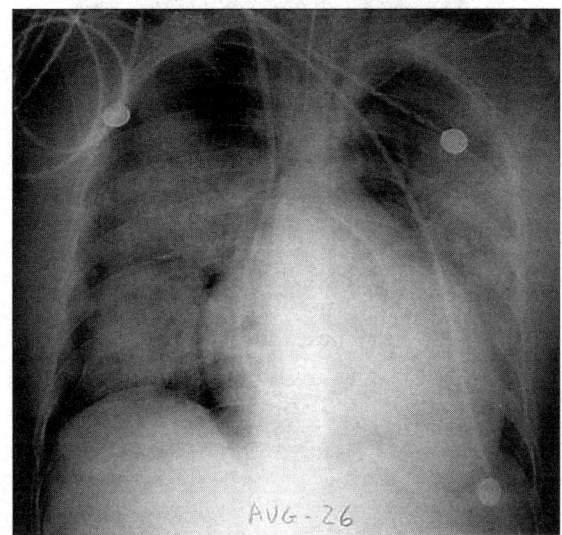

Figure 9 Chest radiograph of a 26-year-old critically ill male patient with pericarditis. (a) The anteroposterior view of the chest demonstrates cardiac enlargement. Diffuse parenchymal consolidations due to increased permeability pulmonary edema are present. A pneumothorax is seen on the right lung. The linear lucencies in the upper mediastinum extending to the soft tissues of the neck indicate the presence of pneumomediastinum. (b) A closer view of the right hemithorax better demonstrates the pleural line of pneumothorax laterally and medially. (Courtesy of Dr. K. Malagari.)

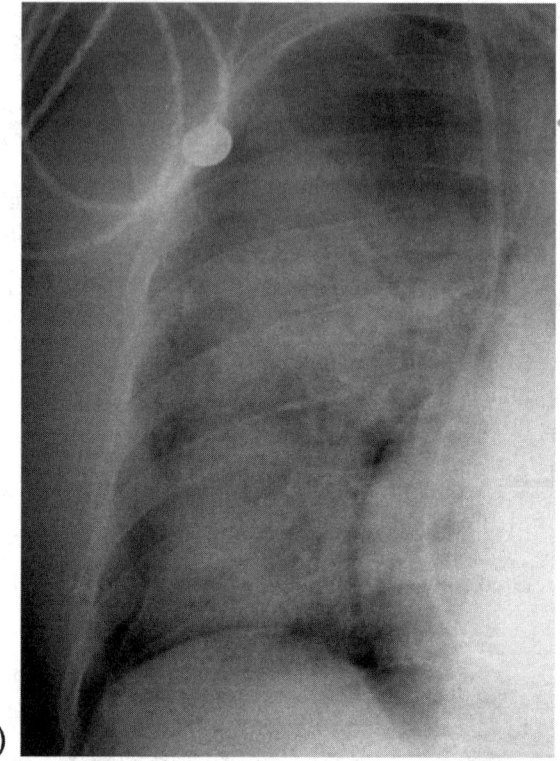

Figure 9 Continued.

the pleural air. However, time delay in chest tube insertion may be associated with increased mortality (27). Once the tube is inserted, it is connected with an underwater seal drainage system with the option of applying suction. The presence of a well-functioning chest tube does not exclude the coexistence of a loculated tension pneumothorax. In this case adequate level of awareness and computerized tomography may prove safe.

F. Conclusions

Barotrauma (air leak) is the presence of extra-alveolar air in locations where it is not normally seen in patients who are mechanically ventilated. Included in the general category of barotrauma are tension lung cysts, hyperinflated lobe, subpleural air cysts, pulmonary interstitial emphysema, pneumothorax, pneumopericardium, subcutaneous emphysema, pneumomediastinum, pneumoretroperitoneum, and pneumoperitoneum. The main determinant of barotrauma seems to be the end-inspiratory volume (the term volutrauma better reflects the pathogenetic mechanism). The incidence of air leak in the ICU patient is difficult

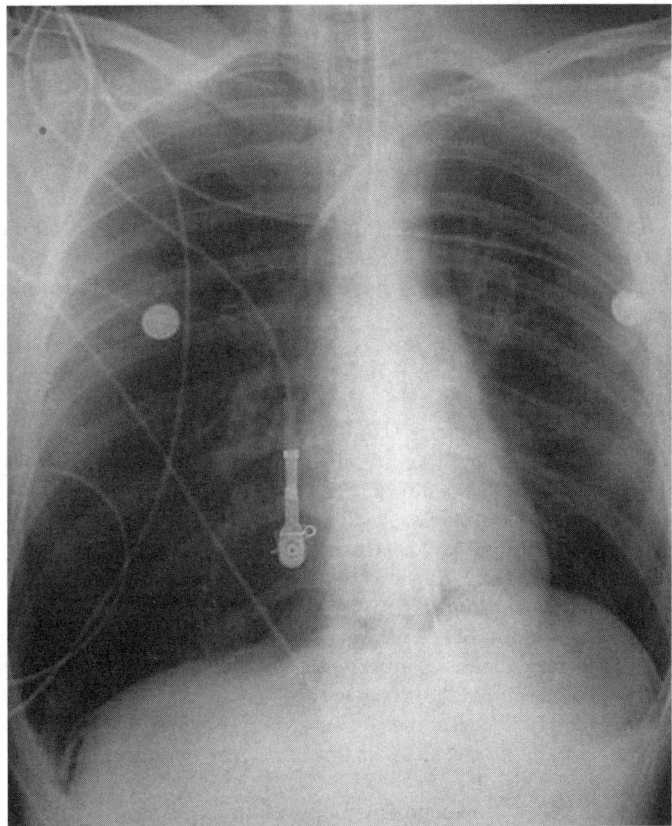

Figure 10 Chest radiograph of a 55-year-old male patient with bilateral pneumothorax. Right-sided pneumothorax is indicated by the visualization of the pleural line above the diaphragm. On the left side pneumothorax is indicated by the increased lucency of the left hemidiaphragm and the double diaphragm sign (the second interface reflects the anterior pleurodiaphragmatic sulcus that is visible by the presence of air at this site). (Courtesy of Dr. K. Malagari.)

to estimate but is not infrequent. Pneumothorax and related conditions in the ICU may go undetected and, when undiagnosed, have the potential to add to morbidity and mortality (tension pneumothorax). Therefore, a high index of suspicion and knowledge of the dynamic of injuries that predispose to barotraumas are imperative. The chest radiograph usually provides diagnostic results but in some cases a chest computed tomography is required. Prophylaxis of barotrauma is necessary in the ICU. Methods to reduce its frequency include measures to decrease alveolar inflation and pressures. Specific treatment modalities for pulmonary barotrauma vary with the type. Pneumothorax constitutes an emergency and requires the immediate placement of chest tubes for decompression.

References

1. Light RW. Pleural Diseases. 4th ed. Philadelphia: Lippincott Williams & Wilkins, 2001.
2. Mattison LE, Coppage L, Alderman DF, Herlong JO, Sahn SA. Pleural effusions in the medical ICU. Prevalence, causes and clinical implications. Chest 1997; 111: 1018–1023.
3. Myers DL. Pleural disease. In: Civetta JM, Taylor RW, Kirby RR, eds. Critical Care. Philadelphia: Lippincott, 1988:1133–1142.
4. Miserocchi G. Physiology and pathophysiology of pleural fluid turnover. Eur Respir J 1997; 10:219–225.
5. Burgess LJ, Maritz FJ, Taljaard JJ. Comparative analysis of the biochemical parameters used to distinguish between pleural transudates and exudates. Chest 1995; 107:1604–1609.
6. Tocino I. Abnormal air and pleural fluid collections. In: Goodman LR, Putman CE, eds. Critical Care Imaging. 3rd ed. Philadelphia: WB Saunders, 1992:137–160.
7. Miller WT Jr, Tino G, Friedburg JS. Thoracic CT in the intensive care unit: assessment of clinical usefulness. Radiology 1998; 209:491–498.
8. Voggenreiter G, Aufmkolk M, Majetschak M, Assenmacher S, Waydhas C, Obertacke U, Nast-Kolb D. Efficiency of chest computed tomography in critically ill patients with multiple traumas. Crit Care Med 2000; 28(4):1033–1039.
9. Rozycki GS, Pennington SD, Feliciano DV. Surgeon-performed ultrasound in the critically care setting: its use as an extension of the physical examination to detect pleural effusion. J Trauma 2001; 50:636–642.
10. Lichtenstein D, Hulot J-S, Rabiller A, Tostivint I, Meziere G. Feasibility and safety of ultrasound-aided thoracentesis in mechanically ventilated patients. Intensive Care Med 1999; 25:955–958.
11. Yeston NS, Grotz RL, Loiacono LA. Important intensive care unit procedures. In: Civetta JM, Taylor RW, Kirby RR, eds. Critical Care. Philadelphia: Lippincott-Raven Publishers, 1997:553–581.
12. LeMense GP, Strange C, Sahn SA. Empyema thoracis. Therapeutic management and outcome. Chest 1995; 107:1532–1537.
13. Strange C. Pleural complications in the intensive care unit. Clin Chest Med 1999; 20:317–327.
14. Sahn SA. Management of complicated parapneumonic effusions. Am Rev Respir Dis 1993; 148:813–817.
15. Hillerdal G. Chylothorax and pseudochylothorax. Eur Respir J 1997; 10:1157–1162.
16. Pingleton SK. Complications of acute respiratory failure. Am Rev Respir Dis 1988; 137:1463–1493.
17. Dreyfuss D, Saumon G. Ventilator-induced lung injury. Lessons of experimental studies. Am J Respir Crit Care Med 1998; 157:294–323.
18. Dreyfuss D, Saumon G. Barotrauma is volutrauma, but which volume is the one responsible? Intensive Care Med 1992; 18:139–141.
19. Parker JC, Hernandez LA, Peevy KJ. Mechanisms of ventilator-induced lung injury. Crit Care Med 1993; 21:139–141.
20. Dreyfuss D, Saumon G. Role of tidal volume, FRC and end-inspiratory volume in the development of pulmonary edema following mechanical ventilation. Am Rev Respir Dis 1993; 148:1194–1203.

21. Weg JG, Anzueto A, Balk RA, Wiedemann HP, Pattishal EN, Schork MA, Wagner LA. The relation of pneumothorax and other air leaks to mortality in the acute respiratory distress syndrome. N Engl J Med 1998; 338:341–346.
22. Macklin MT, Macklin CC. Malignant interstitial emphysema of the lungs and mediastinum as an important occult complication in many respiratory disease and other conditions: an interpretation of the clinical deterioration in light of the laboratory experiment. Medicine 1984; 23:281–287.
23. Tocino IM, Miller MH, Fairfax WR. Distribution of pneumothorax in the supine and semirecumbent critically ill adult. Am J Roentgenol 1985; 144:901–905.
24. Marglin SI, Rowberg AH, Godwin JD. Preliminary experience with portable digital imaging for intensive care radiology. J Thorac Imag 1990; 5:49–54.
25. Lichtenstein D, Meziere G, Biderman P, Gepner A. The comet-tail artifact: an ultrasound sign ruling out pneumothorax. Intensive Care Med 1999; 25:383–388.
26. Lichtenstein D, Meziere G, Biderman P, Gepner A. The "lung point": an ultrasound sign specific to pneumothorax. Intensive Care Med 2000; 26:1434–1440.
27. Brown DL, Kirby RR. Pulmonary barotrauma. In: Civetta JM, Taylor RW, Kirby RB, eds. Critical Care. 3rd ed. Philadelphia: Lippincott-Raven Publishers, 1997: 1959–1967.

41

Pleural Effusions in Gastrointestinal Tract Diseases

EPAMINONDAS N. KOSMAS
University of Athens
and Sotiria Chest Diseases Hospital
Athens, Greece

VLASIS S. POLYCHRONOPOULOS
Sismanoglion General Hospital
Athens, Greece

I. General Considerations

Diseases of the gastrointestinal (GI) tract may cause either transudative or exudative pleural effusions. Transudative pleural effusions occur when the systemic factors influencing the formation and absorption of pleural fluid are altered so that pleural fluid accumulates. In the majority of the cases, the transudative pleural effusion is related causally with cirrhosis and ascites. Exudative pleural effusions related to GI diseases are usually secondary to acute or chronic diseases and conditions affecting pancreas, liver and biliary tract, esophagus, or hernias, or they represent a complication of abdominal surgery. A particular category of exudative pleural effusions is the metastatic invasion of pleura attributed to abdominal neoplasms. Table 1 shows the GI diseases associated with transudative, exudative, or malignant pleural effusions.

Since the etiology of pleural effusion is very often a challenge to diagnose, the clinician must always keep in mind the possibility of abdominal disease in any pleural effusion of undetermined origin.

Table 1 Gastrointestinal Tract Diseases Associated with Pleural Effusions

Transudative
  Hepatic hydrothorax (cirrhosis, ascites)
  Hepatic chylothorax
  Retroperitoneal fibrosis
Exudative
  Acute pancreatitis
  Pancreatic abscess
  Pancreatic pseudocyst (chronic pancreatic effusion)
  Pancreatic ascites
  Subphrenic abscess
  Intrahepatic abscess
  Parasitic liver abscess (amebiasis, echinococcosis)
  Intrasplenic abscess
  Esophageal rupture
  Diaphragmatic hernia
  Biliary tract disorders
  After abdominal surgery
  After endoscopic variceal sclerotherapy
  After liver transplantation
Malignant
  Stomach
  Colon
  Pancreas
  Liver
  Cholangiocarcinoma

II. Transudative Pleural Effusion

A. Hepatic Hydrothorax

A transudative pleural effusion may complicate the clinical course of hepatic cirrhosis, in which case it is called hepatic hydrothorax. Pleural effusions secondary to hepatic cirrhosis occur rarely (5–6%) and usually coexist with ascites (1). Several studies with large series of cirrhotic patients have confirmed the coexistence of ascitic and pleural fluid (2,3). Even when ascites is not clinically evident in patients with cirrhosis and a pleural transudate, ascitic fluid can almost always be demonstrated with ultrasonography (4).

The pleural effusion in patients with cirrhosis and ascites is right-sided in two thirds of patients, but may also be left-sided or bilateral (1–3).

Pathogenesis and Pathophysiology

Patients with advanced cirrhosis and portal hypertension often show an abnormal extracellular fluid volume regulation, which results in accumulation of fluid, as ascites, pleural effusion, or edema. This abnormality in volume regulation is associated with significant changes in the splachnic and renal circulation that induce sodium and water retention (5). Plasma oncotic pressure is low in patients with cirrhosis, mainly due to hypoalbuminemia, and one might speculate that this is the principal pathophysiological mechanism of pleural fluid accumulation. Nowadays, decreased plasma oncotic pressure is not considered the predominant cause of pleural effusion in cirrhotic patients. The accumulation of fluid in the pleural space appears to be caused by a movement of the ascitic fluid from the peritoneal cavity into the pleural cavity.

It is a subject for discussion whether this transfer of fluid from the peritoneal to the pleural cavity is a result of either a direct movement through diaphragmatic pores/defects or a transfer through the diaphragmatic lymphatic system. When Johnston and Loo (2) injected intravenously radiolabeled albumin, they detected albumin first in the ascitic fluid and then in the pleural fluid. When they injected the labeled protein intraperitoneally, the concentration of protein was greater in pleural fluid than in the plasma; when the same material was injected intrapleurally, the radiolabeled albumin was detected in the plasma before it appeared in ascitic fluid. They concluded that the pleural effusion in cirrhotic patients with ascites originates from the passage of ascitic fluid from the peritoneal to the pleural cavity through the lymphatic vessels of the diaphragm. Two decades later, Datta et al. (6) reported completely different findings, since they observed that when labeled protein was injected intraperitoneally in patients with ascites and pleural effusion, the protein was picked up by the lymphatic system in the diaphragm, after which it moved across the mediastinal lymphatic vessels towards the venous system, and therefore protein did not enter the pleural cavity.

On the other hand, when Lieberman et al. (3) induced pneumoperitoneum by introducing air into the peritoneal cavity of five patients with cirrhosis, ascites and pleural effusion, they observed in all patients the development of hydropneumothorax during the first 2 days after the introduction of air. Moreover, when they performed thoracoscopy in their patients, they saw air bubbles coming through diaphragm, probably through diaphragmatic microdefects. In postmortem examination, diaphragmatic defects were demonstrated in two of their patients. In a more recent study, Mouroux et al. (7) visualized the diaphragmatic defects in the diaphragm during thoracoscopy. Hence, these investigators, along with the Datta study, disputed the diaphragmatic lymphatic system being the channel of fluid passage from the peritoneal to pleural cavity. These studies documented that the pleural effusion arises from the passive movement of fluid from the peritoneal to the pleural space through defects or pores in the diaphragm. The role of these defects in the pathogenesis of hepatic hydrothorax explains satisfactorily why hydrothorax is much more common on the right side than on the left side. It is thought that cirrhosis-related pleural transudate is more common on the right hemithorax because the right hemidiaphragm is more likely to have embryological developmental defects (8). Recent scintigraphic studies (9–12) with intraperitoneal injection of technetium-99m sulfur colloid have verified the above theory by providing evidence of a one-way flow of fluid from the peritoneal to pleural cavity, even in the rare cases of hepatic hydrothorax without ascitic fluid (13–15).

The pathophysiological basis of this theory relies on the increased intraabdominal pressure caused by the presence of ascitic fluid. The increased intraabdominal pressure poses a stretch pressure on the diaphragm, thus causing microscopic defects or magnifying preexisting defects. In addition, the increased intraabdominal pressure acts as the driving pressure, which leads to the transfer of fluid from the peritoneal to the pleural cavity through these diaphragmatic defects. According to Light's experience (1), the cardinal mechanism is the direct movement of the fluid through diaphragmatic defects or pores. He observed that when chest tubes were placed in order to relieve dyspnea from large pleural effusions, the amount of ascitic fluid decreased rapidly.

Clinical Features and Diagnosis

The clinical picture of a patient with hepatic hydrothorax is one of the cirrhotic patient with ascites. In case of frequent large effusion, patients may be dyspneic. It has to be noted that the amount of pleural fluid is usually large and may occupy the entire hemithorax, probably because the movement of the fluid from the abdomen to the pleural space is continued until the equilibration of pleural and peritoneal pressures. Light et al. measured the pleural pressures in patients with pleural effusions secondary to ascites and found them to be higher than in patients with other transudative pleural effusions (16). The diagnosis of hepatic hydrothorax is easy and is based on thoracentesis and abdominal paracentesis. Both fluids are transudates, and although the pleural fluid protein tends to be higher than the ascitic fluid protein level, it is still below 3.0 g/dL, while the pleural fluid lactate dehydrogenase (LDH) is low. Occasionally the fluid is bloody, and the patient may have a poor coagulation profile due to cirrhosis. The differential cell count may be variable with predominance either of polymorphonuclear leukocytes or lymphocytes. Pleural effusion related to pancreatic ascites will be excluded by the measurement of amylase levels, while cytological examination of both fluids should be always performed in order to rule out malignant disease.

As mentioned above, when hepatic hydrothorax is suspected in a patient with large pleural effusion and cirrhosis but without clinically evident ascites, abdominal ultrasonography should be performed which may reveal the presence of ascitic fluid (4). Intraperitoneal injection of Tc-99m and radionuclide scintigraphy of peritoneal and pleural cavities may facilitate diagnosis in cases of a nondiagnostic ultrasound and may help with respect to treatment decision (13–15).

In patients with cirrhosis, ascites, and pleural effusion, it is important to be aware of the possibility of pleural infection. Xiol et al. (17) reported on 24 episodes of spontaneous bacterial empyema in 16 out of 120 patients (13%) admitted with a diagnosis of hepatic hydrothorax. In 14 of the 24 cases of bacterial pleuritis, there was a concomitant spontaneous bacterial peritonitis.

The term bacterial pleuritis is preferred to the term bacterial empyema, since in most of the cases the pleural fluid was not frank pus. Diagnosis of bacterial pleuritis in a patient with cirrhosis and ascites is established when pneumonia is excluded, when there is a positive culture of the pleural fluid along with a neutrophil count of >250 cells/mm^3, or even a negative culture along with a neutrophil count of >500 cells/mm^3. Pathogenic agents usually include *Escherichia coli*, *Enterococcus* species, *Streptococcus* species, and *Streptococcus pneumoniae* (17). The treatment of bacterial pleuritis is an appropriate antibiotic according to bacterial susceptibility; placement of a chest tube is not indicated.

Treatment

The treatment of hepatic hydrothorax should be directed toward the therapeutic measures for ascites, since hydrothorax originates from the transfer of ascitic fluid into the pleural cavity. The patient should be started on a low-salt diet and should be given diuretics, with the more appropriate combination being furosemide (40–160 mg daily) and spironolactone (100–400 mg daily) (18). Therapeutic thoracenteses are of temporary benefit since the pleural fluid usually reaccumulates rapidly.

While the majority of patients respond satisfactorily to salt restriction and the administration of diuretics, some do not respond well and continue to have symptoms, such as dyspnea, due to the persistence of large pleural effusion and ascites. In such patients, liver transplantation or alternatively implantation of a transjugular intrahepatic portal systemic shunt (TIPS) should be considered. Many recent studies (9,19–23) have addressed the issue of the beneficial effects of TIPS in patients with refractory hepatic hydrothorax. All studies proved the effectiveness and safety of the procedure, documenting a significant advantage with respect to treatment and survival rates in those patients assigned to TIPS as compared to those assigned to serial thoracenteses.

Another alternative treatment option is videothoracoscopy with an attempt to close the diaphragmatic defects and to perform pleurodesis. Aerosolized talc pleurodesis at the time of thoracoscopy has been proven effective in controlling recurrence of the pleural effusion (24). Mouroux et al. (25) reported their results in 8 patients; diaphragmatic defects were found and closed in 6 out of the 8 patients, while talc pleurodesis was performed in all patients. In all patients the combination was proved effective. In a more recent study (26) of 18 patients who were subjected to thoracoscopy combined with talc insufflation, the results are not so encouraging in comparison with the results of the Mouroux study. In a minority of patients (28%) the diaphragmatic defects were detected and closed, while the whole procedure was successful only in 48% of patients. However, videothoracoscopy remains an acceptable alternative method when neither liver transplantation nor TIPS is available or feasible. It has to be mentioned here that talc use for pleurodesis has been associated recently with the development of acute respiratory distress in approximately 5% of patients, with a mortality rate of about 1%.

A successful surgical repair of hepatic hydrothorax in the absence of ascites has been reported (27). The method consists of induction of pneumoperitoneum in order to identify possible defects in the diaphragm and of direct suture of the defect.

B. Cirrhotic Chylothorax

Chylothorax is a rare and apparently underappreciated manifestation of cirrhosis, resulting from transdiaphragmatic passage of chylous ascites. In one series of 809 patients, 24 patients had pleural effusions being chylothoraces. Five of these patients (20%) were found to have liver cirrhosis (28). Cirrhotic chylous effusions were transudates with distinct biochemical fluid characteristics (significantly lower protein, LDH, and cholesterol levels as compared to chylous effusions resulting from other causes).

C. Retroperitoneal Fibrosis

Reports from Japan have identified cases of retroperitoneal fibrosis associated with transudative pleural effusions (29,30). Retroperitoneal fibrosis is considered as an extremely rare cause of pleural effusion, and the possible pathophysiological mechanism appears to be the extrahepatic portal vein obstruction.

III. Exudative Pleural Effusion

As mentioned above, exudative pleural effusions may arise as a manifestation during the clinical course of various GI diseases, acute or chronic, affecting the pancreas, liver, biliary tract, esophagus, hernias, intraabdominal abscesses, or as a complication of various surgical and other invasive procedures (Table 1).

A. Pancreatic Diseases

Acute Pancreatitis

The introduction of the computed tomography (CT) scan in everyday clinical practice revealed that many cases of acute pancreatitis may be associated with the presence of a pleural effusion, with usually minimal findings on chest x-ray, given that the amount of pleural fluid is usually small. Lankisch et al., in a series of 133 consecutive patients admitted in hospital due to acute pancreatitis, reported that about 50% of them had a pleural effusion on CT scan during the first 3 days of admission (31). The effusion is usually bilateral (75%) or left-sided (16%). In the vast majority of the patients, pleural cavity contains a small amount of fluid. In one series of 539 patients from Italy (32), 77 patients (14%) had a pleural effusion (44% bilateral, 32% left-sided, and 24% right-sided). Maringhini et al. (33) have also reported a 20% incidence of pleural effusion among patients with acute pancreatitis.

The presence of pleural effusion in patients with acute pancreatitis has been correlated with a more severe clinical course and poor outcome of the pancreatic disease. Heller et al. (34) studied 116 patients with mild pancreatitis and 19 patients with severe pancreatitis. The incidence of pleural effusion was much higher in the group of severe pancreatitis as compared with that in the group of patients with mild pancreatitis (84% vs. 8.5%, respectively). Similarly, Talamini et al. (32) studied 539 patients and found that the presence of a pleural effusion along with serum creatinine within the first 24 hours of admission were correlated with mortality risk, with a diagnosis of necrotizing pancreatitis and with the risk of developing infected necrosis. In another series of 100 patients (33), it has been documented that the presence of ascitic and pleural fluids were accurate independent predictors of severity of acute pancreatitis.

The pathophysiological mechanism of exudative pleural effusion during the clinical course of acute pancreatitis seems to be the transdiaphragmatic transfer, via the diaphragmatic lymphatic vessels, of the exudative fluid produced during the acute inflammatory process of pancreas and diaphragm (35). This pancreatic exudate enters the lymphatic vessels on the peritoneal side of the diaphragm toward the pleural side of the diaphragm. The increased content of the fluid in pancreatic enzymes contributes to the formation of pleural effusion by increasing the permeability of lymphatic vessels, resulting in the leakage of the fluid into the pleural cavity, and by obstructing the pleural lymphatics and decreasing the pleural lymphatic flow (36). The diaphragm itself participates in the acute pancreatitis-induced inflammation, and this is because of the proximity between pancreas and diaphragm.

The clinical presentation of patients with acute pancreatitis and pleural effusion is usually dominated by the abdominal symptoms, such as pain, nausea, and vomiting. Occasionally, patients report symptoms indicative of respiratory disease, such as pleuritic chest pain and/or dyspnea. The chest radiography may reveal a small or moderate pleural effusion, an elevation of the diaphragm, and, possibly, infiltrates located in the lung base (37).

Differential diagnosis consists of pneumonia or pulmonary embolism complicated by pleural effusion. The diagnosis is usually established by demonstrating a high serum amylase or lipase level in a patient with abdominal pain, nausea, or vomiting. When the diagnosis of acute pancreatitis is confirmed and the pleural effusion is symptomless and of small or moderate size, thoracentesis should not be performed. Thoracentesis, either for diagnostic or for therapeutic reasons, should be restricted to providing relief from dyspnea due to a large effusion and for the exclusion of empyema in a febrile patient.

The pleural fluid is an exudate, with high protein and LDH levels, and is occasionally serosanguineous or even bloody. The glucose level is similar to that of the blood, and polymorphonuclear leukocytes predominate with respect to the differential white blood cell count. Pleural fluid amylase in patients with acute pancreatitis and pleural effusion is usually higher than the serum amylase and remains elevated for a longer period in comparison with the serum amylase (36–38). Fluid levels of phospholipase A_2 are also high in patients with acute pancreatitis (39), while the fluid levels of trypsinogen activation peptide are low (40).

In the vast majority of patients with acute pancreatitis and a small- or moderate-size effusion, there is not indication for additional treatment beyond the treatment of acute pancreatitis. Therapeutic thoracentesis and pleural fluid drainage is indicated only for large effusions causing dyspnea or for empyema due to superinfection. The pleural effusion usually resolves spontaneously as the acute pancreatitis subsides. In the case of nonresolving effusion within 2–3 weeks, one must consider the possibility of a pancreatic abscess or pseudocyst (37). A beneficial effect of oral administration of high-dose octreotide has been reported (41).

Pancreatic Abscess

In most cases, acute pancreatitis responds to therapy within 10–14 days. When the clinical course of acute pancreatitis is not favorable and 14–21 days after the initiation of medical treatment with an initial response the patient becomes febrile with recurrence of abdominal pain and peripheral blood leukocytosis, the formation of a pancreatic abscess must be suspected (42). Pancreatic abscess must also be suspected in the case of nonresponding pancreatitis, even if the patient is receiving the appropriate treatment (42). Whenever there is a suspicion of a pancreatic abscess development, abdominal ultrasonography and CT scanning must be performed without delay. It is important to mention that the mortality rate in undrained pancreatic abscesses is very high (~100%); therefore, the need for immediate diagnostic confirmation and surgical drainage is essential and urgent (36,42). Pleural effusion is a frequent finding in patients with pancreatic abscess. Miller et al. (42), in their series of 63 patients with pancreatic abscess, have reported an incidence rate of 38% with respect to the presence of a pleural effusion. The pleural fluid amylase level is high, but there is a lack of data concerning pleural fluid characteristics in patients with pancreatic abscess (37).

Pancreatic Pseudocyst and Chronic Pancreatic Pleural Effusion

A pancreatic pseudocyst (implying that this is not a cyst with true walls) represents a collection of fluid with high pancreatic enzyme content, usually situated within the pancreas. Pancreatic pseudocysts may result from acute pancreatitis and rarely (5%) are followed with a pleural effusion (43). According to Rockey and Cello in their review on pancreatic pseudocysts (43), pleural effusions are relatively uncommon.

The primary mechanism for the development of pleural effusion in patients with a chronic pseudocyst is the formation of a pancreatic-pleural fistula between the pancreas and the pleural space (37,43). Once fluid enters the pleural cavity, the pancreatic-pleural fistula is likely to result in a massive effusion. A secondary mechanism is the passage of the pseudocyst fluid into the mediastinum through the esophageal or aortic hiatus. This passage may result in the formation of a mediastinal pseudocyst, decompression into one or both pleural spaces (37,44–47), or an enzymatic mediastinitis (48). An extremely rare complication of a pancreatic pseudocyst is the formation of a pancreatic-bronchial fistula (49).

General symptoms, such as malaise, fatigue, and weight loss, and respiratory symptoms, such as chest pain and dyspnea, usually dominate the clinical picture in these patients (43,48,50). Uchiyama et al. (50), in one series of 113 patients, documented that the cardinal complaints were dyspnea (42%) and chest pain (29%), while the frequency of upper abdominal pain was impressively low (23%) for a disease affecting the upper abdomen. The lack of abdominal symptoms may be attributed to the fact that the pancreatic-pleural fistula decompresses the pseudocyst. The effusion, as mentioned above, is usually large or even massive, occupying the entire hemithorax. It usually affects the left hemithorax, but is occasionally right-sided or bilateral (43,50). It is important to note that the diagnosis of chronic pancreatic pleural effusion is frequently missed because of the lack of typical abdominal symptoms and the absence of prior pancreatic disease.

The diagnosis should be suspected in any case of a patient who looks chronically ill and who has a large or even massive pleural effusion, particularly left-sided. A good proportion of patients have a history of prior pancreatic disease or abdominal trauma (37). However, many patients have no such a history. The more useful laboratory test for establishing the diagnosis is the measurement of pleural fluid amylase. Pleural fluid amylase levels are remarkably increased (usually >1000 U/L), whereas serum amylase may be within normal or near-normal levels (37). It has to be mentioned here that the specificity of high amylase in pleural fluid is not 100%; therefore, one must think of other causes of high amylase levels in the fluid, such as malignant pleural effusions or esophageal diseases (38,51). Measurement of amylase isoenzymes on pleural fluid appears to be helpful in the differential diagnosis between malignant and pancreatic effusion, since with malignant effusions the amylase is of the salivary rather than the pancreatic type (52). Peripheral blood eosinophilia (>500 cells/ mm^3) was found in 21 patients (17%) in one series of 122 cases with chronic pancreatitis (53). Eosinophilia frequently developed in association with severe damage to neighboring organs (pleural effusion, pericarditis, ascites), as well as in association with pancreatic pseudocyst (53).

CT scanning of the chest and abdomen usually establishes the diagnosis, revealing both the pancreatic pseudocyst and the pancreatic-pleural fistula (37, 47–49,54). Endoscopic retrograde cholangiopancreatography (ERCP) plays an important role in the evaluation and management of patients with that kind of fistula. The greatest utility for ERCP is to define preoperatively the precise anatomical relationship between the fistula and the adjacent structures, such as the pancreas, the diaphragm, and the pleura (37,47–49,54).

The initial treatment of patients with a pancreatic pseudocyst and a pleural effusion is usually nonsurgical. It has to be noted that a therapeutic thoracentesis is not helpful since the fluid has the tendency to reaccumulate rapidly (50). The concept of conservative treatment is to reduce pancreatic secretions in order to achieve regression of the pseudocyst and functional closure of the fistula (55). The insertion of a nasogastric tube is required in all patients, and intravenous hyperalimentation is given. The administration of somatostatin or octreotide, a synthetic analogue of somatostatin, have shown benefit in some patients (56,57). It is known that somatostatin exerts an inhibitory action on pancreatic exocrine secretion (43). If the above conservative treatment fails, the treatment of choice is surgical.

Surgical intervention should be considered whenever the patient remains symptomatic and the pleural effusion persists after 2 weeks of treatment. Approximately 50% of patients, particularly those with more severe pancreatic disease, require surgery (37). The preoperative assessment consists of ERCP and abdominal CT scan, which are helpful in planning the appropriate surgical procedure. Recently, some patients have been successfully treated by placing stents in the pancreatic duct at the time the ERCP is performed (58,59). Depending on the location of the pseudocyst within the pancreas and of the duct with the leak, different procedures are available, such as distal pancreatectomy, direct anastomosis between the leak and a jejunal loop or internal drainage of the cyst into the stomach or into a jejunal loop (37,60–62). In an attempt to avoid the surgical procedure, some investigators have tried to drain the pseudocyst percutaneously under CT guidance (63,64). A catheter is inserted through the anterior abdominal wall, the stomach, and the pseudocyst, and it accomplishes drainage from the cyst into the stomach. Lang et al. reported a success rate of 77% in their series of 26 patients (64). However, there are not many available data in the literature regarding percutaneous drainage. In addition, Brelvi et al. (65) introduced nasopancreatic drainage, a novel approach for treating internal pancreatic fistulas and pseudocysts.

The prognosis of these patients is usually favorable, with a mortality rate of approximately 5% (43). In patients with chronic pleural effusions secondary to pancreatic pseudocystic disease, pleural thickening is a probable complication and decortication may be needed. Sometimes the pleural thickening resolves gradually over months and watchful waiting is necessary prior to deciding upon decortication. Clinicians must be aware of unusual manifestations of pancreatic pseudocysts, such as mediastinal extension of the pseudocyst, obstructive jaundice, intraperitoneal rupture, pancreatic ascites, pancreaticobronchial fistula, and massive hemorrhage due to the development of a false aneurysm in a branch of the celiac axis in the wall of the pseudocyst, since they require different surgical management (62). One very uncommon complication of pancreatic pleural effusion is the development of a bronchopleural fistula. In this situation, a chest tube should be inserted immediately to drain the pleural space and to protect the lung from the enzymatic fluid (36).

Pancreatic Ascites

The development of pancreatic ascites is attributed to leakage of fluid from a pseudocyst directly into the peritoneal cavity via an internal pancreatic fistula and is characterized by high amylase and protein levels (66). Some patients happen to have a defect in their diaphragm, and they subsequently develop large pleural effusion as a result of the flow of fluid from the peritoneal cavity in the same manner that pleural effusion develops secondary to cirrhotic ascites. Approximately 20% of patients with pancreatic ascites have a pleural effusion (66). Over one half of patients had no history of inflammatory pancreatic disease (67). However, a history of chronic alcoholism is associated with the syndrome of pancreatic ascites (68,69).

Common symptoms of this syndrome are intermittent abdominal pain, nausea, vomiting, and considerable weight loss, which occurs despite fluid retention (68). Patients complain of dyspnea whenever the pleural effusion is large. The diagnosis of pancreatic ascites is made if amylase and protein levels of the peritoneal and pleural fluid are high (66,67). Serum amylase is usually, but not always, elevated (67). Hypoalbuminemia is common as well (68). The internal pancreatic fistula is successfully demonstrated in most instances by ERCP (67). The treatment of pancreatic ascites is the same as for pancreatic pseudocyst and chronic pancreatic pleural effusion, except serial abdominal paracenteses rather than serial therapeutic thoracenteses are performed. Initial treatment is nonoperative (nasogastric suction, hyperalimentation, administration of somatostatin or octreotide), with a success rate of 32–48% (67,69–71). In an attempt to determine risk factors for failure of conservative treatment, Parekh and Segal studied 23 patients with pancreatic ascites or effusion (70). They observed that serum sodium and albumin levels were significantly lower and the ratio of fluid total protein to serum total protein was significantly higher in the group that failed to heal in response to conventional medical therapy. In addition, they found that patients with severe pancreatitis did not respond to nonsurgical treatment, implying that patients with advanced pancreatic disease should be selected for early surgery (70).

When nonoperative medical therapy fails, surgery is performed to drain or to resect the internal fistula (71), with an overall success rate of 82% (67). In one series of 49 patients (71), conservative treatment was successful in 18, while the remaining 31 patients were assigned to surgical treatment. The different surgical procedures chosen were internal pancreatic drainage, external pancreatic drainage, and distal pancreatectomy with fistula resection. It seems that internal pancreatic drainage was the ideal surgical treatment for patients with pancreatic ascites and/or pleural effusion that did not respond to medical treatment (71). An alternative choice is endoscopic placement of a stent across the pancreatic duct disruption (72).

B. Subphrenic Abscess

The vast majority of subphrenic abscesses result from abdominal surgical procedures, such as splenectomy, gastrectomy, exploratory laparotomy, laparoscopic cholecystectomy, etc. (73–75). However, the incidence of subphrenic abscess formation following an abdominal surgical procedure is relatively small;

Sanders states that in a total of 1566 abdominal operations, only 1% are followed by a subphrenic abscess (74). The time interval between the surgical procedure and the development of a subphrenic abscess is usually 1–3 weeks, but can be as long as 5–6 months. Rarely, a subphrenic abscess may develop without any surgical procedure in the abdomen as a result of gastric, appendiceal, or duodenal perforation, diverticulitis, cholecystitis, pancreatitis, or trauma (76). In such patients, the diagnosis may be missed because of the atypical clinical picture.

Pleural effusion is a common manifestation, occurring in about 60–80% of patients with a subphrenic abscess, and is usually small to moderate in size, although it sometimes may be large enough to occupy a large part of the hemithorax (74,76,77).

Carter and Brewer proposed as a possible pathogenetic mechanism the transfer of abscess material from the subphrenic inflamed location into the pleural cavity via the diaphragmatic lymphatics (77). However, there is doubt as to that theory, since culture of pleural fluid is rarely positive. There is a general belief that the pathogenesis of subphrenic abscess-induced pleural effusion is probably related to inflammation of the diaphragm. This inflammation probably increases permeability of the capillaries in the diaphragmatic pleura and causes the accumulation of pleural fluid (37).

The clinical symptoms and signs of patients with subphrenic abscess and pleural effusion are due to the abdominal and chest disease. As reported in one series of 125 cases, 44% of patients had exclusively chest findings, with the pleuritic chest pain being the dominant symptom (77). Patients may have no abdominal symptoms at the time of presentation. The majority of patients with a postoperative subphrenic abscess have fever, leukocytosis, and abdominal pain or tenderness (76,77), but not all patients have characteristic symptoms or signs (37).

The diagnosis of subphrenic abscess should be considered whenever the patient develops a pleural effusion several days or weeks after an abdominal operation or when the patient has an exudative polymorphonuclear effusion of otherwise undetermined cause. Examination of the pleural fluid usually reveals a polymorphonuclear type of exudate. The white blood cell count of the fluid may approach 30,000–50,000 cells/mm^3, but the pH and glucose level remain above 7.20 and 60 mg/dL, respectively, and it is very uncommon for the pleural fluid to be infected (37). However, there are occasional case reports of empyema formation (75).

Radiographic examination usually reveals the presence of the pleural fluid and additional radiographic findings include basal pneumonitis, compression atelectasis, or elevation of the diaphragm on the affected side. The pathognomonic radiological finding is an air-fluid level below the diaphragm outside the gastrointestinal tract. The patient must be in upright and lateral decubitus position for the best demonstration (73). Sometimes a displacement of intraabdominal viscera can be noticed on radiographs. Barium enema is sometimes helpful in demonstrating the extraluminal location of gas leakage or displacement of normal structures. Abdominal CT scan is the best imaging procedure to establish the diagnosis (78). CT scan is more sensitive and has the advantage over other methods (gallium scanning, ultrasonography) of detecting the precise anatomical location and magnitude of the abscess, whereas ultrasound examination is technically difficult in the left upper abdominal quadrant because of overlying lung, ribs, and gas in the GI tract.

Optimal treatment consists of the administration of broad-spectrum antibiotics (usually against more than one organism, such as *E. coli*, *Staphylococcus aureus*, and anaerobes) and drainage, either percutaneously under CT guidance or surgically. Sepsis is the most common and most life-threatening complication of subphrenic abscess. In a series of 125 patients with a subphrenic abscess (77), 23% of the patients had positive blood cultures, and in those patients the mortality rate was impressively high, approaching 93%. However, even in nonseptic abscesses, the mortality rate is still high, ranging from 20 to 45% (73,76,77). This unfavorable prognosis is mainly due to delayed diagnosis or even a lack of diagnosis. It is important to consider the possibility of a subphrenic abscess in every patient presenting with exudative pleural effusion containing predominantly polymorphonuclear leukocytes and particularly when this picture follows an abdominal surgical procedure.

C. Intrahepatic Abscess

About 20% of patients with a liver abscess present pleural effusion, with the same mechanism as the subphrenic abscess (37). Half of the patients have a history of hepatolithiasis or other hepatobiliary disease, while the remaining 50% have not known disease predisposing to the development of a liver abscess (79). There are occasional reports of liver abscesses with right-sided pleural effusions manifested during the clinical course of disseminated infections from various pathogens, such as *Mycobacterium tuberculosis* (80) or *Corynebacterium afermentans lipophilum* (81).

Since the mortality rate is quite high, nearly 100%, in patients with untreated intrahepatic abscesses, clinicians should be very careful when evaluating a right-sided exudative pleural effusion with predominance of polymorphonuclear leukocytes (37). In a multivariate analysis of risk factors in 73 patients with pyogenic liver abscess and overall mortality rate 19%, it was revealed that clinical jaundice, pleural effusion, bilobar abscess, profound hypoalbuminemia, hyperbilirubinemia, hypertransaminasemia, elevated serum alkaline phosphatase level, and marked leukocytosis were associated with a higher mortality rate (82). Most patients have anorexia and fever accompanied by chills, while abdominal pain is common but frequently not localized to the right upper quadrant. In the majority of cases, there is an enlargement and tenderness of the liver (79).

Laboratory tests may reveal leukocytosis, anemia, and elevated alkaline phosphatase and bilirubin levels. Because none of the above tests is invariably present, the diagnosis of pyogenic liver abscess is best established by an abdominal CT scan and alternatively by an abdominal ultrasound study.

Abdominal CT scanning may detect abscesses and fluid-filled intrahepatic lesions of small diameter. Since not all the fluid-filled lesions are pyogenic liver abscesses (differential diagnosis includes cysts, hematomas, hemangiomas, amebic abscesses), diagnosis can be established definitely by percutaneous aspiration under CT or ultrasound guidance.

Treatment consists of the administration of parenteral antibiotics and drainage of the abscess. CT-guided or ultrasound-guided percutaneous needle aspiration is the procedure of choice for draining the abscess (79,83,84). Persistent fever, pain and tenderness in the right upper quadrant, and leukocytosis are the indications for multiple aspirations (84). Laparotomy is indicated either when aspiration has failed or when there are signs of peritonitis and clinical deterioration (79).

D. Parasitic Liver Abscess

Amebic liver abscess is the most common extraintestinal site of infection by *Entamoeba histolytica*. In turn, pleural-pulmonary amebiasis is the most common complication of amebic liver abscess and usually is attributed to erosion of the abscess through the diaphragm to involve the pleural space or lung parenchyma (85,86). The mortality rate varies between 2 and 3% (87). There have been efforts to define possible prognostic factors in large series (87,88) in terms of both clinical and laboratory indices. The presence of jaundice, large or multiple abscesses, acute abdomen, liver failure, sepsis, dyspnea, alterations in hematocrit, prothrombin time, albumin, LDH, urea nitrogen, and pleural effusion have been recognized as predictors of severity (87,88).

The significance and severity of a pleural effusion in patients with amebic liver abscesses varies from mild cases of "sympathetic" transudates to more severe cases of amebic empyema and formation of hepatobronchial fistula. Transudative "sympathetic" pleural effusions and atelectasis are common accompaniments of liver abscesses and do not indicate extension of disease. Patients with pleural-pulmonary complications have an exudative effusion and present with cough, pleuritic pain, and dyspnea. Empyema due to rupture of the abscess into the pleural cavity presents with sudden respiratory distress, fever, and pain and has a substantial mortality. In some instances, a hepatobronchial fistula forms and has been associated with spontaneous drainage of the hepatic abscess.

The diagnosis of amebiasis-induced pleural effusion is suggested by the discovery of "chocolate sauce" or "anchovy paste" appearance of the pleural fluid. *Entamoeba histolytica* is usually demonstrable in the pleural fluid. Abdominal ultrasonography serves as a useful diagnostic aid (89).

Treatment consists of metronidazole 750 mg per os 3 times a day for 5–10 days plus diloxanide furoate 500 mg 3 times a day for 10 days for intraluminal infection. Chloroquine has been used as well (89). Severe cases require, in addition to amebicidal treatment, either percutaneous aspiration or surgical drainage of pus, especially in those patients with ruptured abscesses (87). Patients with abscesses that rupture into the thoracic cavity must be treated by either thoracotomy or needle aspiration (87).

The hydatid cysts of *Echinococcus granulosus* form in the liver in 50–70% of patients and in the lung in 20–30% of patients. Pleural disease develops when either a hepatic or a parenchymal lung cyst ruptures into the pleural space (85). The patient develops an acute illness with severe chest pain, dyspnea, and sometimes shock secondary to severe allergic reactions to parasitic antigens suddenly released. The diagnosis is established by recognition of daughter cysts in the pleural fluid. Optimal treatment is surgical resection to drain the pleural space and removal of the original cyst.

E. Splenic Abscess

Intrasplenic abscess is actually a very unusual clinical entity. Approximately 20 cases were reported in U.S. hospitals during the period 1950–1990. Most presented with an associated left-sided pleural effusion (90,91). Splenic abscess, although a rare clinical entity, may occur de novo in septic ICU patients and is associated with significant mortality. In the majority of patients, the splenic suppurative disease arises from primary hematogenous dissemination of infection, such as endocarditis (92). Various pathogens have been identified, such as *Candida albicans, Streptococcus viridans, E. coli, Citerobacter freundii, Enterobacter*, and *S. aureus* (91,92). Particularly vulnerable populations include patients who suffer from chronic hemolytic anemia or sickle cell anemia (90). Mortality rate ranges between 40 and 50%.

Fever is usually present, accompanied by chills and vomiting (92). Left upper quadrant tenderness and leukocytosis appear in almost all patients (92). The diagnosis is not easily made, since not all the patients with a splenic abscess complain of a localized pain or tenderness in the left upper quadrant. The presence of a left-sided pleural effusion with thrombocytosis is a combination of findings suggestive of the disease (91). Unexplained thrombocytosis in a septic patient with persistent left pleural effusion is suggestive of splenic abscess. The diagnosis can be made with an abdominal CT scan or ultrasonography and can be confirmed by fine needle aspiration (92,93).

The treatment of choice consists of splenectomy plus antibiotics (93), while an alternative approach is the catheter drainage (93).

F. Esophageal Rupture

Esophageal perforation is a rare clinical emergency in which, if no early diagnosis and treatment are made, the mortality rate may be as high as 100% (94,95). Rupture of esophagus most commonly is a complication of esophagoscopy, particularly when there is an attempt to dilate an esophageal stricture or to remove a foreign body (96). Keszler and Buzna, in one series of 108 consecutive patients with esophageal perforation, reported that 67% of the events occurred as a complication of an esophagoscopic procedure (96). However, esophageal perforation is a rare complication of esophagoscopy, since the reported incidence of perforation following an esophagoscopic examination is below 1% (94). Importantly, the endoscopist usually does not realize that the esophagus has been perforated. Other, less frequent causes of an esophageal rupture include the insertion of a Blakemore tube for esophageal varices, foreign bodies, chest trauma, chest surgery, gastric intubation, and carcinomas (37,94). Finally, spontaneous rupture of the lower part of esophagus may occur as a complication of vomiting (Boerhaave's syndrome).

The mediastinum is a sterile compartment of human body, and the entrance of oropharyngeal and esophageal contents contaminates this sterile area and produces acute mediastinitis. When the mediastinal pleura ruptures, a pleural effusion develops, frequently complicated by pneumothorax. Most morbidity from esophageal rupture is the result of infection of the mediastinum and pleural space by microorganisms of the oropharyngeal bacterial flora (97).

Clinical manifestations of esophageal rupture depend on the cause of perforation. As mentioned above, in cases of "iatrogenic" perforation, endoscopists usually do not realize the trauma they have caused. Such patients usually report persistent chest or epigastric pain within several hours of the procedure. Patients with spontaneous (noniatrogenic) rupture of the esophagus, usually give a history of vomiting and chest pain, followed by a sensation of tearing or bursting in the lower part of the chest or the epigastrium. Chest pain is very strong and often not relieved by opiates. Hematemesis is present frequently, and dyspnea may be a prominent symptom (98). Subcutaneous emphysema is usually a late complication of esophageal rupture (98). Very rarely, the appearance of symptoms is not so dramatic and patients may have only mild distress.

Pleural effusion, often left-sided, is present in about 60% of patients with esophageal rupture, and pneumothorax is present in about 25% (94). In a retrospective 15-year chart review, chest x-ray was abnormal in all patients, with findings of pleural effusion and/or pneumothorax (99). Diagnosis of esophageal rupture must be made as soon as possible because of the high mortality rate (60%). A patient who appears acutely ill, has an exudative left-sided pleural effusion, and reports a history of an endoscopic esophageal procedure or vomiting, esophageal cancer, etc. should be very carefully evaluated for esophageal rupture. Examination of the pleural fluid is very helpful because it is characterized by a high amylase level (particularly of the salivary isoenzyme), low pH, and the presence of squamous epithelial cells and sometimes of ingested food particles.

High amylase levels appear to be the best indication of esophageal rupture (51,98). The origin of the amylase is salivary rather than pancreatic because the saliva, with its high amylase content, enters the pleural space through the defect in the esophagus (100). Pleural fluid pH is usually decreased. Dye and Laforet (101) concluded that a pleural fluid pH below 6.0 is highly suggestive of esophageal rupture. Low pH was traditionally attributed to the leakage of acidic gastric contents through the esophageal tear towards pleural space. Reports from Good et al. demonstrated that leukocyte metabolism may be the major contributing factor to the low pleural fluid pH in these patients (102), since patients with severe pleural infections and an intact esophagus frequently have a pleural pH below 6.0. Squamous epithelial cells are usually found in pleural fluid of patients with esophageal perforation, since these cells enter the pleural cavity through the esophageal perforation. Eriksen documented the presence of these cells in all of 14 such patients (103). The demonstration of food in the pleural fluid is the pathognomonic finding of esophageal perforation (104).

Simple chest radiography may be of help, since it reveals the pleural effusion and/or the pneumothorax, and it may reveal a mediastinal widening or the presence of air (pneumomediastinum) within the mediastinal compartments. Contrast radiological studies of the esophagus establish the diagnosis of esophageal perforation by detecting an esophageal disruption. Hexabrix, a water-soluble agent (320 mg/mL), is preferred to barium, because the latter, once it leaks into the mediastinum or pleural space, produces a marked inflammatory reaction in the pleura. Gastrographin or Hexabrix are not known to produce this reaction, but the former may cause bronchospasm (105). Contrast studies are positive in about 85% of patients, but when the perforation is small or has already closed spontaneously, the esophagogram may not be diagnostic. A chest CT scan may facilitate the diagnosis if the contrast studies are not helpful. The morphological alterations seen on chest CT that are suggestive of esophageal rupture include the presence of extraesophageal air, periesophageal fluid, and esophageal wall thickening, while occasionally the site of perforation may be visible.

The treatment for esophageal rupture and pleural effusion or pneumothorax (or pneumomediastinum) is surgical. Mediastinotomy with repair of the esophageal perforation and drainage of the pleural cavity and mediastinum is the surgical procedure of choice. Parenteral antibiotics should be given to treat mediastinitis and pleural infection. It is important to perform the operation as soon as possible, because any delay may increase the mortality rate.

G. Abdominal Surgical Procedures

Small pleural effusion is a usual finding following abdominal operations, particularly of the upper abdomen. According to George and Light, about 50% of patients develop small pleural effusions within 48–72 hours after a surgical procedure (106). Moreover, Nielsen et al. reported a more frequent incidence (about 70%) of pleural effusion after upper abdominal surgery (107).

Since in the majority of cases (80%) the pleural effusion is small, fluid is detected only in the lateral decubitus position. A larger and usually left-sided effusion may follow splenectomy. Thoracentesis is performed only when the thickness of the fluid layer is more than 10 mm on decubitus film. In about 80% of cases, the fluid is exudative and without any other characteristic findings. Other causes of postoperative pleural effusion are a pulmonary embolism, a respiratory infection with parapneumonic effusion, a postoperative atelectasis, and a subphrenic abscess. The majority of effusions occur within the first 72 hours after the abdominal surgery and resolve spontaneously.

H. Diaphragmatic Hernia

Diaphragmatic hernias can either cause or mimic a pleural effusion. When the hernia is strangulated, a pleural effusion is usually present.

Hernias through the diaphragm should be suspected whenever an apparent pleural effusion has an atypical shape or location. The presence of air in the herniated intestine is the diagnostic clue. The possibility of a strangulated diaphragmatic hernia should always be considered in patients with left pleural effusion and signs of an acute abdominal trauma. At least 90% of these hernias are traumatic and occur in the left side, because the liver protects the right hemidiaphragm (108). Strangulation may occur months or even years after a car accident, which is usually the cause of abdominal trauma.

Pleural fluid, almost always present, is a serosanguineous exudate, with predominantly polymorphonuclear leukocytes. The diagnosis is suggested by the presence of an air-fluid level in the left pleural space. Sometimes contrast imaging studies of the gastrointestinal tract (i.e., barium enema) are necessary to establish the diagnosis.

The treatment is imperative and consists of immediate surgical operation to prevent gangrene of the strangulated viscera (108).

I. Variceal Sclerotherapy

Endoscopic variceal sclerotherapy is nowadays the main form of treatment for patients who present with a hemorrhage from ruptured esophageal varices. The incidence of pleural effusion after the above procedure seems to depend on the sclerosant that has been used. Saks et al. report pleural effusions in 50% of 38 such patients in which 5% sodium morrhuate was used as a sclerosing agent (109). Similar are the results of Bacon et al. (48% of 65 patients) (110), who used the same sclerosant as in the Saks study. In contrast, Parikh et al. (111), who used absolute alcohol as the sclerosant, reported an incidence of pleural effusion in only 19% of 31 patients. Most of the effusions are small with no predilection for the right or left pleural cavity. Sometimes, bilateral pleural effusions have been observed.

Pathogenesis of the pleural effusion is probably related to the extravasation of the sclerosant into the esophageal mucosa, which results in an intense inflammatory reaction affecting the mediastinum and the pleura (110). Pleural fluid is usually exudative and no treatment is necessary, unless the fluid persists more than 1–2 days, the patient is febrile, and more than 25% of the hemithorax is occupied in chest x-ray. In such cases, a thoracentesis is necessary in order to rule out an infection or an esophagopleural fistula, especially if the fluid amylase level is high. An alternative method, endoscopic ligation of esophageal varices, significantly reduced the adverse effects associated with sclerotherapy, such as pyrexia, retrosternal pain, and pleural effusion (112).

J. Bilious Pleural Effusion

Bilious pleural effusion is a rare complication of biliary tract disorders and occurs only when there is a fistula from the biliary tract to the pleural space. The most common cause is a thoracoabdominal trauma, while less frequent causes include a parasitic (i.e., echinococcus), liver disease, suppurative complications of biliary tract obstruction, postoperative strictures of bile ducts, percutaneous biliary drainage, or the stent placement for an obstructed biliary system (113, 114). Very rarely, the biliary-pleural fistula is large enough to allow the passage of gallstones into the pleural cavity.

The instillation of bile into the pleural space produces an inflammatory reaction. The diagnosis should be suspected in any patient with an obstructed biliary system who presents a pleural effusion. Interestingly, the pleural fluid does not necessarily appear to be bile. Although the fluid bilirubin level may be lower than that anticipated, the ratio of the pleural fluid to serum bilirubin usually is greater than 1.0 in these patients (37).

The optimal treatment is the reestablishment of normal biliary drainage. In most cases of bilious pleural effusion, the treatment of choice consists of decortication of pleural space (113). It should be remembered that the incidence of empyema is high in these patients (about 50%), so clinicians should be aware of this complication to treat it effectively.

K. Pleural Effusion Following Liver Transplantation

Most patients who undergo a liver transplantation develop a postoperative pleural effusion. The frequency varies from 75 to 95% of patients, according to various studies (115,116). The pleural effusion usually develops within 72 hours of transplantation, usually is right-sided or bilateral, but in this case the amount of fluid on the right side is greater than that of the left side.

Pleural effusion following liver transplantation may be large and may cause respiratorysymptoms. Bilik et al. (117) reported that in 48 children who were recipients of a liver transplant, a large pleural effusion manifested in 23 and required the placement of chest tubes.

The pathogenesis of the liver transplant–induced pleural effusion is unclear as of yet. It has been suggested that the effusion may be due to irritation or injury of the right hemidiaphragm during the operation. The effusion gradually increases during the first 3 postoperative days and then gradually resolves within several weeks to several months. Patients with continuously enlarging effusions should be evaluated for subdiaphragmatic pathology (i.e., hematomas, abscesses, etc.). The pleural effusion can be prevented effectively if a fibrin sealant is sprayed on the undersurface of the diaphragm at the time of transplantation (118).

IV. Metastatic Pleural Effusions

Carcinoma of any organ can metastasize to the pleura. However, carcinomas of the lung, breast, ovary, and lymphomas account for approximately 80% of malignant pleural effusions (119). In approximately 6–7% of patients with malignant pleural effusions, the primary site is unknown when the diagnosis of malignant pleural effusion is first established. Neoplasms of the GI tract are recognized as rare causes of malignant pleural effusions. Carcinoma of the stomach is relatively more common, accounting for 1–3% of metastatic effusions, while colon carcinoma and pancreatic carcinoma are even more rare (less than 1% of malignant effusions) (120,121). Malignant effusions due to invasion of pleura from hepatocellular carcinoma (122) or cholangiocarcinoma (123) are extremely rare. The most common symptoms reported by patients with malignant pleural effusions are dyspnea, chest pain, weight loss, malaise, anorexia, and symptoms attributable to the tumor itself. Chest radiography is essential in revealing the pleural effusion. The size of the effusion usually is large, with the fluid occupying the entire hemithorax. Malignant disease is the most common cause of a massive pleural effusion.

The pleural fluid usually is an exudate. Most pleural effusions that meet exudative criteria by LDH level but not by the protein level are malignant. The presence of bloody fluid (red blood cell count >100,000 cells/mm^3) suggests malignant pleural disease. The predominant cells in the pleural fluid differential white cell count of these effusions are lymphocytes in about 45% and other mononuclear cells in about 40%. Pleural fluid eosinophilia is very uncommon.

In most cases, positive cytological examination of the fluid establishes the diagnosis. Pleural biopsy has a moderate diagnostic yield ranging from 40 to 74%, which may improve with thoracoscopy or open thoracotomy. However, these diagnostic procedures, if positive, establish the diagnosis of the pleural involvement by an adenocarcinoma, and they are not helpful in indicating the adenocarcinoma primary site. Immunohistochemical staining of the fluid may be of help, while the measurement of tumor markers in the fluid has no utility. Consequently, when clinicians face the challenge of diagnosing a pleural effusion secondary to adenocarcinoma of unknown primary site, they must perform an abdominal CT scan, contrast radiological examination of stomach and colon, gastroscopy, and colonoscopy. The palliative treatment of malignant pleural effusions, depending on the site of primary tumor and the symptoms, consists of repeated therapeutic thoracenteses, systemic chemotherapy, placement of chest tubes, chemical pleurodesis with intrapleural injection of a sclerosing agent, pleuroperitoneal shunt, and pleurectomy.

The prognosis in patients with malignant pleural effusions is not good, although it obviously varies according to the histological features of the tumor. The prognosis is worse if the pleural fluid glucose level is below 60 mg/dL or the pleural fluid pH is less than 7.30 (124). Low fluid glucose level and low fluid pH indicates that the patient has a high tumor burden in his pleural space. In a relatively recent series, the mean survival was 5 months with GI cancer (124).

References

1. Light RW. Transudative pleural effusions. In: Light RW, ed. Pleural Diseases. Philadelphia: Lippincott, Williams & Wilkins, 2001:96–107.
2. Johnston RF, Loo RV. Hepatic hydrothorax: studies to determine the source of the fluid and report of thirteen cases. Ann Intern Med 1964; 61:385–401.
3. Lieberman FL, Hidemura R, Peters RL, Reynolds TB. Pathogenesis and treatment of hydrothorax complicating cirrhosis with ascites. Ann Intern Med 1966; 64:341–351.
4. Rubinstein D, McInnes IE, Dudley FJ. Hepatic hydrothorax in the absence of clinical ascites: diagnosis and management. Gastroenterology 1985; 88:188–191.
5. Cardenas A, Gines P. Pathogenesis and treatment of fluid and electrolyte imbalance in cirrhosis. Semin Nephrol 2001; 21:308–316.
6. Datta N, Mishkin FS, Vasinrapee P, Niden AH. Radionuclide demonstration of peritoneal-pleural communication as a cause for pleural fluid. JAMA 1984; 13:210–252.
7. Mouroux J, Hebuterne X, Perrin C, Venissac N, Benchimol D, Rampal P, Richelme H. Treatment of pleural effusion of cirrhotic origin by videothoracoscopy. Br J Surg 1994; 81:546–547.
8. Lazaridis KN, Frank JW, Krowka MJ, Kamath PS. Hepatic hydrothorax: pathogenesis, diagnosis and management. Am J Med 1999; 107:262–267.
9. Degawa M, Hamasaki K, Yano K, Nakao K, Kato Y, Sakamoto I, Nakata K, Eguchi K. Refractory hepatic hydrothorax treated with transjugular intrahepatic portosystemic shunt. J Gastroenterol 1999; 34:128–131.
10. Schuster DM, Mukundan S Jr, Small W, Fajman WA. The use of the diagnostic radionuclide ascites scan to facilitate treatment decision for hepatic hydrothorax. Clin Nucl Med 1998; 23:16–18.
11. Mittal BR, Maini A, Das BK. Peritoneopleural communication associated with cirrhotic ascites: scintigraphic demonstration. Abdom Imaging 1996; 21:69–70.
12. Park CH, Pham CD. Hepatic hydrothorax: scintigraphic confirmation. Clin Nucl Med 1995; 20:278–280.
13. Kakizaki S, Katakai K, Yoshinaga T, Higuchi T, Takayama H, Takagi H, Nagamine T, Mori M. Hepatic hydrothorax in the absence of ascites. Liver 1998; 18:216–220.
14. Daly JJ, Potts JM, Gordon L, Buse MG. Scintigraphic diagnosis of peritoneopleural communication in the absence of ascites. Clin Nucl Med 1994; 19:892–894.
15. Benet A, Vidal F, Toda R, Siurama R, De Virgala CM, Richart C. Diagnosis of hepatic hydrothorax in the absence of ascites by intraperitoneal injection of 99m-Tc Fluor colloid. Postgrad Med 1992; 68:153–154.
16. Light RW, Jenkinson SG, Minh V, George RB. Observations on pleural pressures as fluid is withdrawn during thoracentesis. Am Rev Respir Dis 1980; 121:799–804.
17. Xiol X, Castellvi JM, Guardiola J, Sese E, Castellote J, Perello A, Cervantes X, Iborra MJ. Spontaneous bacterial empyema in cirrhotic patients: a prospective study. Hepatology 1996; 23:719–723.
18. Runyon BA. Care of patients with ascites. N Engl J Med 1994; 330:337–342.
19. Rossle M, Ochs A, Gulberg V, Siegerstetter V, Holl J, Deibert P, Olschewski M, Reiser M, Gerbes AL. A comparison of paracentesis and transjugular intrahepatic

portosystemic shunting in patients with ascites. N Engl J Med 2000; 342:1701–1707.
20. Gordon FD, Anastopoulos HT, Crenshaw W, Gilchrist B, McEniff N, Falchuk KR, LoCicero J III, Lewis WD, Jenkins RL, Trey C. The successful treatment of symptomatic, refractory hepatic hydrothorax with transjugular intrahepatic portosystemic shunt. Hepatology 1997; 25:1366–1369.
21. Haskal ZJ, Zuckerman J. Resolution of hepatic hydrothorax after TIPS placement. Chest 1994; 106:1293–1295.
22. Strauss RM, Martin LG, Kaufman SL, Boyer TD. Transjugular intrahepatic portal systemic shunt for the management of symptomatic cirrhotic hydrothorax. Am J Gastroenterol 1994; 89:1520–1522.
23. Conklin LD, Estrera AL, Weiner MA, Reardon PR, Reardon MJ. Transjugular intrahepatic portosystemic shunt for recurrent hepatic hydrothorax. Ann Thorac Surg 2000; 69:609–611.
24. Vargas FS, Milanez JR, Filomeno LT, Fernandez A, Jatene A, Light RW. Intrapleural talc for the prevention of recurrence in benign or undiagnosed pleural effusions. Chest 1994; 106:1771–1775.
25. Mouroux J, Perrin C, Venissac N, Blaive B, Richelme H. Management of pleural effusion of cirrhotic origin. Chest 1996; 109:1093–1096.
26. Milanez de Campos JR, Filho LO, Werebe EC, Sette H Jr, Fernandez A, Filomeno LT, Jatene FB. Thoracoscopy and talc poudrage in the management of hepatic hydrothorax. Chest 2000; 118:13–17.
27. Yaguchi T, Harada A, Sakakibara T, Kamatsu Y, Yoshida S, Yokoi K, Murakami H, Fukuhara Y. A successful surgical repair of the hepatic hydrothorax using pneumoperitoneum: report of a case. Surg Today 1999; 29:795–798.
28. Romero S, Martin C, Hernandez L, Verdu J, Trigo C, Perez-Mateo M, Alemany L. Chylothorax in cirrhosis of the liver: analysis of its frequency and clinical characteristics. Chest 1998; 114:154–159.
29. Gatanaga H, Ohnishi S, Miura H, Kita H, Matsuhashi N, Kodama T, Minami M, Okudaira T, Imawari M, Yazaki Y. Retroperitoneal fibrosis leading to extrahepatic portal vein obstruction. Intern Med 1994; 33:346–350.
30. Sassa H, Kondo J, Tsuboi H, Sone T, Tsubone M. A case of idiopathic retroperitoneal fibrosis with chronic pericarditis. Intern Med 1992; 31:414–417.
31. Lankisch PG, Droge M, Becher R. Pleural effusions: a new negative prognostic parameter for acute pancreatitis. Am J Gastroenterol 1994; 89:1849–1851.
32. Talamini G, Uomo G, Pezzilli R, Rabitti PG, Billi P, Bassi C, Cavallini G, Pederzoli P. Serum creatinine and chest radiographs in the early assessment of acute pancreatitis. Am J Surg 1999; 177:7–14.
33. Maringhini A, Ciambra M, Patti R, Randazzo MA, Dardanoni G, Mancuso L, Termini A, Pagliaro L. Ascites, pleural, and pericardial effusions in acute pancreatitis. A prospective study of incidence, natural history and prognostic role. Dig Dis Sci 1996; 41:848–852.
34. Heller SJ, Noordhoek E, Tenner SM, Ramagopal V, Abramowitz M, Hughes M, Banks PA. Pleural effusion as a predictor of severity in acute pancreatitis. Pancreas 1997; 15:222–225.
35. Gumaste V, Singh V, Dave P. Significance of pleural effusion in patients with acute pancreatitis. Am J Gastroenterol 1992; 87:871–874.
36. Kaye MD. Pleuropulmonary complications of pancreatitis. Thorax 1968; 23:297–306.

37. Light RW. Pleural effusion secondary to diseases of the gastrointestinal tract. In: Light RW ed. Pleural Diseases. Philadelphia: Lippincott, Williams & Wilkins, 2001:226–240.
38. Light RW, Ball WC. Glucose and amylase in pleural effusions. JAMA 1973; 225: 257–260.
39. Makela A, Kuusi T, Nuutinen P, Schroder T. Phospholipase A2 activity in body fluids and pancreatic tissue in patients with acute necrotising pancreatitis. Eur J Surg 1999; 165:35–42.
40. Mayer JM, Rau B, Siech M, Berger HG. Local and systemic zymogen activation in human acute pancreatitis. Digestion 2000; 62:164–170.
41. Karakoyunlar O, Sivrel E, Tanir N, Denecli AG. High-dose octreotide in the management of acute pancreatitis. Hepatogastroenterology 1999; 46:1968–1972.
42. Miller TA, Lindenauer SM, Frey CF, Stanley JC. Proceedings: pancreatic abscess. Arch Surg 1974; 108:545–551.
43. Rockey DC, Cello JP. Pancreaticopleural fistula. Report of 7 patients and review of the literature. Medicine 1990; 69:332–344.
44. Standaert L, Verstappen G, Malbrain H, Van Bosstraeten B, Kerremans R, Eggermont E, Casteels-Van Daele M. Hemorrhagic pleural effusion and mediastinal mass: presenting symptoms in a child with pseudocyst of the pancreas. J Pediatr Gastroenterol Nutr 1983; 2:329–331.
45. Ahmad N, Auld CD, Lawrence JR, Watson GD. Pancreatic mediastinal pseudocyst: report of two cases simulating intrathoracic disease. Scott Med J 1991; 36:146–147.
46. Zeilender S, Turner MA, Glauser FL. Mediastinal pseudocyst associated with chronic pleural effusions. Chest 1991; 99:1318–1319.
47. Lee DH, Shin DH, Kim TH, Park SS, Park KN, Lee JH. Mediastinal pancreatic pseudocyst with recurrent pleural effusion. Demonstration by endoscopic retrograde cholangiopancreatogram and subsequent computed tomography scan. J Clin Gastroenterol 1992; 14:68–71.
48. Iacono C, Procacci C, Frigo F, Andreis IA, Cesaro G, Caia S, Bassi C, Pederzoli P, Serio G, Dagradi A. Thoracic complications of pancreatitis. Pancreas 1989; 4:228–236.
49. Izbicki JR, Wilker DK, Waldner H, Rueff FL, Schweiberer L. Thoracic manifestations of internal pancreatic fistulas: report of five cases. Am J Gastroenterol 1989; 84:265–271.
50. Uchiyama T, Suzuki T, Adachi A, Hiraki S, Izuka N. Pancreatic pleural effusion: case report and review of 113 cases in Japan. Am J Gastroenterol 1992; 87:387–391.
51. Branca P, Rodriguez RM, Rogers JT, Ayo DS, Moyers JP, Light RW. Routine measurement of pleural fluid amylase is not indicated. Arch Intern Med 2001; 161:228–232.
52. Kramer MR, Saldana MJ, Cepero RJ, Pitchenik AE. High amylase levels in neoplasm-related pleural effusion. Ann Intern Med 1989; 110:567–569.
53. Tokoo M, Oguchi H, Kawa S, Homma T, Nagata A. Eosinophilia associated with chronic pancreatitis: an analysis of 122 patients with definite chronic pancreatitis. Am J Gastroenterol 1992; 87:455–460.
54. Bronner MH, Marsh WH, Stanley JH. Pancreaticopleural fistula: demonstration by computed tomography and endoscopic retrograde cholangiopancreatography. J Comput Tomogr 1986; 10:167–170.

55. Closset J, Gelin M. The management of pancreatic ascites and pancreaticopleural effusion. Acta Gastroenterol Belg 2000; 63:269–270.
56. Pederzoli P, Bassi C, Falconi M, Albrigo R, Vantini I, Micciolo R. Conservative treatment of external pancreatic fistulae with parenteral nutrition along or in combination with continuous intravenous infusion of somatostatin, glucagon or calcitonin. Surg Gynecol Obstet 1986; 163:428–432.
57. Singh P, Holubka J, Patel S. Acute mediastinal pancreatic fluid collection with pericardial and pleural effusion. Complete resolution after treatment with octreotide acetate. Dig Dis Sci 1996; 41:1966–1971.
58. Safadi BY, Marks JM. Pancreatic-pleural fistula: the role of ERCP in diagnosis and treatment. Gastrointest Endosc 2000; 51:213–215.
59. Hastier P, Rouquier P, Buckley M, Simler JM, Dumas R, Delmont JP. Endoscopic treatment of wirsungo-cysto-pleural fistula. Eur J Gastroenterol Hepatol 1998; 10:527–529.
60. Kotsis L, Agocs L, Kostic S, Vadasz P. Transdiaphragmatic cyst-jejunostomy with Roux-en-Y loop for an exclusively mediastinal pancreatic pseudocyst. Scand J Thorac Cardiovasc Surg 1996; 30:181–183.
61. Tsang TM, Tam PK. Pancreatic pleural effusion: an indication for emergency distal pancreatectomy and Roux-en-Y pancreatico-jejunostomy. J Pediatr Surg 1995; 30:1632–1633.
62. Christensen NM, Demling R, Mathewson C Jr. Unusual manifestations of pancreatic pseudocysts and their surgical management. Am J Surg 1975; 130:199–205.
63. Faling LJ, Gerzof SG, Daly BD, Pugatch RD, Snider GL. Treatment of chronic pancreatic pleural effusion by percutaneous catheter drainage of abdominal pseudocyst. Am J Med 1984; 76:329–333.
64. Lang EK, Paolini RM, Pottmeyer A. The efficacy of palliative and definitive percutaneous versus surgical drainage of pacreatic abscesses and pseudocysts. South Med J 1991; 84:55–64.
65. Brelvi ZS, Jonas ME, Trotman BW, Dodda G, DaCosta JA, Cho KC, Sundaram NK, Kim KH. Nasopancreatic drainage: a novel approach for treating internal pancreatic fistulas and pseudocysts. J Assoc Acad Minor Phys 1996; 7:41–46.
66. Lipsett PA, Cameron JL. Internal pancreatic fistula. Am J Surg 1992; 163:216–220.
67. Cameron JL, Kieffer RS, Anderson WJ, Zuidema GD. Internal pancreatic fistulas: pancreatic ascites and pleural effusions. Ann Surg 1976; 184:587–593.
68. Hotz J, Goebell H, Herfarth C, Probst M. Massive pancreatic ascites without carcinoma. Report of three cases. Digestion 1977; 15:200–216.
69. Uchiyama T, Yamamoto T, Mizuta E, Suzuki T. Pancreatic ascites—a collected review of 37 cases in Japan. Hepatogastroenterology 1989; 36:244–248.
70. Parekh D, Segal I. Pancreatic ascites and effusion. Risk factors for failure of conservative therapy and the role of octreotide. Arch Surg 1992; 127:707–712.
71. da Cunha JE, Machado M, Bacchela T, Penteado S, Mott CB, Jukemua J, Pinotti HW. Surgical treatment of pancreatic ascites and pancreatic pleural effusion. Hepatogastroenterology 1995; 42:748–751.
72. Kochhar R, Goenka MK, Nagi B, Singh K. Pancreatic ascites and pleural effusion treated by endoscopic pancreatic stent placement. Indian J Gastroenterol 1995; 14:106–107.

73. Connell TR, Stephens DH, Carlson HC, Brown ML. Upper abdominal abscess: a continuing and deadly problem. Am J Roentgenol 1980; 134:759–765.
74. Sanders RC. Post-operative pleural effusion and subphrenic abscess. Clin Radiol 1970; 21:308–312.
75. Kelty CJ, Thorpe JA. Empyema due to spilled gall stones during laparoscopic cholecystectomy. Eur J Cardiothorac Surg 1998; 13:107–108.
76. Sherman NJ, Davis JR, Jesseph JE. Subphrenic abscess: a continuing hazard. Am J Surg 1969; 117:117–123.
77. Carter R, Brewer LA. Subphrenic abscess: a thoracoabdominal clinical complex. Am J Surg 1964; 108:165–174.
78. Alexander ES, Proto AV, Clark RA. CT differentiation of subphrenic abscess and pleural effusion. Am J Roentgenol 1983; 145:47–51.
79. Chu KM, Fan ST, Lai EC, Lo CM, Wong J. Pyogenic liver abscess. An audit of experience over the past decade. Arch Surg 1996; 131:148–152.
80. Roy R, Goyal RK, Gupta N. Tuberculous liver abscess. J Assoc Physicians India 2000; 48:241–243.
81. Dykhuisen RS, Douglas G, Weir J, Gould IM. *Corynebacterium afermentans* subsp. *Lipophilum*: multiple abscess formation in brain and liver. Scand J Infect Dis 1995; 27:637–639.
82. Lee KT, Sheen PC, Chen JS, Ker CG. Pyogenic liver abscess: multivariate analysis of risk factors. World J Surg 1991; 15:372–377.
83. Wong KP. Percutaneous drainage of pyogenic liver abscesses. World J Surg 1990; 14:492–497.
84. Baek SY, Lee MG, Cho KS, Lee SC, Sung KB, Auh YH. Therapeutic percutaneous aspiration of hepatic abscesses: effectiveness in 25 patients. AJR Am J Roentgenol 1993; 160:799–802.
85. Light RW. Pleural diseases. Dis Mon 1992; 28:263–331.
86. Lyche KD, Jensen WA, Kirsch CM, Yenokida GG, Maltz GS, Knauer CM. Pleuropulmonary manifestations of hepatic amebiasis. West J Med 1990; 153:275–278.
87. Chuah SK, Chang-Chien CS, Sheen IS, Lin HH, Chiou SS, Chiu CT, Kuo CH, Chen JJ, Chiu KW. The prognostic factors of severe amebic liver abscess: a retrospective study of 125 cases. Am J Trop Med Hyg 1992; 46:398–402.
88. Munoz LE, Botello MA, Carillo O, Martinez AM. Early detection of complications in amebic liver abscess. Arch Med Res 1992; 23:251–253.
89. Tony JC, Martin TK. Profile of amebic liver abscess. Arch Med Res 1992; 23:249–250.
90. Sarr MG, Zuidema GD. Splenic abscess: presentation, diagnosis and treatment. Surgery 1982; 92:480–485.
91. Ho HS, Wisner DH. Splenic abscess in the intensive care unit. Arch Surg 1993; 128:842–848.
92. Green BT. Splenic abscess: report of six cases and review of the literature. Am Surg 2001; 67:80–85.
93. Tikkakoski T, Siniluoto T, Paivansalo M, Taavitsainen M, Leppanen M, Dean K, Koivisto M, Suramo I. Splenic abscess. Imaging and intervention. Acta Radiol 1992; 33:561–565.
94. Michel L, Grillo HC, Malt RA. Operative and nonoperative management of esophageal perforations. Ann Surg 1981; 194:57–63.

95. Reeder LB, DeFilippi VJ, Ferguson MK. Current results of therapy for esophageal perforation. Am J Surg 1995; 169:615–617.
96. Keszler P, Buzna E. Surgical and conservative management of esophageal perforation. Chest 1981; 80:158–162.
97. Maulitz RM, Good JT Jr, Kaplan RL, Reller RB, Sahn SA. The pleuropulmonary consequences of esophageal rupture: an experimental model. Am Rev Respir Dis 1979; 120:363–367.
98. Abbott OA, Mansour KA, Logan WD Jr, Hatcher CR Jr, Symbas PN. Atraumatic so-called "spontaneous" rupture of the esophagus. J Thorac Cardiovasc Surg 1970; 59:67–83.
99. Lemke T, Jagminas L. Spontaneous esophageal rupture: a frequently missed diagnosis. Am Surg 1999; 65:449–452.
100. Sherr HP, Light RW, Merson MH, Wolf RO, Taylor LL, Hendrix TR. Origin of pleural fluid amylase in esophageal rupture. Ann Intern Med 1972; 76:985–986.
101. Dye RA, Laforet EG. Esophageal rupture: diagnosis by pleural fluid pH. Chest 1974; 66:454–456.
102. Good JT Jr, Antony VB, Reller LB, Maulitz RM, Sahn SA. The pathogenesis of the low pleural fluid pH in esophageal rupture. Am Rev Respir Dis 1983; 127:702–704.
103. Eriksen KR. Oesophagopleural fistula diagnosed by microscopic examination of pleural fluid. Acta Chir Scand 1964; 128:771–777.
104. Drury M, Anderson W, Heffner JE. Diagnostic value of pleural fluid cytology in occult Boerhaave's syndrome. Chest 1992; 102:976–978.
105. Ginai AZ. Experimental evaluation of various available contrast agents for use in the gastrointestinal tract in case of suspected leakage: effects on pleura. Br J Radiol 1986; 59:887–894.
106. Light RW, George RB. Incidence and significance of pleural effusion after abdominal surgery. Chest 1976; 69:621–626.
107. Nielsen PH, Jensen SB, Olsen AD. Postoperative pleural effusion following upper abdominal surgery. Chest 1989; 96:1133–1135.
108. Aronchick JM, Epstein DM, Gefter WB, Miller WT. Chronic traumatic diaphragmatic hernia: the significance of pleural effusion. Radiology 1988; 168:675–678.
109. Saks BJ, Kilby AE, Dietrich PA, Coffin LH, Krawitt EL. Pleural and mediastinal changes following endoscopic injection sclerotherapy of esophageal varices. Radiology 1983; 149:639–642.
110. Bacon BR, Bailey-Newton RS, Connors AF Jr. Pleural effusions after endoscopic variceal sclerotherapy. Gastroenterology 1985; 88:1910–1914.
111. Parikh SS, Amarapurkar DN, Dhawan PS, Kalro RH, Desai HG. Development of pleural effusion after sclerotherapy with absolute alcohol. Gastrointest Endovasc 1993; 39:404–405.
112. Tsugawa K, Hashizume M, Migou S, Kishihara F, Kawanaka H, Tomikawa M, Tanoue K, Sugimashi K. Endoscopic ligation of oesophageal varices compared with injection sclerotherapy in primary biliary cirrhosis. Eur J Gastroenterol Hepatol 2000; 12:1111–1115.
113. Ivatury RR, O'Shea J, Rohman M. Post-traumatic thoracobiliary fistula. J Trauma 1984; 24:438–441.
114. Delco F, Domenigheti G, Kauzlaric D, Donati D, Mombelli G. Spontaneous

biliothorax (thoracobilia) following cholecystopleural fistula presenting as an acute respiratory insufficiency. Chest 1994; 106:961–963.
115. Spizarny DL, Gross BH, McLoud T. Enlarging pleural effusion after liver transplantation. J Thorac Imaging 1993; 8:85–87.
116. Afessa B, Gay PC, Plevak DJ, Swensen SJ, Patel HG, Krowka MJ. Pulmonary complications of orthotopic liver transplantation. Mayo Clin Proc 1993; 68:427–434.
117. Bilik R, Yellen M, Superina RA. Surgical complications in children after liver transplantation. Pediatr Surg 1992; 27:1371–1375.
118. Uetsuji S, Komada Y, Kwon AH, Imamura A, Takai S, Kamiyama Y. Prevention of pleural effusion after hepatectomy using fibrin sealant. Int Surg 1994; 79:135–137.
119. Sahn SA. Malignant pleural effusions. In: Fishman AP, ed. Fishman's Pulmonary Diseases and Disorders. New York: McGraw-Hill, 1998:1429–1438.
120. Spriggs AI, Boddington MM. The Cytology of Effusions. 2d ed. New York: Grune & Stratton, 1968.
121. Anderson CB, Philpott GW, Ferguson TB. The treatment of malignant pleural effusions. Cancer 1974; 33:916–922.
122. Falconieri G, Zanconati F, Colautti I, Duoline S, Bonifacio-Gori D, DiBonito L. Effusion cytology of hepatocellular carcinoma. Acta Cytol 1995; 39:893–897.
123. Tamai M, Tanimura H, Yamaue H, Tsunoda T, Iwahasi M, Nakai T, Sugimoto Y, Asae M, Sasaki M, Aoki Y. Nasobiliary drainage for spontaneous bile peritonitis due to cholangiocarcinoma. Nippon Geka Hokan 1991; 60:195–202.
124. Sanchez-Armengol A, Rodriguez-Panadero F. Survival and talc pleurodesis in metastatic pleural carcinoma, revisited. Report of 125 cases. Chest 1993; 104:1482–1485.

42

Pleural Effusions in Pulmonary Embolism

LUIS PUENTE-MAESTU

Hospital General Universitario
 Gregorio Marañón
Madrid, Spain

VICTORIA VILLENA

Hospital Universitario 12 de Octubre
Madrid, Spain

I. Introduction

Pulmonary embolism (PE) is responsible for approximately 20 deaths per 100,000 inhabitants per year in the United States (1–3). Untreated PE is associated with an overall mortality rate of approximately 30%, although more than half is due to underlying conditions like cancer and myocardial infarction (4,5), which can be decreased to between 2 and 8% with the institution of appropriate treatment(6–8).

Most of the deaths due to PE occur within the first few hours of the event (6,9). Although the majority of patients with a PE live beyond these first few hours, it is apparent from long-term studies that, if untreated, recurrent PE, possibly with fatal consequences, is common in this population (7). It is, therefore, imperative that effective therapy be instituted after a thromboembolic event. However, it has been reported than only 30% of patients with PE at autopsy had received the diagnosis before death (10), and it is estimated that 5% of patients undergoing autopsies (11,12) had died of undiagnosed PE. Thus, many deaths can be prevented by a more accurate diagnosis of this condition (2).

Pleural effusion visible in the chest radiography occurs in 10–50% of patients with PE (13–20), thus, it may be a clue for PE diagnosis. Furthermore, among the patients of the International Cooperative Pulmonary Embolism Registry (ICOPER), 36% of the 39 patients diagnosed with PE at autopsy who had a chest radiograph had a pleural effusion (20). In studies conducted in Worcester, Massachusetts (2), and Olmsted County, Minnesota (3), the incidence of venous thromboembolism was 1 case per 1000 inhabitants per year. Symptomatic PE occurs in approximately 30% of the patients with deep venous thrombosis, but if one counts the asymptomatic events, some 50–60% of the patients with deep venous thrombosis may develop PE (21). From these data and the reported prevalence of pleural effusion around 25% (13–20) a fair amount of pleural effusions can be expected to be due to PE. To give only an example, more pleural effusions should be expected to be due to PE than to lung cancer (22). In striking contrast with those estimations, most clinicians feel that PE is an infrequent cause of pleural effusion (23). Furthermore, several series studying the prevalence of the different causes of pleural effusions find PE to be an uncommon cause, with figures lower than 6% of the effusions studied, in spite of different epidemiological contexts and durations of collection of the series (24–29). Possible explanations for the discrepancy are that PE is not often considered in undiagnosed pleural effusions, that pleural effusions related to PE are attributed to other causes easier to recognize when several concomitant potential causes are present (e.g., heart failure, atelectasis, or infection), or that postmortem diagnoses are not included in these series, which might underestimate the number of cases due to PE. For example, in an autopsy series of 290 patients with congestive heart failure and pleural effusions, 60 (21%) had pulmonary emboli (30).

The decision to pursue more invasive procedures or simply observe a patient with undiagnosed pleural effusion requires clinical judgment that is guided by the patient's presentation. Minimal disservice will be done to a patient if a diagnosis of metastatic malignancy to the pleura is not established for a few weeks; however, missing the diagnosis of acute pulmonary embolism can lead to significant morbidity and mortality in that period of time. Thus, in every patient with pleural effusion in which pulmonary thromboembolism is clinically probable, the diagnosis of PE should be sought.

II. Mechanisms

In the normal pleural space, there is a steady state in which the rate of the formation of liquid matches the rate of absorption. Therefore, pleural fluid starts to accumulate when either an increase in entry rate or a reduction in exit rate occurs. It is likely that both mechanisms contribute, since the absorbing pleural lymphatics have a large reserve capacity to deal with excess pleural liquid (31) and an isolated decrease in exit rate is unlikely to be the sole cause because the normal entry rate is low. Even if the exit of liquid ceased entirely, accumulation of fluid would take many days to become evident. As an example, at a normal entry rate in the pleural space of 0.01 ml/kg per h, only 15–20 mL would accumulate per day if the exit were completely shut off (31).

Potential mechanisms operating in PE include:

1. An increase in entry rates of liquid by increase in capillary permeability or by elevated hydrostatic pressures in pulmonary and systemic veins, and perhaps by lowering pleural pressure due to atelectasis.
2. Pulmonary embolism might also decrease exit rates of pleural liquid by increasing the systemic venous pressure (hindering lymphatic drainage) or perhaps by decreasing pleural pressure (hindering lymphatic filling). In one study, the calculated lymphatic flow for patients with pulmonary embolism was 0.18 mL/kg/h, which is only slightly lower than the maximal exit rate measured for sheep (0.28 mL/kg/h) (32).

Bynum and Wilson (33) studied the characteristics of pleural fluids associated with PE, and apparently 24% of the effusions were transudates (33). In a recent series (34) when all three Light's criteria to differentiate exudates from transudates (24) were employed, all the effusions associated with PE fell into the exudate category. The transudative effusions associated with PE described by Bynum and Wilson (33) had a protein ratio higher than what would be expected if the only source of fluid were the ultrafiltration from capillaries of the systemic circulation of the pleural membranes due to increased microvascular pressures. Thus, if they indeed were transudates, most of the liquid must had come from another source, such as the leakage of interstitial fluid of the lung (35). In the normal state, lung interstitial liquid has a lung-to-plasma protein concentration ratio of 0.7, but with increased flow due to increased pulmonary microvascular pressures, this ratio falls to 0.4–0.5 (36) which approximates to the characteristics described (33).

The most relevant mechanisms by which PE can produce exudates is the increase in the permeability of the capillaries of the lung by ischemia or more probably by release of inflammatory mediators such as vascular endothelial growth factor from the platelets of the thrombi (37). The excess of interstitial fluid so formed will leak into the pleural space throughout the visceral pleura (38). Apparently visceral pleura capillaries are supplied by bronchial circulation (39), and thus inflammatory mediators released into the pulmonary circulation do not influence them. It is possible, however, that inflammatory mediators released by the ischemia of the adjacent lung could affect visceral pleura capillaries.

As many as 65% of the pleural effusions associated with PE have a bloody appearance (33,34). The passing of red cells into the pleural space seems to be related, at least in part, to the existence of an adjacent pulmonary infarction, as indicated by the fact that 88% of the patients with infiltrates suggestive of infarction had bloody effusions (33). However, up to 30% of the pleural effusions associated with PE without apparent pulmonary infiltrates in chest x-ray also were bloody in appearance (33).

III. Clinical Picture

A. Epidemiology and Natural History

The incidence of PE increases with age; for each year increase in age its incidence doubles (2,3,40,41). Three quarters of the cases of PE occur in people older than 50 years and approximately 90% in those older than 40 years (41). Prospective series find a male predominance in venous thromboembolic episodes (2,3). Interestingly, though, retrospective reports of cases of PE find a slight female predominance (40,41). The available experience regarding pleural effusions associated with PE is limited, but it also appears that effusions due to PE are more frequent in patients older than 40 years and particularly in those older than 50 (26,27). It has to be noted, however, that in this range of ages the most prevalent cause recognized of exudative and transudative effusions are neoplasms and heart failure, respectively (24–27) (see Sec. I). Two series have described a male predominance in pleural effusions due to PE (27,34). The value of that finding is questionable, though, due to the small number of cases on which it is based.

Pleural effusion has been found in 10–50% of patients with PE (13–20). It was seen in 23% of the 2,322 patients included in the ICOPER who had chest radiographs (20) and it occurred more often when acute PE followed certain surgical procedures [e.g., general abdominal surgery (33%)] than others [e.g., orthopedic surgery (19%)]. Nevertheless, these differences may reflect the incidence of common radiographic abnormalities after specific surgical procedures, rather than different chest abnormalities caused by PE. The delay between initial presentation and thoracentesis in the study of Romero et al. (34) was 6.8 ± 5.2 days and between thoracentesis and the diagnosis of PE 2 ± 3 days.

In the absence of complications, pleural effusions tend to reach their maximum size early. In the only study to our knowledge aimed specifically at describing the clinical picture of pleural effusions associated with PE (14), the maximal size had been reached on the first chest radiograph in 57 of the 62 (92%) pleural effusions attributed to PE, and in only 2 (2%) did its size increase after the third day. In those two cases other causes (i.e., infection in one and recurrence of the PE in the other) were thought responsible for the late increase in effusion.

The course of resolution of these effusions has not been extensively studied. In the series of Bynum and Wilson (14), while 18 of 25 (72%) pleural effusions without parenchymal infiltrates resolved in less than 7 days, in all 31 patients with associated parenchymal consolidation effusions persisted longer than 7 days. This might reflect, at least in part, the larger size at the onset of effusions associated with pulmonary infarctions. No data are reported on the time resolution of the cases that persisted for more than 7 days (14). Thus, if an effusion increases after the third day, recurrent pulmonary embolism, hemothorax from anticoagulation, secondary infection, or an alternate diagnosis should be suspected (14,42,43).

Most effusions secondary to PE evolve to complete resolution; however, some can leave minimal sequels. In one study in which 58 angiographically proven pulmonary infarcts in 32 patients were followed by chest radiography, 9

(16%) showed pleural diaphragmatic adhesions and 6 (10%) localized pleural thickening. In all cases the features had improved when compared with the original abnormality (44).

The two main acute complications of pleural effusions associated to PE are infection (14) and hemothorax (42,43). Both are rare, presenting in less than 1% of the cases (14). The worst, because of its high mortality, is massive hemothorax. Its causes are not clear; it may be spontaneous, secondary to anticoagulation therapy or, likely, to both. The clinical picture consists of a sudden or rapid deterioration of the hemodynamic status of the patient, marked increase in the size of the pleural effusion, that usually fills the whole hemithorax, and secondary deterioration of the respiratory function (42,43). The hematocrit is frequently lower than previous values, although not as much as would be expected by the hemodynamic repercussion (42,43). The pleural fluid is frank blood (42,43). Hematocrit values that equal those of the blood are almost the rule. At autopsy massive unilateral hemothorax and evidence of parenchymal necrosis are seen (43,44). The term acute rupture of pulmonary infarction has been proposed for those cases in which parenchymal necrosis is evident (43). Acute hemothorax must be distinguished from recurrent embolism and from bleeding from other sources. The evident increase in the effusion on the chest radiography points toward this complication and the analysis of the fluid confirms its bloody nature. The treatment consists of immediate withdrawal of thrombolytic or anticoagulant medication, reposition of volume with fresh blood, and drainage of the pleural space (42,43). Emergency surgical intervention can be considered, although its utility has not been proven.

Another rare pleural complication after pulmonary infarction is the development of persistent, usually small, left-sided or bilateral pleural effusions (45,46). The effusions are associated with the classical signs and symptoms of the post–cardiac injury syndrome (47) (i.e., chest pleuritic in nature, but possibly oppressive precordial, pericardial rub, fever, leukocytosis, an elevated erythrocyte sedimentation rate, and variable combinations of pulmonary infiltrates and pleural or pericardial effusions). The clinical picture may mimic the radiographic manifestations of congestive heart failure, pulmonary embolism, or pneumonia. The effusions are hemorrhagic in 70% of cases and frankly bloody in 30% (45,46,48). The pleural fluid pH and glucose are normal, and the leukocyte differential reveals a predominance of polymorphonuclear leukocytes during the acute phase and mononuclear cells later in the course (45,46,48). Patients with post–cardiac injury syndrome typically present one week or more after a primary event such as a pulmonary infarction. In one report, for example, 65% of affected patients presented within 3 months and 100% within 12 months (49). In the post–pulmonary infarction syndrome, the delay from the embolic episode has not been well defined, but it may appear as early as 3 days after the PE event (45). The response to treatment with glucocorticoid for both postcardiac and postpulmonary syndromes is dramatic (45,46), but it would probably respond to nonsteroidal anti-inflammatory agents as well, since the majority of patients with post–cardiac injury syndrome (in whom glucocorticoids are relatively contraindicated) respond well to the initiation of aspirin (650 mg every 4–6 hours), ibuprofen (400–600 mg every 6 hours), or naproxen (375–500 mg every 12 hours) (50). The pathogenesis of this post–pulmonary infarction syndrome is unclear.

B. Clinical Manifestations

There is little information on whether patients with PE and pleural effusions present a different clinical picture than patients with PE but without pleural effusion. The available information suggests that chest pain on the side of the effusion is more common when PE has an associated pleural effusions (14,51). In one study of patients without prior cardiopulmonary disease who had a PE diagnosed by arteriography (52), pleural effusion was present in 67 of 119 (56%) of those patients who reported a syndrome of "pulmonary infarction or hemorrhage" (defined as pleuritic pain or hemoptysis as presentation symptoms). On the other hand, 6 of 31 (19%) of those reporting isolated dyspnea and none of the 5 (0%) patients with circulatory collapse had pleural effusion. In apparent contrast with this later figure, since it might be expected that death would occur predominantly in patients with circulatory collapse, the data of the ICOPER showed that 11 of the 39 (36%) patients diagnosed with PE at autopsy who had antemortem chest radiographs had pleural effusion (20). Nevertheless, death could have been caused by recurrence of the PE and not by a first episode causing the pleural effusion.

Effusions secondary to pulmonary embolism generally are small and occupy less than one third of the hemithorax, but they can be of any size (13–21,34). On plain chest radiographs they usually are unilateral, even in the presence of bilateral pulmonary emboli. Only 1 of 62 cases (2%) in the series of Bynum and Wilson (14) and 8 of 60 (13%) in the series of Romero et al. (34) presented bilateral effusion. Similar figures are reported in other series (24–27). It has been described, however, that in computed tomographs up to 75% of the effusions are bilateral (19). Pleural effusion may occur independently of the presence of visible infarction. In one series of the pleural effusions associated with PE, 55% of the patients showed an ipsilateral parenchyma infiltrate on the chest radiography. Interestingly, in those cases with associated infiltrates, the pleural effusions tended to be larger and persist for longer periods (14). Romero et al. (34) found pulmonary infiltrates suggestive of pulmonary infarction in 8 of the 60 patients studied (13%). In contrast, Talbot et al. (53) found associated infiltrates in 95% of the cases. Among the 119 patients reported by Stein and Henry (52) who had "pulmonary hemorrhage or infarction" as presenting syndrome, 56 had pleural effusion and 43 pleural-based opacities. Thus, a maximum of 63% of the cases could have had both. This figure is in accordance with the data reported by Bynum and Wilson (14). To our knowledge there are no specific data on the frequency of the combination of pleural effusion with other common radiographic signs associated with PE (i.e., cardiac enlargement, elevated hemidiaphragm, enlargement of pulmonary arteries, atelectasis, pulmonary congestion, oligemia) and their value to lead one to suspect PE in pleural effusions of difficult diagnosis.

C. Pleural Fluid Characteristics

There are few reports about the pleural fluid characteristics of effusions (33,34). In addition, the reported characteristics of pleural fluid associated with PE are quite variable (33,34).

Among the 26 patients of Bynum and Wilson (33), 24% of effusions were transudates (33). Nevertheless, pleural fluid lactate dehydrogenase (LDH) was not measured in all cases (33). In the series of Romero et al. (34) using all three Light's criteria for differentiating transudate from exudates (which include pleural effusion–to–plasma LDH ratio) (24), all effusions were classified as exudates.

A blood-tinged or bloody-appearing fluid has been reported in more than half of cases (33,34). The blood cell count is >10,000 cells/mm^3 in 66–73% of patients, and it is >100,000 cells/mm^3 in 15–18% of patients (33,34).

The white blood cell count ranges from <100 cells/mm^3 to >50,000 cells/mm^3 (33,34). A polymorphonuclear leukocyte predominance has been found in 60% of patients (33,34). Nevertheless, more than 80% lymphocytes may be found in 15% of patients (33). Pleural eosinophilia (> 10% eosinophils) has been also reported in around 20% of these patients (34,54). In addition, a higher mesothelial cell score in comparison to other effusions has been also found (34).

The characteristics though to be "typical" of pleural effusions due to PE, i.e., bloody exudates with a predominance of polymorphonuclear leukocytes, were seen only in 7 patients (27%) in the study of Bynum and Wilson (33).

IV. Diagnosis

The diagnostic value of pleural effusion in patients suspected of having a PE has been analyzed in several studies. Worsley et al. (17) looked at the predictive value of different radiological signs in 1063 patients involved in the Prospective Investigation of Pulmonary Embolism Diagnosis (PIOPED). The population consisted of patients in which PE was clinically suspected. Pleural effusions were noted in 47% of 383 and 39% of 680 patients with and without pulmonary embolism, respectively. Pleural effusion was a poor predictor of PE (17). In a subsample of 500 patients of the Prospective Investigative Study of Acute Pulmonary Embolism Diagnosis (PISA-PED), pleural effusion was seen in 45% of 202 patients with PE and 35% of 298 patients without PE. While the difference was statistically significant, again the specificity as diagnostic criterion for PE was low (55). Of patients diagnosed with PE by helical computed tomography, pleural effusions were seen in 16 of 28 (57%) patients with PE and in 36 of 64 (56%) patients without PE. Interestingly, by computed tomography the effusions were predominantly bilateral in both groups (75% of patients with PE and 72% of the group without PE) (19). In a different population of subjects, i.e., young patients who presented with acute chest pain, McNeil et al. (51) found that the presence of pleural effusion increased the likelihood of PE.

A few studies have looked at the predictive value for PE of the size of the effusion in patients in which PE had been clinically suspected, but the information produced is contradictory. While Goldberg et al. (56), in a retrospective study, reported that 43% of those with large pleural effusions actually had PE versus 28% and 30% of those with small pleural effusions and without pleural effusions, respectively, neither Talbot et al. (53) nor Shah et al. (19) (the latter using helical computed tomography) found that the size of the effusion discriminated between patients with and without PE. Furthermore, in the series of Talbot et al. (53), small effusions were more frequent in patients with PE than patients without PE.

The characteristics of pleural fluids associated with PE are quite variable (33). The pattern believed to be more specific, i.e., a blood-tinged exudate rich in polymorphonuclear leukocytes, occurs only in about 25% of cases, but the diagnostic value of this pattern has not been studied. Furthermore, an excessive reliance on the finding of blood-tinged pleural fluid can be misleading since 35–70% of the effusions associated with PE did not present this characteristic (23,33,34). Even in the presence of adjacent infarction, 12% of the effusions may not be blood stained (33). Thus, the characteristics of the fluid will not be helpful in a majority of cases, nevertheless, a thoracentesis is generally indicated to narrow the differential diagnosis.

Pulmonary embolism, therefore, should be a diagnostic consideration in every patient with an acute, unilateral pleural effusion, whether it is an exudate or a transudate, especially if small or medium in size or if associated with acute chest pain of pleuritic characteristics. Pleural effusions due to PE do not enlarge after the third day of presentation (14). If the effusion increases after the third day, recurrent pulmonary embolism, secondary infection of an alternate diagnosis should be suspected. Although PE is seldom the cause of significant bilateral pleural effusions in plain chest radiographs (14), in one series of bilateral effusions without enlarged cardiac shadow, 10 of 78 cases (13%) were diagnosed with PE (57). Particular caution is needed with effusions thought to be due to heart failure, since in certain circumstances a significant proportion of them can be due to or may have a concomitant PE (30,57).

A. Clinical Evaluation

The decision as to whether to further study a pleural effusion to exclude or confirm a pulmonary embolism should be based on the associated clinical picture. The most commonly reported symptoms, signs, and predisposing conditions found in several large cohorts are described in Table 1 (15,16,55,58). However, the frequency of many of these symptoms and signs is similar in patients who are though to have a PE do not (15,16,55). The PIOPED showed that among patients with PE the most frequent symptoms were dyspnea and chest pain and the most frequent signs tachycardia and tachypnea (15,16). The

Table 1 Incidence of Symptoms, Signs, and Predisposing Conditions in Patients with PE

	Incidence (%)
Symptoms	
Dyspnea	75–80
Pleuritic pain	44–74
Fainting or syncope	13–26
Cough	11–53
Hemoptysis (rarely massive)	9–30
Signs	
Tachypnea	70–92
Tachycardia	24–44
Fourth heart sound	24–34
Accentuated pulmonary component of the second heart sound	23–53
Rales	18–51
Signs of lower extremity deep venous thrombosis	17–32
Cyanosis	16–19
Fever	7–43
Preexisting diseases	
Cardiac or pulmonary diseases	33–38
Malignant neoplasm	6–10
Predisposing risk factors	
Immobilization	55–59
Surgery	40
Previous venous disease	34–43
Bone fracture of lower extremities	23

Source: Refs. 15,16,55,58.

prevalence of these symptoms and signs did not differ significantly from those patients who turned out not to have PE (15,16). Dyspnea, tachypnea, or pleuritic chest pain were present in 97% of the patients with confirmed PE (16). Miniati et al. (55) found that dyspnea and chest pain of sudden onset and fainting were significantly more frequent in patients with PE than in patients with suspected PE who did not have PE, while dyspnea of gradual onset, orthopnea, and fever were significantly more frequent in patients with suspected PE who did not have PE than in true positive cases with PE. At least one of the risk factors listed in Table 1 was present in 81% of patients with PE, but was also present in 69% of patients without PE (55). Immobilization, history of venous disease, and bone fractures of lower extremities prevailed significantly in patients with confirmed PE. However, the history of risk factors was of little value in discriminating patients with PE from patients without PE (55).

In conclusion, only a minority of patients with PE have no important clinical manifestation of the disease. However, no single symptom or sign or combination of them is sufficient to diagnose PE; in spite of their lack of specificity, combinations of symptoms, signs, and abnormalities or other simple

B. Laboratory Abnormalities

Routine laboratory findings including arterial blood gases are nonspecific (15,55,59,60). Arterial blood gases usually reveal hypoxemia, hypocapnia, and respiratory alkalosis, but 10–20% of patients with PE have an arterial oxygen pressure higher than 80 mmHg (15,55). Furthermore, the criterion that is considered most sensitive, the alveolar-arterial gradient for oxygen, was normal (i.e., <15 mmHg) in the 6% of patients with PE from the PIOPED study (15). In another recent study in patients referred to a tertiary hospital where it was found that 16% of 49 patients who had a positive diagnosis of PE had a normal alveolar-arterial gradient for oxygen (59). Neither of the subgroups presenting with or without dyspnea mean arterial oxygen pressures were significantly different between the PE and non-PE patients (59). In contrast, Egermayer et al. (60) found that arterial oxygen pressure higher than 80 mmHg had a negative predictive value of 97% for PE. The differences between the studies could have resulted from the type of population analyzed. In the PIOPED the frequency of normal alveolar-arterial gradient for oxygen in patients diagnosed with PE increased from 6 to 14% when the patients had no history or evidence of preexisting cardiac or pulmonary disease (15). The sensivity of arterial blood gases may depend on the age of the subjects as well. In one retrospective study 29% of patients less than 40 years old had arterial oxygen pressure higher than 80 mmHg compared with 3% in the older group (61). In another retrospective study of elderly patients, only 2.5% of 75 patients with confirmed PE had an arterial oxygen pressure higher than 75 mmHg (62).

The combination of an arterial oxygen pressure higher than 80 mmHg and a negative rapid red blood cell agglutination testing (SimpliRED) was useful in excluding all 40 patients with PE in an study of 517 subjects in which PE had been clinically suspected; however, only approximately 20% of the patients not diagnosed with PE met this criterion. Blood gas analysis may not be necessary if a D-dimer concentration lower than 500 ng/mL is found (see below). In fact only 2 of 49 (0.8%) patients with a negative SimpliRED had a PE (60).

Thus, arterial blood gas alterations are nonspecific, and in general patients with and without PE cannot be distinguished on the basis of either arterial oxygen pressure or alveolar-arterial gradient abnormalities (15,55,59,60). Most experience suggests that the sensitivity of arterial blood gas analysis is not high enough to rule out PE, although the sensitivity appears to increase with the age of the patient and the presence of underlying cardiac or pulmonary diseases. Even so, arterial blood gas analysis is necessary to initially assess the severity and, hence, to determine the most appropriate diagnostic approach (see multimodality algorithms). Besides a sudden deterioration of arterial blood gases in the context of a patient with acute respiratory symptoms (dyspnea, chest pain, fainting, or tachypnea), when both the symptoms and the abnormal alveolar-arterial gradient for oxygen cannot be explained by an alternative cause, especially if accompanied by risk factors for PE, there is a high clinical probability of PE (63). Physicians' clinical judgment has proven successful in assigning meaningful pretest probability in patients with suspected PE (64,65).

C. Electrocardiogram

Electrocardiogram is often abnormal, but the most frequent findings are generally nonspecific ST and T-wave changes, especially in V_1–V_4 leads (66). Other frequent abnormalities are tachycardia and atrial fibrillation (15,41,55,66,67). Seventy percent of patients without preexisting cardiovascular disease in PIOPED presented an abnormal electrocardiogram. The most common abnormalities (49%) were non-specific ST segment and T-wave changes (16). In the Urokinase Pulmonary Embolism Trial, electrocardiographic abnormalities were demonstrated in 87% of patients with massive or submassive PE. Only 26% had manifestations of right ventricle overload [t-wave inversion in right precordial leads, S1Q3/S1Q3T3, transient right bundle branch block, P-wave pulmonale or pseudoinfarction (S1S2S3)] (67). In the PISA-PED, right ventricular overload was seen in 50% of the patients with PE and 12% of the subjects without PE (55).

In summary, electrocardiogram often presents unspecific abnormalities, but it can be helpful in the integrative interpretation of pretest probability of PE.

D. Chest Radiography

Only around 10–25% of chest radiographs were interpreted as normal in a large series of patients with PE (17,20,41,53,55). The most frequent changes described in prospective studies are described in Table 2. In the study of Worsley et al. (17), the most common chest radiographic finding was atelectasis and/or parenchymal areas of increased opacity; however, the prevalence was not significantly different from that in patients without PE. Oligemia (Westermark sign), prom-

Table 2 Chest Radiographic Abnormalities Associated with Acute Pulmonary Embolism

Abnormality	Incidence (%)
Cardiac enlargement	27–61
Pleural effusion	23–45
Elevated hemidiaphragm	20–62
Pulmonary artery enlargement	16–19
Atelectasis	18–32
Infiltrate	12–17
Oligemia	8–45
Pulmonary infarction	5–15
Pulmonary congestion	1–14
Amputation of pulmonary artery	<1–15

Source: Refs. 17,20,53,55.

inent central pulmonary artery (Fleischner sign), pleural-based area of increased opacity (Hampton hump), vascular redistribution, pleural effusion, elevated diaphragm, and enlarged hilum were poor predictors of PE. Miniati et al. (55) found that amputation of hilar artery, oligemia, or consolidations compatible with infarction were present in 45, 36, and 15% of patients with PE, respectively. These abnormalities occurred only in 1% of patients without PE. They were good predictors of PE when associated with certain symptoms. Other radiographic findings such as elevated hemidiaphragm, atelectasis, and pleural effusion had much lower specificity. Interstitial edema was found in 9% of patients without PE and 1% of those with PE. Using helical computed tomography, no radiological sign, with the exception of wedge sapped infiltrates, differentiated between effusions due to PE and those due to other causes (19).

Thus, although chest radiographs are essential in the investigation of suspected PE, their main value is to exclude diagnoses that clinically mimic PE, to aid in the integrative interpretation of pretest probability of PE and of the ventilation-perfusion scan. The signs considered more specific are rare in most series, and their predictive value is not proven.

E. Clinical Evaluation Probability Assessment

With the information discussed above, clinicians appear to be able to assign meaningful probabilities for PE prior to specific tests. In PIOPED, for example, clinical probabilities were rated as low (0–19%), intermediate (20–79%), or high (80–100%). Among patients determined clinically to have a high probability of disease prior to lung scanning, 67% were found to have PE; in contrast, only 9% of those assigned a low probability had it, but intermediate probabilities were assigned in the majority of patients (64%) (64). In another large multicentric trial, the PISA-PED, a standardized diagnostic protocol was used, and a clinical probability of PE was assigned out of three alternatives: very likely (90%), possible (50%), or unlikely (10%). PE was diagnosed in only 9% of the patients with unlikely clinical presentation and in 91% of those in whom the disease was considered likely on clinical grounds. Again, the majority of patients had intermediate probabilities (65). Similar findings were noted in other large prospective studies (68,69). Miniati et al. (55) analyzed 500 patients of the PISA-PED and found that at least one of three symptoms (sudden onset dyspnea, chest pain, or fainting) was present in 96% of the patients with PE compared with 59% of the patients without PE. At least one of these three symptoms was associated with one or more of the following abnormalities: electrocardiographic signs of right ventricle overload, radiographic signs of oligemia amputation of the hilar artery, or pulmonary consolidation compatible with infarction in 81% of the patients with PE and only 7% of the patients without PE. Using this criterion (association of at least one sign with one of electrocardiographic or radiologic abnormalities mentioned above) in a validation group of 250 in which the prevalence of PE was 42%, the sensitivity for PE was 84% and the specificity 95%. However, in this study the frequency of findings like oligemia, consolidation suggestive of infarction, and amputation of hilar artery was quite high compared with other series (20,41,53). Another algorithm was based on the combination of three blocks of information: (1) several symptoms or signs and radiological, arterial blood gases or electrocardiographic abnormalities, (2) the clinician assessment of the likelihood of an alternative diagnosis, and (3) the presence of risk factors used to classify patients in three groups (high, moderate, or low) as to pretest probability of PE. The scheme was applied to 1239 patients with suspected PE; PE was ultimately documented in 3% of patients with a low pretest probability, 28% with a moderate pretest probability, and 78% with a high pretest probability (70). In contrast with this experience, the ability of clinicians, either subjectively or by using standardized clinical models, to estimate meaningful pretest probabilities for PE has been questioned in a recent study (71).

Thus, the systematic assessment of the clinical probability after careful consideration of risk factors, presentation, and screening laboratory test is recommended. PE is very unlikely in those not presenting any important clinical manifestation of the disease. In the remainder, the assessment of a pretest clinical probability will be helpful for the subsequent diagnostic work-up.

F. D-dimer

Levels of D-dimer higher than 500 ng/mL are detectable in nearly all patients with PE with accurate assays (72). An elevated D-dimer is nonspecific, however, and it is commonly present in hospitalized patients limiting its usefulness in such patients (72). A meta-analysis of 11 studies pooling 1337 patients revealed a negative predictive value of D-dimer assay for PE of 94%. This finding suggests that further testing may not be necessary if a D-dimer concentration could be accurately and rapidly determined to be lower than 500 ng/mL (73). Most [but not all (74)] latex tests are not sufficiently accurate, whereas the ELISA is complex and takes several hours, thus the development of inexpensive rapid tests has renewed the interest in D-dimer. Rapid, semiquantitative red blood cell agglutination testing (SimpliRED) that detects D-dimer by an antibody reaction causing agglutination of the patient's own red cells using whole blood has been tested in two trials involving 1177 (75) and 517 (60) patients, respectively. In the first study patients with a low pretest probability and a negative D-dimer by SimpliRED had a 99% negative predictive value (74). In the second a negative SimpliRED assay had a negative predictive value of 98%, regardless of the pretest probability (60). Another rapid, automated, quantitative assay (Liatest) has been shown to have a negative predictive value of 100% (76).

This experience suggest that a D-dimer lower than 500 ng/mL or a negative SimpliRED test will allow to exclude PE when the clinical probability is low, but the D-dimer assay may be insufficient as a stand-alone test in patient populations with a high prevalence of PE (77,78). Low D-dimer levels have been found in only about 25% of patients without PE, and it is unlikely to be helpful in patients with recent surgery (within 3 months) or with malignancy, since so few of these patients have D-dimer levels below 500 ng/mL (73).

Another important consideration with D-dimer is that, despite promising data, practical experience may be difficult to generalize since test accuracy varies largely depending on the methodology (79).

G. Lung Scanning

Lung scanning is probably the most frequently used test to aid in the diagnosis of PE in patients in whom a careful physical examination and routine diagnostic tests have failed to reveal a specific diagnosis to explain the pulmonary symptoms.

Three prospective studies, involving a considerable number of patients, on ventilation/perfusion scanning in the diagnosis of PE (64,80,81) have established the value of this technique. In the study of Hull et al. (80) a high-probability scan had a positive predictive value of 86%, but occurred in only 58% of patients with angiographically proven PE. In patients with low-probability scans the prevalence of PE was between 25 and 36%, depending on the size of the defect. In a subsequent study Hull and Raskob (81) analyzed prospectively in 483 patients with clinically suspected PE with two different methods of interpretation. High-probability scans had a sensitivity and specificity of 57–53% and 90–92%, respectively, with each of the methods. Approximately 25% of patients with low-probability scans had a PE. In the PIOPED study (64), only 14 of 480 patients (3%) who did not have evidence of PE on angiography had high-probability ventilation/perfusion scans (specificity 97%). The false-positive rate of high-probability lung scans was 14%. Many of these false positives had either residual vascular defects from prior pulmonary emboli or cancer with vascular involvement. Excluding patients with prior pulmonary embolism, for example, reduced the false-positive rate for high probability scans to 9%. The sensitivity of high-probability scans was 41%. Of 239 patients with low-probability scans and a definite angiographic diagnosis, 39 (16%) had pulmonary embolism. With the initial "normal" criterion for ventilation/perfusion lung scan, 5 of 57 patients (9%) had false negatives. These few cases of emboli were actually near-normal scans with marginal defects, not fully normal scans. Thus, from the three studies quoted it can be concluded that (1) a normal perfusion lung scan virtually excludes the diagnosis of PE, (2) if the patient has no previous history of PE, a high-probability lung scan indicates a high likelihood of emboli, particularly in patients with a high clinical suspicion, (3) the majority of patients have nondiagnostic patterns (i.e., low or intermediate probability), and (4) the concept of "low-probability" ventilation/perfusion is misleading because of the fairly high frequency of PE on patients exhibiting this scan pattern (82), but the combination of a low-probability scan with a low probability on clinical grounds was associated with 4% of false negatives in the PIOPED, most of them with small emboli (64). It was concluded that further testing might not be needed to exclude emboli in such patients.

A different interpretation of lung scanning was tested in 890 patients in the PISA-PED study (65). A set of criteria defined four categories of perfusion lung scan-normal, near normal, abnormal compatible with pulmonary embolism (PE+), and abnormal not compatible with pulmonary embolism (PE−). It is important to point out that single wedge-shaped segmental perfusion defects, which have not been found to be consistent predictors of PE (83), were included in the PE+ category. Normal or near-normal scans occurred in 220 patients who did not undergo further testing. A definitive diagnosis was established in 563 of the 670 patients with abnormal scans, in 173 based on follow-up results, and the remainder on pulmonary angiography. Of the 347 patients with PE, 320 had a PE+ scan (sensitivity of 92%). On the other hand, 192 of the 216 patients in whom PE was excluded had a PE− scan (specificity of 89%). The predictive values of the PE+ and PE− scans were 93% and 88%, respectively. When clinical pictures assessed as very likely or possible for PE were combined with a PE+ perfusion scan, the PE prevalences were 99% and 93%, respectively. Three percent of the patients who had an unlikely clinical evaluation associated with a PE− scan had a confirmed PE. These three "diagnostic" patterns were observed in 76% of the patients. Thus, this strategy appears to be superior to PIOPED results since the proportion of undiagnosed patients is reduced to 25%, but the study populations differed. In the PISA-PED 24% of the patients had normal scans compared with 2% in the PIOPED. The authors argue that certain lesions frequently associated with PE, like atelectasis and infiltrates (17), which have an effect not only upon the perfusion but also on the ventilation, hinder the interpretation of ventilation/perfusion scans with the PIOPED criteria. Also, the scattered radiation from previously administered 99mTc particles may decrease the accuracy of the washout phase of the ventilation scan, particularly if 99mTc is used for the ventilation scan (84).

Chest radiographs are used to evaluate lung scans for PE in patients with pleural effusions. Mobile effusions may gravitate to different regions of the pleural space, depending upon the position of patients, and thus apparent defects can be seen in different locations than the effusion in the chest radiograph when each is performed in different positions (85). In addition, pleural effusion may enter the major fissures when the patients lie down. In moderate or large effusions a therapeutic thoracentesis before ventilation/perfusion scan has been recommended (85), measuring the pleural fluid pressure in order to aspirate as much fluid as possible (86). Following the criteria of Biello et al. (87) for the interpretation of defects in lung scans corresponding with radiological abnormalities, Goldberg et al. (56) found that 45% of patients with matched ventilation-perfusion defects of the same size as the effusion were angiographically positive for PE. They concluded that matched ventilation/perfusion scans corresponding to radiologically evident pleural effusions are of intermediate probability for PE. Thus, they did not recommend revision of the traditional lung interpretative criteria based upon pleural effusions.

The positive predictive value of high-probability and normal ventilation-perfusion scans is not affected by the presence of underlying cardiac or respiratory disease, although the frequency of nondiagnostic scans is increased, especially in COPD patients (88,89).

As discussed above, up to 70% of patients present with combinations of clinical and lung ventilation/perfusion scan that cannot confirm or exclude the diagnosis of pulmonary emboli with certainty (64,80,81). They generally should undergo pulmonary angiography to definitively establish or exclude the diagnosis, but this technique is not readily available, and in many settings the majority of these patients are managed without a definitive diagnosis, potentially exposing them to the risks of unnecessary anticoagulation or undertreatment of acute PE (90). Because of this multimodality noninvasive strategies have been proposed. They will be discussed below.

H. Noninvasive Multimodality Algorithms

Because lung scan is often inconclusive and high-quality angiography is not widely available, interest has turned to strategies based in noninvasive tests for lower extremity venous thrombosis, the refinement of the clinical assessment of pretest probability of PE, or D-dimer determination. These approaches are only considered appropriate, however, if the patient is stable (i.e., hemodynamically stable and without severe hypoxemia).

Compared to venography, color-flow Doppler with compression ultrasound (duplex ultrasound venography) has high sensitivity (89–100%) and specificity (89–100%) for the detection of a first episode of proximal deep venous thrombosis (91). Impedance plethysmography (IPG) offers lower sensitivity, similar specificity, is portable, and its cost is lower in comparison to duplex venous ultrasonography (92). One strategy, therefore, is that, in patients with intermediate clinical or scan probabilities, a positive venous study would justify anticoagulation. The question though is what to do with those with a negative leg study. Hull et al. (93) studied 1564 patients with suspected PE and adequate cardiopulmonary reserve with ventilation/perfusion scan and serial impedance plethysmography performed over 2 weeks. Anticoagulation was withheld in 627 patients with nondiagnostic lung scans and negative serial impedance plethysmography, and only 12 (1.9%) developed a deep venous thrombosis on long-term follow-up compared with 0.7% of patients with normal lung scans and 5.5% patients with high-probability scans who received anticoagulation therapy. Wells et al. (94) prospectively studied 1239 patients with suspected PE. They used defined criteria for pretest probability and a defined diagnostic algorithm of ventilation/perfusion scanning, duplex ultrasonography of the legs, contrast venography, and pulmonary angiography. With their strategy only 46 patients (3.7%) required venography or pulmonary angiography, and only 6 of 1022 patients (0.6%) considered negative for PE by the algorithm had thromboembolic events during the 3-month follow-up period. The same group of investigators has published a similar model in which a negative SimpliRED D-dimer assay coupled with a low clinical likelihood of pulmonary embolism effectively excluded the diagnosis of PE (95).

Perrier et al. (96) prospectively studied 918 outpatients referred to the hospital because deep venous thrombosis or PE was suspected. They, too, utilized defined criteria for pretest clinical probability of both conditions and a diagnostic algorithm based on D-dimer measurement, compression ultrasonography of the legs of ventilation/perfusion scanning, duplex ultrasonography of the legs, contrast venography, and pulmonary angiography. The novelty was that ultrasonography of the legs was performed before ventilation/perfusion scanning. A D-dimer lower than 500 ng/mL (by a rapid ELISA) ruled out venous thromboembolism in 286 patients (31%). Evidence of deep venous thrombosis was found in 157 (17%). Lung scan was diagnostic in 80 (9%). PE was excluded also in patients with a negative duplex leg ultrasonography and low or intermediate clinical probability of deep venous thrombosis [236 (26%)] and patients with low clinical probability for PE, and nondiagnostic lung scan [107 (12%)]. Pulmonary angiography was done in 50 (5%) and phlebography in 2 (less than 1%) of the patients. The 3-month risk of thromboembolic events was 1.8% in those in whom PE was excluded.

A different group devised an algorithm based upon 500 consecutive patients of the PISA-PED and then validated it in an additional 250 consecutive patients (55). Pretest probability was based upon the presence of sudden onset dyspnea, chest pain, or syncope, as well as certain electrocardiographic or radiographic findings. This probability was combined with the results of a perfusion scan (without accompanying ventilation images) to yield a final estimate of the likelihood of PE. Of the 750 patients studied, 167 (21%) had a normal perfusion scan and were not further studied. Of the remaining 583, the diagnostic criteria employed would have classified 271 (36%) as having PE with a specificity of 98% and 187 as not having PE (25%) with a specificity of 99%. With this approach, however, some 18%, still need pulmonary angiography for diagnosis. The prevalence of PE was low in this study.

The effectiveness of noninvasive strategies at reducing angiography rates is higher when the PE prevalence is low. False-positive venous ultrasound studies (~3%) would result in overuse of anticoagulation. Another limitation is that a negative single noninvasive study does not exclude PE and that to improve sensitivity, serial noninvasive studies of the leg veins may be needed. The cost-effectiveness of these approaches has been questioned. It is dependent on the local cost of the various diagnostic tests and the availability of alternatives (i.e., pulmonary angiography of quality).

I. Pulmonary Angiography

This is the definitive diagnostic technique in PE. A negative pulmonary angiogram seems to exclude clinically relevant pulmonary embolism. Mortality is <0.5% and morbidity about 5%, usually related to catheter insertion or contrast reactions (64,97).

J. Helical Computed Tomography

The role of this technique for diagnosing acute PE is the subject of particularly intense debate. Initial reports suggested that it had a very high sensitivity (95%)

(98), but subsequently sensitivities as low as 53% even for segmental or larger emboli have been found (99,100). The specificity, however, has been generally above 90% (101). The wide range of sensitivities among the studies published may be due to differences in patient selection, extent of pulmonary emboli, technology, and reader experience. Thus, generalization of the operating characteristics of CT angiography quoted in published studies to one's local environment must be undertaken with care (101). In addition, none of the studies published so far meet all the methodological criteria for adequately evaluating the value of a diagnostic test. Reader experience appears to be necessary to avoid false-positive CT scans and to achieve high specificity (101). Despite the low sensitivities reported in some series, one nonrandomized trial of 1015 patients with suspected PE found that patients with a negative CT angiogram had a similarly low (1%) risk of subsequent PE during 3 months of follow-up as those with a negative ventilation/perfusion lung scan (102). These values compare favorably with conventional angiography. Two large multicenter trials (conducted by the European Society of Thoracic Radiology and by several of the PIOPED centers) evaluating helical computed tomography against angiography are currently on course in different phases of development. Potential additional benefits of helical computed tomography are its ability to help in the diagnosis of competing diseases (19,100) and to image the subdiaphragmatic deep veins (including the legs) at the same session (103).

Thus, while helical computed tomograph is gaining acceptance for the diagnosis of pulmonary emboli, the paucity of high-quality clinical trials employing the test renders its value incompletely proven at the present time.

K. Magnetic Resonance Angiography

Technological advances, including respiratory gating, ultrafast techniques performed during breath holding, and the use of gadolinium, offer promise for an expanded role of magnetic resonance imaging. Preliminary studies show sensitivities between 98% and 70% with high specificity (104,105). Magnetic resonance imaging is also useful for studying the venous systems of the pelvis and lower extremities.

V. Conclusion

Pleural effusions due to PE are frequently not recognized as such. There are no specific clinical or radiological features, and pleural fluid characteristics are quite variable. Therefore, PE should be considered in every patient with an acute unilateral pleural effusion even if it is a transudate. The decision whether to pursue more invasive procedures or simply observe a patient with undiagnosed pleural effusion requires clinical judgment that is guided by the patient's presentation. Pleuritic chest pain, dyspnea, tachypnea or fainting, the likelihood of alternative diagnosis, and the association to other radiological and electrocardiographic alterations will allow us to decide on the basis of the clinical probability for PE. PE is very unlikely in those not presenting any important clinical manifestation of the disease. If PE is suspected and if the patient is stable, the combination of clinical assessment, lung scanning, D-dimer testing, and venous ultrasound will confirm or exclude acute pulmonary emboli in many patients. In other cases, pulmonary angiography remains the gold standard for diagnosis. Helical computed angiography shows promise as a noninvasive test for pulmonary embolism, where the experience required to optimally obtain and interpret images is available.

References

1. Dismuke SE, Wagner EH. Pulmonary embolism as a cause of death. The changing mortality in hospitalized patients. JAMA 1986; 255:2039–2042.
2. Anderson FA Jr, Wheeler HB, Goldberg RJ, Hosmer DW, Patwardhan NA, Jovanovic B, Forcier A, Dalen JE. A population-based perspective of the hospital incidence and case-fatality rates of deep vein thrombosis and pulmonary embolism: the Worcester DVT Study. Arch Intern Med 1991; 151:933–938.
3. Silverstein MD, Heit JA, Mohr DN, Petterson TM, O'Fallon WM, Melton LJ III. Trends in the incidence of deep venous thrombosis and pulmonary embolism. A 25 yr population based study. Arch Intern Med 1998; 158:585–593.
4. Barritt DW, Jordon SC. Anticoagulant drugs in the treatment of pulmonary embolism: A controlled trial. Lancet 1960; 1:1309–1313.
5. Kanis JA. Heparin in the treatment of pulmonary thromboembolism. Thromb Diath Haemorrh 1974; 32:519–527.
6. Alpert JS, Smith R, Carlson J, Ockene IS, Dexter L, Dalen JE. Mortality in patients treated for pulmonary embolism. JAMA 1976; 236:1477–1480.
7. Carson JL, Kelley MA, Duff A, Weg JG, Fulkerson WJ, Palevsky HI, Schwartz JS, Thompson BT, Popovich J Jr, Hobbins TE, et al. The clinical course of pulmonary embolism. N Engl J Med 1992; 326:1240–1245.
8. Douketis JD, Kearon C, Bates S, Duku EK, Ginsberg JS. Risk of fatal pulmonary embolism in patients with treated venous thromboembolism. JAMA 1998; 279:458–462.
9. Donaldson GA, Williams C, Scanell J. A reappraisal of the application of the Trendelenburg operation to massive fatal embolism. N Engl J Med 1963; 268:171.
10. Goldhaber SZ, Hennekens CH, Evans DA, Newton EC, Godleski JJ. Factors associated with correct antemortem diagnosis of major pulmonary embolism. Am J Med 1982; 73:822–826.
11. Morgenthaler TI, Ryu JW. Clinical characteristics of fatal pulmonary embolism in a referral hospital. Mayo Clin Proc 1995; 70:417–424.
12. Stein PD, Henry JW. Prevalence of acute pulmonary embolism among patients in a general hospital and at autopsy. Chest 1995; 108:978–981.
13. Moser KM. Pulmonary embolism. Am Rev Respir Dis 1977; 115:829–852.
14. Bynum LJ, Wilson JE. Radiographic features of pleural effusions in pulmonary embolisms. Am Rev Respir Dis 1978; 117:829–834.
15. Stein PD, Terrin ML, Hales CA, Palevsky HI, Saltzman HA, Thompson BT, Weg JG. Clinical, laboratory, roentgenographic and electrocardiographic findings in pa-

tients with acute pulmonary embolism and no pre-existing cardiac or pulmonary disease. Chest 1991; 100:598–603.
16. Stein PD, Saltzman HA, Weg JG. Clinical characteristics of patients with acute pulmonary embolism. Am J Cardiol 1991; 68:1723–1724.
17. Worsley DF, Alavi A, Aronchick JM, Chen JT, Greenspan RH, Ravin CE. Chest radiographic findings in patients with acute pulmonary embolism: observations from the PIOPED study. Radiology 1993; 189:133–136.
18. Coche EE, Müller NL, Kim K. Acute pulmonary embolism: ancillary findings at helical CT. Radiology 1998; 207:753–758.
19. Shah AA, Davis SD, Gamsu G, Intriere L. Parenchyma and pleural findings in patients with and without acute pulmonary embolism detected at helical CT. Radiology 1999; 211:147–153.
20. Elliott CG, Goldhaber SZ, Visani L, DeRosa M. Chest radiographs in acute pulmonary embolism. Results from the International Cooperative Pulmonary Embolism Registry. Chest 2000; 118:33–38.
21. Moser KM, Fedullo PF, LitteJohn JK, Crwford R. Frequent asymptomatic pulmonary embolism in patients with deep venous thrombosis. JAMA 1994; 271:223–225.
22. Olsen JH. Epidemiology of lung cancer. In: Spiro SG, ed. Carcinoma of the Lung. Sheffield, UK: European Respiratory Journals Ltd., 1995:1–18.
23. Griner PF. Bloody pleural fluid following pulmonary infarction. JAMA 1967; 202:123–125.
24. Light RW, MacGregor MI, Luchsinger PC, Ball WC Jr. Pleural effusions: the diagnostic separation of transudates and exudates. Ann Intern Med 1972; 77:507–613.
25. Storey DD, Dines DE, Coles DT. Pleural effusion: a diagnostic dilemma. JAMA 1976; 236:2183–2186.
26. Marel M, Zrustova M, Stasny B, Light RW. The incidence of pleural effusion in a well-defined region: epidemiologic study in central Bohemia. Chest 1993; 104:1486–1489.
27. Valdés L, Álvarez D, Valle JM, Pose A, San José E. The etiology of pleural effusions in an area with high incidence of tuberculosis. Chest 1996; 109:158–162.
28. Preterman TA, Speicher CE. Evaluating pleural effusions: a two stage laboratory approach. JAMA 1984; 252:1051–1053.
29. Mattison LE, Copagge L, Alderman F, Herlong JO, Sahn SA. Pleural effusion in the medical ICU: prevalence, causes and clinical implications. Chest 1997; 111:1018–1023.
30. Race GA, Scheifley CH, Edward JE. Hydrothorax in congestive heart failure. Am J Med 1957; 22:83–89.
31. Broaddus VC, Wiener-Kronish JP, Berthiaume Y, Staub NC. Removal of pleural liquid and protein by lymphatics in awake sheep. J Appl Physiol 1988; 64:384–390.
32. Stewart PB. The rate of formation and lymphatic removal of fluid in pleural effusions. J Clin Invest 1963; 42:258–262.
33. Bynum LJ, Wilson JE II. Characteristics of pleural effusions associated with pulmonary embolism. Arch Intern Med 1976; 136:159–162.
34. Romero Candeira S, Hernández Blasco L, Soler MJ, Muñoz A, Aranda I. Biochemical and cytological characteristics of pleural effusions secondary to pulmonary embolism. Chest 2002; 121:465–469.
35. Light RW. Diseases of the pleura. Curr Opin Pulm Med 1995; 1:313–317.

36. Erdmann AJ III, Vaughan TR Jr, Brigham KL, Woolverton WC, Staub NC. Effect of increased vascular pressure on lung fluid balance in unanesthetized sheep. Circ Res 1975; 37:271–284.
37. Cheng D, Rodriguez RM, Perkett EA, Rogers J, Bienvenu G, Lappalainen U, Light RW. Vascular endothelial growth factor in pleural fluid. Chest 1999; 116:760–765.
38. Wiener-Kronish JP, Broaddus VC, Albertine KH, Gropper MA, Matthay MA, Staub NC. Relationship of pleural effusions to increased permeability pulmonary edema in anesthetized sheep. J Clin Invest 1988; 82:1422–1429.
39. Albertine KH, Wiener-Kronish JP, Roos PJ, Staub NC. Structure, blood supply, and lymphatic vessels of the sheep's visceral pleura. Am J Anat 1982; 165:277–294.
40. Stein P, Huang H, Afzal A, Noor HA. Incidence of acute pulmonary embolism in a general hospital. Chest 1999; 116:909–913.
41. Goldhaber SZ, Visan L, DeRosa M for ICOPER. Acute pulmonary embolism: clinical outcomes in the International Cooperative Pulmonary Embolism Registry (ICOPER). Lancet 1999; 353:1386–1389.
42. Simon H, Daggett WM, DeSanctis R. Hemothorax as a complication of anticoagulant therapy in the presence of pulmonary infarction. JAMA 1969; 208:1830–1834.
43. Wick MR, Ritter JH, Schuller D. Ruptured pulmonary infarction: a rare, fatal complication of thromboembolic disease. Mayo Clin Proc 2000; 75:639–642.
44. McGoldrick PJ, Rudd TG, Figley MM, Wilheim JP. What becomes of pulmonary infarcts. AJR 1979; 133:1039–1045.
45. Sklaroff HJ. The post-pulmonary infarction syndrome. Am Heart J 1979; 98:772–776.
46. Jerjes-Sanchez C, Ibarra-Perez C, Ramirez-Rivera A, Padua-Gabriel A, González-Carmona VM. Dressler-like syndrome after pulmonary embolism and infarction. Chest 1987; 92:115–117.
47. Dressler W. The post-myocardial infarction syndrome: a report of forty-four cases. Arch Intern Med 1959; 103:28.
48. Stelzner TJ, King TE Jr, Antony VB, Sahn SA. The pleuropulmonary manifestations of postcardiac injury syndrome. Chest 1983; 84:383–387.
49. Welin L, Vedin A, Wilhelmsson C. Characteristics, prevalence, and prognosis of postmyocardial infarction syndrome. Br Heart J 1983; 50:140–145.
50. Khan AH. The postcardiac injury syndromes. Clin Cardiol 1992; 15:67–72.
51. McNeil BJ, Hessel SJ, Branch WT. Measures of clinical efficacy: 3, The value of lung scan in the evaluation of lung patients with pleuritic chest pain. J Nucl Med 1976; 17:163–164.
52. Stein P, Henry JW. Clinical characteristics of patients with acute pulmonary embolism stratified according to their presenting syndromes. Chest 1997; 112:74–79.
53. Talbot S, Worthington BS, Roebuck EJ. Radiographic signs of pulmonary embolism and pulmonary infarction. Thorax 1973; 28:198–203.
54. Adelman M, Albelda SM, Gottlieb J, Haponik EF. Diagnostic utility of pleural fluid eosinophilia. Am J Med 1984; 77:915–920.
55. Miniati M, Prediletto R, Formichi B, Marini G, Tonelli L, Allescia G, Pistolesi M. Accuracy of clinical assessment in the diagnosis of pulmonary embolism. Am J Respir Crit Care Med 1999; 158:864–871.
56. Goldberg SN, Richardson DD, Palmer EL, Scott JA. Pleural effusion and ven-

tilation/perfusion scan interpretation for acute pulmonary embolus. J Nucl Med 1996; 37:1310–1313.
57. Rabin CB, Blackman NS. Bilateral pleural effusions. Its significance in association with a heart of normal size. J Mt Sinai Hosp 1957; 24:45–63.
58. Bell WR, Simon TL, DeMets DL. The clinical features of submassive and massive pulmonary emboli. Am J Med 1977; 62:355–360.
59. Rodger MA, Carrier M, Jones GN, Rasuli P, Raymond F, Djunaedi H, Wells PS. Diagnostic value of arterial blood gas measurement in suspected pulmonary embolism. Am J Respir Crit Care Med 2000; 162:2105–2108.
60. Egermayer P, Town GI, Turner JG, Heaton DC, Mee AL, Beard ME. Usefulness of D-dimer, blood gas, and respiratory rate measurements for excluding pulmonary embolism. Thorax 1998; 53:830–834.
61. Green RM, Meyer TJ, Dunn M, Glassroth J. Pulmonary embolism in younger adults. Chest 1992; 101:1507–1511.
62. Massoti L, Ceccarelli E, Capelli R, Barbesi L, Forconi S. Arterial blood gas analysis and alveolar-arterial oxygen gradient in diagnosis and prognosis of elderly patients with suspected pulmonary embolism. J Gerontolog 2000; 12:M761–M764.
63. Hyers TM. Venous thromboembolism. Am J Respir Crit Care Med 1999; 159: 1–14.
64. The PIOPED Investigators. Value of the ventilation/perfusion scan in acute pulmonary embolism. Results of the prospective investigation of pulmonary embolism diagnosis (PIOPED). JAMA 1990; 263:2753–2759.
65. Miniati M, Pistolesi M, Marini G, DiRicco G, Formichi B, Predileto R, Allescia G, Tonelli L, Sostman HD, Giuntini C. Value of perfusion lung scan in the diagnosis of pulmonary embolism: results of the Prospective Investigative Study of Acute Pulmonary Embolism Diagnosis (PISA-PED). Am J Respir Crit Care Med 1996; 154:1387–1393.
66. Ferrari E, Imbert A, Chevalier T, Mihoubi A, Morand P, Baudoy M. The ECG in pulmonary embolism: predictive value of negative T waves in precordial leads-80 case reports. Chest 1997; 111:537–543.
67. The Urokinase Pulmonary Embolism Trial: a national cooperative study. Circulation 1973; 47(suppl II):1–108.
68. Perrier A, Bounameaux H, Morabia A, de Mooerlose P, Slosman D, Didier D, Unger PF, Junod D. A diagnosis of pulmonary embolism by a decision analysis-based strategy including clinical probability, D-dimer levels, and ultrasonography: a management study. Arch Intern Med 1996; 156:531–536.
69. Stein PD, Henry JW, Gottschalk A. The addition of clinical assessment to stratification according to prior cardiopulmonary disease further optimizes the interpretation of ventilation/perfusion lung scans in pulmonary embolism. Chest 1993; 104:1472–1476.
70. Wells PS, Ginsberg JS, Anderson DR, Kearon C, Gent M, Turpie AG, Bormanis J, Weitz J, Chamberlain M, Bowie D, Barnes D, Hirsh J. Use of a clinical model for safe management of patients with suspected pulmonary embolism. Ann Intern Med 1998; 129:997–1005.
71. Sanson BJ, Lijmer JG, Mac Gillavry MR, Turkstra F, Prins MH, Buller HR. Comparison of a clinical probability estimate and two clinical models in patients with suspected pulmonary embolism. ANTELOPE-Study Group. Thromb Haemost 2000; 83:199–203.
72. Goldhaber SZ, Simons GR, Elliott CG, Haire WD, Toltzis R, Blacklow SC,

Doolittle MH, Weinberg DS. Quantitative plasma D-Dimer levels among patients undergoing pulmonary angiography for suspected pulmonary embolism. JAMA 1993; 270:2819–2822.
73. Bounameaux H, de Moerloose P, Perrier A, Reber G. Plasma measurement of D-dimer as diagnostic aid in suspected venous thromboembolism: an overview. Thromb Haemost 1994; 71:1–6.
74. Bates SM, Grand'Maison A, Johnston M, Naguit I, Kovacs MJ, Ginsberg JS. A latex D-dimer reliably excludes venous thromboembolism. Arch Intern Med 2001; 161:447–453.
75. Ginsberg JS, Wells PS, Kearon C, Anderson D, Crowther M, Weitz JI, Bormanis J. Sensitivity and specificity of a rapid whole-blood assay for D-dimer in the diagnosis of pulmonary embolism. Ann Intern Med 1998; 129:1006–1011.
76. Oger E, Leroyer C, Bressollette L, Monent L, Le Moigne E, Bizais Y, Amiral J, Grimaux M, Clavier J, ill P, Abgrall JF, Mottier D. Evaluation of a new, rapid and quantitative D-dimer test in patients with suspected pulmonary embolism. Am J Respir Crit Care Med 1998; 158:65–70.
77. Lee AY, Julian JA, Levine MN, Weitz JI, Kearon C, Wells PS, Ginsberg JS. Clinical utility of a rapid whole-blood D-dimer assay in patients with cancer who present with suspected acute deep venous thrombosis. Ann Intern Med 1999; 131:417–423.
78. Farrell S, Hayes T, Shaw M. A negative SimpliRED D-dimer assay result does not exclude the diagnosis of deep vein thrombosis or pulmonary embolus in emergency department patients. Ann Emerg Med 2000; 35:121–125.
79. Becker DM, Philbrick JT, Bachhuber TL, Humphries JE. D-dimer testing and acute venous thrombosis. A shortcut to accurate diagnosis? Arch Intern Med 1996; 156:939–946.
80. Hull RD, Hirsh CJ, Carter CJ, Raskob GE, Gill GJ, Jay RM, Leclerc JR, David M, Coates G. Diagnostic value of ventilation-perfusion lung scanning, in patients with suspected pulmonary embolism. Chest 1985; 88:819–828.
81. Hull RD, Raskob GE. Low_probability lung scan findings: a need for change. Ann Intern Med 1991; 114:142–143.
82. Bone RC. The low-probability scan. A potentially lethal reading. Arch Itern Med 1993; 153:2621–2622.
83. Tapson VF, Carroll BA, Davidson BL, Elliot CG, Fedullo PF, Hales CA, Hull RD, Hyers TM, Leeper KV, Morris TA, Moser KM, Raskob GE, Shure D, Sostman HD, Thompson BT. The diagnostic approach to acute venous thromboembolism. Am J Respir Crit Care Med 1999; 160:1043–1066.
84. Stein PD, Gottschalk A. Critical review of ventilation-perfusion scans in acute pulmonary embolism. Prog Cardiovasc Dis 1994; 37:13–24.
85. Light RW. Pleural Diseases. 4th ed. Philadelphia: Lippincott Williams & Wilkins, 2001.
86. Villena V, Lopez-Encuentra A, Pozo F, De-Pablo A, Martin-Escribano P. Measurement of pleural pressure during therapeutic thoracentesis. Am J Respir Crit Care Med 2000; 162:1534–1538.
87. Biello DR, Mattar AG, McKnight RC, Siegel BA. Ventilation-perfusion studies in suspected pulmonary embolism. AJR Am J Roentgenol 1979; 133:1033–1037.
88. Stein PD, Coleman RE, Gottchalk A, Saltzman HA, Terrin ML, Weg JG. Diagnostic utility of ventilation/perfusion lung scans in acute pulmonary embolism is not diminished by pre-existing cardiac or pulmonary disease. Chest 1991; 100:604–606.

89. Ieneke Hartmann JC, Petronella Hagen J, Christian Melissant F, Pieter Postmus E, Martin H. Prins on behalf of the ANTELOPE Study Group. Diagnosing acute pulmonary embolism. Effect of chronic obstructive pulmonary disease on the performance of D-dimer testing, ventilation/perfusion scintigraphy, helical computed tomographic angiography and conventional angiography. Am J Respir Crit Care Med 2000; 162:2232–2237.
90. Khorasani R, Gudas TF, Nikpoor N, Polak JF. Treatment of patients with suspected pulmonary embolism and intermediate-probability lung scans: is diagnostic imaging underused? Am J Roentgenol 1997; 169:1355–1357.
91. Kearon C, Ginsberg JS, Hirsh J. The role of venous ultrasonography in the diagnosis of suspected deep venous thrombosis and pulmonary embolism. Ann Intern Med 1998; 129:1044–1049.
92. Wells PS, Hirsh J, Anderson DR, Lensing AW, Foster G, Kearon C, Weitz J, Cogo A, Prandoni P, Minuk T, et al. Comparison of the accuracy of impedance plethysmography and compression ultrasonography in outpatients with clinically suspected deep venous thrombosis. Thromb Haemost 1995; 74:1423–1427.
93. Hull RD, Raskob GE, Ginsberg A, Panju AA, Brill-Edwards P, Coates, Pireo GF. A noninvasive strategy for the treatment of patients with suspected pulmonary embolism. Arch Intern Med 1994; 154:289–297.
94. Wells PS, Ginsberg JS, Anderson DR, Kearon C, Gent M, Turpie AG, Bormanis J, Weitz J, Chamberlain M, Bowie D, Barnes D, Hirsh J. Use of a clinical model for safe management of patients with suspected pulmonary embolism. Ann Intern Med 1998; 129:997–1005.
95. Wells PS, Anderson DR, Rodger M, Ginsberg JS, Kearon C, Gent M, Turpie AG, Bormanis J, Weitz J, Chamberlain M, Bowie D, Barnes D, Hirsh J. Derivation of a simple clinical model to categorize patients probability of pulmonary embolism: increasing the models utility with the SimpliRED D-dimer. Thromb Haemost 2000; 83:416–420.
96. Perrier A, Desmarais S, Miron MJ, de Moerloose P, Lepage R, Slosman D, Didier D, Unger PF, Patenaude JV, Bounameaux H. Non-invasive diagnosis of venous thromboembolism in outpatients. Lancet 1999; 353:190–195.
97. Stein PD, Athanasoulis C, Alavi A, Greenspan RH, Hales CA, Saltzman HA, Vreim CE, Terrin ML, Weg JG. Complications and validity of pulmonary angiography in acute pulmonary embolism. Circulation 1992; 85:462–468.
98. Remy-Jardin M, Remy J, Wattinne L, Giraud F. Central pulmonary thromboembolism: diagnosis with volumetric CT with the single-breath-holding technique- comparison with pulmonary angiography. Radiology 1992; 185:381–387.
99. Drucker EA, Rivitz SM, Shepard JA, Boiselle PM, Trotman-Dickenson B, Welch TJ, Maus TP, Miller SW, Kaufman JA, Waltman AC, McLoud TC, Athanasoulis CA. Acute pulmonary embolism: Assessment of helical CT for diagnosis. Radiology 1998; 209:235–241.
100. Garg K, Welsh CH, Feyerabend AJ, Subber SW, Russ PD, Johnston RJ, Durham JD, Lynch DA. Pulmonary embolism: diagnosis with spiral CT and ventilation-perfusion scanning- correlation with pulmonary angiographic results or clinical outcome. Radiology 1998; 208:201–208.
101. Rathbun SW, Raskob GE, Whitsett TL. Sensitivity and specificity of helical computed tomography in the diagnosis of pulmonary embolism: a systematic review. Ann Intern Med 2000; 132:227–232.
102. Goodman LR, Lipchik RJ, Kuzo RS, McAuliffe TL, O'Brien DJ. Subsequent

pulmonary embolism: risk after a negative helical CT pulmonary angiogram. Prospective comparison with scintigraphy. Radiology 2000; 215:535–542.
103. Loud PA, Katz DS, Klippenstein DL, Shah RD, Grossman ZD. Combined CT venography and pulmonary angiography in suspected thromboembolic disease: diagnostic accuracy for deep venous evaluation. Am J Roentgenol 2000; 174:61.
104. Meaney JF, Weg JG, Chenevert TL, Stafford-Johnson D, Hamilton BH, Prince MR. Diagnosis of pulmonary embolism with magnetic resonance angiography. N Engl J Med 1997; 336:1422–1427.
105. Gupta A, Frazer CK, Ferguson JM, Kumar AB, Davis SJ, Fallon MJ, Morris IT, Drury PJ, Cala LA. Acute pulmonary embolism: diagnosis with MR angiography. Radiology 1999; 210:353–359.

43

Pleural Effusions Secondary to Fungal, Nocardial, and Actinomycotic Infection

MARK WOODHEAD

Manchester Royal Infirmary
Manchester, England

I. Introduction

The infections covered in this section are nowhere common and sometimes geographically isolated in their occurrence. The majority of these infections have their greatest pulmonary impact in the lung parenchyma, with pleural involvement occurring rarely and usually secondary to the parenchymal pathology.

There are two clinical and pathogenetic groupings: those "pathogenic" fungi that cause infections in the immunocompetent as well as the immunocompromised (e.g., histoplasmosis, actinomycosis) and those that are of low pathogenicity and are unusual other than as "opportunists" in hosts with depressed host defense (e.g., aspergillus, candida, cryptococcus). In almost all cases pleural effusion occurs because of direct infection of the pleural space in the form of empyema. Most such infections are difficult to treat, and, particularly in the latter group, outcome is poor. This is partly because of the difficulty in treatment, but also because of the nature of underlying pathology and immune suppression. In a study of 67 patients with fungal empyema the mortality was 73% (1). The frequency of each fungal species is shown in Table 1. In this study only 10% of cases had no significant underlying condition, with malignant disease (49%), diabetes mellitus (16%), long-term steroid use (15%), liver cirrhosis (12%), and organ transplantation (6%) the most common underlying conditions. In 84% of cases the fungal empyema was judged to be nosocomial in origin.

Table 1 Fungi Isolated from 73 Pleural Effusion Specimens from 67 Patients[a] with Fungal Empyema in Taiwan

Fungal isolate	Number (%)
Candida species	47 (64)
C. albicans	28 (38)
C. tropicalis	13 (18)
C. parapsilosis	2 (3)
C. guilliermondii	2 (3)
C. humicola	1 (1)
C. famata	1 (1)
Torulopsis glabrata	13 (18)
Aspergillus species	9 (12)
Cryptococcus species	3 (4)
Rhizopus species	1 (1)

[a] Some had more than one species isolated.
Source: Ref. 1.

II. *Aspergillus* Species

Aspergillus infection of the lung is unusual in the absence of a breakdown of the host defenses. This breakdown may be local (e.g., due to damage to lung tissue caused, e.g., by previous *Mycobacterium tuberculosis* infection) or generalized due to some form of immune suppression. The type of alteration of host defense determines the type of aspergillus infection. At one end of the spectrum aspergillus may be found as a colonist in minimally damaged airways. In some individuals an allergic immune response to the aspergillus will lead to allergic bronchopulmonary aspergillosis. Local damage to the lung parenchyma may lead to local intra cavitary saprophytic growth of fungal mycelia as a mycetoma or aspergilloma. Two clinicopathological manifestations of aspergillus infection occur with generalized immune suppression. Rarely an aspergillus tracheobronchitis occurs, but more commonly invasive pulmonary aspergillosis (IPA) of the lung parenchyma is found. Aspergillus involvement of the pleura is uncommon and is only described as a complication of local damage to the lung parenchyma, with or without aspergilloma, and as a complication of IPA. In each situation the common pathogenic factor appears to be the occurrence at some point of a bronchopleural fistula. This may occur due to direct pleural invasion by aspergillus infection, by rupture of chronically damaged lung, or be iatrogenic. Iatrogenic pleural aspergillosis may be as a consequence of treatment directed at pulmonary aspergillosis [e.g., surgery or pleural instrumentation either at intercostal drainage or the percutaneous instillation of antifungal agents for the treatment of intracavitary aspergilloma (2)] or following surgery for other lung disease [e.g., lung cancer, pneumothorax (3)]. Most older studies refer to pleural involvement following tuberculous lung damage, either due to the disease itself or following artificial pneumothorax used in treatment (4,5), while more recent studies more commonly relate to IPA as a consequence of immunosuppression. Aspergillus pleural effusion has been described as a complication in AIDS (6).

The absolute frequency of pleural involvement depends on the sensitivity of the method used for detection and also the origin of the patients. Many studies do not make a clear distinction between pleural thickening and effusion. While a computed tomography (CT) study of patients with pneumonia after lung transplantation found a frequency of pleural effusions of 63% in eight patients with aspergillus pneumonia (7) and a study of 3284 unselected autopsies found pleural involvement in 22% of 18 patients with various forms of pulmonary aspergillosis (8), these figures probably overestimate the frequency encountered in clinical practice. Pleural effusion was seen on chest radiograph in only one of 30 (3%) patients with aspergilloma pulmonary infection following lung transplantation (9), in only one of 87 (1%) cases of IPA in hematology patients (10) and was not commented on in a study of 595 cases of IPA of diverse origin in another (11). Local pleural thickening close to an aspergilloma within a lung cavity is a common phenomenon, but the development of pleural effusion as a consequence of this appears to be unusual (5).

Clinical presentations are diverse and may be acute with sudden onset of pleuritic chest pain and cough (12) or hemoptysis (3) or indolent with weeks or months of weight loss, malaise, fevers, and cough (5,13). Clinical presentation may occur shortly after breach of the visceral pleura where this is traumatic, e.g., as a postoperative complication. However, this may, even in these circumstances, be delayed for months as in the two cases reported to have occurred 4 and 6 months after percutaneous instillation of antifungal agents into an intrapulmonary mycetoma (2). Where it occurs as a complication of structural lung disease, presentation may be up to 25 years after the pleura was originally breached (3,5). In these circumstances it is not clear whether the original pleural breach was responsible for the introduction of aspergillus into the pleural space or whether (as appears more likely) a subsequent clinically unrecognized breach occurred.

Radiographic appearances may be of an uncomplicated pleural effusion or a hydro(pyo)pneumothorax (14) (Fig. 1). Underlying lung disease (e.g., old tuberculous changes, bullae, aspergilloma, or consolidation due to IPA) may also be visible. On CT these appearances will be confirmed and in addition the pleura is usually seen to be thickened and may be nodular. Movement of the nodules with gravity when the CT is repeated in the prone position may confirm the presence of intrapleural mycetoma as in intracavitary disease (15,16). In those cases complicating chronic lung disease serial chest radiographs may reveal slowly progressing pleural thickening (3,5).

Laboratory investigations may show nonspecific abnormalities such as anemia and high erythrocyte sedimentation rate. Examination of pleural fluid usually reveals pus, which is odorless unless concomitant bacterial infection is present. The fluid has the characteristics of an exudate, and cytological examination usually shows over 80% neutrophils. Using specific antifungal stains,

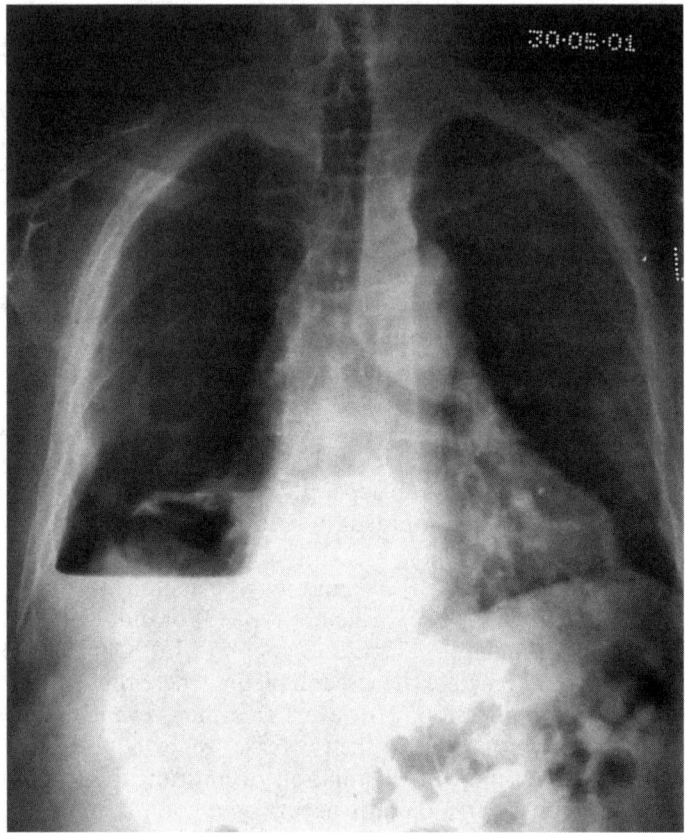

Figure 1 Patient with underlying Wegener's granulomatosis on cyclophosphamide with remission and on maintenance corticosteroids presents 9 months later with "pneumonia" and an empyema from which there is a pure growth of *Aspergillus fumigatus*. The *Aspergillus* infection had almost completely destroyed the right lung, leaving a pyopneumothorax. This chest radiograph was taken after response to itraconazole, but in the presence of a bronchopleural fistula, coinfected with β-hemolytic streptococci. (Courtesy of Dr. David Denning.)

mycelia may be seen in the aspirated fluid, which on culture will be confirmed as aspergillus. Fungi may, however, be scanty, and multiple pleural fluid samples require examination before the diagnosis can be excluded (13). In some patients aspergillus may also be found in sputum. In the immunocompetent where pleural involvement complicates chronic parenchymal involvement, aspergillus precipitating antibodies may be present in high titer in the peripheral blood (4). Pleural biopsy may show nonspecific or granulomatous inflammation and may or may not contain fungal hyphae. *Aspergillus fumigatus* is the most common fungal species identified, followed by *Aspergillus flavus* and *Aspergillus niger*. The frequency of coincident bacterial pleural infection is not clear and may have been reduced by the widespread use of broad-spectrum antibiotics. Older publications suggest from 70% to 25% (1,4,15), but these may be overestimates. *Staphylococcus aureus*, *Klebsiella*, *Pseudomonas*, and *Mycobacterium* are the most commonly reported coincident bacterial infections (4,14,15).

Guidelines for antifungal therapy in aspergillus infection are available in other texts and will not be repeated here (17). A combination of pleural drainage and antifungal treatment is the cornerstone of treatment, but a consensus on the best method of pleural drainage is not available. Patients affected by aspergillus effusion/empyema generally have comorbid conditions that render them unfit for surgery, but closed drainage may not be adequate, especially where pleural infection is complicated by local aspergillus osteomyelitis of the ribs (14). Closed tube drainage accompanied by local pleural instillation of antifungal agents (nystatin or amphotericin) has been reported to be successful (1,4,12). Most reports, however, describe operative surgical drainage of the pleural cavity, accompanied variably by decortication, pleurectomy, pneumonectomy, omentoplasty, and myoplasty (3,5,14,15,18). Complication rates are about 50%, with recurrent empyema and hemorrhage being prominent. Death occurred postoperatively in 10% of 19 patients in the literature where those with pleural disease were separately defined (3,5,13,18).

III. *Candida* and *Torulopsis* Species

Lung infection (as opposed to colonization) by organisms of these two genera is extremely rare. They are normal colonists of the gastrointestinal tract and occur more frequently in the presence of chronic disease and following broad-spectrum antibiotic therapy. In a study of fungal empyemas, these two organisms were the most common cause accounting for 82% of cases (Table 1) (1). In 84% of cases the fungal empyema was judged to be nosocomial in origin, chronic underlying disease was present in 90%, and 60% had received prior broad spectrum antibiotics. Occasionally candida empyema may complicate subdiaphragmatic disease (19) or gastrointestinal tract pathology (20,21). *Candida albicans* occurs most frequently, followed by *Candida tropicalis* and *Torulopsis glabrata* (Table 1). As for aspergillus, drainage of the pleural space and antifungal therapy are required in treatment. Intrapleural instillation of fluconazole was reported to be successful in two patients (1).

IV. *Pneumocystis carinii*

Pleural involvement in pneumocystosis is very rare, with pleural effusions unrecorded in early radiographic series (22). While the association of this infection with pneumothorax in 4–5% of cases (23,24) is now well recognized, the occurrence of pleural effusion remains a rare phenomenon. It has only been documented in those receiving aerosolized pentamidine and appears to be a complication of subpleural *P. carinii* infection (25,26). While usually associated with *P. carinii* pneumonia, it may occur without apparent lung involvement (26). Bronchopleural fistula was present in four of seven cases described up to 1993 (25,26).

P. carinii may be seen in pleural fluid with appropriate staining (26). Pleural fluid–to–serum LDH ratio is >1, but protein level may be below 3 g/dL and glucose levels and pH normal. Neutrophils or monocytes may predominate in the fluid (25).

Drug treatment is as for *P. carinii* pneumonia. Tube drainage has been described, but the necessity for this is unknown (26).

V. *Cryptococcus* Species

Cryptococcus neoformans is an ubiquitous soil fungus. It is rarely found in the human lung. It can occur as a commensal organism or can cause infection, mainly in the immunocompromised, but also rarely in the immunocompetent. Lung infection can occur in isolation or be a manifestation of disseminated disease, the latter usually involving the meninges. Radiographically it is usually manifest as consolidation or isolated pulmonary nodule(s).

Pleural effusion is unusual, especially in the immunocompetent (27). In the non–HIV-immunocompromised it was reported in 23% of 13 patients with *C. neoformans* pulmonary infection in one study (28). A review of eight studies in the HIV-positive, each containing 18 patients or less, found pleural effusion in 14% of 92 cases. A study of 37 such patients in Rwanda found pleural effusion in only 5%. Isolated pleural effusion due to *C. neoformans* appears not to have been described, but a single such case of empyema due to *Cryptococcus albidus* (with coincident mucormycosis) has been described (29). Examination of pleural fluid may yield cryptococcal antigen or the organism on culture.

Treatment is of the underlying cryptococcal infection, which may be successful without the need for therapeutic pleural drainage (30).

VI. *Mucor* Species

These include *rhizopus*, *absidia*, and *mucor*. Disease caused by these saprophytic fungi is rare, usually occurs in the immunocompromised, and presents as rhinocerebral or pulmonary disease. In the lung it may be confined to the airways or be invasive. Pleuritic chest pain is common, and pleural friction rubs may be heard. Pleural effusion may occur (31) and may be unilateral or bilateral (32).

VII. *Histoplasma capsulatum*

Histoplasma capsulatum is a soil-living fungus which is endemic to certain geographic regions, especially the eastern United States, South and Central

America, Southeast Asia, and India. Infection occurs through inhalation of microconidia from the mycelial form of the organism. The clinical pattern of illness varies according to the innoculum size and host factors, which include immune status. Illness may be acute or chronic. As many as 50% of infections may be asymptomatic (33).

Pleural thickening due to fibrosis is common in the chronic fibrocavitary form of the infection, but pleural effusion is very uncommon (34,35). The true frequency in patients presenting with clinical illness is probably close to the 0.4% found in a series of 269 cases reported in 1976 (36). Other series of more selected groups of patients report frequencies of 3.6% (37) and 6.3% (38). Pleural effusion may be more common in those with histoplasma pericarditis with a frequency of 44% in a small series of 16 such patients (39).

Pleural effusion may be asymptomatic (40), may occur in both the presence and absence (35) of underlying lung involvement, and may be blood-stained (41) or empyematous (38). The infrequency of pleural effusion means that it is often investigated by surgical drainage and pleural biopsy. Pleural examination may show fibrosis (35) or subpleural granulomata (36).

In the absence of pleural fibrosis, resolution, either spontaneously or with treatment (33), normally occurs, but tube drainage or surgery may be required.

VIII. Blastomyces dermatitidis

B. dermatitidis is another soil-living fungus that occurs in southeastern North America and is reported less commonly from Central and South America and occasionally from Africa and elsewhere. As with histoplasmosis, infection is acquired by inhalation and the clinical manifestations are varied. Many cases of infection are asymptomatic. Pleural effusion appears to be more common than with histoplasmosis. It was reported in 6% of 517 cases in seven series (42–48) ranging from 0% (43,44) to 20% (46) of cases in individual series (45). Large effusions have occasionally been reported (49,50).

In three patients pleural fluid was described to have a high protein content with normal glucose and raised cell count, with neutrophils predominating (45). The pleura may contain noncaseating granulomatous inflammation, and yeasts may be visible (50).

IX. Coccidioides immitis

Coccidioidomycosis is a systemic fungal infection caused by *C. immitis*, which is usually self-limiting. It is endemic in the south western United States and parts of South and Central America. Outbreaks occur when the fungus is liberated from soil in dust storms, natural disasters and earth excavation. The majority of infections are asymptomatic, and most symptomatic cases have a flu-like illness.

Occasionally a chronic fibrocavitary lung infection develops and extrapulmonary dissemination can occur. Pleural effusion is most unusual, but rupture of pulmonary cavities into the pleural space leading to pyopneumothorax has been recorded (51).

X. Paracoccidioides brasiliensis

P. brasiliensis is a fungus endemic to South and Central America. Primary infection usually occurs in childhood, with chronic adult infection occurring due to reactivation or reinfection. Pleural effusion has been described in primary infection in a child (52), but is unusual. The chronic form is associated with midzone interstitial lung shadowing and nodules that may cavitate, but pleural involvement is very unusual and was not recorded in a study of the CT appearances in 43 cases (53).

XI. Sporothrix schenkii

S. schenkii is another soil fungus with worldwide distribution that occasionally causes human disease. This nearly always involves the skin, but primary lung infection can occur and disseminated disease can affect the lung. Consolidation and nodular (sometimes cavitating) shadowing occurs and pleural effusion has been reported (54). Of two cases where the pleural fluid characteristics were described, both were exudates—one with a mononuclear cell infiltrate and the other with a frank empyema containing granulocytes.

XII. Actinomyces israelii

Both *Actinomyces* and *Nocardia* are gram-positive bacteria which share a number of characteristics with the fungi (e.g., branching and mycelium formation). *Actinomyces* is a normal commensal organism of the oropharynx which primarily causes disease in the cervico-dental region. Only 15% of cases are said to involve the thorax.

Disease characteristics are dependent on chronicity when the organism's unusual capacity to ignore anatomical boundaries and to directly invade contiguous tissues becomes manifest. In the thorax, early infection typically affects the lower lobes and lung periphery and takes the form of consolidation. The overlying pleura becomes fibrosed and thickened, and local intrapleural abscesses and empyema may occur (55). Pleural shadowing typically occurs in one third of cases (56) and, notwithstanding the above comments, may occur in isolation (57). A wavy periosteal reaction in the overlying ribs was said to be typical, but appears to be an unusual feature in recent reports (56). Direct invasion of contiguous tissues includes the chest wall (56,58,59), the diaphragm (60,61) and the mediastinum (62) (Fig. 2).

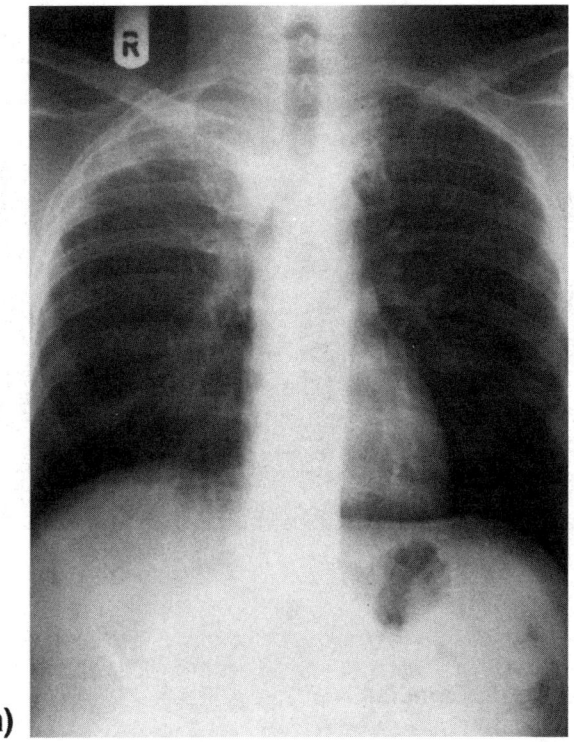

(a)

Figure 2 Patient with *Actinomyces israelii* lung infection. In addition to acute respiratory symptoms, the patient had a typical pustular overlying skin rash due to direct skin invasion and neurological features due to spinal cord compression. (a) Chest radiograph of right upper lobe pneumonia with pleural involvement. (b) CT scan showing direct invasion of adjacent structures including pleura, chest wall, contralateral lung, and spinal canal.

Clinical features are nonspecific, with cough, sputum, fever, chest pain, weight loss, dyspnea, hemoptysis, and night sweats all being common. Symptom chronicity may mimic tuberculosis and the capacity for tissue invasion, neoplasia.

Diagnosis is based on isolation of the usual causative species, *A. israelii*, on culture from lung secretions or pleural fluid, but may be suspected from the presence of typical "sulfur granules" in pus or tissue including pleura (63). These particles are composed of an outer ring of neutrophils surrounding a central core of bacterial filaments. Concomitant infection with other microorganisms is not infrequent.

Treatment is with penicillin or other β-lactam antibiotics. Pleural drainage and/or surgery may be required, but does not appear to be mandatory (64).

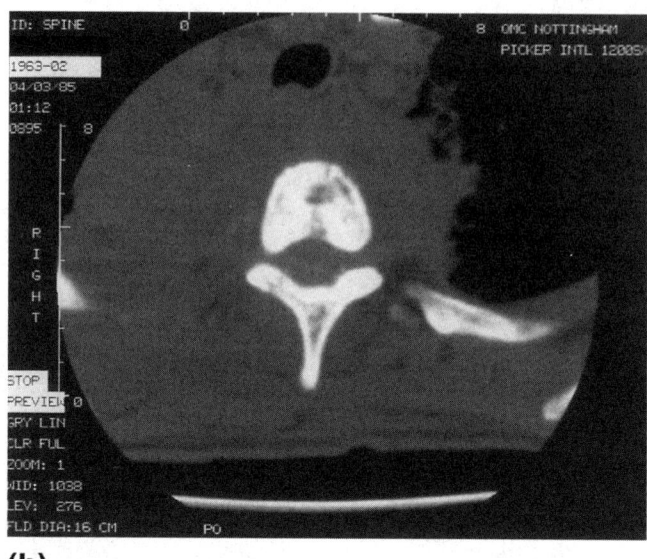
(b)

Figure 2 Continued.

XIII. *Nocardia* Species

Nocardia bacteria are common commensal organisms in soil and water. Infection is acquired by inhalation, and in two thirds or more of cases pulmonary involvement occurs. Dissemination occurs frequently, and the organism has a predilection for involving the brain. Although the organism is gram-positive, it is also weakly acid-fast, which may lead to misdiagnosis as tuberculosis (65). *Nocardia asteroides* is the most common disease-causing species, with other species (e.g., *Nocardia brasiliensis, Nocardia farcinica*) varying in frequency, probably according to their environmental prevalence. Infection usually occurs in the frankly immunocompromised, but those with mildly compromised host defenses [e.g., chronic steroid intake or bronchiectasis (66)] can be affected and ~10% of cases are immunocompetent. Pathologically the infection can lead to suppuration or granulomatous inflammation depending on the integrity of the host immune response. This variability in pathology is in part responsible for the variable clinical and radiographic presentation. Cough and sputum, which may be blood-stained, are typically associated with fever and leukocytosis. Consolidation or nodules, which may be multiple, are typical radiographic features, with cavitation occurring frequently (67–69). Pleural changes may be seen in 12% (68) to 90% (69) of cases, but many studies are of small numbers of patients and often do not distinguish clearly between pleural thickening and fluid. Isolated empyema may occur (70) and simultaneous infection with other organisms [e.g., *Pneumocystis carinii* (71)] has been reported. Direct spread into contiguous structures has been described, but appears to be less common than with *Actinomyces* infection.

Diagnosis is based on identification of the causative organism in affected tissues including pleural fluid and pleura. The bacterium grows slowly, and cultures should be kept for 3 weeks if *Nocardia* is suspected.

Appropriate antibiotics (sulfonamides) are the mainstay of treatment, but drainage and/or surgery may be required when the pleura is affected. Antibiotic therapy should be continued for a minimum of 3 months and possibly for as long as one year (67). The mortality may be as high as 80% in those with cerebral involvement, but in isolated pulmonary disease cure is usually achievable.

References

1. Ko SC, Chen KY, Hsueh PR, Luh KT, Yang PC. Fungal empyema thoracis: an emerging clinical entity. Chest 2000; 117:1672–1678.
2. Nakanishi Y, Wakamatsu K, Nomoto Y, Kawasaki M, Takayama K, Yatsunami J, et al. Empyema following the percutaneous instillation of antifungal agents in patients with aspergillosis. Intern Med 1996; 35:657–659.
3. Endo S, Sohara Y, Murayama F, Yamaguchi T, Hasegawa T, Fuse K. Late pleuropulmonary aspergillosis after the treatment of pneumothorax: report of three cases. Surg Today 1999; 29:1125–1128.
4. Krakowka P, Rowinska E, Halweg H. Infection of the pleura by *Aspergillus fumigatus*. Thorax 1970; 25:245–253.
5. Hillerdal G. Pulmonary aspergillus infection invading the pleura. Thorax 1981; 36:745–751.
6. Staples CA, Kang EY, Wright JL, Phillips P, Muller NL. Invasive pulmonary aspergillosis in AIDS: radiographic, CT, and pathologic findings. Radiology 1995; 196:409–414.
7. Collins J, Muller NL, Kazerooni EA, Paciocco G. CT findings of pneumonia after lung transplantation. AJR Am J Roentgenol 2000; 175:811–818.
8. Barth PJ, Rossberg C, Koch S, Ramaswamy A. Pulmonary aspergillosis in an unselected autopsy series. Pathol Res Pract 2000; 196:73–80.
9. Diederich S, Scadeng M, Dennis C, Stewart S, Flower CD. *Aspergillus* infection of the respiratory tract after lung transplantation: chest radiographic and CT findings. Eur Radiol 1998; 8:306–312.
10. Yeghen T, Kibbler CC, Prentice HG, Berger LA, Wallesby RK, McWhinney PH, et al. Management of invasive pulmonary aspergillosis in hematology patients: a review of 87 consecutive cases at a single institution. Clin Infect Dis 2000; 31:859–868.
11. Patterson TF, Kirkpatrick WR, White M, Hiemenz JW, Wingard JR, Dupont B, et al. Invasive aspergillosis. Disease spectrum, treatment practices, and outcomes. I3 Aspergillus Study Group. Medicine (Baltimore) 2000; 79:250–260.
12. Albelda SM, Gefter WB, Epstein DM, Miller WT. Bronchopleural fistula complicating invasive pulmonary aspergillosis. Am Rev Respir Dis 1982; 126:163–165.

13. Kearon MC, Power JT, Wood AE, Clancy LJ. Pleural aspergillosis in a 14 year old boy. Thorax 1987; 42:477–478.
14. Meredith HC, Cogan BM, McLaulin B. Pleural aspergillosis. AJR Am J Roentgenol 1978; 130:164–166.
15. Costello P, Rose RM. CT findings in pleural aspergillosis. J Comput Assist Tomogr 1985; 9:760–762.
16. Winer-Muram HT, Scott RL, Eastridge CE, Salazar JE. Pleural aspergillosis diagnosed by computerized tomography. South Med J 1987; 80(9):1193–1194.
17. Stevens DA, Kan VL, Judson MA, Morrison VA, Dummer S, Denning DW, et al. Practice guidelines for diseases caused by *Aspergillus*. Infectious Diseases Society of America. Clin Infect Dis 2000; 30:696–709.
18. Wex P, Utta E, Drozdz W. Surgical treatment of pulmonary and pleuropulmonary *Aspergillus* disease. Thorac Cardiovasc Surg 1993; 41:64–70.
19. Malik S, Giacoia GP. *Candida tropicalis* empyema associated with acquired gastro- pleural fistula in a newborn infant. Am J Perinatol 1989; 6:347–348.
20. Duffner F, Brandner S, Opitz H, Klier R, Grote EH. Primary *Candida albicans* empyema associated with epidural hematomas in craniocervical junction. Clin Neuropathol 1997; 16:143–146.
21. Weber KH, Wehmer W. Candida-Pleuraempyem nach Tonsillektomie. [Thoracic empyema due to *Candida* after tonsillectomy]. Munch Med Wochenschr 1970; 112: 2170–2173.
22. DeLorenzo LJ, Huang CT, Maguire GP, Stone DJ. Roentgenographic patterns of *Pneumocystis carinii* pneumonia in 104 patients with AIDS. Chest 1987; 91:323–327.
23. Leoung GS, Feigal DW, Montgomery AB, Corkery K, Wardlaw L, Adams M, et al. Aerosolized pentamidine for prophylaxis against *Pneumocystis carinii* pneumonia. The San Francisco community prophylaxis trial. N Engl J Med 1990; 323:769–775.
24. Pastores SM, Garay SM, Naidich DP, Rom WN. Review: pneumothorax in patients with AIDS-related *Pneumocystis carinii* pneumonia. Am J Med Sci 1996; 312:229–234.
25. Horowitz ML, Schiff M, Samuels J, Russo R, Schnader J. *Pneumocystis carinii* pleural effusion. Pathogenesis and pleural fluid analysis. Am Rev Respir Dis 1993; 148:232–234.
26. Jayes RL, Kamerow HN, Hasselquist SM, Delaney MD, Parenti DM. Disseminated pneumocystosis presenting as a pleural effusion. Chest 1993; 103:306–308.
27. Nunez M, Peacock JE, Chin R. Pulmonary cryptococcosis in the immunocompetent host. Therapy with oral fluconazole: a report of four cases and a review of the literature. Chest 2000; 118:527–534.
28. Aberg JA, Mundy LM, Powderly WG. Pulmonary cryptococcosis in patients without HIV infection. Chest 1999; 115:734–740.
29. Horowitz ID, Blumberg EA, Krevolin L. *Cryptococcus albidus* and mucormycosis empyema in a patient receiving hemodialysis. South Med J 1993; 86:1070–1072.
30. Fukuchi M, Mizushima Y, Hori T, Kobayashi M. Cryptococcal pleural effusion in a patient with chronic renal failure receiving long-term corticosteroid therapy for rheumatoid arthritis. Intern Med 1998; 37:534–537.
31. Bartrum RJ, Watnick M, Herman PG. Roentgenographic findings in pulmonary mucormycosis. Am J Roentgenol Radium Ther Nucl Med 1973; 117:810–815.

32. McAdams HP, Rosado-de-Christenson M, Strollo DC, Patz EF. Pulmonary mucormycosis: radiologic findings in 32 cases. AJR Am J Roentgenol 1997; 168: 1541–1548.
33. George RB, Penn RL. Histoplasmosis. In: Sarosi GA, Davies SF, eds. Fungal Diseases of the Lung. New York: Raven Press, 1993:39–50.
34. Brewer PL, Himmelwright JP. Pleural effusion due to infection with histoplasma capsulatum. Chest 1970; 58:76–79.
35. Gluckman TJ, Corbridge T. Isolated pleural effusion with pleural fibrosis in a patient with subacute progressive disseminated histoplasmosis. Clin Infect Dis 1998; 26:1477–1478.
36. Connell JV, Muhm JR. Radiographic manifestations of pulmonary histoplasmosis: a 10-year review. Radiology 1976; 121:281–285.
37. Straus SE, Jacobson ES. The spectrum of histoplasmosis in a general hospital: a review of 55 cases diagnosed at Barnes Hospital between 1966 and 1977. Am J Med Sci 1980; 279:147–158.
38. Sutaria MK, Polk JW, Reddy P, Mohanty SK. Surgical aspects of pulmonary histoplasmosis. A series of 110 cases. Thorax 1970; 25:31–40.
39. Picardi JL, Kauffman CA, Schwarz J, Holmes JC, Phair JP, Fowler NO. Pericarditis caused by *Histoplasma capsulatum*. Am J Cardiol 1976; 37:82–88.
40. Swinburne AJ, Fedullo AJ, Wahl GW, Farnand B. Histoplasmoma, pleural fibrosis, and slowly enlarging pleural effusion in an asymptomatic patient. Am Rev Respir Dis 1987; 135:502–503.
41. Kilburn CD, McKinsey DS. Recurrent massive pleural effusion due to pleural, pericardial, and epicardial fibrosis in histoplasmosis. Chest 1991; 100:1715–1717.
42. Blastomycosis Cooperative study of the Veterans Administartion. Blastomycosis I: a review of 198 collected cases in Veterans Administration hospitals. Am Rev Respir Dis 1964; 89:659–672.
43. Sarosi GA, Hammerman KJ, Tosh FE, Kronenberg RS. Clinical features of acute pulmonary blastomycosis. N Engl J Med 1974; 290:540–543.
44. Rabinowitz JG, Busch J, Buttram WR. Pulmonary manifestations of blastomycosis. Radiological support of a new concept. Radiology 1976; 120:25–32.
45. Kinasewitz GT, Penn RL, George RB. The spectrum and significance of pleural disease in blastomycosis. Chest 1984; 86:580–584.
46. Sheflin JR, Campbell JA, Thompson GP. Pulmonary blastomycosis: findings on chest radiographs in 63 patients. AJR Am J Roentgenol 1990; 154:1177–1180.
47. Patel RG, Patel B, Petrini MF, Carter RR, Griffith J. Clinical presentation, radiographic findings, and diagnostic methods of pulmonary blastomycosis: a review of 100 consecutive cases. South Med J 1999; 92:289–295.
48. Vasquez JE, Mehta JB, Agrawal R, Sarubbi FA. Blastomycosis in northeast Tennessee. Chest 1998; 114:436–443.
49. Failla PJ, Cerise FP, Karam GH, Summer WR. Blastomycosis: pulmonary and pleural manifestations. South Med J 1995; 88:405–410.
50. Wiesman IM, Podbielski FJ, Hernan MJ, Sekosan M, Vigneswaran WT. Thoracic blastomycosis and empyema. JSLS 1999; 3:75–78.
51. Galgiani JN, Catanzaro A, Cloud GA, Johnson RH, Williams PL, Mirels LF, et al. Comparison of oral fluconazole and itraconazole for progressive, nonmeningeal coccidioidomycosis. A randomized, double-blind trial. Mycoses Study Group. Ann Intern Med 2000; 133:676–686.
52. Benard G, Orii NM, Marques HH, Mendonca M, Aquino MZ, Campeas AE, et al.

Severe acute paracoccidioidomycosis in children. Pediatr Infect Dis J 1994; 13: 510–515.
53. Funari M, Kavakama J, Shikanai-Yasuda MA, Castro LG, Bernard G, Rocha MS, Cerri GG, Muller NL. Chronic pulmonary paracoccidioidomycosis (South American blastomycosis): high-resolution CT findings in 41 patients. AJR Am J Roentgenol 1999; 173:59–64.
54. Fields CL, Ossorio MA, Roy TM. Empyema associated with pulmonary sporotrichosis. South Med J 1989; 82:910–913.
55. Bates M, Cruickshank G. Thoracic actinomycosis. Thorax 1957; 12:99–124.
56. Kinnear WJ, MacFarlane JT. A survey of thoracic actinomycosis. Respir Med 1990; 84:57–59.
57. Merdler C, Greif J, Burke M, Sasson E. A Campus, Primary actinomycotic empyema. South Med J 1983; 76:411–412.
58. Varkey B, Landis FB, Tang TT, Rose HD. Thoracic actinomycosis. Dissemination to skin, subcutaneous tissue, and muscle. Arch Intern Med 1974; 134:689–693.
59. Webb WR, Sagel SS. Actinomycosis involving the chest wall: CT findings. AJR Am J Roentgenol 1982; 139:1007–1009.
60. Thompson AJ, Carty H. Pulmonary actinomycosis in children. Pediatr Radiol 1979; 8:7–9.
61. Zeebregts CJ, van der Heyden AH, Ligtvoet EE, Wagenaar JP, Hoitsma HF. Transphrenic dissemination of actinomycosis. Thorax 1996; 51:449–450.
62. O'Sullivan RA, Armstrong JG, Rivers JT, Mitchell CA. Pulmonary actinomycosis complicated by effusive constrictive pericarditis. Aust N Z J Med 1991; 21:879–880.
63. Legum LL, Greer KE, Glessner SF. Disseminated actinomycosis. South Med J 1978; 71:463–465.
64. Skoutelis A, Petrochilos J, Bassaris H. Successful treatment of thoracic actinomycosis with ceftriaxone. Clin Infect Dis 1994; 19:161–162.
65. Olson ES, Simpson AJ, Norton AJ, Das SS. Not everything acid fast is *Mycobacterium tuberculosis*—a case report. J Clin Pathol 1998; 51:535–536.
66. Cremades MJ, Menendez R, Santos M, Gobernado M. Repeated pulmonary infection by *Nocardia asteroides* complex in a patient with bronchiectasis. Respiration 1998; 65:211–213.
67. Conant EF, Wechsler RJ. Actinomycosis and nocardiosis of the lung. J Thorac Imaging 1992; 7:75–84.
68. Buckley JA, Padhani AR, Kuhlman JE. CT features of pulmonary nocardiosis. J Comput Assist Tomogr 1995; 19:726–732.
69. Yoon HK, Im JG, Ahn JM, Han MC. Pulmonary nocardiosis: CT findings. J Comput Assist Tomogr 1995; 19:52–55.
70. Brechot JM, Capron F, Prudent J, Rochemaure J. Unexpected pulmonary nocardiosis in a non-immunocompromised patient. Thorax 1987; 42:479–480.
71. Soubani AO, Ibrahim I, Forlenza S. Simultaneous nocardial empyema and *Pneumocystis carinii* pneumonia as an initial manifestation of HIV infection. South Med J 1993; 86:1318–1319.

44

Pleural Effusions in Parasitic Infections

SEMRA BILAÇEROĞLU

Izmir Training and Research Hospital for Thoracic Medicine and Surgery
Izmir, Turkey

I. Introduction

With or without involvement of the adjacent lung, pleural disease secondary to parasitic infections constitutes a significant percentage of pleural disorders in underdeveloped and developing countries, whereas it is uncommon in developed parts of the world since high standards of food preparation and waste disposal have rendered parasitic diseases uncommon. However, as global travel, transportation, and trade increase, it appears to be that the incidence of parasitic pleural disorders can increase in developed areas, too (1,2).

Furthermore, in appropriate epidemiological exposures, malignancy, acquired immunodeficiency syndrome (AIDS), immunosuppression, solid organ, bone marrow or stem cell transplantations, neutropenia, corticosteroid treatment, and malnutrition are common coinducers of parasite replication and will increase the frequency of pleural disorders due to parasitic infections, which might be latent in an immunocompetent state. Thus, parasitosis should be considered in any pleural effusion of unclear cause whether epidemiological risk factors are present or not (2–6).

II. Amebiasis

A. Ecology and Epidemiology

This disease, caused by a cosmopolitan protozoan, *Entamoeba histolytica*, is the third leading parasitic cause of death in developing countries and is one of the important health risks to which travelers are exposed. Entamoebas, existing practically in every country in the world, cause infection in 20–30% of people living in the tropical areas and in up to 5% of those in temperate climate countries in south and southeastern Asia, South Africa, Mexico, South America, the Middle East, and some parts of the United States (e.g., California) (7,8).

B. Pathogenesis

The infectious quadrinucleate cyst of *E. histolytica* (Fig. 1), ingested by humans, converts to eight daughter trophozoites, which later colonize intestines, particularly the proximal colon. Commensal and potentially invazive uninucleate trophozoites (Fig. 2) can proliferate and migrate via portal circulation to the liver. Cytolytic enzymes released by the trophozoites cause hepatic abscesses and related complications. The cysts that some trophozoites revert to and pass in the stool complete the life cycle of the parasite. Trophozoites passed in the stool are not infectious (1,2,7–9).

Although in some cases ameba may have entered the respiratory system by direct inhalation (9) or by transcoelomic migration in the peritoneal cavity (8) before giving rise to pulmonary and/or pleural pathology, it has been generally

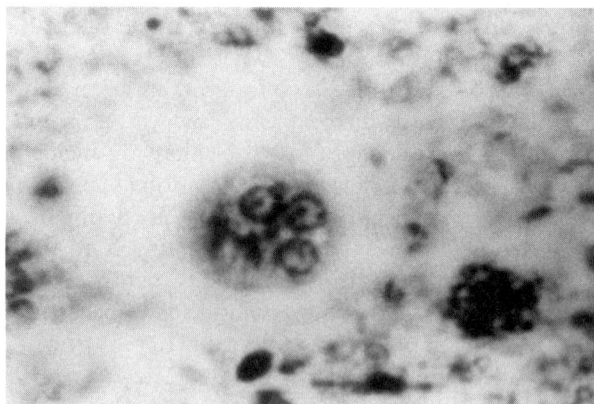

Figure 1 A quadrinucleate, mature *Entamoeba histolytica* cyst of 12–20 μm diameter in stool specimen. (Courtesy of Department of Parasitology, Chiang Mai University, Chiang Mai, Thailand.)

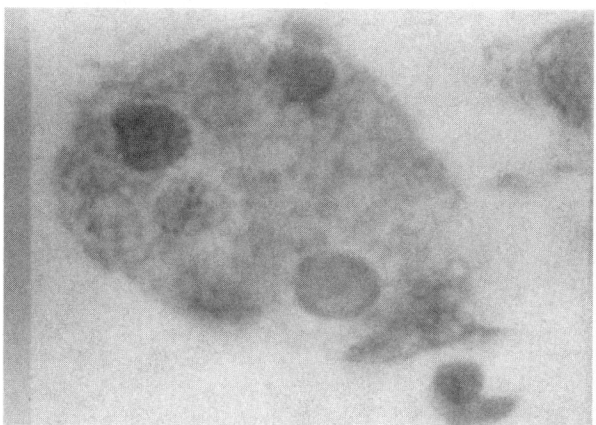

Figure 2 An invasive uninucleate trophozoite of *Entamoeba histolytica* containing erythrocytes and bacteria. (Courtesy of P. Caramello, Carlo Denegri Foundation, Torino, Italy.)

accepted that amebic infestation, once established in the intestinal tract, can spread further through three main channels:

1. Through the portal circulation to liver, then directly by perforation subdiaphragmatically or across the diaphragm to pleural space, lungs, and pericardial space
2. Through the general circulation, invading the inferior vena cava and from there giving metastases to lungs, brain, spleen, etc.
3. Through the lymphatic stream locally (then to the inferior vena cava) or through the thoracic duct to the superior vena cava and thereafter to lungs, brain, spleen and genitourinary tract (2,7,9)

The most frequent form of dissemination in intestinal amebiasis is to the liver by portal system. Hepatic abscess formed by coalescing microabscesses as a result of host response of polymorphonuclear leukocytes and amebic proteolytic enzymes occurs in 5–20% of the cases and is mostly located in the right lobe of the liver (Fig. 3). Cell-mediated immune defense mechanisms probably have a role in limiting invasive disease and recurrence.

An amebic liver abscess can appear concurrently with colitis, but more frequently there is no evidence or history of recent intestinal infection by *E. histolytica*; likewise, less than 50% have amebic cysts in their stool (2,7–9).

C. Clinical Manifestations

Amebic Liver Abscess

An amebic liver abscess involves the right lobe 85% of the time and the left about 30%; right and left thoracic complications occur proportionally.

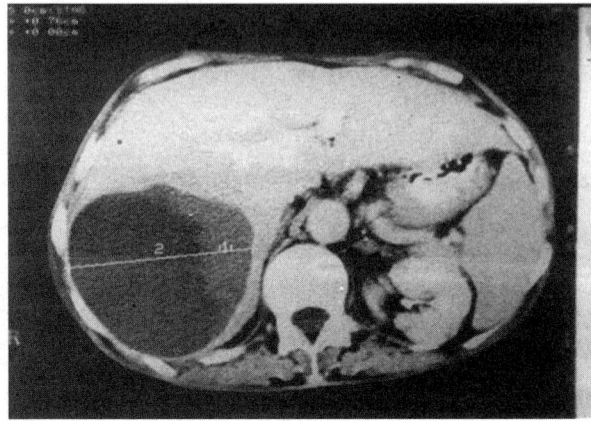

Figure 3 Amebic liver abscess in the right lobe of the liver. Higher-density area inside the abscess may be due to hemorrhage.

By the time the abscess breaches the diaphragm (Fig. 4), there can be an acute onset (less than 10 days) with abdominal pain in the right upper quadrant and fever or a subacute onset with weight loss, and less than half of the patients having fever or abdominal pain. Abdominal pain can be referred to the shoulder and accompanied by a nonproductive cough. Physical examination may reveal exquisite point tenderness over liver, hepatomegaly, and dullness and rales at the right lung base. The presence of peritonitis or a pericardial friction rub indicates extension of infection beyond liver and increased mortality.

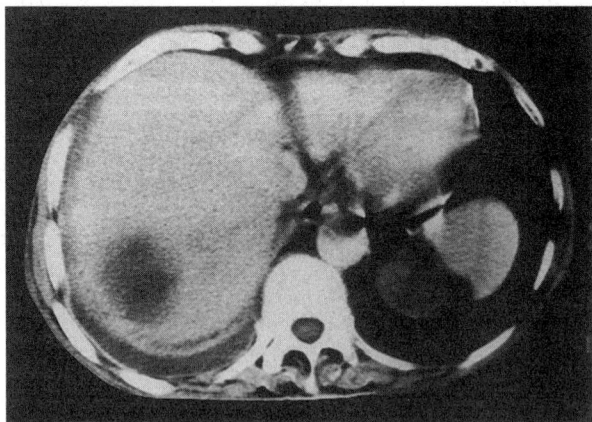

Figure 4 Upper pole of the amebic liver abscess in Figure 3 has breached the diaphragm and ruptured into the pleural space, resulting in right pleural empyema.

Laboratory findings include leukocytosis without eosinophilia in 80%, mild anemia in more than half, elevated erythrocyte sedimentation rate, alkaline phosphatase, and transaminase levels, and decreased serum cholesterol and albumin levels in most patients; hyperbilirubinemia is usually present in the setting of severe disease or peritonitis (2,8,9).

Pleuropulmonary Manifestations

Thoracic repercussions of amebiasis occurring in 25–35% of the cases with liver involvement are:

1. Reactive, sympathetic dry pleurisy or pleural effusion
2. Pyothorax (Figs. 4, 5)
3. Pneumothorax
4. Pyopneumothorax
5. Reactive, fistulous (Fig. 5), or metastatic pneumonitis
6. Fistulous or metastatic lung abscess (Fig. 6)
7. Subdiaphragmatic abscess
8. Reactive or pyogenic pericardial effusion

Pleuropulmonary involvement, mostly right sided and developing in 15–20%, is the most common complication of amebic liver abscess (1,2,7,9).

Sympathetic pleural effusion accompanying amebic liver abscess, but not an extension of the disease, is more frequently (30–34%) seen than an amebic empyema (18–22%) due to rupture of an amebic abscess through the diaphragm into the pleural space. The incidence of sympathetic pleural effusion appears to be underestimated since many cases are missed owing to the small amount of the

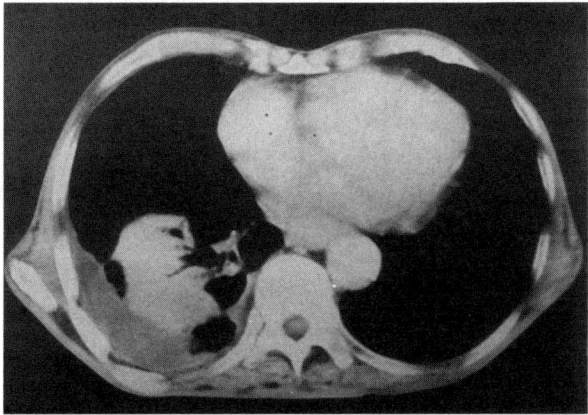

Figure 5 Right pleural empyema and fistulous pneumonitis secondary to the rupture of the amebic liver abscess shown in Figures 3 and 4. The patient coughed up chocolate-sauce sputum after rupture of the abscess.

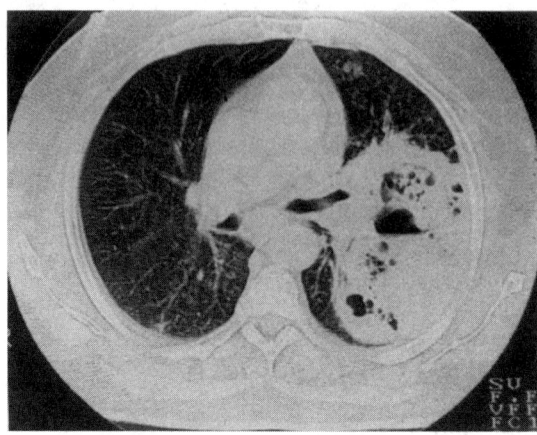

Figure 6 Metastatic amebic abscess in the left lung of an AIDS patient with intestinal amebiasis.

effusion escaping attention on physical examination and chest roentgenograms (9–13). Sympathetic pleural effusion usually causes dry or mucus-producing cough and pleuritic chest pain that may be referred to the shoulder or scapular area; a tender enlarged liver is palpated in most patients. Usually, a small- to moderate-sized pleural effusion, elevation of the ipsilateral hemidiaphragm, plate-like atelectasis, and pneumonitis are the radiological findings. Sometimes pleural effusion may be large enough to cause respiratory distress. Pleural effusion in this setting is a sterile exudate without amebas and bacteria, but its characteristics are not defined in detail. The pleural effusion accompanying an amebic liver abscess should be examined to distinguish a reactive effusion from amebic empyema, which requires aggressive therapy. All pleural effusions, particularly right-sided ones, without obvious explanation should be investigated for amebiasis (1,2,9,11,13).Direct or contiguous extension of an amebic liver abscess comprises about 65–75% of all amebic pleuropulmonary complications: pulmonary abscess extending directly from the liver abscess (18–37%), bronchohepatic fistula with little pulmonary involvement (20–21%), and empyema extending from the liver abscess (15–25%) (Figs. 3–5). Hematogenous pleuropulmonary involvement occurs in less than 25% of the cases (2,7,9) (Fig. 6).

Transdiaphragmatic rupture is generally accompanied with a sudden worsening of pain and a sharp and tearing sensation in the right upper quadrant of the abdomen or lower hemithorax. Rapidly progressing respiratory distress, sepsis, and sometimes hyperdynamic shock follow these symptoms. Rupture into the pleural space, right-sided in more than 90% of cases and occuring when there is no adhesion, between the lung and diaphragm, causes a frequently massive pleural effusion, totally opacifying the hemithorax and leading to mediastinal shift to the contralateral side. Pleural empyema due to rupture of the liver abscess portends a substantial mortality (15–35%). Symptoms may develop more gradually in patients presenting with subacute or chronic clinical picture.

Simultaneous rupture into the airways, hepatobronchial fistula (8–30%), is usually followed by the expectoration of hemoptysis-like chocolate-sauce sputum, but the sputum, like amebic pus in liver abscess or pleural space, may vary in color (7,9,11,14,15). Reactive inflammatory or direct invasive involvement of the pulmonary parenchyma and the pleural space may occur simultaneously in 14–33% of cases with amebic liver abscess, about 10–21% presenting the invasive form (8,9,11,13,16,17) (Figs. 3–5).

Concomitant rupture into pleural and pericardial cavities occurs rarely (0.2%) but carries a mortality rate of 74–100% (7,9,11,14,15). About 10–30% of amebic liver abscesses develop in the left lobe of the liver and may lead to reactive or invasive pericardial effusion (5%), left pleural effusion, and/or left lung involvement. Mostly fatal invasive pericardial effusion is encountered in only 1% of liver abscesses (7,8,11,14,17,18).

Pneumothorax or pyopneumothorax may infrequently complicate a rupturing amebic liver abscess. Since the abscess causes an inflammatory reaction and local thickening in the pleura before rupture, pneumothorax is uncommon even in patients with hepatobronchial fistulas (Fig. 5). Pneumothorax almost always indicates the presence of a bronchopleural fistula. Furthermore, air may rarely enter the pleural space from the liver abscess with a hepatoenteric fistula. Superinfection with gas-forming organisms may cause air in the amebic empyema (7,9,19).

D. Diagnosis

An unequivocal diagnosis is made when motile amebic trophozoites (Fig. 2) can be demonstrated in the amebic pus of the liver, pleural fluid, sputum, or pericardial effusion; however, this can usually be accomplished in less than 10% (10–30%) of the cases even when the most sensitive saline wet mount is used. Both over- and underdiagnoses are common since demonstration of trophozoites is technically difficult. Amebic pus contains few cells and is usually sterile until bacterial superinfection ensues. Concomitant biopsy of the wall of the liver abscess may increase the diagnostic yield since active trophozoites live in the capsule.

Distinctive anchovy paste or chocolate-sauce pleural fluid—thick, opaque, and usually reddish-brown in color—strongly suggests the diagnosis of amebic abscess. Amebic pus is composed largely of liquefied liver. Nevertheless, the color of the fluid may vary from dark brown, green, yellow, or pink, to white (1,7,9,11,12).

In a greater number of cases, the diagnosis of pleural or other thoracic amebiasis is made on the basis of the consistent clinical and radiological aspects and response to a therapeutic trial for amebiasis. A wide variety of serological tests, detecting serum antiamebic antibodies and positive in up to 95–99% of patients, confirm the diagnosis in extraintestinal disease (complement fixation, indirect hemagglutination, amebic gel diffusion tests and immunofluorescent techniques, etc.). However, in acute presentations of less than 7 days, serological studies may be negative, and after a resolved infection it may also take up to 10 years for serology to revert to negative, an important problem in endemic areas. Though slightly less sensitive, immunodiffusion tests are advantageous over the most sensitive method, indirect hemagglutination, since they revert to negative more quickly, in 6–12 months (7,9,11,13).

Chest radiograms are usually sufficient to show and suggest thoracic involvement by amebiasis. However, imaging of the liver by ultrasonography (USG) or computed tomography (CT) is required to reveal and delineate the extent of intrahepatic, subphrenic, or splenic abscesses but can rarely distinguish an amebic abscess from a pyogenic abscess, infected hydatid cyst, hematoma, biloma, cystic or necrotic tumor and infected or hemorrhagic cyst. USG or CT may also be needed in some radiologically and clinically atypical thoracic involvements (1,2,7,10,19,20) and may be helpful in the diagnosis of amebic liver abscess at an early stage or later when a complication is suspected. Both techniques can also help to indicate and safely perform percutaneous therapeutic aspiration. Although therapeutic response can be followed up by both techniques, USG is less costly, and can image some locations better (10,20–23).

Thoracic amebiasis can masquerade as tuberculosis, pyogenic empyema, pyogenic lung abscess, pneumonia, and malignant disease. Chronic cough, hemoptysis, and fever can occur in all of these conditions. The diagnostic work-up can be further confounded by similar geographic distribution of amebiasis and tuberculosis (11,13,16).

E. Treatment

More than 80% of the cases of amebic liver abscess can be managed with a 10- to 14-day course of intravenous or oral metronidazole. Generally, metronidazole at 750 mg three times a day for 10 days is the treatment of choice. In cases of suspected amebic liver abscess, treatment should be started before diagnostic confirmation since, once diagnosed, amebiasis is a treatable disease, but when untreated it is often fatal (2,7,10,11,13,24).

Although more toxic, emetine and dehydroemetine are occasionally used for critically ill patients or those with frequently fatal complications (i.e., rupture into the pericardium or peritoneum) since these drugs are considered by some physicians to give a more rapid response than metronidazole. Chloroquine, less effective for extraintestinal amebiasis, might be preferred in a pregnant patient who is not critically ill. It is given at a dose of 600 mg base daily for the first 2 days, followed by 300 mg daily for 3–10 weeks.

All four of the above-mentioned drugs are more effective for tissue-dwelling amebas. Metronidazole is the most effective of the four for intestinal disease, with an eradication rate of 85%. Thus, a course of luminal amebicide (i.e., iodoquinol, 650 mg three times a day for 20 days, or paromomycin for 10 days) should follow metronidazole treatment (2,7,8,13,24).

Most patients show good, immediate clinical response to metronidazole within 48–72 hours. Some authors defend a treatment change to dehydroemetine and chloroquine if there is no clinical improvement after 72–96 hours (24). However, bacterial superinfection, occurring in up to 33% of cases with pleural disease, may be a possible explanation for unresponsiveness to metronidazole (1,2,7,13).

A sympathetic, reactive pleural effusion almost always warrants no additional therapy other than that performed for the amebic liver abscess. Only if the effusion is large enough to cause respiratory distress can therapeutic thoracentesis be performed to control symptoms; a single tap will be sufficient (1,2,11,13). In case of transdiaphragmatic rupture, percutaneous drainage of both the liver abscess and the pus in pleural or pericardial space must be performed in addition to antiamebic drug therapy. Large chest tubes recommended for drainage in the past (11,13,17) have been effectively replaced by 12–14 F small tubes in the last decade (25).

Concomitant bacterial infection of the pleural space in amebic empyema should be treated with appropriate antibiotics (1,2,7,13). Not infrequently, rapid development of a thick pleural peel can require an open drainage procedure or decortication. If the lung fails to reexpand in 10 days, decortication should be performed whether there is bacterial superinfection or not. At decortication operation, the visceral pleura is found to be covered by a thick membrane that can be easily stripped off (12,13,17,26).

The prognosis of amebiasis, even with transdiaphragmatic rupture, is good if the patient is not too debilitated initially or if the diagnosis is not delayed (2,11–13). The mortality rate of 2.4–4.2% in amebic liver abscess is higher in patients with complications and with underlying disorders such as diabetes mellitus, AIDS, immunosuppression, etc. Jaundice, large or multiple abscesses, acute abdomen, liver failure, and sepsis in addition to alterations in prothrombin time, activated partial thromboplastin time, total bilirubin, albumin, blood urea nitrogen, lactate dehydrogenase, and leukocytes should alert the clinician to suspect complications in order to reduce morbidity and mortality (6,7,27,28).

III. Echinococcosis

Tissue infestation with the larval form of a tapeworm of *Echinococcus* species causes two main types of echinococcosis: hydatid or unilocular cyst disease caused by *Echinococcus granulosus* and alveolar cyst disease caused by *Echinococcus multilocularis*. Alveolar disease, uncommonly encountered, rarely involves thoracic structures, whereas more prevalent cystic hydatid disease constitutes almost all of the echinococcal thoracic involvements. The pleura can be involved primarily, but more frequently it is involved secondarily by spread from the liver or lungs. Human infection with the larvae of this cestode is one of the most important helminthic pulmonary diseases (1,2,29–32).

A. Ecology and Epidemiology

Cystic hydatid disease is seen most commonly in rural sheep- and cattle-farming areas. It is particularly prevalent in Latin America (Argentina, Uruguay, Chile), the southwestern United States, Australia, New Zealand, parts of Africa, the Middle East (Lebanon), and eastern and southern Europe (Greece and Turkey). Close contact with dogs and urban residence near slaughterhouses where dogs access animal viscera increase the risk of infection with this parasite (29,30–33). The rare alveolar hydatid disease found mostly in northern forest areas of Europe, Asia, North America, and Arctic regions is transmitted by wild canines (30,31).

In developing countries and among children where hygiene usually tends to fail, ingestion of weeklong-viable eggs from dog feces is the frequent route of infection with echinococcosis. Human infection has been decreased significantly through strict and scrupulous hygiene in rural areas of many developed countries, even though sheep and dog infections have stayed at 10–20% in these areas (2,30,32).

B. Pathogenesis

Because of the circulatory anatomy, the most common site for the development of hydatid cysts is the liver, followed by the lung. A rim of compressed host tissue, the pericyst, lies external to the laminated membrane. The 1–2 mm thick, tough and acellular laminated membrane surrounds the hydatid cyst. The germinal membrane lying beneath the laminated membrane gives rise to protoscolices that contain a double row of hooklets (Fig. 7). The protoscolices accumulating inside the cyst form the hydatid sand and give rise to either adult tapeworms or new hydatid cysts. Occasionally, in addition to watery fluid and hydatid sand, the cyst may also contain daughter cysts (Fig. 8) similar in structure to the mother cyst (2,30).

C. Clinical Manifestations

Primary involvement of the pleura with hydatid disease is rare since the pleura is a well-vascularized tissue (30,31,34–38). When a hepatic, pulmonary, or on rare occasions splenic cyst ruptures into the pleural space, there is a danger of secondary pleural hydatidosis by seeding with protoscolices and daughter cysts. Most frequently, daughter cysts get implanted on pleura and form multiple and sandwiched groups of cysts between thickened pleural layers (Fig. 9). Small secondary cysts grown from hydatid sand and floating freely in the pleural fluid, hydatidothorax, is another form of secondary pleural hydatidosis (Fig. 10). In a third presentation, younger cysts together with granulomas developed against hydatid elements pave the pleura. This so-called hydatid pleural granulomatosis

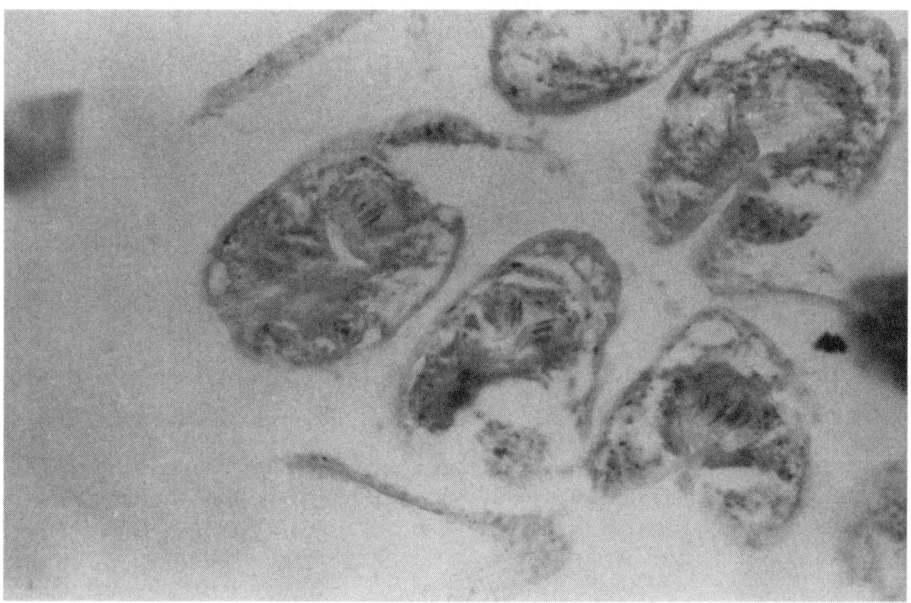

Figure 7 Protoscolices in pleural fluid after rupture of a pulmonary hydatid cyst. Note the hooklets in the protoscolices.

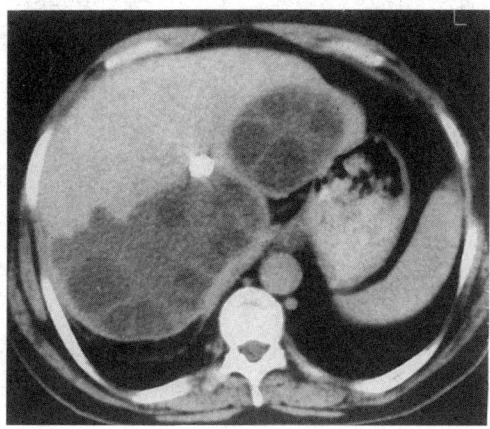

Figure 8 Daughter cysts in the mother cysts of the liver. Note the calcification in the wall of the larger cyst.

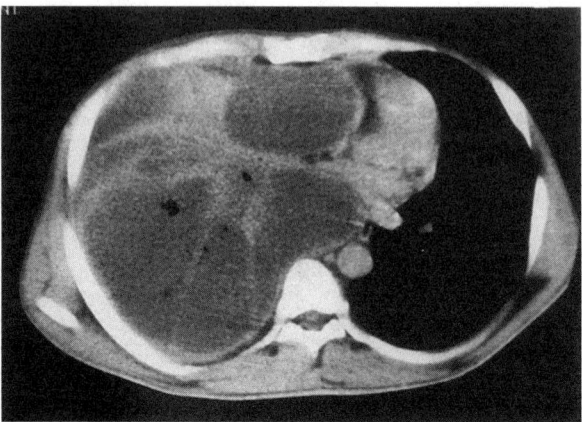

Figure 9 Secondary right pleural hydatidosis shifting the heart to the contralateral side. Multiple, sandwiched groups of pleural cysts with air inside some, indicating bronchopleural fistula.

(Fig. 11) can lead to marked pleural thickening, requiring decortication (29,30,34,36,38,39).

Liver cysts involve the thorax 3–7% of the time, and less than 5% of hepatic or pulmonary hydatid cysts rupture into the pleural space. Following rupture, secondary hydatidosis in the thorax occurs in about 10% of cases (36,38,40). A tendency for bacterial superinfection that destroys the parasite (30,34) and the relative rarity of daughter cysts in pulmonary and hepatic cysts (41) make the pleura a less likely site for secondary hydatidosis. It appears that

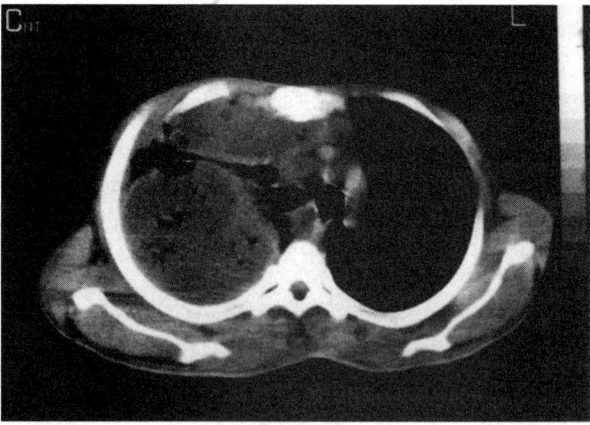

Figure 10 Hydatidothorax: two small secondary cysts floating in the anterior loculation of right empyemic pleural fluid. There is air in both anterior and posterior loculations, indicating bronchopleural fistula.

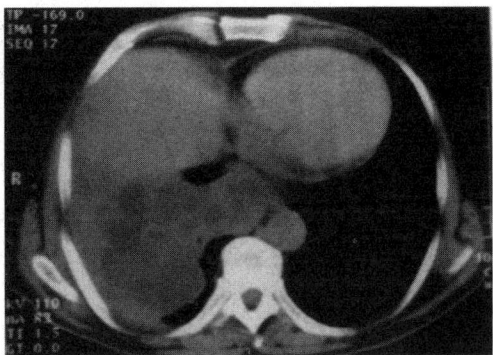

Figure 11 Hydatid pleural granulomatosis: pleural thickening due to younger cysts and antihydatid granulomas paving the right basal face of the pleura.

the more consistent is the tissue carrying the mother cyst, the higher is the number of daughter cysts produced. Thus, many daughter cysts can develop in bone but few in liver and almost none in lung (41). Secondary hydatidosis seems to involve the pleura less frequently than the peritoneum. Pleural seeding due to spills at surgery is uncommon even when there is no superinfection (2,32).

Intact cysts are usually asymptomatic and without any clinical manifestations. However, an intact cyst can cause pleural reaction and exudative pleural effusion in approximately 5% of the patients with a hepatic or pulmonary hydatid (Figs. 12, 13). Most patients with pleural involvement experience chest pain, dyspnea, fever, and cough. The characteristics of this reactive, sympathetic pleural fluid have not been determined (32,42).

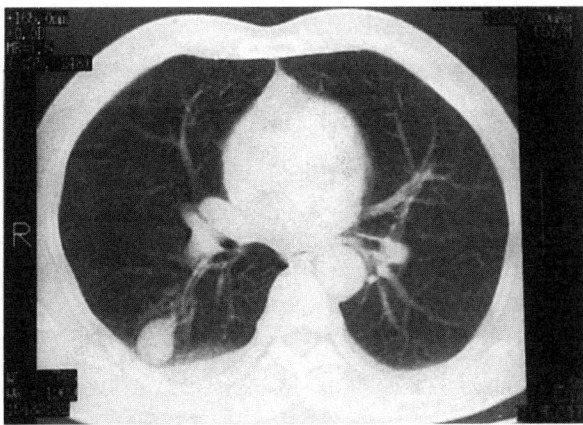

Figure 12 Intact hydatid cyst in the right lung and the accompanying sympathetic pleural effusion.

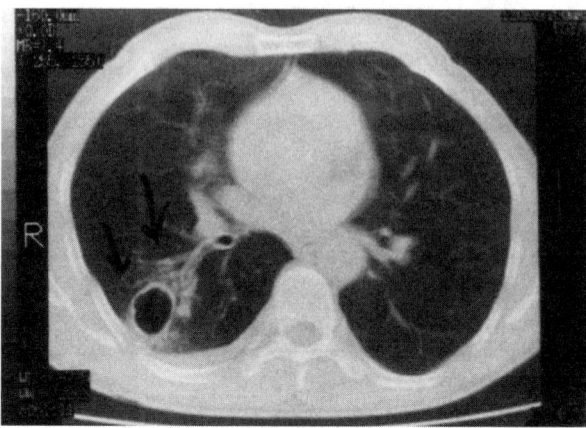

Figure 13 Rupture of the hydatid cyst in Figure 12 into the airways. Right sympathetic pleural effusion shows no change in amount.

A pleural effusion tends to develop more commonly when a pulmonary or hepatic cyst is superinfected or becomes an abscess (Fig. 14). In the early stages, the infected hydatid high in the liver or peripherally located in the lung may cause inflammation of the adjacent pleura and may later rupture into the pleural space. Local pleural obliteration due to chronic reactive pleuritis may result in rupture only into the lung and/or airways without any rupture into the pleural space (32,34,36,43).

Rupture of a hepatic, pulmonary, or rarer splenic hydatid cyst into the above-mentioned thoracic structures usually renders the patient acutely ill, with sudden tearing chest pain, dyspnea, and shock due to antigenic challenge to the body. Anaphylaxis, pleural or pulmonary implantation of daughter cysts, and

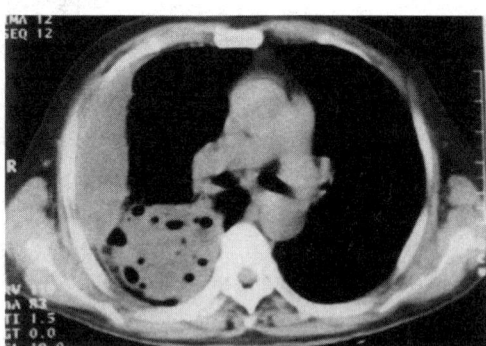

Figure 14 An infected pulmonary hydatid cyst that has turned into an abscess and accompanying loculated pleural empyema on the right. Note the air-filled cavities of daughter cysts that have ruptured into the airways.

biliary-bronchial and/or bronchopleural fistula in hepatic cysts and bronchopleural fistula in pulmonary or splenic cysts can develop (34,35,39,44,45).

Simultaneous rupture into the airways occurs in about half of hepatic cysts rupturing into the pleural space (Fig. 15). Rupture into the airways is characterized by the expectoration of large quantities of pus and/or cyst contents, which may be pieces of laminated membrane resembling the white of a hard-boiled egg, daughter cysts, often compared with grapes, and/or watery cyst liquid with a salty taste. Hemoptysis may accompany the expectorated substances. Bronchospasm, urticaria, or anaphylaxis can follow the rupture into the airways (33,34,39,44). Simultaneous rupture of a pulmonary cyst into the airways and pleural space is mostly accompanied by a bronchopleural fistula and pneumothorax or more commonly hydropneumothorax with cyst contents (Fig. 16). This hydropneumothorax may readily become infected to form pyopneumothorax (35-37) (Fig. 10).

In some cases, pulmonary hydatid cysts may rupture solely into the pleural cavity or solely into airways (30,35). After cyst contents are partly or completely discharged into the bronchial tree and air enters the cyst cavity, it may then become incarcerated or become secondarily infected and form an abscess (30,46) (Fig. 14).

Sterile hepatic, pulmonary, or splenic cysts can rupture into the pleural space, lung, or airways owing to the mechanical effect on the diaphragm by the enlarging cyst, positive abdominal and negative thoracic pressures, the vacuum-like action of diaphragmatic movements, the slow but steady action of pericystium growth, trauma, cough, or the force of respiration (29,30,45,47) (Figs. 13, 17, 18).

Pleural inflammation or pleural effusion can also accompany rare thoracic presentations of hydatid disease such as hydatid cysts of the chest wall (48,49)

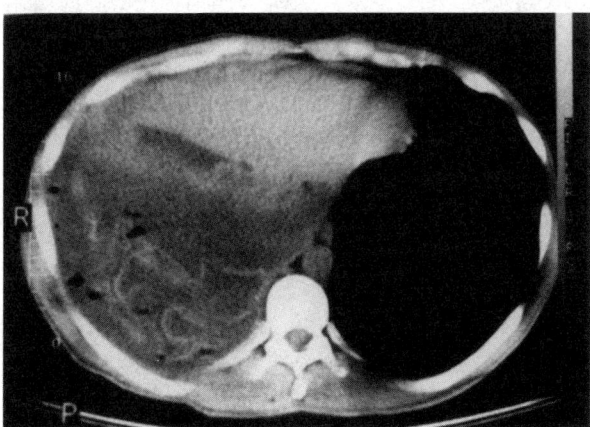

Figure 15 Simultaneous rupture of a hepatic hydatid cyst into pleural space and airways. Pieces of laminated membrane and air are seen in the pleural fluid.

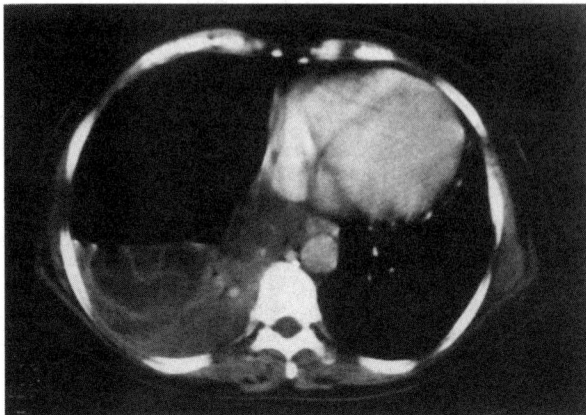

Figure 16 Tension hydropneumothorax with floating cyst contents. Simultaneous rupture of a pulmonary hydatid cyst into the pleural space and airways have occurred. The heart is shifted to the contralateral side by tension pneumothorax resulting from bronchopleural fistula.

and diaphragm (50,51) (Fig. 19). Unusual chyliform pleural effusion can also develop in hepatothoracic hydatid disease (52).

D. Diagnosis

Demonstration of echinococcal protoscolices with hooklets, free hooklets, or laminated membrane in the pleural fluid or biopsy specimen establishes the

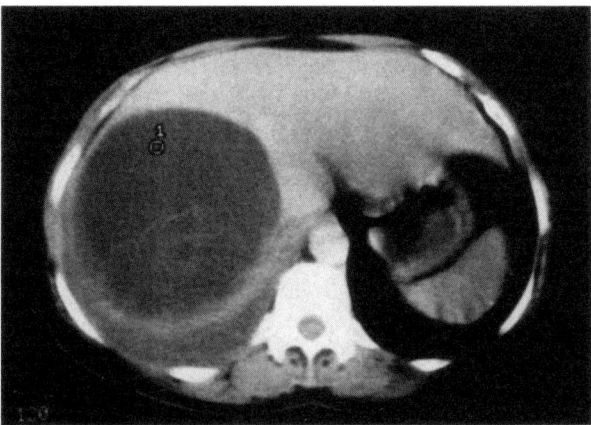

Figure 17 A sterile hepatic hydatid cyst rupturing into the pleural space and causing pleural effusion. Ill-defined posterior margin and the floating membranes in the cyst indicate rupture.

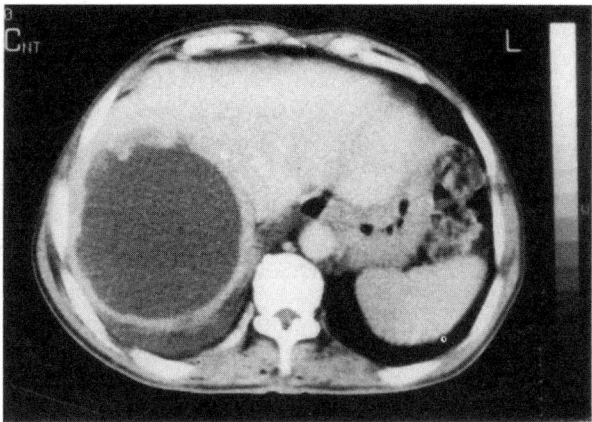

Figure 18 A sterile hepatic hydatid cyst rupturing into the pleural space and causing pleural effusion; irregular anterior and lateral contour due to collapsing is a sign of rupture. Note the prominent pericyst area medially and calcification on the anteromedial margin.

diagnosis of pleural hydatid disease (53–55). Protoscolices and hooklets are acid-fast on Ziehl-Neelsen stain. Sputum (45,55) or bronchoscopic specimens (33,56) from a patient with ruptured cyst or the fluid aspirated from a cyst itself (57) may also contain the diagnostic fragments of the cyst.

Peripheral blood eosinophilia, although it may be high immediately after cyst rupture, is not reliable in diagnosis (47). Eosinophils can frequently be found in the pleural fluid unless it is secondarily infected (34,45,53).

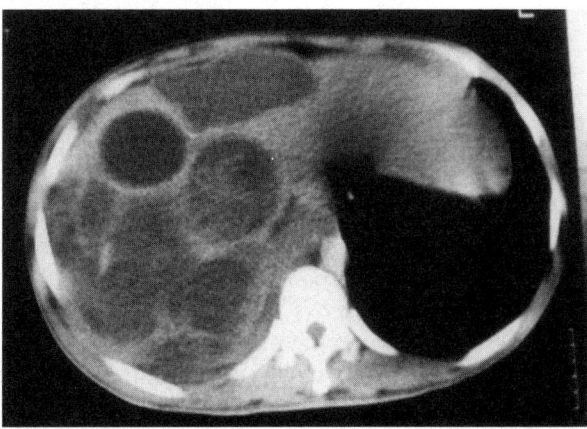

Figure 19 Secondary hydatidosis of the right hemidiaphragm.

Hydatid disease suspected on the basis of imaging studies [chest radiogram, USG, CT scan, or magnetic resonance imaging (MRI)] is usually confirmed by specific enzyme-linked immunosorbent assay (ELISA) or Western blot serology, confirming exposure to the parasite (30). Serology is highly sensitive (80–100%) and specific (88–96%) for liver cysts but less sensitive for unruptured lung cysts (50–56%) or other organ involvement (25–56%). It is suggested that in the lung, little antigen escapes to stimulate antibody formation since the cyst is so completely separated from the lung tissue (2,30,31). An ELISA for antigen detection is highly accurate for aspirated fluid of intact cysts, but its accuracy for ruptured or infected cysts or spilled cyst fluid is not well established (58). Serological cross-reactions with other worms, particularly cysticercus, can occur (59).

The Casoni skin test is positive in about 75% of the patients with hydatid disease and the Weinberg complement-fixation test in a higher percentage (31,39). However, the skin test reaction, once acquired, remains positive for life even when the cyst is surgically removed. Likewise, the Weinberg complement-fixation test may remain positive for 2 years after elimination of the infection (31). Not infrequently, serological and skin tests yield false-negative results as well as false-positive ones, creating confusion. Assays using recombinant *Echinococcus* antigens and that may provide higher specificity for diagnosis are under development (30).

Imaging remains more sensitive than skin testing and serodiagnosis for the hydatid disease. There may be false-negative cases with negative serological result but with typical appearance on imaging studies (2,30,39,59,60). Conventional chest radiography has been the mainstay of the diagnostic workup for hydatid disease of the lungs, usually coupled with Casoni's skin test and serological test for antibodies. However, this combination may not establish a definitive diagnosis in a considerable number of cases, owing to conditions mimicking hydatid cysts of the lung (carcinomas, benign tumors, inflammatory masses, metastasis, and solid or fluid-filled cysts) on imaging studies or false-positive and false-negative results obtained by skin and serological tests (30,46,60).

On chest radiogram most patients with hydatid disease of the lungs have multiple round cystic lesions. The majority of the cases are unruptured at the lung bases and at the posterior segments. A small single cyst has the appearance of a coin lesion. Multiple cysts may suggest metastatic cancer. Large cysts take a complex shape as they are indented and folded by adjacent structures. The sharp edge of the cyst can become blurred by the alterations in the surrounding tissue. Calcification of the cyst wall or internally may be present. A fluid-fluid level is produced by the hydatid sand in the cyst fluid.

When the cyst is disrupted, peculiar radiological signs appear and can at times confuse and mislead the physician. When air enters between the pericyst and cyst wall, a crescent of air separates the cyst from an outer rim, creating the crescent sign. If air enters the cyst cavity, the crescent of air arches over a cavity with air-fluid level; this is called the double arc sign. Crumpled endocystic membranes of the further collapsed cyst floating on the air-fluid level in a cavity constitutes the water lily sign, which can also be seen in a hydropneumothorax (2,40,41,59) (Fig. 16).

CT scanning is superior to plain radiography in elucidating the cystic nature of the hydatid disease in the lungs or other thoracic structures such as the pleural space and chest wall besides providing a road map for accurate localization in planning of surgical treatment. The fluid density of an intact cyst, air-fluid density of a ruptured cyst, and "solid" density of a complicated cyst are revealed by CT. CT scan can be of value in determining the presence of cysts in areas difficult to visualize with plain chest radiographs, especially in the posterior and anterior costophrenic angles. Determination of wall thickness of the cyst is more accurate with CT than other modalities (46,60). CT is also beneficial in diagnosing, locating, and determining the extent of cysts in the liver, spleen, or other parts of the body (30,32). Furthermore, it can be employed to guide percutaneous treatment of hepatic cysts (61).

In addition to classical crescent (meniscus), double arc (cumbo's), water lily (camalote) signs, and calcification in the wall or inner part of the cyst, the recently described inverse crescent sign and signet ring sign can be shown by CT. The inverse crescent sign is a crescent-like rim of air at the lower end of the cyst, with an appearance morphologically opposite of the crescent sign. A zone of pericystic fibrosis and distortion of lung-cyst interface on the upper end of the cyst causes separation of the cyst membranes by air dissection only from the posterior aspect. This bleb of air dissecting into the wall of the cyst, giving it the shape of a ring, is called a signet ring sign and can be a harbinger of impending cyst rupture (60).

The presence of intact daughter cysts and collapsed daughter cyst membranes or evacuated daughter cysts are other CT findings that aid in the diagnosis (2,46). High (solid) CT density of a complicated cyst results from fibrosis or infection and attracts a differential diagnosis of tumors, infarcts, etc. Inadvertent transthoracic aspiration can be attempted in these cases if serological methods are negative or not performed because of not considering hydatid cyst in the differential diagnosis. In addition, the cyst wall can be thick owing to infection and should not negate a diagnosis of hydatid disease (46,60).

USG is an inexpensive, noninvasive, and easily accessible method in the diagnosis of echinococcosis in liver, spleen, and many other organs. However, its use in thoracic echinococcosis is limited to disease in or contiguous to the chest wall (62,63). That it can show the inner structure and density of the cyst better than CT can help in differentiation of cystic and alveolar hydatid diseases, in the recognition of complicated cysts, and in the staging of the cysts by the inner density (62–65). USG is extensively used in guiding the percutaneous treatment of hydatid cysts (64–66).

MRI can be useful in the diagnosis of some selected cases of echinococcosis that cannot be elucidated with initial chest radiography, USG, or CT studies: e.g., vertebral (67), soft tissue (68), cardiovascular (69), central nervous system cysts (70), and some cases of alveolar disease (71). Complicated cysts, vitality of the cysts, and proximity to and differentiation from vascular and neural structures are some infrequent indications for MRI study (72,73).

Alveolar hydatid disease, which is more aggressive, is tumorlike in appearance on imaging studies (Fig. 20) and accounts for the "metastatic behavior" of the sections of the parasite. Serology combined with characteristic imaging studies is an alternative means of establishing the diagnosis (30,74–78).

E. Treatment

Progress in the medical treatment of echinococcosis is still inadequate; thus, optimal treatment of symptomatic disease is by surgical resection to remove the cyst in toto. When a hepatic or pulmonary cyst ruptures into the pleural space, immediate thoracotomy is recommended to remove the parasite from the site of original cyst, to close the bronchopleural fistula, and to reexpand the lung immediately (29,36,39,43). The patient may be treated perioperatively with an antihelminthic active against *Echinococcus* cysts (albendazole, mebendazole) to prevent intraoperative dissemination of daughter cysts (30).

The role of additional medical therapy with hydatid surgery is controversial and has not been clearly determined (2). Medical therapy for inoperable cysts with either albendazole or mebendazole provided improvement in 55–79% and cure in 29% of patients (30). In patients with hydatid disease that cannot be cured or effectively palliated by surgery, or following inadequately treated rupture, albendazole is the treatment of choice: three or more cycles of 400 mg of albendazole bid for 4 weeks, followed by a 2-week rest period without therapy. Unpredictable hepatitic toxic reaction can occur at any time during albendazole therapy. It appears to be more effective for pulmonary than abdominal disease (1,2,30). The alternative agent, mebendazole, is given at a dose of 50–70 mg/kg/

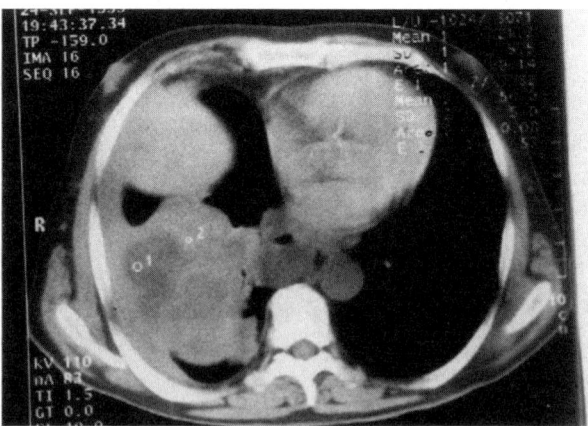

Figure 20 Tumor-like alveolar hydatid disease of the lung causing pleural effusion and thickening. Note the invasive behavior of the disease centrally and peripherally and different densities in the alveolar hydatid mass.

day for several months (2,30). Response to drug therapy depends on the cyst size and location.

IV. Paragonimiasis

Paragonimiasis is a parasitic disease caused by the trematode *Paragonimus westermani*, *Paragonimus miyazakii*, *Paragonimus africanus*, or other species of *Paragonimus*, which is called the lung fluke. The disease, also called endemic hemoptysis, pulmonary distomiasis, or oriental lung fluke disease, is distributed over three continents. It is endemic in certain areas of eastern and southeastern Asia (Japan, Korea, Taiwan, Manchuria, Central China, and the Philippines), the Indian subcontinent, West Africa, and several parts of Central and South America. It is known as a tropical disease but can occur in temperate areas as well. Cases have been diagnosed in North Americans as well as Indo-Chinese refugees and immigrants (2,79–81).

Paragonimus has an interesting life cycle. The worms migrate from intestines to peritoneum, diaphragm, pleural space, and the lung. They may migrate through or occasionally stay in the pleura (2,80–82). Pleuropulmonary paragonimiasis is characterized by the migration of a juvenile worm in the early stage and by formation of cysts around the worm later on.

A. Ecology and Epidemiology

Traditional eating habits play an important role in the epidemiology of human paragonimiasis. Human infection is sporadic and rare in some parts of the world, although animal paragonimiasis is endemic in these areas, e.g., Nepal, Bangladesh, Assam, Korea, Samoa, west and central Africa, Brazil, Peru, eastern United States, and Canada. Human infection is frequently seen in east Asian countries since raw crab or crayfish is eaten and crab juice is added into traditional medicines (2,83,84).

Contamination of hands and utensils with metacercariae can cause human infection in some endemic areas where crabs and crayfish are never eaten raw. Metacercaria are viable for 20 days in cold water, 5 days in warm water, and a month in a refrigerated crab. Pickling and brief freezing does not kill them, but drying and deep freezing do (2,85). Outbreaks can occur during civil disturbances and wars since being compelled to eat raw crab, crayfish, or shrimp, or displacements from nonendemic to endemic areas can occur more frequently at these times (81,86,87).

B. Pathogenesis

Once ingested, the metacercaria excyst in the duodenum as larvae which later bore through the intestinal wall and enter the peritoneal cavity. They migrate upward in the peritoneal cavity, bore through the diaphragm and pleura, and enter the lung, where they finally lodge (79,85,88). Compatibility of the species and its host determine the success of paragonimus in reaching the lungs. *P. westermani* is the most human-adapted species and migrates directly through the diaphragm and causes intrathoracic disease in 98% of the cases (85). Other species may enter the lungs via the liver or may lodge in other sites. There can be larva migrans manifesting with transient and migratory subcutaneous nodules with some species or pleuropulmonary manifestations with others (89). Although brain is the most frequently involved ectopic site (85), any organ (gastrointestinal tract, skeletal muscles, diaphragm, pericardium, anterior mediastinum, hilar lymph nodes, etc.) can be involved (83,85,86,88).

When larvae are multiple, they tend to migrate into the lung after maturing and mating, whereas a single larva usually remains in the pleural space (85). Mature flukes about $7–12 \times 4–7$ mm encapsulate within the parenchyma of the lung and live in small pulmonary cavities, usually close to bronchioles. Multiple worms, eggs, and brown necrotic debris are found in these cavities, which are connected by burrows. Ischemic infarction after obstruction of an arteriole or a vein by a worm or eggs and expansion of the small airway by intraluminal parasite are possible mechanisms for these worm cysts. An inflammatory and fibrotic layer surrounds the cavity. When the cystic space is filled with hemorrhagic fluid and surrounded by pericystic consolidation, it appears as a mass (79,80,85,88).

The *Paragonimus* worm may discharge its eggs into pleural space (81) or may become buried within the thickened pleura (88). However, not much is known about the pleural pathophysiology. Eosinophilic inflammation (90) or chronic inflammation with no remarkable number of eosinophils (91) has been reported on pleural biopsies. As pleural paragonimiasis becomes chronic, pleural thickening can develop and form a restrictive peel (90).

The relationship between immunity and paragonimiasis has not been established. However, corticosteroid treatment may render the worms larger and more numerous (85).

C. Clinical Manifestations

Paragonimiasis causes diarrhea and abdominal pain and sometimes urticaria as the early symptoms after a 2- to 15-day incubation period. Thoracic symptoms, particularly cough productive of brownish sputum and chest pain, begin 1–2 weeks later. The condition may evolve to a picture of chronic bronchitis or bronchiectasis with profuse expectoration (79,89,92). However, cases may infrequently present with constitutional symptoms of fatigue, fever, and malaise instead of gastrointestinal symptoms and develop pleural or pulmonary disease after a month. Constitutional and pulmonary symptoms may persist until a specific diagnosis is established (2,83,88).

Generally, paragonimiasis does not cause systemic illness; the patient's overall health is good despite the extension of the lesions on the chest radiograph. Most light and moderate infections are asymptomatic and detected during screening for tuberculosis or other diseases (81,93). There may be low-grade fever and slight hemoptysis. The flukes tunneling across the pleura into the lung cause pleuritic pain (85,88,92).

The incidence of pulmonary involvement is 83–92% (80,94) and that of pleural involvement 1–69%(2,80,85,95). This wide variation in the incidence of pleural involvement may be ascribed to the species or strain of fluke, the state of the host, and particularly nonperformance of immunodiagnostic methods and reliance mostly on sputum examination. However, in mainly pleural involvement of paragonimiasis, the eggs mostly are not in the sputum but in pleural fluid or pleural biopsy (81,91,92,96).

In studies with large series, in endemic areas, or in susceptible risk groups, pleural disease has been found to be common (80,95,96). In a Korean study, 43 (61%) of 71 cases of pleuropulmonary paragonimiasis had pleural disease; 28% had unilateral pleural effusion, 8% bilateral pleural effusion, 8% unilateral hydropneumothorax, 8% bilateral hydropneumothorax, and 7% pleural thickening (80). In another study from Japan 69% of 13 cases (95) and in a third study from United States 48% of 25 Indochinese refugees with paragonimiasis had pleural effusions (96). Non-Asian cases develop the disease from ingesting infected crayfish (83) or crabs (97). Pleural effusion can be massive in half of the patients (96).

D. Diagnosis

The diagnosis of paragonimiasis should be considered in patients with an East Asian origin or a history of recent travel to East Asia, a family history of paragonimiasis, and consumption and handling of raw or undercooked freshwater crabs, crayfish, or shrimps. Most exposure to paragonimiasis has been familial (83,85,86,96). A cough productive of brown or blood-tinged sputum is the most frequently occurring symptom in paragonimiasis caused by *P. westermani*: numerous golden-brown *P. westermani* eggs give sputum a brown color (88,98). At times, patients may complain about fishy odor of their sputa (90).

On chest radiographs, pulmonary involvement accompanies pleural disease in most cases with pleural paragonimiasis (96). Nevertheless, some cases of pleural paragonimiasis may present only with a nonspecific pleural effusion or basal thickening, or even a normal chest radiograph (2,80,81). Initially, diffuse or focal patchy or masslike air-space consolidations (52%), usually in the middle and lower lung zones, are the areas of hemorrhagic pneumonitis caused by migrating larvae. Within the consolidated lung, round cystic areas 5–15 mm in diameter and consisting of either fluid or gas can be seen on CT scan. At this stage, pleural effusion or pneumothorax is frequently seen. Peripherally located linear shadows 2–4 mm thick and 2–7 cm long frequently adjacent to these consolidated areas are more prominent in patients with pleural effusion. On CT, these linear lesions are suggestive of worm tracks. Variable-sized nodules (25%) appear as the consolidations resolve and maturing worms settle down (Fig. 21). Later the nodules change into 5–30 mm cystic lesions (46%), which are surrounded by linear radiating lesions. The appearance of pleuropulmonary

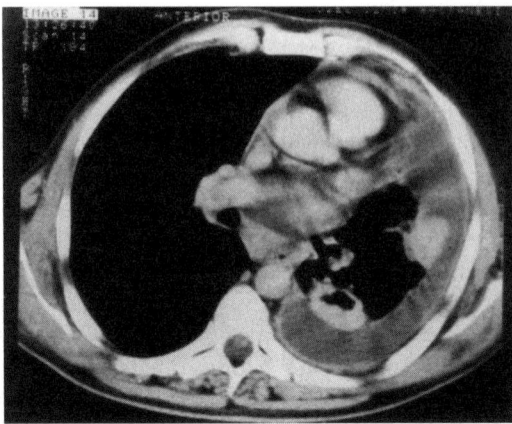

Figure 21 Two peripheral pulmonary nodules, pleural effusion and thickening in paragonimiasis. Note the cavitation in one nodule and hypodense areas in the other, the peripheral linear lesions, and the displacement of mediastinum to the left.

lesions on radiographs varies with the stage of the infection and the surrounding tissue reaction (80,87,94,96,99).

The diagnosis of paragonimiasis is definitely made by demonstration of characteristic brown operculated eggs in the sputum, stool, fluid from bronchoscopic lavage, biopsy specimens, or pleural fluid (84,86,91,98) (Fig. 22). The examination of a 24-hour specimen of sputum previously processed with NaOH

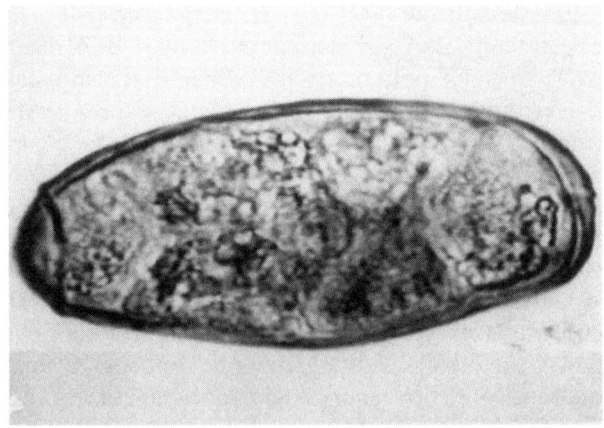

Figure 22 A *Paragonimus westermani* egg in stool sediment: 80–100 by 40–60 μm, golden brown and with a thick shell and prominent operculum. (Courtesy of P. Caramello, Carlo Denegri Foundation, Torino, Italy.)

or hypochlorite is more sensitive than that of direct smears (84,85,91). Sputum examination provides higher diagnostic yield in those with active pulmonary infiltrates but lower yield in those with pleural disease (91,92,96).Although specific, egg detection rates in sputum have been reported to be low (28–50%) (80,98,99). Stool can reveal ova in a substantial fraction of patients with negative sputum and negative serology (84–86). Eggs can be detected in the pleural fluid of only a small group with pleural involvement (81,91,96). Pleural fluid is an opaque and yellow exudate and frequently has cholesterol crystals. Low pleural glucose (<10 mg/dL) and pH (<7.10), high lactic dehydrogenase (>1000 IU/dL) and protein levels (>6 g/dL), a white cell count of <2000/mm^3, and significant eosinophilia varying up to >80% are the characteristics of the fluid (81,82,91, 96). Charcot-Leyden crystals can be found in the pleural or pulmonary worm cysts (81,82,88,96). The only other disease with eosinophilic, low-pH, and low-glucose exudate is Churg-Strauss syndrome (100). Peripheral eosinophilia, although frequent, is unreliable as in all helminthiases (2,98,101).

The sensitivity of serological tests is about 80–90%, and serology becomes negative within a year after cure (79,80,85,88). Complement fixation test, widely used in the past (88), has been replaced by enzyme-linked immunosorbent assay (ELISA), which is highly sensitive (92%) and specific in detecting anti-*Paragonimus* antibodies. Antibody levels drop to normal range 4–24 months after successful treatment (80,99,102). Higher serological titers have been shown in patients with sputum and stool negative for ova than in those positive for ova (96). Pleural fluid IgE levels were determined to be elevated and higher than the simultaneous serum IgE levels in pleural paragonimiasis. Furthermore, parasite-specific IgE and IgG measured by ELISA have also been found to be significantly higher in pleural fluid than in serum, suggesting the potential diagnostic usefulness of parasite-specific IgE and IgG and indicating the production of these antibodies in the pleural space (82,103).

Immediate hypersensitivity to *Paragonimus* antigens, shown by a skin test, can be highly sensitive; however, it stays positive for many years and is not available worldwide. Serological and skin tests may be confusing owing to some cross-reactivity with other fluke infections: e.g., schistosomiasis, fascioliasis, and clonorchiasis (82,85,100).

Distinguishing between paragonimiasis and tuberculosis can be difficult owing to simultaneous endemicity of both diseases in the same areas, similar clinical presentations (80,96), absence of examination for *Paragonimus* eggs or *Paragonimus*-specific serological tests (81), and presence of epithelioid tubercles and granulomas as a response to allergic and toxic factors in tissues involved by paragonimiasis (88). However, the patient with paragonimiasis will appear healthier and less wasted than a tuberculous patient with the same degree of disease (79,85). Furthermore, the apices and hilar lymph nodes are unlikely to be involved in paragonimiasis, and lower lung zones and periphery are more likely to be involved than in tuberculosis (80,94,96). Pulmonary infiltrates in paragonimiasis are poorly defined and change rapidly with time; cysts invariably have a smooth inner margin and a typical ring shadow. After treatment, residual fibrosis and emphysematous change are virtually absent in paragonimiasis. Subpleural linear opacities are common in paragonimiasis and are unusual in tuberculosis. Marked residual pleural fibrosis is unusual in paragonimiasis, even in chronic disease, although in the active stage there can be pleural thickening to some extent (80,94,96). Examination of pleural fluid is also useful in distinguishing paragonimiasis and tuberculosis. A tuberculous effusion will always have a higher pH and glucose and lower LDH and lower protein levels than a paragonimus effusion (1,2,81,96).

E. Treatment

The standard treatment for paragonimiasis is praziquantel given orally in a dosage of 25 mg/kg body weight three times per day for 1–3 days (1,2,79,86,92). A one-day course at this dosage will be curative in about 70% of patients with paragonimiasis, a 2-day course in 90%, and a 3-day course in almost 100% (1,2,79,83,92,96). Nausea and vomiting are the main toxic side effects of the drug. It may also cause urticaria or anaphylaxis within the first week after treatment, especially in the presence of heavy parasite burden (2,86).

Bithionol 30–50 mg/kg given on alternate days for 10–15 doses is an alternative for patients unable to tolerate praziquantel. However, frequent toxic gastrointestinal side effects and anaphylactoid reactions of Bithionol can also limit therapy (85,89,91,92,97).

Even asymptomatic or lightly infected patients are advised to be treated with at least praziquantel to prevent pulmonary fibrosis and cerebral paragonimiasis (2).

The pleural surfaces may become thickened as paragonimiasis becomes chronic or if empyema complicates the disease. The drugs cannot be effective since they cannot pass through the thickened pleura. Thoracotomy with decortication may be necessary in these cases (1,81,90,104). Chest tube drainage may be required in some patients with a pleural effusion due to irritating effect of the parasite or its ova acting like foreign bodies; in these patients, medical treatment usually fails (81).

V. Pneumocystosis

The incidence of pneumocystosis has risen associated with the appearance of human immunodeficiency virus (HIV) infection in the 1980s (2,105,106). *Pneumocystis carinii*, related to fungi, is mainly transmitted by an airborne route and deposited in the alveoli. The trophozoite initiates an eosinophilic alveolar exudate and interstitial edema (105). Pneumocystosis tends to develop in states of impaired cellular immunity: immunodeficiency, malignancy, immunosuppressive therapy, and transplantations (105,107–110). In adult HIV patients, $\leq 200/mm^3$ CD4 cells has strong predictive value for pneumocystosis (105,111). The clinical picture may vary from an asymptomatic state to adult respiratory distress syndrome (105,108,110). Besides the typical diffuse pulmonary inter-

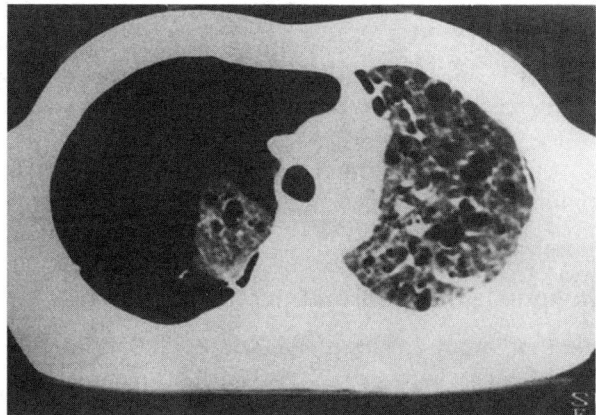

Figure 23 Right pneumothorax secondary to cystic upper lobe lesions in an AIDS patient with *Pneumocystis carinii* pneumonia.

stitial or ground-glass infiltrates (106), there may be atypical findings: normal chest films, pleural effusions, unilateral infiltrates, nodules, cavities, pneumatoceles, lymphadenopathy, and microcalcifications (1,2,105,107,112). The incidence of atypical infiltrates and spontaneous pneumothoraces increases during recovery or prophylaxis with aerosol pentamidine. Pneumothorax has also been associated with cavitary disease (2,105,113,114) (Fig. 23). Pleural effusion, rarely dominating the clinical picture, may be reactive or due to involvement by *P. carinii*. The incidence of pleural effusion increases in advanced and generalized pneumocystosis or underlying disease (106,107,113) (Fig. 24). High-resolution

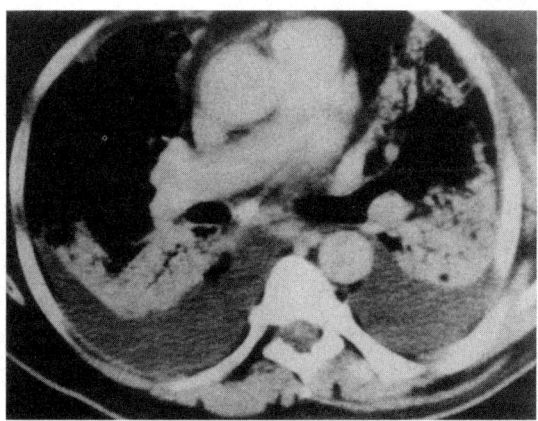

Figure 24 Bilateral pleural effusions and diffuse consolidations in a leukemic patient with *Pneumocystis carinii* pneumonia.

CT and gallium scans of the chest are helpful in cases with normal or equivocal chest radiographs (105,115). Demonstration of *P. carinii* trophozoites or cysts in sputum, bronchial or bronchoalveolar lavage fluid, pleural fluid, or lung biopsy specimens confirms the diagnosis (105,107,116,117). Trimethoprim-sulfamethoxazole is the treatment of choice (15–20 and 75–100 mg/kg/day, respectively, for 14–21 days). Aerosolized pentamidine or dapsone is used for prophylaxis in trimethoprim-sulfamethoxazole intolerance (105,118).

VI. Nematode (Roundworm) Infections

A. Simple Pulmonary Eosinophilia (Loeffler's Syndrome)

Pulmonary migration of the larvae of many helminths, but mostly the roundworms *Ascaris lumbricoides*, hookworms (*Necator americanus* and *Ancylostoma duodenale*), or *Strongyloides stercoralis*, causes pulmonary eosinophilia that is characterized by transient respiratory symptoms (low-grade fever, nonproductive cough, mild to severe dyspnea, and occasionally hemoptysis) associated with eosinophilic, migratory, and transient pulmonary infiltrations, and eosinophilia in sputum and peripheral blood. Pulmonary eosinophilia is an immunological reaction to larvae rather than direct involvement by them (119–123). The roundworms *Trichuris trichiura* (2) and *Trichinella spiralis* (2,124,125) and the tapeworms *Taenia saginata* and *Taenia solium* (2,126) can also cause this syndrome, although they lack a pulmonary migratory phase (2,124–126).

Rarely, eosinophilic pleural effusion manifesting with pleuritic chest pain can accompany pulmonary eosinophilia. Pleuropulmonary involvement is transient (2,119,123). It is usually asymptomatic or with mild symptoms in the presence of frequently and uninterrupted contact in endemic areas since a high degree of natural tolerance develops. The incidence of Loeffler's syndrome has been found to be about 0.25% in an endemic region in Columbia (122).

B. Strongyloidiasis

Massive invasion of the lungs and other tissues by *S. stercoralis* larvae may occur with autoinfection, particularly in immunocompromised host. This hyperinfection strongyloidiasis has been described in patients with leukemia, lymphoma, diabetes mellitus, lepramatous leprosy, HIV infection, mental retardation, and also in those from tropical areas and treated with corticosteroids (120,127–129). In these cases of hyperinfection, larvae of *S. stercoralis* can be found in pleural effusions (127–129), sputum (129,130), bronchial aspiration or bronchoalveolar lavage fluids (130,131) as well as feces (120,129,130), tissues (129,131), and other body fluids (129,130) (Fig. 25). In some cases pleural fluid can be sterile or infected with gram-negative aerobes (2).

Treatment is thiabendazole at 25 mg/kg twice a day for 2 days (maximum 3 g/day). However, in hyperinfection syndrome, treatment should last 2–3 weeks (2,120).

Pleural Effusions in Parasitic Infections 879

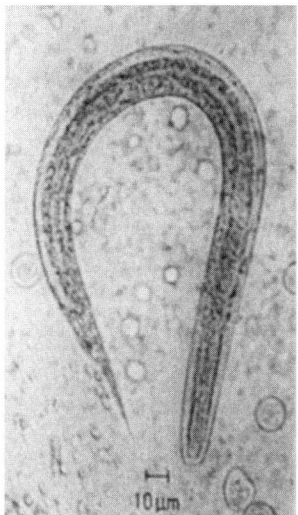

Figure 25 A 0.25–0.3 mm long rhabditiform larva of *Strongyloides stercoralis* in stool specimen. (Courtesy of Department of Parasitology, Chiang Mai University, Chiang Mai, Thailand.)

C. Ascariasis

Rarely, a mature *A. lumbricoides* worm can lodge itself in the pleural cavity passing through a bronchopleural fistula associated with tuberculous pyopneumothorax (132). Very infrequently, relapsing pneumothorax can also occur because of the mechanical inflammatory action of *A. lumbricoides* larvae in pleuropulmonary tissue (133). A rare case, severe pericardial effusion leading to cardiac tamponade due to involvement with *A. lumbricoides*, has been reported (134). The treatment of choice for ascariasis and hookworm infection is mebendazole 100 mg twice daily for 3 days (120).

D. Trichinellosis (Trichinosis, Trichiniasis) and Trichuriasis

In trichinellosis pericardial effusion can also develop (10%) when the heart is involved (135). There is no satisfactory treatment for trichinosis; oral thiabendazole, mebendazole, or albendazole may be tried (120). Mebendazole or albendazole is effective for trichuriasis.

E. Tropical Pulmonary Eosinophilia

Tropical pulmonary eosinophilia, similar to ordinary pulmonary eosinophilia, is a disease syndrome caused by a reaction to migrating microfilariae in tissues, especially in the lungs. It is probably due to immunological hyperresponsiveness to the human filarial parasites *Wuchereria bancrofti*, *Brugia malayi*, or the dog heartworm *Dirofilaria immitis*, which are transmitted by mosquitoes in Africa, south and southeast Asia, and the South Pacific, areas endemic for filariasis. Former residents of endemic areas may have the disease a year after emigration (136–141).

Patients have recurrent episodes of paroxysmal dry cough, dyspnea, and wheezing. Weight loss, malaise, and anorexia are frequently seen. Scattered wheezes or crackles are heard on physical examination. Some patients may have hepatomegaly and lymphadenopathy. Fluctuation of symptoms over many months is characteristic (137,138).

Chest radiograph may occasionally be noýmal at the time of presentation but usually reveals scattered reticulonodular or interstitial opacities, consolidations, pulmonary nodules, and more rarely hilar adenopathy, and pleural effusion (136,137,139,141). Pleural disease can be bilateral (136–140) (Fig. 26).

Microfilariae are absent in the blood, sputum, pleural fluid, or bronchoscopic specimens owing to intense immune response. Examination of stool and urine for ova and parasites is also unrewarding. Peripheral blood eosinophilia at very high levels (>3000 eosinophils/mm^3; up to 90% of the leukocyte differential) is almost always present. Serum (>1000 U/mL) and pleural fluid IgE levels are significantly elevated. High titers of filarial-specific IgE and IgG antibodies in the serum are measured by complement fixation and hemagglutination techniques (2,138–140). Moderate protein levels and predominance of eosinophils (up to 50% of the leukocyte differential) are characteristic of the pleural fluid (136–140). In most cases lung biopsy is not needed. The diagnosis can be established by serology and a successful response to therapy with diethylcarbamazine, which is given orally in a dose of 3 mg/kg three times daily for 2 weeks (2,138–

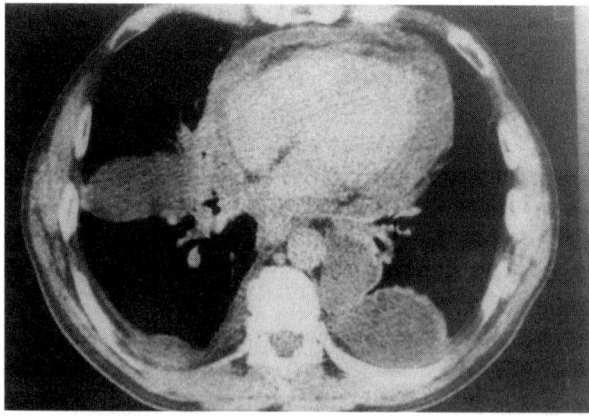

Figure 26 Pericardial and bilateral loculated pleural effusions in a patient with tropical pulmonary eosinophilia. Pulmonary lesions were patchy reticulonodular and interstitial (not shown here).

140). Although in most cases the chest radiograph clears in a few weeks, some cases may have persistent clinical, radiological, and functional abnormalities due to chronic low-grade alveolitis. In such cases it is prudent to repeat the course of treatment with diethylcarbamazine (138,141). In some of these resistant cases corticosteroids are given since bronchospasm due to eosinophilic inflammation can be severe (140).

F. Filariasis

In filariasis, pleural involvement can also be seen without tropical pulmonary eosinophilia. Microfilariae of *D. immitis* (142), *W. bancrofti* (143–146), and Loa Loa (147) have been occasionally demonstrated in pleural effusion or pleural biopsy specimens. The pleural fluid is exudative and occasionally blood-tinged (142,143,146).

W. bancrofti very rarely causes mediastinal lymphadenitis and associated vena caval syndrome, which can facilitate the development of a transudative pleural effusion (144). Chylothorax due to thoracic lymphatic obstruction caused by involvement of thoracic lymph nodes by Bancroftian filariasis has been encountered in a few cases (148,149).

Another rare and unusual occurence of pleural effusion in filariasis is associated with cor pulmonale secondary to pulmonary fibrosis, which is a sequela of tropical pulmonary eosinophilia in Brugian filariasis (150). The dog heartworm *D. immitis* can occasionally (4.1%) cause bloody pleural effusion in humans (151) since the dead filariae cause local pulmonary vasculitis and infarcts besides intravascular or pulmonary granulomas preferentially located in the lower lobes (142,152) (Fig. 27). Radiographically, pulmonary granulomas appear as solitary or multiple nodules or masses, which are cavitated in the presence of infarction (142,153) (Fig. 28). In many cases with pleuropulmonary dirofilariasis, diagnosis must be confirmed by histology since radiographically

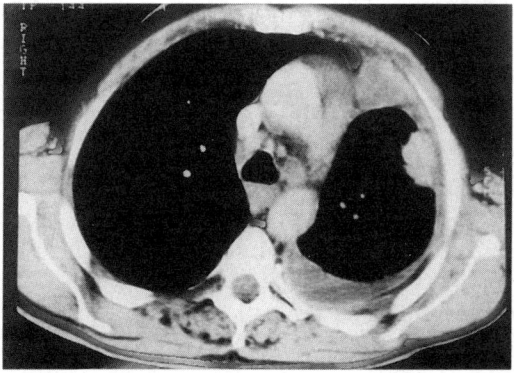

Figure 27 Left pulmonary nodule, pleural effusion and thickening, and aorticopulmonary lymphadenopathy in dirofilariasis. Note the shift of the mediastinum to the left.

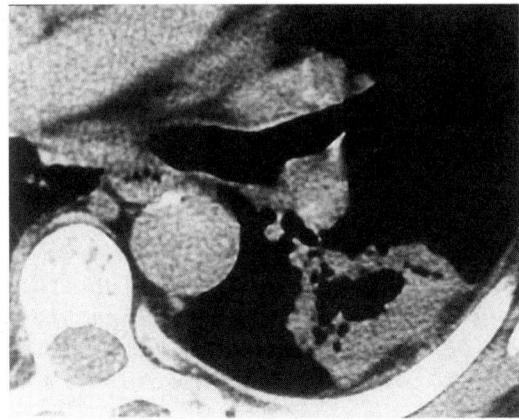

Figure 28 A peripheral, cavitated pulmonary mass mimicking malignant tumor in dirofilariasis. There is minimal, local pleural thickening.

they can initiate and be confused with malignant disease (142,153). Pleural thickening is uncommon in filariasis; 12.5% of 24 cases with human dirofilariasis have been reported to present with pleural thickening (142) (Fig. 27). Pneumothorax secondary to filariasis has not been reported, although it can occur in cats (154) and dogs (155) infected with *D. immitis*. However, in human dirofilariasis the necrotic cavitated subpleural masses can potentially lead to pneumothorax.

VII. Parasitoses with Unlocated Parasites

In some parasitic infections, whether pleural reactions are due to the parasite in the pleural space or due to systemic immune reaction is not clear since the parasite cannot be determined in pleuropulmonary specimens.

A. Toxocariasis

Toxocariasis, visceral larva migrans, is caused mainly by the roundworm *Toxocara canis* or infrequently by *Toxocara catis*. Humans, most commonly children, are inadvertently infected by ingesting the eggs in the feces of dog or cat, the main host. In heavy infestations, eosinophilia, hepatomegaly, fever, wheezing, and cough occur (141,156). Lung involvement is seen in 32–44% of cases (156). Pleuritis has been reported in just a few cases (157–159). Bilateral (157,158) and bloody eosinophilic (157) pleural effusions can occur. Diagnosis is by serology. Visceral larva migrans is usually a self-limited disease, and specific treatment is rarely necessary. In acute cases, a short course of corticosteroids reduces morbidity and mortality, but preventive measures are more important (2,141,156,159).

B. Anisakiasis

Anisakis is another family of roundworms causing pleural effusion but not demonstrated in pleural fluid or other thoracic specimens (2,156,160). The main host is a marine vertebrate, and the intermediate hosts a crustacean or a fish. Ingestion of undercooked or raw crustaceans or fish starts the infestation in humans (156). As larvae bore through the stomach or intestinal wall, patients complain of intense abdominal pain, which may be associated with urticaria and eosinophilic pleural effusion (160,161) with pleural thickening (160). Serology aids in diagnosis (160,161), but the only effective treatment, endoscopic removal of the larvae from the gut, definitely establishes the diagnosis (156).

C. Capillariasis

The roundworm *Capillaria philippinensis* is a parasite causing severe diarrhea, malabsorption, and protein-losing enteropathy. It can multiply rapidly by autoinfection. Bilateral pleural effusions associated with ascites and edema can develop possibly owing to hypoalbuminemia (162). Mebendazole 200 mg orally twice daily for 20 days or albendazole is the treatment of choice.

D. Hypodermiasis

The larvae of the parasitic flies *Hypoderma bovis* and *Hypoderma lineata* cause a subcutaneous creeping eruption after hatching and boring into and through the skin. Hypodermiasis occurs in Europe as well as in the tropics. The usual hosts are cattle. An eosinophilic pleural effusion and pericarditis can develop. It is not clear whether the effusions are due to systemic immune reaction or the presence of parasite in pleural cavity. There is no drug treatment; removal of the larvae from the parasitized tissue may be helpful (2,163,164).

VIII. Schistosomiasis

Schistosomiasis, a common tropical disease, rarely causes pleural disease accompanying a lung lesion (2,165,166). Pleural effusion (Fig. 29), pneumothorax, or pleural adherence to the aorta causing aortic aneurysm can occur during severe lung disease (2,165,166). Pleural effusion can potentially occur secondary to pulmonary or portal hypertension and ascites and hydronephrosis developing as sequelas of schistosomiasis (167) (Fig. 30). Pneumonitis during larval migration or posttreatment Loeffler-like pneumonitis can be accompanied by pleural effusion (168). Schistosoma eggs have been shown in bronchoalveolar lavage fluid, sputum, and ascitic fluid but not in pleural fluid (167,168).

Treatment of choice is praziquantel administered as two oral doses of 20 mg/kg body weight in one day for individuals with *S. mansoni* or *S. haemotobium* infection. In subjects with schistosomiasis japonica, praziquantel is administered as 20 mg/kg body weight three times for one day (167). Exudative polyserositis

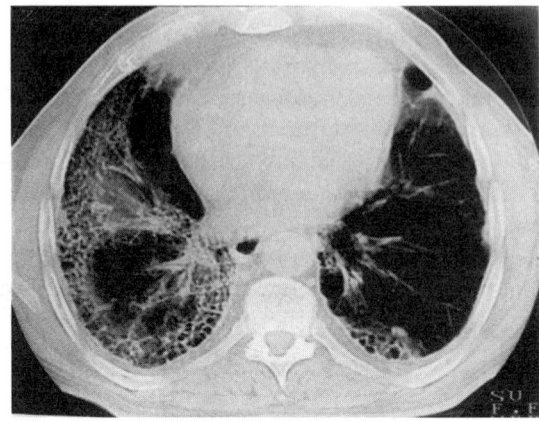

Figure 29 Bilateral pulmonary fibrosis, minimal pleural effusion, and thickening in chronic schistosomiasis.

including pleural, pericardial, and peritoneal effusions can follow praziquantel therapy in schistosomiasis (169).

IX. Incidentally Found Parasites in the Pleura

Some parasites access the pleura but do not cause any disease.

A. Pentastomiasis

Human infestation is seen mostly in Central Africa and Malaysia (2,170,171).

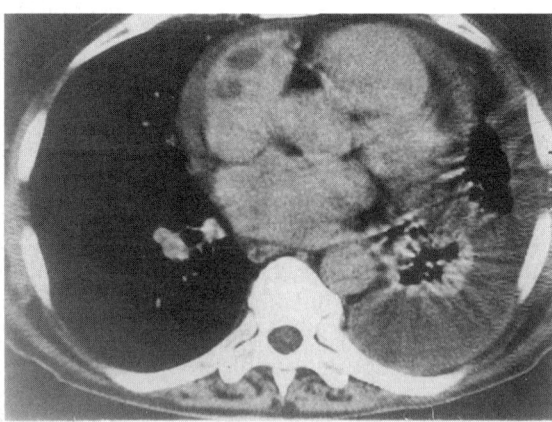

Figure 30 Pericardial and left pleural effusion, cardiomegaly, and right atrial thrombi in a patient with schistosomiasis.

B. Mansonellosis

The filariae *Mansonella ozzardi* and *Mansonella perstans* may be found incidentally in the pleural space. The adults live in serous body cavities. *M. perstans* is endemic in Africa, New Guinea, and South America and *M. mozzardi* in Central and South America and the Caribbean (2,172,173).

X. Miscellaneous Parasitoses Rarely Causing Pleural Effusion

There have been case reports of pleural effusions due to trichomoniasis (174–176), toxoplasmosis (177,178), microsporidiosis (179), sporotrichosis (180,181), leishmaniasis (182,183), fasciolasis (184,185), and malaria (186,187).

In malaria, uni- or bilateral pleural effusions may accompany pulmonary edema and are due to increased permeability and plasma leakage (1,186) (Fig. 31). Rarely, an isolated massive pleural effusion without pulmonary edema can occur (187).

Empyema (175,176) and nonempyemic exudative pleural effusion (174) in trichomoniasis, pneumothorax (188), exudative pleural effusion (177), and pleuropericarditis (178) in toxoplasmosis, empyema (181) and nonempyemic exudative pleural effusion (180) in sporotrichosis, uni- (182,183) or bilateral (189) exudative pleural effusions in leishmaniasis, and eosinophilic exudative pleural effusion (185) and pyopneumothorax (190) in fasciolasis have been reported.

Pleural involvement in almost all of the above-mentioned parasitic infections is encountered in patients with AIDS (177,179,182,183,188,189), malignancy and immunocompromised states (176,178), and in alcoholics (174,175,

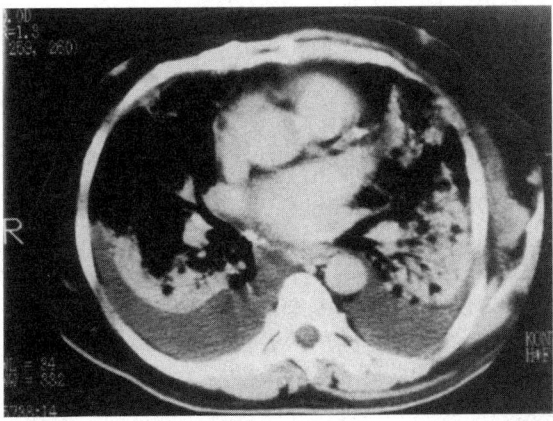

Figure 31 Pulmonary edema and bilateral pleural effusions due to increased permeability in malaria.

180). In most of these reported cases, pulmonary involvement accompanies pleural disease (174,175,177,179,181) and the parasites have been shown in the pleural fluid (174,176,180,189), bronchoalveolar lavage fluid (179), transbronchial lung biopsy specimen (179), sputum (180), and open lung biopsy specimens (180).

References

1. Light RW. Pleural effusion due to parasitic infection. In: Light RW, ed. Pleural Diseases. 4th ed. Philadelphia: Lippincott Williams & Wilkins, 2001:204–209.
2. Roberts PP. Parasitic infections of the pleural space. Semin Respir Infect 1988; 3:362–382.
3. Fishman JA. HIV infection and opportunistic pulmonary infections in AIDS. In: Fishman AP, Elias JA, Fishman JA, Grippi MA, Kaiser LR, Senior RM, eds. Fishman's Pulmonary Diseases and Disorders. 3rd ed. New York: McGraw-Hill, 1998:2105, 2115.
4. Fishman JA. Pulmonary infections in neutropenia and cancer. In: Fishman AP, Elias JA, Fishman JA, Grippi MA, Kaiser LR, Senior RM, eds. Fishman's Pulmonary Diseases and Disorders. 3rd ed. New York: McGraw-Hill, 1998:2126–2127.
5. Fishman JA. Introduction: pulmonary infection in special hosts. In: Fishman AP, Elias JA, Fishman JA, Grippi MA, Kaiser LR, Senior RM, eds. Fishman's Pulmonary Diseases and Disorders. 3rd ed. New York: McGraw-Hill, 1998:2098–2099.
6. Hung CC, Chen PJ, Hsieh SM, Wong JM, Fang CT, Chang SC, Chen MY. Invasive amoebiasis: an emerging parasitic disease in patients infected with HIV in an area endemic for amoebic infection. AIDS 1999; 13:2421–2428.
7. Ravdin JI. Entamoeba histolytica (amebiasis). In: Mandell GL, Bennett JE, Dolin R, eds. Mandell, Douglas, and Bennett's Principles and Practice of Infectious Diseases. 5th ed. Philadelphia: Churchill Livingtone, 2000:2798–2807.
8. Perez-Tamayo R, Brandt H. Amebiasis. In: Marcial-Rojas RA, ed. Pathology of Protozoal and Helminthic Diseases with Clinical Correlation. Huntington, New York: Robert E. Krieger, 1975:145–180.
9. Herrera-Llerandi R. Thoracic repercussions of amebiasis. J Thorac Cardiovasc Surg 1966; 52:361–375.
10. Lyche KD, Jensen WA, Kirsch CM, Yenokida GG, Maltz GS, Knauer CM. Pleuropulmonary manifestations of hepatic amebiasis. West J Med 1990; 153:275–278.
11. Ibarra-Perez C. Thoracic complications of amebic abscess of the liver: report of 501 cases. Chest 1981; 79:672–677.
12. Ibarra-Perez C, Selman-Lama M. Diagnosis and treatment of amebic empyema. Report of eighty-eight cases. Am J Surg 1977; 134:283–287.
13. Cameron EW. The treatment of pleuropulmonary amebiasis with metronidazole. Chest 1978; 73:647–650.
14. Agrawal BV, Somani PN, Khanna MN, Srivastava PK, Jha BN, Verma SP. Amebic pericardial effusion: a rare complication of amebic liver abscess. Am Surg 1975; 41:373–377.

15. Adeyemo AO, Aderounmu A. Intrathoracic complications of amoebic liver abscess. J R Soc Med 1984; 77:17–21.
16. Kennedy D, Sharma OP. Hemoptysis in a 49-year-old man. An unusual presentation of a sporadic disease. Chest 1990; 98:1275–1278.
17. Verghese M, Eggleston FC, Handa AK, Singh CM. Management of thoracic amebiasis. J Thorac Cardiovasc Surg 1979; 78:757–760.
18. Fadlalla AH, Mathew KS. Unusual presentation of amoebic liver abscess. Trop Geogr Med 1989; 41:69–72.
19. Radin DR, Ralls PW, Colletti PM, Halls JM. CT of amebic liver abscess. AJR 1988; 150:1297–1301.
20. Hoffner RJ, Kilaghbian T, Esekogwu VI, Henderson SO. Common presentations of amebic liver abscess. Ann Emerg Med 1999; 34:351–355.
21. Verhaegen F, Poey C, Lebras Y, Iscain P, Guiot S, Lyonnet P, Dupare B. X-ray computed tomographic tests in the diagnosis and treatment of amebic liver abscess. J Radiol 1996; 77:23–28.
22. vanSonnenberg E, Mueller PR, Schiffman HR, Ferucci JT, Casola G, Simeone JF, Cabrera OA, Gosink BB. Intrahepatic amebic abscesses: indications for and results of percutaneous catheter drainage. Radiology 1985; 156:631–635.
23. Salzano A, Rossi E, Carbone M, Mondillo F, De Rosa A, Tuccillo M, Capuona N, Nunziata A. Suburban amebiasis: the diagnostic aspects via computed tomography and echography and percutaneous treatment of amebic liver abscesses. Radiol Med (Torino) 2000; 99:169–173.
24. Badalamenti S, Jameson JE, Reddy KR. Amebiasis. Curr Treat Options Gastroenterol 1999; 2:97–103.
25. Baijal SS, Agarwal DK, Roy S, Choudhuri G. Complex ruptured amebic liver abscesses: the role of percutaneous catheter drainage. Europ J Radiol 1995; 20:65–67.
26. Rasaretnam R, Paul AT, Yoganathan M. Pleural empyema due to ruptured amoebic liver abscess. Br J Surg 1974; 61:713–715.
27. Chuah SK, Chang-Chien CS, Sheen IS, Lin HH, Chiou SS, Chiu CT, Kuo CH, Chen JJ, Chiu KW. The prognostic factors of severe amebic liver abscess: a retrospective study of 125 cases. Am J Trop Med Hyg 1992; 46:398–402.
28. Munoz LE, Botello MA, Carillo O, Martinez AM. Early detection of complications in amebic liver abscess. Arch Med Res 1992; 23:251–253.
29. Pinna AD, Marongiu L, Cadoni S, Luridiana E, Nardello O, Pinna DC. Thoracic extension of hydatid cysts of the liver. Surg Gynecol Obstet 1990; 170:233–238.
30. King CH. Echinococcosis (hydatid and alveolar cyst disease). In: Mandell GL, Bennett JE, Dolin R, eds. Mandell, Douglas, and Bennett's Principles and Practice of Infectious Diseases. 5th ed. Philadelphia: Churchill Livingtone, 2000:2962–2963.
31. Poole JB, Marcial-Rojas RA. Echinococcosis. In: Marcial-Rojas RA, ed. Pathology of Protozoal and Helminthic Diseases with Clinical Correlation. Huntington, New York: Robert E. Krieger, 1975:635–656.
32. Bastani B, Dehdashti F. Hepatic hydatid disease in Iran, with review of the literature. Mt Sinai J Med 1995; 62:62–69.
33. Tor M, Atasalihi A, Altuntas N, Sulu E, Senol T, Kir A, Baran R. Review of cases with cystic hydatid lung disease in a tertiary referral hospital located in an endemic region: a 10 year's experience. Respiration 2000; 67:539–542.
34. Yacoubian HD. Thoracic problems associated with hydatid cyst of the dome of the liver. Surgery 1976; 79:544–548.

35. Bakir F. Serious complications of hydatid cyst of the lung. Am Rev Respir Dis 1967; 96:483–493.
36. Ozer Z, Cetin M, Kahraman C. Pleural involvement by hydatid cysts of the lung. Thorac Cardiovasc Surg 1985; 33:103–105.
37. Agrawal RL, Jain SK, Gupta SC, Agrawal DK, Ahmad KR, Nandi D. Hydropneumothorax secondary to hydatid lung disease. Indian J Chest Dis Allied Sci 1993; 35:93–96.
38. Rakower J, Milwidsky H. Hydatid pleural disease. Am Rev Respir Dis 1964; 90:623–631.
39. Xanthakis DS, Katsaras E, Efthimiadis M, Papadakis G, Varouchakis G, Aligizakis C. Hydatid cyst of the liver with intrathoracic rupture. Thorax 1981; 36:497–501.
40. Balikian JP, Mudarris FF. Hydatid disease of the lungs: a roentgenologic study of 50 cases. AJR 1974; 122:692–707.
41. Sarkissian S. Hydatid disease of the thorax. In: Emerson P, ed. Thoracic Medicine. London: Butterworth, 1981:555–565.
42. Jerray M, Benzarti M, Garrouche A, Klabi N, Hayouni A. Hydatid disease of the lungs. Study of 386 cases. Am Rev Respir Dis 1992; 146:185–189.
43. Dogan R, Yuksel M, Cetin G, Suzer K, Alp M, Kaya S, Unlu M, Moldibi B. Surgical treatment of hydatid cysts of the lung: report on 1055 patients. Thorax 1989; 44:192–199.
44. Hadley MD. Occult hydatid disease presenting as a spontaneous pneumothorax. Br J Radiol 1985; 58:770–772.
45. Barzilai A, Pollack S, Kaftori JK, Sourdry M, Barzilai D. Splenic echinococcal cyst burrowing into left pleural space. Chest 1977; 72:543–545.
46. Gouliamos AD, Kalovidouris A, Papailiou J, Vlahos L, Papavasiliou C. CT appearance of pulmonary hydatid disease. Chest 1991; 100:1578–1581.
47. Aytac A, Yurdakul Y, Ikizler C, Olga R, Saylan A. Pulmonary hydatid disease: report of 100 patients. Ann Thorac Surg 1977; 23:145–151.
48. Rami-Porta R, Bravo-Bravo JL, Aroca-Gonzalez MJ, Alix-Treuba A, Serrano-Munoz F. Tumours and pseudotumours of the chest wall. Scand J Thorac Cardiovasc Surg 1985; 19:97–103.
49. Oguzkaya F, Akcali Y, Kahraman C, Emirogullari N, Bilgin M, Sahin A. Unusually located hydatid cysts: intrathoracic but extrapulmonary. Ann Thorac Surg 1997; 64:334–337.
50. De Vega DS, Vasquez E, Calvo E, Tamames S, Tamames S. Hydatid cyst of the diaphragm. Apropos of a case. J Chir (Paris) 1991; 128:76–78.
51. Kabiri H, Al Aziz S, El Maslout A, Benosman A. Diaphragmatic hydatidosis: report of a series of 27 cases. Rev Pneumol Clin 2001; 57:13–19.
52. Carel RS, Schey G, Bruderman I. Chyliform pleural effusion. An unusual manifestation of hepatothoracic echinococcus cysts. Chest 1975; 68:598–599.
53. Jacobson ES. A case of secondary echinococcosis diagnosed by cytologic examination of pleural fluid and needle biopsy of pleura. Acta Cytol 1973; 17:76–79.
54. al Karawi MA, Mohamed AR, el Tayeb BO, Yasawy MI. Unintentional percutaneous aspiration of a pleural hydatid cyst. Thorax 1991; 46:859–860.
55. Vercelli-Retta J, Manana G, Reissenweber NJ. The cytologic diagnosis of hydatid disease. Acta Cytol 1982; 26:159–168.
56. Saygi A, Oztek I, Guder M, Sungun F, Arman B. Value of fiberoptic bronchoscopy in the diagnosis of complicated pulmonary unilocular hydatidosis. Eur Respir J 1997; 10:811–814.

57. Salama H, Farid Abdel-Wahab M, Strickland GT. Diagnosis and treatment of hepatic hydatid cysts with the aid of echo-guided percutaneous cyst puncture. Clin Infect Dis 1995; 21:1372–1376.
58. Craig PS, Bailey W, Nelson GS. A specific test for the identification of cyst fluid samples from suspected human hydatid infections. Trans R Soc Trop Med Hyg 1986; 80:256–257.
59. Case records of the Massachusetts General Hospital. Weekly clinicopathological exercises. Case 45-1987. A 16-year-old girl with hepatic and pulmonary masses after a sojourn in Bolivia. N Engl J Med 1987; 317:1209–1218.
60. Koul PA, Koul AN, Wahid A, Mir FA. CT in pulmonary hydatid disease: unusual appearances. Chest 2000; 118:1645–1647.
61. Pelaez V, Kugler C, del Carpio M, Correa D, Lopez E, Larrieu E, Guangiroli M, Molina J. Treatment of hepatic cysts by percutaneous aspiration and hypertonic saline injection: results of a cooperative work. Bol Chil Parasitol 1999; 54:63–69.
62. von Sinner WN. Ultrasound, CT and MRI of ruptured and disseminated hydatid cysts. Eur J Radiol 1990; 11:31–37.
63. von Sinner WN. New diagnostic signs in hydatid disease: radiography, ultrasound, CT and MRI correlated to pathology. Eur J Radiol 1991; 12:150–159.
64. Ustunsoz B, Akhan O, Kamiloglu MA, Somuncu I, Ugurel MS, Cetiner S. Percutaneous treatment of hydatid cysts of the liver. AJR 1999; 172:91–96.
65. Haddad MC, Sammak BM, Al-Karawi M. Percutaneous treatment of heterogeneous predominantly solid echopattern echinococcal cysts of the liver. Cardiovasc Intervent Radiol 2000; 23:121–125.
66. Tan A, Yakut M, Kaymakcioglu N, Ozerhan IH, Cetiner S, Akdeniz A. The results of surgical treatment and percutaneous drainage of hepatic hydatid disease. Int Surg 1998; 83:314–316.
67. Tsitouridis I, Dimitriadis AS. CT and MRI in vertebral hydatid disease. Eur Radiol 1997; 7:1207–1210.
68. Garcia-Diez AI, Ros Mendoza LH, Villacampa VM, Cozar M, Fuertes MI. MRI evaluation of soft tissue hydatid disease. Eur Radiol 2000; 10:462–466.
69. Kotoulas GK, Magoufis GL, Gouliamos AD, Athanassopoulou AK, Roussakis AC, Koulocheri DP, Kalovidouris A, Vlahos L. Evaluation of hydatid disease of the heart with magnetic resonance imaging. Cardiovasc Intervent Radiol 1996; 19:187–189.
70. Peter JC, Domingo Z, Sinclair-Smith C, de Villiers JC. Hydatid infestation of the brain: difficulties with computed tomography diagnosis and surgical treatment. Pediatr Neurosurg 1994; 20:78–83.
71. Reuter S, Nussle K, Kolokythas O, Haug U, Rieber A, Kern P, Kratzer W. Alveolar liver echinococcosis: a comparative study of three imaging techniques. Infection 2001; 29:119–125.
72. Singh S, Gibikote SV. Magnetic resonance imaging signal characteristics in hydatid cysts. Australas Radiol 2001; 45(2):128–133.
73. Ramos G, Orduna A, Garcia-Yuste M. Hydatid cyst of the lung: diagnosis and treatment. World J Surg 2001; 25:46–47.
74. Bhatia G. Echinococcus. Semin Respir Infect 1997; 12:171–186.
75. Bressen-Hadni S, Vuitton DA, Bartholomot B, Heyd B, Godart D, Meyer JP, Hrusovsky S, Becker MC, Mantion G, Lenys D, Miguet JP. A twenty-year history of alveolar echinococcosis: analysis of a series of 117 patients from Eastern France. Eur J Gastroenterol Hepatol 2000; 12:327–336.

76. Tuzun M, Hekimoglu B. Pictorial essay. Various locations of cystic and alveolar hydatid disease. CT appearances. J Comput Assist Tomogr 2001; 25:81–87.
77. Peleg H, Best L, Gaitini D. Simultaneous operation for hydatid cysts of right lung and liver. J Thorac Cardiovasc Surg 1985; 90:783–787.
78. Paterson HS, Blyth DF. Thoracoscopic evacuation of dead hydatid cyst. J Thorac Cardiovasc Surg 1996; 111:1280–1281.
79. Mahmoud AAF. Lung flukes—paragonimiasis. In: Mandell GL, Bennett JE, Dolin R, eds. Mandell, Douglas, and Bennett's Principles and Practice of Infectious Diseases. 5th ed. Philadelphia: Churchill Livingstone, 2000:2955.
80. Im J-G, Whang HJ, Kim WS, Han MC, Shim Y-S, Cho S-Y. Pleuropulmonary paragonimiasis: radiologic findings in 71 patients. AJR 1992; 159:39–43.
81. Minh V-D, Engle P, Greenwood JR, Prendergast TJ, Salness K, St. Clair R. Pleural paragonimiasis in a Southeast Asian refugee. Am Rev Respir Dis 1981; 124:186–188.
82. Yokogawa M, Kojima S, Araki K, Tomioka H, Yoshida S. Immunoglobulin E: raised levels in sera and pleural exudates of patients with paragonimiasis. Am J Trop Med Hyg 1976; 25:581–586.
83. Pachucki CT, Levandowski RA, Brown VA, Sonnenkalb BH, Vruno MJ. American paragonimiasis treated with praziquantel. N Engl J Med 1984; 311:582–583.
84. Beland JE, Boone J, Donevan RE, Mankiewicz E. *Paragonimus* (the lung fluke): report of four cases. Am Rev Respir Dis 1969; 99:261–271.
85. Yokogawa M. *Paragonimus* and paragonimiasis. Adv Parasitol 1969; 7:375–387.
86. Johnson RJ, Jong EC, Dunning SB, Carberry WL, Minshew BH. Paragonimiasis: diagnosis and the use of praziquantel in treatment. Rev Infect Dis 1985; 7:200–206.
87. Swanik R, Harinsuta C. Pulmonary paragonimiasis. An evaluation of roentgen findings in 38 sputum-positive patients in an endemic area in Thailand. Am J Roentgenol 1959; 81:236–244.
88. Chung CH. Human paragonimiasis (pulmonary distomiasis, endemic hemoptysis). In: Marcial-Rojas RA, ed. Pathology of Protozoal and Helminthic Diseases with Clinical Correlation. Huntington, New York: Robert E. Krieger, 1975:504–533.
89. Zhong HL, He LY, Xu ZB, Cao WJ. Recent progress in studies of *Paragonimus* and paragonimiasis. Control in China. Chin Med J 1981; 94:483–494.
90. Dietrick RB, Sade RM, Pak JS. Results of decortication in chronic empyema with special reference to paragonimiasis. J Thorac Cardiovasc Surg 1981; 82:58–62.
91. Johnson JR, Falk A, Iber C, Davies S. Paragonimiasis in the United States: a report of nine cases in Hmong immigrants. Chest 1982; 82:168–171.
92. Singh TS, Mutum SS, Razaque MA. Pulmonary paragonimiasis. Clinical features, diagnosis and treatment of 39 cases in Manipur. Trans R Soc Trop Med Hyg 1986; 80:967–971.
93. Roque FT, Ludwick RW, Bell JC. Pulmonary paragonimiasis: a review with case reports from Korea and the Philippines. Ann Intern Med 1953; 38:1206–1221.
94. Mukae H, Taniguchi H, Matsumoto N, Iiboshi H, Ashitani J, Matsukura S, Nawa Y. Clinicoradiologic features of pleuropulmonary *Paragonimus westermani* on Kyusyu Island, Japan. Chest 2001; 120:514–520.
95. Nawa Y. Recent trends of paragonimiasis westermani in Miyazaki Prefecture, Japan. Southeast Asian J Trop Med Public Health 1991; (suppl 22):342–344.
96. Johnson RJ, Johnson JR. Paragonimiasis in Indochinese refugees: roentgenographic findings with clinical correlations. Am Rev Respir Dis 1983; 128:534–538.
97. Sharma OP. The man who loved drunken crabs: a case of pulmonary paragonimiasis. Chest 1989; 95:670–672.

98. Uchiyama F, Morimoto Y, Nawa Y. Reemergence of paragonimiasis in Kyushu, Japan. Southeast Asian J Trop Med Public Health 1999; 30:686–691.
99. Shim Y-S, Cho S-Y, Han Y-C. Pulmonary paragonimiasis: a Korean perspective. Semin Respir Med 1991; 12:35–45.
100. Erzurum SE, Underwood GA, Hamilos DL, Waldron JA. Pleural effusion in Churg-Strauss syndrome. Chest 1989; 95:1357–1359.
101. Nakamura-Uchiyama F, Onah DN, Nawa Y. Clinical features of paragonimiasis cases recently found in Japan: parasite-specific immunoglobulin M and G antibody classes. Clin Infect Dis 2001; 32:E171–E175.
102. Cho SY, Hong ST, Rho YH, Choi S, Han YC. Application of micro-ELISA in serodiagnosis of human paragonimiasis. Korean J Parasitol 1981; 19:151–156.
103. Ikeda T, Oikawa Y, Owhashi M, Nawa Y. Parasite-specific Ig E and Ig G levels in the serum and pleural effusion of paragonimiasis westermani patients. Am J Trop Med Hygiene 1992; 47:104–107.
104. Tomita M, Matsuzaki Y, Nawa Y, Onitsuka T. Pulmonary paragonimiasis referred to the department of surgery. Ann Thorac Surg 2000; 6(5):295–298.
105. Walzer PD. *Pneumocystis carinii*. In: Mandell GL, Bennett JE, Dolin R, eds. Mandell, Douglas and Bennett's Principles and Practice of Infectious Diseases. 5th ed. Philadelphia: Churchill Livingstone, 2000:2781–2795.
106. Cooper NB, Kenny W. Pulmonary complications in AIDS: the radiographic manifestations. J Med Assoc Ga 1989; 78:197–200.
107. Armbruster C, Hassl A, Vetter N. Differential diagnosis of ascites and abscess forming hepatitis in AIDS patients with reference to the first patient with microsporidia infection in Austria. Wien Klin Wochenschr 1992; 104:753–756.
108. Russian DA, Levine SJ. *Pneumocystis carinii* pneumonia in patients without HIV infection. Am J Med Sci 2001; 321:56–65.
109. Mansharamani NG, Balachandran D, Vernovsky I, Garland R, Koziel H. Peripheral blood CD4+ T-lymphocyte counts during *Pneumocystis carinii* pneumonia in immunocompromised patients without HIV infection. Chest 2000; 118:712–720.
110. Gluck T, Geerdes-Fenge HF, Straub RH, Raffenberg M, Lang B, Lode H, Scholmerich J. *Pneumocystis carinii* pneumonia as a complication of immunosuppressive therapy. Infection 2000; 28:227–230.
111. Easterbrook PJ, Yu LM, Goetghebeur E, Boag F, McLean K, Gazzard B. Ten-year trends in CD4 cell counts at HIV and AIDS diagnosis in a London HIV clinic. AIDS 2000; 14:561–571.
112. Ewig S, Bauer T, Schneider C, Pickenhain A, Pizzulli L, Loos U, Luderitz B. Clinical characteristics and outcome of *Pneumocystis carinii* pneumonia in HIV-infected and otherwise immunosuppressed patients. Eur Respir J 1995; 8:1548–1553.
113. Light RW, Hamm H. Pleural disease and acquired immune deficiency syndrome. Eur Respir J 1997; 10:2638–2643.
114. Pastores SM, Garay SM, Naidich DP, Rom WN. Review: pneumothorax in patients with AIDS-related *Pneumocystis carinii* pneumonia. Am J Med Sci 1996; 312:229–234.
115. Gruden JF, Huang L, Turner J, Webb WR, Merrifield C, Stansell JD, Gamsu G, Hopewell PC. High-resolution CT in evaluation of clinically suspected *Pneumocystis carinii* pneumonia in AIDS patients with normal, equivocal, or nonspecific radiographic findings. AJR Am J Roentgenol 1997; 169:967–975.

116. Kroe DM, Kirsch CM, Jensen WA. Diagnostic strategies for *Pneumocystis carinii* pneumonia. Semin Respir Infect 1997; 12:70–78.
117. Schaumberg TH, Schnapp LM, Taylor KG, Golden JA. Diagnosis of *Pneumocystis carinii* infection in HIV-seropositive patients by identification of *P carinii* in pleural fluid. Chest 1993; 103:1890–1891.
118. Wilkin A, Feinberg J. *Pneumocystis carinii* pneumonia: a clinical review. Am Fam Physician 1999; 60:1699–1708, 1713–1714.
119. Goyal SB. Intestinal strogyloidiasis manifesting as eosinophilic pleural effusion. South Med J 1998; 91:768–769.
120. Mahmoud AAF. Intestinal nematodes (roundworms). In: Mandell GL, Bennett JE, Dolin R, eds. Mandell, Douglas, and Bennett's Principles and Practice of Infectious Diseases. 5th ed. Philadelphia: Churchill Livingstone, 2000:2938–2942.
121. Shibuya T. Eosinophilic response in parasitic diseases. Nippon Rinsho 1993; 51:825–831.
122. Spillman RK. Pulmonary ascariasis in tropical communities. Am J Trop Med Hyg 1975; 24:791–800.
123. Zykiewicz Z, Chetkowski A. Loeffler's syndrome in the form of pneumonia with eosinophilic exudative pleurisy. Gruzlica 1970; 38:261–265.
124. Boushy SF, North LB, Helgason AH. Thoracoscopy: technique and results in eighteen patients with pleural effusion. Chest 1978; 74:386–389.
125. Januszkiewicz J. Involvement of the respiratory system in trichinosis. Przegl Epidemiol 1967; 21:307–316.
126. Duran A, Grassin F, Richardi G, Curtet M. Loeffler's syndrome: is taeniasis responsible? Rev Pneumol Clin 1992; 48:279–281.
127. Emad A. Exudative eosinophilic pleural effusion due to *Strongyloides stercoralis* in a diabetic man. South Med J 1999; 92:58–60.
128. Oya H, Mori S, Tsuchihashi H, Kurono A, Mizoguchi A, Kawabata M, Arimura K, Osame M. A case of pleuritis caused by strongyloides in a carrier of T-cell lymphoma virus type I (HTLV-I). Nihon Kokyuki Gakkai Zasshi 1998; 36:262–267.
129. Chacin-Bonilla L. Systemic strongyloidiasis. Review. Invest Clin 1991; 32:131–145.
130. Wehner JH, Kirsch CM. Pulmonary manifestations of strongyloidiasis. Semin Respir Infect 1997; 12:122–129.
131. Kinjo T, Tsuhako K, Nakazato I, Ito E, Sato Y, Koyanagi Y, Iwamasa T. Extensive intra-alveolar hemorrhage caused by disseminated strongyloidiasis. Int J Parasitol 1998; 28:323–330.
132. Sen MK, Chakrabarti S, Ojha UC, Daima SR, Gupta R, Suri JC. Ectopic ascariasis: an unusual case of pyopneumothorax. Indian J Chest Dis Allied Sci 1998; 40:131–133.
133. Santini M, Baldi A, Vicidomini G, Di Marino MP, Baldi F. Relapsing pneumothorax due to *Ascaris lumbricoides* larvae. Monaldi Arch Chest Dis 1999; 54:328–329.
134. Papadopoulos GS, Eleftherakis NG, Thanopoulos BD. Cardiac tamponade in a child with ascariasis. Cardiol Young 2000; 10:539–541.
135. Lazarevic AM, Neskovic AN, Goronja M, Golubovic S, Komic J, Bojic M, Popovic AD. Low incidence of cardiac abnormalities in treated trichinosis: a prospective study of 62 patients from a single source outbreak. Am J Med 1999; 107:18–23.
136. Boornazian JS, Fagan MJ. Tropical pulmonary eosinophilia associated with pleural effusions. Am J Trop Med Hyg 1985; 34:473–475.

137. Maini VK, Bhatia AS, Singh AP. Atypical radiological presentation of tropical pulmonary eosinophilia. Indian J Chest Dis Allied Sci 1994; 36:45–48.
138. Grove DI. Tissue nematodes (trichinosis, dracunculiasis, filariasis). In: Mandell GL, Bennett JE, Dolin R, eds. Mandell, Douglas, and Bennett's Principles and Practice of Infectious Diseases. 5th ed. Philadelphia: Churchill Livingstone, 2000:2943–2949.
139. Singh RS, Sridnar MS, Bhaskar CJ. Tropical pulmonary eosinophilia presenting as eosinophilic pleural effusion. Indian J Chest Dis Allied Sci 1992; 34:225–229.
140. Oyamada Y, Funae O, Kamegaya Y, Soejima K, Nakamura H, Mori S, Yamaguchi K, Kanazawa M, Okusawa E, Yamasawa F. A case of tropical eosinophilia associated with pleural effusion. Nihon Kyobu Shikkan Gakkai Zasshi 1995; 33:451–455.
141. Chitkara RK, Sarinas PS. Dirofilaria, visceral larva migrans, and tropical pulmonary eosinophilia. Semin Respir Infect 1997; 12:138–148.
142. Milanez de Campos JR, Barbas CS, Filomeno LT, Fernandez A, Minamoto H, Filho JV, Jatene FB. Human pulmonary dirofilariasis: analysis of 24 cases from Sao Paulo, Brazil. Chest 1997; 112:729–733.
143. Walter A, Krishnaswami H, Cariappa A. Microfilariae of *Wuchereria bancrofti* in cytologic smears. Acta Cytol 1983; 27:432–436.
144. Seetharaman ML, Bahadur P, Shrinivas V, Subbarao KS. Filarial mediastinal lymphadenitis: another cause of superior vena caval syndrome. Chest 1988; 94:871–872.
145. Aggarwal J, Kapila K, Gaur A, Wali JP. Bancroftian filarial pleural effusion. Postgrad Med J 1993; 69:869–870.
146. Hira PR, Lindberg LG, Ryd W, Behbehani K. Cytologic diagnosis of bancroftian filariasis in a nonendemic area. Acta Cytol 1988; 32:267–269.
147. Klion AD, Eisenstein EM, Smirniotopoulos TT, Neumann MP, Nutman TB. Pulmonary involvement in loiasis. Am Rev Respir Dis 1992; 145:961–963.
148. Goh KL, Tan HW, Loh TG, Yap S. Chylothorax due to filariasis—a case report. Singapore Med 1986; 27:173–176.
149. Freundlich IM. The role of lymphangiography in chylothorax. A report of six cases. Am J Roentgenol Radium Ther Nucl Med 1975; 125:617–627.
150. Quah BS, Anuar AK, Rowani MR, Pennie RA. Cor pulmonale: an unusual presentation of tropical eosinophilia. Ann Trop Pediatr 1997; 17:77–81.
151. Yamakami Y, Mizunoe S, Yamagata E, Hiramatsu K, Yamasaki T, Nagai H, Hashimoto A, Nasu M. Pulmonary dirofilariasis associated with pleural effusion. Nihon Kokyuki Gakkai Zasshi 1998; 36:560–563.
152. Moorhouse DE, Abrahams EW, Stephens BJ. Human pulmonary dirofilariasis associated with pleural effusion. Med J Aust 1976; 2:902–903.
153. Umeki S, Yagi S, Higuma S, Nakashima M, Tsukiyama K, Soejima R. Clinical investigation of pulmonary dirofilariasis with unusual abnormalities on chest roentgenograms. Nihon Kyobu Shikkan Gakkai Zasshi 1989; 27:1274–1282.
154. Smith JW, Scott-Moncrieff JC, Rivers BC. Pneumothorax secondary to *Dirofilaria immitis* infection in two cats. J Am Vet Med Assoc 1998; 213:91–93.
155. Busch DS, Noxon JO. Pneumothorax in a dog infected with *Dirofilaria immitis*. J Am Vet Med Assoc 1992; 201:1983.
156. Nash TE. Visceral larva migrans and other unusual helminth infections. In: Mandell GL, Bennett JE, Dolin R, eds. Mandell, Douglas, and Bennett's Principles and Practice of Infectious Diseases. 5th ed. Philadelphia: Churchill Livingstone, 2000:2965–2969.

157. Herry I, Philippe B, Hennequin C, Danel C, Lejeunne C, Meyer G. Acute life-threatening toxocarial tamponade. Chest 1997; 112:1692–1693.
158. Jeanfaivre T, Cimon B, Tolstuchow N, de Gentile L, Chabasse D, Tuchais E. Pleural effusion and toxocariasis. Thorax 1996; 51:106–107.
159. Bruart J, Remacle P, Henneghien C, Jonckheer J. Pleural effusion and toxocara canis. Rev Mal Respir 1987; 4:35–37.
160. Kobayashi A, Tsuji M, Wilbur DL. Probable pulmonary anisakiasis accompanying pleural effusion. Am J Trop Med Hyg 1985; 34:310–313.
161. Matsuoka H, Nakama T, Kisanuki H, Uno H, Tachibana N, Tsubouchi H, Horii Y, Nawa Y. A case report of serologically diagnosed pulmonary anisakiasis with pleural effusion and multiple lesions. Am J Trop Med Hyg 1994; 51:819–822.
162. Ahmed L, el-Dib NA, el-Boraey Y, Ibrahim M. Capillaria philippinensis: an emerging parasite causing severe diarrhea in Egypt. J Egypt Soc Parasitol 1999; 29:483–493.
163. Uttamchandani RB, Trigo LM, Poppiti RJ Jr, Rozen S, Ratzan KR. Eosinophilic pleural effusion in cutaneous myiasis. South Med J 1989; 82:1288–1291.
164. Mathieu ME, Wilson BB. Myiasis. In: Mandell GL, Bennett JE, Dolin R, eds. Mandell, Douglas, and Bennett's Principles and Practice of Infectious Diseases. 5th ed. Philadelphia: Churchill Livingstone, 2000:2976–2979.
165. Feldman C, Kallenbach J, Sutej P, Lewis M, Goldstein B. Diffuse interstitial pulmonary fibrosis and spontaneous pneumothorax associated with *Schistosoma haematobium* infestation of the lungs. S Afr Med J 1986; 69:138–139.
166. Vanker EA. Aortic aneurysm caused by schistosomiasis. Thorax 1986; 41:890–891.
167. Mahmoud AAF. Trematodes (schistosomiasis) and other flukes. In: Mandell GL, Bennett JE, Dolin R, eds. Mandell, Douglas, and Bennett's Principles and Practice of Infectious Diseases. 5th ed. Philadelphia: Churchill Livingstone, 2000:2950–2955.
168. Abdulla MA, Hombal SM, al-Juwaiser A. Detection of *Schistosoma mansoni* in bronchoalveolar lavage fluid—a case report. Acta Cytol 1999; 43:856–858.
169. Azher M, el-Kassimi FA, Wright SG, Mofti A. Exudative polyserositis and acute respiratory failure following praziquantel therapy. Chest 1990; 98:241–243.
170. Guardia SN, Sepp H, Scholten T, Morava-Protzner I. Pentastomiasis in Canada. Arch Pathol Lab Med 1991; 115:515–517.
171. Drabick JJ. Pentastomiasis. Rev Infect Dis 1987; 9:1087–1094.
172. Bartoloni A, Cancrini G, Bartalesi F, Marcolin D, Roselli M, Arce CC, Hall AC. *Mansonella ozzardi* infection in Bolivia: prevalence and clinical associations in the Chaco region. Am J Trop Med Hyg 1999; 61:830–833.
173. Goljan J, Nahorski W, Tomaszewski R, Felczak-Korzybska I, Gorski J. Diagnosing and treatment of skin filariases based on own observations. Int Marit Health 2000; 51:51–61.
174. Radosavljevic-Asic G, Jovanovich D, Radovanovich D, Tucakovic M. Trichomonas in pleural effusion. Eur Respir J 1994; 7:1906–1908.
175. Walzer PD, Rutherford I, East R. Empyema with *Trichomonas* species. Am Rev Respir Dis 1978; 118:415–418.
176. Shiota T, Arizono N, Morimoto T, Shimatsu A, Nakao K. *Trichomonas tenax* empyema in an immunocompromised patient with advanced cancer. Parasite 1998; 5:375–377.
177. Goodman PC, Schnapp LM. Pulmonary toxoplasmosis in AIDS. Radiology 1992; 184:791–793.

178. Guignard E, Picon L, Bacq Y, Choutet P, Thanh Hai Duong. Toxoplasmic pleuropericarditis associated with Hodgkin's disease. Rev Med Interne 1988; 9:473–476.
179. Weber R, Kuster H, Keller R, Bachi T, Spycher MA, Briner J, Russi E, Luthy R. Pulmonary and intestinal microsporidiosis in a patient with the acquired immunodeficiency syndrome. Am Rev Respir Dis 1992; 146:1603–1605.
180. Pluss JL, Opal SM. Pulmonary sporotrichosis: review of treatment and outcome. Medicine (Baltimore) 1986; 65:143–153.
181. Fields Cl, Ossorio MA, Roy TM. Empyema associated with pulmonary sporotrichosis. South Med J 1989; 82:910–913.
182. Miller RF, Howling SJ, Reid AJ, Shaw PJ. Pleural effusions in patients with AIDS. Sex Transm Infect 2000; 76:122–125.
183. Munoz-Rodriguez FJ, Padro S, Pastor P, Rosa-Re D, Valls ME, Miro JM, Gatell JM. Pleural and peritoneal leishmaniasis in an AIDS patient. Eur J Clin Microbiol Infect Dis 1997; 16:246–248.
184. Arjona R, Riancho JA, Aguado JM, Salesa R, Gonzalez-Macias J. Fasciolasis in developed countries: a review of classic and aberrant forms of the disease. Medicine (Baltimore) 1995; 74:13–23.
185. Corredoira JC, Perez R, Casariego E, Varela J, Lopez MJ, Torres J. Eosinophilic pleural effusion caused by *Fasciola hepatica*. Enferm Infecc Microbiol Clin 1990; 8:258–259.
186. Cayea PD, Rubin E, Teixidor HS. Atypical pulmonary malaria. AJR Am J Roentgenol 1981; 137:51–55.
187. Sirivichayakul C, Chanthavanich P, Chokejindachai W, Pengsaa K, Kabkaew K, Saelim R. Pleural effusion in childhood falciparum malaria. Southeast Asian J Trop Med Public Health 2000; 31:187–189.
188. Libanore M, Bicocchi R, Sighinolfi L, Ghinelli F. Pneumothorax during pulmonary toxoplasmosis in an AIDS patient. Chest 1991; 100:1184.
189. Chenoweth CE, Singal S, Pearson RD, Betts RF, Markovitz DM. Acquired immunodeficiency syndrome-related visceral leishmaniasis presenting in a pleural effusion. Chest 1993; 103, 648–649.
190. Vives L, Gaillemin C, Recco P, Seguela JP. Pyopneumothorax as the first and main manifestation of *Fasciola hepatica* distomatosis. Nouv Presse Med 1980; 9:48.

45

Iatrogenic and Rare Pleural Effusions

MARIA PLATAKI
University Hospital of Heraklion
Heraklion, Crete, Greece

DEMOSTHENES BOUROS
Demokritos University of Thrace
Medical School
and University Hospital
of Alexandroupolis
Alexandroupolis, Greece

I. Iatrogenic Pleural Effusions

In some cases diagnostic or therapeutic interventional techniques or even physicians themselves are responsible for the accumulation of pleural fluid. Several causes of iatrogenic pleural effusions are listed in Table 1. In this chapter pleural effusions due to central venous catheter or nasogastric tube misplacement, translumbar aortography, or rupture of mammary prosthesis are discussed. Other causes are discussed in other chapters of this book.

A. Vascular Erosion by Central Venous Catheters

Percutaneous insertion of indwelling central venous catheters is widely used as an important therapeutic procedure in a wide range of medical problems (1). A major complication of central venous catheterization that is not well recognized is vascular erosion and resultant hydrothorax, sometimes with delayed catheter migration. The incidence of this complication appears to be approximately 0.4–1.0% of catheter placements (1), but it may be higher considering that some cases remain unrecognized. The diagnosis should be suspected if new cardiopulmonary symptoms, enlarging pleural effusions, or mediastinal widening appear after the insertion of a central venous catheter. Roentgenographic detection of

Table 1 Iatrogenic Causes of Pleural Effusion

Vascular erosion by central venous catheters
Perforation of pleura with a nasogastric tube
Translumbar aortography
After mammaplasty
Secondary to pharmaceutical agents
Radiation therapy
Endoscopic esophageal sclerotherapy
Ovarian hyperstimulation syndrome
Fluid overload
Coronary artery bypass surgery
Abdominal surgery

extravascular extravasation of radiocontrast after injection of intravenous contrast material or thoracentesis demonstration of either milky fluid in patients receiving intravenous fat emulsions or a pleural fluid/serum glucose ratio greater than 1 confirms the presence of erosion. Inability to withdraw blood from the catheter supports the possibility of catheter perforation, but free-flowing return does not exclude the diagnosis (2). Large-bore or left-sided central venous catheter placement increases the risk of this complication (3).

Duntley et al. reviewed 34 reports describing 61 patients with catheter-induced vascular erosion and hydrothorax (1). The median time from catheter insertion to vascular perforation was 2.0 days (range 1–60 days), although 50% of erosions occurred in the first 2 days of catheter placement. The route of catheterization was left-sided in 74% and right-sided in 26%. Pleural effusions were present in 79% of patients at presentation, being unilateral on either side of the catheter insertion site in 69% of patients and bilateral in 31%. Pleural fluid volume was usually large, occupying one third to one half of a hemithorax. Pleural fluid was described as clear, milky, serous, serosanguineous, or hemorrhagic. Milky pleural fluid is diagnostic in patients receiving intravenous fat emulsions without other causes of chylothorax (4). When hyperosmolar hyperalimentation fluids, such as TPN, drain into the pleural cavity, tension hydrothorax may develop, leading to serious and acute problems (5). In the review by Duntley et al., however, glucose concentrations in the pleural fluid were relatively low compared with the infused solutions, since normal pleura rapidly uptakes or presents a negligible barrier for glucose transit into serum (1). All patients who had blood glucose concentrations measured had a pleural fluid-to-serum glucose ratio greater than 1, suggesting the value of this ratio in detecting central venous catheter erosion. Although always in the transudative range, protein concentration may vary depending on the protein content of infused fluids, the infusion rate, the degree of pleural inflammation and altered permeability induced by hyperosmolar solutions, and the presence of pleural hemorrhage. Progressive mediastinal widening was also a characteristic roentgenographic finding.

The onset of signs and symptoms of hydrothorax may present a delay from 0 to 60 days. Symptoms may appear suddenly with rapid progression or as a nonspecific discomfort with an indolent evolution. Dyspnea was present in 82% of the patients, chest pain in 46%, cough in 2%, whereas 10% of the patients were asymptomatic.

Delays in diagnosis ranged from 0 to 11 days, and attribution of symptoms and roentgenographic findings to other cardiopulmonary abnormalities was not uncommon. Misdiagnosis or delayed diagnosis contributed to patient morbidity and mortality. There was 12% mortality directly attributable to venous perforation (1).

Early detection of catheter erosion is important because the catheter should be removed immediately and therapeutic thoracentesis should be performed in patients with serious respiratory compromise. Hemothorax requires the insertion of a chest tube, and if the bleeding persists exploratory thoracotomy may be necessary.

B. Perforation of Pleura with a Nasogastric Tube

Enteral tube feeding is an attractive alternative to intravenous alimentation for nutritional support. Small-bore, silicone nasoenteric feeding tubes are increasingly utilized in the critically ill patient to provide nutritional support. The metallic-weighted tips and stiffening-introducing stylets create the potential for misplacement with potentially serious consequences, changing the spectrum of complications seen with previously used larger nasogastric tubes. Although perforation of the esophagus by a nasogastric tube or an intracranial tube has only been reported sporadically, malpositioning of nasogastric tubes in the tracheobronchial tree appears to be more common (6–13). All pleuropulmonary complications are the result of inadvertent passage of tubes into the tracheobronchial tree with eventual perforation into the lung and pleural space. Guide wires used to aid passage may contribute to this complication (11,12). In a report by Bankier et al., the incidence of abnormal tube positioning in the tracheobronchial tree in an 11-month period in intensive care unit patients who received nasogastric tubes was 0.8% (14/1700) (6). In 4 of these 14 patients the nasogastric tubes perforated the bronchial tree and the pleura. All 4 patients suffered subsequent pneumothoraces that had to be drained by chest tubes. None of these patients had alimentary feeding over the malpositioned nasogastric tube. In all patients supine or semi-erect frontal chest radiographs accurately demonstrated that the nasogastric tube was malpositioned in the tracheobronchial tree. Sabga et al. reported a case of inadvertent administration of activated charcoal in water into the right lung and pleural cavity of a 51-year-old man treated for a salicylate overdose due to misplacement of the nasogastric tube (9). A mild chemical pneumonitis and a sterile empyema developed. Charcoal-stained fluid drained through a thoracostomy tube for 8 weeks. Major underlying factors favoring tube malpositioning include depressed sensorium, impaired gag reflex, recent endotracheal intubation, decreased laryngeal sensitivity, and neuromuscular blocking drugs (6,8). The presence of cuffed tracheostomy or endotracheal tubes does not prevent this occurrence (10). The traditional criteria for proper tube placement, like insufflation of air with sounds heard over the region of the stomach or aspiration of fluid, are suboptimal in critically ill patients. Therefore, institution of nasogastric tubes should be performed according to strict guidelines, which include radiographic confirmation of desired position, especially before feedings are initiated, limited and supervised use of stylets, and a need for special precautions in patients who are obtunded or receiving intubated respiratory assistance (6,9–12).

C. Translumbar Aortography

A hemorrhagic pleural effusion may also complicate translumbar aortography resulting from blood leaking from the aorta in the pleural space (14). Therapeutic thoracentesis is indicated in this case. Surgical intervention is not necessary because usually the leak stops spontaneously. Moreover, irritation of the pleural space from extravasated contrast medium may lead to an exudative effusion.

D. Mammaplasty-Induced Pleural Effusion

There are three case reports of rupture of a silicone bag mammary prosthesis leading to silicone migration to the pleura and the development of a pleural effusion (15–17). Hirmand et al. present a case of silicone particles found in the pleural space of a patient 20 years after bilateral augmentation mammaplasty with silicone gel implants (15). When the patient experienced pain in the upper back, a ruptured left implant was found and a left pleural effusion developed subsequently. Analysis of the pleural effusion fluid by scanning electron microscopy suggested the presence of silicone. In the case described by Stevens et al. an oily layer was observed on the top of the aspirated pleural fluid from a patient with a ruptured implant, which was consistent with the presence of silicone gel in the aspirate (16). The findings of the pleural biopsy in this patient were suggestive of a foreign body reaction. In both cases the effusion did not recur after thoracentesis and further pulmonary complications or other symptoms have not developed.

II. Yellow Nail Syndrome

The yellow nail syndrome, first described in 1964 by Samman and White in 13 patients, consists of a triad of yellow nails, lymphedema, and respiratory tract illness, which is rarely present at initial presentation. Pleural effusion is usually a late manifestation and does not regress spontaneously. Respiratory manifestations include pleural effusions, bronchiectasis, recurrent pneumonias, bronchitis, or sinusitis.

It is considered to be a rare clinical condition. Until 1986 only 97 cases of this syndrome had been reported (18). Women are afflicted about twice as often as men, and the age of onset varies from birth to the eighth decade, with the median age being 40 years (18,19). In a review of 96 patients, yellow nails were the presenting manifestation in 37% and lymphedema in 34% (18). Yellow nails were present in 89% of the cases, lymphedema in 80%, and pleural effusion in 36% of all cases (18). Patients may develop pericardial effusion (20–23) or chylous ascites and intestinal lymphangiectasia (20,24,25). There are reports of prenatal manifestation of this disorder as nonimmune fetal hydrops with patients' mothers having yellow nail syndrome (26,27).

There is an autosomal dominant transmission of the disorder (26,28). The etiology of the syndrome remains obscure, but the pathogenesis seems to involve a congenital defect of the lymphatics. In most patients lymphangiograms of the lower extremity demonstrate hypoplasia of at least some lymphatic vessels and impaired lymphatic flow (19). Edema can be pitting or nonpitting and may be confined to the fingertips.

There seems to be an association of the syndrome with recent lower respiratory tract infections, chronic pulmonary infections, and chronic sinus infections (29,30). There is a hypothesis that lower respiratory tract infections or pleural inflammation cause further damage to already impaired but adequate lymphatic vessels (31). The lymphatic drainage becomes insufficient and a pleural effusion develops. Histological study of the pleura in a patient with the syndrome showed that it was thickened with fibrosis and chronic inflammatory infiltrates. The lymphatic capillaries in the visceral pleura were dilated (32). Lewis et al. reported that a biopsy of the parietal pleura revealed abnormally dilated lymphatics, neogenesis of lymphatic channels, and edematous tissues in some areas (33). Runyon et al. measured the pleural fluid turnover by radioiodized albumin to trace the efflux of fluid by lymphatics (34). The pleural lymphatic flow was low in comparison to previous estimates in a variety of other conditions. However, Mambretti-Zumwalt et al. report that the albumin turnover rate in the pleural fluid is not greatly decreased in patients with the syndrome (35).

Affected nails are thickened, excessively curved along both axes, very slow growing with yellowish-gray hue. Cuticle and lunula are usually absent, and onycholysis is frequently evident (25). Women frequently cover their unsightly nails with opaque nail polish, which may obscure the finding from the unwary clinician (36).

Pleural effusions are usually recurrent after a thoracentesis, are bilateral in 50% of cases, and vary in size (19,37). The pleural fluid is exudative with ≥200 nucleated cells per mm^3, predominantly lymphocytic (>80%) (19,38). The glucose is equivalent to serum, and the pH approximates 7.40. There have been cases of the syndrome complicated by an empyema (39,40) and cases associated with cancer and immunodeficiency disease (41–43). However, no direct relationship has been found between the syndrome and malignancies, immunological disorders, endocrine abnormalities, or connective tissue disease.

There is no specific causative treatment for the syndrome. Following thoracentesis, fluid typically recurs over a few days to several months. Chemical pleurodesis, open pleural abrasion, pleurectomy, or pleuroperitoneal shunting may be applied to control the symptomatic pleural effusion (33,44–46). The new oral antifungal drugs may be of value in the treatment of the yellow nail syndrome (36). Local steroid injections and oral vitamin E have been reported to be successful in treating the yellow nails. Spontaneous partial or complete recovery of nail abnormalities occurs in 30% of patients, who may experience occasional relapses. Lymphedema and pleural effusions are persistent, and spontaneous recovery has not been reported.

III. Uremia

Uremic pleuritis has been recognized as a complication of uremia since 1836 (47). Hopps and Wissler reported an incidence of fibrinous pleuritis as high as 20% in patients who died of uremia (48). This pleuritis can become evident as pleuritic chest pain with pleural rubs (49), pleural effusion (49–56), or pulmonary restriction (51,53,57,58). Uremia-associated serosal injury may allow transudation of fluid into the pleural space, but the specific pathogenesis of uremic pleural effusion is not clear (54). The mechanism of pleural effusion and restrictive fibrosis is considered to be similar to that of hemorrhagic and constrictive pericarditis seen in uremia.

The incidence of uremic pleural effusion in patients receiving long-term hemodialysis is reported to be 1–58% (50,52,59). There has not been found a relationship between the level of uremia and the development of a pleural effusion (50). Patients may be asymptomatic or may present with fever (15–50%), chest pain (30–31%), cough (35%), and dyspnea (20%) (50,52,55). Up to 88% of patients may also have cardiomegaly (52). Pleural effusions are bilateral in 50% of patients (52,56) and may be massive (50,56).

Uremic patients have increased susceptibility to many causes of pleural effusion. Uremic pleural effusion should be considered when common etiologies of effusions such as volume overload, congestive heart failure, infection, and malignancy have been excluded (53,54).

Pleural effusions are common in patients receiving long-term hemodialysis. Coskun et al. reported pleural effusion as a thoracic CT finding in 51% of 117 uremic patients (60). Jarratt and Sahn found an incidence of pleural effusions in adult hospitalized patients receiving long-term hemodialysis of 21% (52). Pleural effusions resulted from heart failure in 46% and nonheart failure causes in 54%. Uremic pleurisy (16%), parapneumonic effusion (15%), and atelectasis (11%) accounted for most of the noncardiac failure causes.

Pleural fluid neopterin levels can be used to differentiate uremic pleural effusions from other causes of effusion (61). In a study of 93 patients, neopterin levels were strikingly elevated in patients with uremic pleural effusion compared to tuberculous, malignant, parapneumonic, and other kinds of effusions (61).

A uremic pleural effusion is characterized as a necrotizing fibrinous exudate that is often hemorrhagic with a paucity of nucleated cells that are predominantly lymphocytes (50–56). In a series of 8 patients with uremic pleuritis, the mean pleural fluid pH was 7.37 ± 0.03, the number of nucleated cells $1231 \pm 379/\mu L$ with $22\pm7\%$ neutrophils, the total protein 3.9 ± 0.2 g/dL, the LDH level 163 ± 33 IU/L, and the glucose PF/S ratio 1.8 ± 0.1 (52). Pleural tissue obtained by open or closed biopsy showed chronic fibrosing pleuritis (50–53,55–58).

Uremic pleuritis generally responds to continued hemodialysis (50,54). In a study of 14 patients, the effusions resolved with continued dialysis in 4–6 weeks after thoracentesis in 11 patients and recurred in 3 patients (50). The prognosis is usually good, but fatal cases have also been reported (55,56).

The fibrosing pleuritis may be severe enough to cause disabling restriction and warrant decortication (51,53,57,58). Decortication of the chest wall and the lung can be carried out safely with minimal bleeding producing restoration of pulmonary function and clinical improvement (57,58). Surgical decortication should be considered in cases with a severe clinical course when uremic pleurisy is complicated by progressive pleural thickening and pulmonary restriction.

IV. Trapped Lung

The term trapped lung describes persistent atelectasis with failure of the lung to reexpand following evacuation of a chronic pleural effusion. It most commonly results from the development of a fibrous peel over the visceral pleura in the setting of chronic pleural inflammation (62). The initial pleural inflammation is usually due to pneumonia or hemothorax, but also it may be caused by spontaneous pneumothorax, thoracic operations including coronary artery bypass surgery (63), uremia (57,58), or collagen vascular disease. An ongoing malignant process in the pleural space may also produce a thick visceral pleural peel (62). The peel restricts expansion of the underlying lung parenchyma, generating higher negative pleural pressures within the pleural space. The negative pleural pressure in turn leads to increased pleural fluid formation despite decreased pleural fluid absorption and the development of a chronic pleural effusion. Negative initial pleural pressures and/or rapid changes in the pressures as fluid is withdrawn during thoracentesis are suggestive of trapped lung (64,65). One characteristic of the pleural effusion with trapped lung is that the amount of fluid remains stable from one study to another and after thoracentesis reaccumulates rapidly to its previous level (66).

Patients may exhibit dyspnea at rest or with exertion, cough, or they may be asymptomatic. Symptoms of acute pleural inflammation are absent, but the patient may give a history of fever or pleuritic chest pain in the past. Dyspnea in the setting of trapped lung is likely multifactorial and due not only to restrictive ventilatory dysfunction caused by the pleural peel, but also to physiological changes attributable to the effusion (62). These may include distention of the thoracic cavity, dysfunction of the affected hemidiaphragm, and decreased lung compliance and atelectasis. Patients with trapped lung fail to demonstrate full lung reexpansion despite complete drainage of the pleural effusion. However, they may exhibit symptomatic improvement because of partial lung reexpansion and improvement in these physiological parameters (62).

The pathognomonic radiographic sign of trapped lung is the pneumothorax ex vacuo or suction pneumothorax, a small to moderate-sized air collection in the pleural space after evacuation of the effusion, often seen in association with a visibly thickened visceral pleural surface (67,68).

The pleural fluid is usually borderline exudate (69). The ratio of pleural fluid to serum protein is about 0.5, and the ratio of the pleural fluid LDH level to the serum LDH level is about 0.6. The pleural fluid glucose level is normal and the pleural fluid white blood cell count (WBC) is usually less than $1000/mm^3$, with the differential WBC revealing predominantly mononuclear cells (69).

The diagnosis of trapped lung requires pleurectomy with decortication (57,58,62,63). In cases of malignant pleural effusion in patients with short life expectancy, therapeutic options include repeated thoracentesis, long-term thoracostomy drainage, small-bore indwelling pleural catheters, and pleuroperitoneal shunting (62,70). In asymptomatic or minimally symptomatic patients a surgical procedure is not indicated, and such patients with trapped lung syndrome should be observed.

V. Therapeutic Radiation Exposure

Radiation exposure can cause pleural effusion by two mechanisms: radiation pleuritis and systemic venous hypertension or lymphatic obstruction from mediastinal fibrosis (71). In animals, thoracic radiation causes at an early stage actinic pneumonia and a small pleural effusion. Later on lung changes regress completely and a large pleural effusion appears, probably due to lymphatic block (72). Bachman and Macken followed 200 patients treated with between 4000 and 6000 rads to the hemithorax for breast carcinoma (73). Eleven patients (5.5%) developed pleural effusions with no other obvious explanation, which were attributed to radiation. In all cases the pleural effusion developed within 6 months of completing radiation therapy and concomitant radiation was also present. Most pleural effusions were small, but at least one occupied nearly 50% of the hemithorax. Hietala and Hahn performed chest roentgenograms regularly before and a long time after radiotherapy in 157 patients with breast cancer (74). Radiation-induced parenchymal changes were demonstrated in 73% of the patients and pleural effusions in about 10%. The radiation-induced pleural effusion had no special characteristics, with one exception—it occurred simultaneously with radiation-induced parenchymal infiltrates. The pleural fluid characteristics, however, have not been well described. In a study of two cases of pleuritis by radiation, pleural fluid was found to be a hemorrhagic exudate with multiple reactive mesothelial cells with vacuole formation within the cytoplasm and nuclei (75). In 4 of the 11 patients followed by Bachman and Macken, the fluid gradually disappeared spontaneously in 4–23 months (73). In the rest of the patients, the fluid gradually decreased in size over the follow-up period of 10–40 months.

The pleural effusions associated with radiation pleuritis and mediastinal fibrosis tend to occur 1–2 years following intensive (4000–6000 rads) mediastinal radiation (71). Mechanisms for development of pleural effusion as a late complication of radiation therapy include constrictive pericarditis (with or without tamponade), superior vena cava obstruction, and lymphatic obstruction, all complications of mediastinal fibrosis (71,76,77). Rodriguez-Garcia et al. described a patient with recurrent massive pleural effusions 8 years after mediastinal therapy for Hodgkin's disease (71). The pleural fluid was a serohemorrhagic exudate without malignant cells, and thoracoscopy showed diffuse thickening of the pleura. There is a report of a patient developing bilateral pleural effusion 19 years after thoracic irradiation for Hodgkin's disease (77). The pleural liquid was an exudate with lymphocytic predominance, and thoracoscopy revealed enlarged lymphatic channels in the visceral pleura.

VI. Drowning

Pleural effusion is a common finding both in saltwater and in freshwater drownings. Morild reviewed the files from 133 cases of drowning examined at his institute in the years 1987–1991 (78). Increased pleural fluid was present in 71 (53.4%) of the cases. The mean amount of fluid observed was 432.8 mL while the maximum amount was 3000 mL. According to this study the time spent in water is correlated to the production of pleural fluid. There are drowning cases, however, in which a large volume of pleural fluid has been found although the victim had only been in the water for a short time and cases in which no increased amount of fluid is present although the body had been in the water for a considerable time. In this study, for example, one victim spent only 6–7 minutes in the water but had 900 mL of pleural fluid. The reason for this is unknown. It was also found that more pleural fluid is produced in saltwater than in freshwater drowning. Salt water is hyperosmolar and will lead to plasma leaking out of the capillaries into the alveolar spaces, whereas in freshwater drowning water will leak into the capillaries and cause a hemodilution. After death the gradual breakdown of membranes and the degradation of lung surfactant phospholipids will possibly also add to the leak of fluid through the lungs into the pleural cavities. However, there must be other factors than just passive leak of fluid from the alveolar spaces that contribute to the formation of pleural fluid after drowning. More experimental studies are necessary in order to determine the mechanisms contributing to pleural fluid accumulation after drowning.

VII. Amyloidosis

Although amyloidosis of the respiratory tract is well recognized, pleural involvement is considered to be uncommon and has been rarely reported in the literature. However, this could be due to not considering this diagnosis in patients presenting with pleural effusions and multiorgan disease (79). Pleural biopsy specimens, which can be obtained by percutaneous needle biopsy (79–83), thoracoscopic (84,85) or open lung biopsy, require special staining with Congo red and/or crystal violet to detect amyloid deposition. This is likely to contribute to the underdiagnosis of pleural involvement in patients with systemic amyloidosis.

Pleural effusions can be large, unilateral or bilateral, and occasionally recurrent. Usually they are transudative (79–82), and the cause is most often congestive heart failure due to cardiac amyloid involvement. Other explanations for pleural effusions include nephritic syndrome, liver failure, and direct pleural deposition with amyloid. There are cases where exudative pleural effusions with pleural amyloidosis are reported (79,80,82,86,87). The mechanism of the production of an exudative effusion is unknown, but it could be due to obstruction of the lymphatics in the parietal pleura by the amyloid deposition or it could be that previous diuretic treatment has changed the characteristics of the effusion (82). Macroscopic examination of the parietal pleura during thoracoscopy in a patient with primary amyloidosis and pleural involvement revealed a diffuse inflammation and light brown deposits that were covered with nodules (85).

VIII. Milk of Calcium Pleural Collections

Milk of calcium is a colloidal suspension of calcium crystals, which can accumulate in cystic spaces such as renal, adrenal, or breast cysts producing a characteristic finding of half-moon contour on radiography. Im et al. described five patients with milk of calcium pleural collections (88). The diagnosis was based on needle aspiration in four patients and the presence of fat-calcium level on computed tomography (CT) in one. The concentration of calcium in the aspirated fluid was greater than 500 mg/dL. Four patients had a previous history of pleurisy. Homogeneous increased opacity with a double contour at the interface with the lung was a characteristic radiographic finding. CT showed that the lateral contour was the margin of the milk of calcium and the medial contour was the margin of the thickened visceral pleura facing the lung. On CT milk of calcium collection appeared as a homogeneous area of increased attenuation.

IX. Pleural Effusion in Electrical Injury

The most common visceral lesions associated to electrical burns are cardiac lesions. Pulmonary compromise is rare (89). However, when the entry or exit ports are the thoracic wall, pleural effusion, hemothorax, and pneumonitis may occur (89,90). The pleural fluid is an exudate that resolves gradually (90).

X. Mediastinal Cysts

The rupture into the pleural cavity of a benign cystic teratoma of the mediastinum is a rare complication that leads to pleural fluid formation (91–97). Several explanations have been given for the tendency to rupture of mediastinal teratomas, including ischemia due to tumor enlargement, infection, or erosion from the digestive enzymes derived from the tumor tissues (91). Choi et al. reported that out of 17 cases of surgically resected mediastinal teratomas, preoperative rupture was found in 7 (92). Pleural effusion was seen in 4 of the 7 (57%) ruptured masses, at the ipsilateral ruptured sites in 2 cases, and bilaterally in the other 2 cases. The authors assumed that the pleural effusion resulted from either spillage of internal components of a mass or from an inflammatory reaction to the extravasated contents. There are cases of pleural fluid formation following the rupture of benign mediastinal teratomas in which levels of carcinoembryonic antigen, CA-125, CA19-9, and amylase are elevated (91,93,97). Cobb et al. reported that the examination of the pleural fluid after the rupture of an anterior mediastinal benign cystic teratoma showed the presence of squamous and columnar epithelial cells, hairs, calcospherites (calcium deposits), keratinous material, and cholesterol against an inflammatory background (94). Mediastinal bronchogenic cysts presenting with serofibrinous or serosanguineous pleural fluid have also been described (98). These pleural effusions were probably related to an inflammatory reaction of the pleura to the bronchogenic cyst. Such inflammation could be due to the large size of the masses, perhaps with the onset of rupture.

XI. Whipple's Disease

Although the main manifestation of Whipple's disease is gastrointestinal, it is a systemic disorder, and pulmonary involvement is a frequent but not well-known finding (99). Involvement of the lung as a site of this disease was reported in Whipple's first description in 1907 (100). The lung and the pleura may be affected both before and after the development of diarrhea (101,102). Pleural effusion is reported less often than chronic nonproductive cough, dyspnea, and pleuritic chest pain (101). In cells from pleural effusions, *Tropheryma whippelii*–specific amplification products were found by PCR (103). In a report by Riemer et al. an exudative bilateral pleural effusion in a patient with Whipple's disease subsided after 3 months of antibiotic therapy (99).

XII. Syphilis

Pleural effusion is rarely formed in syphilis patients. Zaharopoulos and Wong described a case of a 68-year-old man with secondary syphilis who concomitantly suffered from left lower lobe pneumonia with associated pleuritis (104).

Cytological examination of the pleural fluid was diagnostic of syphilis, not only by the characteristic cytomorphology but also by demonstration of spirochetes by the May-Grunwald-Giemsa and Steiner staining methods. Cattini et al. also reported a case of pleurisy diagnosed in a patient with tertiary syphilis (105). The spirochetes were discovered in the pleuritic exudate.

References

1. Duntley P, Siever J, Korwes ML, Harpel K, Heffner JE. Vascular erosion by central venous catheters. Clinical features and outcome. Chest 1992; 101:1633–1638.
2. Kollef MH. Fallibility of persistent blood return for confirmation of intravascular catheter placement in patients with hemorrhagic thoracic effusions. Chest 1994; 106:1906–1908.
3. Mukau L, Talamini MA, Sitzmann N. Risk factors for central venous catheter-related vascular erosions. J Parenter Enteral Nutr 1991; 15:513–516.
4. Wolthuis A, Landewe RB, Theunissen PH, Westerhuis LW. Chylothorax or leakage of total parenteral nutrition? Eur Respir J 1998; 12:1233–1235.
5. Bennet MR, Chaudhry RM, Owens GR. Elevated pleural fluid glucose: a risk for tension hydrothorax. South Med J 1986; 79:1287–1289.
6. Bankier AA, Wiesmayr MN, Henk C, Turetschek K, Winkelbauer F, Mallek R, Fleoschmann D, Janata K, Herold CJ. Radiographic detection of intrabronchial malpositions of nasogastric tubes and subsequent complications in intensive care unit patients. Intensive Care Med 1997; 23:406–410.
7. Miller KS, Tomlinson JR, Sahn SA. Pleuropulmonary complications of enteral tube feedings. Two reports, review of the literature, and recommendations. Chest 1985; 88:230–233.
8. Roubenoff R, Ravich WJ. Pneumothorax due to nasogastric feeding tubes. Report of four cases, review of the literature, and recommendations for prevention. Arch Intern Med 1989; 149:184–188.
9. Sabga E, Dick A, Lertzman M, Tenenbein M. Direct administration of charcoal into the lung and pleural cavity. Ann Emerg Med 1997; 30:695–697.
10. McWey RE, Curry NS, Schabel SI, Reines HD. Complications of nasoenteric feeding tubes. Am J Surg 1988; 155:253–257.
11. Hand RW, Kempster M, Levy JH, Rogol PR, Spirn P. Inadvertent transbronchial insertion of narrow-bore feeding tubes into the pleural space. JAMA 1984; 251:2396–2397.
12. Schorlemmer GR, Battaglini JW. An unusual complication of naso-enteral feeding with small-diameter feeding tubes. Ann Surg 1984; 199:104–106.
13. Balogh GJ, Adler SJ, VanderWoude J, Glazer HS, Roper C, Weyman PJ. Pneumothorax as a complication of feeding tube placement. Am J Roentgenol 1983; 146:1275–1277.
14. Bilbrey GL, Hedberg CL. Hemorrhagic pleural effusion secondary to aortography: a case report. J Thorac Cardiovasc Surg 1967; 54:85–89.
15. Hirmand H, Hoffman LA, Smith JP. Silicone migration to the pleural space associated with silicone-gel augmentation mammaplasty. Ann Plast Surg 1994; 32:645–647.

16. Stevens UM, Burdon JG, Niall JF. Pleural effusion after rupture of silicone bag mammary prosthesis. Thorax 1987; 42:825–826.
17. Taupmann RE, Adler S. Silicone pleural effusion due to iatrogenic breast implant rupture. South Med J 1993; 86:570–571.
18. Nordkild P, Kromann-Andersen H, Struve-Christensen E. Yellow nail syndrome-the triad of yellow nails, lymphedema and pleural effusions. A review of the literature and a case report. Acta Med Scand 1986; 219:221–227.
19. Beer DJ, Pereira W Jr, Snider GL. Pleural effusion associated with primary lymphedema: a perspective on the yellow nail syndrome. Am Rev Respir Dis 1978; 117:595–599.
20. Malek NP, Ocran K, Tietge UJ, Maschek H, Gratz KF, Trautwein C, Wagner S, Manns MP. A case of the yellow nail syndrome associated with massive chylous ascites, pleural and pericardial effusions. Z Gastroenterol 1996; 34:763–766.
21. Morandi U, Golinelli M, Brandi L, Ruggiero C, Stefani A, Lodi R. "Yellow nail syndrome" associated with chronic recurrent pericardial and pleural effusions. Eur J Cardiothorac Surg 1995; 9:42–44.
22. Coche G, Chalaoui J, Jeanneret A, Sylvestre J. Yellow nail syndrome. Apropos of a case. A review of the main radiologic manifestations. J Radiol 1986; 67:435–437.
23. Paradisis M, Van Asperen P. Yellow nail syndrome in infancy. J Paediatr Child Health 1997; 33:454–457.
24. Desrame J, Bechade D, Patte JH, Jean R, Karsenti D, Coutant G, Algayres JP, Daly JP. Yellow nail syndrome associated with intestinal lymphangiectasia. Gastroenterol Clin Biol 2000; 24:837–840.
25. Duhra PM, Quigley EM, Marsh MN. Chylous ascites, intestinal lymphangiectasia and the 'yellow-nail' syndrome. Gut 1985; 26:1266–1269.
26. Govaert P, Leroy JG, Pauwels R, Vanhaesebrouck P, Praeter C, Van Kets H, Goeteyn M. Perinatal manifestations of maternal yellow nail syndrome. Pediatrics 1992; 89:1016–1018.
27. Slee J, Nelson J, Dickinson J, Kendall P, Halbert A. Yellow nail syndrome presenting as non-immune hydrops: second case report. Am J Med Genet 2000; 93:1–4.
28. Herbert FA, Bowen PA. Hereditary late-onset lymphedema with pleural effusion and laryngeal edema. Arch Intern Med 1983; 143:913–915.
29. Nakielna EM, Wilson J, Ballon HS. Yellow-nail syndrome: report of three cases. Can Med Assoc J 1976; 115:46–48.
30. Venencie PY, Dicken CH. Yellow nail syndrome: report of five cases. J Am Acad Dermatol 1984; 10:187–192.
31. Emerson PA. Yellow nails, lymphedema, and pleural effusions. Thorax 1966; 21: 247–253.
32. Solal-Celigny P, Cormier Y, Fournier M. The yellow nail syndrome. Light and electron microscopic aspects of the pleura. Arch Pathol Lab Med 1983; 107:183–185.
33. Lewis M, Kallenbach J, Zaltzman M, et al. Pleurectomy in the management of massive pleural effusion associated with primary lymphoedema: demonstration of abnormal pleural lymphatics. Thorax 1983; 38:637–639.
34. Runyon BA, Forker EL, Sopko JA. Pleural-fluid kinetics in a patient with primary lymphedema, pleural effusions, and yellow nails. Am Rev Respir Dis 1979; 119: 821–825.

35. Mambretti-Zumwalt J, Seidman JM, Higano N. Yellow nail syndrome: complete triad with pleural protein turnover studies. South Med J 1980; 73:995–997.
36. Baran R. The new oral antifungal drugs in the treatment of the yellow nail syndrome. Br J Dermatol 2002; 147:189–191.
37. Hiller E, Rosenow EC III, Olsen AM. Pulmonary manifestations of the yellow nail syndrome. Chest 1972; 61:452–458.
38. D'Alessandro A, Muzi G, Monaco A, Filiberto S, Barboni A, Abbritti G. Yellow nail syndrome: does protein leakage play a role? Eur Respir J 2001; 17:149–152.
39. Lodge JP, Hunter AM, Saunders NR. Yellow nail syndrome associated with empyema. Clin Exp Dermatol 1989; 14:328–329.
40. Angelillo VA, O'Donohue WJ Jr. Yellow nail syndrome with reduced glucose level in the pleural fluid. Chest 1979; 75:83–85.
41. Levillain C, Faux N, Taillandier J, Dumont D, Fixy P, Manigand G. Yellow-nail syndrome. Review of the literature apropos of 2 cases associated with cancer. Ann Med Interne 1984; 135:440–443.
42. Guin JD, Elleman JH. Yellow nail syndrome. Possible association with malignancy. Arch Dermatol 1979; 115:734–735.
43. Chernosky ME, Finley VK. Yellow nail syndrome in patients with acquired immunodeficiency disease. J Am Acad Dermatol 1985; 13:731–736.
44. Jiva TM, Poe RH, Kallay MC. Pleural effusion in yellow nail syndrome: chemical pleurodesis and its outcome. Respiration 1994; 61:300–302.
45. Glazer M, Berkman N, Lafair JS, Kramer MR. Successful talc slurry pleurodesis in patients with nonmalignant pleural effusion. Chest 2000; 117:1404–1409.
46. Brofman JD, Hall JB, Scott W, Little AG. Yellow nails, lymphedema and pleural effusion. Treatment of chronic pleural effusion with pleuroperitoneal shunting. Chest 1990; 97:743–745.
47. Bright R. Tabular view of the morbid appearance in 100 cases connected with albuminous urine, with observations. Guys Hosp Rep 1836; 1:380–400.
48. Hopps HC, Wissler RW. Uremic pneumonitis. Am J Pathol 1955; 31:261–273.
49. Nidus BD, Matalon R, Cantacuzino D, Eisinger RP. Uremic pleuritis: a clinicopathological entity. N Engl J Med 1969; 281:255–256.
50. Berger HW, Rammohan G, Neff MS, Buhain WJ. Uremic pleural effusion. A study in 14 patients on chronic dialysis. Ann Intern Med 1975; 82:362–364.
51. Galen MA, Steinberg SM, Lowrie EG, Lazarus JM, Hampers CL, Merrill JP. Hemorrhagic pleural effusion in patients undergoing chronic hemodialysis. Ann Intern Med 1975; 82:359–361.
52. Jarratt MJ, Sahn SA. Pleural effusions in hospitalized patients receiving long-term hemodialysis. Chest 1995; 108:470–474.
53. Maher JF. Uremic pleuritis. Am J Kidney Dis 1987; 10:19–22.
54. Krishnan M, Choi M. A case of uremia-associated pleural effusion in a peritoneal dialysis patient. Semin Dial 2001; 14:223–227.
55. Horita Y, Noguchi M, Miyazaki M, Tadokoro M, Taura K, Watanabe T, Nishiura K, Harada T, Ozono Y, Kohno S. Prognosis of patients with rounded atelectasis undergoing long-term hemodialysis. Nephron 2001; 88:87–92.
56. Yoshii C, Morita S, Tokunaga M, Yatera K, Hayashi T, Imanaga T, Segawa K, Wang KY, Kido M. Bilateral massive pleural effusions caused by uremic pleuritis. Intern Med 2001; 40:646–649.
57. Gilbert L, Ribot S, Frankel H, Jacobs M, Mankowitz BJ. Fibrinous uremic pleuritis: a surgical entity. Chest 1976; 67:53–56.

58. Rodelas R, Rakowski TA, Argy WP, Schreiner GE. Fibrosing uremic pleuritis during hemodialysis. JAMA 1980; 243:2424–2425.
59. Isoda K, Hamamoto Y. Uremic pleuritis—clinicopathological analysis of 26 autopsy cases. Bull Osaka Med School 1984; 30:73–80.
60. Coskun M, Boyvat F, Bozkurt B, Agildere AM, Niron EA. Thoracic CT findings in long-term hemodialysis patients. Acta Radiol 1999; 40:181–186.
61. Chiang CS, Chiang CD, Lin JW, Huang PL, Chu JJ. Neopterin, soluble interleukin-2 receptor and adenosine deaminase levels in pleural effusions. Respiration 1994; 61:150–154.
62. Pien GW, Gant MJ, Washam CL, Sterman DH. Use of an implantable pleural catheter for trapped lung syndrome in patients with malignant pleural effusion. Chest 2001; 119:1641–1646.
63. Lee YC, Vaz MAC, Ely KA, McDonald EC, Thompson PJ, Nesbitt JC, Light RW. Symptomatic persistent post-coronary artery bypass graft pleural effusions requiring operative treatment. Chest 2001; 119:795–800.
64. Light RW, Jenkinson SG, Minh VD, George RB. Observations on pleural fluid pressures as fluid is withdrawn during thoracentesis. Am Rev Respir Dis 1980; 121:799–804.
65. Villena V, Lopez-Encuentra A, Pozo F, De-Pablo A, Martin-Escribano P. Measurement of pleural pressure during therapeutic thoracentesis. Am J Respir Crit Care Med 2000; 162:1534–1538.
66. Moore PJ, Thomas PA. The trapped lung with chronic pleural space, a cause of recurring pleural effusion. Mil Med 1967; 132:998–1002.
67. Boland GW, Gazelle GS, Girard MJ, Mueller PR. Asymptomatic hydropneumothorax after therapeutic thoracentesis for malignant pleural effusions. Am J Roentgenol 1998; 170:943–946.
68. Chang YC, Patz EF, Goodman PC. Pneumothorax after small-bore catheter placement for malignant pleural effusion. Am J Roentgenol 1996; 166:1049–1051.
69. Light RW. Pleural effusion due to miscellaneous diseases. In: Light RW, ed. Pleural Diseases. 4th ed. Philadelphia: Williams & Wilkins, 2000:271–283.
70. Genc O, Petrou M, Ladas G, Goldstraw P. The long-term morbidity of pleuroperitoneal shunts in the management of recurrent malignant effusions. Eur J Cardiothorac Surg 2000; 18:143–146.
71. Rodriguez-Garcia JL, Fraile G, Moreno MA, Sanchez-Corral JA, Penalver R. Recurrent massive pleural effusion as a late complication of radiotherapy in Hodgkin's disease. Chest 1991; 100:1165–1166.
72. Down JD, Tarbell NJ. Pitfalls in the assessment of late lung damage in irradiated mice: complications related to pleural effusion [letter]. Int Radiat Biol 1989; 55:473–478.
73. Bachman AL, Macken K. Pleural effusions following supervoltage radiation for breast carcinoma. Radiology 1959; 72:699–709.
74. Hietala SO, Hahn P. Pulmonary radiation reaction in the treatment of carcinoma of the breast. Radiography 1976; 42:225–230.
75. Fentanes de Torres E, Guevara E. Pleuritis by radiation: reports of two cases. Acta Cytol 1981; 25:427–429.
76. Whitcomb ME, Schwarz M. Pleural effusion complicating intensive mediastinal radiation therapy. Am Rev Respir Dis 1971; 103:100–107.
77. Morrone N, Gama e Silva Volpe VL, Dourado AM, Mitre F, Coletta EN. Bi-

lateral pleural effusion due to mediastinal fibrosis induced by radiotherapy. Chest 1993; 104:1276–1278.
78. Morild I. Pleural effusion in drowning. Am J Forensic Med Pathol 1995; 16:253–256.
79. Kavuru MS, Adamo JP, Ahmad M, Mehta AC, Gephardt GN. Amyloidosis and pleural disease. Chest 1990; 98:20–23.
80. Knapp MJ, Roggli VL, Kim J, Moore JO, Shelburne JD. Pleural amyloidosis. Arch Pathol Lab Med 1988; 112:57–60.
81. Vilaseca J, Cuevas J, Fresno M, Tor J, Guardia J, Bacardi R. Systemic amyloidosis in cystic fibrosis. Am J Dis Child 1981; 135:667.
82. Romero Candeira S. Amyloidosis and pleural disease. Chest 1991; 100:292–293.
83. Maeno T, Sando Y, Tsukagoshi M, Suga T, Endo M, Seki R, Ooyama Y, Yamagishi T, Kaneko Y, Kanda T, Iwasaki T, Kurabayashi M, Nagai R. Pleural amyloidosis in a patient with intractable pleural effusion and multiple myeloma. Respirology 2000; 5:79–80.
84. Astoul P, Cheikh R, Cabanot C, Vialette JP, Vestri R, Boutin C. Pleural amyloidosis: thoracoscopic diagnosis and physiopathological approach. Rev Mal Respir 1992; 9:629–631.
85. Bontemps F, Tillie-Leblond I, Coppin MC, Frehart P, Wallaert B, Ramon P, Tonnel AB. Pleural amyloidosis: thoracoscopic aspects. Eur Respir J 1995; 8:1025–1027.
86. Graham DR, Ahmad D. Amyloidosis with pleural involvement. Eur Respir J 1988; 1:571–572.
87. Case 48-1977. Case records of the Massachusetts General Hospital: weekly clinico-pathological exercises. N Engl J Med 1977; 297:1221–1228.
88. Im JG, Chung JW, Han MC. Milk of calcium pleural collections: CT findings. J Comput Assist Tomogr 1993; 17:613–616.
89. Goldenberg DC, Bringel RW, Fontana C, Teixeira TL, DeAlmeida PC, DeFaria JC, Ferreira MC. Pulmonary lesion in electric injury: report of a case. Rev Hosp Clin Fac Med Sao Paulo 1996; 51:15–17.
90. Baxter CR. Present concepts in the management of major electrical injury. Surg Clin North Am 1970; 50:1401–1418.
91. Hiraiwa T, Hayashi T, Kaneda M, Sakai T, Namikawa S, Kusagawa M, Kusano I. Rupture of a benign mediastinal teratoma into the right pleural cavity. Ann Thorac Surg 1991; 51:110–112.
92. Choi SJ, Lee JS, Song KS, Lim TH. Mediastinal teratoma: CT differentiation of ruptured and unruptured tumors. Am J Roentgenol 1998; 171:591–594.
93. Matsubara K, Aoki M, Okumura N, Menju T, Nigami H, Harigaya H, Baba K. Spontaneous rupture of mediastinal cystic teratoma into the pleural cavity: report of two cases and review of the literature. Pediatr Hematol Oncol 2001; 18:221–227.
94. Cobb CJ, Wynn J, Cobb SR, Duane GB. Cytologic findings in an effusion caused by rupture of a benign cystic teratoma of the mediastinum into a serous cavity. Acta Cytol 1985; 29:1015–1020.
95. Krishnan S, Statsinger AL, Kleinman M, Bertoni MA, Sharma P. Eosinophilic pleural effusion with Charcot-Leyden crystals. Acta Cytol 1983; 27:529–532.
96. Robinson LA, Rikkers LF, Dobson JR. Benign mediastinal teratoma masquerading as a large multiloculated pleural effusion. Ann Thorac Surg 1994; 58:545–548.

97. Ashour M, El-Din Hawass N, Adam KA, Joharjy I. Spontaneous intrapleural rupture of mediastinal teratoma. Respir Med 1993; 87:69–72.
98. Khalil A, Carette MF, Milleron B, Grivaux M, Bigot JM. Bronchogenic cyst presenting as mediastinal mass with pleural effusion. Eur Respir J 1995; 8:2185–2187.
99. Riemer H, Hainz R, Stain C, Dekan G, Feldner-Busztin M, Schenk P, Muller C, Sertl K, Burghuber OC. Severe pulmonary hypertension reversed by antibiotics in a patient with Whipple's disease. Thorax 1997; 52:1014–1015.
100. Whipple GH. A hitherto undescribed disease characterized anatomically by deposits of fat and fatty acids in the intestinal mesenteric lymphatic tissues. Bull Johns Hopkins Hosp 1907; 18:382–391.
101. Symmons DPM, Sheperd AN, Boardman PL, Bacon PA. Pulmonary manifestations of Whipple's disease. Q J Med 1985; 220:497–504.
102. Pollock JJ. Pleuropulmonary Whipple's disease. South Med J 1985; 78:216–217.
103. Muller C, Stain C, Burghuber O. Tropheryma whippelii in peripheral blood mononuclear cells and cells of pleural effusion. Lancet 1993; 341:701.
104. Zaharopoulos P, Wong J. Cytologic diagnosis of syphilitic pleuritis: a case report. Diagn Cytopathol 1997; 16:35–38.
105. Cattini GC, Greco N, Tosto L, Falcieri E, Biagini G. Syphilitic pleuritis. Description of a clinical case. Minerva Med 1983; 74:337–342.

46

Management of the Undiagnosed Persistent Pleural Effusion

RICHARD W. LIGHT

Vanderbilt University
and Saint Thomas Hospital
Nashville, Tennessee, U.S.A.

I. Introduction

On occasion a patient will have a persistent pleural effusion that remains undiagnosed. In this chapter I will assume that the pleural effusion persists after the initial diagnostic workup, which includes measurement of a pleural fluid marker for tuberculosis such as adenosine deaminase (ADA) or gamma interferon.

II. Diseases That Cause Undiagnosed Persistent Pleural Effusions

When a patient with a persistent undiagnosed pleural effusion is encountered, the first thing to be considered is the list of the diseases most likely to be associated with this condition (Table 1). The first question to answer in a patient with a persistent undiagnosed pleural effusion is whether the effusion is a transudate or an exudate. For the past several decades this differentiation has been made by measuring the levels of protein and lactate dehydrogenase (LDH) in the pleural

Table 1 Diseases Most Likely to Produce Persistent Undiagnosed Pleural Effusion

Transudative pleural effusions
  Congestive heart failure
  Cirrhosis
  Nephrotic syndrome
  Urinothorax
  Myxedema
  Cerebrospinal fluid leaks to the pleura
Exudative pleural effusions
  Malignancy
  Pneumonia (especially anaerobic)
  Tuberculosis
  Fungal infection
  Pancreatic pseudocyst
  Intra–abdominal abscess
  Post–coronary artery bypass graft surgery
  Postcardiac injury syndrome
  Pericardial disease
  Meigs' syndrome
  Rheumatoid pleuritis
  Lupus erythematosus
  Drug-induced pleural disease
  Asbestos pleural effusion
  Yellow nail syndrome
  Uremia
  Trapped lung
  Chylothorax
  Pseudochylothorax

fluid and in the serum (Light's criteria). If one or more of the following criteria are met, the patient has an exudative pleural effusion (1):

1. Pleural fluid protein/serum protein >0.5
2. Pleural fluid LDH/serum LDH >0.6
3. Pleural fluid LDH >two-thirds the normal upper limit for serum

Light's criteria are very sensitive at identifying exudates, but they also identify about 15% of transudative pleural effusions as being exudative pleural effusions (2,3). Usually, the transudates that are misclassified only minimally meet the exudative criteria, e.g., the protein ratio is 0.52 or the LDH ratio is 0.63. If the pleural fluid LDH is more than the upper limit for the serum LDH or if the protein level is more than 4.0 g/dL, the patient does not have a transudate. These transudates, which are misclassified as exudates, can be classified correctly if the difference between the albumin levels in the serum and the pleural fluid is measured. If this gradient is greater than 1.2 g/dL, the exudative classification by

Light's criteria can be ignored because almost all such patients have a transudative pleural effusion (3). The albumin gradient alone should not be used to separate transudates from exudates because, by itself, it will misidentify approximately 13% of exudates as transudates (3).

A. Transudative Pleural Effusions

Congestive Heart Failure

Congestive heart failure is the most common cause of pleural effusion (4). At times in patients with persistent pleural effusion, it is not obvious that the heart failure is the cause of the effusion. Certainly symptoms of congestive heart failure such as dyspnea on exertion, orthopnea, paroxysmal nocturnal dyspnea, and nocturia should be sought when the history is taken. In addition, signs of congestive heart failure such as basilar rales, S3 gallop, distended neck veins, and pedal edema should be sought during the physical examination. If the patient clinically has congestive heart failure but the initial pleural fluid analysis reveals an exudate that just barely meets Light's criteria, the difference between the pleural fluid and serum albumin should be measured as detailed above. If this gradient is above 1.2 g/dL, the effusion can be attributed to the congestive heart failure. If the patient has a transudative effusion but does not have obvious heart failure, further investigations of cardiac function such as echocardiography are indicated.

Cirrhosis with Hepatic Hydrothorax

If the patient has overt cirrhosis and massive ascites, the diagnosis of hepatic hydrothorax is easy. However, if the patient does not have ascites, the diagnosis of hepatic hydrothorax may be difficult to establish. In 1998, Kakizaki and associates reviewed the literature and were able to find 28 cases of hepatic hydrothorax without ascites (5). Of these 28 cases, 27 were on the right side. The only left-sided effusion occurred in a patient who had a tear in the left diaphragm as a result of a splenectomy. The mean serum albumin in these 28 cases was 2.7 g/dL with a range of 1.9–3.6 g/dL (5). The explanation for the pleural effusion in the absence of overt ascites is that the patients have defects in their diaphragm. When fluid is present in the peritoneal space, it flows immediately into the pleural space because the pleural pressure is negative compared to the peritoneal pressure. This diagnosis can be established by demonstrating radioactivity in the thorax after the intraperitoneal injection of technetium 99m (^{99m}Tc)-sulfur colloid (6).

Nephrotic Syndrome

Another cause of a chronic transudative pleural effusion is the nephrotic syndrome. More than 20% of patients with the nephrotic syndrome have pleural effusions, which are usually bilateral (7). Therefore, all patients with chronic transudative pleural effusions should be evaluated for proteinouria and hypoproteinemia. It should be remembered that the incidence of pulmonary emboli is high with the nephrotic syndrome (8), and this possibility should be considered in all patients with the nephrotic syndrome and a pleural effusion.

Urinothorax

A transudative pleural effusion can result when there is retroperitoneal urinary leakage secondary to urinary tract obstruction or trauma with subsequent dissection of the urine into the pleural space (9,10). This diagnosis is easy if it is considered as the pleural fluid looks and smells like urine. Confirmation of the diagnosis can be made by demonstrating that the pleural fluid creatinine is greater than the serum creatinine (11). The pleural fluid with urinothorax may also have a low glucose and a low pH. The only other instances in which a transudative pleural effusion has a low glucose or low pH is when there is systemic hypoglycemia or acidosis, respectively.

Cerebrospinal Fluid Leak to the Pleura

On rare occasions cerebrospinal fluid (CSF) can collect in the pleural space and produce a pleural effusion. This most commonly occurs following ventriculopleural shunting (12), but can also occur after penetrating injuries and fractures of the thoracic spine and following thoracic spinal surgery (13,14). The diagnosis should be suggested by the appearance of the pleural fluid, which appears to be CSF. The protein levels are usually very low. The diagnosis can be confirmed by radionuclide cisternography (14).

B. Exudative Pleural Effusions

Malignant Pleural Effusion

There is no doubt that malignancy causes more persistent undiagnosed exudative pleural effusions than any other cause. However, it should be emphasized that there is no huge hurry to establish this diagnosis since (1) the presence of the effusion indicates that the patient has metastases to the pleura and the malignancy cannot be cured surgically, (2) most malignant pleural effusions are due to tumors that cannot be cured with chemotherapy, and (3) there is no evidence that attempts to create a pleurodesis early improve the quality of the patient's life.

Most patients who have a pleural malignancy usually have other characteristics suggesting malignancy. For example, in the series of 211 patients reported by Poe and coworkers (15), the needle biopsy of the pleura was negative in 29 patients who were eventually proven to have malignant pleural effusions. However, all of these patients were strongly suspected of having a malignant effusion by clinical criteria such as weight loss, constitutional symptoms, or a history of a previous cancer (15).

When patients with pleural effusions due to the most common types of tumors are analyzed, some interesting observations can be made. The tumor that causes the highest number of pleural effusions is lung cancer (4). When patients with lung cancer are first evaluated, about 15% have a pleural effusion (16), but 50% of patients with disseminated lung cancer develop a pleural effusion (4). The tumor that causes the second highest number of pleural effusions is breast cancer (4). Patients with breast carcinoma rarely present with pleural effusion. The mean interval between the diagnosis of the primary tumor and the appearance of a pleural effusion is 2 years (17). Hematological malignancies (lymphomas and leukemias) cause the third highest number of malignant pleural effusions (4). Approximately 10% of patients with Hodgkin's lymphoma and 25% of patients with non-Hodgkin's lymphoma have pleural effusions at presentation. Those that do almost invariably have intrathoracic lymph node involvement (18). If the patient has AIDS and cutaneous Kaposi' sarcoma, the likely diagnosis is a pleural effusion due to Kaposi's sarcoma. This diagnosis is usually established at bronchoscopy, which demonstrates erythematous or violaceus macules or papules in the respiratory tree (19).

There are several primary tumors of the pleura that should be considered if the patient has an undiagnosed pleural effusion. If the patient has a history of asbestos exposure, mesothelioma should be considered. Thoracoscopy or thoracotomy is usually necessary to make this diagnosis (4). If the patient has AIDS and has a lymphocytic pleural effusion with a very high LDH level, the diagnosis of primary effusion lymphoma is likely (20). This diagnosis can usually be established with pleural fluid cytology and flow cytometry (4). If the patient received an artificial pneumothorax many years previously, a likely diagnosis is pyothorax-associated lymphoma (21).

Parapneumonic Effusion

The diagnosis of parapneumonic effusion is easy in the patient with an acute febrile illness, purulent sputum, and pulmonary infiltrates. On occasion, however, particularly with anaerobic infections, the patient may present with a chronic illness. In one study of 47 patients with anaerobic parapneumonic effusions, the median duration of symptoms before presentation was 10 days and 60% of the patients had substantial weight loss (mean 29 pounds) (22). Therefore, if the patient has a chronic illness with predominantly neutrophils in their pleural fluid, it is imperative to obtain anaerobic cultures of the pleural fluid. Since patients with actinomycosis and nocardiosis at times have a chronic pleural effusion with predominantly neutrophils, cultures for these organisms should be obtained in patients with chronic neutrophilic pleural effusions.

Tuberculous Pleural Effusion

Throughout the world, tuberculosis remains one of the principal causes of pleural effusion. It is important to make this diagnosis, since if the patient has pleural tuberculosis and is not treated, the effusion will resolve but the patient will have a greater than 50% chance of developing active pulmonary or extrapulmonary tuberculosis over the following 5 years (23). Therefore, all patients with a chronic undiagnosed pleural effusion should be evaluated for tuberculosis. The easiest way to do this is to measure the pleural fluid level of adenosine deaminase or gamma interferon. If the level of adenosine deaminase is below 40 IU/L or the level of gamma interferon is below 140 pg/mL, the diagnosis can be excluded. In one study Ferrer et al. followed 40 patients with a chronic undiagnosed pleural effusion and a pleural fluid ADA level below 43 IU/L for a mean of 5 years, and none developed tuberculosis (24).

Fungal Pleural Effusions

Fungal disease is responsible for a very small percentage of pleural effusions (4). However, at times blastomycosis and coccidioidomycosis may cause a chronic lymphocytic pleural effusion (4). Accordingly, cultures for fungi should be obtained in the patient with a chronic undiagnosed pleural effusion with predominantly lymphocytes in the pleural fluid. It is unknown whether the lymphocytic effusions due to fungal diseases have a high ADA.

Chronic Pancreatic Pleural Effusion

This is one diagnosis that should always be considered in a patient with a chronic undiagnosed pleural effusion. Some patients with a pancreatic pseudocyst will develop a direct sinus tract between the pancreas and the pleural space (25). The sinus tract will decompress the pancreas, and therefore the patient presents with symptoms usually referable only to the chest. The patient with a chronic pancreatic pleural effusion is usually chronically ill and looks like he or she has cancer. The diagnosis is virtually established if the level of amylase in the pleural fluid is greater than 1000 u/L (25). It is important to consider this diagnosis because the patient can be cured with appropriate surgery.

Intra-abdominal Abscess

Subphrenic, intrahepatic, intrasplenic, and intrapancreatic abscesses are all associated with pleural effusion in a large percentage of patients (4). Patients with intra-abdominal abscess are usually chronically ill with fever and weight loss. The pleural fluid is sterile and contains predominantly neutrophils. The diagnosis can be made with CT scan or ultrasound of the abdomen.

Effusion Post–Coronary Artery Bypass Graft (CABG) Surgery

Approximately 25% of patients who undergo CABG surgery have a pleural effusion that occupies more than 25% of their hemithorax 28 days postoperatively (26). The primary symptom (if any) of a patient with a post-CABG pleural effusion is dyspnea; chest pain and fever are distinctly unusual (26). The pleural fluid in these patients is an exudate characterized by a lymphocyte predominance and an LDH approximately equal to the upper limit of normal for serum (27). Although the pleural fluid is similar to the pleural fluid in patients with tuberculous pleuritis, these two entities may be differentiated by the pleural fluid level of ADA—the ADA level is below 40 U/L in patients with the post-

CABG effusion (28). On rare occasions these effusions can persist for years (29), and one must not be too aggressive in pursuing a diagnosis if the pleural fluid findings are as expected.

Postcardiac Injury Syndrome (PCIS)

PCIS, also known as Dressler's syndrome, is characterized by the development of fever, pleuropericarditis, and parenchymal pulmonary infiltrates in the weeks following trauma to the pericardium or myocardium (30). PCIS has been reported following myocardial infarction, cardiac surgery, blunt chest trauma, percutaneous left ventricular puncture, pacemaker implantation, and angioplasty. PCIS differs from pleural effusion post-CABG surgery because fever and chest pain invariably occur with the PCIS and are rare post-CABG. Following cardiac injury, symptoms usually develop between the first and third week, but can develop any time between 3 days and 1 year (30). The pleural fluid is frankly bloody in about 30% of patients, and the differential cell count may reveal predominantly neutrophils or mononuclear cells depending upon the acuteness of the process (31).

Pericardial Disease

Approximately 25% of patients who have a pericardial effusion will have a concomitant pleural effusion (32). In patients with inflammatory pericarditis, the majority of the associated pleural effusions are unilateral and left-sided (32). The characteristics of the pleural fluid seen in conjunction with pericardial disease are not well described (4). The possibility of pericardial effusion should be evaluated in any patient with cardiomegaly and an isolated left pleural effusion.

Approximately 60% of patients with constrictive pericarditis will have a concomitant pleural effusion (33). The associated pleural effusion is bilateral and symmetrical in the majority. In one report of four patients with constrictive pericarditis, the pleural fluid was transudative in one and exudative in three (33). We recently reported one patient with constrictive pericarditis who had a pleural fluid protein of 4.0 g/dL (34). When a patient is seen with edema and an exudative pleural effusion, the diagnosis of constrictive pericarditis should be considered. It is important to realize that echocardiography may be normal in the patient with constrictive pericarditis and that cardiac catheterization may be necessary to establish the diagnosis (34).

Meigs' Syndrome

Meigs' syndrome is the constellation of a benign pelvic neoplasm associated with ascites and pleural effusion in which surgical extirpation of the tumor results in permanent disappearance of the ascites and pleural effusion (4). The pleural fluid is an exudate with a relatively low cell count, which at times may have an elevated CA125 (35). The importance of Meigs' syndrome is that not all patients with a pelvic mass, ascites, and a pleural effusion have metastatic disease.

Rheumatoid Pleuritis

Chronic pleural effusion may be a manifestation of rheumatoid pleuritis, and the diagnosis is usually straightforward. Classically, the effusion occurs in older males who have subcutaneous nodules. The pleural fluid is an exudate with a low glucose, a low pH, and a high LDH. The first manifestation of rheumatoid disease is virtually never a pleural effusion (4).

Systemic Lupus Erythematosus

In contrast to rheumatoid pleuritis, patients with systemic lupus erythematosus (SLE) may present with a pleural effusion. The possibility of drug-induced lupus should always be considered in the patient with an undiagnosed pleural effusion. Drugs that are most commonly implicated in drug-induced lupus are hydralazine, procainamide, isoniazid, phenytoin, and chlorpromazine (4). The diagnosis of systemic lupus erythematosus with pleural involvement is based on the usual criteria for the diagnosis of lupus. Measurement of the pleural fluid ANA levels (36) or performance of LE preparations on the pleural fluid (4) does not assist in the diagnosis.

Drug-Induced Pleural Disease

When a patient is evaluated with a chronic undiagnosed pleural effusion, the list of drugs that the patient is taking should be carefully reviewed as the ingestion of certain drugs can lead to the development of a pleural effusion. The primary drugs associated with the development of a pleural effusion are nitrofurantoin (a urinary antiseptic), dantrolene (a muscle relaxant), and the ergot alkaloids such as bromocriptine, which are used to treat Parkinson's disease (4). Other drugs that have been reported to induce pleural effusions include methysergide, amiodarone, procarbazine, methotrexate, clozapine, dapsone, metronidazole, mitomycin, isotretinoin, propylthiouracil, simvastatin, warfarin, and gliclazide (4).

Asbestos Pleural Effusion

Exposure to asbestos can lead to the development of an exudative pleural effusion. In one series of 1135 asymptomatic asbestos workers, the prevalence of pleural effusion was 3% (37). In this series all patients developed effusions within 20 years of the initial exposure and many had done so within 5 years of the initial exposure (37). The prevalence of pleural effusion was directly related to the total asbestos exposure. Patients with asbestos pleural effusions are usually asymptomatic (37,38). The effusion tends to last several months and then clears, leaving no residual disease. The pleural fluid is an exudate and can contain predominantly neutrophils or mononuclear cells (38). If a patient with a pleural effusion has a history of asbestos exposure and is asymptomatic, the patient can probably be observed to determine if the effusion disappears spontaneously.

Yellow Nail Syndrome

The yellow nail syndrome consists of the triad of deformed yellow nails, lymphedema, and pleural effusions (4). The three separate entities may become manifest at widely varying times. The pleural effusions are bilateral in about 50% of patients and vary in size from small to massive (4). Once a pleural effusion has occurred with this syndrome, it tends to persist and recur rapidly after a thoracentesis. The pleural fluid is usually a clear yellow exudate with a normal glucose level and predominantly lymphocytes in the pleural fluid differential. The pleural fluid LDH tends to be low relative to the pleural fluid protein level.

Uremia

The prevalence of pleural effusions with uremia is approximately 3% (39). As many as 50% of patients on long-term hemodialysis have a pleural effusion (40). There is not a close relationship between the degree of uremia and the occurrence of a pleural effusion (39). More than 50% of the patients are symptomatic, with fever (50%), chest pain (30%), cough (35%), and dyspnea (20%) being the most common symptoms (39). The pleural fluid is an exudate, and the differential usually reveals predominantly lymphocytes (39). Tests of renal function should be obtained in every patient with an undiagnosed exudative effusion.

Trapped Lung

When there is intense inflammation in the pleural space, a fibrous peel may form over the visceral pleura. This peel can prevent the underlying lung from expanding, and therefore the lung is said to be trapped (41). The initial event producing the pleural inflammation is usually a pleural infection or a hemothorax, but it can be a spontaneous pneumothorax, thoracic operations (particularly CABG surgery) (29), uremia, or collagen vascular disease. The pleural fluid is usually clear yellow and is a borderline exudate with predominantly mononuclear cells. The diagnosis can be made by measuring the pleural pressure while fluid is withdrawn during a thoracentesis. If the initial pleural pressure is below -10 cmH$_2$O or if the pleural pressure falls more than 20 cmH$_2$O per 1000 mL fluid removed, the diagnosis is confirmed provided that the patient does not have bronchial obstruction (41).

Chylothorax and Pseudochylothorax

When pleural fluid is found to be milky or very turbid, the possibility of a chylothorax or a pseudochylothorax should be considered. When turbid fluid is found, the first step is to centrifuge the fluid. If the supernatant remains turbid, then the turbidity is due to a high lipid content in the pleural fluid and the patient has a chylothorax or a pseudochylothorax.

Chylothorax is usually easy to differentiate from pseudochylothorax on clinical grounds. Patients with a chylothorax have an acute illness and their pleural surfaces are normal on CT scan. In contrast, patients with a pseudochylothorax usually have had a pleural effusion for more than 5 years and their pleural surfaces are markedly thickened on CT scan. Measurement of the lipid levels in the pleural fluid is also useful in distinguishing these two conditions. Pleural fluid from a chylothorax has a triglyceride level above 110 mg/dL and the ratio of the pleural fluid to serum cholesterol is less than 1.0. In contrast, fluid from a pseudochylothorax has cholesterol crystals and/or a cholesterol above 200 mg/dL and higher than the simultaneous serum level (4).

III. Tests to Consider for Patients with Persistent Undiagnosed Pleural Effusion

A. History

Certain points in the patient's history should receive special attention if the patient has a persistent undiagnosed pleural effusion. If a patient has a transudative pleural effusion, particular attention should be paid to symptoms of congestive heart failure such as dyspnea on exertion, orthopnea, paroxysmal nocturnal dyspnea, and nocturia. In addition, historical evidence of cirrhosis, alcoholism, or chronic hepatitis should be sought with the possibility of a hepatic hydrothorax in mind. A history of trauma or surgery to the thoracic spine should be sought with the diagnosis of a cerebrospinal fluid leak in mind.

If the patient has a exudative pleural effusion, a history of malignancy should be sought. Malignant pleural effusions have been known to develop as long as 20 years after the primary tumor was diagnosed (42). A history of exposure to asbestos should be sought, as this would suggest mesothelioma or an asbestos pleural effusion. A history of fever suggests a chronic anaerobic, tuberculous, or fungal infection or an intra-abdominal abscess. A history of alcoholism or previous pancreatic disease raises the possibility of a chronic pancreatic pleural effusion. A history of CABG surgery or myocardial trauma suggests a post-CABG pleural effusion or postcardiac injury syndrome, respectively. A history of rheumatoid disease raises the possibility of rheumatoid pleuritis. The patient should be questioned carefully regarding the medications they are taking to determine whether they a taking a medication that causes a pleural effusion or is associated with drug-induced lupus erythematosus. The patient should be questioned carefully about previous pleural problems, which raise the likelihood of a pseudochylothorax or a trapped lung.

B. Physical Examination

In the patient with the chronic undiagnosed pleural effusion, it is worthwhile to repeat a careful physical examination. If the patient has a transudative pleural effusion, signs of congestive heart failure such as basilar rales, an S3 gallop, or distended neck veins should be sought. In addition, evidence of ascites should be carefully sought. The presence of pedal edema suggests congestive heart failure, cirrhosis with hepatic hydrothorax, nephrotic syndrome, pericardial disease, or the yellow nail syndrome.

If the patient has an exudative effusion, a careful search for lymphadenopathy or other masses, which would suggest malignancy, is indicated. In women a careful breast examination and a careful pelvic examination should be done to evaluate these locations for masses. Abdominal tenderness suggests an intra-abdominal abscess. Distant heart sounds, a pericardial friction rub, and/or Kussmaul's sign (increased jugular venous pressure that increases during inspiration) suggest pericardial disease. Ascites and a pelvic mass raise the possibility of Meigs' syndrome. Deformed joints and subcutaneous nodules make rheumatoid pleuritis likely. The presence of yellow nails establishes the diagnosis of the yellow nail syndrome.

C. Laboratory Examinations

Several blood tests should be routinely obtained in patients with a persistent undiagnosed pleural effusion. The level of albumin and globulin should be measured to determine whether the patient has cirrhosis or the nephrotic syndrome, and liver function tests should be obtained to ascertain if there is chronic hepatitis. Additionally, I also obtain a CBC with differential. A serum anti-nuclear antibody test should be obtained with the diagnosis of systemic lupus erythematosus in mind. A BUN and creatinine should be obtained to evaluate the possibility of uremia.

Several special tests on the pleural fluid are also indicated. The cheapest test is to smell the pleural fluid. If the pleural fluid smells like urine, the patient probably has a urinothorax, while if the pleural fluid smells feculent, the patient probably has an anaerobic pleural infection. As mentioned previously, either the ADA or the gamma interferon should be measured in the pleural fluid to assess whether the patient has pleural tuberculosis. Flow cytometry on the pleural fluid is indicated if lymphoma is suspected (43). If the pleural fluid is milky or cloudy, it should be centrifuged, and if the supernatant remains milky or cloudy, the pleural fluid should be sent for measurement of cholesterol and triglycerides. Every time a thoracentesis is performed in a patient with a persistent undiagnosed pleural effusion, a pleural fluid LDH level should be determined. If this LDH tends to decrease with time, the pleural process is resolving and one can be conservative in one's approach to the patient. Alternatively, if the LDH is increasing with time, the process is getting worse and one should be aggressive in pursuing a diagnosis (4).

D. Imaging Procedures

Most patients with an undiagnosed persistent pleural effusion should have a spiral CT scan of the chest. With the spiral CT, the diagnosis of pulmonary emboli can be established (44). In addition, parenchymal infiltrates and masses and mediastinal lymphadenopathy can be identified. Moreover, the thickening of the pleura can be demonstrated. Lastly, pericardial thickening and pericardial effusions can be identified on the CT scan. While the patient is receiving the CT scan, it is reasonable to obtain abdominal cuts also. These can demonstrate abdominal masses, lymphadenopathy, and ascites. An echocardiogram is indicated if congestive heart failure is suspected but is not definitely established and if a pericardial effusion is suspected. It is important to remember that the echocardiogram may not reveal any abnormality if the patient has constrictive pericarditis (34). If constrictive pericarditis is suspected, the patient should undergo right heart catheterization.

E. Needle Biopsy of the Pleura

For the past 50 years, most cases of tuberculous pleuritis have been diagnosed with needle biopsy of the pleura. However, in the past 10 years it has been demonstrated that markers for tuberculosis obtained from the pleural fluid such as the ADA or the gamma interferon are very efficient at establishing this diagnosis. The other diagnosis that can be established with needle biopsy of the pleura is pleural malignancy. However, in most series cytology is much more sensitive in establishing the diagnosis. Moreover, if the cytology of the fluid is negative, the pleural biopsy is usually nondiagnostic. In one series of 118 patients from the Mayo Clinic who had malignancy involving the pleural but negative pleural fluid cytology, the needle biopsy of the pleura was positive in only 20 (17%) patients (45). Since thoracoscopy is diagnostic in more than 90% of patients with pleural malignancy and negative cytology, it is the preferred diagnostic procedure in patients with a cytology-negative pleural effusion who are suspected of having pleural malignancy. Needle biopsy of the pleura is indicated if the patient has an undiagnosed pleural effusion that is not improving and thoracoscopy is not available. Needle biopsy of the pleura is also indicated if pleural tuberculosis is suspected and a pleural fluid marker for tuberculosis is unavailable or equivocal (4).

F. Thoracoscopy

When one is dealing with patients with pleural effusions, thoracoscopic procedures should be used only when less invasive diagnostic methods such as thoracentesis with cytology and markers for tuberculosis have not yielded a diagnosis. In the series of 620 patients reported by Kendall and coworkers (46), only 48 (8%) required thoracoscopy for a diagnosis. The final diagnoses in these 48 patients were malignancy 24, parapneumonic effusion 7, rheumatoid pleural effusion 4, congestive heart failure 3, and pulmonary interstitial fibrosis 2. In 8 patients no diagnosis was established with the combination of the clinical presentation and thoracoscopy; 6 of the patients were subsequently diagnosed as having malignancy (mesothelioma 3, adenocarcinoma 3) (46).

In general, if the patient has malignancy, thoracoscopy will establish the diagnosis in about 90% (47–49). The diagnosis of tuberculous pleuritis can also be established with thoracoscopy (50,51). It should be emphasized, however, that thoracoscopy rarely establishes the diagnosis of benign disease other than tuberculosis (52). One advantage of thoracoscopy in the diagnosis of pleural disease is that pleurodesis can be performed at the time of the procedure. In general, thoracoscopy is indicated in the patient with an undiagnosed pleural effusion who is not improving spontaneously, provided that the patient has a significant likelihood of malignancy or tuberculosis.

G. Bronchoscopy

Bronchoscopy can be diagnostically useful in patients with pleural effusion if the patient has one of the following four characteristics (53), otherwise bronchoscopy is not indicated.

1. A pulmonary infiltrate is present on the chest radiograph or the chest CT. If an infiltrate is present, particular attention should be paid to the area with the infiltrate at the time of bronchoscopy.
2. Hemoptysis is present. The presence of hemoptysis in the patient with a pleural effusion increases the likelihood of malignancy with an endobronchial lesion or pulmonary embolus. The former can be diagnosed with bronchoscopy.
3. The pleural effusion is massive. The most common cause of a massive pleural effusion is malignancy, particularly lung cancer, and this diagnosis can be established at bronchoscopy. The other two leading causes of massive pleural effusion are hepatic hydrothorax and tuberculous pleuritis; these diagnoses cannot be established with bronchoscopy.
4. The mediastinum is shifted toward the side of the effusion. With this finding, an obstructing endobronchial lesion is probably responsible, and this can be identified and biopsied at bronchoscopy.

H. Open Biopsy

In many institutions open thoracotomy with direct biopsy of the pleura has been replaced by video-assisted thoracoscopy. If both procedures are available, thoracoscopy is usually preferred because it is associated with less morbidity. The primary indication for open pleural biopsy is progressive undiagnosed pleural disease in an institution where thoracoscopy is not available.

One should realize that even with an open biopsy of the pleura, a diagnosis is not always obtained. In one study the experience at the Mayo Clinic between 1962 and 1972 with open pleural biopsy for undiagnosed pleural effusion was reviewed. They found that no diagnosis was established at open biopsy in 51 patients (54). Thirty-one of the patients had no recurrence of their pleural effusion. However, 13 of these 51 patients were eventually found to have malignant disease (lymphoma 6, mesothelioma 4, other malignancy 3). In another study of 21 patients subjected to open pleural biopsy for undiagnosed pleural effusion, no diagnosis was obtained in 7 (33%) (55).

References

1. Light RW, MacGregor MI, Luchsinger PC, Ball WC Jr. Pleural effusions: the diagnostic separation of transudates and exudates. Ann Intern Med 1972; 77:507–514.
2. Romero S, Candela A, Martin C, Hernandez L, Trigo C, Gil J. Evaluation of different criteria for the separation of pleural transudates from exudates. Chest 1993; 104:399–404.
3. Burgess LJ, Maritz FJ, Taljaard JJ. Comparative analysis of the biochemical parameters used to distinguish between pleural transudates and exudates. Chest 1995; 107:1604–1609.
4. Light RW. Pleural Diseases. 4th ed. Baltimore: Lippincott, Williams and Wilkins, 2001.
5. Kakizaki S, Katakai K, Yoshinaga T, Higuchi T, Takayama H, Takagi H, Nagamine T, Mori M. Hepatic hydrothorax in the absence of ascites. Liver 1998; 18:216–220.
6. Daly JJ, Potts JM, Gordon L, Buse MG. Scintigraphic diagnosis of peritoneopleural communication in the absence of ascites. Clin Nuclear Med 1994; 19:892–894.
7. Cavina C, Vichi G. Radiological aspects of pleural effusions in medical nephropathy in children. Ann Radiol Diagn 1958; 31:163–202.
8. Llach F, Arieff Al, Massry SG. Renal vein thrombosis and nephrotic syndrome: a prospective study of 36 adult patients. Ann Intern Med 1975; 83:8–14.
9. Belie JA, Milan D. Pleural effusion secondary to ureteral obstruction. Urology 1979; 14:27–29.
10. Sulcate JR. Urinothorax. report of 4 cases and review of the literature. J Urol 1986; 135:805–808.
11. Stark D, Shades J, Baron RL, Koch D. Biochemical features of urinothorax. Arch Intern Med 1982; 142:1509–1511.
12. Beach C, Manthey DE. Tension hydrothorax due to ventriculopleural shunting. J Emerg Med 1998; 16:33–36.
13. Monla-Hassan J, Eichenhorn M, Spickler E, Talati S, Nockels R, Hyzy R. Duropleural fistula manifested as a large pleural transudate: an unusual complication of transthoracic diskectomy. Chest 1998; 114:1786–1789.
14. Gupta SM, Frias J, Garg A, Herrera NE. Aberrant cerebrospinal fluid pathway. Detection by scintigraphy. Clin Nucl Med 1986; 11:593–594.
15. Poe RH, Israel RH, Utell MJ, et al. Sensitivity, specificity, and predictive values of closed pleural biopsy. Arch Intern Med 1984; 144:325–328.
16. Naito T, Satoh H, Ishikawa H, Yamashita YT, Kamma H, Takahashi H, Ohtsuka M, Hasegawa S. Pleural effusion as a significant prognostic factor in non-small cell lung cancer. Anticancer Res 1997; 17:4743–4746.
17. Apffelstaedt JP, Van Zyl JA, Muller AG. Breast cancer complicated by pleural effusion: patient characteristics and results of surgical management. J Surg Oncol 1995; 58:173–175.

18. Romano M, Libshitz HI. Hodgkin disease and non-Hodgkin lymphoma: plain chest radiographs and chest computed tomography of thoracic involvement in previously untreated patients. Radiol Med (Torino) 1998; 95:49–53.
19. Huang L, Schnapp LM, Gruden JF, Hopewell PC, Stansell JD. Presentation of AIDS-related pulmonary Kaposi's sarcoma diagnosed by bronchoscopy. Am J Respir Crit Care Med 1996; 153:1385–1390.
20. Ascoli V, Scalzo CC, Danese C, Vacca K, Pistilli A, Lo Coco F. Human herpes virus-8 associated primary effusion lymphoma of the pleural cavity in HIV-negative elderly men. Eur Respir J 1999; 14:1231–1234.
21. Taniere P, Manai A, Charpentier R, Terdjman P, Boucheron S, Cordier JF, Berger F. Pyothorax-associated lymphoma: relationship with Epstein-Barr virus, human herpes virus-8 and body cavity-based high grade lymphomas. Eur Respir J 1998; 11:779–783.
22. Bartlett JG, Finegold SM. Anaerobic infections of the lung and pleural space. Am Rev Respir Dis 1974; 110:56–77.
23. Roper WH, Waring JJ. Primary serofibrinous pleural effusion in military personnel. Am Rev Respir Dis 1955; 71:616–634.
24. Ferrer JS, Munoz XG, Orriols RM, Light RW, Morell RB. Evolution of idiopathic pleural effusion. A prospective, long-term follow-up study. Chest 1996; 109:1508–1513.
25. Rockey DC, Cello JP. Pancreaticopleural fistula. Report of 7 patients and review of the literature. Medicine 1990; 69:332–344.
26. Light RW, Rogers JT, Moyers JP, Lee YCG, Rodriguez RM Prevalence and clinical course of pleural effusions at 30 days post coronary artery bypass surgery. Am J Med. In press.
27. Sadikot RT, Rogers JT, Cheng D-S, Moyers P, Rodriguez RM, Light RW. Pleural fluid characteristics of patients with symptomatic pleural effusion after coronary artery bypass graft surgery. Arch Intern Med 2000; 160:2665–2668.
28. Lee YCG, Rogers JT, Rodriguez RM, Miller KD, Light RW. Adenosine deaminase levels in nontuberculous lymphocytic pleural effusions. Chest 2001; 120:356–361.
29. Lee YC (Gary), Vaz MAC, Ely KA, McDonald EC, Thompson PJ, Nesbitt JC, Light RW. Symptomatic persistent post-coronary artery bypass graft pleural effusions requiring operative treatment. Clinical and histologic features. Chest 2001; 119:795–800.
30. Light RW. Pleural effusions following cardiac injury and coronary artery bypass graft surgery. Sem Respir Crit Care Med, 2001. In press.
31. Steizner TJ, King TE Jr, Antony VB, Sahn SA. The pleuropulmonary manifestations of the postcardiac injury syndrome. Chest 1983; 84:383–387.
32. Weiss JM, Spodick DH. Association of left pleural effusion with pericardial disease. N Engl J Med 1983; 308:696–697.
33. Tomaselli G, Gamsu G, Stulbarg MS. Constrictive pericarditis presenting as pleural effusion of unknown origin. Arch Intern Med 1989; 149:201–203.
34. Sadikot RT, Fredi JL, Light RW. A 43-year-old man with a large recurrent right-sided pleural effusion. Chest 2000; 117:1191–1194.
35. Timmerman D, Moerman P, Vergote I. Meigs' syndrome with elevated serum CA 125 levels: two case reports and review of the literature. Gynecol Oncol 1995; 59:405–408.
36. Wang DY, Yang PC, Yu WL, Kuo SH, Hsu NY. Serial antinuclear antibodies titre in pleural and pericardial fluid. Eur Respir J 2000; 15:1106–1110.

37. Epler GR, McLoud TC, Gaensler EA. Prevalence and incidence of benign asbestos pleural effusion in a working population. JAMA 1982; 247:617–622.
38. Hillerdal G, Ozesmi M. Benign asbestos pleural effusion: 73 exudates in 60 patients. Eur J Respir Dis 1987; 71:113–121.
39. Berger HW, Rammohan G, Neff MS, Buhain WJ. Uremic pleural effusion: a study in 14 patients on chronic dialysis. Ann Intern Med 1975; 82:362–364.
40. Coskun M, Boyvat F, Bozkurt B, Agildere AM, Niron EA. Thoracic CT findings in long-term hemodialysis patients. Acta Radiol 1998; 40:181–186.
41. Light RW, Jenkinson SG, Minh V, George RB. Observations on pleural pressures as fluid is withdrawn during thoracentesis. Am Rev Respir Dis 1980; 121:799–804.
42. Fentiman IS, Millis R, Sexton S, Hayward JL. Pleural effusion in breast cancer: a review of 105 cases. Cancer 1981; 47:2087–2092.
43. Moriarty AT, Wiersema L, Snyder W, Kotylo PK, McCloskey DW. Immunophenotyping of cytologic specimens by flow cytometry. Diag Cytopath 1993; 9:252–258.
44. Goodman PC. Spiral CT for pulmonary embolism. Semin Respir Crit Care Med 2000; 21:503–510.
45. Prakash URS, Reiman HM. Comparison of needle biopsy with cytologic analysis for the evaluation of pleural effusion: analysis of 414 cases. Mayo Clin Proc 1985; 60:158–164.
46. Kendall SW, Bryan AJ, Large SR, Wells FC. Pleural effusions: is thoracoscopy a reliable investigation? A retrospective review. Respir Med 1992; 86:437–440.
47. Hucker J, Bhatnagar NK, al-Jilaihawi AN, Forrester-Wood CP. Thoracoscopy in the diagnosis and management of recurrent pleural effusions. Ann Thorac Surg 1991; 52:1145–1147.
48. Menzies R, Charbonneau M. Thoracoscopy for the diagnosis of pleural disease. Ann Intern Med 1991; 114:271–276.
49. Hansen M, Faurshou P, Clementsen P. Medical thoracoscopy, results and complications in 146 patients: a retrospective study. Respir Med 1998; 92:228–232.
50. de Groot M, Walther G. Thoracoscopy in undiagnosed pleural effusions. S Afr Med J 1998; 88:706–711.
51. Emad A, Rezaian GR. Diagnostic value of closed percutaneous pleural biopsy vs pleuroscopy in suspected malignant pleural effusion or tuberculous pleurisy in a region with a high incidence of tuberculosis: a comparative, age-dependent study. Respir Med 1998; 92:488–492.
52. Daniel TM. Diagnostic thoracoscopy for pleural disease. Ann Thorac Surg 1993; 56:639–640.
53. Chang S-C, Perng RP. The role of fiberoptic bronchoscopy in evaluating the causes of pleural effusions. Arch Intern Med 1989; 149:855–857.
54. Ryan CJ, Rodgers RF, Unni KK, Hepper NC. The outcome of patients with pleural effusion of indeterminate cause at thoracotomy. Mayo Clin Proc 1981; 56:145–149.
55. Douglass BE, Carr DT, Bernatz PE. Diagnostic thoracotomy in the study of "idiopathic" pleural effusion. Am Rev Tuberc 1956; 74:954–957.

47

Hemothorax

PAUL E. VAN SCHIL, PHILIPPE G. JORENS, and PATRIQUE SEGERS

University of Antwerp
and University Hospital of Antwerp
Edegem, Antwerp, Belgium

I. Introduction

Hemothorax is defined as accumulation of a significant amount of blood in the pleural space. By pure visualization of pleural fluid, it is clinically difficult to judge the amount of blood, and usually this is overestimated (1). For a hemothorax, the hematocrit of the pleural fluid should be at least 50% that of the peripheral blood (2). A massive hemothorax is defined as the accumulation of more than 800 mL of blood (3). It should be noted that the pleural space can contain up to 6 L of blood (4). On chest x-ray the amount is considered significant when there is opacification of either diaphragmatic dome or when the depth of blood on the lateral decubitus film exceeds 2 cm at its deepest point (5). In one prospective study on the value of the computed tomography (CT) in blunt chest trauma, hemothorax was defined on CT scan as an intrapleural collection of fluid equivalent to blood (30–100 Hounsfield units) with a thickness of more than 10 mm (6). Immediate insertion of a chest drain is the best prophylaxis against pleural space complications (4). The latter, listed in Table 1, result from an inadequately drained hemothorax.

A clotted or retained hemothorax is defined as a persisting or residual bloody effusion obscuring 25% or more of the lung field after 3 days (5). An

Table 1 Pleural Space Complications of Hemothorax

Clotted or retained hemothorax
Empyema
Persisting pleural effusion
Fibrothorax, trapped lung

empyema is present when there is pus or an infected clot in the pleural cavity. This occurs in 5–10% of cases after tube thoracostomy (5,7). The first phase is exudative, followed by the fibrinopurulent stage when there are fibrin deposits with loculation of fluid (8). When this is not adequately treated, a pleural peel develops—the organizing phase (9).

A persisting pleural effusion is an exudative pleuritis and occurs in more than 10% of cases after removal of the chest tubes. Such effusions are usually nonbloody, and most resolve spontaneously without pleural space sequelae (1). A thoracentesis should be performed to rule out infection.

The incidence of fibrothorax is 1% after hemothorax. A dense fibrous peel develops on the lung surface, leading to a trapped lung, inhibiting lung expansion. In such cases decortication is necessary (4).

II. Etiology

Possible causes of hemothorax are listed in Table 2. Blunt or penetrating trauma is most frequently encountered (Fig. 1). Sources of bleeding include the chest wall, lung, diaphragm, blood vessels, and mediastinum. Abdominal causes, such as lacerations of spleen or liver with an associated diaphragmatic injury, can also give rise to a hemothorax (3). Rib fractures should not be considered to be minor injuries. In a series of 711 patients with rib fractures, a hemo- or pneumothorax was found in 32% of patients, and 26% had a lung contusion (10). Mortality was higher than 10% in this series. In our own recent series of 187 thoracic trauma patients, hemothorax was diagnosed in 55 patients (29.4%) (11). Associated injuries where present in 40 patients (72.7%). Rib fractures were associated with hemothorax in 35.3% of patients, with pneumothorax in 42.1%, and with lung contusion in 60.1% (11).

In the nontraumatic group, pleural tumors and complications of anticoagulant therapy are most frequent (12). A large hemothorax in a patient with hemophilia is shown in Figure 2. Rupture of pleural adhesions may occur in recurrent pneumothorax. In children the most common cause of hemothorax is also trauma, which may occur as a complication of subpleural arteriovenous malformations and malignancy (8).

Table 2 Causes of Hemothorax

Traumatic
   Blunt trauma
   Penetrating trauma
Iatrogenic
   Puncture of subclavian artery or vein
   Thoracentesis
   Puncture or biopsy of pleural or pulmonary lesions
   Transbronchial biopsy
   Cardiac or thoracic surgery
Nontraumatic
   Pleural tumors (primary—metastatic)
   Complication of anticoagulation therapy
   Bleeding disorder such as hemophilia, thrombocytopenia
   Lung metastases
   Rupture of pleural adhesions
   Pleural endometriosis
   Leaking aortic dissection or aneurysm
   Arteriovenous malformations
   Pancreatic pseudocyst

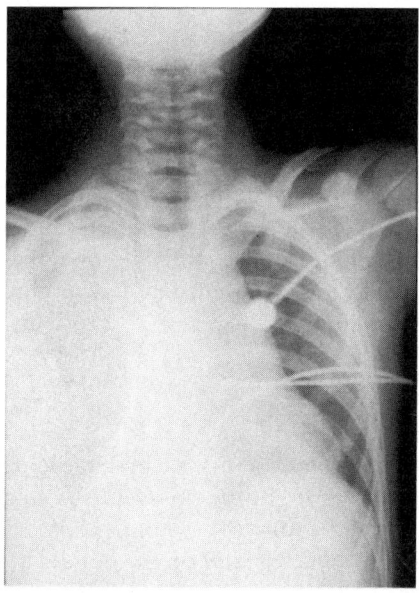

Figure 1 Massive hemothorax in a 10-year-old boy after penetrating injury of the subclavian artery.

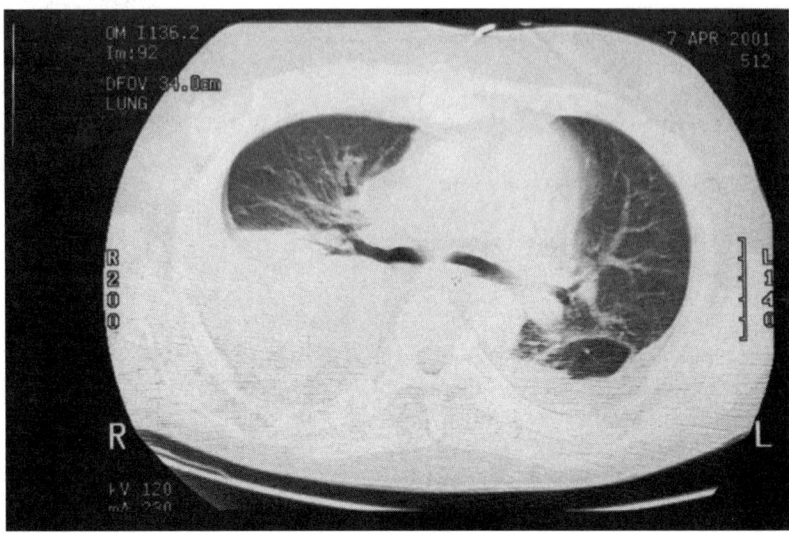

Figure 2 CT scan demonstrating right hemothorax in a patient with hemophilia A who underwent cholecystectomy.

III. Clinical Presentation

General symptoms depend on the amount of blood in the pleural space and range from minimal to life-threatening shock. Symptoms and signs are those of bleeding and pleuritis. Less than 250 mL of blood in the pleural space gives only a few symptoms. In case of massive hemothorax, patient will present with tachypnea, tachycardia, pallor, hypotension, and cardiovascular collapse (3). On clinical examination there are diminished or absent breath sounds on the involved side and dullness to percussion. Routine laboratory tests are performed, including hemoglobin, hematocrit, and coagulation tests. In case of severe blood loss, enough blood is matched and general resuscitation measures started to correct the hypovolemic shock.

IV. Diagnosis

In every patient with a thoracic trauma a chest radiograph is obtained, preferentially in the upright position. In the supine position, only a haziness will be present on the involved side. In study of 130 patients with blunt chest trauma, a hemothorax was not diagnosed correctly on the initial chest radiograph in 24% of patients (13). In a more upright position blunting of the costophrenic angle is noted in a small-sized hemothorax. When the amount of blood increases, a dense opacification is found on the affected hemithorax (Figs. 1 and 2) with a possible mediastinal shifting to the contralateral side. In 50% of traumatic cases a pneumothorax is also present. In any case, a follow-up chest radiograph should be taken after 24 hours to judge the specific evolution (12). When no upright chest radiograph can be obtained or in case of doubt, ultrasonography is helpful to determine the amount of blood in the pleural space. This can be performed by the surgeon or emergency physician during the initial evaluation of the chest trauma patient (14). The accuracy of ultrasound examination in penetrating thoracic wounds has been reported to be as high as 97.3% (15).

Early after trauma, differential diagnosis should be made with diaphragmatic injury and atelectasis for which thoracic CT scanning may be helpful.

As cost is a major concern nowadays, the value of routine CT scanning of the chest in hemodynamically stable patients is disputed (15). However, in a study of 103 patients with blunt chest trauma, thoracic CT scanning provided additional information in 65% of cases (6). CT was especially valid in detecting lung contusions, pneumo- and hemothorax. The specific findings on CT had direct consequences in early trauma management in 42% of the total study population, mostly regarding chest tube placement and respiratory care. CT was also helpful in diagnosing a diaphragmatic rupture, pericardial fluid, and misplaced chest tubes. Compared to historical controls, use of CT resulted in less cases of respiratory failure and ARDS and also in a reduced mortality (6). So, CT scanning of the chest can be recommended in the initial diagnostic work-up in severe chest trauma, except in patients who are hemodynamically unstable or when there is an indication for urgent surgical intervention. Especially in persisting or recurrent pleural effusions for which a precise diagnosis should be obtained, thoracentesis is indicated with puncture of the pleural fluid, if necessary under ultrasonographic or CT guidance. Hematocrit, glucose, and protein contents should be determined and a specimen also sent for bacteriological examination to rule out an empyema. Thoracentesis should be considered a diagnostic procedure and is not indicated for treatment of hemothorax (3).

V. Treatment

Depending on the clinical stage of the patient, general measures are taken for resuscitation and to correct hypovolemia. Hemodynamically unstable patients are taken to the operating room at once. Therapeutic options for hemothorax and its complications are listed in Table 3.

A. Tube Thoracostomy

Early drainage of every hemothorax by a chest tube is indicated to obtain a complete lung expansion and reduce the incidence of empyema and fibrothorax (4). Approximately 85% of all hemothoraces can be treated by a chest drain only (3). A large-bore tube should be inserted in the fifth intercostal space on the midaxillary line and directed posteriorly to the costophrenic angle (Fig. 3). In case of massive bleeding, an autotransfusion device can be used for rapid processing and reinfusion of blood. Tube thoracostomy provides a precise measure of blood loss

Table 3 Treatment Options for Hemothorax and Its Complications

Tube thoracostomy
Fibrinolytic treatment
Thoracoscopy or VATS
Thoracotomy
 Early: massive or persisting blood loss
 Late: clotted hemothorax, empyema, fibrothorax

and its evolution over time (16). By apposing the pleural surfaces, bleeding from the pulmonary parenchyma or pleural lacerations usually stops spontaneously, as a natural tamponade is created (12,16). In an experimental study of massive hemothorax chest tube clamping did not decrease hemorrhage or mortality and did not improve hypotension (17). For these reasons clamping is not recommended in the treatment of a large hemothorax.

By applying suction to the drains, chest tube duration can be decreased, potentially leading to a shorter length of hospital stay (18). When drainage becomes less than 50 mL over 6 hours the chest tubes should be removed as they can serve as conduits for pleural infection and subsequent empyema (5). Prophylactic antibiotics seem to be indicated as they reduce the incidence of empyema and pneumonia in patients with chest tubes for traumatic hemopneumothoraces (19,20). However, the precise dosage and optimal duration remain to be determined.

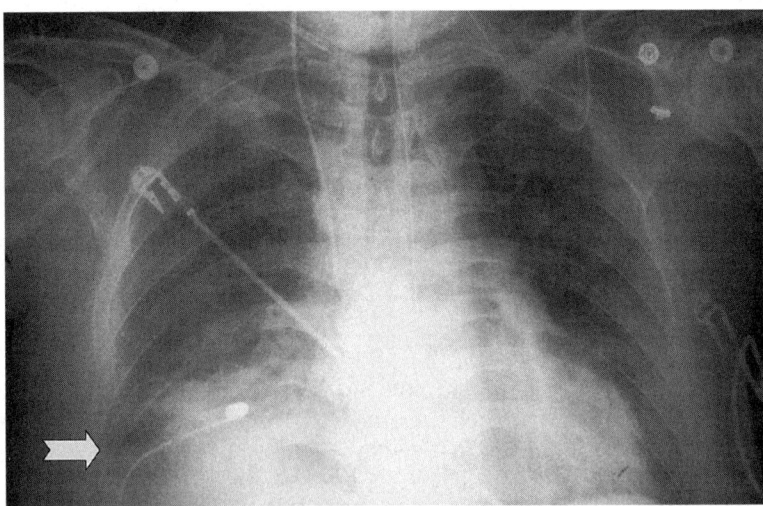

Figure 3 Insertion of a basal chest tube (arrow) in the patient with hemophilia A.

In a retrospective study of 57 chest drains, the overall complication rate was 30%, but there was only one major complication, an empyema thoracis (21). No insertional complications were encountered. However, in another retrospective study the overall complication rate was significantly higher for chest tubes inserted on the inpatient ward as compared to the emergency department or operating room (22).

A short-period treatment aiming at removing the chest tube within 24 hours combined with early mobilization was evaluated in 1845 patients, 7.5% of whom had a blunt chest trauma (5). In total, 91% of patients could be treated by a tube thoracostomy only, and hospital stay was less than 48 hours in 82% of the patients, a remarkable achievement. General principles of treatment included early mobilization, adequate analgesia, and vigorous physiotherapy. In this study, the failure rate of conservative treatment without chest drain was 26%. Empyema was found to occur more frequently in patients with a significantly larger mean drainage time or an increased volume of blood loss (5).

B. Fibrinolytic Treatment

When a residual clotted hemothorax develops, there is an ongoing controversy as to whether this should be treated conservatively or more aggressively by a thoracotomy. Pleural blood can be absorbed spontaneously, but adverse sequelae of an incomplete evacuation may develop (Table 1), favoring a more aggressive approach (14). Intrapleural fibrinolytic treatment is a relatively new therapeutic option, which can be applied by the chest tubes, avoiding a thoracotomy in most cases. The first use of streptokinase in hemothorax was described in 1949 (23). In 1987, the use of urokinase, which is nonantigenic and nonpyrogenic but more expensive, was reported for treatment of extravascular hematomas (24). For treatment of clotted, loculated, or delayed hemothorax, fibrinolytic treatment was utilized in 24 patients, 4 of whom had infected hemothoraces (25). Streptokinase (250,000 IU) or urokinase (100,000 IU) was diluted in 100 mL saline solution and injected through the chest tube, which was clamped for 4 hours. Daily drainage was recorded; the chest tubes were removed when drainage was less than 50 mL over 24 hours. The mean period of time between diagnosis and fibrinolytic treatment was 11.6 days. Complete response, defined as resolution of symptoms with complete drainage of fluid and no residual space radiographically, was obtained in 63% of patients. A partial response with resolution of symptoms but a small remaining pleural cavity was noted in 29%. Only two patients (8%) were nonresponders and underwent decortication. Mean hospital stay was 17 days. There were no complications related to fibrinolytic treatment (25).

In a prospective study of 48 patients with a pleural effusion, of whom 14 had a hemothorax, the overall success rate of fibrinolytic treatment with repeated doses of 250,000 IU of streptokinase was 92% (26).

Moulton et al. described 118 patients with a complicated pleural fluid collection treated with instillation of urokinase. Overall success rate was 94%

without any complications (27). Fibrinolytic treatment seems very effective for treatment of a clotted hemothorax when it is applied within 10 days of injury. Otherwise, organization of the clot leads to a fibrous peel and fibrothorax, necessitating a decortication by thoracotomy, at least 4–5 weeks later (12). At the present time there is no consensus on the duration of fibrinolytic treatment, the amount and frequency of instillation, and the precise assessment of response.

C. Thoracoscopy or VATS

As most patients with a hemothorax can be treated by a thoracic drain, only 10–20% need operative intervention. These represent a high-risk group (3). Video-assisted thoracic surgery (VATS) or thoracoscopy is a new, less invasive treatment modality which can replace thoracotomy in selected cases. Its use in penetrating chest injuries was described in 1946 (28). VATS uses minimal incisions, possibly reducing postoperative pain and hospital stay (29). It offers a complete visualization of the pleural cavity; blood can be evacuated and the source of bleeding determined (14). Contraindications for VATS are hemodynamically unstable patients who should proceed immediately to sternotomy or thoracotomy, suspected great vessel or cardiac injury, obliteration of the pleural space, which renders the introduction of the thoracoscope impossible, and inability to tolerate single lung ventilation (9,30). In this respect, a VATS procedure should be performed within 5 days of the original injury to avoid developing fibrosis from an organizing bloody effusion. Current indications for VATS in thoracic trauma are continued chest tube bleeding in stable patients, clotted hemothorax early after the injury, evaluation of the diaphragm to rule out traumatic rupture, repair of pulmonary lacerations, evaluation of a persistent air leak, and possible mediastinal injuries (9,15,31).

In a study of 58 patients with residual traumatic hemothorax, chest radiograph taken on the second day after injury was compared to CT scanning of the thorax (7). Chest x-ray was found to be unreliable, with an incorrect interpretation in 48%. In 31% of the patients, the chest x-ray–based decision for treatment was changed from operative to nonoperative management and vice versa. So, CT scanning added more diagnostic information and is considered the gold standard according to which to make decisions. Arbitrarily, a volume of 500 mL of blood was chosen as the cut-off value for performing a thoracoscopic procedure (32). Early thoracoscopic evacuation of retained blood was found to be safe and effective.

In another prospective randomized trial, 39 patients with retained hemothoraces were randomized between a second tube thoracostomy and a VATS procedure (33). In the VATS group duration of tube drainage, total hospital stay and costs were reduced. Although VATS represents a more complex and expensive approach, it may be a more efficient and economical strategy for treatment of traumatic retained hemothoraces.

Complications occur in less than 10% of VATS procedures, of which atelectasis is most common (34). Conversion rates of VATS up to 24% are described, so patients should always be prepared for thoracotomy (30). Also in the management of posttraumatic empyema, VATS has been successfully performed (35), but it should be reserved for early cases before the organizing phase sets in.

D. Thoracotomy

With the advent of fibrinolytic treatment and thoracoscopic procedures, the number of thoracotomies will probably be reduced in the management of traumatic hemothorax. No precise criteria for intervention have been established (12). An initial blood loss of more than 1.5 L or a persisting blood loss of more than 250 mL per hour for 3 consecutive hours is generally regarded as an indication for urgent exploration by sternotomy or thoracotomy, especially in unstable patients (1,3,14). In our series of 55 hemothoraces an urgent thoracotomy was performed in 6 patients or (10.9%) (11).

Although there is a trend towards nonoperative or delayed treatment in patients with aortic rupture and severe associated lesions, suspected aortic injury with a massive left-sided hemothorax is still an indication for urgent left thoracotomy and repair (15). Rare cases of traumatic aortic dissection without complications can be treated conservatively (36). Other indications for immediate thoracotomy are cardiac tamponade, evidence of a major bronchial rupture, sucking chest wounds, and injury of the aortic arch vessels (12,16). Cardiac injuries are mostly approached by sternotomy.

In case of bleeding from the lung parenchyma, selective ligation of bleeding vessels is advocated after placement of long vascular clamps or staplers to the entrance and exit sites of injured lobes. This technique is known as pulmonotomy or pulmonary tractotomy (14,15). A so-called trauma pneumonectomy is performed in cases of massive bleeding by stapling of the pulmonary hilum, but carries a high mortality (37,38).

Emergency room thoracotomy is mainly indicated in penetrating injuries with recent cardiac arrest or massive blood loss, but overall survival rates are less than 10% (15,39). Contra-indications are penetrating trauma with no signs of life on the accident scene and blunt trauma without signs of life on arrival in the emergency department.

Late indications for thoracotomy after traumatic injuries include clotted hemothorax, empyema, and fibrothorax. A retained or clotted hemothorax 7–10 days after injury is no longer an indication for fibrinolytic treatment or thoracoscopy due to organization of the clot. Open thoracotomy is necessary to open up the different loculations, drain the effusion, and remove the fibrous peel to obtain a complete lung expansion (3). Empyema in the organizing phase should also be treated by thoracotomy to allow full evacuation of all purulent collections and debridement of devitalized tissue (16). In case of fibrothorax or trapped lung, a decortication is performed. Good results have been described even if the fibrothorax has been present for 10 years or more (2,12).

E. Treatment of Nontraumatic Hemothorax

In case of a nontraumatic hemothorax, treatment depends on the underlying disorder. Pulmonary arteriovenous malformations are treated by embolization or surgical resection and ligation (8). Coagulation disorders are corrected by administration of specific blood products. Anticoagulation is stopped or reduced in case of a significant hemothorax occurring as complication of overzealous anticoagulant therapy.

Treatment of recurrent pneumothorax, endometriosis, and diagnosis of pleural tumors can usually be made by thoracoscopy (40,41). A leaking aortic aneurysm or dissection is an indication for thoracotomy or sternotomy with repair by an interposition graft (42). Iatrogenic hemothorax requires insertion of a chest drain. Only in cases of massive or persistent bleeding is a thoracotomy indicated for repair of the bleeding vessel or lung lesion.

VI. Conclusion

The most common cause of hemothorax is chest trauma. For precise diagnosis in severe chest injury, CT of the thorax is recommended. Most hemothoraces can be adequately treated by insertion of a chest drain, which provides the best prophylaxis against pleural space complications. Thoracotomy is only indicated in cases of massive or persistent bleeding. A clotted or retained hemothorax early after injury is an indication for fibrinolytic treatment or thoracoscopy. Complete drainage is necessary to avoid late complications such as empyema or fibrothorax. The latter usually necessitate an open thoracotomy for adequate drainage and removal of the fibrous peel.

References

1. Sahn SS. Diseases of the pleura and pleural space. In: Baum GL, Crapo JD, Celli BR, Karlinsky JB, eds. Textbook of Pulmonary Diseases. Philadelphia: Lippincott-Raven, 1998:1483–1498.
2. Light RW. Diseases of the pleura, mediastinum, chest wall and diaphragm. In: George RB, Light RW, Matthay MA, Matthay RA, eds. Chest Medicine. Philadelphia: Lippincott, 2000:441–477.
3. Owens MW, Chaudry MS, Eggerstedt JM, Smith LM. Thoracic trauma, surgery and perioperative management. In: George RB, Light RW, Matthay MA, Matthay RA, eds. Chest Medicine. Philadelphia: Lippincott, 2000:592–619.
4. Glinz W. Chest Trauma. Diagnosis and Management. Berlin: Springer-Verlag, 1981.
5. Knottenbelt JD, Van der Spuy JW. Traumatic hemothorax—experience of a protocol for rapid turnover in 1,845 cases. S Afr J Surg 1994; 32:5–8.
6. Trupka A, Waydhas C, Hallfeldt KK, Nast-Kolb D, Pfeifer KJ, Schweiberer L.

Value of thoracic computed tomography in the first assessment of severely injured patients with blunt chest trauma: results of a prospective study. J Trauma 1997; 43:405–412.
7. Velmahos GC, Demetriades D, Chan L, Tatevossian R, Cornwell EE, Yassa N, Murray JA, Asensio JA, Berne TV. Predicting the need for thoracoscopic evacuation of residual traumatic hemothorax: chest radiograph is insufficient. J Trauma 1999; 46:65–70.
8. Zeitlin PL. Pleural effusions and empyema. In: Loughlin GM, Eigen H, eds. Respiratory Disease in Children. Baltimore: Williams & Wilkins, 1994:453–463.
9. Lowdermilk GA, Naunheim KS. Thoracoscopic evaluation and treatment of thoracic trauma. Surg Clin North Am 2000; 80:1535–1542.
10. Ziegler DW, Agarwal NN. The morbidity and mortality of rib fractures. J Trauma 1994; 37:975–979.
11. Segers P, Van Schil P, Jorens PG, Van den Brande F. Thoracic trauma: an analysis of 187 patients. Acta Chir Belg 2001; 101:277–282.
12. Light RW. Chylothorax, hemothorax and fibrothorax. In: Murray JF, Nadel JA, eds. Textbook of Respiratory Medicine. Philadelphia: W.B. Saunders Company, 1998:1760–1769.
13. Drummond DS, Craig RH. Traumatic hemothorax: complications and management. Am Surg 1967; 33:403–408.
14. Battistella FD, Benfield JR. Blunt and penetrating injuries of the chest wall, pleura, and lungs. In: Shields TW, LoCicero J III, Ponn RB, eds. General Thoracic Surgery. Philadelphia: Lippincott, 2000:815–831.
15. Feliciano DV, Rozycki GS. Advances in the diagnosis and treatment of thoracic trauma. Surg Clin North Am 1999; 79:1417–1429.
16. Winterbauer RH. Non malignant pleural effusions. In: Fishman AP ed. Fishman's Pulmonary Diseases and Disorders. New York: McGraw-Hill, 1988:1412–1427.
17. Ali J, Qi W. Effectiveness of chest tube clamping in massive hemothorax. J Trauma 1995; 38:59–63.
18. Davis JW, Mackersie RC, Hoyt DB, Garcia J. Randomized study of algorithms for discontinuing tube thoracostomy drainage. J Am Coll Surg 1994; 179:553–557.
19. Gonzalez RP, Holevar MR. Role of prophylactic antibiotics for tube thoracostomy in chest trauma. Am Surg 1998; 64:617–621.
20. Wilson RF, Nichols RL. The EAST practice management guidelines for prophylactic antibiotic use in tube thoracostomy for traumatic hemopneumothorax: a commentary. J Trauma 2000; 48:758–759.
21. Bailey RC. Complications of tube thoracostomy in trauma. J Accid Emerg Med 2000; 17:111–114.
22. Chan L, Reilly KM, Henderson C, Kahn F, Salluzzo RF. Complication rates of tube thoracostomy. Am J Emerg Med 1997; 15:368–370.
23. Tillett WS, Sherry S. The effect in patients of streptococcal fibrinolysin (streptokinase) and streptococcal deoxyribonuclease on fibrinous, purulent and sanguineous pleural exudations. J Clin Invest 1949; 23:173–179.
24. Vogelzang RL, Tobin RS, Burstein S, Anschuetz SL, Marzano M, Kozlowski JM. Transcatheter intracavitary fibrinolysis of infected extravascular hematomas. Am J Roentgenol 1987; 148:378–380.
25. Inci I, Ozcelik C, Ulku R, Tuna A, Eren N. Intrapleural fibrinolytic treatment of traumatic clotted hemothorax. Chest 1998; 114:160–165.
26. Jerjes-Sanchez C, Ramirez-Rivera A, Elizalde JJ, Delgado R, Cicero R, Ibarra-

26. Perez A, Arroliga AC, Padua A, Portales A, Villarreal A, Perez-Romo A. Intrapleural fibrinolysis with streptokinase as an adjunctive treatment in hemothorax and empyema: a multicenter trial. Chest 1996; 109:1514–1519.
27. Moulton JS, Benkert RE, Weisiger KH, Chambers JA. Treatment of complicated pleural fluid collections with image-guided drainage and intracavitary urokinase. Chest 1995; 108:1252–1259.
28. Branco JMC. Thoracoscopy as a method of exploration in penetrating injuries of the chest. Dis Chest 1946; 12:330–335.
29. Heniford BT, Carrillo EH, Spain DA, Sosa JL, Fulton RL, Richardson JD. The role of thoracoscopy in the management of retained thoracic collections after trauma. Ann Thorac Surg 1997; 63:940–943.
30. Lang-Lazdunski L, Mouroux J, Pons F, Grosdidier G, Martinod E, Elkaïm D, Azorin J, Jancovici R. Role of videothoracoscopy in chest trauma. Ann Thorac Surg 1997; 63:327–333.
31. Carrillo EH, Richardson JD. Thoracoscopy in the management of hemothorax and retained blood after trauma. Curr Opin Pulm Med 1998; 4:243–246.
32. Velmahos GC, Demetriades D. Early thoracoscopy for the evacuation of undrained haemothorax. Eur J Surg 1999; 165:924–929.
33. Meyer DM, Jessen ME, Wait MA, Estrera AS. Early evacuation of traumatic retained hemothoraces using thoracoscopy: a prospective randomized trial. Ann Thorac Surg 1997; 64:1396–1401.
34. Krasna MJ, Deshmukh S, McLaughlin JS. Complications of thoracoscopy. Ann Thorac Surg 1996; 61:1066–1069.
35. Sosa JL, Pombo H, Puente I, Sleeman D, Ginzburg E, McKinney M, Martin L. Thoracoscopy in the evaluation and management of thoracic trauma. Int Surg 1998; 83:187–189.
36. Goverde P, Van Schil P, Delrue F, d'Archambeau O, Vanmaele R, Eyskens E. Traumatic type B aortic dissection. Acta Chir Belg 1996; 96:233–236.
37. Wagner JW, Obeid FN, Karmy-Jones RC, Casey GD, Sorensen VJ, Horst HM. Trauma pneumonectomy revisited: the role of simultaneous stapled pneumonectomy. J Trauma 1996; 40:590–594.
38. Baumgartner F, Omari B, Lee J, Bleiweis M, Snyder R, Robertson J, Sheppard B, Milliken J. Survival after trauma pneumonectomy: the pathophysiologic balance of shock resuscitation with right heart failure. Am Surg 1996; 62:967–972.
39. Kaiser LR, DiPierro FW. Thoracic trauma. In: Fishman AP, ed. Fishman's Pulmonary Diseases and Disorders. New York: McGraw-Hill, 1988:1661–1669.
40. Van Schil P, Van Meerbeeck J, Vanmaele R, Eyskens E. Role of thoracoscopy (VATS) in pleural and pulmonary pathology. Acta Chir Belg 1996; 96:23–27.
41. Van Schil PE, Vercauteren SR, Vermeire PA, Nackaerts YH, Van Marck EA. Catamenial pneumothorax caused by thoracic endometriosis. Ann Thorac Surg 1996; 62:585–586.
42. Ochsner J, Ancalmo N. Descending thoracic aortic aneurysm. Chest Surg Clin North Am 1992; 2:291–309.

48

Chylothorax and Pseudochylothorax

PETROS BAKAKOS, MICHAEL TOUMBIS, and ANTONIS RASIDAKIS
Sotiria Chest Diseases Hospital
Athens, Greece

Pleural fluid is occasionally found to be milky, whitish, opalescent, or at least turbid. This appearance is sometimes due to a high lipid content in the pleural fluid. Two different conditions are characterized by the accumulation of high levels of lipid in pleural fluid. In one, chyle enters the pleural space as a result of disruption of the thoracic duct, producing a chylothorax or a chylous pleural effusion. In the second, large amounts of cholesterol or lecithin-globulin complexes accumulate in a long-standing pleural effusion, producing a pseudothylothorax or a chyliform pleural effusion. Apart from the appearance of the pleural fluid, these two conditions have nothing in common. They have completely different prognosis and management.

I. Chylothorax

A. Physiology

Chylothorax is a collection of chylous fluid in the pleural space arising from a disruption of the thoracic duct or one of its major divisions. Although a rare condition, prompt diagnosis and correct treatment are important. In the past, mortality rates were around 50% (1).

Most absorbed fat is conveyed to the blood by the thoracic duct in the form of chylomicrons. The chylomicrons enter the intestinal lacteal vessels and then travel to the cisterna chyli, a lymphatic structure located on the body of the second lumbar vertebra. The thoracic duct, the main tributary of the lymphatic system, is a 2.0–3.0 mm thin-walled structure, varying in length from 37 to 45 cm, which begins at the cisterna chyli. From the cisterna chyli, the thoracic duct traverses the aortic hiatus of the diaphragm on the anterior surface of the vertebral body between the aorta and the azygos vein into the posterior mediastinum. The thoracic duct then ascends extrapleurally in the posterior mediastinum along the right side of the anterior surface of the vertebral column in proximity to the esophagus and the pericardium. Between the level of the 4th and 6th thoracic vertebrae, the duct crosses to the left of the vertebral column and continues cephalad to enter the superior mediastinum between the aortic arch and the subclavian artery and the left side of the esophagus. The thoracic duct then arches above the clavicle and passes anterior to the subclavian artery, vertebral artery, and thyrocervical trunk to terminate in the region of the left jugular and subclavian veins.

The thoracic duct displays considerable variability. There may be a division into two or more branches in more than 40% of individuals (2). These branches may form a plexiform arrangement in the middle of the course of the duct and may terminate separately or as one duct. Occasionally, the duct divides into two branches in its upper portion, which do not rejoin but drain separately, one in the usual fashion and the other reaching the right subclavian vein (3). The proximity to the esophagus, presence of collateral channels, and highly variable course leads to its injury during esophageal and pulmonary resection.

Chylothorax is usually right-sided, since most of the duct is within the right hemithorax. With damage at the level of aorta, the chyle will appear on the left side (4). When the leakage from the duct occurs where it passes over the mid-line, a bilateral chylothorax may arise (5).

The thoracic duct drains the lymphatics of the body, except for the right side of the head and neck, right upper limb, right lung, right side of the heart, and the convex surface of the liver (Fig. 1). Some 95% of transmitted lymph is derived from the gastrointestinal tract and the liver; the remainder originates in skeletal tissue. The thoracic duct contains many valves forcing the chyle in one direction only. There are extensive collateral pathways between various lymphatic vessels and lymphaticovenous anastomoses between the thoracic duct and the azygos, intercostal and lumbar veins, making it possible to ligate the duct without any resulting problems (6).

Chyle separates into three layers: a creamy uppermost layer containing chylomicrons, a milky intermediate layer, and a dependent layer containing cellular elements. Approximately 1500–2500 mL of chyle normally empties into the venous system daily. The flow of lymph through the thoracic duct can be increased to 2–10 times the resting level when a high-fat meal is ingested. Ingestion of liquid also increases the chyle flow, whereas the ingestion of protein or carbohydrates has little effect on lymph flow. Total protein content of chyle is

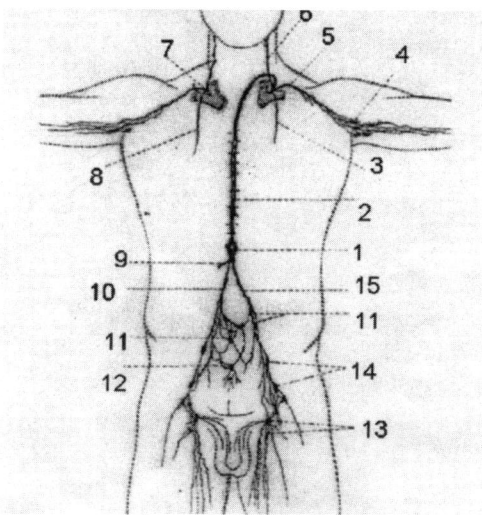

Figure 1 The thoracic duct and the main lymphatic trunks of the human body. 1, Cisterna chyli; 2, thoracic duct; 3, left bronchomediastinal trunk; 4, axillary nodes; 5, left subclavian trunk; 6, left jugular trunk; 7, right lymph duct; 8, right bronchomediastinal trunk; 9, intestinal trunk; 10, right lumbar trunk; 11, lumbar nodes; 12, sacral nodes; 13, superficial inguinal nodes; 14, iliac nodes; 15, left lumbar trunk.

usually >3 g/dL with an albumin-to-globulin ratio of approximately 3:1, and the electrolyte composition is similar to that of serum. Fat-soluble vitamins are also present in chyle. The majority of the lymphocytes in the thoracic duct are T lymphocytes (400–6000 lymphocytes/mm^3) returning to the blood stream. Erythrocytes are also present, numbering between 50 and 600/mm^3. In view of the contents of the thoracic duct lymph (Table 1), it is easy to understand that persistent loss of this fluid would result in nutritional depletion, electrolyte loss, hypolipemia, and lymphopenia (7,8).

Chyle is bacteriostatic and nonirritating and has little propensity to form fibrothorax (9).

B. Etiology

Chylothorax may be classified according to etiology as nontraumatic, postoperative traumatic, nonsurgical traumatic, and congenital (Table 2) (10).

Nontraumatic

Intraluminal obstruction by neoplastic cells or infective organisms and extrinsic obstruction due to lymphadenopathy or local tumor compression can result in chylothorax (11). Nontraumatic chylothorax is an uncommon condition of thoracic or abdominal origin caused by multiple disorders, of which malignancy

Table 1 Features of Lymph Fluid

Relative density	1012–1020
pH	7.4–7.8
Color	Milky, opalescent
Sterile	Yes
Bacteriostatic	Yes
Fat (g/dL)	0.5–3.0
Protein (g/dL)	>3.0
Albumin	1.2–4.2
Globulin	1.1–3.1
Albumin: globulin ratio	3:1
Cell count (per dL)	
Lymphocytes (90% T cells)	40,000–600,000
Erythrocytes	5,000–60,000
Electrolyte concentration (mMol/L)	
Sodium	104–110
Potassium	3.5–5.0
Chloride	85–130

is by far the most frequent (12). More than 50% of chylothoraces are related to tumors involving the mediastinum and invading the thoracic duct. Lymphoma is responsible for 75% of malignancy-associated chylothoraces (13,14). Chylothorax can be the first sign of the lymphoma (6). Recently chylothorax has been reported in patients with AIDS and Kaposi's sarcoma (15,16).

Tuberculosis, filariasis, pancreatic pseudocysts, tuberous sclerosis, amyloidosis, sarcoidosis, cirrhosis, heart failure, yellow nail syndrome, and retrosternal goiter have all been associated with chylothorax. Another rare cause of chylothorax is pulmonary lymphangiomyomatosis, a disease occurring in women of reproductive age that leads to perforation of the thoracic duct (6). Chylothorax may rarely occur after irradiation (17).

Postoperative Traumatic

Trauma is the second leading cause of chylothorax, responsible for approximately 25% of the cases. Surgery is the most common cause of traumatic chylothorax.

Although chylothorax has been reported after almost every type of thoracic operation, certain patients may be predisposed toward postoperative chylothorax. Esophageal resections for carcinoma with mediastinal lymphadenectomy (18) and particularly transhiatal resections are associated with chylothorax in almost 2% of cases (19).

The incidence of chylothorax after cardiovascular operations is about 0.5%. Operations that mobilize the left subclavian artery are more likely to be complicated by chylothorax (20). Chylothorax has also been reported as a com-

Table 2 Causes of Chylothorax

Nontraumatic
  Malignant
    Lymphomas
    Other malignancies
  Benign tumors
  Tuberculosis
  Filariasis
  Tuberous sclerosis
  Amyloidosis
  Sarcoidosis
  Cirrhosis
  Heart failure
  Retrosternal goiter
  Lymphangiomyomatosis
  Yellow nail syndrome
  Pancreatic pseudocysts
  Radiation
Postoperative traumatic
  Surgery of chest
  Head and neck surgery
  Sclerotherapy of the esophagus
  Thrombosis of central veins
Nonsurgical traumatic
  Any accident with damage or stretching of the chest wall or thoracic spine
  Forceful cough, vomiting, weight lifting, or sneezing
Idiopathic
Congenital

plication of esophagoscopy, stellate ganglion blockade, thoracic sympathectomy, high translumbar aortography, cervical node dissection, pneumonectomy, and thrombosis of the jugular and subclavian veins following vein catheterization (21–23). Iatrogenic chylothorax may rarely occur following repeated sclerotherapy for esophageal varices (24).

Nonsurgical Traumatic

Chylothorax may be caused by penetrating and nonpenetrating injuries. Penetrating trauma to the chest, such as gunshot or knife wounds, may disrupt the thoracic duct. Nonpenetrating trauma such as hyperextension of the spine or fracture of a vertebra can also lead to chylothorax. In this circumstance the duct is particularly vulnerable when distended after a meal (25,26). Even everyday stresses such as coughing, sneezing, vomiting, and weight lifting may occasionally produce a chylothorax (27). A chylothorax secondary to closed trauma is usually on the right side, and the site of rupture is in the region of the 9th and 10th thoracic vertebra (25).

Congenital

Chylothorax is the most common cause of pleural effusion in the newborn (28). The etiology is usually unknown, but congenital chylothorax is more often due to malformation of the thoracic duct than trauma at birth (29,30). The thoracic duct may be absent or atretic, or there may be multiple fistulae between the thoracic duct and the pleural space (30). Chylothorax has also been associated with Down's, Turner's, and Noonan's syndromes, tracheoesophageal fistula, and polyhydramnios (7). In childhood, chylothorax is usually a postoperative complication, mainly occurring after cardiothoracic interventions or caused by thrombosis of the left or right subclavian vein (31,32).

Approximately 25% of chylothoraces have no identifiable cause and are labeled as idiopathic. Most cases of idiopathic chylothorax are presumed to be secondary to minor trauma, such as coughing, stretching, or hiccuping after the ingestion of a fatty meal.

C. Clinical Manifestations

The symptoms, physical findings, and roentgenographic features of chylothorax are almost exclusively related to the volume of fluid into the thoracic cavity. Fever and pleuritic chest pain are virtually absent because chyle does not irritate the pleural surface.

Traumatic chylothorax usually develops 2–10 days after trauma. Initially, lymph collects extrapleurally in the posterior mediastinum to form a "chyloma," which may be visible on the chest x-ray as a posterior mediastinal mass (5). The formation of the "chyloma" may be accompanied by a very dramatic clinical event, with acute chest pain causing dyspnea and tachycardia, suggesting myocardial infarction or pulmonary embolism (6). In time, the mediastinal pleura ruptures and chyle enters the pleural space. Hypotension, cyanosis, and dyspnea may develop when the "chyloma" ruptures into the pleural space. There are some rare variations, for instance, chylomediastinum, where the chyle collects in the mediastinum without breaking through the pleura (33) or chylopericardium, where it empties into the pericardial sac (34,35). The local effects of a chyle leak into the pleural cavity include compression of the ipsilateral lung and, if sufficiently voluminous, mediastinal shift, which compromises the contralateral lung and impairs cardiac function.

Neonatal chylothorax usually presents with respiratory distress in the first few days of life. Nearly 50% of the infants have symptoms within the first 24 hours, whereas 75% have symptoms by the end of the first week. Most neonatal chylothoraces are right-sided or bilateral. The appearance of the pleural fluid is serous until feeding with milk has begun (36).

D. Diagnosis

Fluid from a chylothorax looks white, milky, or turbid and is odorless (Table 3). Occasionally it can be blood stained. Effusions with this appearance will be either chylothorax, pseudochylothorax, or empyema. If after centrifugation the supernatant clears, the white color is due to large numbers of white cells and debris and the patient most likely has an empyema. The supernatant of a chylous or a pseudochylous effusion remains opalescent after centrifugation. If the turbidity is due to high levels of cholesterol, it will clear when 1–2 mL of ethyl ether is added to a test tube of the fluid; if the turbidity is due to chylomicrons or lecithin complexes, it will not clear (23).

The best way to establish the diagnosis of chylothorax is to determine the levels of triglycerides in the pleural fluid. Triglyceride levels greater than 110 mg/dL usually indicate a chylothorax. Levels below 50 mg/dL virtually exclude a chylothorax. If the patient has intermediate values (between 50 and 110 mg/dL), a lipid electrophoresis of the pleural fluid should be performed. The presence of chylomicrons establishes the diagnosis of chylothorax (37).

Chylothoraces are usually characterized by a ratio of pleural fluid to the serum triglyceride level of more than 1.0 and a ratio of the pleural fluid to serum cholesterol level of less than 1.0 (12). Cholesterol levels should be measured simultaneously, since high triglyceride levels can also occur in pseudochylothorax (38). The diagnosis may be confirmed by administration of cream or other foodstuff of high fat content by mouth or via the nasogastric tube; this is the most reliable test in the clinical setting. It induces dramatic change in the color and content of the effused fluid owing to the transport of absorbed fat in the lacteal system (39,40).

Table 3 Differences Between Chylothorax and Pseudochylothorax

Characteristics	Chylothorax	Pseudochylothorax
Appearance	Milky	Milky
Odor	Odorless	Odorless
Mechanism	Leakage of lymph	Unknown
Usual etiology	Trauma	Tuberculosis
	Cancer	Rheumatoid arthritis
Presentation	More acute	Chronic
Cholesterol	Low	High
Triglycerides	High	Low
Cholesterol crystals	No	Usually
Chylomicrons on lipoprotein electrophoresis?	Yes	No
Cause of opalescence	Lipid droplets	Cholesterol crystals
Addition of ethyl ether	Opalescence persists	Clearing of opalescence
Creamy layer withstanding	Yes	No

The patient with chylothorax rapidly becomes malnourished and immunocompromised. During prolonged chyle loss the body's reserves of protein (in particular albumin), fat, vitamins, and electrolytes are depleted due to the substantial amounts contained in chyle. Hypovolemia from continued fluid loss may be compounded by hypoproteinemia, which results in transcapillary fluid shifts. Hyponatremia, metabolic acidosis, and hypocalcemia are the most commonly recognized phenomena (26). Prolonged chyle drainage depletes the T-cell population and impairs both cell-mediated immunity, as evidenced by negative intradermal skin testing, and humoral responses to antigen provocation (41). The depletion of the T-cell population caused by prolonged drainage is of benefit in the suppression of transplant rejection states (42,43). Hypoalbuminemia and lymphopenia in conjunction with an altered immune response increase the risk of bacterial and viral infections and sepsis (44).

The clinical picture usually helps in differentiating a chylous from a pseudochylous pleural effusion. Pseudochylous effusions are usually chronic with thickened pleura, and they contain high levels of lecithin-globulin complexes or cholesterol crystals. Chylothoraces are usually acute with no pleural thickening, they do not contain cholesterol crystals, and they have a high level of triglycerides.

Not all chylous effusions have a classic milky appearance. Actually, half of them are bloody or turbid in appearance. The milky aspect can serve as a hint for further investigations. Therefore, a determination of the triglyceride content or a lipoprotein analysis of an exudative fluid of unknown etiology should always be performed (32,37).

Once the diagnosis of chylothorax is established it is important to determine the cause. A computed tomography (CT) scan of the thorax and upper abdomen should be performed to visualize any enlarged lymph nodes or other signs of tumor and to enable scrutiny of the lungs. Since lymphoma is the most common cause of chylothorax and is now treatable with chemotherapy or radiotherapy, every effort should be made to establish the diagnosis.

Lymphangiography provides useful information regarding the site and size of the leak and enables differentiation between thoracic duct damage and anastomotic leaks in the postoperative group. It may also identify complete transection or partial laceration of the duct. It is, however, complex and time-consuming (45,46).

If no cause has been found, the next step is most often thoracic surgery, which is today usually performed by thoracoscopic methods. Biopsies of any suspect area should be taken. Biopsy of the lung, especially any suspicious part seen at CT, should be performed, since this is the best way to diagnose, for instance, a lymphangioleiomyomatosis. This diagnosis is aided by a past medical history of pneumothorax, progressive dyspnea on exertion, and interstitial-type chest x-rays. It should be remembered that chylothorax can be the first sign of a malignant lymphoma, and that even thoracic surgery might not give a definitive diagnosis (6).

E. Treatment

Chylothorax is a debilitating condition to the point of threatening life. The main problem in a patient with chylothorax is malnutrition and immunosuppression. Loss of chyle leads to metabolic disturbances, malnutrition, and immunodeficiency caused by the loss of large amounts of protein, fat, electrolytes, and lymphocytes. Therapeutic efforts should be directed towards correction of the leak rather than simply removing the fluid. With improvements in nutritional support and operative treatment, mortality rate is now low.

There is considerable controversy over the management of chylothorax, in particular the relative merits of conservative measures and the timing of surgical intervention. Some authors advocate a conservative approach, while others favor early operative intervention (47,48). However, most agree that either approach must be considered in the light of the specific etiological type of chylothorax and the patient's general condition (8). Conservative management involves drainage of the pleural cavity, measures that reduce chyle flow and supportive nutrition (Table 4).

Traumatic Chylothorax

In around 50% of patients with traumatic chylothorax, spontaneous healing will occur with conservative treatment. Thus, a trial of such treatment is recommended (11,49).

Efforts to reduce chyle formation are extremely important; these include keeping the patient on bed rest and placing the patient on constant gastric suction with a nasogastric tube and cessation of oral intake. Nutritional status is maintained with parenteral hyperalimentation. This, combined with inhibition of gastrointestinal secretions by somatostatin analogues, reduces the volume of

Table 4 Treatment of Chylothorax

Conservative measures
  Repeated thoracocenteses
  Continuous drainage by tube thoracostomy
  Dietary modifications
    Low-fat diet, medium-chain triglyceride diet
    Total parenteral nutrition
  Pleurodesis
Surgical measures
  Pleuroperitoneal shunt
  Ligation of the thoracic duct
    By thoracoscopy
    By thoracotomy
  Fibrin glue to close the leak in the duct
  Pleurectomy
  Treatment of the underlying disease

chyle and promotes resolution (50). A medium-chain triglyceride diet has also been proposed as a means of providing an oral source of calories to the patient. These triglycerides contain fatty acids with a chain length of fewer than 12 carbon atoms and are absorbed into the portal vein directly. Thus, they enter the circulatory system rather than travel through the thoracic duct. However, long-term use can result in deficiencies of linoleic acid, an essential fatty acid present only in long-chain triglycerides (44,51,52).

In the dyspneic patient management begins with the placement of a chest tube. This permits the underlying lung to remain constantly expanded and allows accurate measurement of the rate of chyle leakage.

An alternative to tube thoracostomy is the pleuroperitoneal shunt, which in principle is a one-way subcutaneous connection between the pleura and the peritoneum with a pump, which can be activated by light pressure (11,53). A thoracoscopically assisted procedure allows more accurate and controlled positioning (54). In this way, the chyle is shunted to the peritoneal cavity and, thus, not removed from the body. Therefore, the patient does not become malnourished or immunocompromised. In the peritoneal cavity the chyle is absorbed without creating significant ascites. Shunted peritoneal fluid passes into the venous system via the right lymphatic duct. However, this procedure has a limited success rate, particularly if the right atrial pressure is raised. Disadvantages also include shunt occlusion, chest wall discomfort, and inconvenience of use because it requires daily pumping and, thus, a cooperative patient (55,56).

Factors that predicted the need for surgical intervention were initial esophageal operation and average daily postoperative chest tube drainage greater than 1000 mL/day for 7 days (18). Exploratory thoracotomy and pleurodesis with a sclerosing agent are the two alternatives. At the time of exploratory thoracotomy an attempt is made to find the leak in the duct and to ligate on both sides of the leak. Due to the rich network of collaterals, there are never any problems with lymph stasis afterwards. If the chylothorax is bilateral, a right thoracotomy should be performed because the duct is more readily approached from that side (57). A preoperative lymphangiography may identify the site of the leak. In addition it can demonstrate accessory ducts and the course of the main duct. Other methods that may help identify the site of leak during operation include feeding the patient a high-fat diet several hours before operation. This will increase the flow of chyle and can assist the surgeon in identifying the leak (18,58). Methylene blue staining of the fat meal has also been used for this purpose but provides little additional information as it also stains the surrounding structures (57). In the event that the duct cannot be identified, mass ligation of the tissue between the aorta and azygous vein may be performed (59).

Chemical pleurodesis is a therapeutic alternative for poor-risk patients that are not surgical candidates. The intrapleural instillation of tetracycline, bleomycin, and talc may result in control of the chylothorax (8,60,61). However, pleurodesis by injecting a material through the chest tube is not generally recommended because of low satisfactory experience. If for some reason the thoracic duct cannot be successfully ligated at thoracotomy, a parietal pleurectomy should be performed to obliterate the pleural space (44).

Video-assisted thoracoscopic surgery (VATS) is now considered an effective tool in the management of persisting postoperative chylothorax since the site of the thoracic duct laceration can be identified in most cases. Its low cost and low morbidity rate suggest an earlier use of VATS in the treatment of postoperative chylothorax. With thoracoscopic, minimally invasive procedures, earlier intervention is now favored by many authors, especially if the patient's nutritional status is already poor (4,62–65).

An innovative method for thoracoscopic scaling of duct leaks with fibrin glue has had wide recognition and has been described in premature neonates as well. Accurate preoperative identification of the damaged point with lymphangiography reduces the quantity of glue required (65–67).

For postesophagectomy chylothorax conservative management is recommended for a maximum of only 2 weeks in the absence of any indication for surgery (e.g., unrelenting effusion, chylothorax with complications, such as incarcerated lung). Surgery is indicated when pleural drainage is greater than 1 L per day for more than 5 days (Table 5) (39,68). Some surgeons favor elective ligation of the thoracic duct during radical surgical procedures in order to prevent chylous fistula. This significantly reduces the mortality rate from chylothorax after esophagectomy (19). The preferred site for elective ligation is in the upper abdomen or lower thorax, where there is more constant anatomy (59).

Nontraumatic Chylothorax

The management of nontraumatic chylothorax poses a challenge to the clinician to identify the cause of the leak (20). A CT scan of the mediastinum should be performed in all patients with nontraumatic chylothorax to ascertain whether mediastinal lymphadenopathy is present.

The initial management of a patient with a nontraumatic chylothorax of unknown cause is similar to that of a patient with traumatic chylothorax. The nutritional status of the patient should be preserved by using parenteral hyperalimentation. In most cases tube thoracostomy is performed or alternatively a pleuroperitoneal shunt is inserted. If the chylothorax is not successfully managed with the initial management or the CT scan of the mediastinum is positive, the patient should undergo exploratory thoracotomy or videothoracoscopy. The

Table 5 Indications for Surgery in Chylothorax

Chyle leak greater than 1 L per day for more than 5 days
Persistent leak for more than 2 weeks despite conservative treatment
Nutritional or metabolic complications
Loculated chylothorax or incarcerated lung

mediastinum should be examined for intrathoracic tumor and the thoracic duct should be ligated.

If the patient is known to have lymphoma or metastatic carcinoma, chylothorax may simply be treated by mediastinal irradiation. In one series mediastinal irradiation adequately controlled the chylothorax for the remainder of the patient's life in 68% of those with lymphoma and in 50% of those with metastatic carcinoma (69). If radiation therapy does not successfully control the chylothorax, then pleurodesis with talc or tetracycline may be effective (8). The general impression is that it is more difficult to achieve a chemical pleurodesis in chylothorax than in malignant pleurisy, probably due to the normal pleura and perhaps a neutralizing effect of the chyle. Alternatively, a pleuroperitoneal shunt may be inserted if the patient is symptomatic. Exploratory thoracotomy is probably not indicated in patients with known lymphoma or metastatic carcinoma in view of the dismal prognosis (69).

In lymphangiomyomatosis, pleurodesis or thoracic duct ligation may control the chylothorax, but the disease is progressive and the prognosis is poor (70). Treatment of the underlying disease is important and will, in some cases, cause the chylothorax to disappear. Example is the use of corticosteroids in sarcoidosis (71).

Congenital Chylothorax

Congenital chylothorax is initially treated conservatively with repeated thoracenteses. It usually resolves after one to three thoracenteses (72). However, if the chylothorax persists after the third aspiration then a pleuroperitoneal shunt should be inserted (56). In most of the patients the chylothorax will be successfully managed and the shunt can be removed after several months. If the shunt cannot adequately control the chylothorax, then thoracotomy with thoracic duct ligation should be considered. Surgery performed as early as 7–10 days after diagnosis of chylothorax certainly shortens hospitalization time. Waiting 2–4 weeks, however, reduces the need for surgical intervention substantially. Delaying surgery in a patient with pertinacious chylothorax > 4 weeks is not recommendable (32).

The standard treatment of chylothorax in pediatric intensive care today includes conservative therapy with fat-free nutrition, total parenteral nutrition and, if this is not successful, operative treatment (pleurodesis, pleuroperitoneal shunt, ligation of the duct).

In children with high central venous pressures, thrombosis of the superior vena cava, or after caval-pulmonary anastomosis, conservative management usually fails (32,56). Somatostatin as treatment of chylothorax has also been described in neonates. The acting mechanism is unknown. On the one hand, it might be a result of vasoconstriction of the vessels in the splanchnic area resulting in reduced intestinal perfusion. On the other hand it is believed that the lymphatic vessels have somatostatin receptors, like the blood vessels in the splanchnic area, and the constriction reduces lymph production. The continuous infusion of somatostatin is a new therapeutic option for treatment of chylothorax and could reduce surgical intervention and hospitalization time, as well as allow earlier enteral feeding (73,74). In severely ill neonates with chylothorax, increasing mean airway pressure by pressure control ventilation and positive end-expiratory pressure should be considered as a therapeutic intervention acting probably in the same way that an increase in mean airway pressure can assist postoperative hemostasis in cardiothoracic patients (75).

Impaired defense mechanisms, nutritional compromise and the presence of indwelling foreign bodies, such as intercostal drains, make the patient vulnerable to life-threatening opportunistic infections.

II. Pseudochylothorax

Pseudochylothorax is the collection of chyliform fluid in the pleural space. The fluid is milky or turbid, caused by high levels of cholesterol or lecithin-globulin complexes. Chylomicrons are, however, not present, and the entity has nothing to do with lymphatic vessels or chyle. Pseudochylothorax is much less common than chylothorax and accounts for approximately 10% of pleural effusions rich in lipids (69).

A. Etiology

Tuberculosis is by far the most frequent cause of pseudochylothorax, accounting for 54% of all cases, with a remarkable association with previous collapse therapy and long-term effusions (76). Patients who have been treated with artificial pneumothorax for pulmonary tuberculosis and who have a chronic pleural effusion secondary to the atelectatic lung are particularly likely to develop a pseudochylothorax (76,77).

Residual pleural effusions after appropriate antituberculous treatment should be closely followed up, because a previous successful drug treatment does not preclude the development of pseudochylothorax (38). The increasing problem with multiresistant forms of tuberculosis might cause a revival of pneumothorax treatment, so pseudochylothorax might also be of interest in the future (6).

Rheumatoid arthritis is a much less common cause of pseudochylothorax (78–80). It is likely that rheumatoid arthritis as a cause of pseudochylothorax will continue to decline, as early diagnosis and precocious and aggressive treatment are the rule.

Other causes are traumatic, i.e., profuse bleeding in the pleura which becomes organized, remnants of poorly treated empyemas, and other diseases with thickened pleura and chronic pleural effusion such as malignancy (6). Paragonimiasis, syphilis, and diabetes may also be associated with pseudochylothorax (81,82). Pseudochylothorax has not been associated with asbestos-related diffuse pleural thickening. Possibly, in this type of pleural fibrosis, the fibrotic tissue contained is too dense, and there is no central pool of fluid, so that conditions for cholesterol pleurisy do not exist (6).

The pathogenesis of pseudochylothorax is not precisely known. Most patients have markedly thickened pleural surfaces and longstanding pleural effusions. The mean duration of the effusion is 5 years until it becomes chyliform, but occasionally it can turn chyliform within 1 year of onset. Typically, pseudochylothorax is seen in fluid, which is encapsulated in a fibrotic area of a grossly thickened pleura. The fibrotic scar tissue, which forms the walls of the chamber, is poorly vascularized, so there is little absorption of any substances in the fluid. It has been supported that the thickened pleura hinders the transfer of cholesterol out of the pleural space, which gradually leads to high cholesterol levels in the fluid. The cholesterol and other lipids are thought to derive from degenerating white and red blood cells in the pleural fluid (76,77). In contrast to the cholesterol in acute exudates, which is mostly bound to low-density lipoproteins (LDL), analysis has shown that there is a predominant binding of the cholesterol to high-density lipoprotein (HDL). This implies that it is derived from serum lipoproteins rather than from cellular debris (38).

It has been hypothesized that the cholesterol that enters the pleural space with acute pleural inflammation becomes trapped in the pleural space and undergoes a change in lipoprotein-binding characteristics (38). It is noteworthy that serum cholesterol levels and systemic cholesterol metabolism are essentially normal in patients with pseudochylothorax. Pseudochylothorax has a tendency to enlarge slowly, probably due to osmotic effects (6). Chyliform pleural effusions are usually unilateral, but bilateral involvement has been reported. Both sides of the chest are affected with equal frequency.

B. Diagnosis

Symptoms are related to the underlying disease or to the impairment of pulmonary function caused by the pleural effusion and the thickened pleura.

The diagnosis of pseudochylothorax is usually not difficult. The clinical picture usually helps in differentiating pseudochylothorax from chylothorax. Pseudochylothorax more often occurs in patients with chronic pleural effusions and thickened pleura, whereas chylothorax is usually acute and the pleura is thin. If after centrifugation of the pleural fluid the supernatant clears, then the white color of the fluid is due to large numbers of white and red blood cells and debris and the patient most likely has an empyema. However, if the supernatant remains opalescent, then the patient has a chylous or chyliform pleural effusion. The fluid should then be examined for the presence of cholesterol crystals. Cholesterol crystals are usually easily recognized as rhomboid structures microscopically. The presence of cholesterol crystals establishes the diagnosis of pseudochylothorax. However, not all patients with pseudochylothorax have cholesterol crystals in their pleural fluid, but most of them have elevated cholesterol levels in the fluid >250 mg/dL and a pleural fluid triglyceride level below 110 mg/dL (77). Addition of 1–2 mL of ethyl ether to the pleural fluid clears the supernatant if opalescence is caused by high cholesterol levels. Factors determining the formation of cholesterol crystals are not clear. Cholesterol crystals have been reported with pleural fluid cholesterol levels below 150 mg/dL, whereas pleural fluids with cholesterol levels above 800 mg/dL have had none (77). Cholesterol levels may also be elevated in chylous pleural effusions (37). If cholesterol crystals are not seen, lipoprotein electrophoresis will confirm the diagnosis.

Pleural biopsy with subsequent culture and histological examination has a low yield for etiological diagnosis, not much higher than fluid culture alone in cases of tuberculosis, and is also a potential source for complications such as secondary empyema. Therefore, if pseudochylothorax of tuberculous origin is suspected, biopsy can be delayed until Lowenstein culture of fluid has proved negative. Adenosine deaminase (ADA) values in pleural fluid are not a major aid for diagnosis of active tuberculous pseudochylothorax and should not be used to sustain any therapeutic decision (82).

C. Treatment

In most cases there is a benign course. Intervention is needed only if the patient has symptoms or if there has been a substantial increase in size (6).

If the patient has symptoms, thoracentecis should be performed, not only to relieve dyspnea but also to prevent complications, which can occur in untreated pseudochylothorax. Complications of pseudochylothorax are respiratory insufficiency, infections (reactivation of tuberculosis, nonspecific infection, fungal infection, particularly *Aspergillus*), and pleurocutaneous or bronchopleural fistulae (Table 6). The peel is often of considerable thickness and in addition calcified, which makes puncture difficult (long needles may be needed). Moreover, the walls around the fluid are stiff, and thus may not adapt easily when the fluid is withdrawn so that a negative pressure can develop if forceful suction is applied. The patient immediately feels this, and further removal of the fluid is painful and meaningless unless air is allowed to enter to equalize the pressures (6). Recurrence is common, and complications may also occur after fluid removal.

Cultures for tuberculosis should always be made on the fluid, since a reactivation of this infection is always possible. Antituberculous treatment

Table 6 Complications of Pseudochylothorax

Respiratory insufficiency
Infections
   Reactivation of tuberculosis
   Nonspecific infection
   Fungal infection
Fistulae: bronchopleural, pleurocutaneous

should be started in patients with isolation of *M. tuberculosis*. Even if the cultures are negative, in a patient who has a history of tuberculosis and has never received antituberculous therapy, a course of chemotherapy should be given.

PPD-positive individuals may also be candidates to receive antimycobacterial treatment if they have progressive effusions (6,82).

Surgical options, such as pulmonary decortication, may be reserved for recurrent symptomatic cases in which medical treatment has proved ineffective and the underlying lung is believed to be functional (82,83).

References

1. Flarer R, Oschsner A. Traumatic chylothorax: a report of a fatal case complicated by a ruptured duodenal ulcer. Surgery 1945; 17:622–623.
2. Cha EM, Sirijintakarn P. Anatomic variation of the thoracic duct and visualization of mediastinal lymph nodes. Radiology 1976; 119:45–48.
3. Kinnaert P. Anatomical variations of the cervical portion of the thoracic duct in man. J Anat 1973; 115:45–52.
4. Janssen JP, Joosten HJ, Postmus PE. Thoracoscopic treatment of postoperative chylothorax after coronary bypass surgery. Thorax 1994; 49:1273.
5. Restoy EG, Cueto FB, Arenas EE, Duch AA. Spontaneous bilateral chylothorax: uniform features of a rare condition. Eur Respir J 1988; 1:872–873.
6. Hillerdal G. Chylothorax and pseudochylothorax. Eur Respir J 1997; 10:1157–1162.
7. Valentine VG, Raffin TA. The management of chylothorax. Chest 1992; 102:586–591.
8. Merrigan BA, Winter DC, O'Sullivan GC. Chylothorax. Br J Surg 1997; 84:15–20.
9. Bower GC. Chylothorax: observations in 20 cases. Dis Chest 1964; 46:464–468.
10. Bessone LN, Ferguson TB, Burford TH. Chylothorax. Collective review. Ann Thorac Surg 1971; 12:527–550.
11. Paes ML, Powell H. Chylothorax: an update. Br J Hosp Med 1994; 51:482–490.
12. Romero S. Nontraumatic chylothorax. Curr Opin Pulm Med 2000; 6:287–291.
13. Fairfax AJ, Mc Nabb WR, Spiro SG. Chylothorax: a review of 18 cases. Thorax 1986; 41:880–885.
14. Mc Farlane RJ, Holman CW. Chylothorax. Am Rev Respir Dis 1972; 105:287–291.
15. Judson MA, Postic B. Chylothorax in a patient with AIDS and Kaposi's sarcoma. South Med J 1990; 83:322–324.
16. Bogner JR, Gross M, Zietz C, Mandel I, Zollner N. Chylothorax as fatal complication in fulminating Kaposi's sarcoma in a patient with AIDS. Klin Wochenschr 1991; 69:134.
17. Mc Williams A, Gabbay E. Chylothorax occurring 23 years post-irradiation: literature review and management strategies. Respirology 2000; 5:301–303.
18. Cerfolio RJ, Allen MS, Deschamps C, Trastek VF, Pairolero PC. Postoperative chylothorax. J Thorac Cardiovasc Surg 1996; 112:1361–1366.
19. Bolger C, Walsh TN, Tanner WA, Keeling P, Hennessy TP. Chylothorax after oesophagectomy. Br J Surg 1991; 78:587–588.

20. Strausser JL, Flye MW. Management of nontraumatic chylothorax. Ann Thorac Surg 1981; 31:520–526.
21. Light RW. Chylothorax and pseudochylothorax. Pleural Diseases. Philadelphia: Lea Febiger, 1990:269–281.
22. Vallieres E, Shamji FM, Todd TR. Post pneumonectomy chylothorax. Ann Thorac Surg 1993; 55:1006–1008.
23. Hughes RL, Mintzer RA, Hidvegi DF, Freinkel RK, Cugell DW. The management of chylothorax. Chest 1979; 76:212–218.
24. Nygaard SD, Berger HA, Fick RB. Chylothorax as a complication of oesophageal sclerotherapy. Thorax 1992; 47:134–135.
25. Thorne PS. Traumatic chylothorax. Tubercle 1958; 39:29–34.
26. Servelle M, Nogues CI, Soulie J, Andrieux JB, Terhedebrugge R. Spontaneous, postoperative and traumatic chylothorax. J Cardiovasc Surg 1980; 21:475–486.
27. Sassoon CS, Light RW. Chylothorax and pseudochylothorax. In: Light RW, ed. Clinics in Chest Medicine: Symposium on Pleural Diseases. Philadelphia: WB Saunders, 1985:163–172.
28. Chernick V, Reed MH. Pneumothorax and chylothorax in the neonatal period. J Pediatr 1970; 76:624–632.
29. van Sraaten HLM, Gerards LJ, Krediet TG. Chylothorax in the neonatal period. Eur J Pediatr 1993; 52:2–5.
30. Randolph JG, Gross RE. Congenital chylothorax. Arch Surg 1957; 74:409–414.
31. Bond SJ, Guzzetta PC, Snyder ML, Randolph JG. Management of pediatric postoperative chylothorax. Ann Thorac Surg 1993; 56:469–473.
32. Buttiker V, Fanconi S, Burger R. Chylothorax in children. Guidelines for diagnosis and management. Chest 1999; 116:682–687.
33. Riquet M, Darse-Derippe J, Saab M, Puyo P, Legmann P, Debesse B. Chylomediastin apres mediastinoscopie: a propos d'une observation. Rev Mal Respir 1993; 10: 473–476.
34. de Winter RJ, Bresser P, Romer JWP, Kromhout JG, Reekers J. Idiopathic chylopericardium with bilateral reflux of chyle. Am Heart J 1994; 127:936–939.
35. Rose DM, Colvin SB, Danilowicz D, Isom OW. Cardiac tamponade secondary to chylopericardium following cardiac surgery: case report and review of the literature. Ann Thorac Surg 1982; 34:333–336.
36. Van Aerde J, Campbell AN, Smyth JA, Lloyd D, Bryan MH. Spontaneous chylothorax in newborns. Am J Dis Child 1984; 138:961–964.
37. Staats BA, Ellefson RD, Budahn LL, Dines DE, Prakash UB, Offord K. The lipoprotein profile of chylous and nonchylous pleural effusions. Mayo Clin Proc 1980; 55:700–704.
38. Hamn H, Pfalzer B, Fabel H. Lipoprotein analysis in a chyliform pleural effusion: implications for pathogenesis and diagnosis. Respiration 1991; 58:294–300.
39. Teba L, Dedhia HV, Bowen R, Alexander JC. Chylothorax review. Crit Care Med 1985; 13:49–52.
40. Marts BC, Naunheim KS, Fiore AC, Pennington DG. Conservative versus surgical management of chylothorax. Am J Surg 1992; 164:532–534.
41. Machleder HI, Paulus H. Clinical and immunological alterations observed in patients undergoing long-term thoracic duct drainage. Surgery 1978; 84:157–165.
42. Fish JC, Sarles HE, Remmers AR Jr, Townsend CM Jr, Bell JD, Flye MW. Renal transplantation after thoracic duct drainage. Ann Surg 1981; 193:752–756.

43. Bell JD, Marshall GD, Shaw BA, Fish JC, Flye MW, Remmers AR Jr, Sarles HE. Alterations in human thoracic duct lymphocytes during thoracic duct drainage. Transplant Proc 1983; 15:677–680.
44. Puntis JW, Roberts JD, Handy D. How should chylothorax be managed? Arch Dis Child 1987; 38:593–596.
45. Sachs PB, Zelch MB, Rice TW, Geisinger MA, Risius B, Lammert GK. Diagnosis and localization of laceration of the thoracic duct: usefulness of lymphangiography and CT. Am J Roentgenol 1991; 157:703–705.
46. Ngan H, Fok M, Wong J. The role of lymphography in chylothorax following thoracic surgery. Br J Radiol 1988; 61:1032–1036.
47. Johnstone DW, Feins RH. Chylothorax. Chest Surg Clin North Am 1994; 4:617–628.
48. Milsom JW, Kron IL, Rheuban KS, Rodgers BM. Chylothorax: an assessment of current surgical management. J Thorac Cardiovasc Surg 1985; 89:221–227.
49. Terzi A, Furlan G, Magnanelli G, Terrini A, Ivic N. Chylothorax after pleuropulmonary surgery: a rare but unavoidable complication. J Thorac Cardiovasc Surg 1994; 42:81–84.
50. Ulibari JI, Sanz Y, Fuentes C, Mancha A, Aramendia M, Sanchez S. Reduction of lymphorrhagia from ruptured thoracic duct by somatostatin. Lancet 1990; 336:258.
51. Martin IC, Marinho LH, Brown AE, Mc Robbie D. Medium chain triglycerides in the management of chylous fistula following neck dissection. Br J Maxillofac Surg 1993; 24:227–230.
52. Jalili F. Medium chain triglycerides and total parenteral nutrition in the management of infants with congenital chylothorax. South Med J 1987; 80:1290–1293.
53. Kitchen ND, Hocken DB, Greenalgh RM, Kaplan DK. Use of the Denver pleuroperitoneal shunt in the treatment of chylothorax secondary to filariasis. Thorax 1991; 46:144–145.
54. Miyamura H, Watanabe H, Eguchi S, Suzuki T. Ligation of the thoracic duct through transabdominal phrenotomy for chylothorax after heart operations (letter). J Thorac Cardiovasc Surg 1994; 107:316.
55. Sade RW, Wiles HB. Pleuroperitoneal shunt for persistent pleural drainage after Fountain procedure. J Thorac Cardiovasc Surg 1990; 100:621–623.
56. Murphy MC, Newman BM, Rodgers BM. Pleuroperitoneal shunts in the management of persistent chylothorax. Ann Thorac Surg 1989; 48:195–200.
57. Robinson CLN. The management of chylothorax. Ann Thorac Surg 1985; 39:90–95.
58. Zoetmulder F, Rutgers E, Baas P. Thoracoscopic ligation of a thoracic duct leakage. Chest 1994; 106:1233–1234.
59. Patterson GA, Todd TRJ, Delarue NC, Ilves R, Pearson FG, Cooper JD. Supradiaphragmatic ligation of the thoracic duct in intractable chylous fistula. Ann Thorac Surg 1981; 32:44–49.
60. Norum J, Aasebo U. Intrapleural bleomycin in the treatment of chylothorax. J Chemother 1994; 6:427–430.
61. Adler RH, Levinsky L. Persistent chylothorax. Treatment by talc pleurodesis. J Thorac Cardiovasc Surg 1978; 76:859–863.
62. Fahimi H, Casselman FP, Mariani MA, van Boven WJ, Knaepen PJ, van Swieten HA. Current management of postoperative chylothorax. Ann Thorac Surg 2001; 71:448–450.
63. Peillon C, D'Hont C, Melki J, Fattouh F, Perrier G, Dujon A, Testart J. Usefulness

of video thoracoscopy in the management of spontaneous and postoperation chylothorax. Surg Endosc 1999; 13:1106–1109.
64. Yeam I, Sassoon C. Hemothorax and chylothorax. Curr Opin Pulm Med 1997; 3:310–314.
65. Graham DD, McGahren ED, Tribble CG, Daniel TM, Rodgers BM. Use of video assisted thoracic surgery in the treatment of chylothorax. Ann Thorac Surg 1994; 57:1507–1511.
66. Akaogi E, Mitsui K, Sohara Y, Endo S, Ishikawa S, Hori M. Treatment of postoperative chylothorax with intrapleural fibrin glue. Ann Thorac Surg 1989; 48:116–118.
67. Inderbitzi RG, Krebs T, Stirneman T, Althaus U. Treatment of postoperative chylothorax by fibrin glue application under thoracoscopic view with the use of local anaesthetic (letter). J Thorac Cardiovasc Surg 1994; 104:209–210.
68. Orringer MB, Bluett M, Deeb GM. Aggressive treatment of chylothorax complicating transhiatal oesophagectomy without thoracotomy. Surgery 1988; 104:720–726.
69. Roy PH, Carr DT, Payne WS. The problem of chylothorax. Mayo Clin Proc 1967; 42:457–467.
70. Taylor JR, Ryu J, Colby TV, Raffin TA. Lymphangioleiomyomatosis: clinical course in 32 patients. N Engl J Med 1990; 323:1254–1260.
71. Jarman PR, Whyte MKB, Sabroe I, Hughes JMB. Sarcoidosis presenting with chylothorax. Thorax 1995; 50:1324–1325.
72. Perry RE, Hodgman J, Cass AB. Pleural effusions in the neonatal period. J Pediatr 1963; 62:838–843.
73. Buettiker V, Hug MI, Burger R, Baenziger O. Somatostatin: a new therapeutic option for the treatment of chylothorax. Intensive Care Med 2001; 27:1083–1086.
74. Rimensberger PC, Muller-Schenker B, Kalangos A, Beghetti M. Treatment of a persistent postoperative chylothorax with somatostatin. Ann Thorac Surg 1998; 66:253–254.
75. Ragosta KG, Alfieris G. Chylothorax: a novel therapy. Crit Care Med 2000; 28:1208–1209.
76. Hillerdal G. Chyliform (cholesterol) pleural effusion. Chest 1985; 88:426–428.
77. Coe JE, Aikawa JK. Cholesterol pleural effusion. Arch Intern Med 1961; 108:763–774.
78. Ferguson GC. Cholesterol pleural effusion in rheumatoid lung disease. Thorax 1966; 21:577–582.
79. Stengel BF, Watson RR, Darling RJ. Pulmonary rheumatoid nodule with cavitation and chronic lipid effusion. JAMA 1966; 198:1263–1266.
80. Lee SS, Trimble R. Rheumatoid arthritis with bloody and cholesterol pleural effusion. Arch Pathol Lab Med 1985; 109:769–771.
81. Johnston JR, Falk A, Iber C, Davies S. Paragonimiasis in the United States. A report of nine cases in Hmong immigrants. Chest 1982; 82:168–171.
82. Garcia-Zamalloa A, Ruiz-Irastorza G, Aguayo FJ, Gurrutxaga N. Pseudochylothorax. Report of 2 cases and review of the literature. Medicine (Baltimore) 1999; 78:200–207.
83. Goldman A, Burford TH. Cholesterol pleural effusion: a report of three cases with a cure by decortication. Dis Chest 1950; 18:586–594.

49

The Pleural Space and Organ Transplantation

MARC A. JUDSON and STEVEN A. SAHN

Medical University of South Carolina
Charleston, South Carolina, U.S.A.

I. Introduction

More than 21,000 solid organ transplants were performed in the United States in 1999 (1). The number of living organ transplant recipients has reached a level where sub-specialists and generalists are involved in the medical management of these patients. In particular, it has become essential for pulmonologists to have a detailed understanding of pulmonary problems associated with organ transplantation.

Several years ago we reviewed the spectrum of pleural disease as it relates to organ transplantation, both before and after the procedure (2). This chapter serves as an update of this review. Pleural considerations of each organ transplant will be reviewed separately, although many of the infectious complications and posttransplant lymphoproliferative disorders (PTLD) relate to the level and duration of immunosuppression and are not organ-specific. Table 1 lists the pleural diseases post-transplantation that are not related to a specific organ transplant.

II. Bone Marrow Transplantation

A. Evaluation of Pleural Disease Pretransplant

Bone marrow transplantation (BMT) is performed for a variety of diseases including aplastic anemia, thalassemias, immunodeficiency and genetic disor-

Table 1 Pleural Disease After Transplantation (Not Organ-Specific)

Pleural effusion
  Infection
    Uncomplicated parapneumonic
    Complicated parapneumonic/empyema
  PTLD with pleural involvement
  Primary effusion lymphoma
  Iatrogenic
    Central venous line
      Pleural effusion
      Hemothorax
      Chylothorax
      Pneumothorax

PTLD = posttransplant lymphoproliferative disorder.
Source: Adapted from Ref. 2.

ders, leukemias, lymphomas, and solid organ malignancies (3). Pleural effusions associated with these diseases should be evaluated by thoracentesis prior to BMT to exclude infection and residual tumor (2).

Pleural effusions are rare at the time of diagnosis in Hodgkin's disease but not uncommon in non-Hodgkin's lymphoma. A review of the literature (4) reported only one (0.3%) of 269 patients with Hodgkin's disease had a pleural effusion at presentation, whereas the incidence of pleural effusion with untreated non-Hodgkin's lymphoma has been reported to be 12–71% (5–7). As Hodgkin's disease progresses, the incidence of pleural effusions increases to 30% in some series (8) and 30–60% at postmortem (9,10). Extrapleural involvement with lymphoma may also be seen with displacement or invasion of the extrapleural fat stripe (11).

Pleural effusions associated with Hodgkin's lymphoma are usually a consequence of lymphatic or venous obstruction from mediastinal adenopathy (12), whereas direct pleural infiltration is the predominant cause in non-Hodgkin's lymphoma (4). Chylous pleural effusions may result from obstruction of the thoracic duct from tumor (6); this is more common with non-Hodgkin's lymphoma than Hodgkin's disease (13).

Because pleural infiltration is a more common cause of pleural effusion in non-Hodgkin's than Hodgkin's lymphoma, the diagnosis of lymphomatous pleural effusion is more easily established with non-Hodgkin's lymphoma. The presence of blood fluid suggests direct pleural involvement, and a transudate is usually seen early in the course of impaired lymphatic pleural space drainage (4). The nucleated cell count is often low, with a predominance of lymphocytes that may approach 100% (14). The pH and glucose are usually normal, but they may be low (10). Cytological examination of the pleural fluid and pleural biopsy have a diagnostic yield of 73–90% in non-Hodgkin's lymphoma (6,15). The combination of immunophenotypic analysis with cytological examination has increased the sensitivity and specificity to as high as 100% for non-Hodgkin's lymphoma (16) so that thoracentesis alone is the diagnostic procedure of choice for this malignancy (7,16,17).

Although thoracentesis needs to be performed in patients with lymphoma prior to BMT to exclude infection, the presence of lymphomatous pleural involvement is not an absolute contraindication to BMT (2,18). However, the presence of pleural involvement portends a greater risk of relapse of Hodgkin's disease after BMT (19). In a study of 100 consecutive patients with Hodgkin's disease receiving autologous BMT, the presence of pleural disease prior to BMT was found to be a poor prognostic factor for disease-free survival. None of 7 patients with pleural disease prior to BMT were free from relapse at 3 years (19). Bone marrow transplantation has also been successfully performed in patients with non-Hodgkin's lymphoma with pleural involvement (20).

Treatment of lymphoma may result in pleural disease. Methotrexate may cause pleurisy (21), pleural effusion (21,22), and pleural thickening (23). In one report, pleurisy occurred in 14 (4%) of 317 patients who received one to several 50 mg intramuscular doses of methotrexate (21). Four (29%) of the 14 patients developed pleural effusions without parenchymal infiltrates. Bleomycin (24,25) has been reported to cause pleural effusion and pleural thickening. These pleural complications have always been associated with an interstitial pneumonitis from bleomycin. A case of massive bilateral pleural effusions has been reported that was thought to be an idiosyncratic reaction from high-dose cyclophosphamide (4200 mg intravenously for 2 consecutive days) with Mesna rescue given as pretreatment prior to BMT (26).

Radiation therapy to the thorax can cause pleural effusions by two mechanisms: (1) radiation pleuritis and (2) systemic venous hypertension, lymphatic obstruction, or constrictive pericarditis from mediastinal fibrosis (4). Ipsilateral pleural effusions have been reported in 6% of patients with breast carcinoma who received radiation therapy (27), all of whom received 4000–6000 rads. The effusions developed between 2 weeks and 6 months after completion of radiation therapy, and all patients had radiation pneumonitis either prior to or simultaneously with the pleural effusion. These effusions lasted a minimum of 4 months to several years. Over time, the amount of fluid remained constant or decreased slightly, and there was an increase in the degree of adhesions and tendency for loculation.

Pleural effusions may also occur 1–2 years after completion of intensive (4000–6000 rads) mediastinal radiation from mediastinal fibrosis that causes constrictive pericarditis, superior vena cava syndrome, or lymphatic obstruction (28). These complications should be considered if other causes of pleural effusion have been excluded and the appropriate time has elapsed between completion of radiation therapy and the development of a pleural effusion.

Pleural effusions may develop prior to BMT from fluid overload secondary to intravenous hydration or infusion of blood products. This is probably a common cause of pleural effusion prior to BMT, although to our knowledge the incidence of pleural effusions from fluid overload has not been determined.

Spontaneous pneumothorax may rarely occur in patients with lymphoma, usually after thoracic radiation (29,30). It is more common with Hodgkin's lymphoma than non-Hodgkin's lymphoma. In one series (29) the incidence of spontaneous pneumothorax in patients with Hodgkin's lymphoma who received thoracic radiation was 2.2% (3 of 138). Most patients received radiation within 3 years of the pneumothorax, and most were younger than 30 years of age (29–32). It has been postulated that pneumothorax develops in these patients from radiation pneumonitis coupled with the presence of subapical blebs that often cause pneumothoraces in tall asthenic individuals (33). Pneumothorax from cytotoxic chemotherapy without radiation occurs much less commonly than from radiation therapy (34,35). It has been proposed that chemotherapy-induced pneumothorax results from rapid tumor lysis leading to tissue necrosis or from rupture of subpleural-based tumor nodules (33).

B. Evaluation of Pleural Disease Posttransplant

Approximately half of BMT recipients develop a pulmonary complication, and half will die of the complication (36,37). Despite these statistics, there are few data available concerning pleural disease after BMT. One study (37) that addressed this issue reported a 16% (9 of 57) incidence of pleural effusion within the first 100 days after BMT. The etiologies of these effusions were not reported in all cases, but more than half (5 of 9) were associated with pneumonia. Causes of pleural disease after BMT are listed in Table 2.

Table 2 Pleural Disease After Bone Marrow Transplantation[a]

Pleural effusion
Hepatic veno-occlusive disease
Recurrent tumor
Iatrogenic
Volume overload
GVHD
Pneumothorax
Obstructive airway disease (chronic GVHD)

[a] See Table 1 for additional pleural diseases associated with transplantation.
GVHD: graft-versus-host disease.
Source: Adapted from Ref. 2.

Noninfectious Causes of Pleural Effusion

We suspect that the most common cause of pleural effusion after BMT is fluid overload because of intravenous overhydration or the need for blood products. These effusions are usually right-sided or bilateral with more fluid in the right pleural space. Thoracentesis is not required if a pleural effusion develops in an appropriate temporal relationship to the intravenous administration of a large volume of fluids and/or blood products, and the patient has no clinical evidence of infection (2).

Because BMT recipients frequently require central venous access and invasive procedures, iatrogenic pleural effusions may occur. A chylothorax has been reported in a BMT recipient as a complication of right subclavian vein thrombosis from a central venous catheter insertion (38).

A syndrome has recently been described of multiorgan failure from a generalized capillary endothelial injury that occurs at the time of engraftment in BMT recipients (39). This syndrome occurs within one week of engraftment and is characterized by fever, rash, hypotension, and edema including ascites and pleural effusions (39,40). Renal and hepatic failure are common (40). This syndrome may occur in autologous and allogeneic BMT recipients (40). It has been proposed that the capillary leak may be the result of release of mediators, proteolytic enzymes, and toxic oxygen metabolites released from leukocytes (40). It is known that leukocytes of patients recovering from BMT have abnormally high oxidative metabolism and often secrete large quantities of cytokines (41). Although there was a report of 29 BMT recipients who developed this syndrome (40) with associated pleural effusions, the frequency of pleural effusions was not noted and pleural fluid characteristics were not reported.

Hepatic veno-occlusive disease (VOD) is a fibrous obliteration of hepatic venules characterized by jaundice, hepatomegaly and/or right upper quadrant pain, ascites, and/or unexplained weight gain (42). VOD occurs in approximately 20% of allogeneic and 5–10% of autologous bone marrow transplantations in which chemotherapy or radiotherapy is used prior to transplantation (42–45). Pleural effusions have been observed in 50% (7 of 14) of BMT recipients who developed VOD after transplantation compared to 3% (1 of 36) of BMT recipients without VOD (iatrogenic pleural effusion) (46). Patients with pleural effusion and VOD had either tachypnea (4/7) or no respiratory signs or symptoms (3/7). It is thought that the pleural fluid probably originates in the peritoneal space because most patients have ascites and none have cardiomegaly (46). The effusions are right-sided or bilateral, with the larger effusion on the right side. VOD usually precedes the development of a pleural effusion by 7 days. VOD lasts from postoperative day 13 to day 29, whereas pleural effusions are present from postoperative day 20 through day 27 (46). Both VOD and the pleural effusions resolve without thoracentesis or tube thoracostomy.

Graft-versus-host disease (GVHD) is a serious complication of allogeneic BMT (47). On occasion, GVHD following BMT is associated with sterile serosal effusions. In a review of 1905 allogeneic BMT recipients, 15 (0.8%) patients were identified who had effusions in two or more of the following cavities: pleural, peritoneal, and pericardial (48). VOD and iatrogenic causes explained 8 of these multiple effusions. The remaining 7 "unexplained" multiple effusions were the result of either acute or chronic GVHD. Five of seven had associated cytomegalovirus (CMV) disease. All the effusions were transudative and developed after engraftment, and in 6 of 7 cases the effusions developed within 100 days of BMT. Four of the patients required chest tube drainage. Most effusions resolved within one month, although they were present at death in 4 patients. An additional case has been reported of a massive pleural and pericardial effusion from chronic GVHD after allogeneic BMT (49). The diagnosis was established by immunophenotypic analysis of pleural fluid lymphocytes.

PTLD may develop early after BMT, and the clinical course is often rapidly progressive with a high mortality (50). The majority of these disorders are of B-cell phenotype and are associated with Epstein-Barr virus (EBV) infection (51). Isolated ascites may occur in BMT patients developing PTLD (52). Recently, a case was reported of isolated pleuroperitoneal effusions from PTLD in a BMT recipient (53). The diagnosis was established by morphological, immunocytological, and molecular studies that demonstrated B-cell origin of the lymphocytes and high titers of EBV.

Isolated pleural effusions may be a manifestation of leukemia relapse after BMT. The diagnosis of pleural relapse can be confirmed by immunophenotyping, cytogenetic, and gene rearrangement studies of pleural lymphocytes obtained by thoracentesis (54,55).

Infectious Causes of Pleural Effusion

The incidence of pleural effusions of an infectious cause after BMT is unknown. One report (37) identified pleural effusions in 16% of 57 BMT recipients within the first 100 days after BMT. Five (39%) of 13 of patients with "nonbacterial, nonfungal pneumonia" had pleural effusions, which included pneumonias characterized as "idiopathic," "unknown," and from CMV, mycobacteria, and *Pneumocystis carinii*. One effusion was a *Candida albicans* empyema that required thoracostomy tube drainage. Other cases of pleural effusions from *Candida* species and other fungi have been reported (56–58). We suspect that bacterial pathogens are responsible for the majority of infectious pleural effusions after BMT despite a lack of evidence in the medical literature.

Pneumothorax

Chronic GVHD after BMT is associated with airflow obstruction. Causes of obstruction include bronchitis, bronchiolitis obliterans, emphysema-like changes, and bronchospasm (36). Spontaneous pneumothorax and pneumomediastinum have been reported in BMT recipients with obstructive airway disease from chronic GVHD (59–63). The pneumothoraces occur after the lung disease progresses to end-stage.

III. Heart Transplantation

A. Evaluation of Pleural Disease Pretransplant

Pulmonary venous hypertension is the major factor for the development of pleural effusions in congestive heart failure (4,64). Chest radiographs of patients with pleural effusions from congestive heart failure typically show cardiomegaly and bilateral small to moderate pleural effusions of relatively equal size, with the right slightly greater than the left. There is usually evidence of pulmonary vascular congestion, and the severity of pulmonary edema usually correlates with the presence of pleural effusions (64). The pleural fluid is transudative with predominantly mesothelial cells and lymphocytes, and it is unusual to observe more than 10% neutrophils. Acute diuretic therapy may cause elevations of pleural fluid total protein and lactate dehydrogenase (LDH) levels as well as pleural fluid–to–serum ratios of total protein and LDH. However, these transudates develop increased protein and LDH concentrations and resemble exudates in only 8–37% of cases (65,66).

Pleural effusions have been observed radiographically in 45 (34%) of 132 potential heart transplant recipients (67), but an analysis of these effusions have not been reported. Ettinger and Trulock (68) stated that a thoracentesis is not mandatory in the pretransplant workup of a patient with congestive heart failure unless the cause of the effusion is unclear or atypical clinical or radiographic features are present. These atypical features include a unilateral effusion, bilateral effusions of disparate size, absence of cardiomegaly, fever, pleuritic chest pain, and an inappropriately low PaO_2 (4). If a thoracentesis is performed, a transudate usually confirms congestive heart failure as the cause of the effusion. Some heart transplant candidates may have pleural effusions with equivocal or exudative characteristics because of diuretic therapy (see above), but other causes of pleural exudates should be excluded by appropriate tests.

B. Posttransplant Considerations

Causes of pleural disease after heart transplantation are listed in Table 3.

Noninfectious Causes of Pleural Effusion

Pleural effusions occur in as many as 78% of cardiac surgical patients during the immediate postoperative period. The majority are small, bilateral, or left-sided and are often associated with atelectasis (69). Pleural effusions may result from congestive heart failure, postsurgical hemorrhage, iced saline cardioplegia solution, and entry of blood through unrecognized pleural tears (69–71).

Pleural effusion has been reported in 8 (9%) of 94 of patients after heart transplantation (72). Of these eight effusions, two were associated with pericarditis, one was malignant, one was iatrogenic, and four were unexplained. Two of the unexplained effusions resolved spontaneously, and the other two demonstrated nonspecific pleural inflammation at autopsy. A patient has been reported who underwent cardiac transplantation for sarcoidosis and developed massive

Table 3 Pleural Diseases After Heart Transplantation[a]

Pleural effusion
  Infection associated with preoperative pulmonary infarction
    Parapneumonic effusion (uncomplicated)
    Empyema
  Cytomegalovirus[b]
  Pericarditis
  Hemothorax/diagnosis secondary to endomyocardial biopsy

[a] See Table 1 for additional pleural diseases associated with transplantation.
[b] Appears to be more common after heart transplantation than after other solid organ transplantations.
Source: Adapted from Ref. 2.

pleural and pericardial effusions within 2 weeks after transplantation (73). The pericardial effusion caused pericardial tamponade that responded to pericardiocentesis but recurred and eventually required a pericardial window. The pleural effusion reaccumulated after thoracentesis and eventually required chemical pleurodesis. The pleural fluid was exudative and lymphocyte-predominant. The etiologies of the pleural and pericardial effusions were never determined.

    Iatrogenic pneumothoraces have been reported in heart transplant recipients. Hemothorax may occur after endomyocardial biopsy to exclude allograft rejection (74). This is a rare complication that occurred only once (0.2%) in a series of 661 endomyocardial biopsies of heart transplant recipients in one series (75), twice (0.6%) out of 339 procedures in another series (76), and in two (0.9%) of 232 patients in a third (the number of biopsies was not reported) (77). A case has been reported of a spontaneous hemothorax 2 weeks after heart transplantation that was treated by tube thoracostomy with evacuation of a large hematoma (78).

    A chylothorax rarely occurs after heart transplantation. These usually occur one to three weeks after transplantation (79,80). It has been postulated that injury to collateral lymphatics in the anterior mediastinal, thymic, or parasternal areas may cause a chylothorax (79). These collaterals may develop after injury from previous cardiac surgery (79), although this complication has been reported in cardiac transplant recipients who have never had a previous procedure (80). If a chest tube is placed, the chylothorax may pose problems in cyclosporine dosing, as the high hydrophobicity of the drug causes accumulation in the lipid-rich chylous fluid that is eliminated via the chest tube. High oral doses or intravenous cyclosporine may be required in these cases (81).

    Primary-effusion lymphoma is a rare tumor that has a distinctive presentation with malignant peritoneal, pericardial, or pleural effusions in the absence of an identifiable tumor mass or nodal involvement (82). This tumor is most common in AIDS patients and is caused by human herpesvirus 8 (HHV-8) (82), which is also the cause of multicentric Castleman's disease and Kaposi's sarcoma. A heart transplant patient has been described who developed Kaposi's sarcoma one year after transplantation and 8 years later developed a pleural effusion from primary-effusion lymphoma (83). The lymphoma was diagnosed by immunophenotypic, genotypic, and ultrastructural studies of pleural fluid lymphocytes obtained from thoracentesis.

Infectious Causes of Pleural Effusion

In a review of respiratory complications of 94 consecutive heart transplant recipients (72), empyemas developed in eight (9%) patients. Bacteria and *Aspergillus* species were the most common pathogens.

The pathogenesis of empyema formation after heart transplantation may involve pulmonary infarction. Pulmonary infarctions often develop in the early postoperative period in heart transplant recipients from inadequate collateral circulation from the pulmonary and bronchial arteries or venous stasis because of heart failure, edema, or infection (84,85). These pulmonary infarcts may become infected from bronchial contamination. The infected infarction may develop into a lung abscess, empyema, and/or bronchopleural fistula (86,87). The infarctions that lead to empyema usually are acute and occur within a week prior to heart transplantation in most cases (86,87).

Empyemas after heart transplantation have been reported from *Salmonella enteritidis* (88), *Pseudomonas paucimobilis* (89), *Streptococcus pneumoniae* (90), *Serratia marcescens* (91), *Pseudomonas aeruginosa* (92) (with *Candida* pericarditis), and *Legionella pneumophila* (93) (with bronchopleural fistula). These empyemas usually occur within 4 months of transplantation. A pleuromediastinal cutaneous fistula is a rare complication of heart transplantation that is associated with pneumothorax and may occur early after the procedure from a sternal wound infection (94).

Pleural effusions associated with CMV pneumonia have been reported in heart transplant recipients (95,96). All these patients eventually had pulmonary infiltrates in addition to the effusions, although in one patient a unilateral effusion preceded bilateral pulmonary infiltrates by 12 days (95). These infections occurred between 1 and 6 months after transplantation, which is the period in which CMV pneumonitis frequently develops (97).

Pneumothorax/Hemothorax

Pneumothoraces have occurred in heart transplant recipients as the result of infectious and iatrogenic complications. Pneumothoraces and bronchopleural fistulas have been reported with empyemas in recipients with preoperative pulmonary infarctions (86,87) and in one recipient with a *L. pneumophila* empyema (93). In a series of 338 endomyocardial biopsies performed after heart transplantation (98), there were 3 (0.9%) pleural complications: one hemothorax from a bioptome passing through the suture line of the superior vena cava, one hemothorax, and one pneumothorax related to venipuncture.

C. Donor Considerations

Because a number of heart transplant candidates are critically ill with unstable hemodynamics and a short life expectancy, attempts have been made to liberalize the donor criteria. One heart transplant group broadened selection criteria for donor hearts to include heart donors with pleural disease (99). Eleven hearts from donors with severe chest trauma, pneumothorax in 5 and hemothorax in 8, were used for heart transplantation. The 1-year actuarial survival of recipients with these allografts was not different from those receiving donor hearts fulfilling standard donor criteria.

IV. Liver Transplantation

A. Evaluation of Pleural Disease Pretransplant

Pleural effusions occur in approximately 5% of patients with cirrhosis in the absence of significant cardiopulmonary disease, and it is referred to as hepatic hydrothorax (100). The fluid is a transudate and most often (70%) right-sided, although it may be bilateral (15%) or unilateral on the left (15%) (101). Hepatic hydrothorax usually occurs with clinical ascites, although it may form in its absence. These effusions are thought to be the result of pleuroperitoneal communications through diaphragmatic defects with the normal fluctuation of intrathoracic pressure with respiration causing unidirectional movement of fluid (102). Thoracentesis reveals a serous transudate with a low nucleated cell count and a predominance of mononuclear cells, a pH > 7.40, a glucose similar to serum, and a low amylase (4). Pleural fluid and ascitic fluid have similar characteristics, with protein and LDH concentrations tending to be slightly higher in pleural fluid (103).

Exclusion of other intrathoracic causes of pleural fluid accumulation, including infection, thromboembolic disease, and metastatic carcinoma, is important in the pretransplant evaluation process, particularly when exudative or hemorrhagic effusions are identified (104). Therefore, a diagnostic thoracentesis should be performed in liver transplant candidates with pleural effusions, especially if the effusions are left-sided or associated with fever or pleuritic chest pain.

In a series of liver transplant recipients (105), pleural effusions were found in 8 (18%) of 44 patients. Four of the effusions were less than 10% of the hemithorax, whereas 4 occupied more than 25%. The mean preoperative arterial oxygen tension of patients with pleural effusions was significantly lower than in patients without effusions (75 ± 14 vs. 88 ± 12 mmHg; $p < 0.05$). The total lung capacity was decreased in 4 (50%) of 8 with preoperative pleural effusion compared to 10 (27%) of 36 without effusion. In another series (106), 7 (39%) of 18 liver transplant recipients had pleural effusions at the time of transplantation. Preoperative ascites was more common in those with pleural effusions (5 of 9, 55%) than in those without ascites (2 of 9, 22%). Preoperative respiratory complications including pleural effusions have been shown by regression analysis to be a significant risk factor for postoperative respiratory complications after liver transplantation (107).

B. Posttransplant Considerations

Causes of pleural disease after liver transplantation are listed in Table 4.

Pleural Effusions in the Early Postoperative Period

Pleural effusions are common in the immediate postoperative period after liver transplantation (108). Data concerning early postoperative pleural effusions after liver transplantation are shown in Table 5. The incidence of pleural effusions after liver transplantation has been reported to be between 23 and 100% within the first week after the operation (105–107,109–117). The effusions are usually isolated right effusions or are bilateral and are rarely isolated to the left pleural space (118). Thoracentesis or tube thoracostomy was required in 0–19% of cases for respiratory embarrassment (105,109–112,115,116). The pleural fluid typically has the characteristics of a transudate (108,110,115). The effusions usually develop and enlarge over the first 3 days to one week after surgery (109,110,112). Most effusions resolve within 2–3 weeks, although occasionally they persist for several months (105,109). In one series (109), 7 (70%) of 10 liver transplant recipients whose effusions were increasing more than 72 hours after surgery had subdiaphragmatic disease (three hematomas, one biloma, and three subphrenic abscesses). Other studies (110,112) have reported that the effusions typically enlarge over the first postoperative week before subsiding.

On the basis of these data, we do not believe that routine thoracentesis is warranted if a pleural effusion develops in the early postoperative period following liver transplantation. However, a thoracentesis is indicated for left-sided effusions, effusions that continue to enlarge beyond the first postoperative week, effusions that persist more than 3 weeks after transplantation, fever without an obvious clinical explanation, or the development of pleuritic chest pain.

Postoperative pleural effusions occur in the majority of pediatric liver transplant recipients as they do in adults (119,120). Pleural effusions may cause respiratory compromise more commonly in the pediatric population, as respi-

Table 4 Pleural Diseases After Liver Transplantation[a]

Pleural effusion
   Transudative effusion (common and early after liver transplantation)[b]
   Subphrenic abscess (uncommon)
   Suprahepatic stenosis of inferior vena cava (rare)

[a] See Table 1 for additional pleural diseases associated with transplantation.
[b] See Table 5.
Source: Adapted from Ref. 2.

Table 5 Pleural Effusion Early After Liver Transplantation

n	Incidence of effusion (%)	Postoperative day	Isolated right effusion (%)	Bilateral effusions (%)	Isolated left effusion (%)	Ref.
300	69	NR	NR	NR	NR	174
18	72	3	62	38	0	108
43	77	7	55	45	0	105
42	95	3	NR	NR	NR	109
14	86	7	71	29	0	110
21	48	NR	NR	NR	NR	111
9	100	NR	33	67	0	112
16	69	NR	NR	NR	NR	114
31	68	NR	NR	NR	NR	113
187	37	NR	NR	NR	NR	116

NR = not reported.
Source: Adapted from Ref. 2.

ratory embarrassment from pleural effusion has been reported in more than 30% of 60 pediatric liver transplant recipients (119). These patients required thoracentesis or tube thoracostomy.

Several mechanisms have been proposed to explain the high incidence of pleural effusions in the early postoperative period after liver transplantation. Surgical trauma, injury to the right hemidiaphragm from right upper abdominal dissection and retraction, perioperative infusion of blood products, residual ascites, hypoalbuminemia, and atelectasis all may contribute to the development of effusions (105,115,116). Operative transection of hepatic lymphatics may also make an important contribution to the development of the effusions. The human liver is connected to the undersurface of the diaphragm by ligaments that contain lymphatics. It has been demonstrated in a swine model (swine and human lymphatics have a similar distribution) (121) that hepatic lymphatics communicate with the visceral pleural lymphatics via the pulmonary ligament (121). When the native liver is removed during liver transplantation, these lymphatics are not ligated but transected. These severed lymphatics connecting the liver to the visceral pleura are then free to deposit lymph. It has been proposed that leakage of lymph from these unattached lymphatics results in the immediate development of ascites and subsequent postoperative right pleural effusions via congenital or acquired diaphragmatic defects (121).

Respiratory compliance may also contribute to the development of pleural effusions after liver transplantation. In one study of 18 liver transplant recipients (106), postoperative respiratory compliance was lower in patients with bilateral effusions than in those with right-sided or no effusions. These authors postulated that the decreased compliance was the result of an increased interstitial volume related to the administration of perioperative blood products and intravenous fluids.

Infectious Causes of Pleural Effusion

It has been proposed that empyema may occur after liver transplantation by contamination of the postoperative right hydrothorax (122). This is consistent with the observation that a postoperative pleural effusion is a risk factor for pneumonia in liver transplant recipients (115). Patients with empyemas after liver transplantation need aggressive management because immunosuppressive medications inhibit inflammatory and immune mechanisms (122).

To our knowledge, only one study has examined the incidence of pleural infections after liver transplantation (123). Five (8%) of 60 liver transplant recipients developed pleural infections. The responsible pathogens were *Aspergillus* species (two cases), *Escherichia coli*, *Enterobacter/Klebsiella* species, and *Toxoplasma gondii*. Pleural infections were responsible for 4% (5 of 139) of the infectious complications in these patients. Pleural effusions in liver transplant recipients have also been described with *Nocardia* species, CMV, non-*Aspergillus* fungi, and *Pneumocystis carinii* (115,117,124,125).

Noninfectious Pleural Disease

Rarely a pleural effusion will be the primary manifestation of lymphoma related to posttransplant lymphoproliferative disorder (PTLD) after liver transplantation (126,127). These usually occur months to years after transplantation. The diagnosis may sometimes be made by cytological and flow cytometric analysis of pleural fluid (126).

A lymphocele is another rare cause of a pleural effusion after liver transplantation (128). These effusions are right-sided and develop several weeks to months after liver transplantation (128). The lymphoceles may be successfully excised at laparoscopy.

Diaphragmatic paralysis after liver transplantation may present with atelectasis, right pleural effusion, and respiratory failure (129). Diaphragmatic plication is usually successful in resolving respiratory failure (129).

A case of a large right pleural effusion has been reported from suprahepatic stenosis of the inferior vena cava 4 months after liver transplantation in a one-year-old girl (130). It was thought that the effusion was secondary to ascites and hepatic hydrothorax. The patient was successfully treated by percutaneous balloon angioplasty of the stenotic segment.

Because liver transplant recipients often undergo invasive procedures such as central line insertions and liver biopsies, iatrogenic complications such as hemothorax and pneumothorax may rarely occur (131–135).

V. Kidney Transplantation

A. Evaluation of Pleural Effusions Pretransplant

Pleural effusions are found in approximately 20% of patients receiving chronic hemodialysis at the time of hospitalization (136). The majority of these effusions are caused by congestive heart failure, uremic pleurisy, atelectasis, and parapneumonic effusions. Patients with parapneumonic effusions and atelectasis are more likely to have unilateral effusions than patients with heart failure. The presence of chest pain was not more frequent in patients with parapneumonic effusions than other non–heart failure effusions, but it was not more common when compared with patients with heart failure effusions (136).

Uremic pleural effusions are usually associated with a fibrinous pleuritis (137). Pleuritic chest pain and cough are presenting complaints in one third of cases, but dyspnea is unusual (138). Pleural friction rubs are common (138,139). The chest radiograph usually shows a moderate pleural effusion that may be unilateral or bilateral, although occasionally the effusion is massive (138,140–142). These effusions are usually serosaganuinous to bloody (138,140); however, the fluid may be serous (138,141). The number of nucleated cells tends to be less than $1500/\mu L$ and is usually lymphocyte-predominant; however a neutrophil predominance and pleural fluid eosinophilia have been reported (138,140). The pleural effusions typically resolve with continued dialysis over several weeks, but they may recur (138). Fibrothorax requiring decortication may complicate these effusions (141–143). Uremic pleural effusions are diagnosed clinically when other causes of exudates, particularly tuberculosis pleurisy, have been excluded. Rare causes of pleural effusions in patients undergoing dialysis include brachiocephalic vein stenosis and/or clot from a previous dialysis catheter placement (144) and "reflux chylothorax" from a clot originating at the dialysis catheter site propagating to the left subclavian vein and obstructing the thoracic duct (145).

It has been suggested (104) that pre–renal transplant evaluation of pleural effusions should exclude disease entities that may cause significant morbidity, particularly tuberculosis, empyema, pulmonary infarction, and malignancy. If hypervolemia is suspected as the cause of the effusion, aggressive dialysis resulting in negative fluid balance may be attempted in lieu of thoracentesis; if the effusion resolves, volume overload is confirmed. Otherwise, pleural fluid should be obtained for routine analysis, cytology, and culture. Pleural tissue should be examined histologically as well as cultured to evaluate for tuberculosis.

There is a paucity of literature describing pleural disease in kidney transplant candidates. One study (146) determined that 10% of diabetic and 4.5% of nondiabetic renal transplant candidates ($p > 0.05$) had pleural effusions on their preoperative chest radiographs. The outcome of these patients compared to patients without effusions was not addressed.

B. Posttransplant Considerations

Causes of pleural disease after kidney transplantation are listed in Table 6.

Noninfectious Causes of Pleural Effusion

Several cases of urinothorax have been reported after renal transplantation (147–150). This complication occurs within 3 weeks of transplantation (147–150). The effusion is usually ipsilateral to the transplanted kidney (147,148), but

Table 6 Pleural Disease After Kidney Transplantation[a]

Pleural effusion
   Urinothorax
   Perirenal lymphocele
   Legionella[b]
   Nocardia[b]

[a] See Table 1 for additional pleural diseases associated with transplantation.
[b] Appears to be more common after kidney transplantation than after other solid organ transplants based on frequent case reports.
Source: Adapted from Ref. 2.

not always (150). Typically the urine output decreases and serum creatinine increases in concert with the development of the pleural effusion. The cause of urinothorax in these cases is ureteral obstruction that requires surgical repair. Renal failure, oliguria, and the urinothorax resolve rapidly after surgical repair of the affected ureter. A urinothorax may diagnosed by pleural fluid analysis revealing a pleural fluid to serum ratio of creatinine that is greater than 1.0; it is the only cause of a low-pH transudate (151).

Cases of PTLD with pleural involvement have been reported after renal transplantation (152–155). T-cell leukemia, anaplastic large cell lymphoma, large-cell (B-cell) lymphoma, and non-Hodgkin's lymphoma have been reported. These tumors have developed 3–8 years after transplantation. The effusions are usually associated with other chest radiographic abnormalities, such as pulmonary nodules or a mediastinal mass. In all cases, the diagnosis of malignancy was made by histological and immunohistochemical analysis of pleural fluid cells obtained by thoracentesis.

Two cases have been described of renal transplant recipients developing a pleural effusion secondary to a perirenal lymphocele 7 and 10 years after transplantation (156,157). We suspect pleural effusion is a rare complication of perirenal lymphocele, as no effusions were described in five studies reporting a total of 47 perirenal lymphoceles after kidney transplantation (158–162). An exudative effusion with 90% lymphocytes was reported in one patient (156). Refractory ascites and pleural effusions resolved after peritoneo-venous shunt placement in one case, whereas in the other case a peritoneo-venous shunt was inadequate to drain the rapidly accumulating pleural fluid (157). Removal of the graft and retransplantation was required, although the kidney had been functioning normally.

One case of skin lesions and pleural effusion from Kaposi's sarcoma in a renal transplant recipient has been reported (163). Human herpesvirus 8 was identified from polymerase chain reaction of a pleural biopsy specimen. One case has been reported of sarcoidosis presenting as a pleural effusion 17 months after renal transplantation (164). Noncaseating granulomas were identified in both pleural and lung tissue. The patient was receiving tacrolimus but not corticosteroids at presentation, and the effusion resolved when after the patient received 20 mg/day of prednisone.

In a retrospective review of the anesthesia complications of 500 consecutive renal transplants (165), one hemothorax occurred as a complication of central line placement. Another recipient developed an idiopathic postoperative pneumothorax.

Infectious Causes of Pleural Disease

As with other organ transplants, pleural infections after renal transplantation usually relate to the level of immunosuppression and are not specific for kidney transplantation.

In a review of 173 kidney transplants recipients (166), pulmonary infections developed in 73 (43%) of 173. Forty-nine (65%) of the infections were caused by bacteria, and 5 (10%) of these were associated with pleural effusions. In a review of 142 renal transplantations in India (167), 27 (19%) of 142 recipients developed pulmonary infection, and bacteria were solely responsible for only 3 (11%) of 27 of these infections. Three (11%) of the 27 had pleural effusions, and all 3 had tuberculosis.

Renal transplantation is a risk factor for *Legionella* pneumonia, and pleural effusions are common (43–90%) in renal transplant recipients who develop *Legionella* pneumonia (168–173). The parapneumonic effusions have been reported to be isolated (174), associated a pulmonary infiltrate (168–172), and initially isolated with subsequent development of an infiltrate (173). The diagnosis of these *Legionella* infections is often made from stains or cultures of pleural fluid (168,169,171,173).

Several cases of *Nocardia* pneumonia with pleural involvement have been reported (175–179). Most occurred within the first 4 months after transplantation or with treatment of graft rejection (175,176,179). Chest radiographs revealed isolated pleural effusions (176) or effusions associated with pulmonary infiltrates (176,178,179).

Tuberculosis can develop in a renal transplant patient from primary infection, reactivation, or from transplantation of an infected graft (180,181). The frequency of these infections after transplantation varies with the prevalence of tuberculosis infection, as 10 (37%) of 27 of all pulmonary infections were attributable to *Mycobacterium tuberculosis* in a review of renal transplants performed in India (167) where tuberculosis is endemic. Infection with bacillus Calmette-Guerin is probably very rare as no cases were reported in a series of 487 renal transplant recipients from South Africa where 21 cases of tuberculosis were reported (181). Tuberculous pleural effusions have been described in some renal transplant recipients (167,180–183).

Pleural effusions have been reported in renal transplant recipients from cryptococcal infections (184,185), and empyemas have been reported from staphylococcal (186) and *Salmonella* species (187). Two cases of pneumothorax from necrotizing pulmonary infections after renal transplantation have been reported (188). The responsible pathogens were not clearly elucidated as both patients were concomitantly treated for *Candida* species and aerobic gram-negative bacilli that were cultured from sputum.

Clinical data suggest that most parapneumonic effusions in renal transplant recipients do not require pleural space drainage as only 3 (1%) of 273 consecutive renal transplants required a surgical procedure to drain the pleural space (189). The procedures used were rib resection, thoracotomy with decortication, and rib resection with decortication (190).

VI. Lung and Heart-Lung Transplantation

A. Pretransplant Considerations

Preexisting pleural disease was initially thought to be a contraindication to lung transplantation (191). This belief was based on reports of frequent postoperative deaths after heart-lung transplantation that were attributed to pleural hemorrhage from lysis of pleural adhesions (192). Because heart-lung transplantation must be performed with cardiopulmonary bypass that requires anticoagulation, the degree of pleural hemorrhage was probably greater in these series than for patients undergoing single lung transplantation who rarely require cardiopulmonary bypass unless they have severe pulmonary hypertension (193). Double lung transplantation is now performed by the sequential single lung technique where during one operation a single lung transplantation is performed followed by a contralateral lung transplantation (194). Therefore, cardiopulmonary bypass is now rarely required for double lung transplantation (195,196). As long as cardiopulmonary bypass can be avoided for lung transplantation, there is only a minimal risk of significant pleural hemorrhage (197). An additional concern is that extensive pleural adhesions may prolong dissection and anesthesia time and may result in severe air leaks that are difficult to control. Although pleural hemorrhage has now become less of a problem after lung transplantation, pleural fibrosis may still increase the risks of the procedure. In one study of 32 cystic fibrosis patients who received lung transplantation, patients with severe pleural disease detected by CT scanning had significantly longer hospital stay (50.5 days vs. 23.3 days; $p < 0.05$) and required mechanical ventilation longer (9.5 ± 13 days vs. 2 ± 2.3 days; $p = 0.06$) than those with minimal pleural disease (198).

The management of pleural disease in a patient with cystic fibrosis considered for lung transplantation is problematic. Because of their chronic suppurative lung disease and life-long requirements for immunosuppression after transplantation, recipients with cystic fibrosis require double lung transplantation (199). Nineteen percent of patients with cystic fibrosis develop at least one pneumothorax by adulthood (200). Pneumothorax may be treated by observation, tube thoracostomy with or without pleurodesis, surgical/thoracoscopic resection of blebs with or without talc poudrage, pleural abrasion, and parietal pleurectomy. The degree and extent of pleurodesis depends upon the procedure that is used. Because pleural hemorrhage and air leaks may occur from lysis of pleural adhesions during lung transplantation, efforts should be made to minimize the extent and degree of pleural fibrosis when selecting a procedure to close a persistent air leak in a potential lung transplant candidate.

It has been recommended that a pneumothorax in a patient with cystic fibrosis being considered for lung transplantation be treated initially with chest tube drainage and observation for as long as 5 days (201,202). If the air leak persists for more than 5 days, it has been suggested that a procedure that minimizes the extent of pleurodesis be attempted, such as thoracotomy or thoracoscopic stapling with apical (limited) talc poudrage. This approach will be successful as 85% of pneumothoraces in cystic fibrosis result from rupture of apical blebs (203). The length of time that the air leak is observed without a surgical procedure should be individualized, as it might be appropriate to wait more than 2 weeks if the air leak is diminishing. Only if the limited pleurodesis procedure fails should diffuse chemical pleurodesis or extensive parietal pleurectomy be considered.

Even if unrestricted chemical pleurodesis or pleurectomy is required, lung transplant is not absolutely contraindicated as several cystic fibrosis patients have undergone successful transplantation after extensive pleural procedures (204–206). In a study comparing lung transplant patients who had previously undergone intrapleural procedures to 18 matched lung transplant recipients who had not had such procedures, there was no statistically significant difference in operating time, blood loss, transfusion requirements, time intubated, and intensive care unit time (206). There was also no difference in spirometry at 6 months and 12 months after transplantation.

B. Early Postoperative Pleural Complications

Pneumothorax, air leak, and pleural effusion are common early postoperative problems after lung transplantation. Most air leaks resolve spontaneously within a few days of lung transplantation; however approximately 10% of lung transplant recipients will have a prolonged air leak lasting at least 2 weeks after surgery (207). Typically these air leaks resolve with tube thoracostomy alone and do not require further intervention (207). Pneumothoraces may occasionally be seen in the early postoperative period because of undersized donor lungs (197,208). These are usually small, insignificant, and resolve within days to weeks.

A pneumothorax may also occur from dehiscence of the bronchial anastomosis (197,209). Total dehiscence is rare and is usually life-threatening as it is extremely difficult to control the air leak and reexpand the allograft. Lesser degrees of bronchial dehiscence occasionally occur (197) and are complicated by air leaks that usually heal with conservative management. Occasionally a pneumothorax will develop in the native lung in the postoperative period after single lung transplantation (210). These are thought to result from positive pressure mechanical ventilation to the diseased native lung.

Pleural effusions are extremely common in the early postoperative period. In one early series of 10 patients there was a 100% incidence of pleural effusion after heart-lung transplantation (211). These effusions are usually small to moderate in size but may rarely be massive (212). Most resolve spontaneously within 14 days after transplantation, although rarely they may increase in volume over the first 3 postoperative weeks (211).

There are several explanations for the development of pleural fluid in the early postoperative period. First, alveolar capillaries have increased permeability during the first few days after transplantation because of allograft ischemia, denervation, and subsequent reperfusion (213). Second, lymphatic flow is severely disrupted from transection of lung lymphatics during the operation. Animal studies have demonstrated that allograft lymphatics are reconstituted and become functional 2–4 weeks after transplantation (214,215), corresponding to the time when pleural effusions resolve after human lung transplantation. Third, pleural effusions are associated with acute lung rejection (216), an event that occurs once in almost all lung transplant recipients and is most common in the second to sixth week after transplant (217). A study of 16 heart-lung transplant recipients (218) demonstrated that new or increased pleural fluid and septal lines were common in patients with acute lung rejection (Table 7). These radiographic findings had a sensitivity of 68%, a specificity of 90%, and an accuracy of 84% for acute lung rejection. Although radiographic findings of new or increased pleural fluid is not diagnostic of acute lung rejection, these findings should heighten the suspicion of rejection if they are observed in the first few weeks to months after transplantation. Furthermore, we propose that a patient with established acute lung rejection does not require investigation of a small-to-moderate sized pleural effusion unless the pleural effusion fails to decrease within 1–2 days after treatment for rejection. The appearance of pleural fluid as a predictor of acute lung rejection has been challenged by some investigators who

Table 7 Radiographic Findings After Heart-Lung Transplantation ($n = 83$)

Radiographic findings	Pathological findings (%)			
	Acute rejection	Infection	Nonspecific	Normal
Pleural fluid				
New or increased[a]	68	6	23	0
Stable	28	53	35	44
Septal lines	76	29	42	11
Air-space disease	44	53	50	44
Normal	0	0	25	33

[a] New or increased pleural fluid and septal lines: sensitivity of 68%, specificity of 90%, accuracy of 84% for acute lung rejection.
Source: Adapted from Ref. 2.

found no correlation between acute lung rejection and the presence of pleural fluid on chest radiograph (219) or chest CT scan (220) in pediatric lung transplant recipients. Fourth, positive fluid balance in the early postoperative period may contribute to the development of pleural effusions, although these effusions often develop while the patient is in extreme negative fluid balance.

The characteristics of the pleural fluid that occurs immediately after lung transplantation has been described in nine successful single lung transplant recipients who had no clinical evidence of infection or rejection (221). The effusions were initially bloody, exudative, and neutrophil-predominant. Over the subsequent 7 days, the percentage of neutrophils and concentration of LDH and protein decreased, whereas the percentage of macrophages and lymphocytes increased. These initial pleural fluid findings were similar to control patients who had undergone nontransplant cardiothoracic surgery. Daily pleural fluid output gradually decreased except in one patient with the pulmonary reimplantation response (213), a form of noncardiogenic pulmonary edema that occurs within 4 days of lung transplantation. This patient required reintubation for respiratory failure, and resolution of his pulmonary edema was paralleled by a decrease in his daily pleural fluid output. We suspect that there was a close correlation between pleural fluid output and lung edema in this patient because of the disruption of lung lymphatics that did not allow for rapid clearance of fluid from the pleural space. Two additional cases have been reported of lung transplantation with graft failure and capillary leak in the immediate postoperative period in which the pleural fluid output was 7 and 10 L/day, respectively (222). Interestingly, both patients had a dramatic decrease in pleural fluid output coupled with marked clinical improvement after administration of C1-esterase inhibitor that was postulated to reverse the capillary leak.

Hemothorax and empyema may also occur in the early postoperative period after lung transplantation (197). These may be associated with airway dehiscence, wound infection, or lysis of pleural adhesions.

An HLA analysis has been done to determine the rate of influx of recipient cells into the pleural space after lung transplantation (223). Donor cells appear to be rapidly cleared from the pleural space, with less than 1% of pleural cells being of donor origin by postoperative day 8.

Pleural fluid analysis has been performed of effusions associated with acute lung rejection (216). The fluid is exudative and often contains more than 90% lymphocytes.

C. Long-Term Postoperative Pleural Complications

In one study of 144 lung transplant recipients (207), pleural complications were found to be less frequent with single lung transplantation (5/53, 9%) than double lung transplantation (25/81, 27%) ($p < 0.05$). All but one of the pleural complications after single lung transplantation were pneumothoraces that persisted more than 14 days. No patient developed an empyema or parapneumonic effusion after single lung transplantation. In contrast, 11 (12%) of 81 double lung transplant recipients developed pleural infections: 7 (8%) empyemas, and 4 (5%) parapneumonic effusions; 3 of the empyemas were fatal. Pleural complications were most common in patients with cystic fibrosis (10/29, 34%) and chronic obstructive pulmonary disease (12/47, 26%).

Parapneumonic effusions are common with pneumonia after lung transplantation, having been reported in 33 (73%) of 45 episodes of pneumonia in one series (224). Pleural effusion was equally common when the pathogen was bacterial, fungal, mycobacterial, or viral.

Empyemas occur commonly after lung transplantation. Several cases of *Burkholderia cepacia* empyema and other *Burkholderia* species have been reported after double lung transplantation for cystic fibrosis (207,225–227); some of these patients developed empyema necessitatis (226). Pathogens causing infected pleural effusions and empyemas after lung and heart-lung transplantation have included *Legionella* species (228), staphylococcal and streptococcal species (229), *Pseudomonas aeruginosa* (212), *Mycobacterium tuberculosis* (230–232), cytomegalovirus (224), *Aspergillus* species (224), and *Candida* species (233).

Rarely, a pleural effusion may result from abnormalities of the pulmonary venous anastomosis, such as thrombosis, kinking, or fibrosis. These abnormalities may cause unilateral or bilateral pulmonary edema with pleural effusions and may mimic allograft rejection, opportunistic infection, or congestive heart failure. Although this complication often occurs in the immediate postoperative period, pleural effusions from pulmonary venous abnormalities has been reported more than a year after lung transplantation (234). As with other solid organ transplants, PTLD may be seen after lung transplantation and is occasionally associated with pleural effusion (235).

An iatrogenic pneumothorax may occur secondary to transbronchial biopsy or percutaneous biopsy for surveillance of rejection or pulmonary infection. In a review of 39 lung transplant centers that perform surveillance bronchoscopy for lung rejection, 95% (37/39) reported a pneumothorax rate of less than 5% of the time and 97% (38/39) reported a frequency of chest tube placement less than 5% of the time (236). In a study of review of 320 transbronchial lung biopsies performed for clinically suspected infection of rejection, 8 of (2.5%) 320 developed a pneumothorax (237). A pneumothorax may also occur from progressive underlying lung disease in the native lung of a single lung transplant recipient (vide infra) or superimposed disorders in the allograft, such as invasive fungal disease.

Pleural fibrosis has been found at autopsy in heart-lung transplant recipients (238). Although this has been attributed to the surgical procedure, an animal study revealed that pleural fibrosis developed in recipients who received allografts but not in those who received an autograft (their own heart-lung bloc) (239). This suggests that surgery was not responsible for the fibrosis, and the investigators suspected that its development was related to chronic rejection.

D. Interpleural Communication After Double Lung and Heart-Lung Transplantation

During the course of a heart-lung transplant, the anterior pleural reflections are severed so that an interpleural communication develops (240–243). Therefore, air or fluid can move between the pleural spaces. Similar interpleural communication has also been observed after heart transplantation and thoracic surgery in patients with previous mediastinotomy (241). Interpleural communication may also occur after bilateral sequential lung transplantation performed through bilateral anterolateral thoracotomies and transverse sternotomy (clamshell) because anterior pleural reflections are also severed with this approach. This phenomenon has been demonstrated to persist for more than 2 years after heart-lung transplantation (240,241), and it is likely permanent.

Awareness of interpleural communication after heart-lung transplantation is important because pleural disease in these recipients should be managed aggressively. Empyemas need to be aggressively and adequately drained so that the infected pleural contents do not spill into the contralateral pleural space. A tension pneumothorax in such recipients is likely to be bilateral and, hence, life-threatening. Usually a single thoracostomy tube is adequate for a heart-lung transplant recipient with bilateral pneumothoraces (244,245). However, a case has been reported where a single chest tube failed to adequately drain a bilateral pneumothoraces in a heart-lung transplant recipient, and a contralateral tension pneumothorax developed (246). The transplant had been performed 2 years previously, and the authors postulated that pleural scar formation had sealed the interpleural communication. Careful radiographic monitoring is therefore recommended when using a single chest tube in this situation.

E. Pleural Considerations in the Contralateral Lung After Single Lung

Transplantation

Pleural complications may develop in the native lung of a single lung transplant recipient. Pneumothorax is the most common complication, and this is not an unexpected finding in patients with end-stage restrictive or obstructive disease. These secondary spontaneous pneumothoraces rarely resolve permanently with tube thoracostomy (247). Thoracoscopic talc poudrage (248) and thoracoscopic partial pleurectomy (2,249) have both been successful long-term.

Donor Considerations

Because potential lung donors may have undergone significant trauma, it is not uncommon for them to have sustained a pneumothorax. Although pneumothorax was initially a contraindication for lung donation, this criterion has been liberalized (250). It is recommended that the extent of the air leak and area of related lung injury be assessed to determine if the lung should be donated (250).

VII. Summary

Pleural disease has important clinical implications both before and after organ transplantation. Pleural effusions are common in candidates for heart, liver, and kidney transplantation. A thoracentesis is not mandatory in these patients but should be performed if clinical or radiographic features suggest that the effusion is not the result of organ failure. Posttransplant pleural infections and PTLD relate to the level and duration of immunosuppression and are not organ-specific. Some posttransplant pleural effusions are organ-specific and are described in the text.

The treatment of pleural disease in potential lung transplant candidates should minimize the extent of pleurodesis. Pleural effusions are to be expected after lung transplantation. Interpleural communication, an expected finding after heart-lung or double lung transplantation, has therapeutic implications.

References

1. United Network for Organ Sharing. 2000 Scientific Registry and Organ Procurement Transplant Network Report.
2. Judson MA, Sahn SA. The pleural space and organ transplantation. Am J Respir Crit Care Med 1996; 153:1153–1165.
3. Armitage JO. Bone marrow transplantation. N Engl J Med 1994; 330:827–838.
4. Sahn SA. The pleura. Am Rev Respir Dis 1988; 138:184–234.
5. Castellano RA, Bellani FF, Gasparini M, Musumeci R. Radiographic findings in previously untreated children with non-Hodgkin's lymphoma. Radiology 1975; 117: 657–663.
6. Xaubert A, Diumenjo MC, Marin A, Montserrat E, Estopa R, Llebaria C, Austi A, Rozman C. Characteristics and prognostic value of pleural effusions in non-Hodgkin's lymphoma. Eur J Respir Dis 1985; 66:135–140.
7. Chaignaud BE, Bonsack TA, Kozakewich HP, Shamberger RC. Pleural effusions in lymphoblastic lymphoma: a diagnostic alternative. J Pediatr Surg 1998; 33:1355–1357.
8. Fischer AMH, Kendell B, Van Leuven BD. Hodgkin's disease: a radiological survey. Clin Radiol 1962; 13:115–127.
9. Wong FM, Grace WJ, Rottino A. Pleural effusions, ascites, pericardial effusions and edema in Hodgkin's disease. Am J Med Sci 1963; 246:678–682.
10. Westling P. Studies of the prognosis in Hodgkin's disease. Acta Radiol (suppl) 1965; 245:5–125.
11. Aquino SL, Chen MYM, Kuo WT, Chiles C. The CT appearance of pleural and extrapleural disease in lymphoma. Clin Radiol 1999; 54:647–650.
12. Au V, Leung AN. Radiologic manifestations of lymphoma of the thorax. AJR 1997; 168:93–98.
13. Wieck JK, Kiely JM, Harrison EG, Carr DT, Scanlon PW. Pleural effusion in lymphoma. Cancer 1973; 31:848–853.
14. Yam LT. Diagnostic significance of lymphocytes in pleural effusion. Ann Intern Med 1967; 66:972–982.

15. Jenkins PF, Ward MJ, Davies P, Fletcher J. Non-Hodgkin's lymphoma, chronic lymphatic leukemia and the lung. Br J Dis Chest 1981; 75:22–30.
16. Bangerter M, Hildebrand A, Griesshammer M. Combined cytomorphologic and immunophenotypic analysis in the diagnostic workup of lymphomatous effusions. Acta Cytol 2001; 45:307–312.
17. Pietsch JB, Whitlock JA, Ford C, Kinney MC. Management of pleural effusions in children with malignant lymphoma. J Pediatr Surg 1999; 34:635–638.
18. Grimwade DJ, Chopra R, King A, Shaw P, Pearce R, Linch DC, Goldstone AH. Detection and significance of pulmonary Hodgkin's disease at autologous bone marrow transplantation. Bone Marrow Transplant 1994; 13:173–179.
19. Poen JC, Hoppe RT, Horning SJ. High-dose therapy and autologous bone marrow transplantation for relapsed/refractory Hodgkin's disease: the impact of involved field radiotherapy on patterns of failure and survival. Int J Radiation Oncol Biol Phys 1996; 36:3–12.
20. Elis A, Blickstein D, Mulchanov I, Manor Y, Radnay J, Shapiro H, Lishner M. Pleural effusion in patients with non-Hodgkin's lymphoma. Cancer 1998; 83:1607–1611.
21. Walden PAM, Michell-Heggs PF, Coppin C, Dent J, Bagshawe KW. Pleurisy and methotrexate treatment. Br Med J 1977; 2:867.
22. Everts CS, Westcott JL, Bragg DG. Methotrexate therapy and pulmonary disease. Radiology 1973; 107:539–543.
23. Urban C, Nirenberg A, Caparros B, Anac S, Cacavio A, Rosen G. Chemical pleuritis as the cause of chest pain following high-dose methotrexate treatment. Cancer 1983; 51:34–37.
24. Pascual RS, Mosher MB, Sikand RS, DeConti RC, Bouhuys AS. Effects of bleomycin on pulmonary function in man. Am Rev Respir Dis 1973; 108:211–217.
25. Holoye PY, Luna MA, Mackay B, Bedrosian CWM. Bleomycin hypersensitivity pneumonitis. Ann Intern Med 1978; 88:47–49.
26. Schaap N, Raymakers R, Schattenberg A, Ottevanger JP, de Witte T. Massive pleural effusion attributed to high-dose cyclophosphamide during conditioning for BMT. Bone Marrow Transplant 1996; 18:247–248.
27. Bachman AL, Macken K. Pleural effusions following supervoltage radiation for breast carcinoma. Radiology 1959; 72:699–709.
28. Whitcomb ME, Schwartz MI. Pleural effusion complicating intensive mediastinal radiation therapy. Am Rev Respir Dis 1971; 103:100–107.
29. Penzer RD, Horak DA, Sayegh HO, Lipsett JA. Spontaneous pneumothorax in patients irradiated for Hodgkin's disease and other malignant lymphomas. Int J Radiation Oncol Biol 1990; 18:193–198.
30. Yellin A, Benfield JR. Pneumothorax associated with lymphoma. Am Rev Respir Dis 1986; 134:590–592.
31. Penniment MG, O'Brien PC. Pneumothorax following thoracic radiation therapy for Hodgkin's disease. Thorax 1994; 49:936–937.
32. Rowinsky EK, Abeloff MD, Wharam MD. Spontaneous pneumothorax following thoracic radiation. Chest 1985; 88:703–708.
33. Melton LJ, Hepper NGG, Offord KD. Influence of height on the risk of spontaneous pneumothorax. Mayo Clin Proc 1981; 56:678–682.
34. Hsu JR, Chang SC, Perng RP. Pneumothorax following cytotoxic chemotherapy in malignant lymphoma. Chest 1990; 98:1512–1513.

35. Stein ME, Shklar Z, Drumea K, Goralnik L, Ben-Arieh Y, Haim N. Chemotherapy-induced spontaneous pneumothorax in a patient with bulky mediastinal lymphoma: a rare oncologic emergency. Oncology 1997; 54:15–18.
36. Krowka MJ, Rosenow EC, Hoagland HC. Pulmonary complications of bone marrow transplantation. Chest 1985; 87:237–246.
37. Noble PW. The pulmonary complications of bone marrow transplantation in adults (clinical conference). West J Med 1989; 150:443–449.
38. Schiller G. Chylothorax as a complication of central venous catheter-induced superior vena cava thrombosis. Bone Marrow Transplant 1992; 9:302.
39. Powels R, Pedrazzini A, Crofts M, Clink H, Millar J, Bhattia G, Perez D. Mismatched family bone marrow transplantation. Semin Hematol 1984; 21:182–187.
40. Cahill RA, Spitzer TR, Mazumder A. Marrow engraftment and clinical manifestations of capillary leak syndrome. Bone Marrow Transplant 1996; 18:177–184.
41. Leino L, Lilius EM, Nkoskelainen J, Pelliniemi TT, Rajamaki A. Neutrophils are responsible for the reappearance of chemiluminescence after allogeneic bone marrow transplantation. Bone Marrow Transplant 1990; 6:391–394.
42. Rollins JB. Hepatic veno-occlusive disease. Am J Med 1986; 81:297–306.
43. Jones JR, Lee KS, Beschorner WE, Vogel VG, Grochow LB, Braine HG. Veno-occlusive disease of the liver following bone marrow transplantation. Transplantation 1987; 44:778–783.
44. Dulley FL, Kanfer EJ, Appelbaum FR, Amos D, Hill RS, Buckner CD, Shulman HM, McDonald GB, Thomas ED. Veno-occlusive disease of the liver after chemoradiotherapy and autologous bone marrow transplantation. Transplantation 1987; 43:870–873.
45. Brugieres L, Hartmann O, Benhamou E, Zafrani ES, Caillaud JM, Patte C, Kalifa C, Flamant F, Lemerle J. Veno-occlusive disease of the liver following high-dose chemotherapy and autologous bone marrow transplantation in children with solid tumors: incidence, clinical course, and outcome. Bone Marrow Transplant 1988; 3:53–58.
46. Ozkaynak MF, Weinberg K, Kohn D, Sender L, Parkman R, Lenarsky C. Hepatic veno-occlusive disease post-bone marrow transplantation in children conditioned with busulfan and cyclophosphamide: incidence, risk factors, and clinical outcome. Bone Marrow Transplant 1991; 7:467–474.
47. Weisdorf D, Haake R, Blazar B, Miller W, McGlave P, Ramsey N, Kersey J, Filipovich A. Treatment of moderate/severe graft-versus-host disease after allogeneic bone marrow transplantation: an analysis of clinical risk factors and outcome. Blood 1990; 75:1024–1030.
48. Seber A, Khan SP, Kersay JH. Unexplained effusions: association with allogeneic bone marrow transplantation and acute or chronic graft-versus-host disease. Bone Marrow Transplant 1996; 17:207–211.
49. Ueda T, Manabe A, Kikuchi A, Yoshino H, Ebihara Y, Ishii T, Yagasaki H, Mitsui T, Hisakawa H, Masunaga A, Tsuji K, Nakahata T. Massive pericardial and pleural effusion with anasarca following allogeneic bone marrow transplantation. Internat J Hematol 2000; 71:394–397.
50. Orazi A, Hromas RA, Neiman RS, Greiner TC, Lee CH, Rubin L, Haskins S, Heerema NA, Gharpure V, Abnour R, Srour EF, Cornetta K. Posttransplantation lymphoproliferative disorders in bone marrow transplant recipients are aggressive diseases with a high incidence of adverse histologic and immunobiologic features. Am J Clin Path 1997; 107:419–429.

51. Papadopoulos EB, Ladanyi M, Emanuel D, Mackinnon S, Boulad F, Carabasi MH, Castro-Malaspina H, Childs BH, Gillio AP, Small TN. Infusions of donor leukocytes to treat Epstein-Barr virus-associated lymphoproliferative disorders after allogeneic bone marrow transplantation. N Engl J Med 1994; 330:1185–1191.
52. Shapiro RS, McClain K, Frizzera G, Gajl-Peczalska KJ, Kersey JH, Blazar BR, Arthur DC, Patton DF, Greenberg JS, Burke B. Epstein-Barr virus associated B cell lymphoproliferative disorders following bone marrow transplantation. Blood 1988; 71:1234–1243.
53. Lechapt-Zalcman E, Rieux C, Cordonnier C, Desvaux D. Posttransplantation lymphoproliferative disorder mimicking a nonspecific lymphocytic pleural effusion in a bone marrow transplant recipient. Acta Cytol 1999; 43:239–242.
54. Dix DB, Anderson RA, McFadden DE, Wadsworth LD. Pleural relapse during hematopoietic remission in childhood acute lymphoblastic leukemia. J Pediatr Hematol Oncol 1997; 19:470–472.
55. Motherby H, Ross B, Kube M, Germing U, Heyll A, Aul C, Braunstein S, Gabbert HE, Bocking A. Pleural carcinosis confirmed by adjuvant cytological methods: a case report. Diagnostic Cytopathol 1998; 19:370–374.
56. Dohmen K, Harada M, Ishibashi H, Taniguchi S, Kudo J, Shimamura R, Niho Y. Ultrasonographic studies on abdominal complications in patients receiving marrow-ablative chemotherapy and bone marrow or blood stem cell transplantation. J Clin Ultrasound 1991; 19:321–333.
57. Merz WG, Sandford GR. Isolation and characterization of a polyene-resistant *Candida tropicalis*. J Clin Microbiol 1979; 9:677–680.
58. Lesire V, Hazouard E, Dequin PF, Delain M, Therizol-Ferly M, Legras A. Possible role of *Chaetomium globosum* in infection after autologous bone marrow transplantation. Intensive Care Med 1999; 25:124–125.
59. Kurzrock R, Zander A, Kanojia M, Vellekoop L, Spitzer G, Jagannath S, Schell S, Peters L, Dicke K. Obstructive lung disease after allogeneic bone marrow transplantation. Transplantation 1984; 37:156–160.
60. Link H, Reinhard U, Niethammer D, Kruger GRF, Waller HD, Wilms K. Obstructive ventilation disorder as a severe complication of chronic graft-versus-host disease after bone-marrow transplantation. Exp Hematol 1982; 10(suppl 10):92–93.
61. Galanis E, Litzow MR, Tefferi A, Scott JP. Spontaneous pneumomediastinum in a patient with bronchiolitis obliterans after bone marrow transplantation. Bone Marrow Transplant 1997; 20:695–696.
62. Suzuki T, Saijo Y, Ebina M, Yaekashiwa M, Minegishi M, Tsuchiya S, Konno T, Ono S, Matsumura Y, Fujimura S, Nukiwa T. Bilateral pneumothoraces with multiple bullae in a patient with asymptomatic bronchiolitis obliterans 10 years after bone marrow transplantation. Bone Marrow Transplant 1999; 23:829–831.
63. Cazzadori A, Di Perri G, Bonora S, Lanzafame M, Allegranzi B, Concia E. Fatal pneumothorax complicating BAL in a bone marrow transplant recipient with bronchiolitis obliterans. Chest 1997; 111:1468–1469.
64. Wiener-Kronish JP, Matthay MA, Callen PW, Filly RA, Gamsu G, Staub NC. Relationship of pleural effusions to hemodynamics in patients with congestive heart failure. Am Rev Respir Dis 1985; 132:1253–1256.
65. Shinto RA, Light RW. Effects of diuresis on the characteristics of pleural fluid in patients with congestive heart failure. Am J Med 1990; 88:23–234.

66. Chakko SC, Caldwell SH, Sfoorza PP. Treatment of congestive heart failure: its effect on pleural fluid chemistry. Chest 1989; 95:798–802.
67. Wright RS, Levine MS, Bellamy PE, Simmons MS, Batra P, Stevenson LW, Walden JA, Laks H, Tashkin DP. Ventilatory and diffusion abnormalities in potential heart transplant recipients. Chest 1990; 98:816–820.
68. Ettinger NA, Trulock EP. Pulmonary considerations of organ transplantation, Part 3. Am Rev Respir Dis 1991; 144:433–451.
69. Carter AR, Sostman HD, Curtis AM, Swett HA. Thoracic alterations after surgery. Am J Roentgenol 1983; 140:475–481.
70. Torsen MK, Goodman LR. Extracardiac complications of cardiac surgery. Semin Roentgenol 1988; 23:32–48.
71. Henry DA, Lolles H, Berberich JJ, Schmetzer V. The post-cardiac surgery radiograph: a clinically integrated approach. J Thorac Imaging 1989; 4:20–41.
72. Schulman LL, Smith CR, Drusin R, Rose EA, Enson Y, Reemtsma K. Respiratory complications of cardiac transplantation. Am J Med Sci 1988; 296:1–10.
73. Lee JT, Durzinsky DS, Wilson WR, Walsh TE. Pericardial tamponade and massive pleural effusion complicating orthotopic heart transplantation. J Cardiovasc Surg 1999; 40:377–379.
74. Aarnio P, Harjula A, Heikkila L, Mattila S. Surgery after heart transplantation. Scand J Thorac Cardiovasc Surg 1990; 24:21–22.
75. Anastasiou-Nana MI, O'Connell JB, Nanas JN, Sorensen SG, Anderson JL. Relative efficiency and risk of endomyocardial biopsy: comparisons in heart transplant and nontransplant patients. Cathet Cardiovasc Diagn 1989; 18:7–11.
76. Grande AM, Minzioni G, Martinelli L, Campana C, Rinaldi M, D'Armini AM, Ragni T, Pederzolli C, Ardemagni E, Pererzolli N, Di Pieri G, Castiglione N, Vigano M. Echo-controlled endomyocardial biopsy in orthotopic heart transplantation with bicaval anastomosis. G Ital Cardiol 1997; 27:877–880.
77. Knisely BL, Mastey LA, Collins J, Kuhlman JE. Imaging of cardiac transplantation complications. Radiographics 1999; 19:321–339.
78. Di Sesa V, Sloss LJ, Cohn LH. Heart transplantation for intractable prosthetic valve endocarditis. J Heart Transplant 1990; 9:142–143.
79. Bowerman RE, Solomon DA, Bognolo D, Brauner LR. Chylothorax: report of a case complicating orthotopic heart transplantation. J Heart Lung Transplant 1993; 12:665–668.
80. Conroy JT, Twomey C, Alpern JB. Chylothorax after orthotopic heart transplantation in an adult patient: a case complicated by an episode of rejection. J Heart Lung Transplant 1993; 12:1071.
81. Repp R, Scheld HH, Bauer J, Becker H, Kreuder J, Netz H. Cyclosporine losses by a chylothorax. J Heart Lung Transplant 1992; 11:397–398.
82. Karcher DS, Alkan S. Human herpesvirus-8-associated body cavity-based lymphoma in human immunodeficiency virus-infected patients: a unique B-cell neoplasm. Hum Pathol 1997; 28:801–808.
83. Jones D, Ballestas ME, Kaye KM, Gulizia JM, Winters GL, Fletcher J, Scadden DT, Aster JC. Primary-effusion lymphoma and Kaposi's sarcoma in a cardiac transplant recipient. N Eng J Med 1998; 339:444:449.
84. Parker BM, Smith JR. Pulmonary embolism and infarction. Am J Med 1958; 24:402–427.
85. Murray JR. The pathogenesis, diagnosis, and treatment of pulmonary embolus. Calif Med 1971; 114:36–43.

86. Young JN, Yazbeck J, Esposito G, Mankad P, Townsend E, Yacoub M. The influence of acute preoperative pulmonary infarction on the results of heart transplantation. J Heart Transplant 1986; 5:120–122.
87. Cavarocchi NC, Carp NZ, Mitra A, McClerkin JB, Elfenbein IB, Alpern JB, Kolff J. Successful heart transplantation in recipients with recent preoperative pulmonary emboli. J Heart Transplant 1989; 8:494–498.
88. Bieber E, Quinn JP, Venezio FR, Miller JB. Team LUCT Salmonella empyema in a heart transplant recipient. J Heart Transplant 1989; 8:262–263.
89. *Pseudomonas paucimobilis* empyema after cardiac transplantation. South Med J 1988; 81:796–798.
90. Amber IJ, Gilbert EM, Schiffman G, Jacobson JA. Increased risk of pneumococcal infections in cardiac transplant recipients. Transplantation 1990; 49:122–125.
91. De Pinto D, Park S, Houck J, Pifarre R. Successful treatment of mediastinitis and empyema in a heart transplant patient: one stage procedure (letter). J Heart Lung Transplant 1993; 12:883–884.
92. Canver CC, Patel AK, Kosolcharoen P, Voytovich MC. Fungal purulent constrictive pericarditis in a heart transplant patient. Ann Thorac Surg 1998; 65:1792–1794.
93. Copeland J, Wieden M, Feinberg W, Salomon N, Hager D, Galagiani J. Legionnaires' disease following cardiac transplantation. Chest 1981; 79:669–671.
94. Knisely BL, Mastey LA, Collins J, Kuhlman JE. Imaging of cardiac transplantation complications. Radiographics 1999; 19:321–339.
95. Rees AP, Meadors M, Ventura HO, Pankey GA. Diagnosis of disseminated cytomegalovirus infection and pneumonitis in a heart transplant recipient by skin biopsy: a case report. J Heart Lung Transplant 1991; 10:329–332.
96. Schulman LL, Reison DS, Austin JH, Rose EA. Cytomegalovirus pneumonitis after cardiac transplantation. Arch Intern Med 1991; 151:1118–1124.
97. Drummer JS, White LT, Ho M, Griffith BP, Hardesty RL, Bahnson HT. Morbidity of cytomegalovirus infection in recipients of heart or heart-lung transplants who receive cyclosporine. J Infect Dis 1985; 152:1182–1191.
98. Grande AM, Minzioni G, Martinelli L, Campana C, Rinaldi M, D'Armini AM, Ragni T, Pederzolli C. Echo-controlled endomyocardial biopsy in orthotopic heart transplantation with bicaval anastomosis. G Ital Cardiol 1997; 27:877–880.
99. Schuler S, Parnt R, Warnecke H, Matheis G, Hetzer R. Extended donor criteria for heart transplantation. J Heart Transplant 1988; 7:326–330.
100. Johnson RF, Loo RV. Hepatic hydrothorax: studies to determine the source of the fluid and report of thirteen cases. Ann Intern Med 1964; 61:385.
101. Krowka MJ, Cortese DA. Pulmonary aspects of chronic liver disease and liver transplantation. Mayo Clin Proc 1985; 60:407–416.
102. Krowka MJ, Cortese DA. Pulmonary aspects of chronic liver disease and liver transplantation. Clin Chest Med 1989; 10:593–616.
103. Lieberman FL, Hidemura R, Peters RL, Reynolds TB. Pathogenesis and treatment of hydrothorax complicating cirrhosis with ascites. Ann Intern Med 1966; 64:341–351.
104. Ettinger NA, Trulock EP. Pulmonary considerations of organ transplantation, Part 1. Am Rev Respir Dis 1991; 143:1386–1405.
105. Afessa B, Gay PC, Plevak DJ, Swensen SJ, Patel HG, Krowka MJ. Pulmonary complications of orthotopic liver transplantation. Mayo Clin Proc 1993; 68:427–434.

106. Tallgren M, Hockerstedt K, Lindgren L. Respiratory compliance during orthotopic liver transplantation. Acta Anaesthesiol Scand 1996; 40:760–764.
107. Hasegawa S, Mori K, Inomata Y, Murakawa M, Yamaoka Y, Tanaka K. Factors associated with postoperative respiratory complications in pediatric liver transplantation from living-related donors. Transplantation 1996; 62:943–947.
108. O'Brien JD, Ettinger NA. Pulmonary complications of liver transplantation. Clin Chest Med 1996; 17:99–114.
109. Spizarny DL, Gross BH, McLoud T. Enlarging pleural effusion after liver transplantation. J Thorac Imaging 1993; 8:85–87.
110. Olutola PS, Hutton L, Wall WJ. Pleural effusion following liver transplantation. Radiology 1985; 157:594.
111. Costello P, Williams CR, Jenkins RW, Jensen WA, Rose RM. The incidence and implications of chest radiographic abnormalities following liver transplantation. J Can Assoc Radiol 1987; 38:90–95.
112. Shieh WB, Chen CL, Wang KL. Respiratory changes and pulmonary complications following orthotopic liver transplantation. Transplant Proc 1992; 24:1486–1488.
113. Cohen JD, Singer P, Keslin J, Shapira Z, Grunberg G, Grozovski E, Shimueli D. Immediate postoperative course and complications of orthotopic liver transplantation: the first 31 adult patients. Transplant Proc 1997; 29:2882.
114. Kim ST, Kim SJ, Park KW, Suh KS, Jung SE, Ha J, Kim YH, Yun IJ, Lee KU. Early experience of liver transplantation at Seoul National University Hospital. Transplant Proc 1996; 26:1695–1696.
115. Golfieri R, Giampalma E, Morselli-Labate AM, d'Arienzo P, Jovine E, Grazi GL, Mazziotti A, Maffei M, Muzzi C, Tancioni S, Sama C, Cavallari A, Gavelli G. Pulmonary complications of liver transplantation: radiological appearance and statistical evaluation of risk factors in 300 cases. Eur Radiol 2000; 10:1169–1183.
116. Duran FG, Piqueras B, Romero M, Carneros JA, de Diego A, Salcedo M, Santos L, Ferreiroa J, Cos E, Clemente G. Pulmonary complications following orthotopic liver transplant. Transpl Int, 1998, S255–S259.
117. Golfieri R, Giampalma E, Sama C, Labate AM, Mazziotti A, Berardi R, Gozzetti G, Gavelli G. Pulmonary complications following orthotopic liver transplant: radiologic patterns and epidemiologic considerations in 100 cases. RAYS 1994; 19:319–338.
118. Adetiloye VA, John PR. Intervention for pleural effusions and ascites following liver transplantation. Pediatr Radiol 1998; 28:539–543.
119. Bilik R, Yellen M, Superina RA. Surgical complications in children after liver transplantation. J Pediatr Surg 1992; 27:1371–1375.
120. Moulin D, Clement de Clety S, Reynaert M, Carlier MA, Veyckmans F, Claus D, Buts JP, de Hemptinne B, Otte JB. Intensive care for children after orthotopic liver transplantation. Intensive Care Med 1989; 15(suppl 1):S71–S72.
121. Collins JD, Discher AC, Shaver ML, Miller TQ. Imagine the hepatic lymphatics: experimental studies in swine. J Natl Med Assoc 1993; 85:185–191.
122. Robinson LA, Moulton AL, Flemming WH, Galbraith TA. Intrapleural fibrinolytic treatment of multiloculated thoracic empyemas. Ann Thorac Surg 1994; 57:803–814.
123. Schroter GP, Hoelscher M, Putnam CW, Porter KA, Starzl TE. Infections complicating orthotopic liver transplantation. Arch Surg 1976; 3:1337–1347.

124. Raby N, Forbes G, Williams R. *Nocardia* infection in patients with liver transplants of chronic liver disease: radiologic findings. Radiology 1990; 174:713–716.
125. Knollmann FD, Maurer J, Bechstein WO, Vogl TJ, Neuhaus P, Felix R. Pulmonary disease in liver transplant recipients. Acta Radiol 2000; 41:230–236.
126. Wolford JF, Krause JR. Post transplant mediastinal Burkitt-type lymphoma. Diagnosis by cytologic and flow cytometric analysis of pleural fluid. Acta Cytol 1990; 34:261.
127. Hoffmann H, Schelette E, Actor J, Medeiros LJ. Pleural posttransplantation lymphoproliferative disorder following liver transplantation. Arch Pathol Lab Med 2001; 125:419–423.
128. Merenda R, Gerunda GE, Neri D, Barbazza F, Barbazza F, Di Marzio E, Meduri F, Valmasoni M, Faccioli AM. Laparoscopic surgery after orthotopic liver transplantation. Liver Transplant 2000; 6:104–107.
129. Smyrniotis V, Andreani P, Muiesan P, Mieli-Vergani G, Rela M, Heaton ND. Diaphragmatic nerve palsy in young children following liver transplantation. Transpl Int 1998; 11:281–283.
130. Zajko AB, Claus D, Clapuyt P, Esquivel CO, Moulin D, Stazl TE, de Ville de Goyet J, Otte JB. Obstruction to hepatic drainage after liver transplantation: treatment with balloon angioplasty. Radiology 1989; 170(3, part 1):763–765.
131. Larson AM, Chan GC, Wartelle CF, McVair JP, Carithers RL, Hamill GM, Kowdley KV. Infection complicating percutaneous liver biopsy in liver transplant recipients. Hepatology 1997; 26:1406–1409.
132. Lovell M, Baines D. Fatal complication from central venous cannulation in a pediatric liver transplant recipient. Pediatr Anaesthes 2000; 10:661–664.
133. Pirenne J, Aerts R, Yoong K, Gunson B, Koshiba T, Fourneau I, Rosakams T, Elias E, Nevens F, Fevery J, Mayer D, Buckels J, Mirza D, McMaster P. Liver transplantation for polycystic kidney disease. Liver Transplant 2001; 7:238–245.
134. Galati JS, Monsour HP, Donovan JP, Zetterman RK, Schafer DF, Langnas AN, Shaw BW, Sorrell MF. The nature of complications following liver biopsy in transplant patients with Roux-en-Y choledochojejunostomy. Hepatology 1994; 20:651–653.
135. Kalayoglu M, D'Alessandro AM, Knechtle SJ, Hoffmann RM, Pirsch JD, Judd RH, Armbrust M, Spaith E, Pilli G, Young CJ, Geffner SR, Odorico JS, Sollinger HW, Belzer FO. Preliminary experience with split liver transplantation. J Am Coll Surg 1996; 182:381–387.
136. Jarratt MJ, Sahn SA. Pleural effusions in hospitalized patients on chronic hemodialysis. Chest 1995; 108:470–474.
137. Hopps HC, Wissler RW. Uremic pneumonitis. Am J Pathol 1955; 31:261–273.
138. Berger HW, Rammohan G, Neff MS, Buhain W. Uremic pleural effusion. A study of 14 patients on chronic hemodialysis. Ann Intern Med 1975; 82:362–364.
139. Nidus BD, Matalon R, Cantacuzino D, Eisinger RP. Uremic pleuritis: a clinicopathological entity. N Engl J Med 1969; 281:874–876.
140. Galen MA, Steinberg SM, Lowrie EG, Lazarus JM, Hampers CL, Merrill JP. Hemorrhagic pleural effusion in patients undergoing chronic hemodialysis. Ann Intern Med 1975; 82:359–361.
141. Rodelas R, Rakowski TA, Argy WP, Schreiner GE. Fibrosing uremic pleuritis during hemodialysis. JAMA 1980; 243:2424–2425.
142. Harnsberger HR, Lee TG, Mukuno DH. Rapid, inexpensive real-time directed thoracentesis. Radiology 1983; 146:545–546.

143. Gilbert L, Ribot S, Frankel H, Jacobs M, Mankowitz BJ. Fibrinous uremic pleuritis: a surgical entity. Chest 1975; 67:53–56.
144. Wright RS, Quinones-Baldrich WJ, Anders AJ, Danovitch GM. Pleural effusion associated with ipsilateral breast and arm edema as a complication of subclavian vein catheterization and arteriovenous fistula formation for hemodialysis. Chest 1994; 106:950–952.
145. Van Veldhuizen PJ, Taylor S. Chylothorax: a complication of a left subclavian vein thrombosis. Am J Clin Oncol 1996; 19:99–101.
146. Heino A. Operative and postoperative non-surgical complications in diabetic patients undergoing renal transplantation. Scand J Urol Nephrol 1988; 22:53–58.
147. Kuzbary Y, Lasher JC, Blumhardt R, Vicks B. Renal transplant extravasation of urine through a chest tube: an unusual appearance on radionuclide imaging. Nucl Med Commun 1984; 5:655–659.
148. Carcillo J, Salcedo JR. Urinothorax as a manifestation of nondilated obstructive uropathy following renal transplantation. Am J Kidney Dis 1985; 5:211–213.
149. Salcedo JR. Urinothorax: report of 4 cases and review of the literature. J Urol 1986; 135:805–808.
150. Kees-Folts D, Cole BR. Ureteral urine leak presenting as a pleural effusion in a renal transplant recipient. Pediatr Nephrol 1998; 12:666–667.
151. Miller KS, Wooten S, Sahn SA. Urinothorax: a cause of low pH transudative pleural effusions. Am J Med 1988; 85:448–449.
152. Hayashi K, Hoshida Y, Ohnoshi K, Kawashima K, Saito S, Matsutomo S, Tagawa S, Mizuta J, Murashima M, Ueno K. Primary pulmonary non-Hodgkin's lymphoma in Japanese renal transplant recipient. Int J Hematol 1993; 57:245–250.
153. Lippman SM, Grogan TM, Ogden DA, Miller TP. Post-transplantation T cell lymphoblastic lymphoma. Am J Med 1987; 82:814–816.
154. Jimenez-Hefferman JA, Viguer JM, Vicandi B, Jimenez-Yuste V, Palacios J, Escuin F, Gamallo C. Posttransplant CD30 (Ki-1)-positive anaplastic large cell lymphoma. Report of a case with presentation as a pleural effuison. Acta Cytol 1997; 41:1519–1524.
155. Levendoglu-Tugal O, Weiss R, Ozkaynak MF, Sandoval C, Lentzner B, Jayabose S. T-cell acute lymphoblastic leukemia after renal transplantation in childhood. J Pediatr Hematol Oncol 1998; 20:548–551.
156. DeCamp MM, Tinley NL. Late development of intractable lymphocele after renal transplantation. Transplant Proc 1988; 20:105–109.
157. Solilinger HW, Starling JR, Oberley T, Glass NR, Belzer FO. Severe "weeping" kidney disease after transplantation: a case report. Transplant Proc 1983; 15:2157–2160.
158. Bear RA, McCallum RW, Cant J, Goldstein MB, Johnson M. Perirenal lymphocyst formation in renal transplant recipients. Urology 1976; 7:581–586.
159. Schweizer RT, Cho S, Kountz SL, Belzer FO. Lymphoceles following renal transplantation. Arch Surg 1972; 104:42–45.
160. Morley P, Barnett E, Bell PRF, Briggs JK, Calman KC, Hamilton DN, Paton AM. Ultrasound in the diagnosis of fluid collections following renal transplantation. Clin Radiol 1975; 26:199–207.
161. Braun WE, Banowsky LH, Straffon RA, Nakamot S, Kiser WS, Popowniak KL. Lymphoceles associated with renal transplantation. Am J Med 1974; 57:714–729.
162. Koehler PR. Injuries and complications of the lymphatic system following renal transplantation. Lymphology 1972; 5:61–67.

163. Gomez-Romain JJ, Ocejo-Vinyals JG, Sanchez-Velasco P, Leyva-Cobian F, Val-Bernal JF. Presence of human herpesvirus 8 DNA sequences in renal transplantation-associated pleural Kaposi's sarcoma. Arch Pathol Lab Med 1999; 12:1269–1273.
164. Schmidt RJ, Bender FH, Chang WWL, Teba L. Sarcoidosis after renal transplantation. Transplantation 1999; 68:1420–1423.
165. Heino A, Orko R, Rosenberg PH. Anaesthesiological complications in renal transplantation: a retrospective study of 500 transplantations. Acta Anaesthesiol Scand 1986; 30:574–580.
166. Vereestrataeten P, DeKoster JP, Vereestrataeten J, Kinnaert P, Van Geertruyden J, Toussaint C. Pulmonary infections after kidney transplantation. Proc Eur Dial Transplant Assoc 1975; 11:300–307.
167. Jha R, Narayan G, Jaleel MA, Sinha S, Bhaskar V, Kashyap G, Rayudu BR, Prasad KN. Pulmonary infections after kidney transplantation. J Assoc Phys India 1999; 47:779–783.
168. Thacker WL, Benson RF, Schifman RB, Pugh E, Steigerwalt AG, Mayberry WR, Brenner DJ, Wilkinson HW. *Legionella tucsonensis* sp. nov. isolated from a renal transplant recipient. J Clin Microbiol 1989; 28:1831–1834.
169. McKinney RM, Wilkenson HW, Sommers HM, Fikes BJ, et al. *Legionella pneumophila* subgroup six: isolation from cases of legionellosis; identification by immunofluorescence staining, and immunological response to infection. J Clin Microbiol 1980; 12:395–401.
170. Bock BV, Kirby BD, Edelstein PH, George WL, Snyder KM, Owens ML, Hatayama CM, Haley CE, Lewis RP, Meyer RD, Finegold SM. Legionnaires' disease in renal-transplant recipients. Lancet 1978; 1:410–413.
171. Marshall W, Foster RS, Winn W. Legionnaires' disease in renal transplant patients. Am J Surg 1981; 141:423–429.
172. Moore EH, Webb WR, Gamsu G, Golden JA. Legionnaires' disease in the renal transplant patient: clinical presentation and radiographic progression. Radiology 1984; 153:589–593.
173. Foster RS, Winn WC, Marshall W, Gump DW. Legionnaires' disease following renal transplantation. Transplant Proc 1979; 11:93–95.
174. Levin AS, Caiaffa-Filho HH, Sinto SI, Sabbaga E, Barone AA, Mendes CM. An outbreak of nosocomial legionnaires' disease in a renal transplant unit in Sao Paulo, Brazil. J Hosp Infect 1991; 18:243–248.
175. Santamaria Saber T, Figueiredo JF, Santos SB, Levy CE, Reis MA, Ferraz AS. Nocardia infection in renal transplant recipient: diagnostic and therapeutic considerations. Rev Inst Med Trop Sao Paulo 1993; 35:417–421.
176. Lovett IS, Houang ET, Burge S, Turner-Warwick M, Thompson FD, Harrison AR, Joekes AM, Parkinson MC. An outbreak of *Nocardia asteroides* infection in a renal transplant unit. Q J Med 1981; 50:123–135.
177. Ochiai T, Ameniya H, Watanabe K, Sato H, Kobayashi A, Takizawa H, Iwasaki Y. Successful treatment of *Nocardia asteroides* infection with minocycline in kidney transplant patients. Jpn J Surg 1982; 8:138–144.
178. Tzamaloukas AH, Ahlin T, Katzestein D, Sterling WA. Association of pulmonary embolism and nocardiosis in renal transplant. Transplantation 1982; 33:569.
179. Arduino RC, Johnson PC, Miranda AG. Nocardiosis in renal transplant recipients undergoing immunosuppression with cyclosporine. Clin Infect Dis 1993; 16:505–512.

180. Lakshiminarayan S, Sahn SA. Tuberculosis in a patient after renal transplantation. Tubercle 1973; 54:72–76.
181. Hall CM, Willcox PA, Swanepoel CR, Khan D, Smit RVZ. Mycobacterial infection in renal transplant recipients. Chest 1994; 106:435–439.
182. Wood M, Wallin JD, O'Neill W. Disseminated tuberculosis in a renal transplant recipient: presentation as an anterior mediastinal mass. South Med J 1983; 76:1577–1579.
183. Malhotra KK, Dash SC, Dhawan IK, Bhuyan UN, Gupta A. Tuberculosis and renal transplantation: observations from an endemic area of tuberculosis. Postgrad Med 1986; 62:359–362.
184. Conces DJ, Vix VA, Traver RD. Pleural cryptococcosis. J Thorac imaging 1990; 5:84–86.
185. Lye WC, Chin NK, Lee YS. Disseminated cryptococcosis presenting with a pleural effusion in a kidney transplant recipient: early diagnosis by pleural biopsy and successful treatment with oral fluconazole (letter). Nephron 1993; 65:646.
186. Spencer CD, Crawford GE. Nontoxic staphylococcal pneumonia with empyema in a renal transplant recipient. West J Med 1982; 136:147–149.
187. Berk MR, Meyers AM, Cassal W, Botha JR, Myburgh JA. Non typhoid salmonella infections after renal transplantation. A serious clinical problem. Nephron 1984; 37:186–189.
188. Poiga JP, Watnick M, Herman PG. Pneumothorax following lung abscess in the renal transplant patient. J Assoc Can Radiol 1973; 24:116–118.
189. Castaneda MA, Garvin PJ. General surgical procedures in renal allograft recipients. Am J Surg 1986; 152:717–721.
190. US Department of Health and Human Services. 1994 Annual Report. Transplant Data: 1988–1993. US Scientific Registry of Transplant Recipients and Organ Procurement and Transplantation Network. US Government Printing Office, Washington, DC, 1994.
191. Egan TM, Kaiser LR, Cooper JD. Lung transplantation. Curr Probl Surg 1989; 26:681–751.
192. Tazelaar HD, Yousem SA. The pathology of combined heart-lung transplantation. Hum Pathol 1988; 19:1403–1416.
193. Bando K, Keenan RJ, Paradis IL, Konishi H, Komatsu K, Hardesty RL, Griffith BP. Impact of pulmonary hypertension on outcome after single-lung transplantation. Ann Thorac Surg 1994; 58:1336–1342.
194. Kaiser LR, Pasque MK, Trulock EP. Bilateral sequential lung transplantation: the procedure of choice for double-lung transplant. Ann Thorac Surg 1991; 52:445–446.
195. Triantafillou AN, Pasque MK, Huddleson CB, Pond CG, Cerza RF, Forstot RM, Cooper JD, Patterson GA, Lappas DG. Predictors, frequency, and indications for cardiopulmonary bypass during lung transplantation in adults. Ann Thorac Surg 1994; 57:1248–1251.
196. De Hoyos A, Demajo W, Snell G, Miller J, Winton T, Maurer JR, Patterson GA. Preoperative prediction for the use of cardiopulmonary bypass in lung transplantation. J Thorac Surg 1993; 106:787–796.
197. Collins J, Kuhlman JE, Love RB. Acute. Life-threatening complications of lung transplantation. Radiographics 1998; 18:21–45.
198. Dusmet M, Winton TL, Kesten S, Maurer J. Previous intrapleural procedures do not adversely affect lung transplantation. Lung Transplant 1996; 15:249–254.

199. Shennib H, Adoumie R, Noirclerc M. Current status of lung transplantation for cystic fibrosis. Arch Intern Med 1992; 152:1585–1588.
200. Panketh ARL, Knight RK, Hodson ME, Batten JC. Management of pneumothorax in adults with cystic fibrosis. Thorax 1982; 37:850–853.
201. Noppen M, Dhondt E, Mahler T, Malfoot A, Dab I, Vineken W. Successful management of recurrent pneumothorax in cystic fibrosis by localized apical thoracoscopic talc poudrage. Chest 1994; 106:262–264.
202. Noyes BE, Orenstein DM. Treatment of cystic fibrosis in the era of lung transplantation. Chest 1992; 101:1187–1188.
203. Rich H, Warwick W, leonard A. Open thoractomy and pleural abrasion in the treatment of spontaneous pneumothorax in cystic fibrosis. J Pediatr Pulmonol 1978; 13:237–242.
204. Madden BP, Hodson ME, Yacoub MH, Alton EW, Barnes PJ, Denison DM, Kay AB, Newman-Taylor A, Geddes DM. Heart-lung transplantation for cystic fibrosis. Br Med J 1992; 304:835–836.
205. Tsang V, Madden BP, Hodson ME, Yacoub MH. Heart-lung transplantation for cystic fibrosis. Pediatr Pulmonol 1990; (suppl 256).
206. Dosanjh A, Jones L, Yuh D, Robbins RC. Pleural disease in patients undergoing lung transplantation for cystic fibrosis. Pediatr Transplantation 1998; 2:283–287.
207. Herridge MS, de Hoyos AL, Chapparro C, Winton TL, Maurer JR. Pleural complications in lung transplant recipients. J Thorac Cardiovasc Surg 1995; 110:22–26.
208. Griffith BP, Zenati M. The pulmonary donor. Clin Chest Med 1990; 11:217–226.
209. Mills NL, Boyd AD, Gheranpong C. The significance of bronchial circulation in lung transplantation. J Thorac Cardiovasc Surg 1970; 60:866–878.
210. Venuta F, Boehler A, Rendina EA, De Giacomo T, Speich R, Schmid R, Coloni GF, Weder W. Complications in the native lung after single lung transplantation. Eur J Cardiovasc Surg 1999; 16:54–58.
211. Chiles C, Guthaner DF, Jamieson SW, Stinson EB, Oyer PE, Silverman JF. Heart-lung transplantation: the perioperative chest radiograph. Radiology 1985; 154:299–304.
212. Raju S, Heath BJ, Warren ET, Hardy JD. Single and double-lung transplantation. Ann Surg 1990; 211:681–693.
213. Siegelman SS, Sinha SBP, Veith FJ. Pulmonary reimplantation response. Ann Surg 1973; 177:30–36.
214. Ruggiero R, Fietsam R, Thomas GA, Muz J, Farris RH, Kowal TA, Myles JL, Stephenson LW, Baciewicz FA. Detection of canine allograft lung rejection by pulmonary lymphoscintigraphy. J Thorac Cardiovasc Surg 1994; 108:253–258.
215. Winter JB, Groen M, Petersen AH, Wildevuur CRH, Prop J. Reduced antibody responses after immunization in rat lung transplants. Am Rev Respir Dis 1993; 147:664–668.
216. Judson MA, Handy JR, Sahn SA. Pleural effusion from acute lung rejection. Chest 1997; 111:1128–1130.
217. Trulock EP. Management of acute lung rejection. Chest 1993; 103:1566–1567.
218. Bergin CJ, Castellino RA, Blank N, Berry GJ, Sibley RK, Starnes VA. Acute lung rejection after heart-lung transplantation: correlation of findings on chest radiographs with lung biopsy results. Am J Roentgenol 1990; 155:23–27.
219. Medina LS, Siegel MJ, Bejarano PA, Glazer HS, Anderson DJ, Mallory GB.

Pediatric lung transplantation: radiographic-histopathologic correlation. Radiology 1993; 187:807–810.
220. Medina LS, Siegel MJ, Glazer HS, Anderson DJ, Sememkovich J, Bejarano PA, Mallory GB. Diagnosis of pulmonary complications associated with lung transplantation in children: value of CT vs. histopathologic studies. Am J Roentgenol 1994; 162:969–974.
221. Judson MA, Handy JR, Sahn SA. Pleural effusions following lung transplantation: time course, characteristics, and clinical implications. Chest 1996; 109:1190–1194.
222. Struber M, Hagl C, Hirt SW, Cremer J, Harringer W, Haverich A. C1-esterase inhibitor in graft failure after lung transplantation. Intensive Care Med 1999; 25:1315–1318.
223. Judson MA, Sahn SA, Hahn AB. Origin of pleural cells after lung transplantation: from donor or recipient?. Chest 1997; 1112:426–429.
224. Collins J, Muller NL, Kazerooni EA, Paciocco G. CT findings of pneumonia after lung transplantation. Am J Roentgenology 2000; 175:811–818.
225. Snell GI, de Hoyos A, Krajden M, Winton T, Maurer JR. *Pseudomonas cepacia* in lung transplant recipients with cystic fibrosis. Chest 1993; 103:466–471.
226. Noyes BE, Michaels MG, Kurland G, Armitage JM, Orenstein DM. *Pseudomonas cepacia* empyema necessitatis after lung transplantation in two patients with cystic fibrosis. Chest 1994; 105:1888–1891.
227. Khan SU, Gordon SM, Stillwell PC, Kirby TJ, Arroliga AC. Empyema and bloodstream infection caused by *Burkholderia gladioli* in a patient with cystic fibrosis after lung transplantation. Pediatr Infect Dis J 1996; 15:637–639.
228. Brooks RG, Hofflin JM, Jamieson SW, Stinson EB, Remington JS. Infectious complications in heart-lung transplant recipients. Am J Med 1985; 79:412–422.
229. Horvath J, Dummer S, Loyd J, Walker B, Merrill WH, Frist WH. Infection in the transplanted and native lung after single lung transplantation. Chest 1993; 104:681–685.
230. Penketh ARL, Higenbottam TW, Hutter J, Coutts C, Stewart S, Wallwork J. Clinical experience in the management of pulmonary opportunist infection and rejection in recipients of heart-lung transplants. Thorax 1988; 43:762–769.
231. Dromer C, Nashef SAM, Velly J, Martigne C, Courand L. Tuberculosis in transplanted lungs. J Heart Lung Transplant, 1993, 924–927.
232. Schulman LL, Scully B, McGregor CC, Austin JHM. Pulmonary tuberculosis after lung transplantation. Chest 1997; 111:1459–1462.
233. Emery RW, Graif JL, Hale K, Eales F, Von Rueden TJ, Pritzker MR, Love K, Arom KV. Treatment of end-stage chronic obstructive pulmonary disease with double lung transplantation. Chest 1991; 99:533–537.
234. Liguori C, Schulman LL, Weslow RG, DiTullio MR, McGregor CC, Smith CR, Homma S. Late pulmonary venous complications after lung transplantation. J Am Soc Echocardiography 1997; 10:763–767.
235. Collins J, Muller NL, Leung AN, McGuinness G, Mergo PJ, Flint JD, Warner TF, Poirier C, Theodore J, Zander D, Yee HT. Epstein-Barr-virus-associated lymphoproliferative disease of the lung: CT and histologic findings. Radiology 1998; 208:749–759.
236. Kukafka DS, O'Brien GM, Furukawa S, Criner GJ. Surveillance bronchoscopy in lung transplant recipients. Chest 1997; 111:377–381.
237. Chan CC, Abi-Saleh WJ, Arroliga AC, Stillwell PC, Kirby TJ, Gordon SM, Petras

RE, Mehta AC. Diagnostic yield and therapeutic impact of flexible bronchoscopy in lung transplant recipients. J Heart Lung Transplant 1996; 15:196–205.
238. Yousem SA, Burke CM, Billingham ME. Pathologic pulmonary alterations in long-term human heart-lung transplantation. Hum Pathol 1985; 16:911–923.
239. Haverich A, Dawkins KD, Baldwin JC, Reitz BA, Billingham ME, Jamieson SW. Long-term cardiac and pulmonary histology in primates following combined heart and lung transplantation. Transplantation 1985; 39:356–360.
240. Engeler CE, Olson PN, Engeler CM, Carpenter BL, Crowe JE, Day DL, Hertz MI, Bolman RM. Shifting pneumothorax after heart-lung transplantation. Radiology 1992; 185:715–717.
241. Wittich GR, Kusnick CA, Starnes VA, Lucas DE. Communication between two pleural cavities after major cardiothoracic surgery: relevance to percutaneous intervention. Radiology 1992; 184:461–462.
242. Paranjpe DV, Wittich GR, Hamid LW, Bergin CJ. Frequency and management of pneumothoraces in heart-lung transplant recipients. Radiology 1994; 190:255–256.
243. Sacks EM, Unger EC. Heart-lung transplantation: postoperative pleural effusion. Am J Roentgenol 1990; 154:1344–1345.
244. Holland SA, Hutton LC, McKenzie FN. Radiologic findings in heart-lung transplantation: a preliminary experience. J Can Assoc Radiol 1989; 40:94–97.
245. Slebos DJ, Elting-Wartan AN, Bakker M, van der Bij W, van Putten JW. Managing a bilateral pneumothorax in lung transplantation using single chest-tube drainage. J Heart Lung Transplant 2001; 19:796–797.
246. Lee YC, McGrath GB, Chin WS, Light RW. Contralateral tension pneumothorax following chest tube drainage of bilateral pneumothoraces in a heart-lung transplant patient. Chest 1999; 116:1131–1133.
247. Spaggiari L, Rusca M, Carbognani P, Cattelani L, Rossini E, Paolucci R, Rizzoli V, Bobbio P. Contralateral spontaneous pneumothorax after single lung transplantation for fibrosis. Acta Biomed Ateneo Parmense 1993; 64:29–31.
248. Venuta F, Rendina EA, Giacomo TD, Ciriaco PP, Rocca GD, Ricci C. Thoracoscopic treatment of recurrent contralateral pneumothorax after single lung transplantation. J Heart Lung Transplant 1994; 13:555–557.
249. Waller DA, Conacher ID, Dark JH. Videothoracoscopic pleurectomy after contralateral single-lung transplantation. Ann Thorac Surg 1994; 57:1021–1023.
250. Shumway SJ, Hertz MI, Petty MG, Bolman RM. Liberalization of donor criteria in lung and heart-lung transplantation. Ann Thorac Surg 1994; 57:92–95.

50

Pharmacokinetics and Pharmacodynamics in Pleural Fluid

IOANNIS LIAPAKIS
University Hospital of Alexandroupolis
Alexandroupolis, Greece

RICHARD W. LIGHT
Vanderbilt University
and Saint Thomas Hospital
Nashville, Tennessee, U.S.A.

**IOANNIS KOTTAKIS and
DEMOSTHENES BOUROS**
Demokritos University of Thrace Medical School
and University Hospital of Alexandroupolis
Alexandroupolis, Greece

I. Introduction

Pharmacokinetics is the study of the quantitative pattern and time course of drug disposition in the body after administration by any route. Pharmacodynamics in turn deals with concentration-effect relationships. To elicit a desirable pharmacological action requires delivering the appropriate concentration of drug to a specific site of action (1). For this purpose, drug pharmacodynamic studies can provide important information to maximize the clinical efficacy of pharmacological agents as well as to minimize their toxicity. In the case of pleural disease, the targeted sites of drug action are the pleural tissue and the pleural fluid. Thus, achieving a clinical relevant pharmacological response depends on the delivery of the drug to the pleural tissue and fluid in sufficient concentrations. However, the pharmacokinetics and pharmacodynamics of drugs in human pleural tissue and fluid have rarely been studied. For example, in the case of pleural infections the role of pleural tissue or pleural fluid antibiotic concentration has been minimally investigated. The limited data available, in support of the importance of the pharmacokinetics of antibiotics in pleural tissues, are mainly derived from experimental animals (2).

To target the pleural cavity, two modes of drug administration can be used: systemic administration and local instillation. Antibiotics are systemically administered for the treatment of complicated parapneumonic effusions, empyema, and tuberculous pleurisy. In the case of complicated parapneumonic effusions it can be hypothesized that higher concentrations can be achieved if the drug is directly injected into in the pleural cavity via a chest tube. At present this type of application is not generally recommended (3), and as a result few pharmacokinetic and pharmacodynamic data referring to the pleural space exist. Fibrinolytics are directly applied in the pleural cavity in the management of loculated pleural effusions, and as a result their pharmacodynamic effects have been studied to some extent. Talc, the tetracyclines and bleomycin are also directly applied in the pleural cavity and used for their fibrosis-inducing effect in the management of malignant pleural effusions. However, as is also the case for fibrinolytics, their pharmacokinetic clearance in the human body following this type of application has not been sufficiently studied.

II. Pharmacokinetics in Pleural Fluid

Systemically administered antibiotics are used in the treatment of pleural infections and especially complicated parapneumonic effusions and empyema. The prescribed antibiotics need to be effective against the specific offending microorganism. Streptococci and staphylococci are the common gram-positive organisms, while *Klebsiella* spp., *Pseudomonas* spp., and *Haemophilus influenzae* are the common gram-negative causative organisms. In addition, up to 15% of parapneumonic effusions are caused by anaerobic bacteria (3). Of importance, empirical therapy needs to be initiated as soon as pleural fluid, sputum, and blood samples have been taken. Second- and third-generation cephalosporins, β-lactam–β-lactamase inhibitor combinations, macrolides, metronidazole, clindamycin, imipenem, aminoglycosides, or aztreonam may be considered (3). In addition to the specifity of the antimicrobial agent for the offending microorganism, its distribution within the body is a critical factor in determining its therapeutic efficacy. If the antimicrobial agent does not enter the site at which the offending microorganism resides, bacterial growth will continue despite in vitro susceptibility of the organism to the drug. In this context, the usefulness of an antimicrobial agent in the treatment of pleural diseases depends on the attainment of adequate drug concentrations within the intrapleural sites of infection (4).

In general, it is believed that antibiotic levels achieved in the pleural fluid following systemic administration are similar to those in serum. However, the evidence supporting this postulation is derived mainly from human studies involving patients with diseases other than empyema. In empyema, changes in permeability caused by thickened pleura (5) and changes in pleural fluid acidity may result in significant differences in the antibiotic level obtained in pleural pus and serum following systemic administration. Low drug concentrations may be the result of poor blood supply through the fibrosed-calcified pleura and/or of binding or inactivation of the drugs by the components of the purulent fluid. In one report, the concentration of rifampin in the pleural fluid was <4% of that in the serum in a case of chronic tuberculous empyema with thickened pleura (containing acidic, purulent fluid) (6). In the particular case, the patient was treated with rifampin, ethambutol, streptomycin, and ofloxacin. The maximum concentration (C_{max}) for ethambutol in the pleural fluid exceeded the C_{max} in serum by 19%, with no observed differences in the time to maximal concentration (T_{max}) in the serum and the pleural fluid. In contrast, the C_{max} in pleural fluid for rifampin, streptomycin, and ofloxacin were only 4, 34, and 48%, respectively, of the C_{max} in serum. For these three drugs, the T_{max} in pleural fluid occurred 8 hours later than in the serum. These findings strongly suggest that in chronic empyema, drug delivery is variable and unreliable.

Overall, the correlation between the pleural fluid and the serum antibiotic levels has been poorly studied. Teixeira et al. (5), in an elegant study using a new rabbit model of empyema, determined the relationships between the pleural fluid and the serum antibiotic levels of metronidazole, penicillin, clindamycin, ceftriaxone, vancomycin, and gentamicin. Drug pharmacokinetics were studied after IV administration. It was found that the penetration of the tested antibiotics into infected pleural fluid varied. Antibiotic penetration was the greatest for penicillin, metronidazole, followed by ceftriaxone, vancomycin, and clindamycin. The degree of penetration was the least for gentamicin. The area under the curve (AUC) pleural fluid: AUC serum ratio for penicillin was >1 as pleural fluid levels remained elevated until 240 minutes despite decreasing serum levels. The time to pleural fluid antibiotic level and serum antibiotic level equilibration was more rapid for penicillin (30–60 min) and metronidazole (60–120 min), followed by ceftriaxone, vancomycin, gentamicin, and finally clindamycin. It should be noted that very high levels of bioactive penicillin remained in the pleural space, despite diminishing serum penicillin levels over time. The pharmacokinetic data for the six different antibiotics are listed in Table 1: the highest ratio of the peak pleural fluid to the peak serum level occurred with metronidazole, and the lowest with gentamicin; the shortest time for peak antibiotic level in the pleural fluid was achieved with metronidazole (15 min), while the longest time was with clindamycin (480 min). These differences in the degree of penetration of antibiotics into the pleural space and the rates of equilibration need be considered when prescribing antibiotics for patients with complicated pleural effusion, although the findings come from animal studies.

Craig (7) found that systemic doses of aminoglycosides are limited by a low therapeutic index, and thus increasing the systemic dose to achieve adequate pleural concentrations may not be appropriate. In contrast, for most penicillins, cephalosporins and quinolones the systemic dose can be increased if necessary to ensure adequate pleural fluid concentrations (7). Thys et al. (8) have reported that the concentration of amikacin in sterile postthoracotomy pleural exudates is variable according to the delay between the injection of the drug and the samplings (8). The ratio of pleural fluid: serum concentration 1, 2, and 4 hours after IV injection of amikacin was 0.6, 0.9, and 1.0 mg/dL, respectively, and after 6 and 8 hours was 1.4 and 1.9, respectively. This implies that the penetration of

Table 1 Pharmacokinetic Data for Six Different Antibiotics in Rabbit Serum and Pleural Fluid

Variables	Metronidazole	Penicillin	Clindamycin	Ceftriaxone	Vancomycin	Gentamicin
Dose	37 mg/kg	24000 U/kg	9 mg/kg	30 mg/kg	15 mg/kg	1 mg/kg
Peak serum level, μg/mL	25.6	12.5	6.8	172	42.9	2.5
Peak fluid level, μg/mL	17.0	3.8	2.9	41.6	9.6	0.3
PF/S ratio	0.7	0.3	0.4	0.2	0.2	0.1
T_{max} serum, min	15	15	30	15	15	15
T_{max} PF, min	15	120	480	240	60	60
AUC PF/S ratio	0.984	2.310	0.743	0.821	0.610	0.496

PF = pleural fluid; S = serum; AUC = area under the curve.
Source: Modified from Ref. 5.

IV-administrated amikacin in the pleural fluid may be satisfactory, a finding supported by the high ratio (80%) of the AUC in the two fluids. Furthermore, the lowest pleural concentration of amikacin observed at 8 hours after the IV injection was greater than the minimal inhibitory concentration (MIC). Since the elimination half-life of amikacin from the pleural fluid is longer than that from the serum, even higher concentrations of amikacin in the pleural space can be expected following multiple dosing. From the above one might deduce that the parenteral (IV) standard dose administration of amikacin is adequate to obtain satisfactory pleural levels of the drug. However, as already mentioned, the pharmacokinetics of antibiotics in pleural tissue and fluid differs depending on the nature of the effusion. Therefore, the pleural and serum amikacin levels observed by Thys et al. (8) cannot be extrapolated to cases of empyema. In particular, in cases of chronic empyema, the aminoglycosides have been found to be especially susceptible to local conditions such as acidic pH < 7.4 (9) or interaction with purulent material; factors that may partially reduce the bioactivity of aminoglycosides in the pleural fluid. In particular, previous in vitro studies (10) have demonstrated that pH and divalent cations influence antimicrobial activity as well as aminoglycoside-modifying enzyme effectiveness: the aminoglycoside MICs can increase up to fivefold at pH < 6.5 and up to eightfold at magnesium, calcium ions, and ferric iron concentrations > 10 mM. The adaptive resistance to aminoglycosides in *Pseudomonas aeruginosa* and other gram-negative bacilli that can cause empyema is greater and more prolonged with higher initial drug concentrations (11).

Pleural fluid acidity is also extremely important for the effectiveness of quinolones and macrolides. Fluoroquinolones have a free carboxyl group that becomes unprotonated at higher pHs. Therefore, less of the antibacterial agent penetrates the cell membrane at a pH of 8 than a pH of 6 (12). These drugs generally tend to accumulate in tissues to the extent that local concentrations usually exceed serum concentrations by a ratio of greater than 2:1 to 3:1 in the bronchial mucosa, 8:1 in epithelial lining fluid, and >25:1 in alveolar macrophages. However, intracellular penetration of a fluoroquinolone agent does not necessarily correlate with its antibacterial activity (13). Ciprofloxacin, compared to newer fluoroquinolones, has the lowest intracellular concentration but exhibits the greatest antibacterial effect. Ciprofloxacin is a fluoroquinolone highly active in vitro against a broad spectrum of gram-negative and gram-positive organisms (14–18). Clinical reports have indicated efficacy and safety in a wide range of bacterial infections (19). Pharmacokinetic studies in humans have shown mean serum concentrations higher than the MICs usually necessary. The serum half-lives range between 3 and 4 hours depending on dose and route of administration, and the absolute bioavailability is approximately 80% (19–21). In addition, the high volume of distribution indicates good tissue penetration (20–22). Furthermore, estimation of ciprofloxacin concentrations in sputum and bronchial mucosa confirmed good penetration into the respiratory tract (23,24).

Bergan (25) recommended that pleural fluid levels and empyema fluid concentrations of ciprofloxacin be in the same order as serum after an interval of 1–2 hours when equilibrium has been established between the blood and pleural cavity compartments. Somewhat higher levels are observed in the pleural fluid than in serum toward the end of the dosage intervals because distribution from the former is slower. Ciprofloxacin levels in pleural tissue correspond to serum concentrations. Furthermore, Morgenroth et al. (26) evaluated the pharmacokinetics of a single 200 mg dose of ciprofloxacin, administered as an intravenous 30-minute infusion, into pleural exudates in patients with empyema. They found that systemically administered ciprofloxacin penetrates well into the pleural fluid of patients with empyema thoracis. The concentrations achieved were well above the MIC of most pathogens normally found in patients with empyema thoracis for a period of approximately 12 hours.

Macrolides, mainly azithromycin and clarithromycin, are acid-stable. This fact, combined with their increased bioavailability and high extracellular concentration, suggests that macrolides may be effective in the treatment of pleural infection (12). However, there are no studies on the pharmacokinetics of macrolides in the pleural effusion. With regard to the use of penicillin and cephalosporins, Taryle et al. (27), using a group of five patients with pleural empyema, nine with uncomplicated parapneumonic effusions, and two with malignant effusions, determined the simultaneous pleural fluid and serum antibiotic concentrations. All patients received either penicillin or a cephalosporin derivative. It was observed that these antibiotics penetrated well into pleural fluid. The PF: serum ratio usually exceeded 0.75, and the absolute pleural fluid concentrations were sufficient in most cases to inhibit the common etiological agents of the uncomplicated parapneumonic effusions and empyema. These findings suggest that standard systemic doses of penicillin and cephalosporins provide adequate pleural fluid concentrations in both empyemas and uncomplicated parapneumonic effusions.

Otero et al. (28) studied the pharmacokinetics of cefoxitin in six healthy volunteers and in five patients with a pleural effusion after administration of a single dose of 30 mg/kg IV infusion. It was shown that the elimination half-life of cefoxitin from pleural fluid was two- to threefold longer than that of serum, which indicates a difference between the kinetic elimination processes of the antibiotic from the two fluids. In this context, the slow elimination of cefoxitin from pleural fluid facilitates its accumulation in this compartment during a multiple-dose regimen.

III. Pharmacodynamics in Pleural Fluid

For systemically administered antibiotics for the treatment of empyema, clinical response depends on the following key parameters (13): (1) time above the MIC (T > MIC) for penicillins and cephalosporins and probably macrolides (with the expecting of azithromycin); (2) area under the inhibitory time curve (AUC/MIC = AUIC) for quinolones. An AUIC below 125 represents inadequate activity, between 125 and 250 is acceptable, and over 250 is optimal. The upper limit of 500 s empiric. Beyond that value the patient is receiving more than twice the drug that is associated with optimal response; (3) peak serum concentration above the minimum inhibitory concentration (C_{max} > MIC) for aminoglycosides.

From a pharmacodynamic perspective, the local instillation of antibiotics has not been proved to be superior to systemic administration in the treatment of empyemas, although direct injection of these drugs into the pleural cavity has been used in an attempt to insure sufficient levels of the drug. For example, the pleural levels of amikacin are extremely high and well sustained, even 8 hours after intrapleural injection. On the negative side, severe intoxication and neuromuscular paralysis with respiratory arrest have been described with intrapleural use of aminoglycosides (8) or other antibiotics.

For directly applied fibrinolytics, many studies have shown that intrapleural fibrinolytic instillation may be an effective and safe mode of treatment of complicated parapneumonic effusions and empyema which minimizes the need for surgical intervention (29). The fibrinolytics used are streptokinase and urokinase. The technique of instillation is not standardized. The success rate ranges from 37.5 to 100%, but it is dependent upon the stage of the pleural effusion. Generally, it is more successful in complicated parapneumonic effusions rather than in empyema. Fibrinolytic agents are more effective if used early in the evolution of parapneumonic effusions before significant collagen is deposited in the pleural space (30), especially if after chest tube placement inadequate evacuation of pleural fluid is noted radiographically with no clinical improvement (31). However, the optimal dosage and timing of intrapleural fibrinolytic therapy still remains to be fully established. Most studies have used single doses of 250,000 IU streptokinase or 100,000 IU urokinase, though a recent study reported good results with single daily doses of 50,000 urokinase (31). Adverse reactions are rare, of allergic type, and more frequent for streptokinase than urokinase. Intravenous use of streptokinase can potentially lead to antistreptokinase antibodies in the blood, which may lead to an allergic reaction if it is readministered later in the patient's life (after an acute myocardial infarction). This has not been systematically studied after intrapleural instillation. A case of acute hypoxemic respiratory failure following intrapleural instillation of both streptokinase and urokinase 24 hours apart for hemothorax has been described (32). Suggestions that intrapleural fibrinolytics may create or reopen a bronchopleural fistula have been made (33,34).

In the case of malignant pleural effusions, intrapleural administration of talc by poudrage or slurry, the tetracyclines (doxycycline or minocycline), or antineoplastic drugs (bleomycin, mitoxantrone, or nitrogen-mustard) is used because these molecules can lead to pleurodesis. None is ideal. Bleomycin is probably less efficacious than are the tetracycline derivatives or talc (35). The injection of the tetracyclines into the pleural space is at times extremely painful (36). The injection of talc can lead to the development of acute respiratory distress syndrome (37,38) and systemic embolization to distant organs (39,40) Accordingly, the search continues for an ideal sclerosing agent. Recent studies have investigated the use of transforming growth factor (TGF-β2) as a pleurodesing agent (41–44). Transforming growth factor-β is unique in that it is the most profibrotic cytokine known, but it also has significant anti-inflammatory properties (45,46). A single intrapleural injection of TGF-β2 can produce effective pleurodesis in rabbits (43) and at a rate faster than talc (41). Importantly, the pleurodesing process does not appear to involve excessive pleural inflammation (41) and, therefore, is not inhibited by corticosteroids (47). Furthermore, no histological abnormalities in extrapulmonary organs have been observed in sheep 2 weeks after TGF-β2 pleurodesis (42). However, the acute effects of intrapleural injection of TGF-β2 and its potential systemic absorption have not been investigated.

IV. Conclusion

Data on the penetration of systemically administered antibiotics in the pleural fluid are limited, and the same applies to their pharmacodynamic effect. In particular, the pharmacokinetics of the antibiotics used in the treatment of complicated effusions differ significantly from one drug to another. Fluoroquinolones accumulate within tissues to the extent that tissue concentrations exceed those in plasma. In this context, fluoroquinolones qualify as a valid option in the therapy of empyema. It needs also to be noted that the free, non–protein-bound fraction of an antibiotic is active against bacteria, and only unbound antibiotic diffuses freely between intravascular and extravascular compartments. Thus, it is the free antibiotic concentrations in plasma and tissues, and not the protein-bound fraction, which is the more relevant parameter for pharmacokinetic/pharmacodynamic correlations. Limited pharmacodynamic data also exist for fibrinolytics and agents that produce pleurodesis, while the pharmacokinetic profile of these agents remains largely unstudied. Because pharmacokinetics and pharmacodynamics relate not only to drug efficacy, but also to drug toxicity, it is important that studies be undertaken with the intent to fully investigate and clarify the pharmacokinetic-pharmacodynamic parameters of all drugs used in the treatment of pleural disease.

References

1. Witek TJ, Schachter EN. Pharmacology and Therapeutics in Respiratory Care. Philadelphia: WB Saunders Company, 1994.
2. Baudouin Byl, Jacobs F, Roucloux I, De Franquen P, Cappello M, Thys J-P. Penetration of meropenem in lung, bronchial mucosa and pleural tissues. Antimicrob Agents Chemother 1999; 43:681–682.
3. Hamm H, Light RW. Parapneumonic effusion and empyema. Eur Respir J 1997; 10:1150–1156.
4. Wong GA, Peirce TH, Goldstein E, Hoeprich PD. Penetration of antimicrobial agents into bronchial secretions. Am J Med 1975; 59:219–223.
5. Teixeira LR, Sasse SA, Villarino MA, Nguyen T, Mulligan ME, Light RW. Antibiotic levels in empyemic pleural fluid. Chest 2000; 117:1734–1739.
6. Elliot AM, Berning SE, Iseman MD, Peloquin CA. Failure of drug penetration and acquisition of drug resistance in chronic tuberculous empyema. Tub Lung Dis 1995; 76:463–467.
7. Craig WA. Interrelationship between pharmacokinetics and pharmacodynamics in determining dosage regimens for broad-spectrum cephalosporins. Diagn Microbiol Infect Dis 1995; 22:89–96.
8. Thys JP, Serruys-Schoutens E, Rocmans P, Herchuez A, Vanderlinden MP, Yourassowsky E. Amikacin concentrations in uninfected postthoracotomy pleural fluid and in serum after intravenous and intrapleural injection. Chest 1984; 85:502–505.
9. Potts EP, Levin DC, Sahn SA. Pleural fluid pH in parapneumonic effusions. Chest 1976; 70:328–331.
10. Nanavaty J, Mortensen JE, Shryock TR. The effects of environmental conditions on the in vitro activity of selected antimicrobial agents against *E. coli*. Curr Microbiol 1998; 36:212–215.
11. Xiong Y-O, Cailon J, Drugeon H, Potel G, Baron D. Influence of pH on adaptive resistance of pseudomonas aeruginosa to aminoglycosides and their postantibiotic effects. Antimicrob Agents Chemother 1996; 40:35–39.
12. Butts JD. Intracellular concentrations of antibacterial agents and related clinical implications. Clin Pharm Concepts 1994; 27:63–84.
13. Wise R. A review of the clinical pharmacology of moxifloxacin, a new 8-methoxyquinolone, and its potential relation to therapeutic efficacy. Clin Drug Invest 1999; 17:365–387.
14. Chin NX, Neu HC. Ciprofloxacin, a quinolone carboxylic acid compound active against aerobic and anaerobic bacteria. Antimicrob Agents Chemother 1984; 25:319–326.
15. Hoogkamp-Korstanje JAA. Comparative in vitro activity of five quinolone deriva-

tives and five other antimicrobial agents used in oral therapy. Eur J Clin Microbiol 1984; 3:333–338.
16. King A, Shannon K, Phillips I. The in vitro activities of enoxacin and ofloxacin compared with that of ciprofloxacin. J Antimicrob Chemother 1985; 15:551–558.
17. Reeves DS, Bywater MJ, Holt HA, White LO. In vitro studies with ciprofloxacin, a new 4-quinolone compound. J Antimicrob Chemother 1984; 13:333–346.
18. Wise R, Andrews JM, Edwards LJ. In vitro activity of Bayer 09867: a new quinolone derivative compared with those of other antimicrobial agents. Antimicrob Agents Chemother 1983; 23:559–564.
19. Schacht P, Bruch H, Chysky V, Hullmann R, Weuta H, Acrieri G. Overall clinical results with ciprofloxacin. 14th International Congress of Chemotherapy, Kyoto, Japan, 1985.
20. Bergan T, Thorsteinsson SB, Solberg R, Bjornskau L, Kolstad IM, Johnsen S. Pharmacokinetics of ciprofloxacin: intravenous and increasing oral doses. Am J Med 1987; 82:97–102.
21. Wise R, Donovan IA. Tissue penetration and metabolism of ciprofloxacin. Am J Med 1987; 82:103–107.
22. Crump B, Wise R, Dent J. Pharmacokinetics and tissue penetration of ciprofloxacin. Antimicrob Agents Chemother 1983; 24:784–786.
23. Honeybourne D, Andrews JM, Ashby JP, Lodwick R, Wise R. Evaluation of the penetration of ciprofloxacin and amoxycillin into the bronchial mucosa. Thorax 1988; 43:715–719.
24. Thys JP, Klastersky J, Jacobs F, Berre J, Gangji D, Hanotte F. Penetration of ciprofloxacin into bronchial secretions and pleural fluid. First International Ciprofloxacin Workshop. Amsterdam: Excerpta Medica, 1986:153–156.
25. Bergan T. Extravascular penetration of ciprofloxacin: a review. Diagn Microbiol Inf Dis 1990; 13:103–114.
26. Mogenroth A, Pfeuffer HP, Seelmann R, Schweisfurth H. Pleural penetration of ciprofloxacin in patients with empyema thoracis. Chest 1991; 100:406–409.
27. Taryle DA, Good JD, Morgan EJ, Reller LB, Sahn SA. Antibiotic concentrations in human parapneumonic effusions. J Antimicrob Chemother 1981; 7:171–177.
28. Otero MJ, Garcia MG, Barrueco M, Dominguez-Gil A, Gomez F, Alvarez JP. Pharmacokinetics of cefoxitin administrated by i.v. infusion to patients with a pleural effusion. Eur J Clin Pharm 1994; 26:389–392.
29. Bouros D, Schiza S, Siafakas NM. Utility of fibrinolytic agents for draining intrapleural infections. Sem Respir Inf 1999; 14:39–47.
30. Sahn SA. Parapneumonic effusions: patholphysiology, diagnosis, and management. American College of Chest Physicians. PCCU, Volume 12, lessons 6, 1997.
31. Bouros D, Schiza S, Siafakas N. Fibrinolytics in the treatment of parapneumonic effusions. Monaldi Arch Chest Dis 1999; 54:258–263.
32. Frye MD, Jarratt M, Sahn SA. Acute hypoxemic respiratory failure following intrapleural thrombolytic therapy for hemothorax. Chest 1994; 105:1595–1596.
33. Bouros D, Schiza S, Panagou P, Drositis J, Siafakas N. Role of streptokinase in the treatment of acute loculated parapneumonic pleural effusions and empyema. Thorax 1994; 49:852–855.
34. Godley PJ, Bell RC. Major hemorrhage following administration of intrapleural streptokinase. Chest 1984; 86:486–487.
35. Walker-Renard PB, Vaughan LM, Sahn SA. Chemical pleurodesis for malignant pleural effusions. Ann Intrern Med 1994; 120:56–64.

36. Light RW, O'Hara VS, Moritz TE, Mc Elhinney AJ, Butz R, Haakenson CM, Read RC, Sasson CS, Eastridge CE, Berger R, Fontenelle LJ, Bell RH, Jenkinson SG, Shure D, Merrill W, Hoover E, Campell SC. Intrapleural tetracycline for the prevention of recurrent spotaneous pneumothorax. JAMA 1990; 264:2224–2230.
37. Milanez de Campos JR, Werebe EC, Vargas FS, Jatene FB, Light RW. Respiratory failure due to insufflated talc. Lancet 1997; 349:251–252.
38. Rehse DH, Aye RW, Florence MG. Respiratory failure following talc pleurodesis. Am J Surg 1999; 177:437–440.
39. Kennedy L, Harley RA, Sahn SA, Strange C. Talc slurry pleurodesis. Pleural fluid and histologic analysis. Chest 1995; 107:1707–1012.
40. Werebe EC, Pazetti R, Milanez de Campos JR. Systemic distribution of talc after intrapleural administration in rats. Chest 1999; 115:190–193.
41. Lee YCG, Texeira LR, Devin CJ. Transforming growth factor-β2 induces pleurodesis significantly faster than talc. Am J Respir Crit Care Med 2001; 163:640–644.
42. Lee YCG, Lane KB, Parker RE. Transforming growth factor-β2 produces effective pleurodesis in sheep with no systemic complications. Thorax 2000; 55:1058–1062.
43. Light RW, Cheng DS, Lee YCG, Rogers J, Davidson J, Lane KB. A single intrapleural injection of transforming growth factor-β2 produces an excellent pleurodesis in rabbits. Am J Respir Crit Care Med 2000; 162:98–104.
44. Lee YCG, Malkerneker D, Devin CJ. Comparing transforming growth factor-β2 and fibronectin as pleurodesing agents. Respirology 2001; 6:281–286.
45. Border W, Noble NA. Transforming growth factor-β2 in tissue fibrosis. N Engl J Med 1994; 331:1286–1292.
46. Lee YCG, Lane KB. The many faces of transforming growth factor-β in pleural diseases. Curr Opin Pulm Med 2001; 7:173–179.
47. Lee YCG, Devin CJ, Texeira LR. Transforming growth factor-β2 induced pleurodesis is not inhibited by corticosteroids. Thorax 2001; 56:643–648.

51

Animal Models in Pleural Investigation

RICHARD W. LIGHT

Vanderbilt University
and Saint Thomas Hospital
Nashville, Tennessee, U.S.A.

I. Pleural Inflammation

Inflammation of the pleural space has been studied by means of the intrapleural injection of several different inflammation-producing agents. Although carrageenan is the agent investigated most extensively, other agents investigated include zymosan (1,2), endotoxin or lipopolysaccharide (LPS) (3,4), antigen-antibody reactions (5), monosodium urate (6), and miconazole (7).

A. Carrageenan

Carrageenan-induced pleurisy in rats or mice has been widely used for many years for the study of pleural inflammation. When 1.2 mL of 0.25% carrageenan is injected into the pleural space of rats, the initial inflammatory response is in the immediate subpleural tissue that contains the blood vessels (8). Then there is a rapid release of white blood cells (WBC) into the pleural space along with the development of an exudative pleural effusion (9). The peak amount of exudative pleural fluid and the peak WBC occur about 16 hours after injection (8). Initially, most of the white blood cells are neutrophils. The number of mononuclear cells peaks at 24 hours when the numbers of mononuclear cells and neutrophils are comparable. By 72 hours postinjection, mononuclear cells account for 90% of the cells. By 96 hours negligible numbers of neutrophils and pleural fluid remain (9). Pleural inflammation has also been studied in mice after the intrapleural administration of carrageenan. They develop inflammatory exudates 4 hours postinjection (10).

This model has been used to investigate the influence of many compounds on this inflammatory reaction. The following are a few examples of the many investigations carried out. The early (<48 h) inflammatory response is depressed by cyclooxygenase inhibitors (aspirin and indomethacin) (8), but the response at 72 hours is influenced much less (9). Corticosteroids decrease the inflammatory response throughout the entire period (8). On a more basic level, Sautebin and associates demonstrated that there was a close correlation between the levels of nitric oxide and prostaglandin E_2 4 hours after the intrapleural injection of carrageenin (11). Scavengers of nitric oxide such as hemoglobin reduced the inflammation and the amount of prostaglandin E_2 in the pleural fluid (11). D'Acquisto and associates (12) demonstrated that there was NF-κB DNA-binding activity in the inflammatory cells that migrated into the pleural cavity at 3 and 6 hours. This activity markedly increased at 24 hours and then decreased at 48 hours after the induction of the inflammation. Frode et al. demonstrated that the intraperitoneal administration of NF-κB inhibitors before the intrapleural injection of carrageenan inhibited the inflammatory response (13). This same group demonstrated that the pro-inflammatory cytokines tumor necrosis factor (TNF)-α and interleukin (IL)-1β, when injected intraperitoneally 5 minutes before carrageenan, augmented the inflammatory response, while antibodies against these two cytokines reduced, in a graded and significant manner, both the exudation and cell migration in the early inflammatory phase while they potentiated or had no effect on the late (48 h) phases of inflammation and fluid exudation (13). In contrast, Cuzzocrea and associates demonstrated that the in vivo depletion of endogenous glutathione pools with L-buthionine-(S,R)-sulfoximine enhances the carrageenan-induced degree of pleural exudation and neutrophil migration (14).

This model has also been used in experiments with knockout mice (mice deficient in certain genes). When IL-6 knockout mice are injected with carrageenan, both the amount of pleural fluid and the pleural fluid WBC fall by 50% as compared with wild-type mice (15). The same reduction in the inflammatory response is obtained if the mice are given anti-IL-6 before the carrageenan treatment (15). It has also been shown that there is a marked reduction in the inflammatory response to carrageenan intrapleurally in mice deficient for the inducible nitric oxide synthetase enzyme, as compared to mice that are not deficient in this gene (10).

B. Zymosan

The intrapleural injection of zymosan also produces an inflammatory exudate. When 0.1 mL of 2% zymosan is injected into the pleural space, the reaction is similar to that induced by carrageenan, with an early neutrophil influx and the maximal accumulation of pleural fluid at 24 hours. The maximal amount of fluid following zymosan and carrageenan are comparable (~1.5 mL) (2,8,16). The levels of TNF-α, IL-1, IL-6, and cytokine-induced neutrophil chemoattractant (CINC) in the pleural fluid all begin to increase after 1–2 hours, preceding the influx of neutrophils, and peak after 4–5 hours (2). The inflammatory response to carrageenan and zymosan are very similar. However, after the intrapleural administration of zymosan, more Evans blue dye (a marker of vascular permeability) accumulates in the pleural cavity than when carrageenan is administered (17). Kikuchi and associates have demonstrated that 5-lipoxygenase inhibitors, but not cyclooxygenase inhibitors (e.g., indomethacin), inhibit the infiltration of leukocytes into the pleural fluid 3 hours after the intrapleural injection of zymosan (16).

C. Lipopolysaccharide or Endotoxin

The injection of endotoxin into the pleural space of mice (5), rats (18), guinea pigs (19), and rabbits (4,20,21) leads to the accumulation of neutrophils in the pleural space at 4 hours, and the accumulation of eosinophils and mononuclear cells at 24 hours, which persist for at least 4 hours (19). This model has been used to study pleural fluid eosinophilia (19). It should be noted that the intrapleural injection of endotoxin does not lead to increased vascular permeability (19).

Although the intrapleural injection of platelet-activating factor (PAF) (22), leukotriene B_4 (22), and bradykinin (23) induces delayed and long-lasting eosinophil infiltration in the rat pleural cavity, none of these appears to be involved in the eosinophil accumulation resulting from endotoxin. Treatment with inhibitors of any of these three cytokines does not prevent the eosinophil accumulation after endotoxin intrapleurally (19). In contrast, dexamethasone and the protein synthesis inhibitor cycloheximide abolish endotoxin-induced eosinophil accumulation (24). It has also been shown that the blockade of nitric oxide biosynthesis prevents endotoxin-induced eosinophil accumulation (25), but that inhibitors of IL-5 do not prevent eosinophil accumulation (19).

In rabbits, the intrapleural injection of endotoxin leads to neutrophil influx into the pleural space, which peaks at 6 hours (4,20). There is also a biphasic increase in the vascular permeability with the first increase 15 minutes after the injection and the second increase 2 hours after the injection (4,20). Broaddus and associates have demonstrated that the neutrophil influx is profoundly inhibited by neutralization of IL-8 (21). Edamitsu and associates have demonstrated that the early neutrophil influx is partly inhibited by anti-TNF-α but not IL-1 receptor antagonists (4). In contrast, the late phase is inhibited by both anti-TNF-α and IL-1 receptor antagonists (4). These investigators also demonstrated that the immediate increase in permeability was inhibited by antihistamines but not by anti-TNF-α or IL-1 receptor antagonists (4). The late increase in vascular permeability was completely inhibited by either the depletion of neutrophils or by anti-TNF-α but not by IL-1 receptor antagonists (4). Fukumoto et al. confirmed these results and also demonstrated that the delayed increase in vascular permeability was due to TNF-α–induced increases in IL-8 (20).

D. Miconazole

One study reported that the intrapleural injection of 1, 2, or 4 mg of the synthetic antifungal imidazole miconazole resulted in an exudative pleural effusion in rats (7). The peak amount of fluid occurs at 9 hours and is dose dependent. The peak cellular influx is at 7 hours and tends to persist for at least 24 hours. At 7 hours most of the cells are neutrophils, while at 24 hours there are about 40% neutrophils, 40% mononuclear cells, and 20% eosinophils. Dexamethasone and to a lesser degree phenylbutazone, but not chlorpheniramine or methysergide, markedly attenuate the fluid formation and leukocyte accumulation.

II. Hypersensitivity Reactions

The pleural space has also been used to study hypersensitivity reactions. Rats are sensitized to ovalbumin with a subcutaneous injection of a mixture containing 50μ g of ovalbumin and 5 mg of aluminum hydroxide (26). Fourteen days after sensitization, 12 μg ovalbumin is injected into the pleural space (26). After the intrapleural injection there is an intense and early leakage of plasma proteins (as show by Evans blue dye leakage), which peaks at 10 minutes and decays precipitously thereafter. Over a 4-hour period approximately 1 mL of pleural fluid accumulates. The total pleural leukocyte count peaks at 24 hours and then declines over the following day. Neutrophils account for most of the cells in the first 24 hours, but thereafter eosinophils and mononuclear cells predominate (26).

This model has been used to study the mechanisms of this allergic hypersensitivity reaction. The administration of systemic corticosteroids blocks the neutrophilic and eosinophilic influx in this model (5). The blockade of endothelin receptor A, but not endothelin receptor B, inhibits the antigen-induced eosinophil and mononuclear cell migration (27). The administration of a bradykinin receptor antagonist blocks the entire response in a dose-dependent manner (28). This model has also been used to show that lipoxin A4 and aspirin-triggered 15-epi-LXA dramatically block the influx of eosinophils into the pleural fluid, while concurrently inhibiting the earlier edema and neutrophil influx (29).

A model of allergic pleurisy has also been developed in mice. In this model, mice are injected subcutaneously on days 1 and 8 with 100 μg ovalbumin and 70μ g of aluminum hydroxide. Then 7–10 days after the last subcutaneous injection, 0.1–10μ g of ovalbumin are injected into the pleural space. In this model there is a dose-dependent recruitment of eosinophils after 48 hours (30). As in the rat model, there is also an early accumulation of leukocytes in the pleural cavity. This model has been used to show that both stem cell factor (SCF) (30) and eotaxin (31) play a major role in the recruitment of eosinophils in allergic pleurisy. In addition, this model has been used to show that the administration of IL-5 monoclonal antibodies prevent the accumulation of eosinophils in the pleural space (18).

III. Pleurodesis

In patients with pneumothoraces or pleural effusions, one frequently wants to fuse the visceral and parietal pleura (pleurodesis) in order to prevent collapse of the lung with pneumothorax or accumulation of pleural fluid with pleural effusions. Animal models have been used to test the effectiveness of various agents for producing a pleurodesis.

A. Rabbit Model

The rabbit has been used more extensively than any other animal in the study of experimental pleurodesis. The primary problem with using the rabbit for a model of pleurodesis is that the rabbit has a thin visceral pleura while humans have a thick visceral pleura. Therefore, it is not obvious that the results of pleurodesis in rabbits can be extrapolated to humans.

Sahn and Good performed the first comprehensive study of pleurodesis when they intrapleurally injected tetracycline (7 mg/kg, 20 mg/kg, 35 mg/kg), hydrochloric acid (0.01 N), quinacrine (10 mg/kg), nitrogen mustard (0.2 mg/kg), bleomycin (1.5 mg/kg), and NaOH (5%) each in a total volume of 2 mL (32). These animals did not have chest tubes but did undergo five diagnostic thoracenteses over the first 6 days so the pleural fluid could be sampled. The intrapleural injection of any of these agents led to an exudative pleural effusion with very similar characteristics. However, when the animals were sacrificed at 30 days, the pleural space was essentially normal in all the animals except those that received 35 mg/kg tetracycline (32). Pleural symphysis involving >75% of the pleural space occurred in 9 of the 10 animals that received this dose of tetracycline. Based on this study tetracycline became the most popular agent for pleurodesis in the 1980s.

In the early 1990s the company that manufactured parenteral tetracycline ceased to produce the compound due to more stringent manufacturing requirements. Accordingly, animal studies were performed to evaluate possible alternative agents. Light and associates (33) demonstrated that minocycline at doses of 7 mg/kg and above produced pleurodesis comparable to tetracycline 35 mg/kg. These investigators did not aspirate the pleural fluid and noted that with doses of 20 mg/kg and higher there was excess mortality due to hemothorax (33). It was subsequently documented that doxycycline 10 mg/kg was effective at producing a pleurodesis but also produced a hemothorax in a significant proportion of study animals (34). Subsequently, Wu and coworkers demonstrated that if small chest tubes were implanted in the rabbits at the time that they received the minocycline intrapleurally, the hemothoraces did not develop and the excess mortality was prevented (35). In this publication the chest tubes were kept in place with thoracic vests. However, subsequently these investigators demonstrated that a better way to keep the chest tubes in place was to tunnel the tubing under the skin and draw the proximal end out through the skin posteriorly and superiorly between the two scapulae (36). The exterior end of the catheter is plugged with a stub adaptor with a Luer lock fitted. Air or liquid can be aspirated through a self-sealing injection site fitting with a Luer lock (36).

There have been multiple other studies evaluating the efficacy of other agents in producing a pleurodesis. It has been shown that the intrapleural administration of talc slurry effectively produces a pleurodesis in rabbits, but the dose necessary to produce a satisfactory pleurodesis in rabbits (400 mg/kg) is much larger than the dose that is normally recommended for humans on a mg/kg basis (37). The pleurodesis that results from talc develops slowly and the pleurodesis at 28 days is much better than the pleurodesis at 14 days (38). The pleurodesis that results from this large dose of talc is less complete than the pleurodesis that results from tetracycline derivatives (37) or silver nitrate (39). The addition of thymol iodide to the talc does not lead to a better pleurodesis (40). If the rabbits are given systemic corticosteroids concomitantly, the effectiveness of the pleurodesis is decreased (41).

Recent studies have demonstrated that the intrapleural administration of 2 mL of 0.5% silver nitrate produces an excellent pleurodesis in rabbits (42). The pleurodesis resulting from this dose of silver nitrate is equivalent to that resulting from 35 mg/kg tetracycline (39) and better than that resulting from talc 400 mg/kg (42,43). The pleurodesis following silver nitrate intrapleurally persists for at least one year (43).

The ability of several antineoplastic agents to produce a pleurodesis in rabbits has also been investigated. Although bleomycin is used in humans with malignant pleural effusions to produce a pleurodesis, it is ineffective in rabbits at doses up to 3.0 IU/kg (32,44). In rabbits the best antineoplastic agent for producing a pleurodesis appears to be nitrogen mustard (0.8 mg/kg) (45). Mitoxantrone is also effective in producing a pleurodesis, but at the doses necessary to produce a pleurodesis, cardiac toxicity develops and the animals develop congestive heart failure (46,47). Interestingly, the intrapleural injection of mitoxantrone leads to much more pleural inflammation than does the intrapleural injection of the tetracycline derivatives (46). The intrapleural injection of dacarbazine or cytarabine does not produce a pleurodesis (45).

The mechanism of pleurodesis is not definitely known, and it may vary from agent to agent (48). It has been thought that the initial event in the production of a pleurodesis is an injury to the pleura because the intrapleural injection of all the agents listed above produces an acute exudative pleural effusion. However, the factors that dictate whether the inflammatory response will resolve or will proceed to pleural fibrosis are not known. It has been shown that the intrapleural administration of tetracycline results in the local elaboration of IL-8 and monocyte chemotactic protein-1 (MCP-1) (49). The pleurodesis resulting from talc slurry but not that resulting from tetracycline derivatives is partially inhibited by blocking antibodies to TNF-α (36) and corticosteroids (50).

Cytokines are probably involved in producing a pleurodesis. In our first experiment to assess this hypothesis, we injected IL-8 by itself or with talc to see if it would facilitate the creation of a pleurodesis. We found that IL-8 had no effect on the production of the pleurodesis (unpublished data). We next turned our attention to transforming growth factor (TGF)-β. We demonstrated that the intrapleural injection of TGF-β_2 would produce a pleurodesis in a dose-dependent manner, with a dose of 1.67μ g/kg producing an excellent pleurodesis (51). The intrapleural injection of TGF-β_2 also led to the production of large amount of exudative pleural fluid, but the WBC count and the lactate dehydrogenase (LDH) level in the fluid were much lower than in the fluid resulting from either talc slurry or tetracycline derivatives administered intrapleurally (51). These observations suggested that TGF-β_2 stimulated the mesothelial cells to produce collagen without requiring injury to the pleura. We subsequently showed that the pleurodesis that resulted from TGF-β_2 occurred much faster than that which occurred following talc (52) and that the pleurodesis that occurs following intrapleural TGF-β_2 is not inhibited by corticosteroids (53). I feel confident that the future for pleurodesis lies in its production by the intrapleural injection of cytokines.

B. Dog Model

There have been several studies of pleurodesis utilizing dogs. However, dogs, like rabbits, have a thin visceral pleura, so extrapolating results in dogs to humans may not be possible. Bresticker and associates performed bilateral thoracotomies on mongrel dogs and subjected the animals to mechanical dry gauze abrasion, chemical sclerosis with 500 mg tetracycline, talc poudrage with 1 g, Nd:YAG laser photocoagulation or argon beam electrocoagulation of the parietal pleural (54). When the animals were sacrificed at 30 days, the mechanical abrasion and the talc were found to produce the best pleurodesis and were virtually equivalent. Jerram and associates reported that mechanical abrasion was significantly better than 1 g talc slurry at producing a pleurodesis (55). Colt and associates compared the pleurodesis resulting from dry gauze abrasion, thoracoscopic mechanical abrasion using a commercially available stainless-steel grooved burr abrader, thoracoscopic talc insufflation (4 g), and instillation of talc slurry (5 g) at 30 days. They reported that the talc poudrage was the best followed by mechanical abrasion (56). The differing results in the above studies may be related to the vigor with which the mechanical abrasion was performed or the amount of talc used.

C. Pig Model

There have also been several articles in which pleurodesis has been studied in pigs, a species that has a thick pleura similar to humans. Whitlow and associates compared the pleurodesis that results from 3 g of insufflated talc and 300 mg of minocycline administered during thoracoscopy and reported that the insufflated talc produced the superior pleurodesis (57). Cohen and associates reported that the pleurodesis resulting from the insufflation of 5 g of talc or the instillation of 5g of talc as a slurry was virtually identical (58).

D. Sheep Model

There has been one pleurodesis study in sheep, another species with a thick pleura like humans. Lee and associates demonstrated that the intrapleural administration of TGF-β_2 produced an excellent pleurodesis in sheep (59) as it had in rabbits (51). There were two significant differences in the results with sheep and the results with rabbits. First, the dose of TGF-β_2 necessary for pleurodesis in the rabbits (2.5μ g/kg) was much larger than the dose necessary for pleurodesis in sheep (0.25μ g/kg). Second, in sheep the pleurodesis could be accomplished without the side effect of producing large amounts of pleural fluid. These studies demonstrate that the species used has a significant influence on the results for pleurodesis.

IV. Asbestos

Clinically, pleural effusions develop in patients who have been exposed to asbestos. The exposure usually occurs many years before the appearance of the pleural effusion. Attempts have been made to duplicate this asbestos pleural effusion in animals. Shore and associates demonstrated that the administration of 5 mL of 1% crocidolite asbestos suspension (60) into the pleural spaces of rabbits resulted in a pleural effusion of 1.5 mL at 4 hours. The neutrophil count in the pleural fluid of animals given asbestos was higher than that in animals given saline, as was the chemotactic activity. It was subsequently shown that IL-8 was responsible for much of the chemotactic activity (61). However, it is not clear what relationship this model has to the asbestos effusion in man since the time course is so different.

Using a similar model, Sahn and Antony (62) demonstrated that the intrapleural injection of 150 mg of UICC chrysotile B asbestos into rabbits resulted in a pleural effusion that persisted at least 30 days. The peak cellular influx (WBC = 27,000 cells/mm^3) occurred at 24 hours when there were predominantly neutrophils in the pleural fluid. By 72 hours macrophages were the predominant cells, while at 120 hours lymphocytes were the predominant cells. The animals developed pleural plaques by 7 days, and the pleural plaques were fully developed by 28 days. If the animals were made neutropenic before the asbestos was injected, there was never a macrophage influx. Moreover, the neutropenic animals did not develop pleural plaques, but rather developed marked fibrosis of the pleural space (62).

V. Tuberculosis

There are two types of animal models related to tuberculosis and pleural disease. In the hypersensitivity model, an animal is sensitized to tuberculous protein. Subsequently a pleural effusion results when tuberculous protein is injected into the pleural space. In the BCG model, bacillus Calmette-Guerin (BCG) is injected directly into the pleural space. If nonimmunized guinea pigs are given *Mycobacterium tuberculosis* intrapleurally, they die of generalized tuberculosis within 4-6 weeks (63).

A. Hypersensitivity Model

Allen and Apicella (64) first developed this model, in which guinea pigs were immunized with a footpad injection of 0.2 mL of complete Freund's adjuvant containing 1 mg killed H37Ra tubercle bacilli/mL, emulsified with an equal volume of isotonic saline. Then 3-5 weeks after immunization, tuberculin PPD in a total volume of 0.5 mL was injected intrapleurally. This resulted in a pleural effusion with a maximal volume of 4 mL at 24 hours with a protein concentration of 3.8 g/dL. In nonimmunized animals, the intrapleural injection of PPD led to much smaller effusions. There was no clear relationship between the amount of PPD injected and the size of the effusion once a threshold amount of PPD was given. The hypersensitivity and the capacity to form pleural effusions could be transferred passively with cells from a sensitized animal (64). This experiment was the first conclusive evidence that the pleural effusion with tuberculosis could be due to hypersensitivity.

Using this same model, Leibowitz and associates (65) subsequently demonstrated that neutrophils were the predominant cells in the early stages of the effusion (<6 h), while at 24 hours lymphocytes and macrophages were the predominant cells. They also demonstrated that the effusion could be completely suppressed if the animals were treated with antilymphocyte serum (ALS) (65). Moreover, after treatment with ALS, the ability to produce a pleural effusion with the intrapleural injection of PPD paralleled the return of the positive skin reaction. These studies provided additional evidence that delayed hypersensitivity is responsible for the effusion.

B. BCG Model

In this model, first described by Widstrom and Nilsson (66), guinea pigs are immunized by the intracutaneous injection of 0.4 mg BCG into the left thigh. This injection causes a small necrotizing skin reaction. Three weeks postinjection, the animals have a positive skin test to PPD. Then 2 mg of BCG is injected into the pleural space. This protocol results in a larger effusion (mean 8 mL), which is maximal in size at about 14 days and has, for the most part, disappeared by 21 days. Again in this model neutrophils were the predominant cells in the first 24 hours, but lymphocytes were the predominant cells after 5 days. If the animals are made neutropenic, then the accumulation of pleural fluid and inflammatory cells is decreased (67). A similar model in which guinea pigs were immunized with a low-virulence strain of *M. tuberculosis* was described by Paterson in 1917 (63).

VI. Empyema

There are a limited number of good human studies on the treatment of parapneumonic effusion and empyema (68). One reason for this is that there is tremendous diversity in patients who have parapneumonic effusions and empyema. In order to compensate for this diversity, patients should be stratified according to the severity of their illness (69). However, once stratification is accomplished, a given medical center sees only a few patients in each category per year. Therefore, good studies take a long time or they need to be multicentered. Unfortunately, multicentered studies are expensive and difficult.

In view of the above, one would think that there would be many studies in animals to help answer questions such as (1) What is the role of therapeutic thoracentesis in the management of parapneumonic effusions? (2) What is the role of fibrinolytics in the management of loculated parapneumonic effusions? (3) Is the penetration of all antibiotics into the pleural space similar? (4) Is there a role for intrapleural antibiotics in the management of pleural infections? Surprisingly, there has been little work done with experimental empyema. Producing an empyema in an animal is somewhat difficult. If *Staphylococcus aureus*, *Escherichia coli*, or *Bacteroides fragilis* are injected into the pleural space of guinea pigs, the animals either survive without developing empyema or die of overwhelming sepsis (70).

To my knowledge four different models of experimental empyema have been described.

A. Direct Injection into Dogs

The first model was described by Graham and Bell in 1918 (71). They injected 30 mL of pure broth cultures of a virulent strain of hemolytic streptococci into the pleural cavity. The first dog injected with this broth died in about 12 hours and had 200 cc of serofibrinous fluid which contained a myriad of streptococci and a few necrotic leukocytes. This exudate was similar to that recovered from early human cases of streptococcus empyema. They subsequently injected smaller amounts of the broth into the animals. In the primary experiment they injected 20 dogs. Then 4–24 hours after the injection, *open* drainage of the pleural space was established with a chest tube in 10 of the dogs, while the remaining dogs did not receive a chest tube. The dogs were paired, and the stronger dog was selected for the chest tube. Nine of the 10 dogs who received the open drainage died, while only 7 of the 10 dogs without the drainage died. The only dog with the open drainage that survived pulled his chest tube out the day following the operation. The dog that received the chest tube in each pair died sooner than the control dog. This experiment demonstrated that open drainage was detrimental to the dog, and the results were extrapolated to humans and the practice of early open tube drainage of empyemas was discontinued.

B. Rabbits with Turpentine-Induced Pleural Effusions

The second model was developed by Sahn and associates in the late 1970s (72). These investigators induced a sterile pleural effusion in rabbits by the intrapleural injection of turpentine and subsequently injected bacteria into the induced pleural effusion. While the rabbit was lightly anesthetized, an 18-guage catheter was introduced through an incision between the eighth and ninth ribs and 0.3 mL turpentine was injected through the catheter, followed by 0.2 mL of air to clear the catheter dead space. This procedure resulted in the presence of an exudative pleural effusion. To produce their empyema, 1×10^9 *Streptococcus pneumoniae* organisms were injected into the pleural fluid 96 hours after the turpentine was injected (73). Within 3 hours of injection, the pleural fluid pH fell to a mean of 7.05 and the pleural fluid glucose fell to below 46 mg/100 mL. By 6 hours postinjection, the pleural fluid WBC averaged over 75,000/mm^3. Shohet and associates used this model to study empyemas due to *Klebsiella pneumoniae* (74). They injected 10^9 *K. pneumoniae* organisms 96 hours after the turpentine was injected and demonstrated that at 1, 3, and 5 days postinoculation, the pleural fluid glucose was below 10 mg/dL and the pleural fluid pH was below 7.00 (74). However, without therapy the pleural effusions resolved within 10 days, and at autopsy there were no significant findings in the pleural cavity or lungs.

It is problematic when findings from this model are extrapolated to the human. Since the animals fully recover without the administration of antibiotics or chest tubes, treatment interventions in the model cannot be assessed. In addition, although Shohet and coworkers (74) used this model to study the penetration of gentamicin into the pleural space, the pleural thickening induced by the turpentine probably influenced their results.

C. Guinea Pigs with Umbilical Tape

The third model was developed in the mid-1980s to assess the factors that influence the development of an empyema when bacteria are injected into the pleural space (70). This model requires the placement of umbilical tape in the pleural space to act as a foreign body to promote infection. After guinea pigs were anesthetized with an intramuscular injection of ketamine hydrochloride, 55 mg/kg, and acepromazine maleate, 0.5 mg/kg, a small skin incision was made at the level of the sixth to ninth intercostal space and the pleural space was bluntly entered. Then a piece of cotton umbilical tape 1 cm long and 1/8 inch wide was placed in the pleural space.

Using this model it was demonstrated that the development of an empyema is dependent on the organisms injected (70). None of the animals injected with *Bacteroides fragilis* developed empyema, whereas 37% of those injected with *Escherichia coli* and 58% of those injected with *Staphylococcus aureus* developed empyema. The incidence of empyema was significantly greater if both *B. fragilis* and *S. aureus* were injected than if only *S. aureus* was injected (75). These investigators also demonstrated that the more organisms injected into the pleural space, the more likely the animal was to develop an empyema. For example, if 10^8 *S. aureus* organisms were injected, 10/10 animals developed an empyema, while if 10^6 of these organisms were injected, only 5/10 animals developed an empyema (70). If blood was injected with the bacteria, the likelihood of developing an empyema was not increased. Finally, guinea pigs that developed pneumonia were more likely to have an empyema.

The primary problem with this model is that it requires a foreign body in the pleural space, which does not mimic the clinical situation in humans.

D. Rabbits with Bacteria in Agar

The fourth model was developed in the late 1990's by Sasse and co-workers (76). In this rabbit model, *Pasteurella multocida* cultured in agar (rather than broth) were injected into the pleural space of rabbits. Agar rather than broth was used so that the mixture would remain in the pleural space longer. Procaine penicillin G was administered once per day starting 24 hours after the initial injection to prevent death from sepsis. With this model the rabbits developed an empyema; 24 hours postinjection the mean pleural fluid pH was 7.01, mean glucose was 10 mg/dL, mean LDH was 21,000 IU/L, and Gram's stain and culture of the pleural fluid were positive (76). At 96 hours postinjection, the Gram's stain and culture of the pleural fluid were usually negative, but gross pus remained in the pleural space. Ten days postinjection, approximately 50% of the animals had gross pus in their pleural space. Approximately 60% of the rabbits survived for 14 days, and at autopsy most animals had pus in their pleural space.

This model closely mimics the empyema that occurs in humans. The process was not cured with antibiotics alone. The pleural fluid became infected, then loculated and a rind formed over the visceral pleura. This model has been used in an attempt to answer several questions concerning the management of empyema. These investigators first investigated whether therapeutic thoracentesis was a reasonable alternative to tube thoracostomy in the management of rabbits with empyema (77). Rabbits were randomized to receive daily therapeutic thoracentesis starting at 48 hours, chest tubes at 48 hours, or neither therapeutic thoracentesis nor tube thoracostomy (controls). The animals in the chest tube group had their chest tubes attached to a Heimlich valve and had their chest tubes aspirated at 12-hour intervals. In this study the mortality rate in the therapeutic thoracentesis group (0/16) was significantly less ($p = 0.02$) than the mortality rate in the other two groups combined (9/33). When the surviving animals were sacrificed at 10 days, the gross empyema score in the therapeutic thoracentesis group was significantly lower ($p < 0.05$) than that in the chest tube group or the control group (77). This study suggests that there is possibly a role for therapeutic thoracentesis in the management of patients with empyema.

The second question addressed was whether the timing of the chest tube insertion is important in the treatment of empyema. After the injection of *P.*

multocida, rabbits were randomized to receive no chest tube or a chest tube after 24, 48, or 72 hours (Fig. 1) (78). The rabbits that received the chest tube at 24 or 48 hours had significantly better results than did the rabbits that received the chest tube at 72 hours or those that did not receive a chest tube at all (78). This study demonstrates that a relatively short delay in initiating tube thoracostomy adversely affects the outcome in these animals with an empyema.

The third question addressed with this model was whether all antibiotics penetrate empyemic pleural fluid similarly (79). Twenty-four hours after the intrapleural injection of *P. multocida*, Teixeira and coworkers injected either penicillin 24,000 units/kg, clindamycin 9 mg/kg, gentamicin 1 mg/kg, metronidazole 37 mg/kg, vancomycin 15 mg/kg, or ceftriaxone 30 mg/kg intravenously. Antibiotic levels in samples of pleural fluid and serum, collected serially for up to 480 minutes, were determined using a bioassay. In this study the degree to which antibiotics penetrated the pleural fluid was highly variable (79). Metronidazole penetrated most easily, followed by penicillin, clindamycin, vancomycin, ceftriaxone, and gentamicin (Fig. 2). This variance in the penetration of antibiotics into empyemic pleural fluid should be taken into consideration when antibiotic therapy is chosen in patients with empyema.

VII. Malignancy

In general there are two types of experimental models of malignant pleural effusion. In the first type, tumor cells are injected, either intravenously or intra-

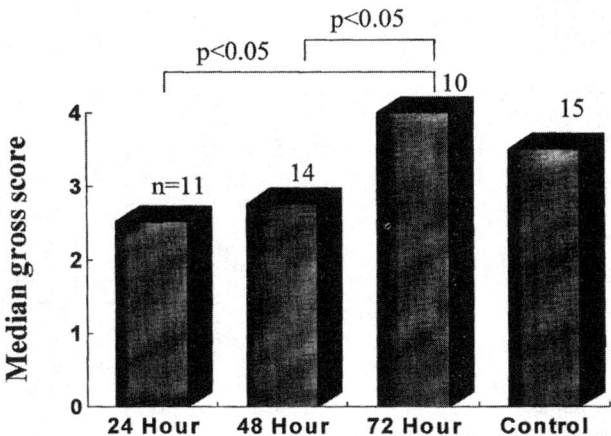

Figure 1 Relationship between gross anatomical score and time of placement of chest tube. A score of 4 indicates pus in the pleural space, 3 = moderate pleural peel without gross pus, 2 = minimal pleural peel, 1 = adhesions between the visceral and parietal pleura, and 0 = normal pleural space. (From Ref. 78.)

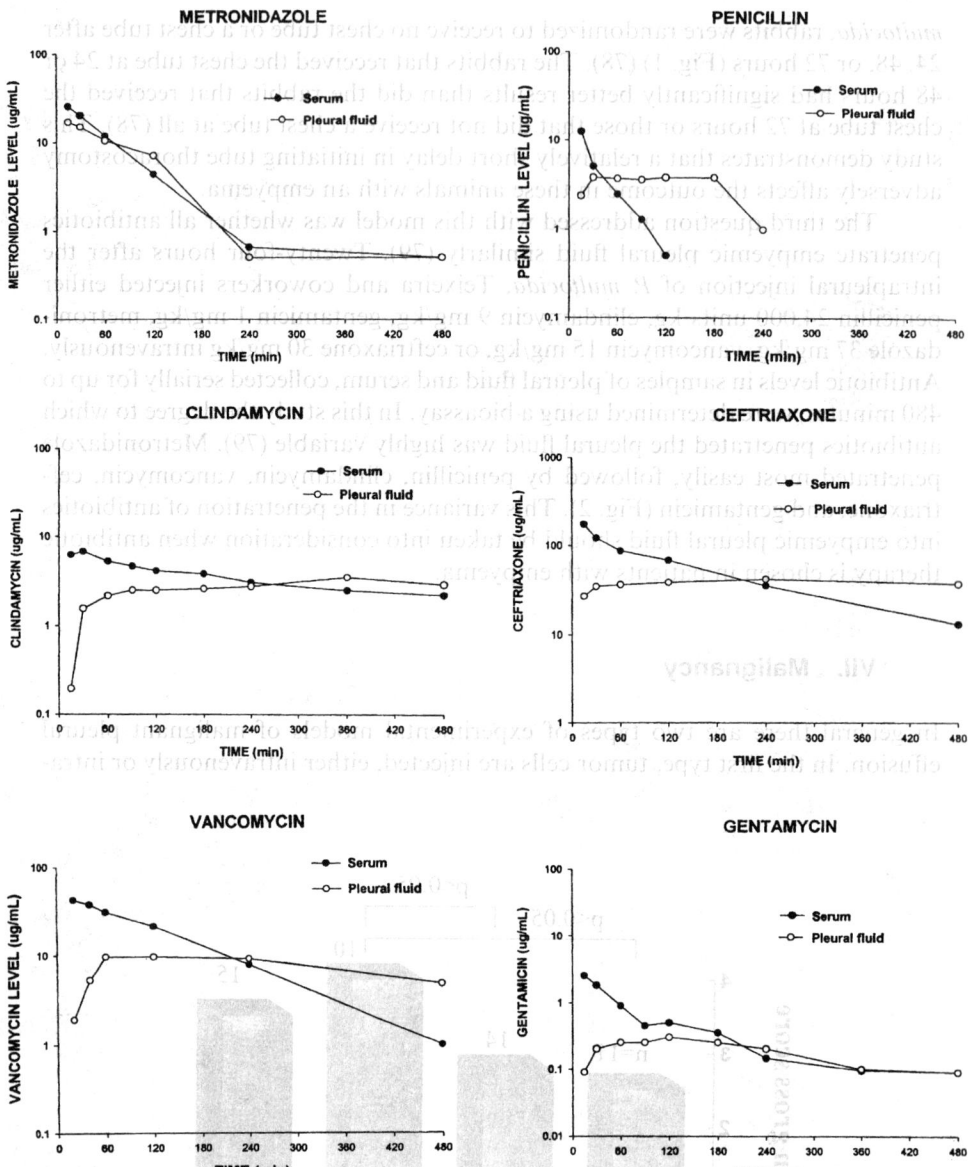

Figure 2 Levels of antibiotics in the serum and pleural fluid after administration of various antibiotics. (From Ref. 79.)

pleurally, into animals that usually have immunological deficiencies to induce disseminated malignancy with pleural effusion. In the second type, animals are exposed to asbestos particles (intrapleurally, inhalational, intratracheal, or intraperitoneally), and malignant mesothelioma subsequently develops.

A. Adenocarcinoma

The Model

Yano and coworkers (80) described a model of malignant pleural effusion in mice. In this model male athymic BALB/c nude mice (Animal Production Area of the National Cancer Institute, Frederick Cancer Research Facility, Frederick, MD) were used. The mice were housed in laminar flow cabinets under specific pathogen-free conditions until they were 6–8 weeks of age.

The human lung adenocarcinoma cell line PC14PE6 and the squamous cell line H226 are maintained in Eagle's minimal essential medium supplemented with 10% phosphate-buffered saline, sodium pyruvate, nonessential amino acids, L-glutamine, two fold vitamin solution, and penicillin-streptomycin in a 10 cm dish and incubated in 5% CO_2–95% room air at 37C°. Cultures were maintained for no longer than 6 weeks after recovery from frozen stocks.

After the cells are harvested, they are washed twice and resuspended in Ca^{2+}- and Mg^{2+}-free Hanks' balanced salt solution (HBSS). Then the tumor cells (1×10^6/300µ L of HBSS) are injected into the lateral tail vein of unanesthetized nude mice. The mice develop colonies of the adenocarcinoma in the lungs as early as week 4 after tumor inoculation, and all recipients develop bloody pleural effusions (80).

Applications

Using the above model, Yano and associates investigated the role of vascular endothelial growth factor (VEGF) in producing the pleural effusions (81). They found that the intravenous injection of PC14, the adenocarcinoma cell line, resulted in multiple lung lesions and invasion of the pleura, and produced a pleural effusion containing high levels of VEGF (82). They also found that the intravenous or intrathoracic injection of H226 cells, the squamous carcinoma cell line, also produced lung lesions. However, there was no invasion of the pleura by these cells, and there were no pleural effusions. The level of expression of VEGF mRNA and protein by the cell lines directly correlated with the amount of pleural effusion. When the PC14 cells were transfected with the antisense VEGF-165 gene, the tumor invasion of the pleura was not altered, but the amount of pleural effusion was decreased. When the H226 cells were transfected with either sense VEGF-165 or sense VEGF-121 genes, their direct implantation, but not their intravenous injection, led to localized vascular hyperpermeability and pleural effusion. This study suggested that in order for a metastatic malignancy to produce a pleural effusion, the tumor must both invade the pleura and express high levels of VEGF (82).

These same researchers then decided to determine if they could block the formation of malignant pleural effusion in their model by administering VEGF inhibitors (81). The inhibitor studied, PTK 787, is a specific inhibitor of a VEGF receptor tyrosine kinase phosphorylation. The administration of PTK 787 at a dose of 100 mg/kg nearly eliminated the formation of pleural effusions, but doses of 10 and 50 mg/kg had no significant effect. PTK 787 appeared to decrease the formation of pleural fluid by reducing vascular permeability rather than by inhibiting tumor growth or pleural invasion. This experiment suggests that PTK 787 or other inhibitors of VEGF could be useful for the treatment of malignant pleural effusions.

In Rats

Ohta and coworkers have developed a model of malignant pleural effusion in rats using the PC-14 adenocarcinoma cell line (83). They reported that the injection of 1×10^7 cells into the thoracic cavity resulted in disseminated malignancy in 8/8 animals and the development of a pleural effusion in 5/8 animals, in which the pleural effusion cytology was positive in 2 (83). Interestingly, these workers showed that intraperitoneal injection of monoclonal anti-human VEGF antibody at a dose of 250μ g twice weekly prevented the development of the pleural effusion but did not affect the dissemination of the tumor (83).

B. Melanoma

Melanoma metastatic to the lung can be produced by injecting murine melanoma cell lines into the lateral tail vein of syngeneic mice (84). In this model, syngeneic mice receive 5×10^4 melanoma cells in a total volume of 0.2 mL. Then 21 days after injection, the mice are sacrificed, the number of lung metastases is determined, and the pleural fluid is quantitated. Using this model, Wang and associates reported that all 20 mice injected with two different cell lines developed lung metastases (84). In addition, 8/10 mice injected with B16-BL6 melanoma cells developed pleural effusions with a median volume of 250 μL, while 9/10 mice injected with B16-F10 melanoma cells developed a pleural effusion with a mean volume of 320 μL. If the melanoma cells were administered to syngeneic mice lacking the gene for nitric oxide synthase II, only about 50% of the animals developed pleural effusions, and those that did had a lower volume (84).

C. Fibrosarcoma

Yasutake and coworkers developed an experimental model of fibrosarcoma with pleural effusion (85). In this model, 1×10^5 Meth A fibrosarcoma cells were injected intrapleurally in syngeneic BALB/c mice. All the injected mice in this model developed pleural fibrosarcoma, and all developed pleural effusions with a mean volume of 733 μL. The mean survival of the injected mice was only 8.7 days after injection. Interestingly, when heat-killed cells of *Lactobacillus casei* were injected on days 3 or 6, the mean survival was increased beyond 40 days and the amount of pleural fluid was only 14 µL (85). Intrapleural injection of antibodies against TNF-a completely eliminated the antitumor effect of the heat-killed cells of *L. casei* (85).

VIII. Asbestos and Mesothelioma

Many papers have been published on the relationship between asbestos and mesothelioma. Wagner in 1962 first reported that the intrapleural administration of chrysotile and crocidolite in rats led to the production of mesothelioma (86). Then Smith and associates in 1965 (87) demonstrated that the intrapleural injection of amosite in hamsters led to the development of mesothelioma. Subsequently, there have been many papers written on the induction of mesotheliomas in animals. Asbestos has been administered intrapleurally, intratracheally, intraperitoneally, and by inhalation. In the following section I will briefly describe the reported results when asbestos is administered by these different routes.

A. Intrapleural Injections

The intrapleural injection of asbestos leads to the development of mesothelioma of the pleural space. The great majority of studies have been performed in rats (86,88–93), although there has been at least one report in hamsters (87). When different asbestos fibers are injected intrapleurally, approximately 30–60% of the animals develop a pleural mesothelioma (89,93). The tumors develop approximately 18 months (89) after the intrapleural injection. There is a dose response, with larger doses being associated with a higher incidence of tumor (93). When different types of asbestos are compared, the intrapleural injection of 25 mg chrysotile or crocidolite produce mesotheliomas in approximately 60%, while the same dose of amosite produces tumors in 35% (94). The main difference in these types of asbestos is that mesotheliomas occur about 200 days later for amosite than for the other two types (94).

The propensity of a fiber type to produce a mesothelioma is dependent to a large extent on its geometric configuration. Long thin fibers appear particularly likely to produce mesothelioma (90). The chemical composition of the asbestos fiber also influences whether its intrapleural injection will induce a mesothelioma. Monchaux and associates demonstrated that if more than 80% of the magnesium was leached from chrysotile fibers, the proportion of pleural mesotheliomas was dramatically lower than with untreated chrysotile (91). If pleural inflammation is induced by the intrapleural injection of carrageenan several months after the initial injection of asbestos, the rate of pleural mesothelioma more than doubled (95).

The most potent inducer of pleural mesothelioma of all the fibers tested is erionite (88,96). Wagner and coworkers injected 20 mg of Oregon erionite, Karain Rock fiber, chrysotile or nonfibrous zeolite intrapleurally, and the incidence of mesothelioma was as follows: erionite 40/40 (100%), Karain Rock fiber 38/40 (95%), chrysotile 19/40 (48%), and nonfibrous zeolite 2/40 (5%) (96). Erionite in the air has been implicated in the epidemic of mesotheliomas in Turkey (97).

If normal mesothelial cells are treated in vitro with chrysotile fibers, mesotheliomas will develop rapidly when these cells are injected subcutaneously into nude mice. Fleury-Feith and associates demonstrated that when untreated cells were injected, tumors developed in 3/5 animals at a median of 22 weeks after injection. However, if the cells were treated repeatedly with chrysotile, tumors develeped in 5/5 animals at a median of only 1 week after injection (98).

B. Inhaled Asbestos

There have also been numerous reports of the effects of inhaled asbestos on rats (99–105), and one in baboons (106). In general it is more difficult to produce tumors by the inhalation of asbestos than it is by intrapleural administration. Wagner and associates exposed rats to asbestos clouds 5 days per week for 7 hours per day for one year (104). Even when asbestos is administered with such intensive regimens, the incidence of mesothelioma is less than it is after one intrapleural (105) or one intraperitoneal injection (102) of asbestos. When rats are given inhaled asbestos for one year, less than 10% develop mesothelioma, but approximately 30% develop lung tumors (104). Multivariate analysis of multiple inhalational experiments have shown that the measure most highly correlated with tumor incidence is the concentration of structures ≥ 20 μm (99). Potency appears to increase with increasing length, with structures longer than 40μ m being about 500 times more potent than structures between 5 and 40μ m (99). When different types of asbestos are compared, chrysotile is less potent than amphiboles in inducing mesothelioma, but comparable in producing lung tumors (99). The agent most efficient at inducing mesothelioma after inhalation is erionite. Wagner and associates demonstrated that the inhalation of Oregon erionite induced mesotheliomas in 27 of 28 (96%) rats and decreased the mean survival time from 738 to 504 days (96).

It has also been demonstrated that inhaled asbestos can induce mesotheliomas in primates. Webster and associates exposed baboons 6 hours daily for 5 days a week to amosite asbestos, except for 3 weeks of the year when the chamber had to be serviced (106). The animals were exposed up to 900 days. Five of 10 animals developed malignant mesothelioma, and the remaining animals all developed asbestosis (106).

C. Intratracheal Injections

There have also been a few reports on the effects of asbestos administered intratracheally in hamsters (107,108), dogs (109), and monkeys (108). Obviously, it is less burdensome to administer the asbestos intratracheally than to do inhalational treatments nearly daily for a year or more. However, in general it is difficult to induce mesotheliomas with intratracheal asbestos. Pylev administered 10 mg of chrysotile twice, separated by a month, and reported that only one of 41 animals developed a malignant mesothelioma, although 25% of the hamsters developed a malignant lung tumor (107). Pylev also tried to induce tumors in three monkeys with the intratracheal administration of 400–600 mg asbestos and reported that no tumors developed during 17–22 months of follow-up (107). Adachi and associates (108) administered amosite and crocidolite asbestos (2 mg/dose) intratracheally once a week for 5 weeks to Syrian hamsters and observed them for the following 2 years. Only one of the 40 animals that were exposed developed a mesothelioma. The study with the highest incidence of mesothelioma after intratracheal asbestos was reported by Humphrey and co-workers (109). These workers administered crocidolite, 4.75 mg/kg/week, for 3 weeks during each of 4 years to 10 dogs. Seven of the dogs also smoked nine cigarettes per day, 5 days per week. They reported that pleural mesothelioma developed in 6 of the 10 animals (60%), including 2 of the 3 that did not smoke (109). The animals with the mesotheliomas died between 6.5 and 9 years after the initial exposure. Four of the animals with mesothelioma had concomitant adenocarcinomas.

D. Intraperitoneal Injections

There have been many studies on the induction of mesothelioma by the intraperitoneal injection of asbestos. In general, it takes a smaller amount of asbestos intraperitoneally than intrapleurally to produce a mesothelioma (88). Tumors appear soon after the intraperitoneal injection of asbestos in rats (~9–10 months) compared to intrapleural injections (~18 months) (89). Moreover, the order in which fibers induce mesotheliomas is the same after intrapleural and intraperitoneal injection. Namely, erionite is the most potent, followed by chrysotile, crocidolite, and then amosite (88). Interestingly, silicon carbide is more potent at inducing peritoneal mesotheliomas than are any of the asbestos types (110).

The length of the fiber appears to be important in producing mesothelioma after intraperitoneal injections as well as intrapleural injections (111). When animals develop malignant peritoneal mesotheliomas after the intraperitoneal injection of asbestos, the first manifestation is the development of ascites (112). The ascitic fluid can then be injected into other animals so that the antitumor effects of different chemotherapeutic agents can be assessed (113).

References

1. Imai Y, Hayashi M, Ohishi S. Key role of complement activation and platelet-activating factor in exudate formation in zymosan-induced rat pleurisy. Jpn J Pharmacol 1991; 57:225–232.
2. Utsunomiya I, Ito M, Ohishi S. Generation of inflammatory cytokines in zymosan-induced pleurisy in rats: TNF induces IL-6 and cytokine-induced neutrophil chemoattractant (cinc) in vivo. Cytokine 1998; 10:956–963.

3. Silva AR, Larangeira AP, Pacheco P, Calixto JB, Henriques MG, Bozza PT, Castro-Faria-Neto HC. Bradykinin down-regulates LPS-induced eosinophil accumulation in the pleural cavity of mice through type 2-kinin receptor activation: a role for prostaglandins. Br J Pharmacol 1999; 127:569–575.
4. Edamitsu S, Matsukawa A, Ohkawara S, Takagi K, Nariuchi H, Yoshinaga M. Role of TNF alpha, IL-1, and IL-1ra in the mediation of leukocyte infiltration and increased vascular permeability in rabbits with LPS-induced pleurisy. Clin Immunol Immunopath 1995; 75:68–74.
5. Pasquale CP, Lima MC, Bandeira-Melo C, Cordeiro RS, Silva PM, Martins MA. Systemic and local dexamethasone treatments prevent allergic eosinophilia in rats via distinct mechanisms. Eur J Pharmacol 1999; 368:67–74.
6. Aihara S, Murakami N, Tomita T, Naruse T, Namba K. Inhibitory action of indomethacin on neutrophil infiltration in monosodium urate-induced pleurisy in rats. Jpn J Pharmacol 1995; 68:271–277.
7. Hanada S, Sugawara SH, Sertie JA. Miconazole as inflammatory agent. II: time course of pleurisy and drug interference. Gen Pharmacol 1998; 30:791–794.
8. Vinegar R, Truax JF, Selph JL, Voelker FA. Pathway of onset, development, and decay of carrageenan pleurisy in the rat. Fed Proc 1982; 41:942–946.
9. Mielens ZE, Connolly K, Stecher VJ. Effect of disease modifying antirheumatic drugs and nonsteroidal antiinflammatory drugs upon cellular and fibronectin responses in a pleurisy model. J Rheumatol 1985; 12:1083–1087.
10. Cuzzocrea S, Mazzon E, Calabro G, Dugo L, De Sarro A, van De Loo FA, Caputi AP. Inducible nitric oxide synthase-knockout mice exhibit resistance to pleurisy and lung injury caused by carrageenan. Am J Respir Crit Care Med 2000; 162:1859–1866.
11. Sautebin L, Ialenti A, Ianaro A, Di Rosa M. Relationship between nitric oxide and prostaglandins in carrageenin pleurisy. Biochem Pharmacol 1998; 55:1113–1117.
12. D'Acquisto F, Ianaro A, Ialenti A, Iuvone T, Colantuoni V, Carnuccio R. Activation of nuclear transcription factor kappa B in rat carrageenin-induced pleurisy. Eur J Pharmacol 1999; 369:233–236.
13. Frode TS, Souza GE, Calixto JB. The modulatory role played by TNF-alpha and IL-1beta in the inflammatory responses induced by carrageenan in the mouse model of pleurisy. Cytokine 2001; 13:162–168.
14. Cuzzocrea S, Costantino G, Zingarelli B, Mazzon E, Micali A, Caputi AP. The protective role of endogenous glutathione in carrageenan-induced pleurisy in the rat. Eur J Pharmacol 1999; 372:187–197.
15. Cuzzocrea S, Sautebin L, De Sarro G, Costantino G, Rombola L, Mazzon E, Ialenti A, De Sarro A, Ciliberto G, Di Rosa M, Caputi AP, Thiemermann C. Role of IL-6 in the pleurisy and lung injury caused by carrageenan. J Immunol 1999; 163:5094–5104.
16. Kikuchi M, Tsuzurahara K, Naito K. Involvement of leukotriene B4 in zymosan-induced rat pleurisy: inhibition of leukocyte infiltration by the 5-lipoxygenase inhibitor T-0757. Biol Pharm Bull 1995; 18:1302–1304.
17. Sampaio AL, Rae GA, Henriques MG. Participation of endogenous endothelins in delayed eosinophil and neutrophil recruitment in mouse pleurisy. Inflamm Res 2000; 49:170–176.
18. Bozza PT, Castro-Faria-Neto HC, Penido C, Larangeira AP, Silva PM, Martins MA, Cordeiro RS. IL-5 accounts for the mouse pleural eosinophil accumulation triggered by antigen but not by LPS. Immunopharmacology 1994; 27:131–136.

19. Castro-Faria-Neto HC, Penido CM, Larangeira AP, Silva AR, Bozza PT. A role for lymphocytes and cytokines on the eosinophil migration induced by LPS. Mem Inst Oswaldo Cruz 1997; 92(suppl 2):197–200.
20. Fukumoto T, Matsukawa A, Yoshimura T, Edamitsu S, Ohkawara S, Takagi K, Yoshinaga M. IL-8 is an essential mediator of the increased delayed-phase vascular permeability in LPS-induced rabbit pleurisy. J Leukoc Biol 1998; 63:584–590.
21. Broaddus VC, Boylan AM, Hoeffel JM, Kim KJ, Sadick M, Chuntharapai A, Hebert CA. Neutralization of IL-8 inhibits neutrophil influx in a rabbit model of endotoxin-induced pleurisy. J Immunol 1994; 152:2960–2967.
22. Silva PMR, Martins MA, Castro-Faria-Neta HC, Cordeiro RSB, Vargaftig BB. Generation of an eosinophilotactic activity in the pleural cavity of platelet-activating factor-injected rats. J Pharmacol Exp Ther 1991; 257:1039–1044.
23. Pasquale CP, Martins MA, Bozza PT, Silva PMR, Castro-Faria-Neto HC, Pires AL, Cordiero RSB. Bradykinin induces eosinophil accumulation in the rat pleural cavity. Int Arch Allergy Appl Immunol 1991; 95:244–247.
24. Bozza PT, Castro-Faria-Neto HC, Martins MA, Larangeira AP, Perales JE, e Silva PM, Cordeiro RS. Pharmacological modulation of lipopolysaccharide-induced pleural eosinophilia in the rat; a role for a newly generated protein. Eur J Pharmacol 1993; 248:41–47.
25. Ferreira HH, Medeiros MV, Lima CS, Flores CA, Sannomiya P, Autunes E, De Nucci G. Inhibition of eosinophil chemotaxis by chronic blockade of nitric oxide biosynthesis. Eur J Pharmacol 1996; 310:201–207.
26. Lima MC, Martins MA, Perez SA, Silva PM, Cordeiro RS, Vargaftig BB. Effect of azelastine on platelet-activating factor and antigen-induced pleurisy in rats. Eur J Pharmacol 1991; 197:201–207.
27. Sampaio AL, Rae GA, Henriques MM. Role of endothelins on lymphocyte accumulation in allergic pleurisy. J Leukoc Biol 2000; 67:189–195.
28. Bandeira-Melo C, Calheiros AS, Silva PM, Cordeiro RS, Teixeira MM, Martins MA. Suppressive effect of distinct bradykinin B2 receptor antagonist on allergen-evoked exudation and leukocyte infiltration in sensitized rats. Br J Pharmacol 1999; 127:315–320.
29. Bandeira-Melo C, Bozza PT, Diaz BL, Cordeiro RS, Jose PJ, Martins MA, Serhan CN. Cutting edge: lipoxin (LX) A4 and aspirin-triggered 15-epi-LXA4 block allergen-induced eosinophil trafficking. J Immunol 2000; 164:2267–2271.
30. Klein A, Talvani A, Cara DC, Gomes KL, Lukacs NW, Teixeira MM. Stem cell factor plays a major role in the recruitment of eosinophils in allergic pleurisy in mice via the production of leukotriene B4. J Immunol 2000; 164:4271–4276.
31. Klein A, Talvani A, Silva PM, Martins MA, Wells TN, Proudfoot A, Luckacs NW, Teixeira MM. Stem cell factor-induced leukotriene b(4) production cooperates with eotaxin to mediate the recruitment of eosinophils during allergic pleurisy in mice. J Immunol 2001; 167:524–531.
32. Sahn SA, Good JT. The effect of common sclerosing agents on the rabbit pleural space. Am Rev Respir Dis 1981; 124:65–67.
33. Light RW, Wang NS, Sassoon SCH, Gruer SE, Vargas FS. Comparison of the effectiveness of tetracycline and minocycline as pleural sclerosing agents in rabbits. Chest 1994; 106:577–582.
34. Hurewitz AN, Lidonicci K, Wu CL, Reim D, Zucker S. Histologic changes of doxycycline pleurodesis in rabbits. Chest 1994; 106:1241–1245.

35. Wu W, Teixeira LR, Light RW. Doxycycline pleurodesis in rabbits. Comparison of results with and without chest tube. Chest 1998; 114:563–568.
36. Cheng D-S, Rogers J, Wheeler A, Parker R, Teixeira L, Light RW. The effects of intrapleural polyclonal anti-tumor necrosis factor alpha (TNFα) Fab fragments on pleurodesis in rabbits. Lung 2000; 178:19–30.
37. Light RW, Wang N-S, Sassoon CSH, Gruer SE, Oliver D, Vargas FS. Talc slurry is an effective pleural sclerosant in rabbits. Chest 1995; 107:1702–1706.
38. Xie C, Teixeira LR, Wang N-S, McGovern JP, Light RW. Serial observations after high dose talc slurry in the rabbit model for pleurodesis. Lung 1998; 176:299–307.
39. Vargas FS, Teixeira LR, Silva LMMF, Carmo AO, Light RW. Comparison of silver nitrate and tetracycline as pleural sclerosing agents in rabbits. Chest 1995; 108:1080–1083.
40. Xie C, McGovern J, Wu W, Wang N-S, Light RW. Comparisons of pleurodesis induced by talc with or without thymol iodide in rabbits. Chest 1998; 113:795–799.
41. Xie C, Teixeira LR, McGovern JP, Light RW. Systemic corticosteroids decrease the effectiveness of talc pleurodesis. Am J Respir Crit Care Med 1998; 157:1441–1444.
42. Vargas FS, Teixeira LR, Vaz MAC, Carmo AO, Marchi E, Cury PM, Light RW. Silver nitrate is superior to talc slurry in producing pleurodesis in rabbits. Chest 2000; 118:808–813.
43. Vargas FS, Teixeira LR, Antonangelo L, Vas MAC, Carmo AO, Marchi E, Light RW. Experimental pleurodesis in rabbits induced by silver nitrate or talc: 1-year follow-up. Chest 2001; 119:1516–1520.
44. Vargas FS, Wang N-S, Lee HM, Gruer SE, Sassoon CSH, Light RW. Effectiveness of bleomycin in comparison to tetracycline as pleural sclerosing agent in rabbits. Chest 1993; 104:1582–1584.
45. Marchi E, Vargas FS, Teixeira LR, Fagundes DJ, Silva LMMF, Carmo AO, Light RW. Comparison of nitrogen mustard, cytarabine and dacarbazine as pleural sclerosing agents in rabbits. Eur Respir J 1997; 10:598–602.
46. Light RW, Wang N-S, Despars JA, Gruer SE, Sassoon C, Vargas FS. Comparison of mitoxantrone and tetracycline as pleural sclerosing agents in rabbits. Lung 1996; 174:373–381.
47. Vargas FS, Teixeira LR, Antonangelo L, Silva LMMF, Strunz CMC, Light RW. Acute and chronic pleural changes after the intrapleural instillation of mitoxantrone in rabbits. Lung 1998; 176:227–236.
48. Light RW, Vargas FS. Pleural sclerosis for the treatment of pneumothorax and pleural effusion. Lung 1997; 175:213–223.
49. Miller EJ, Kajikawa O, Pueblitz Light RW, Koenig KK, Idell S. Chemokine involvement in tetracycline-induced pleuritis. Eur Respir J 1999; 14:1387–1393.
50. Teixeira LR, Wu W, Light RW. The effect of corticosteroids on pleurodesis induced with doxycycline in rabbits. Chest 1997; 112:137S.
51. Light RW, Cheng DS, Lee YC, Rogers J, Davidson J, Lane KB. A single intrapleural injection of transforming growth factor-β_2 produces excellent pleurodesis in rabbits. Am J Respir Crit Care Med 2000; 162:98–104.
52. Lee YCG, Teixeira LR, Devin CJ, Vaz MA, Vargas FS, Thompson PJ, Lane KB, Light RW. Transforming growth factor-beta(2) induces pleurodesis significantly faster than talc. Am J Respir Crit Care Med 2001; 163:640–644.
53. Lee YCG, Devin CJ, Teixeira LR, Rogers JT, Thompson PJ, Lane KB, Light RW. Transforming growth factor β_2 induced pleurodesis is not inhibited by corticosteroids. Thorax 2001; 56:643–648.

54. Bresticker MA, Oba J, LoCicero J III, Greene R. Optimal pleurodesis: a comparison study. Ann Thorac Surg 1993; 55:364–366.
55. Jerram RM, Fossum TW, Berridge BR, Steinheimer DN, Slater MR. The efficacy of mechanical abrasion and talc slurry as methods of pleurodesis in normal dogs. Vet Surg 1999; 28:322–332.
56. Colt HG, Russack V, Chiu Y, Konopka RG, Chiles PG, Pedersen CA, Kapelanski D. A comparison of thoracoscopic talc insufflation, slurry, and mechanical abrasion pleurodesis. Chest 1997; 111:442–448.
57. Whitlow CB, Craig R, Brady K, Hetz SP. Thoracoscopic pleurodesis with minocycline vs talc in the porcine model. Surg Endosc 1996; 10:1057–1059.
58. Cohen RG, Shely WW, Thompson SE, Hagen JA, Marboe CC, DeMeester TR, Starnes VA. Talc pleurodesis: talc slurry versus thoracoscopic talc insufflation in a porcine model. Ann Thorac Surg 1996; 62:1000–1002.
59. Lee YC (Gary), Lane KB, Parker RB, Ayo D-S, Rogers JT, Diters RW, Thompson PJ, Light RW. Transforming growth factorβ_2 (TGF-β_2) produces effective pleurodesis in sheep with no systemic complications. Thorax 2000; 55:1058–1062.
60. Shore BL, Daughaday CC, Spilberg I. Benign asbestos pleurisy in the rabbit. A model for the study of pathogenesis. Am Rev Respir Dis 1983; 128:481–485.
61. Boylan AM, Ruegg C, Kim KJ, Hebert CA, Hoeffel JM, Pytela R, Sheppard D, Goldstein IM, Broaddus VC. Evidence of a role for mesothelial cell-derived interleukin 8 in the pathogenesis of asbestos-induced pleurisy in rabbits. J Clin Invest 1992; 89:1257–1267.
62. Sahn SA, Antony VB. Pathogenesis of pleural plaques. Relationship of early cellular response and pathology. Am Rev Respir Dis 1984; 130:884–887.
63. Paterson RC. The pleural reaction to inoculation with tubercule bacilli in vaccinated and normal guinea pigs. Am Rev Tuberc 1917; 1:353–371.
64. Allen JC, Apicella MA. Experimental pleural effusion as a manifestation of delayed hypersensitivity to tuberculin PPD. J Immunol 1968; 101:481–487.
65. Leibowitz S, Kennedy L, Lessof MH. The tuberculin reaction in the pleural cavity and its suppression by antilymphocyte serum. Br J Exp Pathol 1973; 54:152–162.
66. Widstrom O, Nilsson BS. Pleurisy induced by intrapleural BCG in immunized guinea pigs. Eur J Respir Dis 1982; 63:425–434.
67. Antony VB, Sahn SA, Antony AC, Repine JE. Bacillus Calmette-Guerin-stimulated neutrophils release chemotaxins for monocytes in rabbit pleural space in vitro. J Clin Invest 1985; 76:1514–1521.
68. Colice GL, Curtis A, Deslauriers J, Heffner J, Light RW, Littenberg B, Sahn S, Weinstein RA, Yusen RD. Medical and surgical treatment of parapneumonic effusions: an evidence-based guideline. Chest 2000; 118:1158–1171.
69. Light RW. Pleural Diseases. 4th ed. Baltimore: Lippincott, Williams and Wilkins, 2001.
70. Mavroudis C, Ganzel BL, Katzmark S, Polk HC Jr. Effect of hemothorax on experimental empyema thoracis in the guinea pig. J Thorac Cardiovasc Surg 1985; 89:42–49.
71. Graham EA, Bell RD. Open pneumothorax: its relations to the treatment of empyema. Am J Med Sci 1918; 156:839–871.
72. Sahn SA, Potts DE. Turpentine pleurisy in rabbits: a model of pleural fluid acidosis and low pleural fluid glucose. Am Rev Respir Dis 1978; 118:893–901.
73. Sahn SA, Taryle DA, Good JT Jr. Experimental empyema: time course and

pathogenesis of pleural fluid acidosis and low pleural fluid glucose. Am Rev Respir Dis 1979; 120:355–361.
74. Shohet I, Yellin A, Meyerovitch J, Rubinstein E. Pharmacokinetics and therapeutic efficacy of gentamicin in an experimental pleural empyema rabbit model. Antimicrob Agents Chemother 1987; 31:982–985.
75. Mavroudis C, Ganzel BL, Cox SK, Polk HC Jr. Experimental aerobic-anaerobic thoracic empyema in the guinea pig. Ann Thorac Surg 1987; 43:295–297.
76. Sasse SA, Causing LA, Mulligan ME, Light RW. Serial pleural fluid analysis in a new experimental model of empyema. Chest 1996; 109:1043–1048.
77. Sasse S, Nguyen T, Teixeira LR, Light RW. The utility of daily therapeutic thoracentesis for the treatment of early empyema. Chest 1999; 116:1703–1708.
78. Sasse S, Nguyen TK, Mulligan M, Wang N-S, Mahutte CK, Light RW. The effects of early chest tube placement on empyema resolution. Chest 1997; 111:1679–1683.
79. Teixeira LR, Sasse SA, Villarino MA, Nguyen T, Mulligan ME, Light RW. Antibiotic levels in empyemic pleural fluid. Chest 2000; 117:1734–1739.
80. Yano S, Nokihara H, Hanibuchi M, Parajuli P, Shinohara T, Kawano T, Sone S. Model of malignant pleural effusion of human lung adenocarcinoma in SCID mice. Oncol Res 1997; 9:573–579.
81. Yano S, Herbst RS, Shinohara H, Knighton B, Bucana CD, Killion JJ, Wood J, Fidler IJ. Treatment for malignant pleural effusion of human lung adenocarcinoma by inhibition of vascular endothelial growth factor receptor tyrosine kinase phosphorylation. Clin Cancer Res 2000; 6:957–965.
82. Yano S, Shinohara H, Herbst RS, Kuniyasu H, Bucana CD, Ellis LM, Fidler IJ. Production of experimental malignant pleural effusions is dependent on invasion of the pleura and expression of vascular endothelial growth factor/vascular permeability factor by human lung cancer cells. Am J Pathol 2000; 157:1893–1903.
83. Ohta Y, Kimura K, Tamura M, Oda M, Tanaka M, Sasaki T, Watanabe G. Biological characteristics of carcinomatous pleuritis in orthotopic model systems using immune-deficient rats. Int J Oncol 2001; 18:499–505.
84. Wang B, Xiong Q, Shi Q, Tan D, Le X, Xie K. Genetic disruption of host nitric oxide synthase II gene impairs melanoma-induced angiogenesis and suppresses pleural effusion. Int J Cancer 2001; 91:607–611.
85. Yasutake N, Matsuzaki T, Kimura K, Hashimoto S, Yokokura T, Yoshikai Y. The role of tumor necrosis factor (TNF)-alpha in the antitumor effect of intrapleural injection of *Lactobacillus casei* strain Shirota in mice. Med Microbiol Immunol (Berl) 1999; 188:9–14.
86. Wagner JC. Experimental production of mesothelial tumours of the pleura by implantation of dusts in laboratory animals. Nature 1962; 196:180–181.
87. Smith WE, Miller L, Churg J, Selikoff IJ. Mesotheliomas in hamsters following intrapleural injection of asbestos. J Mt. Sinai Hosp 1965; 32:1–8.
88. Carthew P, Hill RJ, Edwards RE, Lee PN. Intrapleural administration of fibres induces mesothelioma in rats in the same relative order of hazard as occurs in man after exposure. Hum Exp Toxicol 1992; 11:530–534.
89. Davis JM. Structural variations between pleural and peritoneal mesotheliomas produced in rats by the injection of crocidolite asbestos. Ann Anat Pathol (Paris) 1976; 21:199–210.
90. Jaurand MC, Fleury J, Monchaux G, Nebut M, Bignon J. Pleural carcinogenic potency of mineral fibers (asbestos, attapulgite) and their cytotoxicity on cultured cells. J Natl Cancer Inst 1987; 79:797–804.

91. Monchaux G, Bignon J, Jaurand MC, Lafuma J, Sebastien P, Masse R, Hirsch A, Goni J. Mesotheliomas in rats following inoculation with acid-leached chrysotile asbestos and other mineral fibres. Carcinogenesis 1981; 2:229–236.
92. Van der Meeren A, Fleury J, Nebut M, Monchaux G, Janson X, Jaurand MC. Mesothelioma in rats following intrapleural injection of chrysotile and phosphorylated chrysotile (chrysophosphate). Int J Cancer 1992; 50:937–942.
93. Wagner JC, Berry G, Timbrell V. Mesotheliomata in rats after inoculation with asbestos and other materials. Br J Cancer 1973; 28:173–185.
94. Wagner JC. Tumours in experimental animals following exposure to asbestos dust. Ann Anat Pathol (Paris) 1976; 21:211–214.
95. Wagner JC, Hill RJ, Berry G, Wagner MM. Treatments affecting the rate of asbestos-induced mesotheliomas. Br J Cancer 1980; 41:918–922.
96. Wagner JC, Skidmore JW, Hill RJ, Griffiths DM. Erionite exposure and mesotheliomas in rats. Br J Cancer 1985; 51:727–730.
97. Baris YI, Saracci R, Simonato L, Skidmore JW, Artvinli M. Malignant mesothelioma and radiological chest abnormalities in two villages in central Turkey. An epidemiological and environmental investigation. Lancet 1981; 1:984–987.
98. Fleury-Feith J, Nebut M, Saint-Etienne L, Laurent P, Pinchon MC, Kheuang L, Renier A, Jaurand MC. Occurrence and morphology of tumors induced in nude mice transplanted with chrysotile-transformed rat pleural mesothelial cells. Biol Cell 1989; 65:45–50.
99. Berman DW, Crump KS, Chatfield EJ, Davis JM, Jones AD. The sizes, shapes, and mineralogy of asbestos structures that induce lung tumors or mesothelioma in AF/HAN rats following inhalation. Risk Anal 1995; 15:181–195.
100. Davis JM, Jones AD. Comparisons of the pathogenicity of long and short fibres of chrysotile asbestos in rats. Br J Exp Pathol 1988; 69:717–737.
101. Davis JM, Addison J, Bolton RE, Donaldson K, Jones AD, Smith T. The pathogenicity of long versus short fibre samples of amosite asbestos administered to rats by inhalation and intraperitoneal injection. Br J Exp Pathol 1986; 67:415–430.
102. Davis JM, Addison J, Bolton RE, Donaldson K, Jones AD. Inhalation and injection studies in rats using dust samples from chrysotile asbestos prepared by a wet dispersion process. Br J Exp Pathol 1986; 67:113–129.
103. Johnson NF, Edwards RE, Munday DE, Rowe N, Wagner JC. Pluripotential nature of mesotheliomata induced by inhalation of erionite in rats. Br J Exp Pathol 1984; 65:377–388.
104. Wagner JC, Berry G, Skidmore JW, Timbrell V. The effects of the inhalation of asbestos in rats. Br J Cancer 1974; 29:252–269.
105. Wagner JC, Berry G, Skidmore JW, Pooley FD. The comparative effects of three chrysotiles by injection and inhalation in rats. IARC Sci Publ 1980:363–372.
106. Webster I, Goldstein B, Coetzee FS, vanSittert GC. Malignant mesothelioma induced in baboons by inhalation of amosite asbestos. Am J Ind Med 1993; 24:659–666.
107. Pylev LN. Pretumorous lesions and lung and pleural tumours induced by asbestos in rats, Syrian golden hamsters and *Macaca mulatta* (rhesus) monkeys. IARC Sci Publ 1980; 30:343–355.
108. Adachi S, Kawamura K, Kimura K, Takemoto K. Tumor incidence was not related to the thickness of visceral pleural in female Syrian hamsters intratracheally administered amphibole asbestos or manmade fibers. Environ Res 1992; 58:55–65.
109. Humphrey EW, Ewing SL, Wrigley JV, Northrup WF III, Kersten TE, Mayer JE,

Varco RL. The production of malignant tumors of the lung and pleura in dogs from intratracheal asbestos instillation and cigarette smoking. Cancer 1981; 47:1994–1999.

110. Adachi S, Kawamura K, Takemoto K. A trial on the quantitative risk assessment of man-made mineral fibers by the rat intraperitoneal administration assay using the JFM standard fibrous samples. Ind Health 2001; 39:168–174.

111. Miller BG, Searl A, Davis JM, Donaldson K, Cullen RT, Bolton RE, Buchanan D, Soutar CA. Influence of fibre length, dissolution and biopersistence on the production of mesothelioma in the rat peritoneal cavity. Ann Occup Hyg 1999; 43:155–166.

112. Davis MR, Manning LS, Whitaker D, Garlepp MJ, Robinson BW. Establishment of a murine model of malignant mesothelioma. Int J Cancer 1992; 52:881–886.

113. Holiat SM, Smith WE, Hubert DD, Davis S. Chemotherapeutic trials with hamster mesothelioma 10–24: responses to azacitidine, aziridinylbenzoquinone, cisplatin, and PCNU. Cancer Treat Rep 1981; 65:1113–1115.

INDEX

Abscess
 intra-abdominal, 920
 intrahepatic, 795, 768
 liver, 852
 pancreatic, 790
 parasitic liver, 796
 splenic, 768, 797
 subphrenic, 768, 793, 973
 suprahepatic, 973
Actinomyces israelii, 844
Actinomycosis, 837
ADA, 2, 14, 15, 689, 765, 915, 925
 activity, 690–691
Adenocarcinoma, 5
 applications, 1023
 model, 1023
 in rats, 1024
Adhesions, 1, 5, 9, 15, 18, 412
Agents
 antiarrhythmia, 732
 corynebacterium parvum, 497

[Agents]
 doxycycline, 164, 166, 168, 426, 496
 minocycline, 426, 496
 quinacrine, 497
 sclerosing, 488–489, 496
  bleomycin, 16, 426, 496, 1005
  silver nitrate, 497
  sodium hydroxide, 497
  tetracycline, 426
  TGF-b2, 497
AIDS, 355
Albendazole, 870
Albumin, 238
Algorithms, noninvasive multimodality, 826
Alkaline phosphatases, 39
Amebiasis, 852–859
 pleural effusion, 855–858
 pleuropulmonary manifestations, 855
 radiographic features of, 858
Aminoglycosides, 1000–1001
Amphibole, 546

1035

Amyloid
  primary, 582
  pulmonary, 582
  secondary, 582
  systemic, 582
Amyloidosis, 3, 10, 582, 905–906
Anchovy paste appearance, 796
Anemias
  aplastic, 630
  autoimmune, 630
  Fanconi's, 630
  pleural effusions in, 629
Anesthesia
  general, 5, 16
  local, 2, 5
Angiogenesis, 412
Angiography
  magnetic resonance, 828
  pulmonary, 827
Anisakiasis, 883
Antibiotics, 370, 373
Antibodies
  ANA, 317, 319, 335, 337–338, 603
  ANCA, 319, 609
  anti-histones, H2A, H2B, 337
  anti-paragonimus, 875
  antiphospholipid, 744
  anti-rnp, 602
  c-ANCA, 609
  dsDNA, 603
  SnRNP, 606
  SS-A, 605
  ssDNA, 603
Antigens
  echinococcus, 868
  paragonimus, 875
Antiretroviral,
  therapy, 651
Aortography, 900
ARDS, 73, 160, 1005
  drug-induced, 334
Aretaeus, 2, 4, 14
Aristotle, 1, 3
Asbestos, 2, 9, 11, 17, 19, 20, 518–520, 523, 1016, 1025–1027
  fibers, 546–547, 549, 554
    amosite, 519
    anthophyllite, 519
    chrysotile, 519
    crocidolite, 519, 520
    tremolite, 519
    zeolite, 520
  history of, 545–546
  pathogenesis of, 546
Asbestosis, 520
Ascariasis, 879

Ascites, 87
  pancreatic, 792
Aspergilloma, 838
Aspergillosis,
  allergic bronchopulmonary, 838
  iatrogenic pleural, 838
  invasive pulmonary (IPA), 838–839
Aspergillus, 577, 837–838, 983
  flavus, 840
  fumigatus, 840
  Niger, 840
  tracheobronchitis, 838
Aspiration,
  small catheter, 670
Atelectasis, 289, 297
  round
    clinical presentation of, 559
    epidemiology of, 558
    pathogenesis of, 559
    radiology features of, 560
    treatment of, 560–562
Arteriovenous pulmonary aneurysm, 8
ATPase, 39
AUC, 247
AUIC, 1004
Aztreonam, 1000

Bacteroides, 362
BAPE, 268, 271
Barotrauma, 769
Basal lamina, 26, 28, 32
Benign inflammation, 194
Biochemical parameters, 257
Biopsy
  full thickness, 211
  needle, 137, 142, 147, 159, 211–212, 926
  open, 927
  pleural, 123, 127, 957
  pleural thoracentesis, 131
  surgical, 138
  targeted, 210
Blastomyces dermatitidis, 843
BPF (bronchopleural fistula), 400–402, 404–405, 407–409
  closure of, 406
  initial management of, 405
  postpneumonectomy,
    risk factors for, 404
Bronchiectasis, 900
  post-tuberculous, 355
Bronchitis, 900
Bronchopleural fistula, 81, 84, 154, 156, 162, 165, 693–694, 766
Bronchoscopy, 482, 927
Bullectomy, 671

Index

CABG, 920
Cancer
　ovarian, 257
　pancreatic, 257
Candida, 837
　albicans, 841
　tropicalis, 841
Capacity
　diffuse (DLCO), 555
　forced vital (FVC), 552
Capillariasis, 883
Carboplatin, 538
Carcinoma, 254, 256–257, 259
　adenocarcinoma, 179
　bronchogenic, 254
　choriocarcinoma, 745
　lymphangitic, 271
　metastatic, 270
Cardiac disease, pleural effusion
　pathogenesis of, 722
　prevalence of, 722
Cardiac function, 193
Catecholamines, 746
Catheterization, 165, 176
Catheters, chronic indwelling, 428
cDNA, 62
CEA, 522
Cells
　B cells, 59
　foam, 323
　lupus, 319, 603
　malignant, 60
　mesothelial, 55–58, 178, 412
　neoplastic, 412
　RA, 598
　T cells, 56, 58, 59
Cephalosporins, 1000
Cerebrospinal fluid
　leak to the pleura, 918
Charcot-Leyden crystals, 875
Chemokines,
　C3 component, 57
　CD 14, 56
　CD4, 58
　CD8, 59, 60
　CD 11, 59
　CD18, 59
　CD44, 60
　MCP-1, 58
　MIP-1a, 58
Chemotherapy, 422, 526, 538–540, 625
　antimycobacterial, 694
　　ethambutol, 693
　　isoniazid, 683, 687, 692–694
　　pyrazinamide, 683, 687, 692–694

[Chemotherapy]
　rifampicin, 683, 687, 692–694
　thiacetazone, 693
Chest trauma (multitrauma), 164, 168
Chest tube, 153–167
Chocolate sauce appearance, 796
Cholecalciferol, 680
Cholesterol, 238
Chyle, 944, 951
Chyloma, 948
Chylomicrons, 768, 944
Chylothorax, 339, 571, 580–581, 713–715, 746–747, 767, 898, 923
　after organ transplantation, 964
　causes of, 947
　　congenital, 948
　　nontraumatic, 946
　　nonsurgical traumatic, 947
　　postoperative traumatic, 946
　cirrhotic, 788
　indications for surgery, 953
　neonatal, 948
　pleural fluid of, 949
　symptoms of, 950
Ciprofloxacin, 1003
Cirrhossis, 80, 917
Cis-platin, 538–539
Clindamycin, 1000
Clomiphene, 738
Coagulate, 189, 197
Coagulopathy, 132
Coccidioidomycosis, 843
Coccidioides immitis, 843
Collagen vascular associated (CVD-PF), 584–585
Congestive heart failure, 917
　pleural effusion, 721–722
　　characteristics of, 724–725
Costovertebral gutter, 194
Cryptococcus, 837
　albidus, 842
　neoformans, 842
Cyclophosphamide, 538
Cysts
　daughter, 861
　hydatid, 860, 863–866
　liver, 862
　mediastinal, 907
Cytochrome oxidase, 17
Cytokines
　bFGF, 58
　EGF, 58
　FGF, 58, 61
　GM-CSF, 58
　PDGF, 58
　TGF-β, 55, 56

[Cytokines]
  TNF-a, 54, 55
  VEGF, 58
  VPF, 59
Cytology, 419
Cytoplasm, 30
Cytoplasmic vesicles, 9
Cytospin, 2, 4, 11

D-dimer, 823
Debridement, 5, 6
Decortication 15, 903, 937–938
Desmoplastia, 13
Diaphragm, 1, 4, 6, 12, 18
Disease
  adult-onset Still's, 610
  connective tissue, 595
    mixed, 606
  drug-induced pleural, 922
  Erdheim-Chester disease (ECD), 579–580
  Hodgkin disease, pleural effusions in, 621–623
  hydatid 859, 868
  lung disease, concomitant chronic, 211
  miscellaneous, 609–610
  pericardial, 291, 921
  pleural
    benign asbestos-related, 545
    diagnostic criteria of, 318–319
    drug-induced, 317
    in drug abusers, 344
    history of, 1–15
Distomiasis, pulmonary (see Paragonimiasis)
Doppler, 110, 118
Doxorubicin, 538
Drainage
  chest tube, 153, 169, 170, 189, 219, 222, 707
    risk predictors, 372
    open, 373
    percutaneous, 217–221
    pleural fluid, 75, 155, 158, 161
    short-term chest tube, 428
    succion, 373
Drugs
  ACE inhibitors, 335
  amiloride, 47
  amiodarone, 323, 325
  clozapine, 323
  cyclophosphamide, 328
  ergoline, 323, 325
  hydralizin, 335
  isotretinoin, 323

[Drugs]
  l-tryprofan, 338
  mesalazine, 323, 335
  methyldopa, 335
  practolol, 325
  procainaide, 335
  statins, 335
  sulfasalazine, 323, 335
  ticlopidine, 335
Dyspnea, 4, 5, 158, 167

E. coli, 971, 975
Echinococcosis, 859–871
Echinococcus
  granulosus, 797, 859
  multilocularis, 859
Edema
  alveolar, 45
  drug-induced, 334
  interstitial, 50
  pulmonary, 721–722, 729–730
Effusion
  costopulmonary, 11
  diaphragmatic, 14
  interlobular, 14
  pericardial, 323, 901
  thoracic, 11
Egophonia (see Egophony)
Egophony, 11–13
Elastin, 45
Electron microscopy, 4, 16
Electrocardiogram, 821
Empyema, 1–14, 15–17, 983
  after heart transplantation, 970
  after organ transplantation, 964
  bacterial, 353
    causes of, 354
  biochemical characteristics of, 359
  classification of, 358–359
  fungal, 837
  multiloculated pleural, 353
  mycoplasma hominis, 748
  necessitatis, 3, 766
  pneumonectomy, 221
  postpneumonectomy, 220
    risk factors of, 404
  thoracic, 363
  tuberculous, 686–687, 692–694
Endometriosis, 740
Entamoeba histolytica, 796, 852
Esophageal rupture, 268, 797
Ethambutol, 1001

Fanning equation, 5
Fibrinolysis, 219
Fibrinolytics, 371, 373, 379, 707–708, 937

Fibrogenicity, 546
Fibroma, 741
Fibronectin, 46
Fibrosarcoma, 1024–1025
Fibrosis, 30, 63, 197
    parenchymal, 545
    pleural, 545
    retroperitoneal, 788
Fibrothorax, 95, 98, 118, 936–937
Filariasis, 881
Fistula
    bronchopleural, 665–667
    hepatobronchial, 857
Flow cytometry, 258
Fluoroscopy, 305–308
Fluroquinolones, 1001, 1005
Folded lung, 323
Fontan procedure, 289, 294
Fungal, myelia, 838
Fungi
    opportunists, 837
    pathogenic, 837
    saprophytic, 842
Fungus
    Cryptococcus neoformans, 649
    Pneumocystis carinii, 649, 573, 841, 876–877

Galen 2, 4
Gene therapy, 527
Genes, TSC2, 580
Gentamicin, 1001
Gestational trophoblastic disease, 745
Gonadotropin, human chorionic, 738
Graft-versus-host disease (GVHD), 625, 964, 968
Granulomas, 55, 686
Granulomatosis
    Wegener's, 271, 596, 609
Growth factor
    vascular endothelial (VEGF), 412
Gynecological diseases, 737

Haemophilus influenzae, 362, 645, 1000
Hampton hump, 823
Heaf test, 688
Heart failure, 39, 57, 196
    congestive, 31, 237, 244, 271, 288, 290, 721–722
Hemithorax, 82, 84, 102, 104, 106, 111, 114
Hemopneumothorax, 221–222
    spontaneous, 222
Hemorrhage,
    pleural, 898

Hemothorax, 571, 630, 747, 767, 899, 903
    after heart transplantation, 970
    after organ transplantation, 964
    causes of, 933
    complications of, 932
    drug-induced, 329
    nontraumatic, 940
Hernia, diaphragmatic, 800
Hippocrates, 1, 3, 10, 11, 14
Histoplasma capsulatum, 842
Histoplasmosis, 837
Honeycombing, 578
HTLV-1
    viral DNA, 624
Hyaluronan, 523
Hyaluronic acid, 50, 51
Hydatidothorax, 862
Hydropneumothorax, 14
Hydrothorax, 7, 8, 38, 898–899
    acute, 294
    cardiogenic, 722, 724–727
    hepatic, 289, 291–293, 784
Hypodermiasis, 883

Idiopathic pulmonary fibrosis (IPF), 572–573, 583–585
Immunotherapy, 527
    intrapleural, 205
Infections
    HIV, 678, 878
    opportunistic, 573
Integrins, 43, 56
Intercostal nerve, 22
Interferons
    IFN-γ, 57–59, 132, 144, 680, 690–691
Interleukin
    IL1, 56, 58
    IL6, 56
    IL12, 56
    IL 8, 56, 412
    IL10, 58
    IL12, 58
    IL18, 58
    IL15, 58
Interstitial pneumonitis
    usual (UIP), 583
Interstitial lung disease, 571
    collagen, 571
    idiopathic, 571
    infectious, 571
    occupational, 571
    pleural manifestations of, 586
    smoking-related, 578
    vascular, 571
Intrapleural delivery of drugs,
    complications, 344

Intravascular catheters
  iatrogenic effects of, 297
Itraconazole, 840

Kampmeimer's foci, 33, 35, 36
Karnofsky score, 537
Klebsiella, 362, 1000

LAM, 272
Langerhans' cell histiocytosis (LCH), 571, 577–579
LDH, 239, 247–249
Legionella, 573, 971, 975, 978, 983
Leishmania, 650
Leukemia, acute
  lymphocytic, 623
  nonlymphocytic, 623
  T-cell, 623
Light's criteria, 237, 240–241, 245–249, 758, 916
Lobectomy, 196
Lupus erythematosus, 922, 595–596, 600–604
  drug-induced, 335–339
  risk factors of, 336–337
Lymphadenopathy
  angio-immunoblastic, 607–608
Lymphangeiomyomatosis, pulmonary, 746
Lymphangiograms, 901
Lymphangiography, 950, 952
Lymphangioleiomyomatosis (LAM), 579–582
  benign metastasizing, 581
Lymphatic stomas, 33–37
Lymphatic vessels, 46, 48, 49
Lymphedema, 900
Lymphoma, 256–258
  non-Hodgkin's, 651–652
  pleural effusions in, 621–623
Lymphatic channels, 35

Macroglobulinemia
  Waldenstorm's, 272, 629
Macrolides, 1000
Malignancies, 1022
  hematological, 627–628
Maneuvres,
  Valsava, 747
Mansonellosis, 885
Markers
  B72.3, 259
  Ber-EP4, 259
  Bg-8, 259
  CA 15-3, 260
  CA-19-9, 260, 907

[Markers]
  CA- 72-4, 260
  CA-125, 907
  CA125, 602, 604
  calretinin, 259
  CEA, 260
  cytokeratin, 259
  cytokeratin 19, 260
  Leu-M1, 259
  tumor, 260
  VEGF, 260
Mebendazole, 870
Melanoma, 1024
Mesothelioma, 61, 99–101, 1025–1027
  benign, 517
  in children, 520
  diffuse malignant, 532
  localized malignant pleural tumor, 523
  malignant, 517–527
  prognostic factors, 524
  risk factors for, 521
  staging of, 525
  surgery of, 526
  SV-40, 522
  symptoms, 523–524
  types of, 522
Mesothelium, 24, 45, 48
Metacercaria, 871
Metastases, 100, 102, 106, 123–124
  pleural 412
Metronidazole, 859, 1000
MIC, 1001, 1004
Microbes, 55
Microvilli, 28, 34, 37, 39, 46
Mucor species,
  absidia, 842
  mucor, 842
  rhizopus, 842
Multiple myeloma,
  pleural effusions in, 628–629
Mycetoma, 578, 838
Mycobacterium,
  tuberculosis, 646–648, 677, 678, 686–688
Myxedema, 289, 294–295

Needle
  Abrams, 137, 140
  Cope, 139–140
  Raja, 137, 140
  Tru-cut, 137, 140
Neurofibroblastosis, 747
Nocardia, 844, 971, 975, 978
  asteroides, 846
  brasiliensis, 846
  empyema, 645

Index

[Nocardia]
  farcinica, 846
  species, 645
Non-tuberculous mycobacteria,
  avium, 649
  kansasii, 649

Ofloxacin, 1001
Oncogenes, 259
  CHARAS
  CMYC
  MUC1,2,5AC
Operculated eggs, 874

Pancreatitis
  acute, 788
Paragonimiasis, 871–876
  pleuropulmonary manifestations, 872–873
Paragonimus, 871–872
  africanus, 871
  miyazakii, 871
  westermani, 871, 874
Parapneumonic effusions
  causes of, 704
  management of, 705, 711
  symptoms of, 704
Pentastomiasis, 884
Peptostreptococcus, 362
Perforation
  of pleura, 899
Pericarditis, 970
  acute, 728–729
  chronic constrictive, 729, 731
Perirenal lymphocele, 977
Pharmacodynamics
  definition of, 999
  in pleural fluid, 1004–1006
Pharmacokinetics
  definition of, 999
  in pleural fluid, 1000–1004
Photodynamic therapy, 527, 539–540
Plethysmography
  impedance, 826
Pleura
  cervical, 2, 3, 7
  costal, 2, 7, 8, 10
  diaphragmatic, 2, 4, 9, 12
  mediastinal, 2, 3, 7, 15
  parietal, 24, 26, 28–34, 37
  postoperative changes in, 391–392
  visceral, 4, 7, 12, 13, 15, 22
Pleural abrasion, 232
Pleural biopsy, 124, 128, 419, 686, 689–690
Pleural catheter, 498

Pleural catheterization, 177
Pleural cavity, 23, 26, 37
Pleural drainage unit (PDU) 158, 161–162
Pleural effusion, 571, 578, 582, 737, 837, 840–841, 864–866, 874, 877, 983
  after heart transplantation, 970
  after liver transplantation, 974
  after organ transplantation, 964
  associated with GI diseases, 784
  benign asbestos, 556–558
  benign postpartum, 742
  chest radiation following, 339–343
  in children, 699–706
    early effusions, 339
    late-radiation induced, 339
  chylous, differential diagnosis, 621, 622
  drowning, 905
  drug-induced, 319–325
    prognosis of, 323
  in electrical injury, 906
  exudative, 237–239, 243–248, 253, 917–924
    causes of, 274
    rabbits with turpentine-induced, 1019
    secondary to abdominal and pelvic diseases, 768
  fungal, 649–650
  hemorrhagic, 900
  in HIV, 639
    diagnostic evaluation of, 642–643
    epidemiology of, 640
    infectious causes of, 644
    malignant, 650
  iatrogenic, 966
    causes, 898
  malignant, 309–310, 411–418, 431, 918–919
  mammaplasty-induced, 900
  metastatic, 802
  milk of calcium, 906
  mycobacterial, 646–649
  nonmalignant, 250
  paramalignant,
    causes of, 412
    definition of, 412
  parapneumonic, 353, 749
    classification of, 360
    complicated, 354
    loculated, 354
    pathophysiology, 356
    single, 354
    treatment of, 360
    uncomplicated, 354
  primary lymphoma, 653
  pseudoexudative, 243, 246–247

[Pleural effusion]
  secondary causes of, in ILD, 572
  subpulmonic, 117, 760
  sympathetic, 864
  syphilis, 907
  transudative 287–304
    in ICU, pathogenesis of, 759
  tuberculous, 710, 742, 919
Pleural fibrosis, 983
Pleural fluid
  acidosis, 277
  adenosine deaminase, 272
  amylase, 277
  analysis, 368, 418, 701
    bacteriology, 369
    chemistry, 368
    cytology, 369
  charcoal-stained, 899
  eosinophilia, 277, 319, 323
  lymphocyte predominant, 278
  observation, 272
  tuberculous
    characteristics of, 689
    pH, 425
    glucose, 425
Pleural granulomatosis, hydatid, 863
Pleural hydatidosis, 862
Pleural infection
  postoperative, management of, 394–396
Pleural lavage, 175–180
Pleural lymphatic flow, 48, 49
Pleural plaques, 545, 547–553
  asbestos-related, 551
Pleural thickening, 121, 123, 341, 571, 578, 582, 843, 874
  diffuse, 553
    asbestos-related, 555
  drug-induced, 325
Pleurectomy, 26, 228, 242, 498
  parietal, 429
Pleurisy
  chronic rheumatoid, 272
  lupus, 144
  rheumatoid, 144
  tuberculous, 144–146, 272
  viral, 272
Pleuritic chest pain, 362
  drug-induced, 329–331
Pleuritis, 1, 2, 4, 10, 14
  bacterial, 787
  chemical, 223
  exudative stage, 357
  fibrinopurulent stage, 357
  fibrinous, 601
  lupus, 601–602

[Pleuritis]
  drug-induced, 319
  obliterative, 725
  organizing stage, 358
  radiation, 905, 965
  rheumatoid, 922
  sicca stage, 356
  tuberculous, 677–693
  uremic, 902–903
Pleurocentesis, 131–135, 141, 147–148
Pleurodesis, 177, 185, 422, 489, 490, 513
  in benign effusions, 487–488
  chemical, 505
  contraindications, 427, 428
  in malignant pleural effusions, 479–483
    definition of success, 484
  in pneumothorax, 486–487
    indications of, 488
  side effects/complications, 494–496
    adverse effects of, 423–424
      ARDS, 424
      COPD, 424
      SIRS, 424
  talc, 2, 5, 422, 489–490, 513
Pleuroperitoneal shunt, 428–429, 498
Pleyrodynia, 2, 8
Polyserositis (see Serositis)
Pneumoconiosis, 11
Pneumocystosis, 876
Pneumonectomy, 405–406
  extrapleural, 533
    with adjuvant regional modalities, 539–540
    with adjuvant systemic chemoradiation, 537–539
    reported mortality, 537
    versus pleurectomy/decortication, 535–537
  post, 404
Pneumonia, 732
  actinic, 904
  community acquired (CAP), 643–644
  mycoplasma, 271
  Pneumocystis carinii, 271
  viral, 271
Pneumonitis, 729–730
  drug-induced, 323
  pleural effusion in the context of, 331–334
Pneumothorax, 25, 45, 65, 86, 125–126, 140, 142–143, 176, 189, 198, 215, 571, 577–578, 580, 583, 694, 769–778, 857, 877, 903–904
  after BMT, 966,

Index

[Pneumothorax]
  after heart transplantation, 971
  after heart-lung transplantation, 980
  after lung transplantation, 984
  after transplantation, 964
  classification, 663
  contralateral, 663
  diagnosis of, 668
  drug-induced, 328–329
  hydro, 866
  hydropyo, 839
  iatrogenic, 662, 983
  incidence of, 661
  persistent, 221
  primary, 224
  radiation-induced, 342
  recurrent, therapy of, 672
  secondary, 216, 225
  spontaneous, 224, 226, 228
    primary, 661–663, 672
    secondary, 661, 672
    causes of, 664–665
  symptoms of, 667
  tension
    causes of, 668, 669
    therapy for, 669
  traumatic, 662
Polymyositis/dermatomyositis, 604–605
Pracoccidioides brasiliensis, 844
Praziquantel, 876
Pseudochylothorax, 924
  causes of, 955
  complications of, 957
  definition of, 955
Pseudomediastinum, 771
Pseudomonas aeruginosa, 645
Pseudomonas, 362, 645, 971, 983, 1000
Pulmonary embolism, 80, 238, 271, 732, 811
  pleural fluid, characteristics of, 817
Pyothorax-associated lymphoma, 623

Radiation, 422
  therapeutic, 904
Rheumatoid arthritis, 595–600
  complications of, 599
Rheumatoid pleuropulmonary disease, 355

Sarcoidosis, 289, 296, 571, 574–577
Sarcoma, Kaposi's, 650–651
Schistosomiasis, 883
Shunt, pleuroperitoneal, 952, 954
  contraindications for use of, 509
  evolution of, 505–510
  indications for use of, 508

Sign
  deep sulcus, 774
  Fleischner, 822
  Kussmaul's, 925
  middle lobe step, 761
  pseudotumor, 761
  Westermark, 821
Spondylitis, ankylosing, 605, 606
Starling's law, 758
Streptokinase, 375, 937, 1004
Streptomycin, 749, 1001
Strongyloidiasis, 878
Sulfur granules, 845
Syndrome
  Boerhaave's, 798
  Churg-Strauss, 582, 608, 875
  Dressler's, 730
  drug-induced lupus, 601
  eosinophilia-myalgia, 606–607
  Horner's, 204
  Loeffler's, 878
  Meigs', 741, 921, 925
  myelodysplastic, 625
  nephritic, 906
  nephrotic, 204, 271, 289, 293, 298, 917
  ovarian hyperstimulation (OHSS), 334, 738
  overlap autoimmune, 596
  parenchymal infiltration, 323
  postcardiac injury, 729–331, 815, 921
  postpulmonary infarction, 815
  pseudo-Meigs', 741
  pulmonary infarction/hemorrhage, 816
  Raynaud's, 204
  Richter, 626
  Sjögren's, 605
  vasomotor, 204
  yellow nail, 900, 923

Talc, 159, 166, 168, 186, 197, 672–673
  asbestos-free, 672
Tetracycline, 669, 671, 1005
TGF-b2, 1005
Thalassemias
  pleural effusions in, 629
Thoracentesis, 2, 71–74, 127, 131, 132, 137, 158, 166, 168, 190, 221, 237, 241, 401, 408, 482–483, 498, 515, 523, 532, 690, 701, 901–902, 954
  in CHF pleural effusion, 727–728
  diagnostic, 127, 257, 707
  procedure for, 705
Thoracic duct, 944
Thoracic splenosis, 104–105

Thoracoscopy
 medical, 371, 373, 419, 481, 523, 671, 926–927, 938
  advanced indications of, 198–204
  basic indications of, 191–197
  contraindications of, 190
  complications of, 189
  therapeutic, 217
  indications of, 221
Thoracostomy, 155, 160, 169, 373, 505
 chest tubes, 670, 952
Thoracotomy, 176, 179, 184, 197, 211, 220, 223–224, 227–228, 371, 403, 406–408, 506, 533, 672, 870, 939
 chest tube, 671
 exploratory, 952
 minithoracotomy, 222, 230–231
 open, 373, 380
Torulopsis glabrata, 841
Toxocariasis, 882
Toxoplasma, 975
Transplantation
 bone marrow (BMT), 963–969
  pleural effusion in, 625
 heart, 969
 liver, 802, 972
 kidney, 975
 lung, 579
Transthoracic needle aspiration, 166
Trapped lung, 421, 903–904, 923
Trichinellosis, 879
Triglycerides, 950–952
Trocars, 184–188

Trophozoites, 852, 857
Tropical pulmonary eosinophilia, 879
Tube
 endotracheal, 900
 nasogastric, 899
 thoracostomy, 899
Tuberculosis, 55, 56, 183, 191, 194, 1017
 BCG model, 1017–1018
 hypersensitivity model, 1017
Tumors
 fibrous, 227
 neurogenic, 124
 pleural, 113, 124, 128
  chodromas, 123
  fibromas, 123
  lipomas, 124
  liposarcoma, 91–92
  radiation-induced, 342

Ultrasonography
 guided biopsy, 127
 guided thoracentesis, 125
 pleural effusion, 114–122, 726
 pleural tumors, 123–125
Ultrasound, 111–115, 119, 123, 125–127, 133, 137, 143, 154, 364, 869
Urinothorax, 375, 708, 748, 918, 937, 1004
 after kidney transplantation, 977
Urokinase, 375, 708, 937, 1004

VATS, 371, 373, 402–403, 408, 419, 487, 505, 511, 513, 532–533, 938, 953
 diagnostic, 210–213